PTAEXAM
THE COMPLETE STUDY GUIDE

SCOREBUILDERS

P.O. Box 7242
Scarborough, Maine 04070-7242

Phone: (207) 885-0304
Fax: (207) 883-8377

www.scorebuilders.com

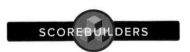

PTAEXAM

THE COMPLETE STUDY GUIDE

SCOTT M. GILES

SCOREBUILDERS

Acknowledgments

Dedication

The new edition of *PTAEXAM: The Complete Study Guide* and every future edition is dedicated to Gwenn Hoyt. Thanks for your years of support, love, and expertise. You are greatly missed for so many reasons.

Special Thanks

Therese Giles, Scorebuilders, Scarborough, Maine

I would like to thank my wife, Traci, for her substantial contributions to all areas of the project. You are a great teammate and, of course, my best friend.

Shawn Paquette, Scorebuilders, Scarborough, Maine

I would like to thank Shawn for his involvement in each of the many phases of this project. Your expanding role in content creation has been an incredible asset for our company.

Thank You

Thanks to the many students from academic programs throughout the country that served as reviewers throughout the project especially Maria Stern, Mary Farnkoff, Lori Joseph, Mayra Zerpa Calderon, Polina Weinstein, Kelly Trancygier, Carly Theriault, Karen Loisel, and Nicole DiBiase.

Lucian Burg, LU Design Studios, Portland, Maine

I would like to thank Lucian for his technical and artistic expertise throughout the creation of the new edition.

Kimberly Mills, Scorebuilders, Scarborough, Maine

I would like to thank Kim for her many contributions throughout virtually all aspects of this project.

Kevin Chugh and Jason Stone, Main Street Computing, East Aurora, New York

I would like to thank Kevin and Jason as well as the entire Main Street Computing team for their technical expertise and making Insight come to life.

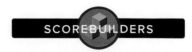

Author's Note

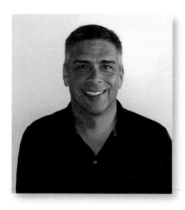

Scott M. Giles PT, DPT, MBA

President, Scorebuilders
Scarborough, Maine

Congratulations on your decision to purchase *PTAEXAM: The Complete Study Guide*. We have been assisting physical therapists and physical therapist assistants with their preparation for the licensing examination for nearly three decades. We take great pride in what we do and believe this edition of *PTAEXAM: The Complete Study Guide* demonstrates our commitment to excellence. Leave no stone unturned in your preparation for this important examination and strive to make your examination score reflect your abilities as a physical therapist assistant. Candidates that have a firm grasp of didactic information combined with a meaningful study plan emphasizing applied knowledge are often richly rewarded on this challenging examination. We are confident that our text will be a valuable component of your comprehensive study program. Although undoubtedly there will be many magical moments in your life, you will never forget the moment when you become licensed as a physical therapist assistant. Best of luck on the examination and in your future career endeavors!

Contributors

This project could not have been completed without the willingness of these contributors to share their clinical expertise. We are indebted to each of you for your individual contributions that have significantly enhanced this edition of *PTAEXAM: The Complete Study Guide*. Thanks for your dedication and desire to assist students with their preparation for this critically important examination.

Therese Giles PT, MS

Shawn Paquette PT, DPT

Michael Fillyaw PT, MS

Daniel Lee PT, DPT, GCS

Holly Daniel PT, MSc

Danielle Cowan PT, DPT, CLT-LANA

Ryan Bailey PT, DPT

Introduction

PTAEXAM: The Complete Study Guide is the most comprehensive resource available for the National Physical Therapy Examination (NPTE-PTA) and sets a new standard for review book excellence. The resource provides candidates with a number of powerful study tools each designed to prepare candidates for the breadth and depth associated with the current NPTE-PTA. A brief description of each unit in the study guide is listed below.

Unit 1–Introduction to the National Physical Therapy Examination (NPTE-PTA)

The unit provides candidates with information on the purpose, development, scoring, and administration of the NPTE-PTA. Candidates are introduced to a systematic approach to answering multiple-choice questions and are exposed to recent developments in item construction. The unit also provides a detailed analysis of each of the system and content outline areas of the NPTE-PTA. By exploring the categories and subcategories of each of these areas, candidates gain a better understanding of the breadth and depth of the current examination and as a result spend less time covering topics that are not clinically relevant. This unit offers a variety of study concepts that candidates can utilize to increase the effectiveness of study sessions.

Unit 2–Academic Review

The unit provides candidates with an efficient method to review didactic information from a physical therapy curriculum. The academic review consists of eight distinct chapters of academic information. The first six chapters consist of academic content in specific system areas (e.g., musculoskeletal) and non-system areas (e.g., equipment, devices, and technologies). Each chapter in the unit includes a description of the physical therapy management of commonly encountered medical diagnoses on the NPTE-PTA. The academic review avoids attempting to cover every aspect of a physical therapist assistant's academic training and instead focuses on the most essential information necessary to maximize examination performance. Since the examination is designed to assess entry-level practice, it is likely that candidates will encounter the information presented in the academic review frequently on the actual examination. Mastery of this information can significantly increase candidates' scores on the NPTE-PTA.

Unit 3–Examinations

The unit includes an answer key for the three, 150 question sample examinations located on our eLearning site **INSIGHT**. Candidates have the option of selecting a full-length examination or creating custom examinations. The examinations were developed based on selected specifications from the current content outline and are designed to expose candidates to the nuances of computer-based testing. Candidates are able to generate a detailed performance analysis summary that identifies current strengths and weaknesses according to system and content outline areas. An answer key includes an explanation specifying why the correct answer is correct and an explanation specifying why each incorrect answer is incorrect. New video explanations provide candidates with the opportunity to watch videos that compare and contrast good, better, and best options for selected examination questions. The answer key also includes a cited resource with page number, an academic focus area, and the assigned system and content outline areas. The examinations provide candidates with the opportunity to refine test taking skills and assess current preparedness for the examination.

*Additional resources to assist candidates with their preparation for the NPTE-PTA are located at the conclusion of the study guide.

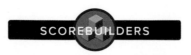

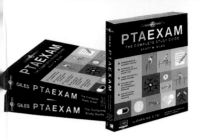

PTAEXAM: The Complete Study Guide
The Gold Standard

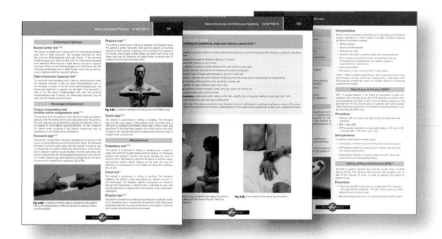

Content is King

The new edition of **PTAEXAM: The Complete Study Guide** is the most comprehensive resource available for the NPTE-PTA. Our academic review section is unparalleled in its breadth and depth and sets a new standard for review book excellence.

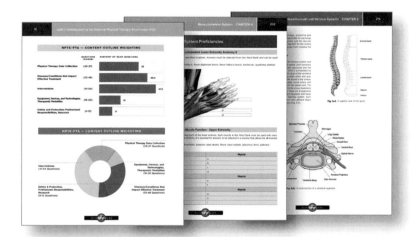

Design, Design, Design

Scorebuilders' products are known for their creative design and innovative features. The new edition of *PTAEXAM: The Complete Study Guide* simply makes a very good thing even better. Break free from traditional encyclopedic resources and feel the power of well conceived design.

A Technology Monster

Scorebuilders has made a massive investment in technology and uses this competitive advantage to provide you with the most realistic testing experience possible. Our eLearning platform **Insight** will amaze you in its level of sophistication. Continuous innovation and commitment to technology widens the gap between **Scorebuilders** and all other licensing companies.

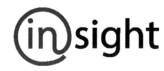

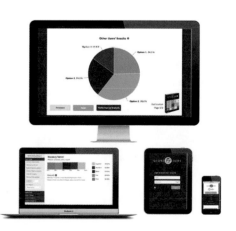

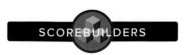

Test Drive the NPTE-PTA

Our sample examination questions are thought provoking, challenging questions designed to be consistent with the specifications and rigor of the NPTE-PTA blueprint. Scorebuilders' questions are consistently reported to be the most realistic questions available for the NPTE-PTA. Use the detailed explanation of answers and videos to refine decision making skills.

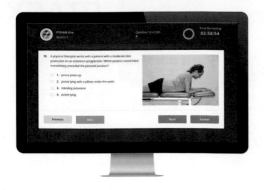

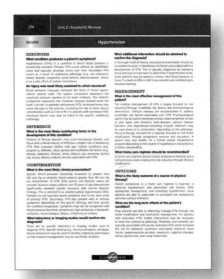

New Clinical Application Templates

Pathology has always been a substantive topic on the NPTE-PTA and the new FSBPT blueprint makes it clear that this fact is not changing. The resource includes Gold, Silver, and Bronze Clinical Application Templates (CATs) which guide candidates through the patient/client management of commonly encountered medical conditions.

Edition Guarantee!

We have always believed that sleep is overrated! As soon as we release a new edition of **PTAEXAM: The Complete Study Guide** we immediately get to work on creating the next edition. Our eLearning site **Insight** includes an Edition Guarantee which delivers updates three times a year to existing users of the current edition.

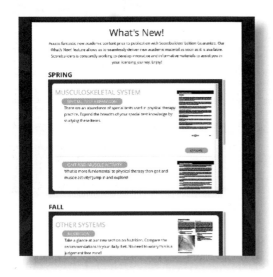

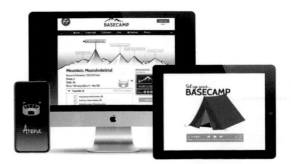

Basecamp - Start Climbing!

Basecamp provides students with an incredibly efficient method to review academic content within **PTAEXAM: The Complete Study Guide**. The content is organized in five distinct Mountains and 120 Trails. Each trail has dedicated assignments, videos, and exams. Our **Arena App** allows **Basecamp** users to access 5,000 content based questions within our competitive games - **King of the Mountain** and **Climb**. A $25 off coupon for **Basecamp** is included within **Insight**. Purchase **Basecamp** today and start climbing!

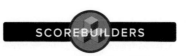

Table of Contents

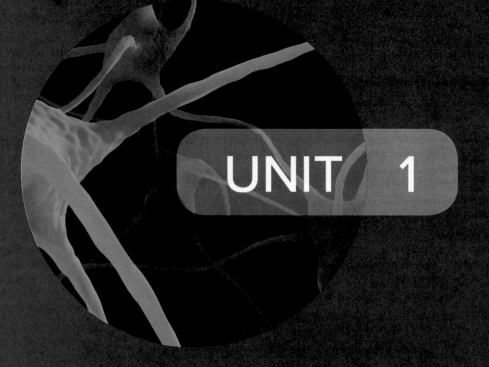

UNIT 1

The National Physical Therapy Examination-PTA

The National Physical Therapy Examination-PTA

The National Physical Therapy Examination (NPTE-PTA) is a 200 question, four hour exam that is the final step required for physical therapist assistants to become licensed practitioners. This unit addresses the application process and the essential information necessary to schedule and take the NPTE-PTA. Candidates are introduced to an approach to answering multiple-choice questions and provided with examples of traditional examination questions and graphically enhanced questions.

A detailed analysis of the **NPTE-PTA Blueprint** provides candidates with a thorough understanding of the relative system and content outline weighting of the examination. This information can assist students to establish a comprehensive study plan consistent with the structure of the NPTE-PTA. Candidates can identify appropriate remedial activities by assessing sample examination performance in specific system and content outline areas.

Study concepts remind candidates that preparing for the NPTE-PTA requires more than simply reviewing academic content and taking sample examinations. Each of the presented study concepts looks at a unique element of the study process such as learning style, automaticity, and time management. Use of this information allows candidates to establish a personalized study plan based on their unique learning needs.

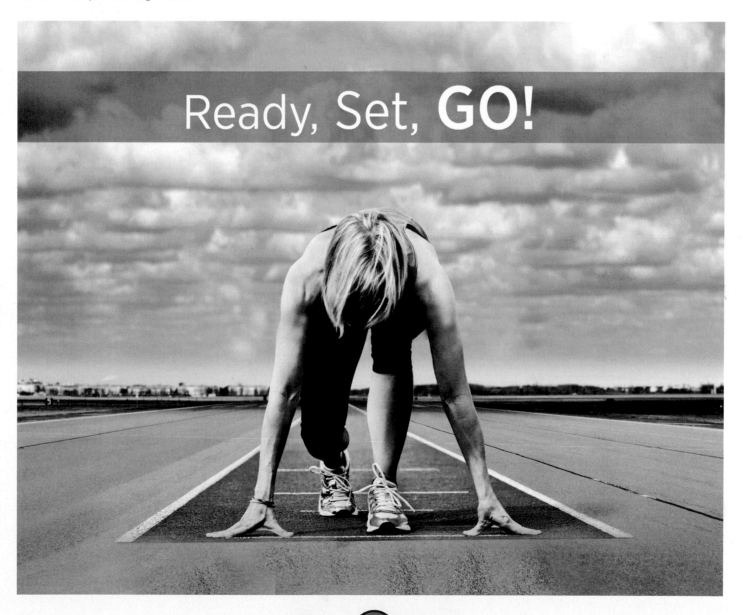

Ready, Set, **GO!**

1

National Physical Therapy Examination-PTA Basics

Scott Giles

CHAPTER 1
National Physical Therapy Examination-PTA Basics

The National Physical Therapy Examination (NPTE-PTA) is a 200 question (150 scored, 50 pre-test), multiple-choice examination designed to determine if candidates possess the minimal competency necessary to practice as physical therapist assistants.

The examination is created under the auspices of the Federation of State Boards of Physical Therapy (FSBPT). According to the *National Physical Therapy Examination Candidate Handbook*, the examination program serves three important purposes:

1. Provide examination services to regulatory authorities charged with the regulation of physical therapists and physical therapist assistants.

2. Provide a common element in the evaluation of candidates so that standards will be comparable from jurisdiction to jurisdiction.

3. Protect the public interest in having only those persons who have the requisite knowledge of physical therapy be licensed to practice physical therapy.

There are two primary methods to obtain a license to practice as a physical therapist assistant in the United States. They are termed examination and endorsement. Licensure by examination is obtained after a candidate meets or exceeds the minimum scoring requirement on the NPTE-PTA and has satisfied all other state requirements. This form of obtaining licensure is the traditional method for candidates seeking initial licensure.

Licensure by endorsement makes it possible for candidates who have already been licensed in a state by virtue of an examination to potentially gain licensure in another state without retaking the examination. Examination scores can be transferred to any physical therapy state licensing agency via the Federation of State Boards of Physical Therapy Score Transfer Service. The web site address for the Federation of State Boards of Physical Therapy is available in the Appendix.

Although the NPTE-PTA is 200 questions, 50 of the questions serve only as pre-test items and are not officially scored. The pre-test items allow new examination questions to be evaluated throughout the year and eliminate lengthy delays in score reporting when new examinations are introduced. Candidates are unable to differentiate between pre-test and scored items on the examination.

The 200 questions are administered to candidates in four sections consisting of 50 questions each. Each section contains scored items and pre-test items, although the number of pre-test and scored items in each section may vary slightly. Candidates have four hours to complete the four sections at their own pace. Since the sections are not timed individually, it is important for candidates to effectively manage their allotted time as they progress through each of the four sections. Candidates have the opportunity to take one scheduled break at the conclusion of section two, immediately prior to beginning section three. Additional unscheduled breaks can be taken at the conclusion of a given section, however, the elapsed time will not stop. If a candidate does not want to take the break or prefers a shorter break, they can end the break by following the directions displayed on the computer screen. Candidates can leave the examination only when either a scheduled or unscheduled break message is displayed on the computer screen. Leaving the testing room while not on a designated break will result in an examination irregularity being reported to the FSBPT.

Candidates are unable to return to previously completed sections once a new section is initiated. The academic content is randomized within each section and scoring is based only on the number of questions a candidate answers correctly out of the 150 scored items. As a result, each of the examinations in *PTAEXAM: The Complete Study Guide* consists of only 150 questions (three sections, each consisting of 50 questions). Candidates will have three hours to complete each of the 150 question sample examinations.

The FSBPT publishes a content outline which describes the specific categories and subcategories of the examination. The categories and subcategories are based on the tasks and roles that comprise the practice of physical therapy. Once established, the content outline remains active for a period of approximately five years. The most recent version was implemented in January of 2018. The five main categories of the examination are listed here, although the entire content outline will be discussed in detail in Chapter 2.

Candidates should attempt to integrate this information in conjunction with the performance analysis summary to accurately identify current strengths and weaknesses and develop appropriate remedial strategies. The computer-based examinations include a number of helpful tools to assist candidates to integrate this information. Candidates should avoid becoming overly excited or depressed based on the results of a given sample examination and use the number of questions answered correctly only as a general indicator of their current level of preparedness. Studying for the examination is much closer to running a marathon than running a sprint. By engaging in meaningful self-assessment activities, candidates can gather valuable information to improve future examination performance.

Examination Content Outline

Physical Therapy Data Collection

Diseases/Conditions that Impact Effective Treatment

Interventions

Equipment, Devices, and Technologies; Therapeutic Modalities

Safety and Protection; Professional Responsibilities; Research and Evidence-Based Practice

According to the FSBPT, the involvement of a large representative group of practicing physical therapists, physical therapist assistants, and other professionals at each stage of examination development ensures that the examinations are relevant to the practice of physical therapy. Individual physical therapists and physical therapist assistants are responsible for writing examination questions. The therapists involved are required to attend item-writing workshops that are taught by experienced testing professionals. Questions, once completed, are analyzed independently to make sure they are reflective of the current examination content outline. Examination questions tend to focus on decision making and not purely rote memorization of fact. Successful candidates on the examination must demonstrate the ability to apply knowledge in a safe and effective manner.

Examination Scoring

The questions on the examination are multiple-choice with four possible answers to each question. Each option is listed as 1, 2, 3, 4. Options such as "none of the above," "all of the above," and "1 and 2 only" are not included on the examination. Candidates are asked to identify the best answer to each of the questions. Each question has only one best answer while the other possible answers serve as distracters. A candidate's score is determined based on the number of scored questions answered correctly. Since there is no penalty for questions answered incorrectly it is imperative that candidates answer all of the available questions. A candidate's cumulative score is termed the total raw score. The maximum total raw score for the NPTE-PTA is 150.

Criterion-referenced scoring is used to determine passing scores on the NPTE-PTA. Passing scores are based on the judgment of selected experts on the minimum number of questions that should be answered correctly by a minimally qualified candidate. Criterion-referenced passing scores are determined independently of candidate performance and are designed to reflect the difficulty level of each examination. For example, if a given examination was judged to be particularly difficult, the criterion-referenced passing score would be lower than the criterion-referenced passing score for another examination that was judged to be less difficult. All state licensing agencies have adopted the FSBPT criterion-referenced passing score and therefore do not individually determine passing scores at the state level. As a result, a passing score for a given examination will always be the same in all jurisdictions.

Since the minimum passing score varies based on the difficulty level of each examination, it is impossible to determine an automatic passing score. Criterion-referenced passing scores often range from 95 - 108. If the criterion-referenced passing score was established as 98 for a given examination, a total raw score of greater than or equal to 98 would be considered a passing score, while a total raw score of less than 98 would be considered a failing score. Within a given examination cycle, criterion-referenced passing scores usually fluctuate in a relatively small range, perhaps by as few as five questions.

An individual examination score is often reported to candidates in the form of a scaled score. Scaled scores range from 200 - 800 with the minimum passing score always being equal to a scaled score of 600. Scaled scores are necessary as a method of equating examinations with different criterion-referenced passing scores. A few state licensing agencies use a slightly different scaled score system where the minimum passing score is equivalent to a scaled score of 75.

Applying for the Examination

The application process officially starts when a candidate's academic program initiates their FSBPT profile. This action results in each candidate receiving an email with specific login information. At this point a candidate can formally complete their FSBPT profile. In addition to registering through the FSBPT, candidates must be approved through the state licensing agency where they intend to practice as a physical therapist assistant. The address, phone number, and web site for each agency is available at the Federation of State Boards of Physical Therapy (FSBPT) web site, www.fsbpt.org. Candidates are not permitted to apply for the examination in more than one jurisdiction at a time. All state licensing agencies offer online registration for the examination through the FSBPT.

Each state licensing agency can establish its own criteria to be eligible to sit for the NPTE-PTA. variety of items may be required as part of the application process. These items often include a photograph, a notarized birth certificate, an official transcript from an accredited school, professional reference letters, and a check or money order for the required application, examination, and licensing fees. After the necessary application forms have been completed, the information is returned along with any necessary fees to the state licensing agency or an identified intermediary. Candidates should recognize that even a small departure from the established eligibility criteria can lead to a significant delay in processing a candidate's application. To avoid such delays, it is prudent to read the application carefully and to inquire as to the status of the application approximately two weeks after the completed application has been submitted.

2020 Dates and Deadlines

Test Date	Registration and Payment Deadline	Jurisdiction Approval Deadline	Seat Reservation Deadline	Scores Reported to Jurisdictions
January 9	December 5*	December 12*	December 26*	January 16
April 7	March 3	March 10	March 24	April 14
July 8	June 3	June 10	June 24	July 15
October 6	September 1	September 8	September 22	October 14

*indicates 2019 date

2021 Dates and Deadlines

Test Date	Registration and Payment Deadline	Jurisdiction Approval Deadline	Seat Reservation Deadline	Scores Reported to Jurisdictions
January 6	December 2*	December 9*	December 23*	January 13
April 6	March 2	March 9	March 23	April 15
July 6	June 1	June 8	June 22	July 13
October 6	September 1	September 8	September 22	October 14

*indicates 2020 date

Some states offer candidates with verifiable employment the opportunity to practice prior to being licensed by issuing a temporary license. Typically, candidates are required to have a completed application on file and have met all other qualifications for licensure before being considered for the temporary license. In most states temporary licenses are revoked if a candidate receives notification that they were unsuccessful on the NPTE-PTA.

In addition to the NPTE-PTA, a significant number of states require candidates to successfully complete a jurisprudence examination. This type of examination is based on the state rules and regulations governing physical therapy practice. The examination can include multiple-choice items, short-answer questions or fill in the blanks. States can administer the examination using computer-based testing or even as a take-home examination.

The NPTE-PTA officially moved from continuous testing to fixed-date testing in 2012. The change was necessitated by the need to substantially reduce or eliminate candidates' ability to gain a score advantage by having advance access to NPTE-PTA questions. The move to fixed-date testing has resulted in the establishment of a number of important dates and deadlines that are critical for all candidates. Candidates taking the NPTE-PTA in 2019 or 2020 must register for one of the four established testing dates.

Candidates are encouraged to visit the FSBPT web site frequently since established dates and/or registration deadlines are subject to change. A dedicated fixed-date testing page has been integrated into the FSBPT web site.

Examination Administration

The examination is offered on computer at over 300 Prometric Testing Centers within the United States. Candidates are encouraged to make an appointment at a Prometric Testing Center as soon as they receive notification from the FSBPT that they are eligible. The move to fixed-date testing has created shortages at selected Prometric Testing Centers on specific fixed dates. As a result, the FSBPT recommends that candidates wait to make travel arrangements until after they have secured a scheduled test date and location.

Many Prometric Testing Centers will offer both a morning and afternoon appointment. When possible, candidates should schedule their examination at a time consistent with their optimal level of functioning. For example, if a candidate tends to be a "morning person," it would be prudent to schedule the examination in the morning. Candidates with significant anxiety may also want a morning appointment in order to avoid worrying about the examination throughout the day. If candidates are not familiar with the exact location of the examination site, it may be desirable to travel to the site before the actual examination date. The trip will provide candidates with an accurate idea of the time necessary to travel to the site and avoid the possibility of getting lost and subsequently being late for the examination.

Within each Prometric Testing Center, candidates can concentrate on the examination without environmental distracters. Private, modular booths provide adequate work space with proper lighting and ventilation. All Prometric Testing Centers are fully accessible and in compliance with the Americans with Disabilities Act. Candidates requesting accommodation for a documented disability must do so through the state licensing agency. Candidates are not limited to the testing centers within the state they are applying for licensure. For example, a candidate that has recently graduated from a physical therapy program in Maine could apply for licensure in California and take the required examination while still residing in Maine.

Candidates must arrive 30 minutes prior to their scheduled appointment with two forms of acceptable identification which include a government issued photo ID and another piece of identification preprinted with a name and a signature. The first and last names on both forms of ID must match the name on the Authorization to Test letter issued by the FSBPT. Candidates are photographed and a digital image of their fingerprint is taken prior to beginning the examination. Candidates cannot bring any electronic devices (e.g., watches, cell phones) or food and drink into the testing area. A locker will be provided to store personal items. Candidates can request headphones if they want to minimize background noise.

It is important to note that computer skills are not necessary with computer-based testing. Prior to beginning the examination, candidates utilize a tutorial that explains topics such as selecting answers and navigating within the examination. Time spent on the computer tutorial does not count toward the allotted time for the actual examination. The tutorial typically takes candidates less than ten minutes and if necessary, candidates can go through the tutorial a second time.

Candidates have the option of entering their answers using a computer keyboard or mouse. Candidates can go back to previously answered or unanswered questions and make any desired changes within a given section of 50 questions. Once a candidate submits a given section, they are unable to return to the questions within the section. Paper and pencil are not permitted in the Prometric Testing Centers, however, candidates are given an erasable note board or an electronic writing board to utilize during the examination.

The FSBPT is responsible for scoring the examination and reporting results to the individual state licensing agencies. According to the FSBPT, score will be reported approximately one week after the test date. This time allows the FSBPT to receive, process, and deliver to jurisdictions several thousand exam score files. The FSBPT reports scores to the candidate and the associated state licensing agency. Candidates receive a free online score report from the FSBPT approximately 10 business days after the examination. The score report offers more detailed information on a candidate's performance in specific content areas.

If a candidate successfully completes the examination, in most cases they have fulfilled the final requirement for licensure. Conversely, if a candidate is unsuccessful on the examination, they are required to reapply to the state licensing agency. With computer-based testing there is no mandatory waiting period before retaking the examination, however, candidates will need to wait until the next fixed date. Some states limit the number of times a candidate can take the examination as well as mandate remedial coursework. In all states, candidates are prohibited from taking the examination more than three times in a 12 month period. The FSBPT has established a six-time lifetime limit on NPTE-PTA attempts.

Candidates that were unsuccessful on the NPTE-PTA can receive feedback from the FSBPT. The performance feedback report compares individual examination performance using the content outline and system categories with the performance of other candidates exposed to the same examination. Additional information on feedback is available through the FSBPT.

Test Taking Skills

Test taking skills are specific skills that allow individuals to utilize the characteristics and format of a selected examination in order to maximize their performance. These skills can be valuable when taking an examination such as the NPTE-PTA. Despite the importance of this topic, very little, if any, academic time is set aside to address test taking skills. The good news is that test taking skills can be learned and that through dedication, desire, and determination, these skills can serve to improve examination performance.

The NPTE-PTA consists of multiple-choice questions with four potentially correct answers to each question. Candidates are instructed to select the "best answer" to complete each question. Before exploring selected test taking strategies, we need to identify the various components of a multiple-choice question. Multiple-choice questions can be dissected into specific identifiable components:

Item

An item refers to an individual multiple-choice question and the corresponding potential answers. The NPTE-PTA contains 150 scored items and 50 pre-test items. Each item consists of a stem and four options. Items may vary in content and length, but should utilize a consistent format.

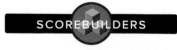

Stem

The stem refers to the statement that asks the question. Typically, the stem conveys to the reader the necessary information needed to respond correctly to the question. In addition to the necessary information, extraneous information may be included in the stem. This information, when not recognized by the candidate as unnecessary, often can serve as a significant distracter.

The stem commonly takes on the form of a complete sentence or an incomplete sentence. The stem can be expressed in a positive or negative form. A positive form requires a candidate to identify correct information, while a negative form requires a candidate to identify incorrect information. It is important to scrutinize each stem, since a single key word such as "NOT," "EXCEPT" or "LEAST" can turn a positive stem into a negative stem. Failure to identify this can lead to the identification of an incorrect answer.

Options

The options refer to the potential answers to the question asked. One option in each item will be the "best answer," while the others are considered distracters. Options can take on a variety of forms, including a single word, a group of words, an incomplete sentence, a complete sentence or a group of sentences. The method for analyzing each option does not change, regardless of form.

Approach for Answering Multiple-Choice Questions

On the NPTE-PTA there are 200 items (150 scored, 50 pre-test) that candidates must answer within a four hour time period. Due to the length of the examination and the time constraints associated with it, candidates need to approach the examination in a systematic and organized fashion. Loss of control during the examination will yield poor results that are not reflective of a candidate's actual knowledge. To assist candidates to minimize the impact of this potential pitfall, we will introduce a systematic approach to utilize when answering sample examination items.

The following six-step approach is recommended as a method for answering examination items:

1. Read the stem carefully to become familiar with the item and to determine the command words that indicate the desired action.

2. Read the stem again and identify relevant words or groups of words based on the identified command words.

3. Attempt to generate an answer to the stem.

4. Examine each option completely before moving to the next option.

5. Attempt to identify the best option.

6. Utilize deductive reasoning strategies.

The six-step approach begins with a candidate reading the stem. Candidates should read the stem initially to become familiar with the item and to determine the command words that indicate the desired action. Once this has been determined, candidates can reread the stem and attempt to extract the necessary components including relevant words or groups of words.

Perhaps the most important step in the six-step approach is to have candidates attempt to generate an answer to each question based on the identified command words. This is the only opportunity a candidate will have to objectively evaluate the question prior to exposing each of the options. Once a candidate exposes the options, they are no longer able to examine the question in a fully objective manner and instead become more likely to have their interpretation of the question influenced by a presented option. If for some reason a candidate is unable to generate a specific answer, they should attempt to think about the general topic and recall related information. Once a possible answer is generated, candidates should then begin to examine each option one at a time. It is important to read the entire option, since one word can often make a potentially correct answer incorrect. If the generated answer is consistent with one of the available options, the candidate should give the option strong consideration, however, since more than one option can be correct, it is imperative to analyze each presented option.

If candidates finish analyzing an item and are still unable to select one of the available options they should consider using a deductive reasoning strategy. Deductive reasoning strategies allow candidates to improve examination scores without direct knowledge of subject matter. This type of strategy should be applied only when candidates are unable to identify the correct response using academic knowledge. Deductive reasoning strategies often allow candidates to eliminate one or more of the potential answers. Elimination of any option significantly increases the probability of identifying the correct answer. On the NPTE-PTA, eliminating one option increases the chance of selecting a correct answer from 25% to 33%. Eliminating two options increases the chance of selecting a correct answer to 50%. On the surface, this may not seem terribly significant, however, on an examination such as the NPTE-PTA, this can often be the difference between a passing and a failing score. Selected deductive reasoning strategies that can be used effectively on the NPTE-PTA are presented.

Absurd options

Many times a multiple-choice item will include an option that is not consistent with what the stem is asking or with the other options. In many cases, this option can be eliminated. Rapid elimination of specific options will allow candidates to spend additional time analyzing other more viable options.

Similar options

When two or more options have a similar meaning or express the same fact, they often imply each other's incorrectness. For this reason, candidates can often eliminate both options.

Obtainable information

There is a great deal of factual material that candidates must sift through when taking the NPTE-PTA. In some instances, the material can provide candidates with valuable information that can assist them when answering other examination questions.

Degree of qualification

Particularly in the sciences, there seems to be many exceptions to general rules. Therefore, specific wording such as "always" or "never" often overqualify an option.

Activity One

In this activity, three sample questions are presented. Candidates should attempt to identify the best answer to each question by utilizing the six-step approach.

An analysis section immediately follows each of the three sample questions. The analysis section begins by showing the sample question with key terms underlined and command words in bold type. A brief narrative follows, which describes how the six-step approach can be applied to the sample question.

An answer key located at the conclusion of the exercise indicates the best answer and an explanation for each question.

Sample Question One

A physical therapist assistant instructs a patient with a Foley catheter in ambulation activities. During ambulation, the therapist should position the collection bag:

1. above the level of the patient's bladder
2. below the level of the patient's bladder
3. above the level of the patient's heart
4. below the level of the patient's heart

Analysis

A physical therapist assistant instructs a patient with a <u>Foley catheter in ambulation activities</u>. During ambulation, the therapist should **position** <u>the collection bag</u>:

1. above the level of the patient's bladder
2. below the level of the patient's bladder
3. above the level of the patient's heart
4. below the level of the patient's heart

A candidate should attempt to generate an answer to the question after reading the stem and identifying the pertinent information and command words. The candidate should then begin to reveal each of the available options one at a time. If a generated answer is consistent with one of the available options, there is a high probability that the answer is correct.

If a candidate was not able to generate an answer, they should expose the first option and give it careful consideration before moving on to the next option. They should progress through the remaining options in a similar manner. Candidates should remember it is possible to have more than one option that satisfactorily answers the question. It is then the candidate's responsibility to select the best answer from the viable options.

Sample Question Two

A physical therapist assistant monitors a patient's pulse after ambulation activities. The therapist notes that at times the rhythm of the pulse is irregular. When assessing the patient's pulse rate, the therapist should measure the pulse for:

1. 10 seconds
2. 15 seconds
3. 30 seconds
4. 60 seconds

Analysis

A physical therapist assistant monitors <u>a patient's pulse after ambulation activities</u>. The therapist notes that <u>at times the rhythm of the pulse is irregular</u>. <u>When assessing the patient's pulse rate</u>, the therapist should **measure the pulse for**:

1. 10 seconds
2. 15 seconds
3. 30 seconds
4. 60 seconds

After reading the question and identifying the pertinent information and command words, a candidate should recognize that it is a significant challenge to generate an exact answer prior to viewing the available options. A candidate should, however, begin to think about the nuances associated with assessing an irregular pulse. The candidate should then expose each of the available options and attempt to identify the correct response.

Although the six-step approach does not directly supply a candidate with the correct response, by carefully reading the stem, a candidate can avoid an unnecessary mistake. In this item, the stem asks the candidate to identify the pulse of a patient with an irregular rhythm. If a candidate does not read the question carefully, they may make an assumption that the question is asking for a traditional measurement of pulse (i.e., regular rhythm).

It is important that a candidate answer each question based only on the given information. By making even small assumptions or by not reading each question carefully, a candidate can make careless mistakes.

Sample Question Three

A physical therapist assistant completes an isokinetic test on an 18-year-old male rehabilitating from a medial meniscectomy. The therapist notes that the patient generates 140 ft/lbs of force using the uninvolved quadriceps at 60 degrees per second. Assuming a normal ratio of hamstrings to quadriceps strength, which of the following would be an acceptable hamstrings value at 60 degrees per second?

1. 64 ft/lbs
2. 84 ft/lbs
3. 114 ft/lbs
4. 116 ft/lbs

Analysis

A physical therapist assistant completes an isokinetic test on an 18-year-old male rehabilitating from a medial meniscectomy. The therapist notes that the patient generates 140 ft/lbs of force using the uninvolved quadriceps at 60 degrees per second. Assuming a normal ratio of hamstrings to quadriceps strength, which of the following would be **an acceptable hamstrings** value at 60 degrees per second?

1. 64 ft/lbs
2. 84 ft/lbs
3. 114 ft/lbs
4. 116 ft/lbs

For the purpose of discussion, let's assume a candidate has no idea of the normal ratio of quadriceps/hamstrings strength at 60 degrees per second. Lack of specific academic knowledge will result in a candidate not being able to identify the correct answer using the first five steps of the six-step approach. However, by utilizing deductive reasoning strategies, a candidate can significantly increase their chances of identifying the best answer without applying direct academic knowledge.

In this item, the stem asks a candidate to identify a value that would be representative of a normal quadriceps/hamstrings ratio at 60 degrees per second. As with many measurements in physical therapy, precise normal values are difficult to ascertain, and therefore often are expressed in ranges. Since options 3 and 4 are so close in value, they likely imply each other's incorrectness and can therefore be eliminated. Although in this example deductive reasoning strategies were not able to identify the correct answer, they were able to eliminate two of the four possible options. By eliminating two options, a candidate now has a 50% chance of identifying the best answer, even without utilizing any direct academic or clinical knowledge.

Activity One – Answer Key

1. Correct Answer: 2

The effect of gravity necessitates the collection bag being below the level of the patient's bladder.

2. Correct Answer: 4

Identification of an "irregular" pulse is an indicator to measure for one full minute. This method will provide the therapist with the most accurate assessment of the patient's actual pulse rate.

3. Correct Answer: 2

A gross estimate of quadriceps:hamstrings ratio is 3:2. Option 2, 84 ft/lbs is therefore the most consistent with the expressed ratio.

Alternate Examination Items

The NPTE-PTA will include a number of graphically enhanced items. Although representing a relatively small percentage of the total examination, candidates need to be comfortable answering this type of item.

Graphically Enhanced Items

Graphically enhanced items consist of figures, diagrams, pictures or other static images that are combined with traditional text in an examination item.

Activity Two

Two graphically enhanced items are presented. Candidates should attempt to identify the best answer to each question. An answer key located at the conclusion of the exercise indicates the best answer and an explanation for each question.

The following image should be used to answer question 1:

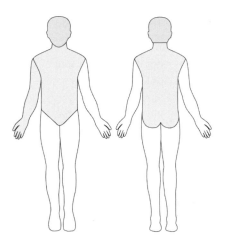

1. A 32-year-old male sustained extensive burns in a house fire. The shaded portion of the body diagrams represents the areas affected by the burns. Using the rule of nines, what percentage of the patient's body was involved?

   1. 40.5%
   2. 44.0%
   3. 49.5%
   4. 54.5%

The following image should be used to answer question 2:

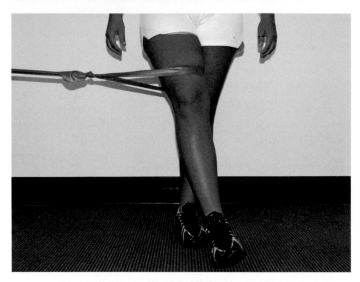

2. A physical therapist assistant instructs a patient to complete an exercise activity using a piece of elastic band as pictured. The patient is a 14-year-old female rehabilitating from a lower extremity injury sustained in a soccer contest. The therapist's primary objective for the activity is to:

   1. strengthen the right hip abductor muscles
   2. strengthen the right hip adductor muscles
   3. stretch the right hip abductor muscles
   4. stretch the right hip adductor muscles

Activity Two – Answer Key

1. Correct Answer: 3

The percentage of the body surface burned in an adult can be calculated using the rule of nines: anterior thorax (18%) + posterior thorax (18%) + head (9%) + anterior arm (4.5%) = 49.5%.

2. Correct Answer: 2

Successful completion of the activity requires the adductor muscles to exert a force greater than the tension supplied by the elastic band while moving into hip adduction. Muscles acting to adduct the hip include the adductor longus, adductor brevis, adductor magnus, and gracilis.

Time Constraints

Like many objective examinations, candidates have a specific allotted time to complete the NPTE-PTA. For physical therapist assistants, the available time is four hours. Since the examination consists of 200 questions, candidates will have 72 seconds available to answer each question. This number, although correct when viewing the examination as a whole, can be misleading. There will be many questions that a candidate will be able to answer in much less than 72 seconds, whereas other questions will take

somewhat longer. The key to success lies in progressing through the examination in a consistent and predictable manner.

Although 72 seconds per question does not seem like a great deal of time, the majority of candidates will have ample time to complete the examination. Despite this fact, it is important to pay attention to the elapsed time during the examination. It also is important to know your test taking history. Are you typically one of the first, one of the last, or somewhere in the middle of individuals completing an examination? This information is important as you plan your test taking strategy. In order to make sure your pace is appropriate during practice sessions and during the actual examination, it is important to formally check on the elapsed time, at a very minimum, when completing each section of 50 questions. This action will allow candidates to assess their progress and modify their pace, if necessary.

Preparing for the Examination

The simple thought of preparing for a comprehensive examination such as the NPTE-PTA can be overwhelming. Many candidates ask themselves how it is possible to prepare adequately for an examination that encompasses up to three years of professional coursework. To further complicate matters, the majority of candidates take the NPTE-PTA shortly after graduation. This can be a very anxious and unsettled time. Candidates often are actively seeking employment or are attempting to adjust to a new job. As a result, it is critical that candidates outline a well conceived and deliberate study plan for the examination.

One of the largest advantages of taking an examination such as the NPTE-PTA is that it does not require candidates to demonstrate mastery of new material. On the surface, this may not seem like a significant advantage, but since candidates are, in effect, only reviewing or relearning previously presented information, their level of attainment should be significantly greater. Many candidates fail to utilize this advantage. Candidates who attempt to learn large quantities of new information, instead of focusing on understanding and applying basic concepts, often do themselves a tremendous disservice. It is true that there undoubtedly will be questions that contain information that was not part of a selected curriculum, but to attempt to study this new information in any significant detail would be a large mistake for most candidates. Instead, candidates should focus on reviewing or relearning basic concepts that are an integral component of all accredited physical therapist assistant programs. It is this type of information that will make up the vast majority of the examination. Individuals who take this common sense approach optimize their chances of success.

Although students typically exhibit mastery of selected material during a scheduled examination, they do not always retain the information for later use. Often times, simply reviewing information is enough for candidates to relearn the material, however, in some cases, a more in-depth approach is necessary. It is recommended that candidates pay particular attention to their practice-oriented professional coursework. Practice-oriented professional coursework includes, but is not limited to, study of the musculoskeletal, neuromuscular, and cardiopulmonary systems. The content outline from the FSBPT clearly demonstrates the need for candidates to also review "other systems" (i.e., integumentary, metabolic and endocrine, gastrointestinal, genitourinary, lymphatic, multi-system). In addition, candidates usually have coursework in patient care skills, physical agents, ethics, education, and evidence-based practice. Each of these topics are important components of the content outline for the NPTE-PTA, although the weighting of each item differs significantly. **Chapter 2** will offer specific information on the relative weighting of each area according to systems and non-systems categories.

Special attention must be taken not to become bogged down in one specific area for any significant amount of time. General concepts that are understood should be scanned quickly, while other concepts that are more difficult for a candidate should be read carefully. Concepts that remain unclear after being reviewed should be written down for future study sessions.

Other foundational coursework encountered earlier in the professional curriculum can be consulted as needed during various study sessions. This type of coursework often includes, but is not limited to anatomy and physiology, neuroanatomy, exercise physiology, and kinesiology. It is important to limit the amount of time spent reviewing this type of foundational coursework. Candidates often can make better use of their allotted time by reviewing coursework encountered later in the curriculum that may be more practice-oriented. By reviewing practice-oriented information, candidates not only keep their studying consistent with the format of the examination, but also at the same time indirectly review much of the information presented in the foundational coursework.

Before beginning to study, develop specific goals for each study session. Ideally, these goals should be established on a weekly basis. Establishing goals will ensure that candidates cover the desired material and will serve as a mechanism to keep them on schedule with their study plan. Candidates should be realistic with the goals they establish and should not attempt to cover more material than is possible in a particular study session.

2

National Physical Therapy Examination-PTA Blueprint

Scott Giles

CHAPTER 2
National Physical Therapy Examination-PTA Blueprint

Perhaps the most valuable piece of information a candidate can utilize when preparing for the NPTE-PTA is the NPTE-PTA Blueprint. The blueprint provides a detailed analysis of each of the content areas of the NPTE-PTA. A thorough understanding of the content outline and system specific weighting will streamline a candidate's preparation. Less time will be spent covering topics that are not clinically relevant to the actual examination and as a result, more time will be available for reviewing and relearning.

This chapter will explore the examination in detail according to the content outline and system specific areas. Each of the sample examinations in *PTAEXAM: The Complete Study Guide* offers candidates the opportunity to view their performance according to five system and five content outline categories. Candidates must be familiar with the content contained in each system and content outline category and use this information to develop remedial plans to improve performance on sample examinations. We will begin with an exploration of the NPTE-PTA Content Outline. All examination information is publicly available from the Federation of State Boards of Physical Therapy.

Content Outline Summary

Content	Questions (Range)	Midpoint (Questions)	Midpoint (Percentage)
Physical Therapy Data Collection	29-37	33	22%
Diseases/Conditions that Impact Effective Treatment	33-48	40.5	27%
Interventions	41-54	47.5	31.67%
Equipment, Devices, and Technologies; Therapeutic Modalities	16-20	18	12%
Safety and Protection; Professional Responsibilities; Research	9-13	11	7.33%

NPTE-PTA — CONTENT OUTLINE WEIGHTING

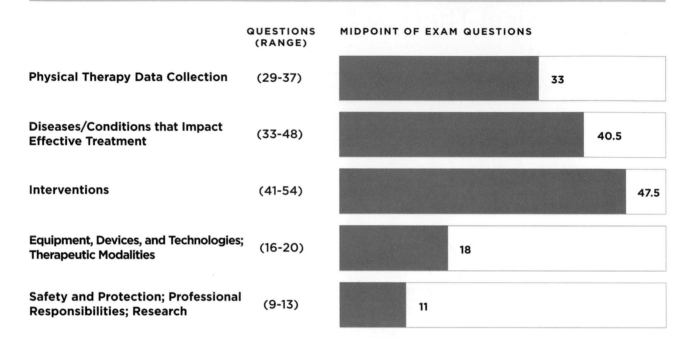

	QUESTIONS (RANGE)	MIDPOINT OF EXAM QUESTIONS
Physical Therapy Data Collection	(29-37)	33
Diseases/Conditions that Impact Effective Treatment	(33-48)	40.5
Interventions	(41-54)	47.5
Equipment, Devices, and Technologies; Therapeutic Modalities	(16-20)	18
Safety and Protection; Professional Responsibilities; Research	(9-13)	11

NPTE-PTA — CONTENT OUTLINE WEIGHTING

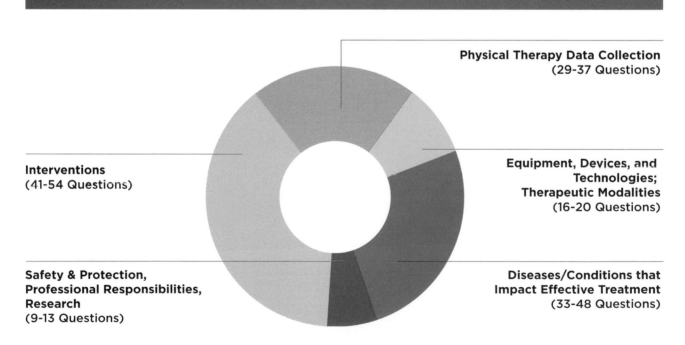

Physical Therapy Data Collection
(29-37 Questions)

Equipment, Devices, and Technologies;
Therapeutic Modalities
(16-20 Questions)

Interventions
(41-54 Questions)

Diseases/Conditions that
Impact Effective Treatment
(33-48 Questions)

Safety & Protection,
Professional Responsibilities,
Research
(9-13 Questions)

Physical Therapy Data Collection
Midrange: 33 Questions (22%)

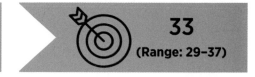

33
(Range: 29–37)

This category refers to knowledge of the types and applications of specific system tests/measures, including outcome measures, according to current best evidence. The category includes the reaction of the specific system to tests/measures. Information covered in these areas supports appropriate and effective patient/client management for rehabilitation, health promotion, and performance across the lifespan.

PHYSICAL THERAPY DATA COLLECTION

	QUESTIONS (RANGE)	MIDPOINT OF EXAM QUESTIONS
Musculoskeletal System	(12-14)	13
Neuromuscular and Nervous Systems	(8-10)	9
Cardiovascular and Pulmonary Systems	(6-8)	7
Other Systems	(3-5)	4

Diseases/Conditions that Impact Effective Treatment
Midrange: 40.5 Questions (27%)

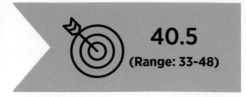

40.5
(Range: 33-48)

This category refers to foundational scientific principles and knowledge of diseases and conditions to support appropriate and effective patient/client management for rehabilitation, health promotion, and performance across the lifespan.

DISEASES/CONDITIONS THAT IMPACT EFFECTIVE TREATMENT

	QUESTIONS (RANGE)	MIDPOINT OF EXAM QUESTIONS
Musculoskeletal System	(9-11)	10
Neuromuscular and Nervous Systems	(8-10)	9
Cardiovascular and Pulmonary Systems	(6-7)	6.5
Other Systems	(10-20)	15

Interventions
Midrange: 47.5 Questions (31.67%)

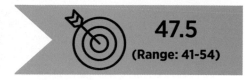

47.5
(Range: 41-54)

This category refers to specific system interventions (including types, applications, responses, and potential complications), according to current best evidence, as well as the impact on the specific system of interventions performed on other systems in order to support appropriate and effective patient/client management for rehabilitation, health promotion, and performance across the lifespan.

INTERVENTIONS

	QUESTIONS (RANGE)	MIDPOINT OF EXAM QUESTIONS
Musculoskeletal System	(15-16)	15.5
Neuromuscular and Nervous Systems	(12-14)	13
Cardiovascular and Pulmonary Systems	(9-11)	10
Other Systems	(5-13)	9

Equipment, Devices, and Technologies
Midrange: 8 Questions (5.33%)

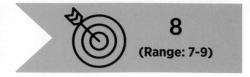

8
(Range: 7-9)

This category refers to the different types of equipment, devices and technologies, use requirements, and/or contextual determinants, according to current best evidence, as well as any other influencing factors involved in the application of equipment, devices, and technologies, in order to support appropriate and effective patient/client management for rehabilitation, health promotion, and performance across the lifespan.

- Assistive and adaptive devices/technologies (e.g., walkers, wheelchairs, adaptive seating systems and positioning devices, mechanical lifts)
- Prosthetic devices/technologies (e.g., lower extremity and upper extremity, microprocessor-controlled prosthetic devices)

Therapeutic Modalities
Midrange: 10 Questions (6.67%)

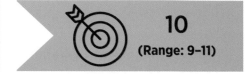

10
(Range: 9–11)

This category refers to the different types of therapeutic modalities, use requirements, and/or contextual determinants, according to current best evidence, as well as any other influencing factors involved in the application of therapeutic modalities, in order to support appropriate and effective patient/client management for rehabilitation, health promotion, and performance across the lifespan.

- Thermal modalities
- Iontophoresis
- Electrotherapy modalities (e.g., neuromuscular electrical stimulation (NMES), transcutaneous electrical nerve stimulation (TENS), functional electrical stimulation (FES), interferential therapy, high-voltage pulsed current)
- Phonophoresis
- Ultrasound modalities
- Mechanical modalities (e.g., mechanical motion devices, traction devices)
- Biofeedback
- Intermittent compression

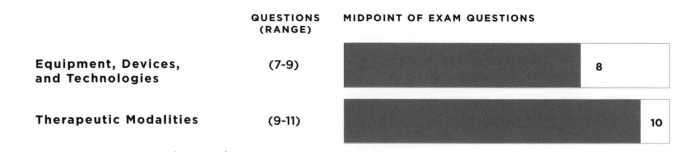

EQUIPMENT, DEVICES, AND TECHNOLOGIES; THERAPEUTIC MODALITIES

	QUESTIONS (RANGE)	MIDPOINT OF EXAM QUESTIONS
Equipment, Devices, and Technologies	(7-9)	8
Therapeutic Modalities	(9-11)	10

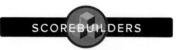

Safety and Protection
Midrange: 5 Questions (3.33%)

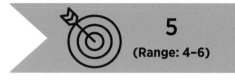

5
(Range: 4–6)

This category refers to the critical issues involved in patient/client safety and protection and the responsibilities of health-care providers to ensure that patient/client management and health-care decisions take place in a secure environment.

- Factors influencing safety and injury prevention (e.g., safe patient handling, fall prevention, equipment maintenance, environmental safety)
- Function, implications, and related precautions of intravenous lines, tubes, catheters, monitoring devices, and mechanical ventilators/oxygen delivery devices
- Emergency preparedness (e.g., CPR, first aid, disaster response)
- Infection control procedures (e.g., standard/universal precautions, isolation techniques, sterile technique)
- Signs/symptoms of physical, sexual, and psychological abuse and neglect

Professional Responsibilities
Midrange: 3.5 Questions (2.33%)

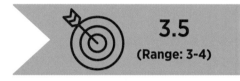

3.5
(Range: 3-4)

This category refers to the responsibilities of health-care providers to ensure that patient/client management and health-care decisions take place in a trustworthy environment.

- Standards of documentation
- Patient/client rights (e.g., ADA, IDEA, HIPAA, patient bill of rights)
- Human resource legal issues (e.g., OSHA, sexual harassment)
- Roles and responsibilities of the physical therapist, physical therapist assistant, other healthcare professionals, and support staff
- Standards of professional ethics
- Standards of billing, coding, and reimbursement
- Obligations for reporting illegal, unethical, or unprofessional behaviors (e.g., fraud, abuse, neglect)
- State and federal laws, rules, regulations, and industry standards set by state and accrediting bodies (e.g., state licensing entities, Joint Commission, CARF, CMS)
- Risk management and quality assurance (e.g., policies and procedures, incident reports, peer chart review)
- Cultural factors and/or characteristics that affect patient/client management (e.g., language differences, disability, ethnicity, customs, demographics, religion)
- Socioeconomic factors that affect patient/client management
- Health information technology (e.g., electronic medical records, telemedicine)

Research and Evidence-Based Practice
Midrange: 2.5 Questions (1.67%)

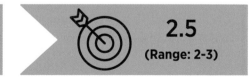

2.5
(Range: 2-3)

This category refers to the knowledge of basic research methods and data collection techniques necessary for interpretation of information sources and practice research to support patient/client management decisions fundamental to evidence-based practice.

- Research methodology and interpretation (e.g., qualitative, quantitative, levels of evidence)
- Data collection techniques (e.g., surveys, direct observation)
- Measurement science (e.g., reliability, validity)
- Techniques for accessing evidence (e.g., peer-reviewed publications, scientific proceedings, guidelines, clinical prediction rules)

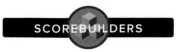

SAFETY AND PROTECTION; PROFESSIONAL RESPONSIBILITIES; RESEARCH

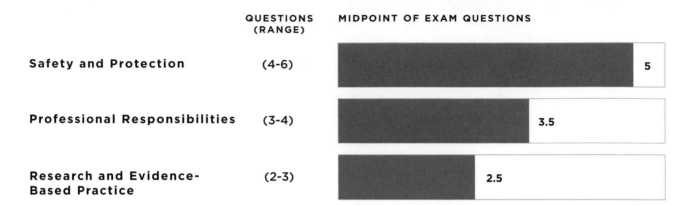

	QUESTIONS (RANGE)	MIDPOINT OF EXAM QUESTIONS
Safety and Protection	(4-6)	5
Professional Responsibilities	(3-4)	3.5
Research and Evidence-Based Practice	(2-3)	2.5

System Summary

Systems	Questions (Range)	Midpoint (Questions)	Midpoint (Percentage)
Musculoskeletal System	36-41	38.5	25.67%
Neuromuscular and Nervous Systems	28-34	31	20.67%
Cardiovascular and Pulmonary Systems	21-26	23.5	15.67%
Other Systems			
Integumentary System	5-10	7.5	5%
Metabolic and Endocrine Systems	5-7	6	4%
Gastrointestinal System	0-4	2	1.33%
Genitourinary System	0-4	2	1.33%
Lymphatic System	3-6	4.5	3%
System Interactions	5-7	6	4%
Non-Systems	Questions (Range)	Midpoint (Questions)	Midpoint (Percentage)
Equipment, Devices, and Technologies; Therapeutic Modalities			
Equipment, Devices, and Technologies	7-9	8	5.33%
Therapeutic Modalities	9-11	10	6.67%
Safety and Protection; Professional Responsibilities; Research			
Safety and Protection	4-6	5	3.33%
Professional Responsibilities	3-4	3.5	2.33%
Research and Evidence-Based Practice	2-3	2.5	1.67%

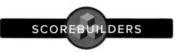

NPTE-PTA — SYSTEM WEIGHTING

	QUESTIONS (RANGE)	MIDPOINT OF EXAM QUESTIONS
Musculoskeletal System	(36-41)	38.5
Neuromuscular and Nervous Systems	(28-34)	31
Cardiovascular and Pulmonary Systems	(21-26)	23.5
Other Systems	(18-38)	28
Non-Systems	(25-33)	29

NPTE-PTA — SYSTEM WEIGHTING

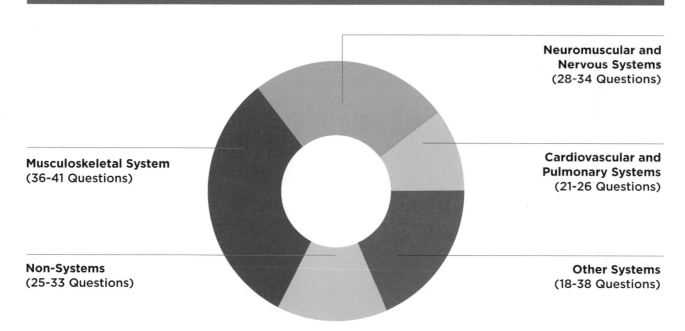

Musculoskeletal System
(36-41 Questions)

Non-Systems
(25-33 Questions)

Neuromuscular and
Nervous Systems
(28-34 Questions)

Cardiovascular and
Pulmonary Systems
(21-26 Questions)

Other Systems
(18-38 Questions)

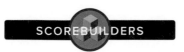

Musculoskeletal System
Midrange: 38.5 Questions (25.67%)

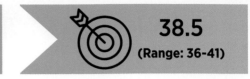

38.5
(Range: 36-41)

Physical Therapy Data Collection: This category refers to knowledge of the types and applications of musculoskeletal system tests/measures, including outcome measures, according to current best evidence. The category includes the reaction of the musculoskeletal system to tests/measures and the mechanics of body movement as related to the musculoskeletal system. Information covered in these areas supports appropriate and effective patient/client management for rehabilitation, health promotion, and performance across the lifespan.

- Musculoskeletal system tests/measures, including outcome measures, and their applications according to current best evidence
- Anatomy and physiology of the musculoskeletal system as related to tests/measures
- Movement analysis as related to the musculoskeletal system
- Joint biomechanics and their applications

Diseases/Conditions that Impact Effective Treatment: This category refers to foundational scientific principles and knowledge of diseases and conditions of the musculoskeletal system to support appropriate and effective patient/client management for rehabilitation, health promotion, and performance across the lifespan.

- Musculoskeletal system diseases/conditions and their pathophysiology to carry out the established plan of care
- Nonpharmacological medical management of the musculoskeletal system (e.g., diagnostic imaging, laboratory test values, other medical tests, surgical procedures)
- Pharmacological management of the musculoskeletal system
- Connective tissue diseases/conditions and their pathophysiology to carry out the established plan of care

Interventions: This category refers to musculoskeletal system interventions (including types, applications, responses, and potential complications), according to current best evidence, as well as the impact on the musculoskeletal system of interventions performed on other systems in order to support appropriate and effective patient/client management for rehabilitation, health promotion, and performance across the lifespan.

- Musculoskeletal system physical therapy interventions and their applications for rehabilitation, health promotion, and performance according to current best evidence
- Anatomy and physiology of the musculoskeletal system as related to physical therapy interventions
- Adverse effects or complications on the musculoskeletal system from physical therapy interventions used on other systems

Neuromuscular and Nervous Systems
Midrange: 31 Questions (20.67%)

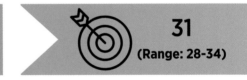

31
(Range: 28-34)

Physical Therapy Data Collection: This category refers to knowledge of the types and applications of neuromuscular and nervous systems tests/measures, including outcome measures, according to current best evidence. The category includes the reaction of the neuromuscular and nervous systems to tests/measures and the mechanics of body movement as related to the neuromuscular and nervous systems. Information covered in these areas supports appropriate and effective patient/client management for rehabilitation, health promotion, and performance across the lifespan.

- Neuromuscular and nervous systems tests/measures, including outcome measures, and their applications according to current best evidence
- Anatomy and physiology of the neuromuscular and nervous systems as related to tests/measures
- Movement analysis as related to the neuromuscular and nervous systems

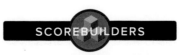

Diseases/Conditions that Impact Effective Treatment: This category refers to foundational scientific principles and knowledge of diseases and conditions of the neuromuscular & nervous systems to support appropriate and effective patient/client management for rehabilitation, health promotion, and performance across the lifespan.

- Neuromuscular and nervous systems (CNS, PNS, ANS) diseases/conditions and their pathophysiology to carry out the established plan of care

- Nonpharmacological medical management of the neuromuscular and nervous systems (e.g., diagnostic imaging, laboratory test values, other medical tests, surgical procedures)

- Pharmacological management of the neuromuscular and nervous systems

Interventions: This category refers to neuromuscular and nervous systems interventions (including types, applications, responses, and potential complications), according to current best evidence, as well as the impact on the neuromuscular and nervous systems of interventions performed on other systems in order to support appropriate and effective patient/client management for rehabilitation, health promotion, and performance across the lifespan.

- Neuromuscular and nervous systems physical therapy interventions and their applications for rehabilitation, health promotion, and performance according to current best evidence

- Anatomy and physiology of the neuromuscular and nervous systems as related to physical therapy interventions, daily activities, and environmental factors

- Adverse effects or complications on the neuromuscular and nervous systems from physical therapy interventions

- Adverse effects or complications on the neuromuscular and nervous systems from physical therapy interventions used on other systems

- Motor control as related to neuromuscular and nervous systems physical therapy interventions

- Motor learning as related to neuromuscular and nervous systems physical therapy interventions

Cardiovascular and Pulmonary Systems
Midrange: 23.5 Questions (15.67%)

23.5
(Range: 21-26)

Physical Therapy Data Collection: This category refers to knowledge of the types and applications of cardiovascular and pulmonary systems tests/measures, including outcome measures, according to current best evidence. The category includes the reaction of cardiovascular and pulmonary systems to tests/measures and the mechanics of body movement as related to the cardiovascular and pulmonary systems. Information covered in these areas supports appropriate and effective patient/client management for rehabilitation, health promotion, and performance across the lifespan.

- Cardiovascular and pulmonary systems tests/measures, including outcome measures, and their applications according to current best evidence

- Anatomy and physiology of the cardiovascular and pulmonary system as related to tests/measures

- Movement analysis as related to the cardiovascular and pulmonary systems (e.g., rib cage excursion, breathing pattern)

Diseases/Conditions that Impact Effective Treatment: This category refers to foundational scientific principles and knowledge of diseases and conditions of the cardiovascular & pulmonary systems to support appropriate and effective patient/client management for rehabilitation, health promotion, and performance across the lifespan.

- Cardiovascular and pulmonary systems diseases/conditions and their pathophysiology to carry out the established plan of care

- Nonpharmacological medical management of the cardiovascular and pulmonary systems (e.g., diagnostic imaging, laboratory test values, other medical tests, surgical procedures)

- Pharmacological management of the cardiovascular and pulmonary systems

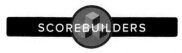

Interventions: This category refers to cardiovascular and pulmonary systems interventions (including types, applications, responses, and potential complications) according to current best evidence, as well as the impact on the cardiovascular and pulmonary systems of interventions performed on other systems in order to support appropriate and effective patient/client management for rehabilitation, health promotion, and performance across the lifespan.

- Cardiovascular and pulmonary systems physical therapy interventions and their applications for rehabilitation, health promotion, and performance according to current best evidence
- Anatomy and physiology of the cardiovascular and pulmonary systems as related to physical therapy interventions, daily activities, and environmental factors
- Adverse effects or complications on the cardiovascular and pulmonary systems from physical therapy interventions
- Adverse effects or complications on the cardiovascular and pulmonary systems from physical therapy interventions used on other systems

Other Systems (overview)
Midrange: 28 Questions (18.67%)

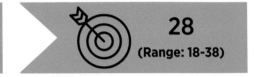

28
(Range: 18-38)

The Other Systems category includes the Integumentary System, Metabolic and Endocrine Systems, Gastrointestinal System, Genitourinary System, Lymphatic System, and System Interactions.

OTHER SYSTEMS

	QUESTIONS (RANGE)	MIDPOINT OF EXAM QUESTIONS
Integumentary System	(5-10)	7.5
Metabolic and Endocrine Systems	(5-7)	6
Gastrointestinal System	(0-4)	2
Genitourinary System	(0-4)	2
Lymphatic System	(3-6)	4.5
System Interactions	(5-7)	6

Integumentary System
Midrange: 7.5 Questions (5%)

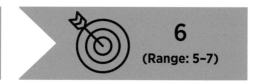

7.5
(Range: 5-10)

Physical Therapy Data Collection: This category refers to knowledge of the types and applications of integumentary system tests/measures, including outcome measures, according to current best evidence. The category includes the reaction of the integumentary system to tests/measures and the mechanics of body movement as related to the integumentary system. Information covered in these areas supports appropriate and effective patient/client management for rehabilitation, health promotion, and performance across the lifespan.

- Integumentary system tests/measures, including outcome measures, and their applications according to current best evidence
- Anatomy and physiology of the integumentary system as related to tests/measures
- Movement analysis as related to the integumentary system (e.g., friction, shear, pressure, and scar mobility)

Diseases/Conditions that Impact Effective Treatment: This category refers to foundational scientific principles and knowledge of diseases and conditions of the integumentary system to support appropriate and effective patient/client management for rehabilitation, health promotion, and performance across the lifespan.

- Integumentary system diseases/conditions and their pathophysiology to carry out the established plan of care
- Nonpharmacological medical management of the integumentary system (e.g., diagnostic imaging, laboratory test values, other medical tests, surgical procedures)
- Pharmacological management of the integumentary system

Interventions: This category refers to integumentary system interventions (including types, applications, responses, and potential complications), according to current best evidence, as well as the impact on the integumentary system of interventions performed on other systems in order to support appropriate and effective patient/client management for rehabilitation, health promotion, and performance across the lifespan.

- Integumentary system physical therapy interventions and their applications for rehabilitation, health promotion, and performance according to current best evidence
- Anatomy and physiology of the integumentary system as related to physical therapy interventions, daily activities, and environmental factors
- Adverse effects or complications on the integumentary system from physical therapy and medical/surgical interventions
- Adverse effects or complications on the integumentary system from physical therapy interventions used on other systems

Metabolic and Endocrine Systems
Midrange: 6 Questions (4%)

6
(Range: 5-7)

Diseases/Conditions that Impact Effective Treatment: This category refers to foundational scientific principles and knowledge of diseases and conditions of the metabolic & endocrine systems to support appropriate and effective patient/client management for rehabilitation, health promotion, and performance across the lifespan.

- Metabolic and endocrine systems diseases/conditions and their pathophysiology to carry out the established plan of care
- Nonpharmacological medical management of the metabolic and endocrine systems (e.g., diagnostic imaging, laboratory test values, other medical tests, surgical procedures)
- Pharmacological management of the metabolic and endocrine systems

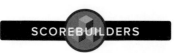

Interventions: This category refers to metabolic and endocrine systems interventions (including types, applications, responses, and potential complications), according to current best evidence, as well as the impact on the metabolic and endocrine systems of interventions performed on other systems in order to support appropriate and effective patient/client management for rehabilitation, health promotion, and performance across the lifespan.

- Metabolic and endocrine systems physical therapy interventions and their applications for rehabilitation, health promotion, and performance according to current best evidence
- Anatomy and physiology of the metabolic and endocrine systems as related to physical therapy interventions, daily activities, and environmental factors
- Adverse effects or complications on the metabolic and endocrine systems from physical therapy interventions
- Adverse effects or complications on the metabolic and endocrine systems from physical therapy interventions used on other systems

Gastrointestinal System
Midrange: 2 Questions (1.33%)

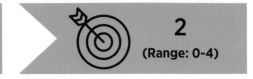

2

(Range: 0-4)

Diseases/Conditions that Impact Effective Treatment: This category refers to foundational scientific principles and knowledge of diseases and conditions of the gastrointestinal system to support appropriate and effective patient/client management for rehabilitation, health promotion, and performance across the lifespan.

- Gastrointestinal system diseases/conditions and their pathophysiology to carry out the established plan of care
- Nonpharmacological medical management of the gastrointestinal system (e.g., diagnostic imaging, laboratory test values, other medical tests, surgical procedures)
- Pharmacological management of the gastrointestinal system

Interventions: This category refers to gastrointestinal system interventions (including types, applications, responses, and potential complications), according to current best evidence, as well as the impact on the gastrointestinal system of interventions performed on other systems in order to support appropriate and effective patient/client management for rehabilitation, health promotion, and performance across the lifespan.

- Gastrointestinal system physical therapy interventions and their applications for rehabilitation, health promotion, and performance according to current best evidence (e.g., positioning for reflux prevention, bowel programs)
- Anatomy and physiology of the gastrointestinal system as related to physical therapy interventions, daily activities, and environmental factors
- Adverse effects or complications on the gastrointestinal system from physical therapy interventions
- Adverse effects or complications on the gastrointestinal system from physical therapy interventions used on other systems

Genitourinary System
Midrange: 2 Questions (1.33%)

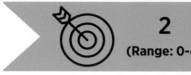

2
(Range: 0-4)

Diseases/Conditions that Impact Effective Treatment: This category refers to foundational scientific principles and knowledge of diseases and conditions of the genitourinary system to support appropriate and effective patient/client management for rehabilitation, health promotion, and performance across the lifespan.

- Genitourinary system diseases/conditions and their pathophysiology to carry out the established plan of care
- Nonpharmacological medical management of the genitourinary system (e.g., diagnostic imaging, laboratory test values, other medical tests, surgical procedures)

Interventions: This category refers to genitourinary system interventions (including types, applications, responses, and potential complications), according to current best evidence, as well as the impact on the genitourinary system of interventions performed on other systems in order to support appropriate and effective patient/client management for rehabilitation, health promotion, and performance across the lifespan.

- Genitourinary system physical therapy interventions and their applications for rehabilitation, health promotion, and performance according to current best evidence (e.g., bladder programs, biofeedback, pelvic floor retraining)
- Anatomy and physiology of the genitourinary system as related to physical therapy interventions, daily activities, and environmental factors
- Adverse effects or complications on the genitourinary system from physical therapy interventions
- Adverse effects or complications on the genitourinary system from physical therapy interventions used on other systems

Lymphatic System
Midrange: 4.5 Questions (3%)

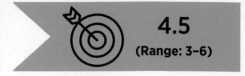

4.5
(Range: 3–6)

Physical Therapy Data Collection: This category refers to knowledge of the types and applications of lymphatic system tests/measures, including outcome measures, according to current best evidence. The category includes the reaction of the lymphatic system to tests/measures and the mechanics of body movement as related to the lymphatic system. Information covered in these areas supports appropriate and effective patient/client management for rehabilitation, health promotion, and performance across the lifespan.

- Lymphatic system tests/measures, including outcome measures, and their applications according to current best evidence
- Anatomy and physiology of the lymphatic system as related to tests/measures
- Movement analysis as related to the lymphatic system (e.g., posture, compensatory movement, extremity range of motion)

Diseases/Conditions that Impact Effective Treatment: This category refers to foundational scientific principles and knowledge of diseases and conditions of the lymphatic system to support appropriate and effective patient/client management for rehabilitation, health promotion, and performance across the lifespan.

- Lymphatic system diseases/conditions and their pathophysiology to establish and carry out a plan of care, including prognosis

Interventions: This category refers to lymphatic system interventions (including types, applications, responses, and potential complications), according to current best evidence, as well as the impact on the lymphatic system of interventions performed on other systems in order to support appropriate and effective patient/client management for rehabilitation, health promotion, and performance across the lifespan.

- Lymphatic system physical therapy interventions and their applications for rehabilitation, health promotion, and performance according to current best evidence
- Anatomy and physiology of the lymphatic system as related to physical therapy interventions, daily activities, and environmental factors
- Adverse effects or complications on the lymphatic system from physical therapy interventions
- Adverse effects or complications on the lymphatic system from physical therapy interventions used on other systems

System Interactions
Midrange: 6 Questions (4%)

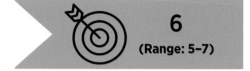

6
(Range: 5-7)

Diseases/Conditions that Impact Effective Treatment: This category refers to foundational scientific principles and knowledge of diseases and conditions involving system interactions to support appropriate and effective patient/client management for rehabilitation, health promotion, and performance across the lifespan.

- Diseases/conditions where the primary impact is on more than one system (e.g., cancer, multitrauma, sarcoidosis, autoimmune disorders, pregnancy) to carry out the established plan of care
- Nonpharmacological medical management of multiple systems (e.g., diagnostic imaging, other medical tests, surgical procedures)
- Pharmacological management of multiple systems, including polypharmacy
- Impact of comorbidities/coexisting conditions on patient/client management (e.g., diabetes and hypertension; obesity and arthritis; dementia and hip fracture)
- Psychological and psychiatric conditions that impact patient/client management (e.g., grief, depression, schizophrenia)
- Dimensions of pain that impact patient/client management (e.g., psychological, social, physiological, neurological, mechanical)

Non-Systems

Equipment, Devices, and Technologies
Midrange: 8 Questions (5.33%)

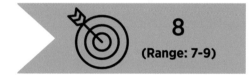

8
(Range: 7-9)

This category refers to the different types of equipment, devices and technologies, use requirements, and/or contextual determinants, according to current best evidence, as well as any other influencing factors involved in the application of equipment, devices, and technologies, in order to support appropriate and effective patient/client management for rehabilitation, health promotion, and performance across the lifespan.

- Assistive and adaptive devices/technologies (e.g., walkers, wheelchairs, adaptive seating systems and positioning devices, mechanical lifts)
- Prosthetic devices/technologies (e.g., lower extremity and upper extremity, microprocessor-controlled prosthetic devices)

Therapeutic Modalities
Midrange: 10 Questions (6.67%)

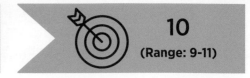

10
(Range: 9-11)

This category refers to the different types of therapeutic modalities, use requirements, and/or contextual determinants, according to current best evidence, as well as any other influencing factors involved in the application of therapeutic modalities, in order to support appropriate and effective patient/client management for rehabilitation, health promotion, and performance across the lifespan.

- Thermal modalities
- Iontophoresis
- Electrotherapy modalities (e.g., neuromuscular electrical stimulation (NMES), transcutaneous electrical nerve stimulation (TENS), functional electrical stimulation (FES), interferential therapy, high-voltage pulsed current)
- Phonophoresis
- Ultrasound modalities
- Mechanical modalities (e.g., mechanical motion devices, traction devices)
- Biofeedback
- Intermittent compression

Safety and Protection
Midrange: 5 Questions (3.33%)

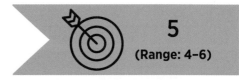

5
(Range: 4–6)

This category refers to the critical issues involved in patient/client safety and protection and the responsibilities of health-care providers to ensure that patient/client management and health-care decisions take place in a secure environment.

- Factors influencing safety and injury prevention (e.g., safe patient handling, fall prevention, equipment maintenance, environmental safety)
- Function, implications, and related precautions of intravenous lines, tubes, catheters, monitoring devices, and mechanical ventilators/ oxygen delivery devices
- Emergency preparedness (e.g., CPR, first aid, disaster response)
- Infection control procedures (e.g., standard/universal precautions, isolation techniques, sterile technique)
- Signs/symptoms of physical, sexual, and psychological abuse and neglect

Professional Responsibilities
Midrange: 3.5 Questions (2.33%)

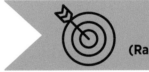

3.5
(Range: 3-4)

This category refers to the responsibilities of health-care providers to ensure that patient/client management and health-care decisions take place in a trustworthy environment.

- Standards of documentation
- Patient/client rights (e.g., ADA, IDEA, HIPAA, patient bill of rights)
- Human resource legal issues (e.g., OSHA, sexual harassment)
- Roles and responsibilities of the physical therapist, physical therapist assistant, other healthcare professionals, and support staff
- Standards of professional ethics
- Standards of billing, coding, and reimbursement
- Obligations for reporting illegal, unethical, or unprofessional behaviors (e.g., fraud, abuse, neglect)
- State and federal laws, rules, regulations, and industry standards set by state and accrediting bodies (e.g., state licensing entities, Joint Commission, CARF, CMS)
- Risk management and quality assurance (e.g., policies and procedures, incident reports, peer chart review)
- Cultural factors and/or characteristics that affect patient/client management (e.g., language differences, disability, ethnicity, customs, demographics, religion)
- Socioeconomic factors that affect patient/client management
- Health information technology (e.g., electronic medical records, telemedicine)

Research and Evidence-Based Practice
Midrange: 2.5 Questions (1.67%)

2.5
(Range: 2-3)

This category refers to the knowledge of basic research methods and data collection techniques necessary for interpretation of information sources and practice research to support patient/client management decisions fundamental to evidence-based practice.

- Research methodology and interpretation (e.g., qualitative, quantitative, levels of evidence)
- Data collection techniques (e.g., surveys, direct observation)
- Measurement science (e.g., reliability, validity)
- Techniques for assessing evidence (e.g., peer-reviewed publications, scientific proceedings, guidelines, clinical prediction rules)

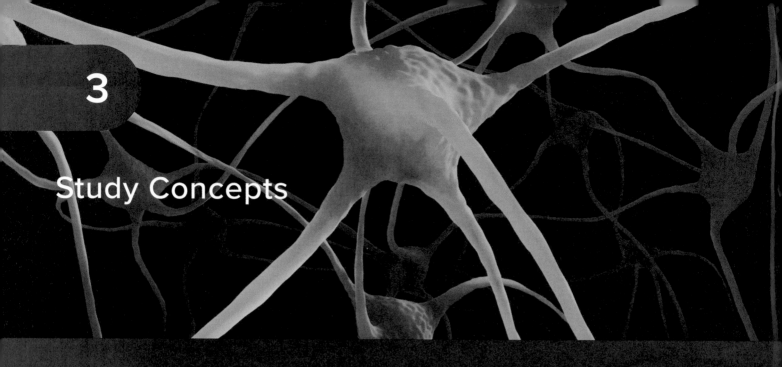

3

Study Concepts

Scott Giles

CHAPTER 3
Study Concepts

The inclusion of Study Concepts in *PTAEXAM: The Complete Study Guide* serves to remind candidates that preparing for the NPTE-PTA requires more than simply reviewing academic content and taking sample examinations.

Each of the presented Study Concepts provides candidates with an idea or concept to potentially integrate into their comprehensive study plan. For example, perhaps a candidate has a strong learning style preference where they tend to favor active learning over passive learning. To date, their study plan has consisted of purely passive activities such as reading the academic review section of a review book and reviewing class notes. Not surprisingly, the candidate has experienced a great deal of difficulty moving through the academic review and class notes and has serious doubts about how much of the material they have retained. In addition, the candidate finds they are unable to concentrate after approximately 90 minutes of studying and typically discontinues the study session at this point.

The presented Study Concept entitled "Learning Styles" offers a number of practical suggestions to assist candidates to identify their own unique learning style and to design study sessions to incorporate these preferences. Study plans that are designed to address decided learning preferences yield a much greater return on investment than generic study plans.

As a second example, consider the Study Concept entitled "Golden Rules." This item explores whether it is possible to develop specific rules that allow candidates to differentiate between two or more plausible options on multiple-choice questions used on the NPTE-PTA. A potential rule would be something like the following: "When choosing between a number of acceptable interventions, always select the most conservative option in an effort to minimize any potential safety risk to the patient."

Potential rules like this are very tempting since they provide candidates with a means to make questions more objective and therefore less amorphous. The problem, however, is that the NPTE-PTA is designed to assess a candidate's ability to make clinical decisions rather than to rely on memorization or simply apply a set of standardized rules. The Study Concept presents a variety of potential rules and walks candidates through a number of clinical scenarios demonstrating why rules are better used as only loose guidelines to consider when answering multiple-choice questions.

Study Concepts	
Study Concept 1	Learning Styles
Study Concept 2	Time Management
Study Concept 3	Levels of Knowledge and Understanding
Study Concept 4	Golden Rules
Study Concept 5	Automaticity
Study Concept 6	Truths and Myths
Study Concept 7	Blood Pressure
Study Concept 8	Lines, Tubes, and Equipment
Study Concept 9	Emergent Conditions
Study Concept 10	Assessment

In truth, many questions on the examination require candidates to make unique judgments based on the exact circumstances presented in the two to four sentences that make up the question stem. Candidates who develop the flexibility to apply clinical information in a wide variety of scenarios are well poised to be successful on the NPTE-PTA.

Enjoy each of the presented Study Concepts and use the notes section to make observations of your present performance related to each of these unique topics.

Study Concept 1: Learning Styles

Studying for a comprehensive examination such as the NPTE-PTA can be a significant challenge for any candidate. Given the volume of information required to be reviewed or relearned, it is critical for candidates to be as efficient as possible as they move through their established study plan. In order to maximize the efficiency of established study sessions, candidates should consider their preferred learning channels.

Perhaps the most critical question to answer relates to your preferred learning style for input and processing. Is your preferred learning style for input and processing more active or passive? Here is a brief description of each style that may assist you to label your individual preference.

ACTIVE LEARNING STYLE – when exposed to new material, a learner who likes to hear it, see it, say it, question it, interact with it, and then keep on doing this. Learners with this style tend to be multisensoral (visual, auditory, tactile/kinesthetic).

PASSIVE LEARNING STYLE – when exposed to new material, a learner who likes to hear it or read it and then keep on doing this. Learners with this style tend to determine the relationship to known material after input and before processing.

It is important to recognize that one learning style is not better than another, but each learning style can come with particular strengths and weaknesses. For example, a candidate who is active for both input and processing may be able to focus intently on the application and utility of ideas, however, may consider details boring and have a short attention span. Conversely, a candidate who is passive for both input and processing may be effective at sequential thinking and focusing on details, but may miss the "big picture."

Please recognize that an individual's learning style varies depending on the situation, however, it is equally important to recognize that most candidates have decided learning style preferences that when harnessed can result in greater efficiency of study sessions.

General Recommendations for Specific Learning Styles

Active learning style

Study sessions should consist of 60-90 minute sessions of interactive study. Study sessions should take place as frequently as possible. Group studying is recommended since multisensory stimulation is difficult to achieve alone. Learning tools should include items such as discussions, simulations, hands-on practice, and role playing.

Passive learning style

Study sessions should be two to three hours in length and focus on large pieces of material. Study sessions should take place three to five times per week. Group studying is recommended periodically with members who are application driven. Learning tools should include items such as lectures, briefings, observations, handouts, texts, and notes.

Awareness of one's learning style will not make an unqualified candidate qualified, however, it can significantly increase the rate of new learning, reviewing, and relearning. A well conceived study plan combined with an awareness of learning style is a powerful one-two combination that can pay significant dividends for candidates on the NPTE-PTA.

NOTES

Study Concept 2: Time Management

Physical therapist assistant students by definition tend to have strong time management skills, however, these skills are severely tested when preparing for the NPTE-PTA. The majority of students take the NPTE-PTA shortly after graduation, which can be a very anxious and unsettled time. Candidates are often actively seeking employment or are attempting to adjust to a new job. They may have relocated to a different residence or perhaps moved to another part of the country.

The thought of preparing for an examination that represents two years of study makes it critical that available study time is spent in areas that will yield the highest return on investment. To illustrate this point, consider the relative systems weighting of the current examination.

System	Midpoint (percentage)
Musculoskeletal System	25.67%
Neuromuscular and Nervous Systems	20.67%
Cardiovascular and Pulmonary Systems	15.67%
Other Systems	18.67%
Non-Systems	19.33%

For example, on a typical examination a candidate will have between 36 and 41 Musculoskeletal system questions and between 21 and 26 Cardiovascular and Pulmonary systems questions. Given the relative weighting of these areas, a typical candidate should spend almost twice as much time studying Musculoskeletal content than Cardiovascular and Pulmonary systems content. The actual percentage of time spent in each area may vary from candidate to candidate, but the relative weighting of the system on the examination should always remain an important variable to consider when determining the necessary breadth and depth in each area. Fortunately, there are a number of specific strategies candidates can utilize to ensure that they make meaningful progress in their study sessions.

Strategy: Master Study Schedule

Develop a master schedule for studying which emphasizes the relative weighting of the Systems and Non-Systems areas on the NPTE-PTA.

Step One – Create a monthly calendar that identifies specific study days and the anticipated duration of each session.

Step Two – Allocate more frequent study sessions and therefore additional study time to systems that are more heavily weighted on the NPTE-PTA.

Step Three – Integrate weekly activities that are designed to maintain a balance in life. These areas may address emotional, intellectual, physical, and social needs.

Step Four – Reassess your progress on a weekly basis and make any necessary changes to the master schedule.

PTAEXAM: The Complete Study Guide offers a great deal of additional information on the NPTE-PTA Blueprint. The blueprint specifies the relative weighting of the Systems and Non-Systems areas and introduces the Content Outline.

NOTES

Study Concept 3: Levels of Knowledge and Understanding

The NPTE-PTA has evolved into an examination that requires candidates to demonstrate their ability to make clinical decisions rather than purely recall factual information. Candidates need to demonstrate solid didactic knowledge of entry-level physical therapy concepts, however, they also need to be able to apply the information in diverse clinical scenarios usually presented in multiple-choice questions of two to four sentences. Candidates who can effectively integrate physical therapy concepts into the various presented scenarios and make informed clinical decisions tend to perform strongly on the examination, while candidates who struggle with this skill tend to perform poorly.

When reviewing academic content, it is important that candidates familiarize themselves with the content at multiple levels of breadth and depth. The following table depicts a hierarchy of knowledge and understanding.

Typically, within a physical therapy academic program, students acquire the information in a hierarchical progression beginning with the lower cognitive levels (i.e., vocabulary level, literal level) and progress over time to higher cognitive levels (i.e., interpretive level, applied level). As candidates begin to prepare for the NPTE-PTA, it is likely that the majority of candidates are comfortable at the vocabulary and literal level, however, there is far greater variability in comfort level at the interpretive and applied levels. Varying levels of comfort may result from exposure or lack thereof to specific subject matter on clinical education experiences or opportunities to develop competence with applied learning activities in the classroom. Regardless of where a candidate is on this spectrum, it is critical that candidates constantly challenge themselves to explore higher level cognitive knowledge as they progress through their academic review.

The presented hierarchy of knowledge and understanding can also be useful for candidates when answering multiple-choice questions. After reading the stem of a given examination question, it may be beneficial for candidates to ask themselves what the question is specifically asking. In this manner, candidates can ensure that their interpretation of the question is consistent with the intended meaning of each question. Failure to interpret the specific meaning of a question often results in a candidate selecting an incorrect response to a multiple-choice item. Test taking mistakes can be extremely harmful on the examination since once this occurs a candidate's examination score is no longer consistent with their true ability. As a candidate's score moves further away from their true ability there is a greater risk of failing the examination.

Applied Level: (How)
Process Analysis, Process Synthesis, Evaluation

Interpretive Level: (Why, When, Which)
Composition, Classification, Example of Purpose

Literal Level: (What, Where)
Characteristics, Background, Location, Function

Vocabulary Level: (Who, What, When)
Names, Definitions

NOTES

Study Concept 4: Golden Rules

We have all used certain rules to help us move through our education such as "I before E, except after C." When preparing for the NPTE-PTA, candidates often look for similar rules that can assist them to make important distinctions between two or more plausible options to a given question. Unfortunately, these types of rules do not exist on the NPTE-PTA since every question relies on the nuances of a particular scenario that is typically conveyed in two to four sentences. Perhaps this is best demonstrated by stating a possible rule and then providing several examples to explore the rule in more detail.

Hypothetical Golden Rule Number One: When confronted with a situation where patient safety is potentially compromised, always contact the referring physician.

RULE BUSTER: Candidates must be vigilant to identify and act on any potential threat to patient safety, but this does not mean that it is always necessary to contact the referring physician. In some cases, it would be appropriate for a physical therapist assistant to minimize the threat to safety themselves. For example, consider the situation where a patient has a sudden and dramatic drop in their systolic blood pressure while working on vertical positioning. In this case, it may only be necessary for the physical therapist assistant to lower the patient toward the horizontal; in other cases contact with the physician would undoubtedly be necessary.

NEW RULE: It depends.

Hypothetical Golden Rule Number Two: When choosing between a number of acceptable interventions, always select the most conservative option in an effort to minimize any potential safety risk to the patient.

RULE BUSTER: Patient safety is a critical component on the NPTE-PTA, but in many cases, it is equally important to weigh the relative benefit of a selected option to achieving a desired patient outcome. How aggressive a therapist should be in a particular situation can only be determined after carefully weighing the relative risk versus the relative reward of each option. It is also important to recognize that all interventions have some degree of risk. If each of the available options to a given question offered no tangible difference in patient outcome, but were considered to be very different in terms of the relative degree of risk, it would then be sensible to select the safest or most conservative option.

NEW RULE: It depends.

Hypothetical Golden Rule Number Three: Physical therapist assistants should always contact the supervising physical therapist prior to changing any aspect of a patient's therapy session.

RULE BUSTER: Physical therapist assistants are licensed personnel in the vast majority of states and tend to have a fairly standardized list of acceptable work activities. Communication between a physical therapist and physical therapist assistant is strongly encouraged, however, in some instances, it may not always be necessary. For example, what about the case where a physical therapist assistant wants to change the sequence of resistive exercises or needs to increase or decrease a weight on an existing progressive resistive exercise? In this case, formal communication with the physical therapist would typically not be necessary since physical therapist assistants are able to engage in ongoing assessment. In other instances, formal communication would be necessary. For example, a physical therapist assistant may want to introduce a new intervention that falls outside the current established plan of care or perhaps identifies several findings that indicate a relevant change in a patient's medical status.

NEW RULE: It depends.

As you can see, the only safe rule to rely on is "it depends." Stated differently, the answer to a given question is always dependent on the specific terms and conditions presented in each clinical scenario. Candidates should attempt to inform future clinical decision making based on their experiences with previous sample examination items, but should avoid becoming inflexible or attempting to develop general rules that apply to all situations.

NOTES

Study Concept 5: Automaticity

On occasion, candidates attempt to complete an academic review by simply taking sample examinations and then reviewing and memorizing the correct answers. This strategy, although potentially helpful, is at best a scattered approach since the scope of the review is dependent solely on the questions asked.

For example, a given series of sample examinations may have a total of eight questions on ultrasound, but it is possible that the questions do not address necessary subject matter such as ultrasound using the underwater technique or explore important concepts such as beam nonuniformity ratio or effective radiating area. This example emphasizes the need for a thorough academic review which allows candidates access to the vast majority of didactic content potentially encountered on the NPTE-PTA.

Consider another example dealing with accessibility standards such as a ramp. Most candidates would quickly recall that the ratio of rise:run is 1:12 or stated differently, each inch of rise requires a minimum of 12 inches of run. Although candidates are likely to be familiar with this concept, they may not be prepared to handle each of the various ways this concept could be tested on the NPTE-PTA.

An examination item could require a candidate to:

- Determine the minimum length of a ramp after being given a specific height in inches or feet

- Determine the minimum height of a ramp after being given a specific length in inches or feet

- Determine if a ramp violates the minimum ADA requirements given a height and length in inches or feet

- Determine a given maximum percentage grade for a ramp (using rise:run formula)

- Determine if a ramp violates the maximum percentage grade given a height and length in inches or feet

- Determine the minimum length of a ramp in inches or feet given the need to safely traverse a height the equivalent of a given number of standard size steps

The examples illustrate both the need to be familiar with specific didactic content and the need to apply the information in different scenarios. In truth, each of the listed examination items related to ramps relies on the same basic formula (i.e., rise:run), but a candidate's ability to answer the question correctly will depend on their ability to recognize this and in some cases, utilize related information (i.e., the relationship of percentage grade to rise:run and the size of a standard step).

Candidates who have this skill are demonstrating automaticity. Automaticity is a test taking term that describes the ability to quickly recall relevant facts, procedures, and routines and apply this information within the context of a clinically-oriented multiple-choice question. As candidates become increasingly comfortable with the academic knowledge and the ability to apply the information via multiple-choice questions, they tend to score higher on sample examinations.

When reviewing completed sample examination items, candidates greatly benefit from considering other possible scenarios related to the same subject matter or topic being tested. In many cases, the incorrect options for a question are often correct for a variation of the question. For example, a question may ask specifically about the testing procedure for a given cranial nerve. In this case, a candidate may identify option 1 as being correct, but upon reviewing the question later may recognize that options 2, 3, and 4 are also correct for different cranial nerves. Given that there are literally thousands of potential questions that could be asked on the NPTE-PTA, candidates who possess greater flexibility with particular subject matter have a greater probability of answering the item correctly.

NOTES

Study Concept 6: Truths and Myths

There are a variety of popular myths that exist in regard to the NPTE-PTA. Most of the myths are simply misinformation that becomes perpetuated over time. The following section addresses some of the more common myths about the current examination and then sets the record straight.

TRUTHS AND MYTHS NUMBER ONE: The NPTE-PTA has several different forms (i.e., versions), each which has a particular emphasis in terms of systems weighting. For example, a given form may emphasize the musculoskeletal system while another may emphasize the neuromuscular and nervous systems.

ANSWER: False

EXPLANATION: Each form of the NPTE-PTA is designed based on the same blueprint. The blueprint provides a targeted number of items in each system and content outline area, however, slight variation is permitted in each area within a specified range. The Federation of State Boards of Physical Therapy publicly disseminates the blueprint that provides detailed information on the current examination.

TRUTHS AND MYTHS NUMBER TWO: When studying for the examination, it is critical to be familiar with multiple academic resources for a selected topic since a given question could require knowledge from a specific resource.

ANSWER: False

EXPLANATION: An examination question would not require a candidate to differentiate between multiple academic sources. For example, different academic resources sometimes have subtle differences in select subject matter such as dermatomes or temperature ranges for physical agents. Instead of focusing on this level of detail, a candidate should become comfortable with a given source and have confidence that if this information is encountered on the examination, their answer will be correct.

TRUTHS AND MYTHS NUMBER THREE: The 50 questions on the NPTE-PTA that are considered pre-test items are clearly identifiable from scored items on the examination.

ANSWER: False

EXPLANATION: The 50 pre-test items are intermingled with 150 scored items to make up the 200 question NPTE-PTA. The pre-test items are not distinguishable from scored items and exist in each of the five sections of the examination.

TRUTHS AND MYTHS NUMBER FOUR: Candidates have exactly one hour to complete each of the four sections of the NPTE-PTA.

ANSWER: False

EXPLANATION: Candidates have a total of four sections, each with 50 questions, to complete on the NPTE-PTA, however, they are not timed independently. The examination clock will begin at 4 hours and count down from this value regardless of the rate at which each of the sections is completed. The examination will conclude when the candidate submits their final section or when the four hours have elapsed.

TRUTHS AND MYTHS NUMBER FIVE: A score of 75% correct is necessary to pass the NPTE-PTA in most states.

ANSWER: False

EXPLANATION: Each form of the examination has an individual criterion-referenced passing score. The passing score may differ by a relatively small amount from form to form. If a particular form was determined to be slightly more difficult than another form, the more difficult form would have a slightly lower criterion-referenced passing score. Individual states do not have the ability to determine passing scores in their respective jurisdictions and instead rely on the established national criterion-referenced passing scores. Recently, criterion-referenced passing scores have been below 75% of the questions answered correctly.

TRUTHS AND MYTHS NUMBER SIX: Scores on subsequent attempts of sample examinations are good indicators of success on the NPTE-PTA.

ANSWER: False

EXPLANATION: Scores on subsequent attempts of a given sample examination are usually better indicators of memory and less accurate as predictors of future performance. Candidates should always review correct and incorrect answers from a given sample examination, however, they should resist the urge to retake the same examination for the purpose of assessing performance.

Study Concept 7: Blood Pressure

Vital signs serve as an important screening tool for physical therapist assistants and should be formally measured for all examinations and then periodically thereafter based on the particular medical diagnosis and specific physical therapy interventions. Given the obvious safety implications associated with measuring and interpreting the results of vital signs, it is critical that candidates have in-depth knowledge of this particular content. This section will present a variety of detailed information related to blood pressure.

- Systolic pressure measures the force exerted against the arteries during the ejection cycle, while diastolic pressure measures the force exerted against the arteries during rest.

- Blood pressure is directly related to cardiac output and peripheral vascular resistance and therefore is an effective non-invasive performance measure of the pumping mechanism of the heart.

- Systolic pressure increases with exertion in a linear progression, often at a rate of 8-12 mm Hg per metabolic equivalent, however, with sustained activity, no further increases typically occur. If systolic pressure does not rise with increasing workload, it may indicate that the functional reserve capacity of the heart has been exceeded.

- Diastolic pressure may increase or decrease a maximum of 10 mm Hg due to adaptive dilation of peripheral vasculature. In a typical clinical setting, the exercise session should be terminated if the systolic pressure exceeds 210 mm Hg or if the diastolic pressure exceeds 110 mm Hg.

- Pulse pressure, which is the difference between systolic and diastolic pressure, generally increases in direct proportion to the intensity of exercise since systolic pressure increases with exercise and diastolic pressure tends to stay the same. In a healthy adult it is common to see a 40-50 mm Hg change in systolic pressure with intense exercise. Excessive pulse pressure may be indicative of stiffening of the aorta secondary to atherosclerosis.

- Normally, systolic blood pressure in the legs is 10-20% higher than the pressure in the arms (brachial artery). This is why in some cases an ankle-brachial index value of greater than 1.0 is still considered to be normal. Blood pressure readings that are lower in the legs as compared to the arms are abnormal and may be indicative of peripheral vascular disease.

- Blood pressure increases during dynamic resistance exercise, such as free weights, machines or isokinetics, and continues to increase as an exercise set progresses. Blood pressure response is higher during weight training that incorporates a concentric and eccentric phase compared to isokinetic exercise. Blood pressure tends to be higher during the concentric phase of the repetition or when the Valsalva maneuver is used.

- With advancing age, the same amount of blood fills the ventricles, but the pumping mechanism is less effective. As a result, the body compensates by increasing blood pressure in an attempt to maintain homeostasis.

- During exercise testing, a systolic blood pressure that fails to increase or decrease with increasing workloads may signal a plateau or decrease in cardiac output.

- Systolic blood pressure normally decreases promptly with the cessation of exercise. As a general guideline, the three-minute post exercise systolic blood pressure should be less than 90% of the systolic blood pressure at peak exercise.

NOTES

Study Concept 8: Lines, Tubes, and Equipment

The NPTE-PTA is designed to protect consumers from unqualified practitioners. Given the purpose of the examination, it is inevitable that candidates will encounter a variety of questions that deal with patients with a significantly compromised medical status.

This section presents information on various types of lines, tubes, and equipment. The purpose is to remind physical therapist assistants of some of the more critical elements to consider when treating patients using these devices. Please remember that this is not an all-inclusive list and additional detail will be provided on the vast majority of items throughout **PTAEXAM: The Complete Study Guide.**

Lines

Arterial Lines (A Line)

- Avoid applying a blood pressure cuff above the infusion site
- Grasp the IV line support pole so the infusion site is at heart level
- Avoid activities that require the infusion site to be above the level of the heart for a prolonged period
- Exercise is possible with the line, but avoid disturbing the apparatus

Swan-Ganz Catheters (Pulmonary Artery Catheters), Central Venous Pressure Catheters, Indwelling Right Atrial Catheters

- Exercise is possible with the line, but mobility may need to be restricted near the catheter insertion

Total Parenteral Nutrition, Hyperalimentation Devices (Intravenous Feeding)

- Alarm sound indicates the fluid source is empty or the system has become unbalanced
- Disruption or disconnection may result in an air embolus
- Shoulder motion on the side of the infusion site may be restricted primarily in flexion and abduction
- Exercise is possible with the line, but mobility may need to be restricted near the catheter insertion

Intracranial Monitoring

- Isometric exercise and the Valsalva maneuver should be avoided since these activities increase intracranial pressure
- Avoid neck flexion, hip flexion greater than 90 degrees, and lying down in a prone position
- Venous drainage is maximal with the head of the bed elevated 30 degrees
- Momentary elevation of intracranial pressure is normal, but sustained increases are not and therefore should be reported

Tubes

Nasogastric Tube (NG Tube)

- Patient will not be able to eat food or drink fluids by mouth while the nasogastric tube is in place
- Enteral feedings can be disconnected temporarily for mobility
- Exercise requiring movements of the head and neck should be avoided, especially forward bending

Gastrostomy Tube (G Tube)

- Distal tubing can inadvertently become caught on items such as furniture and be pulled out
- Enteral feedings should be turned off temporarily prior to and during treatment
- Enteral feedings can be disconnected temporarily for mobility

Urinary Catheters

- Tubes should be placed below the region being drained since the devices rely on gravity
- The collection bag should not be raised above the level of the bladder for any sustained period
- Avoid disrupting, stretching, disconnecting or occluding the tube during exercise

Chest Tubes

- When ambulating, collection bottles should be kept below the level of the inserted tube location
- Monitor the patient for changes in breath sounds before and after intervention
- Avoid pressing directly on the chest tube during mobility activities

Equipment

Mechanical Ventilation

- Alarm may indicate disconnected tube, coughing or change in respiratory pattern
- Develop nonverbal means of communication with the patient
- Patient is at greater risk for developing contractures, skin ulcers, and deconditioning

Supplemental Oxygen Delivery System

- Be aware of signs of respiratory distress (i.e., dyspnea, cyanosis, cramping)
- Monitor SaO_2, PaO_2, and hemodynamics prior to, during, and after physical therapy intervention
- Exercise is possible, but avoid disturbing the tubing

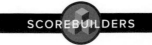

Study Concept 9: Emergent Conditions

According to the Federation of State Boards of Physical Therapy, the NPTE-PTA is designed to assess basic entry-level competence of the licensure candidate who has graduated from an accredited program. The primary purpose of the examination is therefore to protect the public from unqualified practitioners. Given the purpose of the examination, it is reasonable to expect that a high percentage of examination items will deal with safety-related issues including the identification and management of potentially emergent conditions. When encountering this type of question, it is critical that candidates are armed with the necessary knowledge to make informed clinical decisions.

The following provides relevant information on three commonly encountered emergent conditions.

Pulmonary Embolism

DESCRIPTION: A blockage of the pulmonary artery or one of its branches, usually precipitated by a blood clot from a vein (venous thrombus) becoming dislodged from its site of formation. The dislodged blood clot then travels to the arterial blood supply of one of the lungs.

CLINICAL PRESENTATION: Difficulty breathing, chest pain that often mimics a heart attack, rapid pulse; in more severe cases circulatory instability and death

RISK FACTORS: Surgery, long periods of inactivity, increased levels of clotting factor in the blood, and abnormal factors in the vessel wall

DIAGNOSIS: Pulmonary angiography is the most accurate method to diagnose pulmonary embolism, however, because the procedure carries inherent risks to the patient, other diagnostic procedures such as chest x-ray, lung scan, and spiral computerized tomography scan are more commonly utilized.

TREATMENT: Anticoagulant medication such as Heparin and Warfarin

NOTES: Pulmonary embolism remains the leading cause of hospital death in the United States.

Hypovolemic Shock

DESCRIPTION: A life-threatening condition caused by insufficient circulating blood volume. Primary causes include hemorrhage or severe burns.

CLINICAL PRESENTATION: Hypotension due to lack of circulating volume, anxiety, altered mental state, cool and clammy skin, rapid and thready pulse, thirst, and fatigue due to inadequate oxygenation

RISK FACTORS: Exposure to severe trauma or burns

DIAGNOSIS: Primarily through the identification of the described clinical presentation

TREATMENT: Management of suspected shock includes activating the emergency medical system. Positional management includes lying in supine with the legs elevated approximately 12 inches in situations where it is tolerated. Management of confirmed shock includes controlling bleeding and attempting to restore blood volume by providing infusions of balanced salt solutions or blood in more severe cases.

NOTES: There are several other common forms of shock including cardiogenic, septic, and anaphylactic. Cardiogenic shock is characterized by failure of the heart to pump effectively. Management includes oxygen therapy and administering cardiac medications. Septic shock is characterized by an overwhelming infection leading to vasodilation. Management includes restoring intravascular volume and identifying and controlling the source of infection. Anaphylactic shock is characterized by a severe and sometimes fatal reaction to an allergen, antigen or drug which causes vasodilation leading to hypotension and increased capillary permeability. Management includes identifying and removing the causative antigen and administering counter-mediators such as anti-histamine.

Autonomic Dysreflexia

DESCRIPTION: A massive sympathetic discharge that can occur in association with a spinal cord injury or disease. The condition is triggered by a variety of noxious stimuli including bladder distention, urinary tract infection, skin ulcers, and bowel impaction.

CLINICAL PRESENTATION: Sweating above the level of the lesion, flushing of the skin above the level of the lesion, elevated blood pressure, and blurred vision

RISK FACTORS: Patients with spinal cord injuries at and above the T6 level

DIAGNOSIS: Primarily through the identification of the described clinical presentation

TREATMENT: Management of autonomic dysreflexia includes immediate determination and removal of the triggering stimuli. Positional management includes sitting the patient upright to lower the elevated blood pressure below dangerous levels. Tight clothing and stockings should also be removed. If the noxious stimuli cannot be identified, medical management may include vasodilators to assist with symptomatic relief.

NOTES: Prevalence rates for autonomic dysreflexia have been reported ranging from 48-90% of all individuals with spinal cord injuries at T6 and above. The occurrence of autonomic dysreflexia is increased as an individual moves out of spinal shock.

Study Concept 10: Assessment

Candidates must carefully assess their examination performance when taking sample examinations. Each of the sample examinations in **PTAEXAM: The Complete Study Guide** offers candidates the opportunity to view their performance according to five system and five content outline categories. The shaded areas in the tables below will be used in the performance analysis section to express the number of questions answered correctly in each category, the total number of questions in the category, and the percentage of questions correct.

System Specific Summary		
Musculoskeletal System		
Neuromuscular and Nervous Systems		
Cardiovascular and Pulmonary Systems		
Other Systems		
Non-Systems		

Content Outline Summary		
Physical Therapy Data Collection		
Diseases/Conditions that Impact Effective Treatment		
Interventions		
Equipment, Devices, and Technologies; Therapeutic Modalities		
Safety and Protection; Professional Responsibilities; Research		

Candidates should use this information to develop remedial plans to improve performance on sample examinations. Candidates must be familiar with the content contained in each system specific and content outline category and carefully assess how their performance changes over time.

The academic review section of **PTAEXAM: The Complete Study Guide** is arranged according to the exact categories used in the system specific summary and therefore serves as an excellent resource for candidates to utilize when initially remediating deficient areas. In some instances, a candidate may determine that it is necessary to access a more formal academic resource such as a textbook to locate information not covered in the review book. In these situations it is important for candidates to stay focused and avoid purely exploring the textbook since often candidates do not emerge for several hours.

The content outline is less intuitive than the system categories since the content outline is not system based, however, it is still very useful given the detailed information available on the NPTE-PTA Blueprint. For example, a candidate may find that they tend to perform very well on questions within the "Physical Therapy Data Collection" category, but have more difficulty on questions within the "Diseases/Conditions that Impact Effective Treatment" category. By consulting the NPTE-PTA Blueprint, a candidate will quickly realize that the "Physical Therapy Data Collection" category deals primarily with tests and measures, anatomy and physiology, and movement analysis, while the "Diseases/Conditions that Impact Effective Treatment" category deals primarily with diseases/conditions and pathophysiology. The information from the content outline combined with the system information allows candidates to gain greater insight toward their current performance and should assist them to be more specific when selecting appropriate remedial activities.

Candidates are encouraged to look for general trends in their scoring when taking sample examinations and avoid making a definitive statement on their level of competence in any given category based on the results of a single sample examination. This is especially true in a category where there is a smaller number of questions. As the number of questions in each category diminishes, the category becomes less accurate as a predictor of actual performance. In some instances, candidates will have a few glaring areas of deficiency (e.g., "Musculoskeletal" and "Other Systems"), while in other cases, candidates will demonstrate more consistency. Consistency can be a very good thing if the scores are consistent at a very high level (i.e., a high percentage of questions answered correctly in the majority of areas) or more problematic if the scores are consistent at a very low level (i.e., a low percentage of questions answered correctly in the majority of areas).

In summary, studying for the examination is analogous to developing a plan of care for a patient; the more specific the plan of care is for the particular needs of the patient, the better the patient outcome. In terms of preparing for the examination, the more specific a remedial plan is to the particular needs of a given candidate, the better the candidate's outcome.

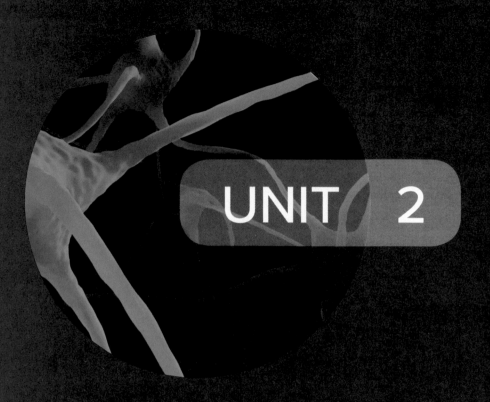

UNIT 2

Academic Review

Academic Review

The academic review section of **PTAEXAM: The Complete Study Guide** provides candidates with a method to review essential didactic information from a physical therapy curriculum. Mastery of this core academic information can significantly increase candidates' scores on the NPTE-PTA.

Each Chapter of the academic review will have unique elements.

Spotlight on Safety

Spotlight on Safety provides candidates with critical safety information related to relevant physical therapy topics. This information is essential on a licensing examination where the ultimate priority is safe and effective patient care.

Consider This

Consider This offers candidates valuable application driven information related to selected academic content. Candidates use this essential information to increase the breadth and depth of their content knowledge.

Motivational Moments

Even with the fantastic design of the academic review section there will be periods of time when a candidate's focus begins to drift and efficiency precipitously declines. To combat this tendency, we periodically insert Motivational Moments into the academic review. These lighthearted breaks allow candidates to look to the future as a licensed physical therapist assistant or perhaps just chuckle or grin!

Essentials

The Essentials section located at the end of each unit provides a summary of critical topics for candidates to reflect on. Ensuring mastery of this material allows candidates to stay focused on big ticket items and provides a valuable repetition loop to commit information to long term memory.

Proficiencies

The proficiencies provide students with an opportunity to determine their competency in a variety of academic areas. The proficiency activities include image identification, matching, sequencing, and fill in the blank. Candidates should carefully assess their proficiency results and use the information to direct remedial activities.

Clinical Application Templates

Clinical Application Templates (CATs) explore the patient/client management for a wide variety of medical conditions. By utilizing CATS candidates can broaden their experience base and as a result be better prepared to answer examination questions.

References

The references provide information on the specific resources used to construct the academic review. Scorebuilders uses a wide variety of resources to ensure that the academic review is consistent with current clinical practice.

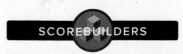

4

Musculoskeletal System

Scott Giles

Musculoskeletal System represents approximately 36 – 41 questions (24% – 27.3%) of the NPTE-PTA.

Contributors

Shawn Paquette
Daniel Lee

CHAPTER 4
Musculoskeletal System

Exercise Physiology

ATP-PC or Phosphagen System

Anaerobic Glycolysis or Lactic Acid System

Aerobic or Oxygen System

Anaerobic Metabolism

ATP-PC System

This energy system is used for ATP production during high intensity, short duration exercise such as sprinting 100 meters. Phosphocreatine decomposes and releases a large amount of energy that is used to construct ATP. There is two to three times more phosphocreatine in cells of muscles than ATP. This process occurs almost instantaneously, allowing for ready and available energy needed by the muscles. The system provides energy for muscle contraction for up to 15 seconds.

The phosphagen system represents the most rapidly available source of ATP for use by the muscle. The energy system is able to function in the described manner since:

- It does not depend on a long series of chemical reactions.
- It does not depend on transporting the oxygen we breathe to the working muscles.
- Both ATP and PC are stored directly within the contractile mechanisms of the muscle.

Anaerobic Glycolysis

This energy system is a major supplier of ATP during high intensity, short duration activities such as sprinting 400 or 800 meters. Stored glycogen is split into glucose, and through glycolysis, split again into pyruvic acid. The energy released during this process forms ATP. The process does not require oxygen. Anaerobic glycolysis results in the formation of lactic acid, which causes muscular fatigue.

This system is nearly 50% slower than the phosphocreatine system and can provide a person with 30 to 40 seconds of muscle contraction. The energy system is able to function in the described manner since:

- It does not require the presence of oxygen.
- It only uses carbohydrates (glycogen and glucose).
- It releases enough energy for the resynthesis of only small amounts of ATP.

Aerobic Metabolism

The aerobic system is used predominantly during low intensity, long duration exercise such as running a marathon. The oxygen system yields by far the most ATP, but it requires several series of complex chemical reactions. This system provides energy through the oxidation of food. The combination of fatty acids, amino acids, and glucose with oxygen releases energy that forms ATP. This system will provide energy as long as there are nutrients to utilize.

Kinesiology

The anatomical position is an erect posture of the body with the face forward, feet pointing forward and slightly apart, arms at the side, and palms forward with fingers and thumbs in extension (Figs. 4-1, 4-2). The position serves as a point of reference for definitions and descriptions of movement including the cardinal planes and associated axes.

Motions are described as occurring in three cardinal planes of the body (frontal, sagittal, transverse). Movement in the cardinal planes occurs around three corresponding axes (anterior-posterior, medial-lateral, vertical).

Frontal plane (coronal)

The frontal (or coronal) plane divides the body into anterior and posterior sections. Motions in the frontal plane, such as abduction and adduction, occur around an anterior-posterior axis.

Sagittal plane

The sagittal plane divides the body into right and left sections. Motions in the sagittal plane, such as flexion and extension, occur around a medial-lateral axis.

Transverse plane

The transverse plane divides the body into upper and lower sections. Motions in the transverse plane, such as medial and lateral rotation, occur around a vertical axis.

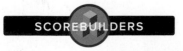

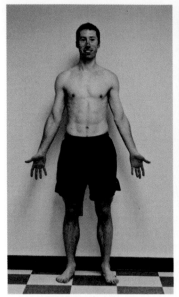
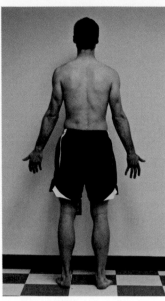

Fig. 4-1 (Left): Anatomical position - anterior view.
Fig. 4-2 (Right): Anatomical position - posterior view.

Classes of Levers[4]

Class 1 Lever

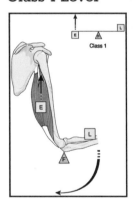

A class 1 lever has the axis of rotation (fulcrum) between the effort (force) and resistance (load). There are very few class 1 levers in the body. A class 1 lever is illustrated with the triceps brachii force on the olecranon with an external counterforce pushing on the forearm. Another example of a class 1 lever is a seesaw.

Class 2 Lever

A class 2 lever has the resistance (load) between the axis of rotation (fulcrum) and the effort (force). The length of the effort arm is always longer than the resistance arm. In most instances, gravity is the effort and muscle activity is the resistance, however, there are class 2 levers where the muscle is the effort when the distal attachment is on a weight bearing segment. An example of a class 2 lever is a wheelbarrow.

Class 3 Lever

A class 3 lever has the effort (force) between the axis of rotation (fulcrum) and the resistance (load). The length of the effort arm is always shorter than the length of the resistance arm. Shoulder abduction with weight at the wrist is a class 3 lever. Class 3 levers usually permit large movements at rapid speeds and are the most common type of lever in the body. An example of a class 3 lever is elbow flexion.

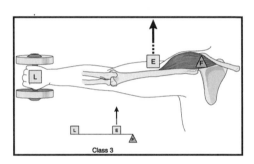

Joint Classification[4,5,6]

Fibrous Joints (Synarthroses)

Fibrous joints are composed of bones that are united by fibrous tissue and are nonsynovial. Movement is minimal to none with the amount of movement permitted at the joint dependent on the length of the fibers uniting the bones.

Suture – (e.g., sagittal suture of the skull)
- Union of two bones by a ligament or membrane
- Immovable joint
- Eventual fusion is termed synostosis

Syndesmosis – (e.g., the tibia and fibula with interosseous membrane)
- Bone connected to bone by a dense fibrous membrane or cord
- Very little motion

Gomphosis – (e.g., a tooth in its socket)
- Two bony surfaces connect as a peg in a hole
- The teeth and corresponding sockets in the mandible/maxilla are the only gomphosis joints in the body
- The periodontal membrane is the fibrous component of the joint

Cartilaginous Joints (Amphiarthroses)

Cartilaginous joints have hyaline cartilage or fibrocartilage that connects one bone to another. These are slightly moveable joints.

Synchondrosis – (e.g., sternum and true rib articulation)
- Hyaline cartilage
- Cartilage adjoins two ossifying centers of bone

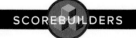

- Provides stability during growth
- May ossify to a synostosis once growth is completed
- Slight motion

Symphysis – (e.g., pubic symphysis)
- Generally located at the midline of the body
- Two bones covered with hyaline cartilage
- Two bones connected by fibrocartilage
- Slight motion

Synovial Joints (Diarthroses)

Synovial joints provide free movement between the bones they join. They have five distinguishing characteristics: joint cavity, articular cartilage, synovial membrane, synovial fluid, and fibrous capsule. These joints are the most complex and vulnerable to injury.

They are further classified by the type of movement and shape of the articulating bones.

Uniaxial joint – one motion around a single axis in one plane of the body
- Hinge (ginglymus) – elbow joint
- Pivot (trochoid) – atlantoaxial joint

Biaxial joint – movement occurs in two planes and around two axes through the convex/concave surfaces
- Condyloid – metacarpophalangeal joint of a finger
- Saddle – carpometacarpal joint of the thumb

Multi-axial joint – movement occurs in three planes and around three axes
- Plane (gliding) – carpal joints
- Ball and socket – hip joint

Joint Receptors[1,4]

Free Nerve Endings

Location	Joint capsule, ligaments, synovium, fat pads
Sensitivity	One type is sensitive to non-noxious mechanical stress; other type is sensitive to noxious mechanical or biochemical stimuli
Primary Distribution	All joints

Golgi Ligament Endings

Location	Ligaments, adjacent to ligaments' bony attachment
Sensitivity	Tension or stretch on ligaments
Primary Distribution	Majority of joints

Golgi-Mazzoni Corpuscles

Location	Joint capsule
Sensitivity	Compression of joint capsule
Primary Distribution	Knee joint, joint capsule

Pacinian Corpuscles

Location	Fibrous layer of joint capsule
Sensitivity	High frequency vibration, acceleration, and high velocity changes in joint position
Primary Distribution	All joints

Ruffini Endings

Location	Fibrous layer of joint capsule
Sensitivity	Stretching of joint capsule; amplitude and velocity of joint position
Primary Distribution	Greater density in proximal joints, particularly in capsular regions

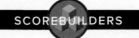

Muscle Physiology[5,6]

Classification of Muscle Fibers	
Type I	**Type II**
Aerobic	Anaerobic
Red	Red/White*
Tonic	Phasic
Slow twitch	Fast twitch
Slow-oxidative	Fast-glycolytic

* Type IIa muscle fibers appear red, while Type IIb muscle fibers appear white

Functional Characteristics of Muscle Fibers	
Type I	**Type II**
Low fatigability	High fatigability
High capillary density	Low capillary density
High myoglobin content	Low myoglobin content
Smaller fibers	Larger fibers
Extensive blood supply	Less blood supply
Large amount of mitochondria	Fewer mitochondria
Examples: marathon, swimming	Examples: high jump, sprinting

Muscle Receptors[6,7]

Muscle Spindle

Muscle spindles are distributed throughout the belly of the muscle. They function to send information to the nervous system about muscle length and/or the rate of change of its length. The muscle spindle is important in the control of posture, and with the help of the gamma system, involuntary movements.

Golgi Tendon Organ

Golgi tendon organs are encapsulated sensory receptors through which the muscle tendons pass immediately beyond their attachment to the muscle fibers. They are very sensitive to tension, especially when produced from an active muscle contraction. They function to transmit information about tension or the rate of change of tension within the muscle.

An average of 10-15 muscle fibers are usually connected in series with each Golgi tendon organ. The Golgi tendon organ is stimulated through the tension produced by muscle fibers. Golgi tendon organs provide the nervous system with instantaneous information on the degree of tension in each small muscle segment.

Muscle Action

Head

Temporomandibular Joint

Depress	Elevate	Protrusion	Retrusion	Side to Side
• Lateral pterygoid	• Temporalis	• Masseter	• Temporalis	• Medial pterygoid
• Suprahyoid	• Masseter	• Lateral pterygoid	• Masseter	• Lateral pterygoid
• Infrahyoid	• Medial pterygoid	• Medial pterygoid	• Digastric	• Masseter
				• Temporalis

Spine

Cervical Intervertebral Joints

Flexion
- Sternocleidomastoid
- Longus colli
- Scalenus muscles

Extension
- Splenius cervicis
- Semispinalis cervicis
- Iliocostalis cervicis
- Longissimus cervicis
- Multifidus
- Trapezius

Rotation and Lateral Bending
- Sternocleidomastoid
- Scalenus muscles
- Splenius cervicis
- Longissimus cervicis
- Iliocostalis cervicis
- Levator scapulae
- Multifidus

Thoracic and Lumbar Intervertebral Joints

Flexion
- Rectus abdominis
- Internal oblique
- External oblique

Extension
- Erector spinae
- Quadratus lumborum
- Multifidus

Rotation and Lateral Bending
- Psoas major
- Quadratus lumborum
- External oblique
- Internal oblique
- Multifidus
- Longissimus thoracis
- Iliocostalis thoracis
- Rotatores

Upper Extremity

Scapula

Elevation
- Upper trapezius
- Levator scapulae

Depression
- Latissimus dorsi
- Pectoralis major
- Pectoralis minor
- Lower trapezius

Protraction
- Serratus anterior
- Pectoralis minor

Retraction
- Trapezius (middle)
- Rhomboids

Upward Rotation
- Trapezius (upper, lower)
- Serratus anterior

Downward Rotation
- Rhomboids
- Levator scapulae
- Pectoralis minor

Shoulder Joint

Flexion
- Anterior deltoid
- Coracobrachialis
- Pectoralis major (clavicular head)
- Biceps brachii

Extension
- Latissimus dorsi
- Posterior deltoid
- Teres major
- Triceps brachii (long head)

Abduction
- Middle deltoid
- Supraspinatus

Adduction
- Pectoralis major
- Latissimus dorsi
- Teres major

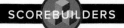

Upper Extremity (continued)

Shoulder Joint (continued)

Horizontal Abduction	Horizontal Adduction	Lateral Rotation	Medial Rotation
• Posterior Deltoid	• Anterior Deltoid	• Teres minor	• Subscapularis
• Infraspinatus	• Pectoralis major	• Infraspinatus	• Teres major
• Teres minor		• Posterior deltoid	• Pectoralis major
			• Latissimus dorsi
			• Anterior deltoid

Elbow Joint / Radioulnar Joint

Flexion	Extension	Supination	Pronation
• Biceps brachii	• Triceps brachii	• Biceps brachii	• Pronator teres
• Brachialis	• Anconeus	• Supinator	• Pronator quadratus
• Brachioradialis			

Wrist Joint

Flexion	Extension	Radial Deviation	Ulnar Deviation
• Flexor carpi radialis	• Extensor carpi radialis longus	• Extensor carpi radialis longus and brevis	• Extensor carpi ulnaris
• Flexor carpi ulnaris	• Extensor carpi radialis brevis	• Flexor carpi radialis	• Flexor carpi ulnaris
• Palmaris longus	• Extensor carpi ulnaris	• Extensor pollicis longus and brevis	

Finger Joints

Flexion	Extension	Abduction	Adduction
• Flexor digitorum profundus and superficialis	• Extensor digitorum communis	• Dorsal interossei	• Palmar interossei
• Flexor digiti minimi (fifth digit)	• Extensor indicis (second digit)	• Abductor digiti minimi (fifth digit)	
• Interossei	• Extensor digiti minimi (fifth digit)		
• Lumbricals			

Thumb Joint

Flexion	Extension	Abduction	Adduction	Opposition
• Flexor pollicis longus and brevis	• Extensor pollicis longus and brevis	• Abductor pollicis longus and brevis	• Adductor pollicis	• Opponens pollicis
• Opponens pollicis	• Abductor pollicis longus			• Flexor pollicis brevis
				• Abductor pollicis brevis
				• Opponens digiti minimi

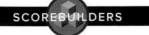

Lower Extremity

Hip Joint

Flexion
- Iliopsoas
- Sartorius
- Rectus femoris
- Pectineus

Extension
- Gluteus maximus and medius
- Semitendinosus
- Semimembranosus
- Biceps femoris

Abduction
- Gluteus medius
- Gluteus minimus
- Piriformis
- Obturator internus
- Tensor fasciae latae

Adduction
- Adductor magnus
- Adductor longus
- Adductor brevis
- Gracilis

Medial Rotation
- Tensor fasciae latae
- Gluteus medius
- Gluteus minimus
- Pectineus
- Adductor longus

Lateral Rotation
- Gluteus maximus
- Obturator externus
- Obturator internus
- Piriformis
- Gemelli
- Sartorius

Knee Joint

Flexion
- Biceps femoris
- Semitendinosus
- Semimembranosus
- Sartorius

Extension
- Rectus femoris
- Vastus lateralis
- Vastus intermedius
- Vastus medialis

Ankle Joint

Plantar Flexion
- Tibialis posterior
- Gastrocnemius
- Soleus
- Peroneus longus
- Peroneus brevis
- Plantaris
- Flexor hallucis

Dorsiflexion
- Tibialis anterior
- Extensor hallucis longus
- Extensor digitorum longus
- Peroneus tertius

Inversion
- Tibialis posterior
- Tibialis anterior
- Flexor digitorum longus

Eversion
- Peroneus longus
- Peroneus brevis
- Peroneus tertius

Toe Joints

Flexion
- Flexor digitorum longus and brevis
- Flexor hallucis longus and brevis
- Flexor digiti minimi brevis
- Quadratus plantae
- Lumbricals

Extension
- Extensor digitorum longus and brevis
- Extensor hallucis longus and brevis
- Lumbricals

Abduction
- Abductor hallucis
- Abductor digit minimi
- Dorsal interossei

Adduction
- Adductor hallucis
- Plantar Interossei

Specific Joints - Upper Extremity

Shoulder[5,7-11]

The shoulder complex is formed by a series of unique articulations including the glenohumeral joint, sternoclavicular joint, acromioclavicular joint, and scapulothoracic articulation.

Articulations

Glenohumeral joint

The glenohumeral joint is formed by the convex head of the humerus and the concave glenoid fossa of the scapula. The glenohumeral joint is a ball and socket synovial joint with three degrees of freedom. The relatively small articular surface of the glenoid fossa in relation to the size of the humeral head, makes the glenohumeral joint inherently unstable.

Glenohumeral Snapshot
Osteokinematic motions: flexion, extension, abduction, adduction, medial rotation, lateral rotation
Loose packed position: 55 degrees abduction, 30 degrees horizontal adduction
Close packed position: abduction and lateral rotation
Capsular pattern: lateral rotation, abduction, medial rotation

Sternoclavicular joint

The sternoclavicular joint is formed by the medial end of the clavicle and the manubrium of the sternum. The joint is a saddle-shaped synovial joint with three degrees of freedom. A fibrocartilaginous disc between the manubrium and clavicle enhances the stability of the joint. The disc acts as a shock absorber and serves as the axis for clavicular rotation.

Sternoclavicular Snapshot
Osteokinematic motions: elevation, depression, protraction, retraction, medial rotation, lateral rotation
Loose packed position: arm resting by the side
Close packed position: maximum shoulder elevation
Capsular pattern: pain at extremes of range of movement

Acromioclavicular joint

The acromioclavicular joint is formed by the acromion process of the scapula and the lateral end of the clavicle. The joint is a plane synovial joint with three degrees of freedom. The acromioclavicular joint functions to maintain the relationship between the scapula and clavicle during glenohumeral range of motion.

Acromioclavicular Snapshot
Osteokinematic motions: anterior tilting, posterior tilting, upward rotation, downward rotation, protraction, retraction
Loose packed position: arm resting by the side
Close packed position: arm abducted to 90 degrees
Capsular pattern: pain at extremes of range of movement

Scapulothoracic articulation

The scapulothoracic articulation is formed by the body of the scapula and the muscles covering the posterior chest wall. Motion consists of sliding of the scapula on the thorax. The articulation is not a true anatomical joint because it lacks the necessary synovial joint characteristics.

Muscle Action

Shoulder flexion: anterior deltoid, coracobrachialis, pectoralis major (clavicular head), biceps brachii

Shoulder extension: latissimus dorsi, posterior deltoid, teres major, triceps brachii (long head)

Shoulder abduction: middle deltoid, supraspinatus

Shoulder adduction: pectoralis major, latissimus dorsi, teres major

Shoulder lateral rotation: teres minor, infraspinatus, posterior deltoid

Shoulder medial rotation: subscapularis, teres major, pectoralis major, latissimus dorsi, anterior deltoid

Shoulder horizontal abduction: posterior deltoid, infraspinatus, teres minor

Shoulder horizontal adduction: anterior deltoid, pectoralis major

Scapula elevation: upper trapezius, levator scapulae

Scapula depression: latissimus dorsi, pectoralis major, pectoralis minor, lower trapezius

Scapula protraction: serratus anterior, pectoralis minor

Scapula retraction: trapezius (middle), rhomboids

Scapula upward rotation: trapezius (upper, lower), serratus anterior

Scapula downward rotation: rhomboids, levator scapulae, pectoralis minor

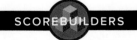

Primary Structures

Acromioclavicular ligaments

The acromioclavicular ligaments surround the acromioclavicular joint on all sides and help to control horizontal movements of the clavicle.

Coracoacromial ligament

The coracoacromial ligament attaches between the coracoid process and acromion and forms a "roof" over the humeral head. This ligament helps to limit superior translation of the humeral head and also helps prevent separation of the acromioclavicular joint.

Coracoclavicular ligament

The coracoclavicular ligament attaches between the coracoid process and the clavicle and consists of two different ligaments: the conoid and trapezoid ligaments. The coracoclavicular ligament acts as the primary support of the acromioclavicular joint, limiting superior translation of the clavicle.

Coracohumeral ligament

The coracohumeral ligament attaches proximally to the coracoid process and splits distally to attach to the greater and lesser tuberosities. This ligament is found between and helps to unite the supraspinatus and subscapularis tendons. It limits inferior translation of the humeral head.

Costoclavicular ligament

The costoclavicular ligament attaches between the medial portion of the clavicle and the first rib. This ligament is the primary supporting ligament for the sternoclavicular joint.

Glenohumeral ligaments

The glenohumeral ligaments consist of the superior, middle, and inferior glenohumeral ligaments. The superior glenohumeral ligament limits adduction of the shoulder as well as lateral rotation with the shoulder in 0-45 degrees of abduction. The middle glenohumeral ligament limits lateral rotation with the shoulder in 45-90 degrees of abduction. The inferior glenohumeral ligament has an anterior and a posterior band that limits lateral rotation and medial rotation, respectively, above 90 degrees of abduction. Between the two bands is an axillary pouch that limits inferior translation when the shoulder is above 90 degrees of abduction.

Glenoid labrum

The glenoid labrum is a fibrocartilaginous structure that serves to deepen the glenoid fossa and increases the size of the articular surface. The glenoid labrum consists of a dense fibrous connective tissue that is often damaged with recurrent shoulder instability.

Joint capsule

The joint capsule arises from the glenoid fossa and the glenoid labrum to blend with the muscles of the rotator cuff. The volume of the joint capsule is twice as large as the size of the humeral head. The capsule is reinforced by the glenohumeral ligaments and the coracohumeral ligament.

Rotator interval

The rotator interval is a space in the anterosuperior shoulder that consists of and is bordered by the coracohumeral ligament, superior glenohumeral ligament, joint capsule, and supraspinatus and subscapularis tendons.

Subacromial bursa

The subacromial bursa extends over the supraspinatus tendon and distal muscle belly, beneath the acromion and deltoid muscle. The bursa facilitates movement of the deltoid muscle over the fibrous capsule of the shoulder joint and supraspinatus tendon. The bursa is often involved with impingement beneath the acromial arch.

Subscapular bursa

The subscapular bursa overlies the anterior joint capsule and lies beneath the subscapularis muscle. Anterior shoulder fullness may indicate articular effusion secondary to distention of the bursa.

Transverse humeral ligament

The transverse humeral ligament attaches between the greater and lesser tubercles of the humerus, spanning over the bicipital groove. This ligament helps to maintain the tendon of the long head of the biceps within the bicipital groove.

Elbow[5,8-10]

The elbow joint is a synovial joint consisting of three bones (i.e., humerus, radius, ulna) and three primary articulations (i.e., radiohumeral, ulnohumeral, proximal radioulnar) enclosed within a single joint capsule. The elbow is classified as a hinge joint formed by the articulation of the ulna with the humerus.

Articulations

Radiohumeral joint

The proximal joint surface of the radiohumeral joint is the ball-shaped capitulum of the distal humerus. The distal joint surface is the concave head of the radius.

Radiohumeral Snapshot
Osteokinematic motions: flexion, extension, pronation, supination
Loose packed position: full extension, supination
Close packed position: 90 degrees flexion, 5 degrees supination
Capsular pattern: flexion, extension, supination, pronation

Ulnohumeral joint

The ulnohumeral joint is formed by the hourglass-shaped trochlea of the humerus and the trochlear notch of the ulna.

Ulnohumeral Snapshot
Osteokinematic motions: flexion, extension
Loose packed position: 70 degrees elbow flexion, 10 degrees supination
Close packed position: extension
Capsular pattern: flexion, extension

Proximal radioulnar joint

The proximal radioulnar joint consists of the concave radial notch of the ulna and the convex rim of the radial head.

Proximal Radioulnar Snapshot
Osteokinematic motions: pronation, supination
Loose packed position: 70 degrees elbow flexion, 35 degrees supination
Close packed position: 5 degrees supination
Capsular pattern: supination, pronation

Muscle Action

Elbow flexion: biceps brachii, brachialis, brachioradialis

Elbow extension: triceps brachii, anconeus

Forearm supination: biceps brachii, supinator

Forearm pronation: pronator teres, pronator quadratus

Primary Structures

Annular ligament

The annular ligament consists of a band of fibers that surrounds the head of the radius. It allows the head of the radius to rotate and retain contact with the radial notch of the ulna.

Anterior ligament

The anterior ligament is capsular in nature and function. It stretches from the radial collateral ligament and attaches above the upper edge of the coronoid fossa, extending to just below the coronoid process.

Cubital fossa

The cubital fossa is a triangular space located at the anterior elbow that is bordered by the brachioradialis, pronator teres, brachialis, and a horizontal line passing through the humeral epicondyles. The cubital fossa contains several structures, including the biceps brachii tendon, median nerve, radial nerve, brachial artery, and median cubital vein.

Cubital tunnel

The cubital tunnel is a space formed by the ulnar collateral ligament, the flexor carpi ulnaris, the medial head of the triceps, and the medial epicondyle. The ulnar nerve runs through the cubital tunnel. The cubital tunnel becomes smallest with the elbow held in full flexion.

Olecranon bursa

The olecranon bursa lies posterior to the olecranon process and is considered the main bursa in the elbow. This bursa commonly becomes inflamed with direct trauma to the elbow due to its superficial position.

Posterior ligament

The posterior ligament resembles the anterior ligament. It blends on each side with the collateral ligaments and is attached to the upper portion of the olecranon fossa, and to just below the olecranon process.

Radial collateral ligament (i.e., lateral collateral ligament)

The radial collateral ligament extends from the lateral epicondyle of the humerus to the lateral border and olecranon process of the ulna and to the annular ligament. It is a fan-shaped ligament that prevents adduction of the elbow joint, and provides reinforcement for the radiohumeral articulation.

Ulnar collateral ligament (i.e., medial collateral ligament)

The ulnar collateral ligament runs from the medial epicondyle of the humerus to the proximal portion of the ulna. The ligament prevents excessive abduction of the elbow joint.

CONSIDER THIS
MECHANISMS OF INJURY FOR ELBOW LIGAMENTS

The ulnar and radial collateral ligaments can become stretched, frayed or torn through the stress of repetitive throwing motions. If the force on the soft tissues is greater than the tensile strength of the structure, tiny tears of the ligaments can develop. Months (and even years) of throwing can cause microtears, degeneration, and finally, rupture of the ligaments. Baseball pitchers are the athletes treated most often for this problem. Tennis, track and field, football, ice hockey, and water polo participants have also been reported to injure the collateral ligaments. A fall on an outstretched arm can lead to collateral ligament rupture, often with associated elbow dislocation.

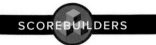

Wrist[5,8,9,10,12]

The wrist complex is formed by the radiocarpal and midcarpal joints. The radiocarpal joint attaches the hand to the forearm. The midcarpal joint is formed by the articulations of the proximal and distal row of carpals.

Articulations

Radiocarpal joint

The proximal joint surface of the radiocarpal joint is formed by the distal radius and the radioulnar articular disc, which connects the medial aspect of the distal radius to the distal ulna. The distal joint surface is formed by the scaphoid, lunate, and triquetrum. The radiocarpal joint has two degrees of freedom. It is encased in a strong capsule reinforced by numerous ligaments shared with the midcarpal joint.

Radiocarpal Snapshot
Osteokinematic motions: flexion, extension, radial deviation, ulnar deviation
Loose packed position: neutral with slight ulnar deviation
Close packed position: extension with radial deviation
Capsular pattern: flexion and extension equally limited

Midcarpal joint

Motion of the wrist results in complex motion between the proximal and distal row of carpals with the exception of the pisiform. The joint surfaces are reciprocally convex and concave.

Muscle Action

Wrist flexion: flexor carpi radialis, flexor carpi ulnaris, palmaris longus

Wrist extension: extensor carpi radialis longus, extensor carpi radialis brevis, extensor carpi ulnaris

Radial deviation: extensor carpi radialis longus and brevis, flexor carpi radialis, extensor pollicis longus, extensor pollicis brevis

Ulnar deviation: extensor carpi ulnaris, flexor carpi ulnaris

Primary Structures

Anatomic snuffbox

The anatomic snuffbox is a depression found on the dorsal surface of the wrist near the distal radius. The snuffbox is bordered by the tendons of the abductor pollicis longus, extensor pollicis brevis, and extensor pollicis longus. This location is often used for palpation of the scaphoid when there is concern for a fracture.

Carpal tunnel

The carpal tunnel is located close to the deep surface of the flexor retinaculum. The median nerve enters the palm through the carpal tunnel. Any condition that significantly reduces the size of the carpal tunnel (e.g., tenosynovitis, inflammation of the flexor retinaculum) may result in compression of the median nerve.

Dorsal radiocarpal ligament

The dorsal radiocarpal ligament is the only major ligament on the dorsal surface of the wrist. The ligament originates on the posterior surface of the distal radius and styloid process of the radius and attaches to the lunate and triquetrum. The ligament serves to limit wrist flexion.

Extensor retinaculum

The extensor retinaculum is a ligamentous structure that crosses the dorsal aspect of the wrist, covering the tendons of the extensor musculature. The retinaculum prevents the tendons from "bowstringing" as the wrist is extended.

Flexor retinaculum

The flexor retinaculum (transverse carpal ligament) is a ligamentous structure that crosses the palmar aspect of the wrist, forming the most anterior aspect of the carpal tunnel. The flexor retinaculum prevents the tendons of the flexor musculature from "bowstringing" as the wrist is flexed. It also serves as an attachment site for the thenar and hypothenar muscles.

Interosseous membrane

The interosseous membrane consists of a dense band of fibrous connective tissue that runs obliquely from the radius to the ulna. The structure spans from the proximal radioulnar joint to the distal radioulnar joint and serves as a stabilizer against axial forces applied to the wrist.

Palmar radiocarpal ligament

The palmar radiocarpal ligament maintains the alignment of the associated joint structures and limits hyperextension of the wrist. The ligament originates from the anterior surface of the distal radius and attaches to the capitate, triquetrum, and scaphoid.

Radial collateral ligament

The radial collateral ligament serves to limit ulnar deviation and becomes taut when the wrist is in extremes of extension and flexion. The ligament originates from the styloid process of the radius and inserts on the scaphoid and trapezium.

Triangular fibrocartilage complex

The triangular fibrocartilage complex is a cartilaginous disc that sits between the ulna, lunate, and triquetrum. The disc provides stability to the wrist joint, connecting the radius and ulna together and allowing for better distribution of forces through the wrist.

Tunnel of Guyon

The tunnel of Guyon is a space that is located between the hook of the hamate, pisiform, palmar carpal ligament, and flexor retinaculum. It provides passage for the ulnar nerve and artery as they enter the hand. Compression of the nerve in this location may result in ulnar tunnel syndrome.

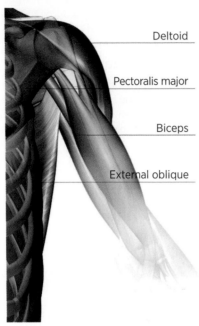

Fig. 4-3: Muscles of the anterior upper limb.

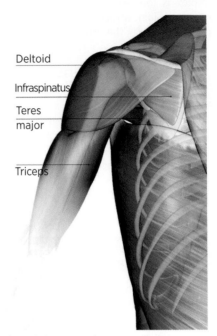

Fig. 4-4: Muscles of the posterior upper limb.

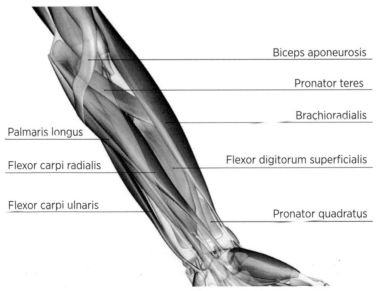

Fig. 4-5: Muscles of the volar surface of the forearm.

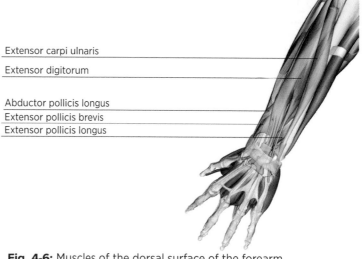

Extensor carpi ulnaris

Extensor digitorum

Abductor pollicis longus
Extensor pollicis brevis
Extensor pollicis longus

Fig. 4-6: Muscles of the dorsal surface of the forearm.

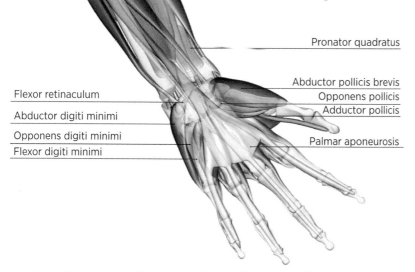

Pronator quadratus

Abductor pollicis brevis
Opponens pollicis
Adductor pollicis

Flexor retinaculum

Abductor digiti minimi

Opponens digiti minimi

Flexor digiti minimi

Palmar aponeurosis

Fig. 4-7: Muscles of the volar surface of the wrist and hand.

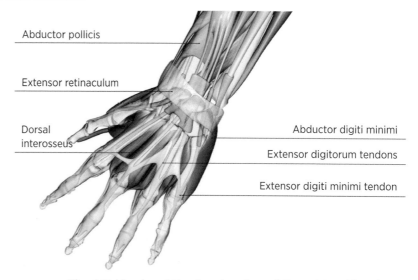

Abductor pollicis

Extensor retinaculum

Dorsal
interosseus

Abductor digiti minimi

Extensor digitorum tendons

Extensor digiti minimi tendon

Fig. 4-8: Muscles of the dorsal surface of the wrist and hand.

Specific Joints - Lower Extremity

Hip[5,8-10]

The hip (iliofemoral) joint is a synovial joint formed by the head of the femur and the acetabulum. The hip is classified as a ball and socket joint with three degrees of freedom.

Articulations

Iliofemoral joint

The proximal joint surface of the iliofemoral joint consists of the acetabulum which is oriented laterally, inferiorly, and anteriorly. The distal joint surface consists of the convex head of the femur.

Iliofemoral Snapshot

Osteokinematic motions: flexion, extension, abduction, adduction, medial rotation, lateral rotation

Loose packed position: 30 degrees flexion, 30 degrees abduction, slight lateral rotation

Close packed position: full extension, medial rotation

Capsular pattern: flexion, abduction, medial rotation (sometimes medial rotation is most limited)

Muscle Action

Hip flexion: iliopsoas, sartorius, rectus femoris, pectineus

Hip extension: gluteus maximus, gluteus medius, semitendinosus, semimembranosus, biceps femoris

Hip abduction: gluteus medius, gluteus minimus, piriformis, obturator internus, tensor fasciae latae

Hip adduction: adductor magnus, adductor longus, adductor brevis, gracilis

Hip medial rotation: tensor fasciae latae, gluteus medius, gluteus minimus, pectineus, adductor longus

Hip lateral rotation: gluteus maximus, obturator externus, obturator internus, piriformis, gemelli, sartorius

Primary Structures

Acetabular labrum

The acetabular labrum consists of a fibrocartilaginous rim attached to the margin of the acetabulum. The structure enhances the depth of the acetabulum.

Articular capsule

A strong articular capsule extends from the rim of the acetabulum to the neck of the femur. The capsule is reinforced by the iliofemoral, pubofemoral, and ischiofemoral ligaments.

Bursae

There are several bursae within the hip region, some of which include the iliopsoas, trochanteric, and ischiogluteal bursae. The iliopsoas bursa is located between the anterior joint capsule and iliopsoas tendon. There are multiple trochanteric bursae, all of which lie between the greater trochanter and the different gluteal muscles. The ischiogluteal bursa is located between the ischium and gluteus maximus.

Femoral triangle

The femoral triangle is a space located in the anterior hip that is bordered by the inguinal ligament, sartorius, and adductor longus. Within this space, the femoral artery and lymph glands can be palpated. The femoral nerve and vein also pass through this space.

Iliofemoral ligament

The iliofemoral ligament consists of a thickened portion of the articular capsule that extends from the anterior inferior iliac spine of the pelvis to the intertrochanteric line of the femur. The structure is considered to be the strongest ligament in the body and serves to prevent excessive hip extension and assists to maintain upright posture.

Ischiofemoral ligament

The ischiofemoral ligament consists of a thickened portion of the articular capsule that extends from the ischial wall of the acetabulum to the neck of the femur. The structure is the weakest of the three ligaments, however, it serves to reinforce the articular capsule.

Ligamentum teres

The ligamentum teres (ligament of the head of the femur) is a ligament that provides a physical attachment between the head of the femur and the inferior rim of the acetabulum. Blood vessels and nerves travel with this ligament in a sheath to the head of the femur. The ligament provides minimal stability to the hip.

Pubofemoral ligament

The pubofemoral ligament consists of a thickened portion of the articular capsule that extends from the pubic portion of the rim of the acetabulum to the neck of the femur. The structure serves to prevent excessive abduction of the femur and limits hip extension.

CONSIDER THIS
COMMON MECHANISMS OF INJURY FOR KNEE LIGAMENTS

Stability of the knee is enhanced by the role of four primary ligaments. The ligaments are capable of functioning in isolation or collectively. Due to the unique function of each ligament, it is possible to identify specific mechanisms of injury often associated with a particular ligamentous injury.

Anterior cruciate ligament (ACL)

The ACL may be injured through a noncontact twisting injury associated with hyperextension and varus or valgus stress to the knee. Other mechanisms for ACL damage include the tibia being driven anteriorly on the femur, the femur being driven posteriorly on the tibia or severe knee hyperextension. Special tests designed to assess the integrity of the ACL include the anterior drawer test, Lachman test, lateral pivot shift test, and Slocum test.

Posterior cruciate ligament (PCL)

The PCL may be injured when the superior portion of the tibia is struck while the knee is flexed. A common example of this occurs in a motor vehicle accident when a passenger's leg collides against the dashboard. Other mechanisms for PCL damage include the tibia being driven posteriorly on the femur, the femur being driven anteriorly on the tibia or severe knee hyperflexion. Special tests designed to assess the integrity of the PCL include the posterior drawer test and posterior sag sign.

Medial collateral ligament (MCL)

The MCL may be injured with a pure valgus load at the knee without rotation. This type of injury is often sustained with contact activities such as a lateral blow to the knee during a football game. Injury to the MCL often involves injury to other knee structures such as the ACL or medial meniscus. A valgus stress test can assess the integrity of the MCL.

Lateral collateral ligament (LCL)

The LCL may be injured with a pure varus load at the knee without rotation. This type of injury is often sustained with contact activities such as a medial blow to the knee. The LCL is rarely completely torn without a concurrent injury to the ACL or PCL. A varus stress test can assess the integrity of the LCL.

Knee[8-12]

The knee joint is a synovial joint consisting of three bones (i.e., femur, tibia, patella) and two primary articulations (i.e., tibiofemoral, patellofemoral) enclosed within a single joint capsule. The knee is classified as a hinge joint, formed by the articulation of the tibia with the femur, with two degrees of freedom.

Articulations

Tibiofemoral joint

The proximal joint surface of the tibiofemoral joint is formed by the convex medial and lateral condyles of the distal femur. The distal joint surface is formed by the concave medial and lateral condyles of the proximal tibia.

Patellofemoral joint

The patellofemoral joint is formed by the convex patella and the concave trochlear groove of the femur. The patella slides superiorly in knee extension and inferiorly in knee flexion. Patella rotation and tilting also occur during knee extension and flexion.

Tibiofemoral Snapshot

Osteokinematic motions: flexion, extension, medial rotation, lateral rotation
Loose packed position: 25 degrees flexion
Close packed position: full extension, lateral rotation of tibia
Capsular pattern: flexion, extension

Muscle Action

Knee flexion: biceps femoris, semitendinosus, sartorius, semimembranosus

Knee extension: rectus femoris, vastus lateralis, vastus intermedius, vastus medialis

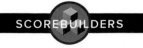

Primary Structures

Anterior cruciate ligament

The ACL runs from the anterior intercondylar area of the tibia to the medial aspect of the lateral femoral condyle in the intercondylar notch. The ACL prevents anterior displacement of the tibia on the femur.

Arcuate ligament complex

The arcuate ligament complex consists of the arcuate ligament, oblique popliteal ligament, lateral collateral ligament, popliteus tendon, and lateral head of the gastrocnemius. The complex assists the cruciate ligaments in controlling posterolateral rotatory instability of the knee and provides support to the posterolateral joint capsule.

Bursae

The knee has several important bursae including the prepatellar bursa, superficial infrapatellar bursa, and deep infrapatellar bursa. The prepatellar bursa lies over the patella and allows for greater freedom of movement of the skin covering the anterior aspect of the patella. The superficial infrapatellar bursa lies between the patellar tendon and skin, while the deep infrapatellar bursa lies between the patellar tendon and the tibia.

Fat pads

There are three fat pads in the knee: quadriceps, prefemoral, and infrapatellar. The infrapatellar fat pad is the one most commonly affected and can be a source of anterior knee pain when it becomes impinged (e.g., Hoffa's syndrome).

Lateral collateral ligament

The LCL runs from the lateral femoral epicondyle to the fibular head. The LCL prevents excessive varus displacement of the tibia relative to the femur.

Medial collateral ligament

The MCL runs from slightly above the medial femoral epicondyle to the medial aspect of the shaft of the tibia. The deep capsular fibers are attached to the medial meniscus. The MCL prevents excessive valgus displacement of the tibia relative to the femur.

Menisci

The medial and lateral menisci are firmly attached to the proximal surface of the tibia. The menisci are thick at the periphery and thinner at their internal unattached edges. Menisci function to deepen the articular surfaces of the tibia where they articulate with the femoral condyles. The menisci function as shock absorbers and contribute to lubrication and nutrition of the joint.

Pes anserine

The pes anserine is the common insertion point for the gracilis, semitendinosus, and sartorius muscles. The pes anserine is located medial and distal to the tibial tuberosity. Pain and/or swelling in this region may indicate the presence of pes anserine bursitis.

Plicae

Plicae are extensions of the synovial membrane that are sometimes found in the anterior knee, most commonly medial to the patella. They do not serve a specific function, though they can be a source of anterior knee pain.

Posterior cruciate ligament

The PCL runs from the posterior intercondylar area of the tibia to the lateral aspect of the medial femoral condyle in the intercondylar notch. The PCL prevents posterior displacement of the tibia on the femur.

Retinacula

The medial and lateral retinacula are ligamentous structures that attach the patella to the femur, tibia, and menisci. The lateral retinaculum is the stronger of the two and plays a larger role in patellar positioning.

Ankle and Foot[8-12]

The ankle and foot are formed by a series of unique articulations including the distal tibiofibular joint, talocrural joint, subtalar joint, midtarsal joint, and forefoot.

Articulations

Distal tibiofibular joint

The distal tibiofibular joint is formed by a fibrous union between the lateral aspect of the distal tibia and the distal fibula.

Talocrural joint

The talocrural joint is formed by the articulations of the distal tibia, talus, and fibula. The joint is a synovial hinge joint with one degree of freedom. The talocrural joint offers significant stability in dorsiflexion, however, it becomes much more mobile with plantar flexion.

Talocrural Snapshot
Osteokinematic motions: dorsiflexion, plantar flexion
Loose packed position: 10 degrees plantar flexion, midway between maximum inversion and eversion
Close packed position: maximum dorsiflexion
Capsular pattern: plantar flexion, dorsiflexion

Subtalar joint

The subtalar joint is formed by three articulations (anterior, middle, posterior) between the talus and calcaneus. The joint has one degree of freedom. The anterior and middle articulations are formed by two convex facets on the talus and two concave facets on the calcaneus. The posterior articulation is formed by a concave facet on the inferior surface of the talus and a convex facet on the body of the calcaneus.

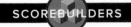

Subtalar Snapshot
Osteokinematic motions: inversion, eversion
Loose packed position: midway between extremes of range of movement
Close packed position: supination
Capsular pattern: limitation of varus range of movement

Midtarsal joint

The midtarsal (transverse tarsal) joint is formed by the talocalcaneonavicular joint and the calcaneocuboid joint. The joint is considered to have two axes, one longitudinal and one oblique. Motions around both axes are triplanar.

Midtarsal Snapshot
Osteokinematic motions: inversion, eversion
Loose packed position: midway between extremes of range of movement
Close packed position: supination
Capsular pattern: dorsiflexion, plantar flexion, adduction, medial rotation

Forefoot

The forefoot consists of the tarsometatarsal joints, metatarsophalangeal joints, and interphalangeal joints.

Muscle Action

Plantar flexion: tibialis posterior, gastrocnemius, soleus, peroneus longus, peroneus brevis, plantaris, flexor hallucis

Dorsiflexion: tibialis anterior, extensor hallucis longus, extensor digitorum longus, peroneus tertius

Inversion: tibialis posterior, tibialis anterior, flexor digitorum longus

Eversion: peroneus longus, peroneus brevis, peroneus tertius

Primary Structures

Anterior talofibular ligament

The anterior talofibular ligament is taut during plantar flexion and resists inversion of the talus and calcaneus. The ligament also resists anterior translation of the talus on the tibia.

Calcaneofibular ligament

The calcaneofibular ligament is an extracapsular ligament that resists inversion of the talus within the midrange of talocrural motion.

Deltoid ligament

The deltoid ligament is formed by the anterior tibiotalar ligament, tibiocalcaneal ligament, posterior tibiotalar ligament, and tibionavicular ligament. The ligament provides medial ligamentous support by resisting eversion of the talus.

Interosseous membrane

The interosseous membrane consists of a strong fibrous tissue that serves to fixate the fibula to the tibia. Distally, the structure blends into the anterior and posterior tibiofibular ligaments and provides additional support at the distal tibiofibular syndesmosis joint.

Ligaments

The majority of the ligaments in the ankle are areas of increased density within the joint capsule. As a result, damage to the ankle ligaments typically produces damage to the joint capsule and irritation of the synovial lining.

Plantar fascia

The plantar fascia is a thick layer of fascial tissue on the plantar aspect of the foot that originates on the calcaneal tuberosity and inserts into the plantar forefoot. The plantar fascia plays a role in supporting the weight of the body and also helps to support the arch of the foot for improved propulsion during gait.

Posterior talofibular ligament

The posterior talofibular ligament resists posterior displacement of the talus on the tibia.

Retinacula

There are several retinacula within the ankle. The major retinaculum is the extensor retinaculum, which lies on the anterior side of the joint. This structure contains the tendons on the extensor musculature and prevents them from "bowstringing" as the ankle dorsiflexes. There is also a flexor retinaculum and a peroneal retinaculum.

Retrocalcaneal bursa

The retrocalcaneal bursa lies just anterior to the Achilles tendon where it attaches into the superior calcaneus and acts as a cushion between the tendon and the bone. Irritation of the bursa, due to trauma or overuse, can result in retrocalcaneal bursitis.

Sinus tarsi

The sinus tarsi is a space located between the inferior talus, superior calcaneus, and anterior portion of the lateral malleolus. This area contains ligaments that can also be injured during a common inversion ankle sprain.

Tensor fasciae latae

Gracilis

Sartorius

Rectus femoris

Vastus lateralis

Vastus medialis

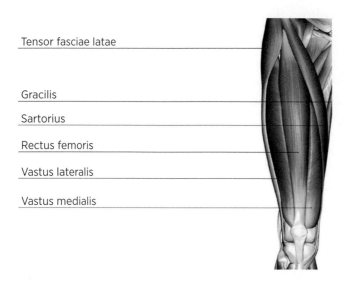

Fig. 4-9: Muscles of the anterior upper leg.

Gluteus maximus

Adductor magnus

Iliotibial tract

Biceps femoris

Semitendinosus

Semimembranosus

Gracilis

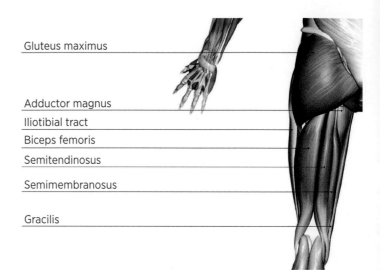

Fig. 4-10: Muscles of the posterior upper leg.

Peroneus longus

Tibialis anterior

Extensor digitorum longus

Extensor hallucis longus

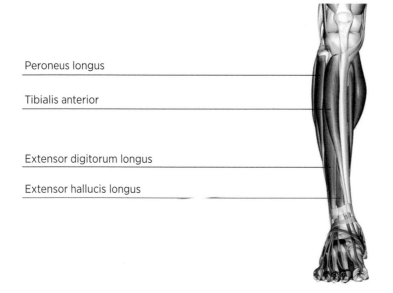

Fig. 4-11: Muscles of the anterior lower leg.

Plantaris

Gastrocnemius medial head

Gastrocnemius lateral head

Soleus

Achilles tendon

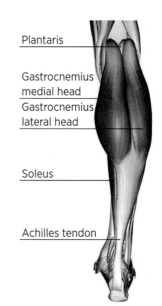

Fig. 4-12: Muscles of the posterior lower leg.

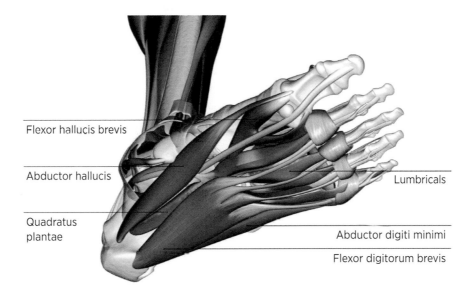

Flexor hallucis brevis

Abductor hallucis

Quadratus plantae

Lumbricals

Abductor digiti minimi

Flexor digitorum brevis

Fig. 4-13: Muscles of the volar surface of the foot.

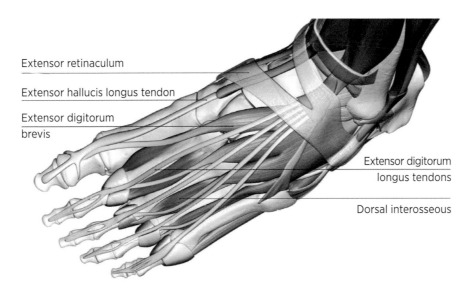

Extensor retinaculum

Extensor hallucis longus tendon

Extensor digitorum brevis

Extensor digitorum longus tendons

Dorsal interosseous

Fig. 4-14: Muscles of the dorsal surface of the foot.

Spine

Cervical Spine[3,10,13,14]

The cervical spine consists of seven cervical vertebrae. The first two, the atlas and axis, are unique. The atlas (C1) supports the weight of the head through two facet joints which form the atlanto-occipital joint. The axis (C2) has a superior projection called the dens. The articulation between the dens and the anterior arch of the atlas forms the atlantoaxial joint.

Articulations

Atlanto-occipital joint

The atlanto-occipital joint is a condylar synovial joint that permits flexion and extension of the cranium. This motion is often noted when nodding the head to say "yes."

Atlantoaxial joints

The atlantoaxial joints are plane synovial joints that permit flexion, extension, lateral flexion, and rotation of the cervical spine. The majority of rotation of the skull on the spinal column occurs at the atlantoaxial joints.

Intervertebral joints

The intervertebral joints are formed by the superior and inferior surfaces of the vertebral bodies and the associated intervertebral disks.

Zygapophyseal joints

The zygapophyseal joints are formed by the right and left superior articular facets of one vertebra and the right and left inferior articular facets of an adjacent superior vertebra.

Muscle Action

Cervical flexion: sternocleidomastoid, longus colli, scalenus muscles

Cervical extension: splenius cervicis, semispinalis cervicis, iliocostalis cervicis, longissimus cervicis, multifidus, trapezius

Cervical rotation and lateral bending: sternocleidomastoid, scalenus muscles, splenius cervicis, longissimus cervicis, iliocostalis cervicis, levator scapulae, multifidus

Primary Structures

Alar ligaments

The alar ligaments attach the dens of the axis to the occipital condyles. These ligaments function to resist flexion, contralateral side bending, and contralateral rotation. They also help to limit sagittal plane translation between the atlas and the occiput.

Anterior longitudinal ligament

The anterior longitudinal ligament limits extension of the spine and reinforces the anterior portion of the intervertebral disks and vertebrae.

Cervical Spine Snapshot

Osteokinematic motions: flexion, extension, lateral flexion, rotation
Loose packed position: midway between flexion and extension
Close packed position: extension
Capsular pattern: lateral flexion and rotation equally limited, extension

Brachial plexus

The brachial plexus arises from the nerve roots of C5 through T1. These nerve roots combine to form trunks, then later divide to form divisions, cords, and finally the peripheral nerves. The nerves that arise from the brachial plexus provide innervation to muscles of the entire upper quarter.

Cruciform ligament

The cruciform ligament has vertical and horizontal portions. The vertical portion connects the dens of the axis to the foramen magnum. The horizontal portion connects the dens with the atlas. This ligament functions to limit upper cervical flexion, as well as translation of the atlas on the axis.

Interspinous ligaments

The interspinous ligaments are located between the spinous processes and serve to limit flexion and rotation of the spine.

Intervertebral disks

Intervertebral disks are formed by a dense layer of collagen fibers and fibrocartilage called the annulus fibrosus as well as a flexible inner layer called the nucleus pulposus. The annulus fibrosus is firmly attached to the adjacent vertebrae and provides tensile strength to the disk during spinal movement. The nucleus pulposus is a gelatinous mass located centrally in the disk. Flexion of a vertebral segment causes the anterior portion of the disk to be compressed and the posterior portion of the disk to be distracted.

Intervertebral foramina

The intervertebral foramina are located in the posterior pillar of each vertebral segment. Spinal nerves and blood vessels exit the spinal canal via the foramina. The size of the intervertebral foramen increases with flexion and contralateral sidebending and decreases with extension and ipsilateral sidebending. Nerve root entrapment can result from closure or narrowing of the intervertebral foramen due to arthritic changes, spurring or narrowing of the intervertebral disks.

Ligamentum flavum

The ligamentum flavum connects the lamina of one vertebra to the

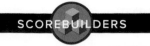

lamina of the vertebra above it. The structure serves to limit flexion and rotation of the spine.

Ligamentum nuchae

The ligamentum nuchae restricts flexion in the cervical spine.

Posterior longitudinal ligament

The posterior longitudinal ligament limits flexion of the spine and reinforces the posterior aspect of the intervertebral disks.

Uncovertebral joints

Also known as the uncinate processes or joints of Luschka, the uncovertebral joints are formed between the lateral projections on the inferior surface of one vertebra and the lateral projections on the superior surface of the vertebra below it. These joints are found between C3 and T1. They function to guide motion in the sagittal plane and limit motion in the other two planes.

Thoracolumbar Spine[3,9,10,14-16]

The thoracic spine consists of 12 vertebrae with long prominent spinous processes. The first ten thoracic vertebrae have articular facets on each transverse process where the ribs articulate. The lumbar spine consists of five vertebrae that provide the primary stability for the low back.

Articulations

Intervertebral joints

The intervertebral joints are formed by the superior and inferior surfaces of the vertebral bodies and the associated intervertebral disks.

Zygapophyseal joints

The zygapophyseal joints are formed by the right and left superior articular facets of one vertebra and the right and left inferior articular facets of an adjacent superior vertebra.

Muscle Action

Thoracolumbar flexion: rectus abdominis, internal oblique, external oblique

Thoracolumbar extension: erector spinae, quadratus lumborum, multifidus

Thoracolumbar rotation and lateral bending: psoas major, quadratus lumborum, external oblique, internal oblique, multifidus, longissimus thoracis, iliocostalis thoracis, rotatores

Primary Structures

Anterior longitudinal ligament

The anterior longitudinal ligament limits extension of the spine and reinforces the anterior portion of the intervertebral disks and vertebrae.

Anterior sacroiliac ligament

The anterior sacroiliac ligament connects the anterior surface of the ilium to the anterior sacrum. It is a thickening of the joint capsule and is considered the weakest of the sacroiliac ligaments.

Thoracolumbar Spine Snapshot

Osteokinematic motions: flexion, extension, lateral flexion, rotation	
Loose packed position: midway between flexion and extension	
Close packed position: extension	
Capsular pattern: lateral flexion and rotation equally limited, extension	

Coccyx

The coccyx articulates with the sacrum and most often consists of four small, fused vertebral bodies. The coccyx does not have a specific purpose and is most often considered an embryological remnant.

Iliolumbar ligament

The iliolumbar ligament connects the posterior portion of the ilium to the transverse process of the L5 vertebra and functions to limit all motions between L5 and S1.

Interosseous sacroiliac ligament

The interosseous sacroiliac ligament connects the sacrum and ilium and is located deep to the posterior sacroiliac ligament. The ligament is strong and functions to resist anterior and inferior movements of the sacrum.

Interspinous ligaments

The interspinous ligaments are located between the spinous processes and serve to limit flexion and rotation of the spine.

Intervertebral disks

Intervertebral disks are formed by a dense layer of collagen fibers and fibrocartilage called the annulus fibrosus as well as a flexible inner layer called the nucleus pulposus. The annulus fibrosus is firmly attached to the adjacent vertebrae and provides tensile strength to the disk during spinal movement. The nucleus pulposus is a gelatinous mass located slightly posterior to the center of the disk in the lumbar spine. Flexion of a vertebral segment causes the anterior portion of the disk to be compressed and the posterior portion of the disk to be distracted.

Intervertebral foramina

The intervertebral foramina are located in the posterior pillar of each vertebral segment. Spinal nerves and blood vessels exit the spinal canal via the foramina. The size of the intervertebral foramen increases with flexion and contralateral sidebending and decreases with extension and ipsilateral sidebending. Nerve root entrapment can result from closure or narrowing of the intervertebral foramen due to arthritic changes, spurring or narrowing of the intervertebral disks.

Ligamentum flavum

The ligamentum flavum connects the lamina of one vertebra to the lamina of the vertebra above it. The structure serves to limit flexion and rotation of the spine.

Lumbar plexus

The lumbar plexus is formed by the nerve roots of T12 and L1-L4. The plexus innervates the anterior and medial muscles of the thigh and the dermatomes of the medial leg and foot. The largest and most important branches of the plexus are the obturator and femoral nerves.

Posterior longitudinal ligament

The posterior longitudinal ligament limits flexion of the spine and reinforces the posterior aspect of the intervertebral disks.

Posterior sacroiliac ligament

The posterior sacroiliac ligament connects the posterior superior iliac spine with the lateral portions of the 3rd and 4th sacral segments. This ligament is strong and its fibers run in multiple directions, eventually combining with the fibers of the sacrotuberous ligament. This ligament functions to limit all sacral motions, especially posterior rotation of the sacrum.

Pubic symphysis

The pubic symphysis is the joint formed between the end of each pubis bone. The ends of the bones are covered with hyaline cartilage with a fibrocartilage disk between them. Motion at this joint is very limited.

Ribs

Ribs 1-10 articulate with the thoracic vertebrae through the costovertebral joints and the costotransverse joints. Ribs 1-7 are attached to the sternum through costal cartilage and ribs 8-10 join with the costal cartilage of ribs 1-7. Ribs 11-12 articulate only with the vertebral bodies of T11-T12, but not the transverse process of the same vertebra. Ribs 11-12 are classified as floating because they do not attach to the sternum or the costal cartilage at their distal end.

Sacral plexus

The sacral plexus is formed by the lumbosacral trunk, the ventral rami of S1-S3, and the descending portion of S4. The plexus supplies the muscles of the buttocks, and through the sciatic nerve, innervates the muscles of the posterior thigh and lower leg.

Sacrospinous ligament

The sacrospinous ligament connects the ischial spine to the lateral sacrum and coccyx, and also has fibers that blend with the fibers of the sacrotuberous ligament. This ligament functions to limit anterior rotation of the sacrum on the pelvis.

Sacrotuberous ligament

The sacrotuberous ligament has several attachment sites, including the posterior superior iliac spine, lateral sacrum, coccyx, and ischial tuberosity. The ligament primarily functions to resist sacral anterior rotation and prevent superior translation of the sacrum.

Sacrum

The sacrum is a broad, thick bone consisting of five fused vertebrae that fixate the spinal column to the pelvis. The main functions of the sacrum are to provide an attachment for the iliac bones and to protect the pelvic organs. The sacrum is attached to the pelvis by strong ligaments forming the sacroiliac joint.

Supraspinous ligament

The supraspinous ligament restricts flexion in the thoracic and lumbar spine.

Thoracolumbar fascia

The thoracolumbar fascia is connected to the spinous processes of the lumbar vertebrae, the posterior superior iliac spines, and the iliac crests. The fascia consists of three layers that separate the lumbar muscles into three different compartments. This structure functions to provide stability to the spine, transmit forces, resist lumbar flexion, and provide a site for muscular attachments.

Musculoskeletal System Screening

Upper Quarter Screening[10,13,17-18]

The upper quarter screen provides a rapid assessment of mobility and neurologic function of the cervical spine and upper extremities. The screen is traditionally performed with the patient in sitting.

The following are components of an upper extremity screening:

Posture

- Postural assessment

Range of Motion

- Active range of motion of the cervical spine
- Active range of motion of the upper extremities
- Passive overpressure of the cervical spine and upper extremities, if the patient does not exhibit signs and symptoms of pathology

Resistive Testing (C1 – T1)	
Resistive Test	**Innervation Level**
Cervical rotation	C1
Shoulder elevation	C2 – C4
Shoulder abduction	C5
Elbow flexion	C5 – C6
Wrist extension	C6
Elbow extension	C7
Wrist flexion	C7
Thumb extension	C8
Finger adduction	T1

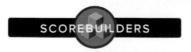

Reflex Testing (C5 – C7)

Reflex Test	Innervation Level
Biceps	C5
Brachioradialis	C6
Triceps	C7

Dermatome Testing (C2 – T1)

Area of Skin	Innervation Level
Posterior head	C2
Posterior-lateral neck	C3
Acromioclavicular joint	C4
Lateral arm	C5
Lateral forearm and thumb	C6
Palmar distal phalanx – middle finger	C7
Little finger and ulnar border of the hand	C8
Medial forearm	T1

Lower Quarter Screening[10,13,18]

The lower quarter screen provides a rapid assessment of mobility and neurologic function of the lumbosacral spine and lower extremities. The screen is traditionally performed with the patient in standing or sitting.

The following are components of a lower extremity screening:

Posture

- Postural assessment

Range of Motion

- Active range of motion of the lumbosacral spine
- Active range of motion of the lower extremities
- Passive overpressure of the lumbosacral spine and lower extremities, if the patient does not exhibit signs and symptoms of pathology

Functional Testing (L4 – S1)

Functional Test	Innervation Level
Heel walking	L4 – L5
Toe walking	S1
Straight leg raise	L4 – S1

Resistive Testing (L1 – S1)

Resistive Test	Innervation Level
Hip flexion	L1 – L2
Knee extension	L3 – L4
Ankle dorsiflexion	L4 – L5
Great toe extension	L5
Ankle plantar flexion	S1

Reflex Testing (L4 – S1)

Reflex Test	Innervation Level
Patella	L4
Achilles	S1

Dermatome Testing (L2 – S5)

Area of Skin	Innervation Level
Anterior thigh	L2
Middle third of anterior thigh	L3
Patella and medial malleolus	L4
Fibular head and dorsum of foot	L5
Lateral and plantar aspect of foot	S1
Medial aspect of posterior thigh	S2
Perianal area	S3 – S5

Pain[5,9,13,18]

Pain Transmission

Nociceptors are free nerve endings present in most types of tissue that are activated by thermal, mechanical or chemical stimuli. They are the terminal portions of two types of afferent neurons, A-delta fibers and C fibers. A-delta fibers transmit detailed information rapidly from peripheral cutaneous structures. C fibers transmit information from deeper tissues (e.g., joints, viscera) and do so more slowly than A-delta fibers. Because of these differences, A-delta fibers are more likely to transmit pain signals that are sharp and localized, while C fibers transmit pain signals that are dull, aching, and diffuse. These nerve fibers send their impulses to the dorsal horn of the spinal cord, where the impulses are then carried to the thalamus via the spinothalamic tracts. The nerve signal is then projected to the sensory cortex to be interpreted and become a conscious pain sensation.

Gate Control Theory

The gate control theory helps to explain the regulation of pain, specifically how other stimuli can help to decrease the sensation of pain. A-delta and C fibers synapse with a secondary neuron, which sends the pain signal to the brain. However, they also synapse with an inhibitory interneuron at this same junction. A-alpha and A-beta fibers provide input to these inhibitory interneurons. Therefore, nerve transmission through the A-alpha and A-beta fibers can stimulate these interneurons to inhibit pain signals to the brain ("closing the gate"). The use of electrical stimulation and massage as interventions work on this theory by stimulating A-alpha and A-beta fibers.

Endogenous Opioids

Pain regulation is also controlled by endogenous opioids known as opiopeptins (also known as endorphins). These substances bind to opioid receptors, which are located throughout the nervous system, resulting in inhibition of pain signals. Opiopeptins have a direct effect on nerve signals by controlling the amount of calcium and potassium that move into and out of the cell during depolarization. They also have an indirect effect on nerve signals by inhibiting the release of GABA, a substance that normally inhibits the activity of structures that help to control pain, such as A-beta fibers.

Numerical Rating Scale

A tool used to assess pain intensity by rating pain on a scale of 0-10 or 0-100. The 0 represents no discernable pain and the 10 or 100 represent the worst pain ever. The information is used as a baseline and should be reassessed at regular intervals in order to monitor progress. This scale is easy to administer, assess, and monitor.

Visual Analogue Scale

A tool used to assess pain intensity using a 10-15 cm line with the left anchor indicating "no pain" and the right anchor indicating "the worst pain you can have." The level of perceived pain is indicated on the line and is reassessed frequently over the course of physical therapy to record changes and progress, and to predict patient outcome. This scale can be highly sensitive if small increments such as millimeters are used to measure the patient's point of pain on the scale. The visual analogue scale is a valid tool if measurements are taken accurately.

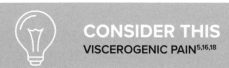
CONSIDER THIS
VISCEROGENIC PAIN[5,16,18]

Viscerogenic pain is pain that results from pathology of an internal organ, which can often refer to a site distant from the organ and mimic common patterns of musculoskeletal pain. Recognizing the pain patterns associated with viscerogenic pain is an important component of the screening process. Viscerogenic pain differs from musculoskeletal pain in many ways. Viscerogenic pain does not change based on movement or positioning of the body part, as would musculoskeletal pain. Because the organs have innervation from multiple spinal cord levels and a low density of nerve receptors, the pain is often diffuse and poorly localized. Additionally, viscerogenic pain may be accompanied by other systemic symptoms, such as nausea, vomiting, weight loss, pallor, profuse sweating, fever, and abnormal vital signs. Common sites for referred viscerogenic pain include the shoulder, scapula, back, chest, pelvis, sacroiliac joint, groin, and hip.

EXAMPLES

Myocardial infarction

The heart is innervated by the C3-T4 spinal segments and thus cardiac pathology can result in referred pain to a variety of areas. A patient having a myocardial infarction may experience pain on the left side of the body in the chest, mid-back, shoulder, arm, neck or jaw.

Kehr's sign

Blood that accumulates in the abdominal cavity, often secondary to rupture of the spleen, can cause irritation of the diaphragm and refer pain to the left shoulder. Pain is referred to this region due to the innervation of the phrenic nerve (i.e., C3-C5). Kehr's sign is positive when pressure to the upper abdomen or supine positioning results in left shoulder pain.

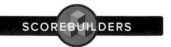

Posture

Good and Faulty Posture: Summary Chart

Good Posture	Part	Faulty Posture
Toes should be straight, that is, neither curled downward nor bent upward. They should extend forward in line with the foot and should not be squeezed together or overlap.	Toes	Toes bend up at the first joint and down at middle joints so that the weight rests on the tips of the toes (hammer toes). This fault is often associated with wearing shoes that are too short. Big toe slants inward toward the midline of the foot (hallux valgus). "Bunion." This fault is often associated with wearing shoes that are too narrow and pointed at the toes.
In standing, the longitudinal arch has the shape of a half dome. Barefoot or in shoes without heels, the feet toe-out slightly. In shoes with heels, the feet are parallel. In walking with or without shoes, the feet are parallel and the weight is transferred from the heel along the outer border to the ball of the foot. In sprinting, the feet are parallel or toe-in slightly. The weight is on the balls of the feet and toes because the heels do not come in contact with the ground.	Foot	Low longitudinal arch or flat foot. Low metatarsal arch, usually indicated by calluses under the ball of the foot. Weight borne on the inner side of the foot (pronation). "Ankle rolls in." Weight borne on the outer border of the foot (supination). "Ankle rolls out." Toeing-out while walking, or while standing in shoes with heels ("slue-footed"). Toeing-in while walking or standing ("pigeon-toed").
Legs are straight up and down. Kneecaps face straight ahead when feet are in good position. Looking at the knees from the side, the knees are straight (i.e., neither flexed or hyperextended).	Knees and Legs	Knees touch when feet are apart (knock-knees). Knees are apart when feet touch (bowlegs). Knee curves slightly backward (hyperextended knee). "Back-knee." Knee bends slightly forward, that is, it is not as straight as it should be (flexed knee). Kneecaps face slightly toward each other (medially rotated femurs). Kneecaps face slightly outward (laterally rotated femurs).
Ideally, the body weight is borne evenly on both feet and the hips are level. One side should not be more prominent than the other as seen from front or back, nor is one hip more forward or backward than the other as seen from the side. The spine does not curve to the left or the right side. (A slight deviation to the left in right-handed individuals and to the right in left-handed individuals is not uncommon. Also, a tendency toward a slightly low right shoulder and slightly high right hip is frequently found in right-handed people, and vice versa for left-handed people.)	Hips, Pelvis, and Spine Back View	One hip is higher than the other (lateral pelvic tilt). Sometimes it is not really higher but appears so because a sideways sway of the body has made it more prominent. (Tailors and dressmakers often notice a lateral tilt because the hemline of skirts or length of trousers must be adjusted to the difference.) The hips are rotated so that one is farther forward than the other (clockwise or counterclockwise rotation).

Good and Faulty Posture: Summary Chart (continued)

Good Posture	Part	Faulty Posture
The front of the pelvis and the thighs are in a straight line. The buttocks are not prominent in back but slope slightly downward. The spine has four natural curves. In the neck and lower back the curve is forward; in the upper back and lowest part of the spine (sacral region) it is backward. The sacral curve is a fixed curve while the other three are flexible.	**Spine and Pelvis Side View**	The low back arches forward too much (lordosis). The pelvis tilts forward too much. The front of the thigh forms an angle with the pelvis when this tilt is present. The normal forward curve in the low back has straightened. The pelvis tips backward as in swayback and flat-back postures. Increased backward curve in the upper back (kyphosis or round upper back). Increased forward curve in the neck. Almost always accompanied by round upper back and seen as a forward head. Lateral curve of the spine (scoliosis); toward one side (C-curve), toward both sides (S-curve).
In young children, up to about the age of 10, the abdomen normally protrudes somewhat. In older children and adults it should be flat.	**Abdomen**	Entire abdomen protrudes. Lower part of the abdomen protrudes while the upper part is pulled in.
A good position of the chest is one in which it is slightly up and slightly forward (while the back remains in good alignment). The chest appears to be in a position about halfway between that of a full inspiration and a forced expiration.	**Chest**	Depressed or "hollow-chest" position. Lifted and held up too high, brought about by arching the back. Ribs more prominent on one side than on the other. Lower ribs flaring out or protruding.
Arms hang relaxed at the sides with palms of the hands facing toward the body. Elbows are slightly bent, so forearms hang slightly forward. Shoulders are level and neither one is more forward or backward than the other when seen from the side. Shoulder blades lie flat against the rib cage. They are neither too close together or too wide apart. In adults, a separation of about 4 inches is average.	**Arms and Shoulders**	Arms held stiffly in any position forward, backward, or out from the body. Arms turned so that palms of hands face backward. One shoulder higher than the other. Both shoulders hiked-up. One or both shoulders drooping forward or sloping. Shoulders rotated either clockwise or counterclockwise. Shoulder blades pulled back too hard. Shoulder blades too far apart. Shoulder blades too prominent, standing out from the rib cage (winged scapulae).
Head is held erect in a position of good balance.	**Head**	Chin up too high. Head protruding forward. Head tilted or rotated to one side.

From Kendall F, McCreary E, Provance P: Muscle Testing and Function. Lippincott, William & Wilkins, Baltimore 1993, p.115-116, with permission.

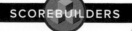

CONSIDER THIS
IDEAL PLUMB LINE ALIGNMENT[10,18]

A plumb line is a tool that consists of a weight suspended at the end of a string to determine verticality. Ideal positioning of selected body parts in relation to the plumb line is described below.

- Slightly posterior to coronal suture
- Through the external auditory meatus
- Through the axis of the odontoid process
- Midway through the tip of the shoulder
- Through the bodies of the lumbar vertebrae
- Slightly posterior to the hip joint
- Slightly anterior to the axis of the knee joint
- Slightly anterior to the lateral malleolus
- Through the calcaneocuboid joint

Although desirable, rarely will a given patient demonstrate ideal alignment with all of the anatomical landmarks listed above. The following pictures provide an example of a patient with "good posture" and a patient with "faulty posture" (Figs. 4-16, 4-17).

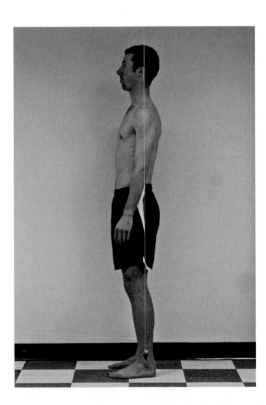

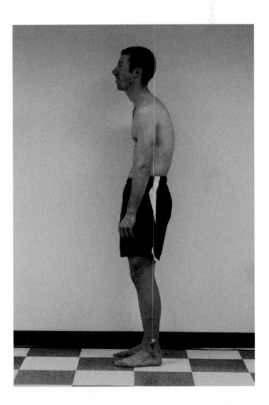

Fig. 4-16: An example of a patient with relatively "good posture" using a plumb line. The image demonstrates several anatomical landmarks in ideal alignment and others that are in close proximity.

Fig. 4-17: An example of a patient with relatively "faulty posture" using a plumb line.

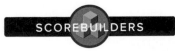

Positioning of a Joint[10]

Loose Packed Position of Joints

Joint	Position
Glenohumeral	55° abduction, 30° horizontal adduction
Ulnohumeral (elbow)	70° flexion, 10° supination
Radiohumeral	Full extension, full supination
Proximal radioulnar	70° flexion, 35° supination
Distal radioulnar	10° supination
Radiocarpal (wrist)	Neutral with slight ulnar deviation
Hip	30° flexion, 30° abduction, slight lateral rotation
Knee	25° flexion
Talocrural (ankle)	10° plantar flexion, midway between maximum inversion and eversion
Subtalar	Midway between extremes of range of movement

Adapted from Magee, DJ: Orthopedic Physical Assessment. W.B. Saunders Company, Philadelphia 2002, p.50, with permission.

Close Packed Position of Joints

Joint	Position
Glenohumeral	Abduction and lateral rotation
Ulnohumeral (elbow)	Extension
Radiohumeral	Elbow flexed 90°, forearm supinated 5°
Proximal radioulnar	5° supination
Distal radioulnar	5° supination
Radiocarpal (wrist)	Extension with radial deviation
Hip	Full extension, medial rotation
Knee	Full extension, lateral rotation of tibia
Talocrural (ankle)	Maximum dorsiflexion
Subtalar	Supination

Adapted from Magee, DJ: Orthopedic Physical Assessment. W.B. Saunders Company, Philadelphia 2002, p.50, with permission.

Descriptions of Specific Positions

	Loose Packed	Close Packed
Stress on joint	Minimal	Maximal
Congruency of joint	Minimal	Full
Ligament position	Great laxity	Full tightness
Joint surface	No volitional separation	Compressed

Common Capsular Patterns of Joints[10]

Joint	Restriction*
Cervical spine	Lateral flexion and rotation equally limited, extension
Glenohumeral	Lateral rotation, abduction, medial rotation
Ulnohumeral	Flexion, extension
Radiohumeral	Flexion, extension, supination, pronation
Proximal radioulnar	Supination, pronation
Distal radioulnar	Full range of movement, pain at extremes of rotation
Radiocarpal (wrist)	Flexion and extension equally limited
Thoracic spine	Lateral flexion and rotation equally limited, extension
Lumbar spine	Lateral flexion and rotation equally limited, extension
Hip	Flexion, abduction, medial rotation (sometimes medial rotation is most limited)
Knee	Flexion, extension
Tibiofibular	Pain when joint stressed
Talocrural	Plantar flexion, dorsiflexion
Subtalar	Limitation of varus range of movement

* Movements are listed in order of restriction.
Adapted from Magee, DJ: Orthopedic Physical Assessment. W.B. Saunders Company, Philadelphia 2002, p.28, with permission

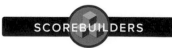

End-Feel[3,20]

Normal End-Feel	Abnormal End-Feel

Normal End-Feel

End-feel is the type of resistance that is felt when passively moving a joint through the end range of motion. Certain tissues and joints have a consistent end-feel and are described as firm, hard or soft. Pathology can be identified through noting the type of abnormal end-feel within a particular joint.

Firm (stretch)

Examples: Ankle dorsiflexion
Finger extension
Hip medial rotation
Forearm supination

Hard (bone to bone)

Example: Elbow extension

Soft (soft tissue approximation)

Examples: Elbow flexion
Knee flexion

Abnormal End-Feel

Abnormal end-feel consists of any end-feel that is felt at an abnormal or inconsistent point in the range of motion or in a joint that normally presents with a different end-feel.

Empty (cannot reach end-feel, usually due to pain)

Examples: Joint inflammation
Fracture
Bursitis

Firm

Examples: Increased tone
Tightening of the capsule
Ligament shortening

Hard

Examples: Fracture
Osteoarthritis
Osteophyte formation

Soft

Examples: Edema
Synovitis
Ligament instability/tear

Muscle Testing

Manual Muscle Testing Grades[2,21]

Zero (0/5)	The subject demonstrates no palpable muscle contraction.		**Fair (3/5)**	The subject completes range of motion against gravity without manual resistance.
Trace (1/5)	The subject's muscle contraction can be palpated, but there is no joint movement.		**Fair Plus (3+/5)**	The subject completes range of motion against gravity with only minimal resistance.
Poor Minus (2-/5)	The subject does not complete range of motion in a gravity-eliminated position.		**Good Minus (4-/5)**	The subject completes range of motion against gravity with minimal-moderate resistance.
Poor (2/5)	The subject completes range of motion in a gravity-eliminated position.		**Good (4/5)**	The subject completes range of motion against gravity with moderate resistance.
Poor Plus (2+/5)	The subject is able to initiate movement against gravity.		**Good Plus (4+/5)**	The subject completes range of motion against gravity with moderate-maximal resistance.
Fair Minus (3-/5)	The subject does not complete the range of motion against gravity, but does complete more than half of the range.		**Normal (5/5)**	The subject completes range of motion against gravity with maximal resistance.

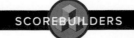

Positioning for Muscle Testing[2,21]

Supine

Abdominals	Anterior deltoid*
Biceps	Brachioradialis
Finger flexors	Finger extensors
Iliopsoas	Infraspinatus
Lateral rotators of shoulder*	Medial rotators of shoulder*
Neck flexors	Pectoralis major
Pectoralis minor	Peroneals
Pronators	Sartorius
Serratus anterior	Supinators
Tensor fasciae latae	Teres minor
Thumb muscles	Tibialis anterior
Tibialis posterior	Toe extensors
Toe flexors	Triceps*
Wrist extensors	Wrist flexors

Sidelying

Gluteus medius (Fig. 4-22)	Gluteus minimus
Hip adductors (Fig. 4-23)	Lateral abdominals

Prone

Back extensors	Gastrocnemius
Gluteus maximus	Hamstrings*
Lateral rotators of the shoulder*	Latissimus dorsi (Fig. 4-20)
Lower trapezius	Medial rotators of the shoulder*
Middle trapezius	Neck extensors
Posterior deltoid*	Quadratus lumborum
Rhomboids	Soleus
Teres major	Triceps*

Sitting

Coracobrachialis	Deltoid* (Figs. 4-18, 4-19)
Hip flexors* (Fig. 4-21)	Lateral rotators of hip (Fig. 4-24)
Medial rotators of hip	Quadriceps (Fig. 4-25)
Upper trapezius	Serratus anterior*

Standing

Ankle plantar flexors	Serratus anterior*

*Indicates multiple acceptable positions for muscle testing

Manual Muscle Testing

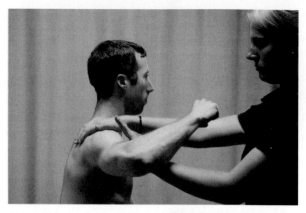

Fig. 4-18: Manual muscle testing of the anterior deltoid.

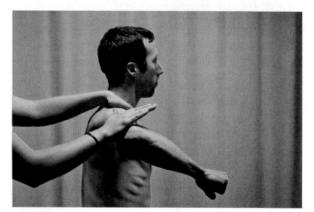

Fig. 4-19: Manual muscle testing of the posterior deltoid.

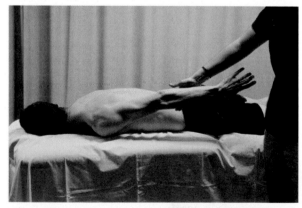

Fig. 4-20: Manual muscle testing of the latissimus dorsi.

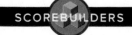

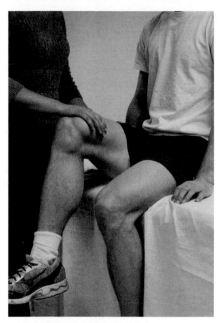

Fig. 4-21: Manual muscle testing of the hip flexors.

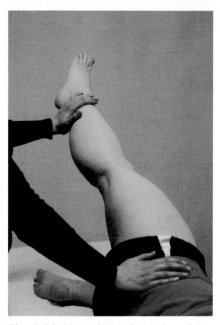

Fig. 4-22: Manual muscle testing of the gluteus medius

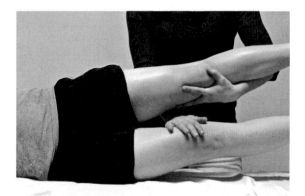

Fig. 4-23: Manual muscle testing of the hip adductors.

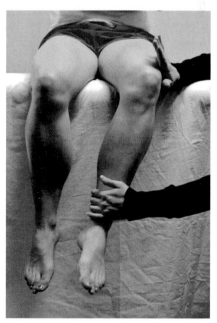

Fig. 4-24: Manual muscle testing of the hip lateral rotators.

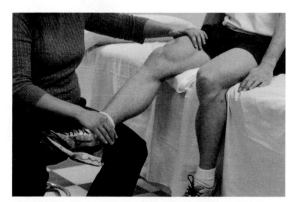

Fig. 4-25: Manual muscle testing of the quadriceps femoris.

Muscle Insufficiency[2,16]

A muscle contraction that is less than optimal due to an extremely lengthened or shortened position of the muscle. There are two types of insufficiency:

Active: when a two-joint muscle is incapable of shortening to the extent required to produce full range of motion at all joints crossed simultaneously

Passive: when a two-joint muscle cannot lengthen to the extent required to allow full range of motion of all joints it crosses simultaneously

Grip[10,18]

Stages of Gripping

1. The hand opens fully, which requires activation of the wrist and finger extensor musculature as well as the hand intrinsics.

2. The fingers position around the object and close to grasp the object, which requires activation of the finger flexor musculature as well as the hand intrinsics.

3. The force of the grasp is modified based on the shape, weight, fragility, and surface characteristics of the object.

4. The object is released by opening the hand, which again requires activation of the extensor musculature.

Types of Grips

A power grip is used when a strong or forceful grip is needed and involves stabilization of the object against the palm of the hand. The fingers are in flexion and the wrist is in ulnar deviation and slight extension. Types of power grips include:

- A cylindrical grasp is characterized by the entire hand wrapping around an object with the thumb on one side and the four fingers on the opposite side of the object. This type of grasp is used for cylindrically shaped objects, such as a soda can.

- A fist grasp is similar to a cylindrical grasp, but involves grasping around a narrower object so that the thumb and fingers overlap. This type of grasp is used for smaller cylindrically shaped objects, such as a hammer.

- A spherical grasp is characterized by the entire hand wrapping around a spherical object. It differs from a cylindrical grasp in that the fingers are separated from one another and there is a greater amount of thumb opposition. This type of grasp is used for spherical objects, such as a baseball.

- A hook grasp is characterized by use of the second and third interphalangeal joints (though it can involve all four fingers) to create a hook to hold an object. A hook grasp is controlled by the forearm flexors and extensors. This type of grasp is used for objects with a handle, such as a pail.

A precision grip (i.e., prehension grip) is used when accurate and precise movements of the hand are needed. This type of grip involves the metacarpophalangeal and interphalangeal joints on the radial side of the hand. Types of precision grips include:

- A digital prehension grip (i.e., three-fingered pinch) is characterized by pulp-to-pulp contact between the thumb,

index finger, and middle finger. This type of grip may be used when holding a pencil.

- A lateral prehension grip is characterized by contact between the thumb and lateral side of the index finger. This type of grip may be used when using a key.

- A tip prehension grip (i.e., tip pinch) is characterized by thumb opposition so that the tip of the thumb contacts the tip of another finger. This type of grip may be used when holding a needle.

Dynamometry[10]

Dynamometry is the process of measuring forces that are doing work. A dynamometer is a device that measures strength through the use of a load cell or spring-loaded gauge. There are various kinds of dynamometers that are used based on treatment objectives. Three types of dynamometry that will be discussed here include the handheld dynamometer that measures grip strength, the handheld dynamometer used to measure strength of the extremities through isometric contraction, and the dynamometer used to measure strength through isokinetic contraction. Handheld dynamometry demonstrates intrarater reliability of > .94. The same dynamometer should be used each session and the same tester should consistently measure the patient.

- **A handheld dynamometer** can be used to assess the grip strength of a patient (Fig. 4-26). Normally, a patient's dominant grip strength is five to ten pounds greater than the non-dominant grip strength. Handheld dynamometry is also used to measure muscle group strength by having the patient exert maximal force against the dynamometer. Portable, non-electric units include a hydraulic or spring-load system and display the force on a gauge. Electrical units use load cells or strain gauges and display force digitally. Grip strength is usually recorded in pounds or kilograms.

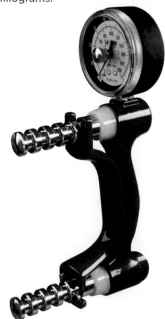

Fig. 4-26: A handheld dynamometer. Courtesy Chattanooga, a DJO Global Company.

- **Isometric dynamometry** measures the static strength of a muscle group without any movement. The extremity is restrained by stabilization straps or stabilized with only verbal instruction (Fig. 4-27).

  Benefits include attaining peak and average force data, reaction time data, rate of motor recruitment, and maximal exertion data. This method is relatively safe, simple to use, easy to interpret data, and cost effective.

  Disadvantages include the inability to convert data to functional activities, as well as the need for caution with patients with acute orthopedic injury, osteoporosis or hernia. This method is contraindicated for patients with fractures and significant hypertension.

- **Isokinetic dynamometry** measures the strength of a muscle group during a movement with constant, predetermined speed. This device will alter the resistance to accommodate for the change in the length-tension ratio and lever arm throughout the entire arc of motion. The muscle group will therefore maximally contract throughout the motion. Common speeds of motion include 60, 120, and 180 degrees per second.

  Benefits include the ability to test the muscle strength at various speeds, the ability to measure the patient's power, and that the patient will never have more resistance than they can handle during the isokinetic testing.

  Disadvantages include the high cost of operation for the device, limitations in patterns of movement, a higher level of understanding required by the patient, and that this method does not truly correlate to function since people do not perform at a constant velocity during daily activities.

Make Test:

A make test is an evaluation procedure where a patient is asked to apply a force against the dynamometer.

Break Test:

A break test is an evaluation procedure where a patient is asked to hold a contraction against pressure that is applied in the opposite direction to the contraction.

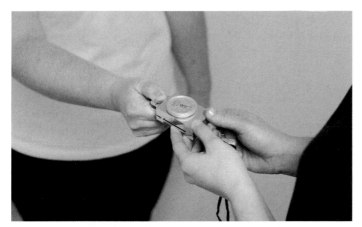

Fig. 4-27: A patient using a pinch grip dynamometer.

Gait

	Standard versus Rancho Los Amigos Terminology[4,22]	
	Standard Terminology	**Rancho Los Amigos Terminology**
Stance Phase (60% of gait cycle)	Heel strike Foot flat Midstance Heel off Toe off	Initial contact Loading response Midstance Terminal stance Pre-swing
Swing Phase (40% of gait cycle)	Acceleration Midswing Deceleration	Initial swing Midswing Terminal swing

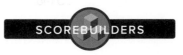

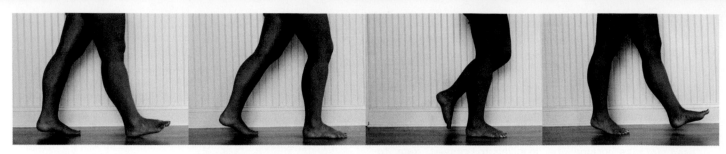

Fig. 4-28: Initial contact   **Fig. 4-29:** Loading response   **Fig. 4-30:** Midstance   **Fig. 4-31:** Terminal stance

Standard Terminology[4,23]

Stance Phase

Heel strike: Heel strike is the instant that the heel touches the ground to begin stance phase.

Foot flat: Foot flat is the point in which the entire foot makes contact with the ground and should occur directly after heel strike.

Midstance: Midstance is the point during the stance phase when the entire body weight is directly over the stance limb.

Heel off: Heel off is the point in which the heel of the stance limb leaves the ground.

Toe off: Toe off is the point in which only the toe of the stance limb remains on the ground.

Swing Phase

Acceleration: Acceleration begins when toe off is complete and the reference limb swings until positioned directly under the body.

Midswing: Midswing is the point when the swing limb is directly under the body.

Deceleration: Deceleration begins directly after midswing, as the swing limb begins to extend, and ends just prior to heel strike.

Rancho Los Amigos Terminology[4,22,23]

Stance Phase

Initial contact: Initial contact is the beginning of the stance phase that occurs when the foot touches the ground (Fig. 4-28).

Loading response: Loading response corresponds to the amount of time between initial contact and the beginning of the swing phase for the other leg (Fig. 4-29).

Midstance: Midstance corresponds to the point in stance phase when the other foot is off the floor until the body is directly over the stance limb (Fig. 4-30).

Terminal stance: Terminal stance begins when the heel of the stance limb rises and ends when the other foot touches the ground (Fig. 4-31).

Pre-swing: Pre-swing begins when the other foot touches the ground and ends when the stance foot reaches toe off (Fig. 4-32).

Swing Phase

Initial swing: Initial swing begins when the stance foot lifts from the floor and ends with maximal knee flexion during swing (Fig. 4-33).

Midswing: Midswing begins with maximal knee flexion during swing and ends when the tibia is perpendicular with the ground (Fig. 4-34).

Terminal swing: Terminal swing begins when the tibia is perpendicular to the floor and ends when the foot touches the ground (Fig. 4-35).

Range of Motion Requirements for Normal Gait[13,23]

Hip flexion:	**0 – 30 degrees**
Hip extension:	**0 – 10 degrees**
Knee flexion:	**0 – 60 degrees**
Knee extension:	**0 degrees**
Ankle dorsiflexion:	**0 – 10 degrees**
Ankle plantar flexion:	**0 – 20 degrees**

Gait and Muscle Activity[10,13,18]

Initial contact: The ankle dorsiflexors place the ankle in dorsiflexion during heel strike and prepare to lower the foot towards the ground. The quadriceps contract to place the knee in extension while the hamstrings help stabilize the knee and prevent hyperextension. The hip extensors and abductors contract to stabilize the trunk and pelvis over the leg.

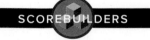

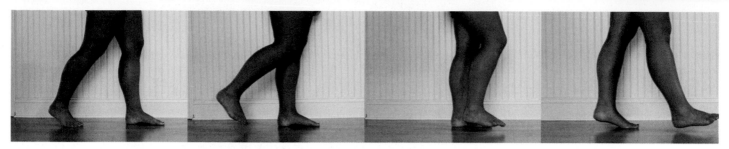

Fig. 4-32: Pre-swing   **Fig. 4-33:** Initial swing   **Fig. 4-34:** Midswing   **Fig. 4-35:** Terminal swing

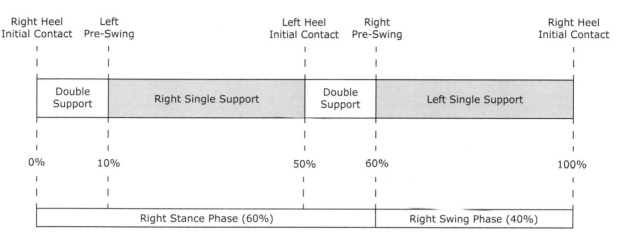

Fig. 4-36: Timing and sequence of the gait cycle.

Loading response: The ankle dorsiflexors act eccentrically to control lowering of the foot towards the ground. The quadriceps contract eccentrically to control knee flexion as the limb accepts the weight of the body. In the latter portion of this phase, the plantar flexors eccentrically control dorsiflexion as the tibia moves over the foot. Simultaneously, the tibialis posterior eccentrically controls pronation of the foot. The quadriceps contraction becomes concentric to draw the femur forward over the tibia. Throughout the loading response phase, the hip extensors contract concentrically to produce hip extension.

Midstance: The plantar flexors continue to act eccentrically to control dorsiflexion as the body moves over the stance limb. Activity in the knee musculature is minimal during this phase, though the quadriceps contract concentrically to continue producing closed chain knee extension. The hip abductor muscles stabilize the pelvis and prevent contralateral hip drop. The iliopsoas also begins to contract eccentrically to control hip extension.

Terminal stance: The plantar flexors begin to work concentrically to aid the foot in its propulsion of the body forward. Knee muscle activity remains limited. The hip abductors continue to stabilize the pelvis and the iliopsoas continues to slow the rate of hip extension.

Pre-swing: The plantar flexors are at their peak activity as the foot "toes off" from the ground. The hamstrings begin to produce knee flexion to prepare for the swing phase, though the momentum of the body also aids in this motion. The iliopsoas begins to work concentrically to produce hip flexion, along with other hip flexors (e.g., rectus femoris, sartorius, adductor longus).

Initial swing: The ankle dorsiflexors contract concentrically to clear the foot from the ground, while the hamstrings assist with foot clearance by flexing the knee. The hip flexors continue to produce hip flexion to advance the limb forward.

Midswing: The ankle dorsiflexors continue to contract concentrically to maintain dorsiflexion. Knee and hip muscle activity are minimal during this phase since forward momentum allows for advancement of the limb.

Terminal swing: The ankle dorsiflexors continue to contract concentrically to maintain dorsiflexion. The ankle invertors also contract concentrically to prepare the foot for initial contact. The quadriceps contract concentrically to place the knee in extension for initial contact, while the hamstrings act eccentrically to control the rate of knee extension. The hip extensors eccentrically slow the rate of hip flexion and prepare the limb for initial contact.

Gait Terminology[4,10]

Base of support: The distance measured between the left and right foot during progression of gait. The distance decreases as cadence increases. The average base of support for an adult is two to four inches.

Cadence: The number of steps an individual will walk over a period of time. The average value for an adult is 110–120 steps per minute.

Degree of toe-out: The angle formed by each foot's line of progression and a line intersecting the center of the heel and second toe. The average degree of toe-out for an adult is seven degrees.

Double support phase: The double support phase refers to the two times during a gait cycle where both feet are on the ground. The time of double support increases as the speed of gait decreases. This phase does not exist with running.

Gait cycle: The gait cycle refers to the sequence of motions that occur from initial contact of the heel to the next consecutive initial contact of the same heel.

Pelvic rotation: Rotation of the pelvis occurs opposite the thorax in order to maintain balance and regulate speed. The average pelvic rotation during gait for an adult is a total of 8 degrees (4 degrees forward with the swing leg and 4 degrees backward with the stance leg).

Single support phase: The single support phase occurs when only one foot is on the ground and occurs twice during a single gait cycle.

Step length: The distance measured between right heel strike and left heel strike. The average step length for an adult is 28 inches (Fig. 4-37).

Stride length: The distance measured between right heel strike and the following right heel strike. The average stride length for an adult is 56 inches (Fig. 4-37).

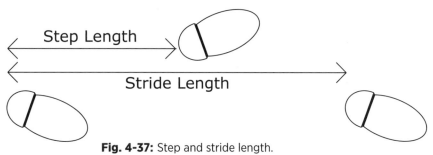

Fig. 4-37: Step and stride length.

Abnormal Gait Patterns[10,23]

Antalgic: A protective gait pattern where the stance time is decreased to avoid weight bearing on the involved side due to pain. This is typically associated with a rapid and shorter swing phase of the uninvolved limb. Causes of antalgic gait include disease (usually bone or joint), joint inflammation, or injuries to muscles, tendons, and/or ligaments.

Ataxic: A gait pattern characterized by staggering and unsteadiness. There is usually a wide base of support and movements are exaggerated.

Cerebellar: A staggering gait pattern seen in cerebellar disease.

Circumduction: A gait pattern characterized by a circular motion to advance the leg during swing phase; this may be used to compensate for insufficient hip or knee flexion or dorsiflexion.

Double step: A gait pattern in which alternate steps are of a different length or at a different rate.

Equine: A gait pattern characterized by high steps; usually involves excessive activity of the gastrocnemius.

Festinating: A gait pattern where a patient walks on toes as though pushed. It starts slowly, increases, and may continue until the patient grasps an object in order to stop.

Hemiplegic: A gait pattern in which patients abduct the paralyzed limb, swing it around, and bring it forward so the foot comes to the ground in front of them.

Parkinsonian: A gait pattern marked by increased forward flexion of the trunk and knees; gait is shuffling with quick and small steps; festinating may occur.

Scissor: A gait pattern in which the legs cross midline upon advancement.

Spastic: A gait pattern with stiff movement, toes seeming to catch and drag, legs held together, and hip and knee joints slightly flexed. Commonly seen in spastic paraplegia.

Steppage: A gait pattern in which the feet and toes are lifted through hip and knee flexion to excessive heights; usually secondary to dorsiflexor weakness. The foot will slap at initial contact with the ground secondary to the decreased control.

Tabetic: A high stepping ataxic gait pattern in which the feet slap the ground.

Trendelenburg: A gait pattern that denotes gluteus medius weakness; excessive lateral trunk flexion and weight shifting over the stance leg.

Vaulting: A gait pattern where the swing leg advances by compensating through the combination of elevation of the pelvis and plantar flexion of the stance leg.

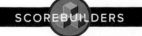

Gait Deviations[10,22,23,25]

Gait Deviations

	Foot slap	Toe down instead of heel strike	Clawing of toes	Heel lift during midstance	No toe off
Ankle and Foot	• Weak dorsiflexors • Dorsiflexor paralysis	• Plantar flexor spasticity • Plantar flexor contracture • Weak dorsiflexors • Dorsiflexor paralysis • Leg length discrepancy • Hindfoot pain	• Toe flexor spasticity • Positive support reflex	• Insufficient dorsiflexion range • Plantar flexor spasticity	• Forefoot/toe pain • Weak plantar flexors • Weak toe flexors • Insufficient plantar flexion range of motion
	Exaggerated knee flexion at contact	**Hyperextension in stance**	**Exaggerated knee flexion at terminal stance**	**Insufficient flexion with swing**	**Excessive flexion with swing**
Knee	• Weak quadriceps • Quadriceps paralysis • Hamstrings spasticity • Insufficient extension range of motion	• Compensation for weak quadriceps • Plantar flexor contracture	• Knee flexion contracture • Hip flexion contracture	• Knee effusion • Quadriceps extension spasticity • Plantar flexor spasticity • Insufficient flexion range of motion	• Flexor withdrawal reflex • Lower extremity flexor synergy
	Insufficient hip flexion at initial contact	**Insufficient hip extension at stance**	**Circumduction during swing**	**Hip hiking during swing**	**Exaggerated hip flexion during swing**
Hip	• Weak hip flexors • Hip flexor paralysis • Hip extensor spasticity • Insufficient hip flexion range of motion	• Insufficient hip extension range of motion • Hip flexion contracture • Lower extremity flexor synergy	• Compensation for weak hip flexors • Compensation for weak dorsiflexors • Compensation for weak hamstrings	• Compensation for weak dorsiflexors • Compensation for weak knee flexors • Compensation for extensor synergy pattern	• Lower extremity flexor synergy • Compensation for insufficient ankle dorsiflexion

Range of Motion

Average Adult Range of Motion - Upper and Lower Extremities; Spine[3]

Upper Extremity	
Shoulder	
Flexion	0-180
Extension	0-60
Abduction	0-180
Medial rotation	0-70
Lateral rotation	0-90
Elbow	
Extension	0
Flexion	0-150
Forearm	
Pronation	0-80
Supination	0-80
Wrist	
Flexion	0-80
Extension	0-70
Radial deviation	0-20
Ulnar deviation	0-30
Thumb	
Carpometacarpal	
Abduction	0-70
Flexion	0-15
Extension	0-20
Opposition	Tip of thumb to base of fifth digit
Metacarpophalangeal	
Flexion	0-50
Interphalangeal	
Flexion	0-80
Digits – Second to Fifth	
Metacarpophalangeal	
Flexion	0-90
Hyperextension	0-45
Proximal interphalangeal	
Flexion	0-100
Distal interphalangeal	
Flexion	0-90
Hyperextension	0-10

Lower Extremity	
Hip	
Flexion	0-120
Extension	0-30
Abduction	0-45
Adduction	0-30
Medial rotation	0-45
Lateral rotation	0-45
Knee	
Flexion	0-135
Ankle (talocrural)	
Dorsiflexion	0-20
Plantar flexion	0-50
Midtarsal (transverse tarsal)	
Inversion	0-35
Eversion	0-15
Subtalar	
Inversion	0-5
Eversion	0-5

Spine	
Cervical Spine	
Flexion	0-45
Extension	0-45
Lateral flexion	0-45
Rotation	0-60
Thoracic and Lumbar Spine	
Flexion	0-80
Extension	0-25
Lateral flexion	0-35
Rotation	0-45

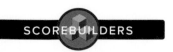

CONSIDER THIS
PROCESS FOR CONDUCTING GONIOMETRIC MEASUREMENT[3]

Goniometric measurement can be reliable (i.e., possessing repeatability of measures) and valid (i.e., meaningful interpretation can be inferred through the measure) when performed by a trained individual following the recommended procedure. The following 12-step process outlines the recommended procedure for conducting goniometric measurement.

1. Place the subject in the recommended testing position.
2. Stabilize the proximal joint segment.
3. Move the distal joint segment through the available range of motion. Make sure that the passive range of motion is performed slowly, the end of the range is attained, and the end-feel is determined.
4. Make a clinical estimate of the range of motion.
5. Return the distal joint segment to the starting position.
6. Palpate bony anatomical landmarks.
7. Align the goniometer.
8. Read and record the starting position. Remove the goniometer.
9. Stabilize the proximal joint segment.
10. Move the distal segment through the full range of motion.
11. Replace and realign the goniometer. Palpate the anatomical landmarks again if necessary.
12. Read and record the range of motion.

Adapted from Norkin and White: Measurement of Joint Motion: A Guide to Goniometry. F.A. Davis Company, Philadelphia, 2003, p.35, with permission.

Goniometric Technique[3,20]

Upper Extremity

Shoulder

Flexion

Patient position: supine

Stabilization: thorax to prevent extension of the spine

End-feel: firm

Axis: acromial process

Stationary arm: midaxillary line of the thorax

Moveable arm: lateral midline of the humerus using the lateral epicondyle of the humerus for reference

Extension

Patient position: prone

Stabilization: thorax to prevent flexion of the spine

End-feel: firm

Axis: acromial process

Stationary arm: midaxillary line of the thorax

Moveable arm: lateral midline of the humerus using the lateral epicondyle of the humerus for reference

Abduction

Patient position: supine

Stabilization: thorax to prevent lateral flexion of the spine

End-feel: firm

Axis: anterior aspect of the acromial process

Stationary arm: parallel to the midline of the anterior aspect of the sternum

Moveable arm: medial midline of the humerus

Adduction

Patient position: supine

Stabilization: thorax to prevent lateral flexion of the spine

End-feel: firm

Axis: anterior aspect of the acromial process

Stationary arm: parallel to the midline of the anterior aspect of the sternum

Moveable arm: medial midline of the humerus

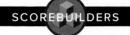

Medial rotation

Patient position: supine with shoulder abducted to 90 degrees and elbow flexed to 90 degrees

Stabilization: distal end of the humerus to maintain the shoulder in 90 degrees of abduction

End-feel: firm

Axis: olecranon process

Stationary arm: parallel or perpendicular to the floor

Moveable arm: ulna using the olecranon process and ulnar styloid process for reference

Lateral rotation

Patient position: supine with shoulder abducted to 90 degrees and elbow flexed to 90 degrees

Stabilization: distal end of the humerus to maintain the shoulder in 90 degrees of abduction

End-feel: firm

Axis: olecranon process

Stationary arm: parallel or perpendicular to the floor

Moveable arm: ulna using the olecranon process and ulnar styloid process for reference

*The supplied stabilization descriptions are for shoulder complex motion. The required stabilization may vary for glenohumeral motions.

Elbow

Flexion (Fig. 4-38)

Patient position: supine

Stabilization: humerus to prevent flexion of the shoulder

End-feel: soft

Axis: lateral epicondyle of the humerus

Stationary arm: lateral midline of the humerus using the center of the acromial process for reference

Moveable arm: lateral midline of the radius using the radial head and radial styloid process for reference

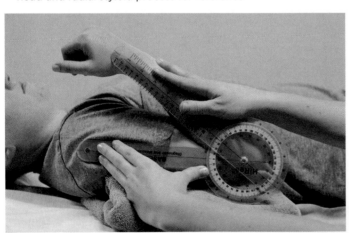

Fig. 4-38: A therapist measuring elbow flexion with a goniometer.

Extension

Patient position: supine

Stabilization: humerus to prevent flexion of the shoulder

End-feel: hard

Axis: lateral epicondyle of the humerus

Stationary arm: lateral midline of the humerus using the center of the acromial process for reference

Moveable arm: lateral midline of the radius using the radial head and radial styloid process for reference

Forearm

Pronation

Patient position: sitting with the elbow flexed to 90 degrees

Stabilization: distal end of the humerus to prevent medial rotation and abduction of the humerus

End-feel: firm or hard

Axis: lateral to the ulnar styloid process

Stationary arm: parallel to the anterior midline of the humerus

Moveable arm: dorsal aspect of the forearm, just proximal to the styloid process of the radius and ulna

Supination

Patient position: sitting with the elbow flexed to 90 degrees

Stabilization: distal end of the humerus to prevent lateral rotation and adduction of the humerus

End-feel: firm

Axis: medial to the ulnar styloid process

Stationary arm: parallel to the anterior midline of the humerus

Moveable arm: ventral aspect of the forearm, just proximal to the styloid process of the radius and ulna

Wrist

Flexion

Patient position: sitting next to a supporting surface with the shoulder abducted to 90 degrees and the elbow flexed to 90 degrees

Stabilization: radius and ulna to prevent supination or pronation

End-feel: firm

Axis: lateral aspect of the wrist over the triquetrum

Stationary arm: lateral midline of the ulna using the olecranon and ulnar styloid process for reference

Moveable arm: lateral midline of the fifth metacarpal

Extension

Patient position: sitting next to a supporting surface with the shoulder abducted to 90 degrees and the elbow flexed to 90 degrees

Stabilization: radius and ulna to prevent supination or pronation

End-feel: firm

Axis: lateral aspect of the wrist over the triquetrum

Stationary arm: lateral midline of the ulna using the olecranon and ulnar styloid process for reference

Moveable arm: lateral midline of the fifth metacarpal

Radial deviation

Patient position: sitting next to a supporting surface with the shoulder abducted to 90 degrees and the elbow flexed to 90 degrees

Stabilization: radius and ulna to prevent supination or pronation

End-feel: firm or hard

Axis: over the middle of the dorsal aspect of the wrist over the capitate

Stationary arm: dorsal midline of the forearm using the lateral epicondyle of the humerus for reference

Moveable arm: dorsal midline of the third metacarpal

Ulnar deviation

Patient position: sitting next to a supporting surface with the shoulder abducted to 90 degrees and the elbow flexed to 90 degrees

Stabilization: radius and ulna to prevent supination or pronation

End-feel: firm

Axis: over the middle of the dorsal aspect of the wrist over the capitate

Stationary arm: dorsal midline of the forearm using the lateral epicondyle of the humerus for reference

Moveable arm: dorsal midline of the third metacarpal

Thumb

Carpometacarpal flexion

Patient position: sitting with the forearm and hand on a supporting surface

Stabilization: carpals, radius, and ulna to prevent wrist motion

End-feel: firm

Axis: over the palmar aspect of the first carpometacarpal joint

Stationary arm: ventral midline of the radius using the ventral surface of the radial head and radial styloid process for reference

Moveable arm: ventral midline of the first metacarpal

Carpometacarpal extension

Patient position: sitting with the forearm and hand on a supporting surface

Stabilization: carpals, radius, and ulna to prevent wrist motion

End-feel: firm

Axis: over the palmar aspect of the first carpometacarpal joint

Stationary arm: ventral midline of the radius using the ventral surface of the radial head and radial styloid process for reference

Moveable arm: ventral midline of the first metacarpal

Carpometacarpal abduction

Patient position: sitting with the forearm and hand on a supporting surface

Stabilization: carpals and second metacarpal to prevent wrist motion

End-feel: firm

Axis: over the lateral aspect of the radial styloid process

Stationary arm: lateral midline of the second metacarpal using the center of the second metacarpophalangeal joint for reference

Moveable arm: lateral midline of the first metacarpal using the center of the first metacarpophalangeal joint for reference

Carpometacarpal adduction

Patient position: sitting with the forearm and hand on a supporting surface

Stabilization: carpals and second metacarpal to prevent wrist motion

End-feel: firm

Axis: over the lateral aspect of the radial styloid process

Stationary arm: lateral midline of the second metacarpal using the center of the second metacarpophalangeal joint for reference

Moveable arm: lateral midline of the first metacarpal using the center of the first metacarpophalangeal joint for reference

Fingers

Metacarpophalangeal flexion

Patient position: sitting with the forearm and hand on a supporting surface

Stabilization: metacarpal to prevent wrist motion

End-feel: firm or hard

Axis: over the dorsal aspect of the metacarpophalangeal joint

Stationary arm: over the dorsal midline of the metacarpal

Moveable arm: over the dorsal midline of the proximal phalanx

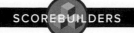

Metacarpophalangeal extension

Patient position: sitting with the forearm and hand on a supporting surface

Stabilization: metacarpal to prevent wrist motion

End-feel: firm

Axis: over the dorsal aspect of the metacarpophalangeal joint

Stationary arm: over the dorsal midline of the metacarpal

Moveable arm: over the dorsal midline of the proximal phalanx

Metacarpophalangeal abduction

Patient position: sitting with the forearm and hand on a supporting surface

Stabilization: metacarpal to prevent wrist motion

End-feel: firm

Axis: over the dorsal aspect of the metacarpophalangeal joint

Stationary arm: over the dorsal midline of the metacarpal

Moveable arm: dorsal midline of the proximal phalanx

Metacarpophalangeal adduction

Patient position: sitting with the forearm and hand on a supporting surface

Stabilization: metacarpal to prevent wrist motion

End-feel: firm

Axis: over the dorsal aspect of the metacarpophalangeal joint

Stationary arm: over the dorsal midline of the metacarpal

Moveable arm: dorsal midline of the proximal phalanx

Proximal interphalangeal flexion

Patient position: sitting with the forearm and hand on a supporting surface

Stabilization: proximal phalanx to prevent motion at the metacarpophalangeal joint

End-feel: soft, firm or hard

Axis: over the dorsal aspect of the proximal interphalangeal joint

Stationary arm: over the dorsal midline of the proximal phalanx

Moveable arm: over the dorsal midline of the middle phalanx

Proximal interphalangeal extension

Patient position: sitting with the forearm and hand on a supporting surface

Stabilization: proximal phalanx to prevent motion at the metacarpophalangeal joint

End-feel: firm

Axis: over the dorsal aspect of the proximal interphalangeal joint

Stationary arm: over the dorsal midline of the proximal phalanx

Moveable arm: over the dorsal midline of the middle phalanx

Distal interphalangeal flexion

Patient position: sitting with the forearm and hand on a supporting surface

Stabilization: middle and proximal phalanx to prevent motion at the proximal interphalangeal joint

End-feel: firm

Axis: over the dorsal aspect of the distal interphalangeal joint

Stationary arm: over the dorsal midline of the middle phalanx

Moveable arm: over the dorsal midline of the distal phalanx

Distal interphalangeal extension

Patient position: sitting with the forearm and hand on a supporting surface

Stabilization: middle and proximal phalanx to prevent motion at the proximal interphalangeal joint

End-feel: firm

Axis: over the dorsal aspect of the distal interphalangeal joint

Stationary arm: over the dorsal midline of the middle phalanx

Moveable arm: over the dorsal midline of the distal phalanx

Lower Extremity

Hip

Flexion (Fig. 4-39)

Patient position: supine

Stabilization: pelvis to prevent posterior tilting

End-feel: soft or firm

Axis: over the lateral aspect of the hip joint using the greater trochanter of the femur for reference

Stationary arm: lateral midline of the pelvis

Moveable arm: lateral midline of the femur using the lateral epicondyle for reference

Extension

Patient position: prone

Stabilization: pelvis to prevent anterior tilting

End-feel: firm

Axis: over the lateral aspect of the hip joint using the greater trochanter of the femur for reference

Stationary arm: lateral midline of the pelvis

Moveable arm: lateral midline of the femur using the lateral epicondyle for reference

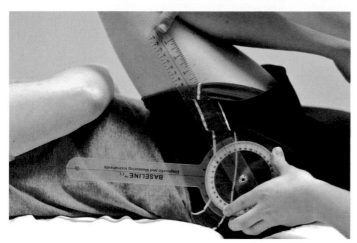

Fig. 4-39: A therapist measuring hip flexion with a goniometer.

Abduction

Patient position: supine

Stabilization: pelvis to prevent lateral tilting and rotation; trunk to prevent lateral flexion

End-feel: firm

Axis: over the anterior superior iliac spine (ASIS) of the extremity being measured

Stationary arm: align with imaginary horizontal line extending from one ASIS to the other ASIS

Moveable arm: anterior midline of the femur using the midline of the patella for reference

Adduction

Patient position: supine

Stabilization: pelvis to prevent lateral tilting

End-feel: firm

Axis: over the anterior superior iliac spine (ASIS) of the extremity being measured

Stationary arm: align with imaginary horizontal line extending from one ASIS to the other ASIS

Moveable arm: anterior midline of the femur using the midline of the patella for reference

Medial rotation

Patient position: sitting

Stabilization: distal end of the femur

End-feel: firm

Axis: anterior aspect of the patella

Stationary arm: perpendicular to the floor or parallel to the supporting surface

Moveable arm: anterior midline of the lower leg using the crest of the tibia and a point midway between the two malleoli for reference

Lateral rotation

Patient position: sitting

Stabilization: distal end of the femur

End-feel: firm

Axis: anterior aspect of the patella

Stationary arm: perpendicular to the floor or parallel to the supporting surface

Moveable arm: anterior midline of the lower leg using the crest of the tibia and a point midway between the two malleoli for reference

Knee

Flexion

Patient position: supine

Stabilization: femur to prevent rotation, abduction, and adduction of the hip

End-feel: soft or firm

Axis: lateral epicondyle of the femur

Stationary arm: lateral midline of the femur using the greater trochanter for reference

Moveable arm: lateral midline of the fibula using the lateral malleolus and fibular head for reference

Extension

Patient position: supine

Stabilization: femur to prevent rotation, abduction, and adduction of the hip

End-feel: firm

Axis: lateral epicondyle of the femur

Stationary arm: lateral midline of the femur using the greater trochanter for reference

Moveable arm: lateral midline of the fibula using the lateral malleolus and fibular head for reference

Ankle (talocrural)

Dorsiflexion

Patient position: sitting with the knee flexed to 90 degrees

Stabilization: tibia and fibula to prevent knee and hip motion

End-feel: firm

Axis: lateral aspect of the lateral malleolus

Stationary arm: lateral midline of the fibula using the head of the fibula for reference

Moveable arm: parallel to the lateral aspect of the fifth metatarsal

Plantar flexion

Patient position: sitting with the knee flexed to 90 degrees

Stabilization: tibia and fibula to prevent knee and hip motion

End-feel: firm or hard

Axis: lateral aspect of the lateral malleolus

Stationary arm: lateral midline of the fibula using the head of the fibula for reference

Moveable arm: parallel to the lateral aspect of the fifth metatarsal

Midtarsal (transverse tarsal)

Inversion (Fig. 4-40)

Patient position: sitting with the knee flexed to 90 degrees

Stabilization: tibia and fibula to prevent knee and hip motion

End-feel: firm

Axis: anterior aspect of the ankle midway between the malleoli

Stationary arm: anterior midline of the lower leg using the tibial tuberosity for reference

Moveable arm: anterior midline of the second metatarsal

Eversion

Patient position: sitting with the knee flexed to 90 degrees

Stabilization: tibia and fibula to prevent knee and hip motion

End-feel: firm or hard

Axis: anterior aspect of the ankle midway between the malleoli

Stationary arm: anterior midline of the lower leg using the tibial tuberosity for reference

Moveable arm: anterior midline of the second metatarsal

Subtalar

Inversion

Patient position: prone with the foot extended over a supporting surface

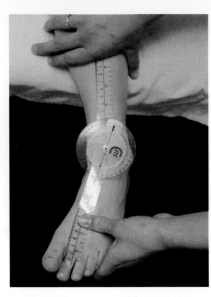

Fig. 4-40: A therapist measuring ankle complex inversion.

Stabilization: tibia and fibula to prevent knee and hip motion

End-feel: firm

Axis: posterior aspect of the ankle midway between the malleoli

Stationary arm: posterior midline of the lower leg

Moveable arm: posterior midline of the calcaneus

Eversion

Patient position: prone with the foot extended over a supporting surface

Stabilization: tibia and fibula to prevent knee and hip motion

End-feel: firm or hard

Axis: posterior aspect of the ankle midway between the malleoli

Stationary arm: posterior midline of the lower leg

Moveable arm: posterior midline of the calcaneus

Spine

Cervical Spine

Flexion

Patient position: sitting with the thoracic and lumbar spine supported

Stabilization: shoulder girdle and chest; the patient's hands should be placed on their knees

End-feel: firm

Axis: over the external auditory meatus

Stationary arm: perpendicular or parallel to the ground

Moveable arm: along the base of the nares or if using a tongue depressor, align the goniometer parallel with the tongue depressor

Extension

Patient position: sitting with the thoracic and lumbar spine supported

Stabilization: shoulder girdle and chest to prevent extension of the thoracic and lumbar spine

End-feel: firm

Axis: over the external auditory meatus

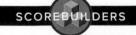

Stationary arm: perpendicular or parallel to the ground

Moveable arm: along the base of the nares, or if using a tongue depressor, align the goniometer parallel with the tongue depressor

Lateral flexion (Fig. 4-41)

Patient position: sitting

Stabilization: shoulder girdle and chest to prevent lateral flexion of the thoracic and lumbar spines

End-feel: firm

Axis: over the spinous process of the C7 vertebra

Stationary arm: with the spinous processes of the thoracic vertebrae so that the arm is perpendicular to the ground

Moveable arm: along the dorsal midline of the head using the occipital protuberance for reference

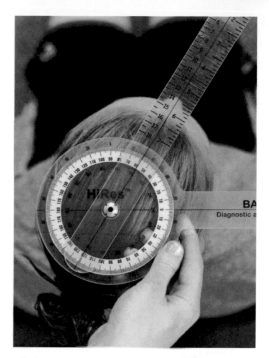

Fig. 4-42: A therapist measuring cervical rotation with a goniometer.

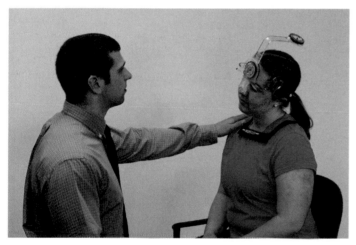

Fig. 4-41: A therapist preparing to measure cervical lateral flexion with a cervical range of motion (CROM) device.

Rotation (Fig. 4-42)

Patient position: sitting with the thoracic and lumbar spine supported

Stabilization: shoulder girdle and chest to prevent rotation of the thoracic and lumbar spines

End-feel: firm

Axis: over the center of the cranial aspect of the head

Stationary arm: parallel to an imaginary line between the two acromial processes

Moveable arm: with the tip of the nose or if using a tongue depressor, align the goniometer parallel with the tongue depressor

Thoracolumbar Spine

Flexion and extension (Fig. 4-43)

Flexion of the thoracic and lumbar spines is most commonly measured with a tape measure instead of a goniometer. The therapist aligns a tape measure between the spinous processes of T1 and S2. The distance is recorded. The patient is then asked

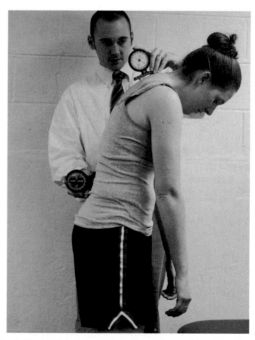

Fig. 4-43: A therapist measuring thoracic and lumbar flexion with a double inclinometer.

to bend forward gradually while the therapist allows the tape measure to unwind. The second distance is recorded. The amount of thoracic and lumbar flexion is determined by calculating the difference between the first and the second measurements. Extension of the thoracic and lumbar spine is measured in a similar manner.

Lateral flexion (Fig. 4-44)

Patient position: standing with the feet shoulder width apart

Stabilization: pelvis to prevent lateral tilting

End-feel: firm

Axis: over the posterior aspect of the spinous process of S2

Stationary arm: perpendicular to the ground

Moveable arm: along the posterior aspect of the spinous process of T1

Rotation

Patient position: sitting on a chair without a back with the feet positioned on the floor for pelvic stabilization

Stabilization: pelvis to prevent rotation

End-feel: firm

Axis: over the center of the cranial aspect of the head

Stationary arm: parallel to an imaginary line between the two prominent tubercles on the iliac crests

Moveable arm: along an imaginary line between the two acromial processes

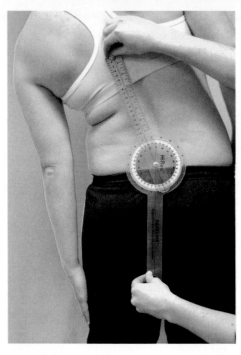

Fig. 4-44: A therapist measuring thoracic and lumbar lateral flexion with a goniometer.

CONSIDER THIS
DOCUMENTATION OF RECORDED MEASURES[3]

Health care providers work in an integrated fashion to deliver patient care. The patient medical record is one of the primary ways that health care providers keep each other informed of current patient status and other relevant information. As a result, it is critical that health care providers document relevant information in the medical record in a timely and accurate manner. Failure to meet this standard potentially results in ineffective medical care and may jeopardize patient safety.

The results of goniometric measurements can be used to illustrate this point. Let's assume that a therapist reviews the medical record of a patient recovering from a motor vehicle accident, in which the patient sustained multiple lower extremity injuries. Upon reviewing the medical record, the therapist determines that in successive notes the patient's right knee range of motion was described as 10-105 degrees and 10-0-105 degrees.

Although the recorded measurements appear extremely similar, they are in fact very different. 10-105 degrees indicates that the patient's range of motion begins at 10 degrees of knee flexion and ends at 105 degrees of knee flexion (95 degrees of total available movement). Conversely, the use of "0" between the starting and ending values indicates the patient has 10 degrees of knee hyperextension and 105 degrees of knee flexion (115 degrees of total available movement).

This type of inaccuracy could cause a variety of potential problems including selecting inappropriate parameters for a device such as a continuous passive motion machine, selecting an inappropriate therapeutic exercise activity based on the patient's available range of motion, and potential reimbursement-related questions concerning the extreme variability in recorded measures.

Special Tests

Special Tests Outline

Upper Extremity

Shoulder

Dislocation

Apprehension test for anterior shoulder dislocation

Apprehension test for posterior shoulder dislocation

Biceps Tendon Pathology

Speed's test

Yergason's test

Rotator Cuff Pathology/Impingement

Drop arm test

Hawkins-Kennedy impingement test

Infraspinatus test

Neer impingement test

Supraspinatus test

Thoracic Outlet Syndrome

Adson maneuver

Allen test

Roos test

Elbow

Ligamentous Instability

Valgus stress test

Varus stress test

Epicondylitis

Cozen's test

Lateral epicondylitis test

Medial epicondylitis test

Neurological Dysfunction

Tinel's sign

Wrist/Hand

Ligamentous Instability

Ulnar collateral ligament instability test

Vascular Insufficiency

Allen test

Capillary refill test **(See Cardiovascular and Pulmonary Systems Unit)**

Neurological Dysfunction

Froment's sign

Phalen's test

Tinel's sign

Miscellaneous

Finkelstein test

Lower Extremity

Hip

Contracture/Tightness

Ely's test

Ober's test

Piriformis test

Thomas test

Tripod sign

90-90 straight leg raise test

Miscellaneous

Craig's test

Patrick's test (FABER test)

Trendelenburg test

Knee

Ligamentous Instability

Anterior drawer test

Lachman test

Lateral pivot shift test

Posterior drawer test

Posterior sag sign

Valgus stress test

Varus stress test

Meniscal Pathology

Apley's compression test

McMurray test

Swelling

Brush test

Patellar tap test

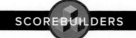

Ankle

Ligamentous Instability

Anterior drawer test

Talar tilt test

Miscellaneous

Homans' sign **(See Cardiovascular and Pulmonary Systems Unit)**

Thompson test

True leg length discrepancy test

Descriptions of Special Tests

Shoulder

Dislocation

Apprehension test for anterior shoulder dislocation[10,26]

The patient is positioned in supine with the arm in 90 degrees of abduction and 90 degrees of elbow flexion. The therapist laterally rotates the patient's shoulder. A positive test is indicated by a look of apprehension or a facial grimace prior to reaching an end point (Fig. 4-45).

Apprehension test for posterior shoulder dislocation[8,10]

The patient is positioned in supine with the arm in 90 degrees of flexion and medial rotation. The therapist applies a posterior force through the long axis of the humerus. A positive test is indicated by a look of apprehension or a facial grimace prior to reaching an end point.

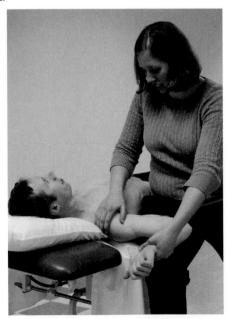

Fig. 4-45: A therapist observing a patient while administering an apprehension test for anterior shoulder dislocation.

Biceps Tendon Pathology

Speed's test[10,26]

The patient is positioned in sitting or standing with the elbow extended and the forearm supinated. The therapist places one hand over the bicipital groove and the other hand on the volar surface of the forearm. The therapist resists active shoulder flexion. A positive test is indicated by pain or tenderness in the bicipital groove region and may be indicative of bicipital tendonitis (Fig. 4-46).

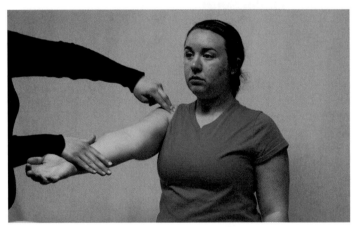

Fig. 4-46: A therapist administering Speed's test. The therapist resists shoulder flexion while palpating the bicipital groove.

Yergason's test[10,13]

The patient is positioned in sitting with 90 degrees of elbow flexion and the forearm pronated. The humerus is stabilized against the patient's thorax. The therapist places one hand on the patient's forearm and the other hand over the bicipital groove. The patient is directed to actively supinate and laterally rotate against resistance. A positive test is indicated by pain or tenderness in the bicipital groove and may be indicative of bicipital tendonitis.

Rotator Cuff Pathology/Impingement

Drop arm test[10,26]

The patient is positioned in sitting or standing with the arm in 90 degrees of abduction. The patient is asked to slowly lower the arm to their side. A positive test is indicated by the patient failing to slowly lower the arm to their side or by the presence of severe pain and may be indicative of a tear in the rotator cuff.

Hawkins-Kennedy impingement test[10]

The patient is positioned in sitting or standing. The therapist flexes the patient's shoulder to 90 degrees and then medially rotates the arm. A positive test is indicated by pain and may be indicative of shoulder impingement involving the supraspinatus tendon (Fig. 4-47).

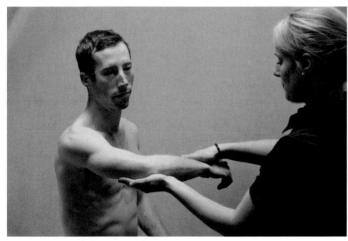

Fig. 4-47: A positive Hawkins-Kennedy impingement test is indicated by the presence of pain.

Infraspinatus test[10,18]

The patient stands with their elbow flexed to 90 degrees and the shoulder in 45 degrees of medial rotation. The patient then resists as the therapist applies a medially directed force to the forearm. Pain or weakness indicates the presence of an infraspinatus strain/tear.

Neer impingement test[10,26]

The patient is positioned in sitting or standing. The therapist positions one hand on the posterior aspect of the patient's scapula and the other hand stabilizing the elbow. The therapist elevates the patient's arm through flexion. A positive test is indicated by a facial grimace or pain and may be indicative of shoulder impingement involving the supraspinatus tendon.

Supraspinatus test[10,13]

The patient is positioned with the arm in 90 degrees of abduction followed by 30 degrees of horizontal adduction with the thumb pointing downward. The therapist resists the patient's attempt to abduct the arm. A positive test is indicated by weakness or pain and may be indicative of a tear of the supraspinatus tendon, impingement or suprascapular nerve involvement.

Thoracic Outlet Syndrome

Adson maneuver[10,26]

The patient is positioned in sitting or standing. The therapist monitors the radial pulse and asks the patient to rotate their head to face the test shoulder. The patient is then asked to extend their head while the therapist laterally rotates and extends the patient's shoulder. A positive test is indicated by an absent or diminished radial pulse and may be indicative of thoracic outlet syndrome.

Allen test[10,26]

The patient is positioned in sitting or standing with the test arm in 90 degrees of abduction, lateral rotation, and elbow flexion. The patient is asked to rotate the head away from the test shoulder while the therapist monitors the radial pulse. A positive test is indicated by an absent or diminished pulse when the head is rotated away from the test shoulder. A positive test may be indicative of thoracic outlet syndrome.

Roos test[10,18]

The patient is positioned in sitting or standing with the arms positioned in 90 degrees of abduction, lateral rotation, and elbow flexion. The patient is asked to open and close their hands for three minutes. A positive test is indicated by the inability to maintain the test position, weakness of the arms, sensory loss or ischemic pain. A positive test may be indicative of thoracic outlet syndrome.

Elbow

Ligamentous Instability

Valgus stress test[8,10]

The patient is positioned in sitting with the elbow in 20 to 30 degrees of flexion. The therapist places one hand on the elbow and the other hand proximal to the patient's wrist. The therapist applies a valgus force to test the medial collateral ligament while palpating the medial joint line. A positive test is indicated by increased laxity in the medial collateral ligament when compared to the contralateral limb, apprehension or pain. A positive test may be indicative of a medial collateral ligament sprain.

Varus stress test[8,10]

The patient is positioned in sitting with the elbow in 20 to 30 degrees of flexion. The therapist places one hand on the elbow and the other hand proximal to the patient's wrist. The therapist applies a varus force to test the lateral collateral ligament while palpating the lateral joint line. A positive test is indicated by increased laxity in the lateral collateral ligament when compared to the contralateral limb, apprehension or pain. A positive test may be indicative of a lateral collateral ligament sprain.

Epicondylitis

Cozen's test[10,18]

The patient is positioned in sitting with the elbow in slight flexion. The therapist places their thumb on the patient's lateral epicondyle while stabilizing the elbow joint. The patient is asked to make a fist, pronate the forearm, radially deviate, and extend the wrist against resistance. A positive test is indicated by pain in the lateral epicondyle region or muscle weakness and may be indicative of lateral epicondylitis.

Lateral epicondylitis test[8,10]

The patient is positioned in sitting. The therapist stabilizes the elbow with one hand and places the other hand on the dorsal aspect of the patient's hand distal to the proximal interphalangeal joint. The patient is asked to extend the third digit against resistance. A positive test is indicated by pain in the lateral epicondyle region or muscle weakness and may be indicative of lateral epicondylitis.

Medial epicondylitis test[8,10]

The patient is positioned in sitting. The therapist palpates the medial epicondyle and supinates the patient's forearm, extends the wrist, and extends the elbow. A positive test is indicated by pain in the medial epicondyle region and may be indicative of medial epicondylitis.

Neurological Dysfunction

Tinel's sign[10,13]

The patient is positioned in sitting with the elbow in slight flexion. The therapist taps with the index finger between the olecranon process and the medial epicondyle. A positive test is indicated by a tingling sensation in the ulnar nerve distribution of the forearm, hand, and fingers. A positive test may be indicative of ulnar nerve compression or compromise.

Wrist/Hand

Ligamentous Instability

Ulnar collateral ligament instability test[10]

The patient is positioned in sitting. The therapist holds the patient's thumb in extension and applies a valgus force to the metacarpophalangeal joint of the thumb. A positive test is indicated by excessive valgus movement and may be indicative of a tear of the ulnar collateral and accessory collateral ligaments. This type of injury is referred to as gamekeeper's or skier's thumb.

Vascular Insufficiency

Allen test[8,10]

The patient is positioned in sitting or standing. The patient is asked to open and close the hand several times in succession and then maintain the hand in a closed position. The therapist compresses the radial and ulnar arteries. The patient is then asked to relax the hand and the therapist releases the pressure on one of the arteries while observing the color of the hand and fingers. A positive test is indicated by delayed or absent flushing of the radial or ulnar half of the hand and may be indicative of an occlusion in the radial or ulnar artery (Figs. 4-48, 4-49).

Neurological Dysfunction

Froment's sign[10,26]

The patient is positioned in sitting or standing and is asked to hold a piece of paper between the thumb and index finger. The therapist attempts to pull the paper away from the patient. A positive test is indicated by the patient flexing the distal phalanx of the thumb due to adductor pollicis muscle paralysis. If at the same time, the patient hyperextends the metacarpophalangeal joint of the thumb, it is termed Jeanne's sign. Both objective findings may be indicative of ulnar nerve compromise or paralysis (Fig. 4-50).

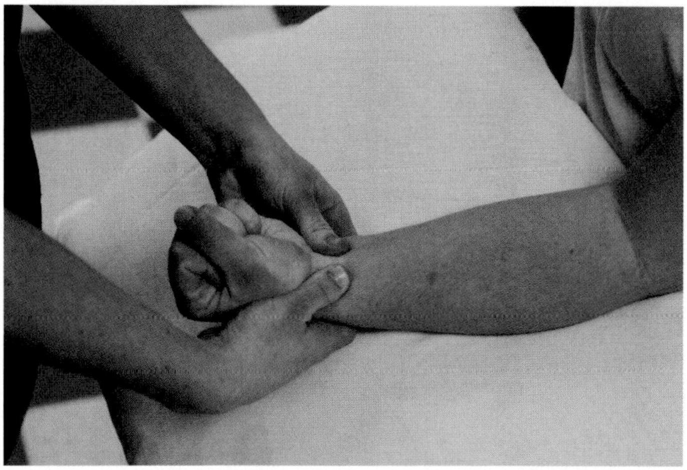

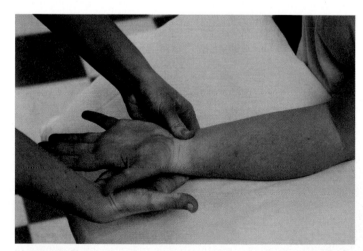

Fig. 4-48: A therapist compresses the radial and ulnar arteries while administering the Allen test.

Fig. 4-49: The therapist releases the radial artery and observes the color of the hand and fingers.

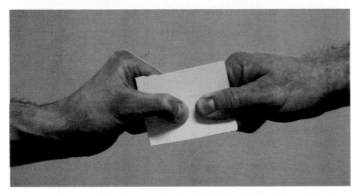

Fig. 4-50: A positive Froment's sign is indicated by the patient flexing the distal phalanx of the thumb due to adductor pollicis muscle paralysis.

Phalen's test[8,10]

The patient is positioned in sitting or standing. The therapist flexes the patient's wrists maximally and asks the patient to hold the position for 60 seconds. A positive test is indicated by tingling in the thumb, index finger, middle finger, and lateral half of the ring finger and may be indicative of carpal tunnel syndrome due to median nerve compression (Fig. 4-51).

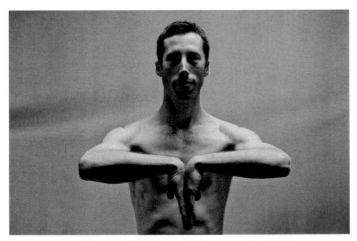

Fig. 4-51: A patient maintains the test position for Phalen's test.

Tinel's sign[10,13]

The patient is positioned in sitting or standing. The therapist taps over the volar aspect of the patient's wrist. A positive test is indicated by tingling in the thumb, index finger, middle finger, and lateral half of the ring finger distal to the contact site at the wrist. A positive test may be indicative of carpal tunnel syndrome due to median nerve compression.

Finkelstein test[10,26]

The patient is positioned in sitting or standing and is asked to make a fist with the thumb tucked inside the fingers. The therapist stabilizes the patient's forearm and ulnarly deviates the wrist. A positive test is indicated by pain over the abductor pollicis longus and extensor pollicis brevis tendons at the wrist and may be indicative of tenosynovitis in the thumb (de Quervain's disease) (Fig. 4-52).

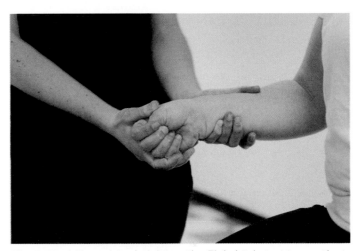

Fig. 4-52: A therapist administers the Finkelstein test to a patient in sitting.

Hip

Contracture/Tightness

Ely's test[10,13]

The patient is positioned in prone while the therapist passively flexes the patient's knee. A positive test is indicated by spontaneous hip flexion occurring simultaneously with knee flexion and may be indicative of a rectus femoris contracture (Fig. 4-53).

Ober's test[10,26]

The patient is positioned in sidelying with the lower leg flexed at the hip and the knee. The therapist moves the test leg into hip extension and abduction and then attempts to slowly lower the test leg. A positive test is indicated by an inability of the test leg to adduct and touch the table and may be indicative of an iliotibial band or a tensor fasciae latae contracture (Fig. 4-54).

Piriformis test[10,13]

The patient is positioned in sidelying with the test leg positioned toward the ceiling and the hip flexed to 60 degrees. The therapist places one hand on the patient's pelvis and the other hand on the patient's knee. While stabilizing the pelvis, the therapist applies a downward (adduction) force on the knee. A positive test is indicated by pain or tightness, and may be indicative of piriformis tightness or compression on the sciatic nerve caused by the piriformis.

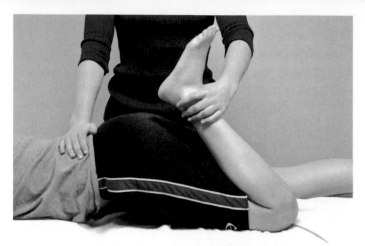

Fig. 4-53: A positive Ely's test is indicated by active hip flexion occurring simultaneously with passive knee flexion.

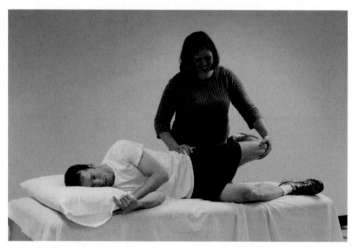

Fig. 4-54: A therapist administers Ober's test by moving the patient's leg into hip extension and abduction, and then attempts to lower the leg towards the table.

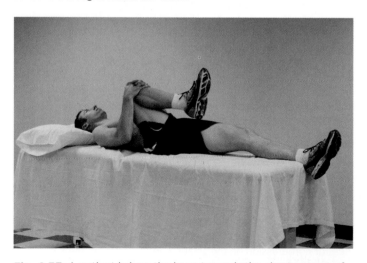

Fig. 4-55: A patient brings the knee towards the chest as part of the Thomas test. A positive test is indicated by the straight leg rising from the table.

Thomas test[10,26]

The patient is positioned in supine with the legs fully extended. The patient is asked to bring one of their knees to the chest in order to flatten the lumbar spine. The therapist observes the position of the contralateral hip while the patient holds the flexed hip. A positive test is indicated by the straight leg rising from the table and may be indicative of a hip flexion contracture (Fig. 4-55).

Tripod sign[10]

The patient is positioned in sitting with the knees flexed to 90 degrees over the edge of a table. The therapist passively extends one knee. A positive test is indicated by tightness in the hamstrings or extension of the trunk in order to limit the effect of the tight hamstrings.

90-90 straight leg raise test[8,10]

The patient is positioned in supine and is asked to stabilize the hips in 90 degrees of flexion with the knees relaxed. The therapist instructs the patient to alternately extend each knee as much as possible while maintaining the hips in 90 degrees of flexion. A positive test is indicated by the knee remaining in 20 degrees or more of flexion and is indicative of hamstrings tightness.

Miscellaneous

Craig's test[10,18]

The patient is positioned in prone with the test knee flexed to 90 degrees. The therapist palpates the posterior aspect of the greater trochanter and medially and laterally rotates the hip until the greater trochanter is parallel with the table. The degree of femoral anteversion corresponds to the angle formed by the lower leg with the perpendicular axis of the table. Normal anteversion for an adult is 8-15 degrees (Fig. 4-56).

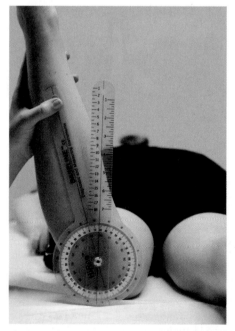

Fig. 4-56: A therapist attempts to quantify the amount of femoral anteversion with a goniometer after administering Craig's test.

Patrick's test (FABER test)[8,10]

The patient is positioned in supine with the test leg flexed, abducted, and laterally rotated at the hip onto the opposite leg. The therapist slowly lowers the test leg through abduction toward the table. A positive test is indicated by failure of the test leg to abduct below the level of the opposite leg and may be indicative of iliopsoas, sacroiliac or hip joint abnormalities.

Trendelenburg test[8,10]

The patient is positioned in standing and is asked to stand on one leg for approximately ten seconds. A positive test is indicated by a drop of the pelvis on the unsupported side and may be indicative of weakness of the gluteus medius muscle on the supported side.

Knee

Ligamentous Instability

Anterior drawer test[8,10]

The patient is positioned in supine with the knee flexed to 90 degrees and the hip flexed to 45 degrees. The therapist stabilizes the lower leg by sitting on the forefoot. The therapist grasps the patient's proximal tibia with two hands, places their thumbs on the tibial plateau, and administers an anterior directed force to the tibia on the femur. A positive test is indicated by excessive anterior translation of the tibia on the femur with a diminished or absent end-point and may be indicative of an anterior cruciate ligament injury (Fig. 4-57).

Lachman test[10,26]

The patient is positioned in supine with the knee flexed to 20-30 degrees. The therapist stabilizes the distal femur with one hand and places the other hand on the proximal tibia. The therapist applies an anterior directed force to the tibia on the femur. A positive test is indicated by excessive anterior translation of the tibia on the femur with a diminished or absent end-point and may be indicative of an anterior cruciate ligament injury (Fig. 4-58).

Lateral pivot shift test[8,10]

The patient is positioned in supine with the hip flexed and abducted to 30 degrees with slight medial rotation. The therapist grasps the leg with one hand and places the other hand over the lateral surface of the proximal tibia. The therapist medially rotates the tibia and applies a valgus force to the knee while the knee is slowly flexed. A positive test is indicated by a palpable shift or clunk occurring between 20 and 40 degrees of flexion and is indicative of anterolateral rotatory instability. The shift or clunk results from the reduction of the tibia on the femur.

Posterior drawer test[8,10]

The patient is positioned in supine with the knee flexed to 90 degrees and the hip flexed to 45 degrees. The therapist stabilizes the lower leg by sitting on the forefoot. The therapist grasps the patient's proximal tibia with two hands, places their thumbs on the tibial plateau, and administers a posterior directed force to the tibia on the femur. A positive test is indicated by excessive posterior translation of the tibia on the femur with a diminished or absent end-point and may be indicative of a posterior cruciate ligament injury.

Posterior sag sign[8,10]

The patient is positioned in supine with the knee flexed to 90 degrees and the hip flexed to 45 degrees. A positive test is indicated by the tibia sagging back on the femur and may be indicative of a posterior cruciate ligament injury.

Valgus stress test[10,13]

The patient is positioned in supine with the knee flexed to 20-30 degrees. The therapist positions one hand on the medial surface of the patient's ankle and the other hand on the lateral surface of the knee. The therapist applies a valgus force to the knee with the distal hand. A positive test is indicated by excessive valgus movement and may be indicative of a medial collateral ligament sprain. A positive test with the knee in full extension may be indicative of damage to the medial collateral ligament, posterior cruciate ligament, posterior oblique ligament, and posteromedial capsule.

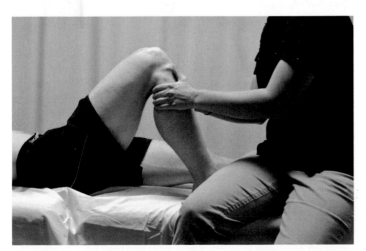

Fig. 4-57: A therapist administers the anterior drawer test to a patient positioned in supine with the hip in 45 degrees of flexion and the knee in 90 degrees of flexion.

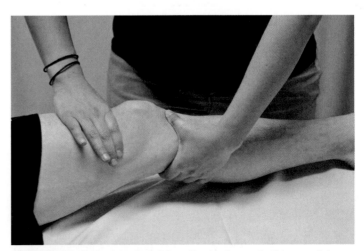

Fig. 4-58: A therapist administers the Lachman test by applying an anterior directed force to the tibia on the femur while stabilizing the distal femur.

Varus stress test[10,13]

The patient is positioned in supine with the knee flexed to 20-30 degrees. The therapist positions one hand on the lateral surface of the patient's ankle and the other hand on the medial surface of the knee. The therapist applies a varus force to the knee with the distal hand. A positive test is indicated by excessive varus movement and may be indicative of a lateral collateral ligament sprain. A positive test with the knee in full extension may be indicative of damage to the lateral collateral ligament, posterior cruciate ligament, arcuate complex, and posterolateral capsule.

Meniscal Pathology

Apley's compression test[10,18]

The patient is positioned in prone with the knee flexed to 90 degrees. The therapist stabilizes the patient's femur using one hand and places the other hand on the patient's heel. The therapist medially and laterally rotates the tibia while applying a compressive force through the tibia. A positive test is indicated by pain or clicking and may be indicative of a meniscal lesion.

McMurray test[8,10]

The patient is positioned in supine. The therapist grasps the distal leg with one hand and palpates the knee joint line with the other. With the knee fully flexed, the therapist medially rotates the tibia and extends the knee. The therapist repeats the same procedure while laterally rotating the tibia. A positive test is indicated by a click or pronounced crepitation felt over the joint line and may be indicative of a posterior meniscal lesion.

Swelling

Brush test[10,22]

The patient is positioned in supine. The therapist places one hand below the joint line on the medial surface of the patella and strokes proximally with the palm and fingers as far as the suprapatellar pouch. The other hand then strokes down the lateral surface of the patella. A positive test is indicated by a wave of fluid just below the medial distal border of the patella and is indicative of effusion in the knee.

Patellar tap test[10,22]

The patient is positioned in supine with the knee flexed or extended to a point of discomfort. The therapist applies a slight tap over the patella. A positive test is indicated if the patella appears to be floating and may be indicative of joint effusion.

Ankle

Ligamentous Instability

Anterior drawer test[8,10]

The patient is positioned in supine. The therapist stabilizes the distal tibia and fibula with one hand, while the other hand holds the foot in 20 degrees of plantar flexion and draws the talus forward in the ankle mortise. A positive test is indicated by excessive anterior translation of the talus away from the ankle mortise and may be indicative of an anterior talofibular ligament sprain.

Talar tilt test[10,22]

The patient is positioned in sidelying with the knee flexed to 90 degrees. The therapist stabilizes the distal tibia with one hand while grasping the talus with the other hand. The foot is maintained in a neutral position. The therapist tilts the talus into abduction and adduction. A positive test is indicated by excessive adduction and may be indicative of a calcaneofibular ligament sprain.

Miscellaneous

Thompson test[8,10]

The patient is positioned in prone with the feet extended over the edge of a table. The therapist asks the patient to relax and proceeds to squeeze the muscle belly of the gastrocnemius and soleus muscles. A positive test is indicated by the absence of plantar flexion and may be indicative of a ruptured Achilles tendon (Fig. 4-59).

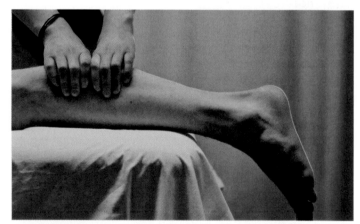

Fig. 4-59: A therapist administers the Thompson test by squeezing the muscle belly of the gastrocnemius and soleus muscles.

True leg length discrepancy test[10]

The patient is positioned in supine with the hips and knees extended, the legs 15 to 20 cm apart, and the pelvis in balance with the legs. Using a tape measure, the therapist measures from the distal point of the anterior superior iliac spines to the distal point of the medial malleoli. A positive test is indicated by a bilateral variation of greater than one centimeter and may be indicative of a true leg length discrepancy.

Osteokinematic and Arthrokinematic Motions

Upper Extremity Joints - Osteokinematic and Arthrokinematic Motion[10,14]

Joint	Resting Position	Convex/Concave	Osteokinematic/ Arthrokinematic Motion
Glenohumeral	55 degrees abduction, 30 degrees horizontal adduction	Convex: humerus Concave: glenoid	Opposite direction
Ulnohumeral	70 degrees flexion, 10 degrees supination	Convex: humerus Concave: ulna	Same direction
Radiohumeral	Full extension, full supination	Convex: humerus Concave: radius	Same direction
Proximal radioulnar	70 degrees flexion, 35 degrees supination	Convex: radius Concave: ulna	Opposite direction
Distal radioulnar	10 degrees supination	Convex: ulna Concave: radius	Same direction
Radiocarpal	Neutral with slight ulnar deviation	Convex: carpals Concave: radius	Opposite direction
Metacarpophalangeal joints of digits 2-5	Slight flexion	Convex: metacarpals Concave: phalanges	Same direction
Proximal and distal interphalangeal joints of digits 2-5	Slight flexion	Convex: proximal phalanges Concave: distal phalanges	Same direction

Lower Extremity Joints - Osteokinematic and Arthrokinematic Motion[10,14]

Joint	Resting Position	Convex/Concave	Osteokinematic/ Arthrokinematic Motion
Hip	30 degrees flexion, 30 degrees abduction, slight lateral rotation	Convex: femur Concave: acetabulum	Opposite direction
Tibiofemoral	25 degrees flexion	Convex: femur Concave: tibia	Same direction
Patellofemoral	25 degrees flexion	Convex: patella Concave: femur	Opposite direction

Lower Extremity Joints - Osteokinematic and Arthrokinematic Motion[10,14] (continued)

Proximal tibiofibular	0 degrees plantar flexion	Convex: tibia Concave: fibula	Same direction
Distal tibiofibular	0 degrees plantar flexion	Convex: fibula Concave: tibia	Opposite direction
Talocrural	10 degrees plantar flexion, midway between maximum inversion and eversion	Convex: talus Concave: tibia and fibula	Opposite direction
Subtalar	Midway between extremes of range of movement	Convex: anterior and middle talus Concave: anterior and middle calcaneus	Same direction
		Convex: posterior calcaneus Concave: posterior talus	Opposite direction
Intermetatarsal	Midway between extremes of range of movement	Convex: more medial metatarsals Concave: more lateral metatarsals	Same direction
Metatarsophalangeal	Neutral	Convex: metatarsals Concave: phalanges	Same direction
Interphalangeal joints of the toes	Slight flexion	Convex: proximal phalanges Concave: distal phalanges	Same direction

Mobilization[14,16]

Mobilization is a passive movement technique designed to improve joint function.

Indications: restricted joint mobility, restricted accessory motion, desired neurophysiological effects

Contraindications: active disease, infection, advanced osteoporosis, articular hypermobility, fracture, acute inflammation, muscle guarding, joint replacement

Grades of Movement

Grade I	Small amplitude movement performed at the beginning of range.
Grade II	Large amplitude movement performed within the range, but not reaching the limit of the range and not returning to the beginning of range.
Grade III	Large amplitude movement performed up to the limit of range.
Grade IV	Small amplitude movement performed at the limit of range.
Grade V	Small amplitude, high velocity thrust technique performed to snap adhesions at the limit of range.

Convex-Concave Rule

Determines the direction of decreased joint gliding and the appropriate direction for the mobilizing force.

Convex surface moving on a concave surface:

- Roll and slide occur in the opposite direction
- Mobilizing force should be applied in the opposite direction of the bone movement

Concave surface moving on a convex surface:

- Roll and slide occur in the same direction
- Mobilizing force should be applied in the same direction as the bone movement

Mobilization Technique

- The patient should have a general understanding of the purpose of mobilization.
- The patient should be completely relaxed during treatment.
- The therapist should be in a comfortable position while performing mobilization activities.
- The therapist's position should allow for optimal control of movement. Explain specific mobilization techniques to the

patient prior to beginning treatment. Complete a general examination of each patient prior to beginning mobilization activities.

• Use gravity to assist with mobilization whenever possible.

• Mobilization activities are usually performed initially with the joint in a loose packed position.

• Maintain contact with the mobilizing hand as close to the joint space as possible.

• Allow one digit to palpate the joint line when possible.

• Mobilize one joint in one direction at a time.

• Use a mobilization belt or wedge to assist with stabilization when necessary.

• Constantly modify mobilization techniques based on individual patient response.

• Compare the quality and quantity of joint play bilaterally.

• Reassess each patient prior to every treatment session.

Therapeutic Exercise[15,16,17,29]

Range of Motion

Range of motion is defined as the amount of mobility available at a single joint, which may be affected by the structure of the joint or the extensibility of soft tissues that surround the joint. Range of motion is classified as passive, active-assisted or active.

Contraindications: Range of motion activities should not be performed when motion is detrimental to the healing of tissues. However, controlled motion within a pain-free range has been shown to be beneficial in the early stages of healing. Increased pain or inflammation are signs that range of motion activities may be too aggressive.

Passive Range of Motion (PROM)

Definition: PROM is movement that is produced by an external force without muscular activation from the patient. PROM is only performed within the available range of motion. Any movement beyond end-range is considered stretching (Figs. 4–60, 4–61).

Indications:

• the patient is unable to physically move the body segment (e.g., comatose, paralyzed)
• the patient is cognitively impaired and unable to move the body segment
• active movement is contraindicated (e.g., post-operative)
• active movement is painful for the patient
• the therapist is preparing the joint for stretching
• the therapist is teaching an active movement to the patient

Benefits:

• improves the mobility of connective tissues and muscles
• prevents joint contracture formation
• improves circulation
• improves synovial fluid movement for cartilage health
• decreases pain
• improves the patient's awareness of movement

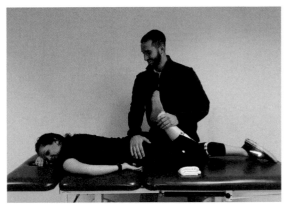

Fig. 4-60: A therapist performs passive knee flexion to stretch the anterior structures of the thigh.

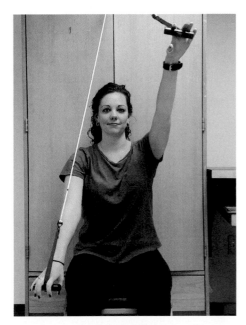

Fig. 4-61: A patient performs passive range of motion of the left upper extremity using an overhead pulley system.

Active-assisted Range of Motion (AAROM)

Definition: AAROM is movement that is produced by the patient through active muscular contraction with some assistance from an external force (Fig. 4-62).

Indications:

- the patient is unable to fully contract a muscle (e.g., paresis, pain)
- full activation of a muscle is contraindicated (e.g., post-operative)
- performed prior to initiating active movement

Benefits:

- improves the mobility of connective tissues and muscles
- prevents joint contracture formation
- improves circulation
- improves synovial fluid movement for cartilage health
- decreases pain
- improves neuromuscular activity
- improves kinesthesia and proprioception

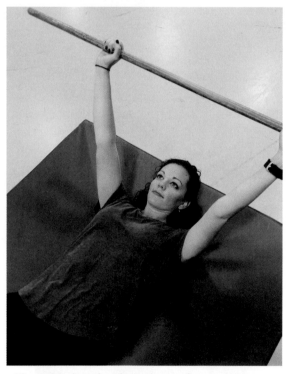

Fig. 4-62: A patient in supine performs active-assisted range of motion of the upper extremities using a dowel.

Active Range of Motion (AROM)

Definition: AROM is movement that is produced by the patient through active muscular contraction without any external assistance (Fig. 4-63).

Indications:

- patient is able to contract a muscle, but demonstrates weakness
- performed prior to initiating resistance training to teach the desired movement

Benefits:

- improves the mobility of connective tissues and muscles
- prevents joint contracture formation
- improves circulation
- improves synovial fluid movement for cartilage health
- decreases pain
- improves neuromuscular activity
- improves kinesthesia and proprioception
- improves strength in very weak muscles (e.g., 3/5 strength)

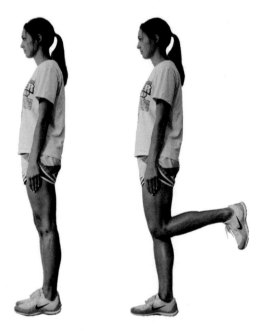

Fig. 4-63: A patient performs active knee flexion in standing.

Stretching

Stretching is a therapeutic technique used to improve joint range of motion and muscle flexibility by increasing the extensibility of the musculotendinous unit and connective tissues.

Indications: decreased joint range of motion or decreased muscle flexibility

Contraindications: acute inflammation, during soft tissue healing (e.g., following a tendon repair), range of motion limited by bone-on-bone contact, recent fracture, hypermobility, hypomobility that allows for improved function (e.g., tenodesis grip), acute pain associated with stretching

Principles of Stretching

Elasticity: The ability of soft tissue to return to its previous length after a stretch is no longer applied.

Viscoelasticity: A time-dependent property of soft tissue that results in resistance to stretch when it is initially applied, but allows for tissue elongation as the stretch is held for longer durations. As with elasticity, the tissue will return to its previous length after the stretch is no longer applied.

Plasticity: A property of soft tissue that allows for tissue elongation even after a stretch is no longer applied.

Stress-strain curve: A graphic representation that depicts the relationship between the amount of force (stress) applied to connective tissue and the amount of deformation (strain) it experiences (Fig. 4-64).

Creep: Due to the viscoelastic property, soft tissue that is stretched for a sustained duration will elongate and not return to its original length after the load has been removed. The principle of creep is the basis for stretching.

Stress-relaxation: The longer a stretching force is maintained, the more the tension within the tissue decreases, therefore less force is required to maintain the same tissue length.

Methods of Stretching

Static stretching

Static stretching (Figs. 4-65, 4-66) involves placing the muscle at its maximal length and holding the position against an external force for a prolonged period of time. Static stretching is characterized by low intensity and long duration. It is considered to be the safest form of stretching and results in the greatest gains in tissue extensibility. This form of stretching leads to less activation of the muscle spindles (as compared to ballistic stretching) and thus less resistance to stretch. Though there is no consensus for the optimal duration of static stretching, 30 seconds is a commonly cited value that has been shown to result in significant range of motion gains.

Ballistic stretching

Ballistic stretching (Fig. 4-67) is characterized by quick, jerky movements that result in a rapid change in muscle length. The muscle is placed near its end of range of motion and then the patient bounces back and forth to place repetitive stretch on the muscle (i.e., high intensity, short duration). Because ballistic stretching occurs quickly, it activates the muscle spindles and results in greater resistance to stretch. Therefore, it is not as effective for improving tissue extensibility, though it may be more effective when preparing the muscles for athletic activity. Additionally, ballistic stretching is more likely to lead to muscle soreness and injury due to the high intensity of stretch force.

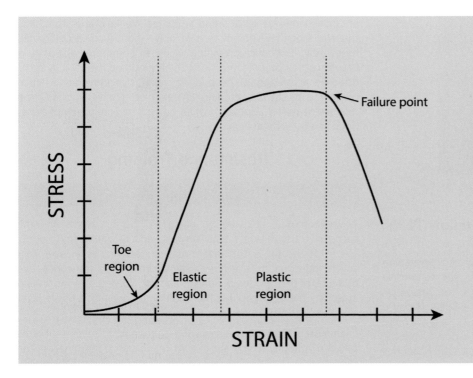

Toe region: Initial stress that results in the wavy collagen fibers becoming straight and aligning with one another.

Elastic region: Added stress to the tissue results in greater deformation, though the tissue returns to its resting length if the stretch force is not maintained. Tissues with greater stiffness will have a steeper slope in this portion of the curve.

Plastic region: The addition of more stress results in permanent deformation even after the stretch force is no longer applied due to the failure of bonds between the collagen fibers.

Fig. 4-64: A stress-strain curve depicting the toe region, elastic region, and plastic region.

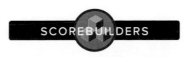

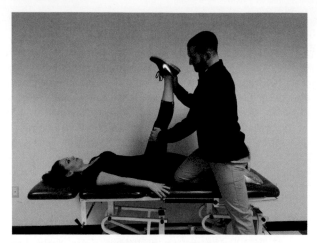

Fig. 4-65: A therapist passively stretching a patient's right hamstrings.

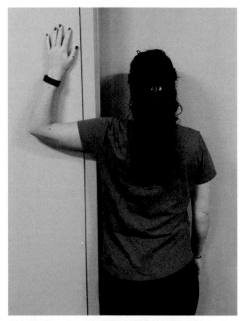

Fig. 4-66: A patient passively stretching the left shoulder using a doorway.

Proprioceptive neuromuscular facilitation (PNF) stretching

PNF incorporates active muscle contractions into stretching techniques. Muscular contraction is thought to lead to muscle relaxation through the principles of autogenic or reciprocal inhibition and results in greater gains in muscle flexibility. Because these techniques exert their effects on muscle fibers, they are more effective at treating range of motion limitations due to muscle spasm as opposed to connective tissue tightness. Other theories for PNF's effects on improved flexibility include increased patient tolerance to the stretch and length changes secondary to the viscoelastic properties of muscle. Because PNF requires active muscular control from the patient, it is not an effective technique for patients with paralysis or spasticity. Common PNF techniques include contract-relax, agonist contraction, and contract-relax with agonist contraction.

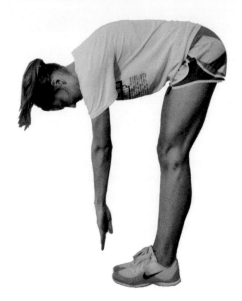

Fig. 4-67: A patient in standing performs ballistic stretching of the hamstrings by quickly assuming the position depicted in the image resulting in a rapid change in muscle length.

Dynamic stretching

Dynamic stretching involves the patient actively moving a body segment to the end of range (but not beyond this limit) while the antagonist muscle relaxes and stretches. Unlike static stretching, the end-range movement is held only briefly and is performed repeatedly. Dynamic stretching is most commonly used as a "warm-up" to prepare the body for athletic activities. It is more effective at preparing the body for explosive movements when compared to static stretching. Dynamic stretching emphasizes a movement based approach, while ballistic stretching emphasizes bouncing movements.

Resistance Training

Muscle Anatomy

A single muscle is made up of several muscle fibers and the connective tissue layers that surround and lie within the muscle. The endomysium is the innermost connective tissue layer that covers individual muscle fibers. The perimysium is the connective tissue layer that groups bundles of muscle fibers (i.e., a fasciculus) together. The epimysium is the outermost connective tissue layer that surrounds the entire muscle.

Each muscle fiber is its own cell and is made up of several subunits called myofibrils, which are in turn made up of sarcomeres. The sarcomere is the smallest unit of a muscle that gives it the ability to contract. Sarcomeres are composed of the myofilaments actin and myosin. The actin and myosin attach to one another and slide together and apart to allow for muscle contraction and relaxation, respectively.

Resistive and Overload Training

Isometric Exercise: Muscular force is generated without a change in muscle length. Isometric exercises are often performed against an immovable object. Submaximal isometric exercises are traditionally used in rehabilitation programs.

Isotonic Exercise: Muscular contraction is generated with the muscle exerting a constant tension. This can also be thought of as muscle movement with a constant load. Isotonic exercises are performed against resistance, often employing equipment such as handheld weights. There are two types of isotonic contractions: concentric and eccentric. A concentric contraction shortens a muscle, while an eccentric contraction lengthens a muscle.

Isokinetic Exercise: Muscular contraction is generated with a constant maximal speed and variable load. In isokinetic exercise, the reaction force is identical to the force applied to the equipment. Cybex, Biodex, and Lido are a few of the companies making isokinetic exercise equipment.

Resistance Training Parameters

Intensity: The intensity of resistance training is often determined by the amount of weight that is being used, which will in turn determine how many repetitions of the exercise can be performed. The amount of weight being used may be expressed as a percentage of the patient's 1 RM (repetition maximum). The intensity chosen will depend on the goals of the training program. If increased strength is the goal, then lower repetitions (e.g., 6-12) of a higher intensity load should be prescribed. If increased endurance is the goal, then higher repetitions (e.g., 20+) of a lower intensity load should be prescribed. When training for power, low repetitions (e.g., 1-3) of a very high intensity load are used.

Volume: The volume is the total amount of work performed and is calculated as the total number of repetitions multiplied by the intensity of the exercise. The total number of repetitions is inversely related to intensity; if heavier weights are used, the patient will be able to perform fewer total repetitions, as is the case when training to increase power or strength. Two to four sets of repetitions is a common exercise prescription, with the number of repetitions within a single set dependent on the goals of treatment (i.e., strength versus endurance).

Frequency: The frequency refers to the number of times per week resistance exercises are performed and is dependent on the intensity and volume of exercise and the fitness level of the individual. For more intense exercise, training should be performed less frequently (e.g., 2-3 times per week). The same applies for patients with a lower overall fitness level. For patients in a rehabilitation program, exercise can be performed several times per day if the intensity and volume of exercise is kept low. Exercise that is performed too frequently may lead to overtraining and a decline in the patient's condition or performance.

Exercise sequence: The general recommendations for exercise sequencing dictate that large muscle groups should be exercised before small muscle groups, multi-joint exercises should be performed before single joint exercises, and high intensity exercises should be performed before low intensity exercises. However, a therapist may choose to disregard these recommendations if they conflict with the rehabilitation goals of a specific patient.

Rest interval: The recovery period between sets will vary depending on the intensity of the exercise. For high intensity exercise, a longer rest interval is needed (e.g., three or more minutes). For low intensity exercise, a shorter rest interval is adequate (e.g., one to two minutes). Patients who have an overall lower fitness level may also need a longer rest interval when compared to more fit individuals.

Open-Chain: Open-chain activities involve the distal segment, usually the hand or foot, moving freely in space. An example of an open-chain activity is kicking a ball with the lower extremity (Fig. 4-68).

Closed-Chain: Closed-chain activities involve the body moving over a fixed distal segment. An example of a closed-chain activity is a squat lift (Fig. 4-69).

Resistance Training Principles

Overload principle

The overload principle states that in order for a muscle to adapt and become stronger, the load that is placed on it must be greater than what it is normally accustomed to. In resistance training, the volume (sets, repetitions) or intensity (resistance) of the exercise can be altered to provide a greater challenge to the muscle.

SAID principle

The SAID principle (Specific Adaptation to Imposed Demands) states that the body will adapt according to the specific type of training that is utilized. To bring about an improvement in a patient's function, the type of training should specifically mirror the desired goal. For example, if a patient needs greater muscular power, the exercises chosen should focus on improving power as opposed to strength or endurance.

Transfer of training principle

The transfer of training principle states that there can be a carryover effect from one exercise or task to another. For example, a patient who performs exercises to improve muscular strength may also see improvements in muscular endurance. However, these carryover effects are far less beneficial than the adaptations that result from more specific training.

Reversibility principle

The reversibility principle states that the adaptations seen with resistance training are reversible if the body is not regularly challenged with the same level of resistance or greater. These reversible effects can begin within 1-2 weeks of stopping an exercise program.

Length-tension relationship

The length-tension relationship is a principle that states that the ability of a muscle to produce force depends on the length of the muscle. A muscle can usually produce a maximal force near its normal resting length. If the muscle is lengthened or shortened, it will likely produce less force.

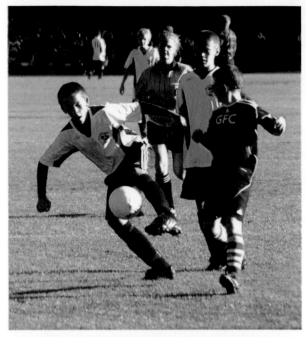

Fig. 4-68: An example of an open-chain exercise.

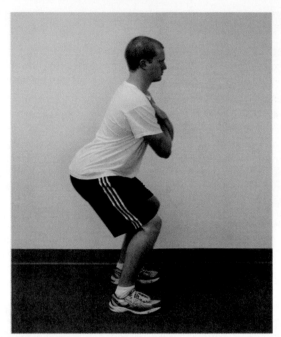

Fig. 4-69: An example of a closed-chain exercise.

Exercise Programs

DeLorme	Protocol	Oxford Technique	Protocol
First Set	10 repetitions x 50% of 10 repetition maximum	First Set	10 repetitions x 100% of 10 repetition maximum
Second Set	10 repetitions x 75% of 10 repetition maximum	Second Set	10 repetitions x 75% of 10 repetition maximum
Third Set	10 repetitions x 100% of 10 repetition maximum	Third Set	10 repetitions x 50% of 10 repetition maximum

Force-velocity relationship

The force-velocity relationship is a principle that states that the speed of a muscle contraction affects the force that the muscle can produce. During a concentric contraction, as the speed of contraction increases, the force of contraction decreases. During an eccentric contraction, as the speed of contraction increases, the force of contraction also increases.

Resistance Training Terminology

Endurance: The ability of a muscle to contract repeatedly against a light external load and resist fatigue over a prolonged period of time.

Moment arm: The linear distance from the axis of rotation to the site of the external load.

Muscle performance: The ability of a muscle to perform work. The components of muscle performance include power, strength, and endurance.

Power: The rate at which work is performed (i.e., work divided by time).

Strength: The greatest amount of force that can be produced within a muscle during a single contraction, which may be assessed clinically by determining a patient's 1 RM (i.e., maximum amount of weight that can be lifted once).

Torque: The ability of an external load to produce rotation around an axis, calculated by multiplying the magnitude of the load by the moment arm.

Work: The magnitude of a load (e.g., weight) multiplied by the distance the load is moved (e.g., range of motion used).

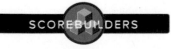

SPOTLIGHT ON SAFETY
POTENTIAL CONSEQUENCES OF RESISTANCE TRAINING[15,16]

Therapists should carefully monitor patients during and following resistance training in order to avoid undesirable training effects. Three of the more common conditions resulting from resistance training include muscle fatigue, delayed-onset muscle soreness, and the Valsalva maneuver.

Muscle fatigue

Muscle fatigue is characterized by the decreasing ability of a muscle to produce force against a load with increasing repetitions. Muscle fatigue is reversible (i.e., strength will improve after a period of rest). The extent of muscle fatigue will depend on the fiber-type distribution within the muscle. Type I (slow-twitch) muscle fibers are able to generate a low level of force for long durations and therefore are very resistant to fatigue, while type II (fast-twitch) muscle fibers produce large amounts of force over short durations and are therefore more prone to fatigue.

While muscle fatigue may occur during a resistance training program, the therapist should be aware of excessive fatigue and avoid working the patient to this point. Signs and symptoms of excessive muscle fatigue include muscle pain and cramping, tremors, movement that becomes slower or jerky, an inability to complete the full movement pattern, and use of substitution patterns. When these signs or symptoms occur, the therapist should decrease the load being lifted or allow the patient to take a rest break. Allowing the patient to continue exercising in the presence of excessive muscle fatigue could lead to further injury.

For some patients, muscle fatigue does not occur in a normal predictable fashion. Patients with certain neuromuscular disorders (e.g., myasthenia gravis, multiple sclerosis) may fatigue more quickly. Pushing these patients to the point of fatigue may actually result in a worsening of their symptoms. Likewise, patients with cardiovascular or pulmonary diseases fatigue more quickly and may need longer recovery periods during exercise. Therapists should be aware of the fatigue patterns associated with different diseases and treat each patient accordingly.

Delayed-onset muscle soreness

Delayed-onset muscle soreness (DOMS) is a specific type of post-exercise soreness that is thought to result from microtrauma to the muscle and its connective tissues that occurs during resistance training. DOMS is most commonly noted in patients who have engaged in high intensity, eccentric strengthening exercises, especially if the patient has recently begun a resistance training program.

DOMS is characterized by tenderness to palpation in the muscle belly or at the muscle-tendon junction, soreness with passive stretching or active contraction of the muscle, and decreased range of motion and strength. These symptoms usually reach their peak two days after exercise and can last for several days. The soreness will diminish with each successive training session as the muscle adapts to higher levels of stress.

It may be possible to minimize the effect of DOMS by slowly increasing the intensity of a new exercise program. Additionally, performing only concentric and isometric exercises significantly reduces the likelihood that DOMS will occur.

Valsalva maneuver

The Valsalva maneuver is a technique that is often used to increase intra-abdominal and intrathoracic pressures during anaerobic activities that require a large effort, such as lifting a heavy box from the floor. The maneuver is performed by forcefully exhaling against a closed glottis, nose, and mouth while simultaneously contracting the abdominal muscles. The increase in internal pressures helps to stabilize the spine during heavy exertion and is therefore employed during powerlifting to help improve performance.

Though the Valsalva maneuver can be useful in certain situations, it leads to undesirable effects on the cardiovascular system. Because of its negative effects, the Valsalva maneuver should be avoided in all patients, but especially for patients with cardiovascular disease (e.g., hypertension, coronary artery disease, stroke), with intervertebral disk pathology or who have recently undergone eye surgery. To avoid using the Valsalva maneuver, patients should be taught to breathe rhythmically and to exhale during the portion of exercise that requires more exertion.

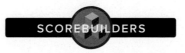

Adaptations to Resistance Training

Strength training	Endurance training
• muscle fiber hypertrophy • fiber type remodeling from IIB to IIA • increased neuromuscular activity (number of motor units, firing rate) • decreased or no change in capillary bed density • decreased mitochondrial density • increased stores of ATP, creatine phosphate, and other energy sources • increased tensile strength of tendons and ligaments • increased bone mineral density • increased lean body mass • decreased body fat percentage	• increased capillary bed density • increased mitochondrial density • increased stores of ATP, creatine phosphate, and other energy sources • increased tensile strength of tendons and ligaments • increased bone mineral density • decreased body fat percentage

Pathology of the Musculoskeletal System

Achilles Tendonitis[18,28,29]

Achilles tendonitis is a repetitive overuse disorder resulting in microscopic tears of collagen fibers on the surface or in the substance of the Achilles tendon. The tendon is most often impacted in an avascular zone located two to six centimeters above the insertion of the tendon.

Etiology - Repetitive overload of the Achilles tendon often caused by changes in training intensity or faulty technique. Patients with limited flexibility and strength in the gastrocnemius and soleus complex and patients with a pronated or cavus foot are at increased risk. Activities frequently associated with Achilles tendonitis include running, basketball, gymnastics, and dancing. A history of Achilles tendonitis increases the likelihood of an Achilles tendon rupture later in life.

Signs and Symptoms - aching or burning in the posterior heel, tenderness of the Achilles tendon, pain with increased activity, swelling and thickening in the tendon area, muscle weakness due to pain, morning stiffness

Treatment - Initially RICE (Rest, Ice, Compression, Elevation), non-steroidal anti-inflammatory medications (NSAIDs), and analgesics as needed. A heel lift and cross training may be used to limit the amount of tensile loading through the tendon. Prevention includes heel cord stretching exercises, use of appropriate soft-soled foot-wear, eccentric strengthening of the gastrocnemius and soleus complex, and avoiding sudden changes in intensity of training pro-grams.

Adhesive Capsulitis[13,28,29]

Adhesive capsulitis results in a loss of range of motion in active and passive shoulder motion due to soft tissue contracture. The condition is caused by adhesive fibrosis and scarring between the capsule, rotator cuff, subacromial bursa, and deltoid.

Etiology - The onset may be related to a direct injury to the shoulder or may begin insidiously. Peak incidence occurs in individuals between 40 and 60 years of age with females being affected more than males. Patients with diabetes have an increased incidence of adhesive capsulitis. The condition is self-limiting and typically resolves in one to two years, although some individuals have residual loss of motion.

Signs and Symptoms - insidious onset of localized pain often extending down the arm, subjective reports of stiffness, night pain, restricted range of motion in a capsular pattern

Treatment - The focus of treatment is on increasing range of motion with glenohumeral mobilization, range of motion exercises, and palliative modalities. The therapist and patient should avoid overstretching and elevating pain since this can result in further loss of motion. Surgical options include suprascapular nerve block and closed manipulation under anesthesia.

Anterior Cruciate Ligament Sprain[8,13,28]

The anterior cruciate ligament (ACL) runs from the anterior intercondylar area of the tibia to the medial aspect of the lateral femoral condyle in the intercondylar notch. The ligament prevents anterior displacement of the tibia in relation to the femur. The extent of the sprain is classified according to the extent of ligament

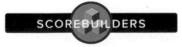

damage. A grade I sprain involves microscopic tears of the ligament, while a grade III sprain indicates a completely torn ligament.

Etiology - Noncontact twisting injury associated with hyperextension, varus or valgus stress to the knee. An ACL sprain often involves injury to other knee structures such as the medial capsule, medial collateral ligament, and menisci.

Signs and Symptoms - The patient may report a loud pop or feeling the knee "giving way" or "buckling" followed by dizziness, sweating, and swelling. Special tests to identify the presence of an ACL tear include the anterior drawer test, Lachman test, and lateral pivot shift test.

Treatment - Initially RICE, NSAIDs, and analgesics as needed. Conservative treatment includes lower extremity strengthening exercises emphasizing the quadriceps and the hamstrings. Surgery is often warranted for a complete ACL tear (grade III). Surgery most often consists of intra-articular reconstruction using the patellar tendon, iliotibial band or hamstrings tendon. A derotation brace may be beneficial for a patient with an ACL deficient knee, however, it has limited benefit for a patient following surgical reconstruction.

Congenital Hip Dysplasia[27,30]

Congenital hip dysplasia, also known as developmental dysplasia, is a condition characterized by malalignment of the femoral head within the acetabulum. The condition develops during the last trimester in utero.

Etiology - cultural predisposition, malposition in utero, environmental and genetic influences

Signs and Symptoms - Clinical presentation includes asymmetrical hip abduction with tightness and apparent femoral shortening of the involved side. Testing for this condition may include the Ortolani's test, Barlow's test, and diagnostic ultrasound.

Treatment - The focus of treatment is dependent on age, severity, and initial attempts to reposition the femoral head within the acetabulum through the constant use of a harness, bracing, splinting or traction. Open reduction with subsequent application of a hip spica cast may be required if conservative treatment fails. Physical therapy may be indicated after cast removal for stretching, strengthening, and caregiver education.

Congenital Limb Deficiencies[27-30]

A congenital limb deficiency is a malformation that occurs in utero, secondary to an altered developmental course. Congenital limb deficiencies are classified as longitudinal or transverse. A longitudinal limb deficiency refers to a reduction or absence of an element or elements within the long axis of the bone. A transverse limb deficiency refers to a limb that has developed to a particular level beyond which no skeletal elements exist.

Etiology - The majority of congenital limb deficiencies are idiopathic or are genetic in origin. Other possible etiologies include poor blood supply, constricting amniotic bands, infection, and maternal drug exposure.

Signs and Symptoms - structural or acquired abnormality of a limb, phantom limb pain

Treatment - The focus of treatment is on symmetrical movements, strengthening, range of motion, weight bearing activities, and prosthetic training when appropriate.

Congenital Torticollis[30-31]

Congenital torticollis, also known as wry neck, is characterized by a unilateral contracture of the sternocleidomastoid muscle. The condition is most often identified in the first two months of life.

Etiology - The cause is unknown, however, it may be associated with malpositioning in utero (e.g., breech) and birth trauma.

Signs and Symptoms - Clinical presentation includes lateral cervical flexion to the same side as the contracture, rotation toward the opposite side, and facial asymmetries.

Treatment - Initially, treatment is conservative with emphasis on stretching, active range of motion, positioning, and caregiver education. Surgical management is indicated when conservative options have failed and the child is over one year of age. A surgical release followed by physical therapy may be indicated for range of motion and proper alignment.

Glenohumeral Instability[8,13,18,28]

Glenohumeral instability refers to excessive translation of the humeral head on the glenoid during active rotation. Instability involves varying degrees of injuries to dynamic and static structures that function to contain the humeral head in the glenoid. Subluxation refers to joint laxity, allowing for more than 50% of the humeral head to passively translate over the glenoid rim without dislocation. Dislocation is the complete separation of the articular surfaces of the glenoid and the humeral head. Approximately 85% of dislocations detach the glenoid labrum (i.e., Bankart lesion).

Etiology - A combination of forces stress the anterior capsule, glenohumeral ligament, and rotator cuff, causing the humerus to move anteriorly out of the glenoid fossa. An anterior dislocation is the most common and is usually associated with shoulder abduction and lateral rotation.

Signs and Symptoms - Subluxation: feeling the shoulder "popping" out and back into place, pain, paresthesias, sensation of the arm feeling "dead," positive apprehension test, capsular tenderness, swelling; Dislocation: severe pain, paresthesias, limited range of motion, weakness, visible shoulder fullness, arm supported by contralateral limb.

Treatment - Initial immobilization with a sling for three to six weeks. RICE and NSAIDs are often utilized in the early phase. Following immobilization, range of motion, and isometric strengthening should be initiated followed by progressive resistive exercises emphasizing the internal and external rotators, as well as the large scapular muscles.

Impingement Syndrome[8,13,18,28]

Impingement syndrome is one of the most common injuries of the shoulder. It is often caused by repetitive microtrauma from upper extremity activity performed above the horizontal plane. Individuals participating in throwing activities, swimming, and racquet sports are particularly susceptible to impingement syndrome.

Etiology - Impingement syndrome is caused by the humeral head and the associated rotator cuff attachments migrating proximally and becoming impinged on the undersurface of the acromion and the coracoacromial ligament.

Signs and Symptoms - discomfort or mild pain deep within the shoulder, pain with overhead activities, painful arc of motion (i.e., 70-120 degrees abduction), positive impingement sign, tenderness over the greater tuberosity and the bicipital groove

Treatment - Initially RICE, NSAIDs, and activity modification. Once tolerated, treatment includes rotator cuff strengthening and scapular stability exercises. Long-term prevention includes continued strengthening of the rotator cuff and scapula stabilizers, along with improved biomechanics related to sport- specific or relevant work activities.

Juvenile Rheumatoid Arthritis[30,31]

Juvenile rheumatoid arthritis (JRA) is the most common chronic rheumatic disease in children and presents with inflammation of the joints and connective tissues. Classification of JRA includes systemic, polyarticular, and oligoarticular.

Etiology - The exact etiology is unknown, however, it is theorized that an external source such as a virus, infection or trauma may trigger an autoimmune response producing JRA in a child with a genetic predisposition.

Signs and Symptoms - The clinical presentation is based on the classification of JRA. Systemic JRA occurs in 10-20% of cases and presents with acute onset, high fevers, rash, enlargement of the spleen and liver, and inflammation of the lungs and heart. Polyarticular JRA accounts for 30-40% of cases and presents with high female incidence, significant rheumatoid factor, and arthritis in more than four joints with symmetrical joint involvement. Oligoarticular (pauciarticular) JRA accounts for 40-60% of cases and affects less than five joints with asymmetrical joint involvement.

Treatment - Pharmacological management to relieve inflammation and pain through NSAIDs, corticosteroids, antirheumatics, and immunosuppressive agents. Physical therapy management includes passive and active range of motion, positioning, splinting, strengthening, endurance training, weight bearing activities, postural training, and functional mobility. Pain management includes the use of modalities such as paraffin, ultrasound, warm water, and cryotherapy. Surgical intervention may be indicated secondary to pain, contractures or irreversible joint destruction.

Lateral Epicondylitis[8,28,29]

Lateral epicondylitis refers to an irritation or inflammation of the common extensor muscles at their origin on the lateral epicondyle of the humerus. Individuals who take part in racquet sports or activities requiring throwing are at the greatest risk for developing lateral epicondylitis.

Etiology - The condition is caused by eccentric loading of the wrist extensor muscles, usually the extensor carpi radialis brevis, resulting in microtrauma. Lateral epicondylitis can be precipitated by poor mechanics or faulty equipment such as a tennis racquet with a handle that is too small or with strings that possess too much tension. The condition is most common in individuals between 30 and 50 years of age.

Signs and Symptoms - Pain is present immediately anterior or distal to the lateral epicondyle of the humerus. Pain typically worsens with repetition and resisted wrist extension.

Treatment - Initially RICE, NSAIDs, and activity modification. Physical therapy should attempt to increase strength, flexibility, and endurance of the wrist extensors. A strap placed two to three inches distal to the elbow joint can reduce muscular tension placed on the epicondyle and may diminish or eliminate patient symptoms.

Legg-Calve-Perthes Disease[30,31]

Legg-Calve-Perthes disease is characterized by degeneration of the femoral head due to a disturbance in the blood supply (i.e., avascular necrosis). The disease is self-limiting and has four distinct stages: condensation, fragmentation, re-ossification, and remodeling.

Etiology - trauma, genetic predisposition, synovitis, vascular abnormalities, infection

Signs and Symptoms - pain, decreased range of motion, antalgic gait, positive Trendelenburg sign

Treatment - Activities are variable based on the clinical presentation, but the primary focus is to relieve pain, maintain the femoral head in the proper position, and improve range of motion. Physical therapy may be required intermittently for stretching, splinting, crutch training, aquatic therapy, traction, and exercise. Orthotic devices and surgical intervention may be indicated depending on classification and severity of the condition.

Medial Collateral Ligament Sprain[8,13,28]

The medial collateral ligament (MCL) runs from slightly above the medial femoral epicondyle to the medial aspect of the shaft of the tibia. An MCL sprain often involves injury to other knee structures such as the ACL or medial meniscus.

Etiology - A contact or noncontact, fixed foot, tibial rotational injury associated with valgus force and external tibia rotation can damage the MCL. This injury is often associated with activities such as football, skiing, and soccer.

Signs and Symptoms - Clinical presentation includes knee pain, swelling, antalgic gait, decreased range of motion, and a feeling of instability. A valgus stress test can be used to assess the integrity of the MCL.

Treatment - Initially RICE, NSAIDs, and analgesics as needed. Conservative treatment includes decreasing inflammation, protecting the knee joint and ligament, range of motion, and strengthening exercises as tolerated. Strengthening exercises gradually become more aggressive and functional activities are introduced. Surgery is rarely required since the MCL is well vascularized.

Meniscus Tear[8,13,18,28]

The medial and lateral menisci are firmly attached to the proximal surface of the tibia. The menisci are thick at the periphery and thinner at their internal unattached edges. The medial meniscus is more commonly injured than the lateral meniscus because it is less mobile due to its attachment to the joint capsule. The incidence of medial meniscal tears increases significantly over time with ACL deficiency. Meniscal injuries are definitively diagnosed by arthroscopy or magnetic resonance imaging.

Etiology - Meniscal injuries are usually associated with fixed foot rotation while weight bearing on a flexed knee. This action produces compression and rotational forces on the meniscus.

Signs and Symptoms - The clinical presentation includes joint line pain, swelling, catching or a locking sensation. Special tests to identify the presence of a meniscus tear include Apley's compression test, bounce home test, and McMurray test.

Treatment - Initially RICE, NSAIDs, and analgesics as needed. Conservative treatment consists of palliative modalities and strengthening exercises. Surgery ranging from a partial meniscectomy to a meniscal repair is often warranted for active individuals. Meniscal repairs are typically performed on tears located on the outer edges of the meniscus due to the increased vascularity. Recent advances in technology have increased the incidence of meniscal transplantation.

Osgood-Schlatter Disease[8,13,29]

Osgood-Schlatter disease, also known as traction apophysitis, is a self-limiting condition that results from repetitive traction on the tibial tuberosity apophysis.

Etiology - The condition is caused by repetitive tension to the patellar tendon over the tibial tuberosity in young athletes. This can result in a small avulsion of the tuberosity and subsequent swelling.

Signs and Symptoms - point tenderness over the patella tendon at the insertion on the tibial tubercle, antalgic gait, pain with increasing activity

Treatment - Conservative treatment focuses on education, icing, flexibility exercises, and eliminating activities that place strain on the patella tendon such as squatting, running or jumping.

Osteoarthritis[29,31]

Osteoarthritis is a chronic disease that causes degeneration of articular cartilage, primarily in weight bearing joints. Subsequent deformity and thickening of subchondral bone occurs resulting in impaired functional status. Any joint may be involved, however, the most commonly affected sites include the hands and weight bearing joints such as the hips and knees.

Etiology - The cause of osteoarthritis is unknown. The condition typically appears during middle age and affects nearly all individuals to some extent by age 70. Osteoarthritis occurs more commonly in men than women up to age 55, however, it is more common in women later in life. Risk factors include being overweight, fractures or other joint injuries, and occupational or athletic overuse.

Signs and Symptoms - Clinical presentation includes gradual onset of pain present at the affected joint, increased pain after exercise, increased pain with weather changes, enlarged joints, crepitus, stiffness, limited joint range of motion, Heberden's nodes, and Bouchard's nodes. Blood tests are not helpful in diagnosing osteoarthritis, although radiographs may show diminished joint space or a bone spur.

Treatment - The goal of treatment is to reduce pain, promote joint function, and protect the joint. Pharmacological management may include acetaminophen, NSAIDs, and corticosteroids. Some patients benefit from viscosupplementation which is administered through a series of injections of hyaluronic acid into the knee. The goal is to improve lubrication of the knee, reduce pain, and improve range of motion. Physical therapy interventions include passive and active range of motion, heating and cooling agents, patient education, strengthening exercises, transcutaneous electrical nerve stimulation, energy conservation, weight loss, body mechanics, joint protection techniques, and bracing. Surgical intervention can range from arthroscopic surgery to total joint arthroplasty.

Osteogenesis Imperfecta[30,31]

Osteogenesis imperfecta is a connective tissue disorder that affects the formation of collagen during bone development. There are four classifications of osteogenesis imperfecta that vary in level of severity.

Etiology - The cause of osteogenesis imperfecta is genetic inheritance with types I and IV considered autosomal dominant traits and types II and III considered autosomal recessive traits.

Signs and Symptoms - pathological fractures, osteoporosis (i.e., brittle bones), hypermobile joints, bowing of the long bones, weakness, scoliosis, impaired respiratory function

Treatment - Management begins at birth with caregiver education on proper handling and facilitation of movement. Physical therapy will focus on active range of motion emphasizing symmetrical movements, positioning, functional mobility, fracture management, and the use of orthotics. In severe cases where ambulation is not realistic, wheelchair prescription and training are indicated.

Patellofemoral Syndrome[8,13,28,29]

Patellofemoral syndrome is a general term describing pain or discomfort in the anterior knee. The condition is often termed chondromalacia patella, which refers to softening of the articular cartilage of the patella.

Etiology - Patellofemoral syndrome is a repetitive overuse disorder resulting from increased force at the patellofemoral joint. Factors associated with increased patellofemoral forces include decreased quadriceps strength, decreased lower extremity flexibility, patellar instability, increased tibial torsion or femoral anteversion. Patients at increased risk for developing patello-femoral syndrome include females, individuals experiencing a growth spurt, runners who have recently increased mileage, and overweight individuals.

Signs and Symptoms - anterior knee pain, pain with prolonged sitting, swelling, crepitus, pain when ascending and descending stairs

Treatment - The focus of treatment is dependent on the contributing factors associated with the abnormal patellar tracking. Possible treatment options include palliative modalities to decrease inflammation and pain, lower extremity flexibility exercises, medial patella glides, biofeedback, and patella taping. Lower extremity strengthening should emphasize the quadriceps and in particular, the vastus medialis oblique, while minimizing patellofemoral compressive forces.

Plantar Fasciitis[13,28,29]

Plantar fasciitis refers to inflammation of the plantar fascia at the proximal insertion on the medial tubercle of the calcaneus. The plantar fascia is a broad structure comprised of connective tissue which spans from the calcaneus to the metatarsal heads. The structure is designed to provide support to the arch of the foot. Excessive tension over time creates chronic inflammation and microtears at the proximal insertion of the plantar fascia.

Etiology - Plantar fasciitis is often associated with an acute injury from excessive loading of the foot or chronic irritation from an excessive amount of pronation or prolonged duration of pronation. The condition is most common in patients between 40 and 60 years of age.

Signs and Symptoms - Clinical presentation includes tenderness at the insertion of the plantar fascia, presence of a heel spur, pain that is worse in the morning or after periods of prolonged inactivity, difficulty with prolonged standing, and pain when walking in bare feet.

Treatment - Initially RICE, NSAIDs, and analgesics as needed. A heel cup, massage using a tennis ball or rolling pin, medial longitudinal arch taping, and joint mobilization may be helpful. Prevention includes heel cord stretching exercises, use of appropriate soft-soled footwear, and avoiding sudden changes in the intensity of training programs. Orthotics may be used to minimize hyperpronation.

Posterior Cruciate Ligament Sprain[8,13,28]

The posterior cruciate ligament (PCL) runs from the posterior intercondylar area of the tibia to the lateral aspect of the medial femoral condyle in the intercondylar notch. The ligament prevents posterior displacement of the tibia in relation to the femur.

Etiology - The most common causes of a PCL injury are landing on the tibia with a flexed knee or hitting a dashboard in a motor vehicle accident with a flexed knee. Isolated PCL tears are not common and often involve other knee structures such as the ACL, MCL, LCL, and menisci.

Signs and Symptoms - The patient may report feeling as if the femur is sliding off the tibia. Swelling and mild pain may be present, but often the patient is asymptomatic. Special tests to identify the presence of a PCL tear include the posterior drawer test and posterior sag sign.

Treatment - Initially RICE, NSAIDs, and analgesics as needed. Physical therapy treatment includes lower extremity strengthening exercises and functional progression. Surgical treatment can occur, however, the procedure is not as evolved as the procedure for the ACL. If surgery is performed, isolated hamstrings exercises are often avoided for a minimum of six weeks.

Rheumatoid Arthritis[31,34,35]

Rheumatoid arthritis is a systemic autoimmune disorder of unknown etiology. The disease presents with a chronic inflammatory reaction in the synovial tissues of a joint that results in erosion of cartilage and supporting structures within the capsule. Onset of rheumatoid arthritis may initially occur at any joint, but it is common in the small joints of the hand, foot, wrist, and ankle. This disease has periods of exacerbation and remission. Rheumatoid arthritis is diagnosed based on the clinical presentation of involved joints, the presence of blood rheumatoid factor, and radiographic changes.

Etiology - The cause of rheumatoid arthritis is unknown. One to two percent of the American population is affected. Women are affected three times more than men and the most common age of onset falls between 40 and 60 years of age.

Signs and Symptoms - onset may be gradual or immediate, symmetrical involvement, pain and tenderness of affected joints, morning stiffness, warm joints, decrease in appetite, malaise, increased fatigue, swan neck deformity (i.e., DIP flexion, PIP hyperextension), boutonniere deformity (i.e., DIP extension, PIP flexion), low grade fever

Treatment - The goal of treatment is to reduce inflammation and pain, promote joint function, and prevent joint destruction and deformity. Pharmacological management includes NSAIDs to reduce inflammation and pain. Corticosteroid medications may be desirable during severe flare-ups or when the patient's condition is not responding to NSAIDs. Disease-modifying antirheumatic medications are slow-acting and take weeks or months to become effective, however, they have the ability to slow the progression of joint destruction and deformity. Physical therapy interventions include passive and active range of motion, heating and cooling agents, splinting, patient education, energy conservation, body mechanics, and joint protection techniques.

Rotator Cuff Tear[16,29,32,33]

The rotator cuff can be torn due to an acute traumatic incident or as a result of a chronic degenerative pathology. Patients 50 years of age and older are particularly susceptible to tears due to chronic degenerative pathology. Rotator cuff tears are classified as partial-thickness or full-thickness. A partial-thickness tear extends through only a portion of the tendon. A full-thickness tear is a complete tear of the tendon. The size of a tear can range from small (1 centimeter or less) to large (more than 5 centimeters).

Etiology - Intrinsic factors associated with rotator cuff tears include impaired blood supply to the tendon, resulting in degeneration. Extrinsic factors include trauma, repetitive microtrauma, and postural abnormalities.

Signs and Symptoms - arm positioned in internal rotation and adduction, point tenderness at the greater tubercle and acromion, marked limitation in shoulder flexion and abduction with upper trapezius recruitment evident, increased tone in anterior shoulder structures

Treatment - Conservative management includes RICE, NSAIDs, and analgesics as needed. The primary focus of therapy is to prevent adhesive capsulitis and strengthen upper extremity musculature. Surgical management to repair the tendon can be arthroscopic, mini-open with arthroscopic assist or a traditional open approach. Following surgery, the patient will be immobilized in a sling. The amount of immobilization time will vary depending on surgeon preference, surgical procedure, and the size of the tear. A large tear may require four to six weeks of immobilization. Physical therapy begins with passive range of motion and gradually moves to active-assisted motion. Active motion and isometric exercises begin once approved by the surgeon. The patient will gradually become functional with activities of daily living and progress to more aggressive strengthening activities. Return to functional activities requiring dynamic overhead motion occurs in 9-12 months.

Scoliosis[13,28,29]

Scoliosis refers to a lateral curvature of the spine. The condition is most often quantified using the Cobb method with a standing radiograph. Scoliosis is often classified as functional, neuromuscular or degenerative. Functional scoliosis results from abnormalities in the body that indirectly impact the spine (e.g., leg length discrepancy, muscle imbalance, poor posture). This type of scoliosis is often referred to as nonstructural scoliosis since the curves are flexible and can be corrected with lateral bending. Neuromuscular scoliosis results from developmental pathology resulting in alterations within the structure of the spine. This type of scoliosis is often observed in patients with cerebral palsy or Marfan syndrome. Degenerative scoliosis occurs due to the normal aging process and is facilitated by changes such as osteophyte formation, bone demineralization, and disk herniation. Neuromuscular and degenerative scoliosis are considered to be forms of structural scoliosis since the curves are inflexible and do not reduce with lateral bending.

Etiology - The development of scoliosis is typically idiopathic. Idiopathic scoliosis is most commonly diagnosed between 10 and 13 years of age. Girls and boys have a similar risk of developing a mild curve (e.g., 10 degrees or less), however, girls have a significantly greater risk of acquiring a curve greater than 30 degrees.

Signs and Symptoms - Shoulder level asymmetry with or without the presence of a rib hump. Pain is not typically associated with the spinal curvature, rather it is a result of the abnormal forces placed on other tissues of the body due to the curvature.

Treatment - The focus of treatment is determined based on the magnitude of the curve and the degree of progression. If the curve is not progressing, generally no formal action is taken. Physical therapy treatment includes muscle strengthening and flexibility exercises, shoe lifts, and bracing. A spinal orthosis is often warranted with a curve that ranges between 25 and 40 degrees. Surgical intervention may be required with curves greater than 40 degrees.

Talipes Equinovarus[30,31]

Talipes equinovarus, also known as "clubfoot," is a deformity characterized by the heel pointing downward and the forefoot turning inward.

Etiology - The cause is unknown, however, theories postulate familial tendency, positioning in utero or a defect in the ovum. This condition accompanies other neuromuscular abnormalities including spina bifida and arthrogryposis, and may result from the lack of movement in utero.

Signs and Symptoms - The clinical presentation includes adduction of the forefoot, varus positioning of the hindfoot, and equinus at the ankle.

Treatment - Medical management begins shortly after birth and includes splinting and serial casting. The goal of intervention is to restore proper positioning of the foot and ankle. Failed management or severe involvement may require surgical intervention and subsequent casting.

Total Hip Arthroplasty[16,18,29,32,36]

Total hip arthroplasty refers to the removal of the proximal and distal joint surfaces of the hip with subsequent replacement by an acetabular component and a femoral implant. The acetabular component is most often press fit into place, although it is occasionally held in place by screws. Bone is removed from the femur with subsequent shaping to accept the femoral stem with the attached prosthetic femoral head. The surgical procedure can utilize an anterolateral, direct lateral or posterolateral approach. The type of approach selected determines the necessary hip precautions post-operatively.

Fixation can be cemented or cementless. Cemented fixation allows weight bearing as tolerated on the involved lower extremity, often immediately, since the cement achieves maximum fixation in approximately 15 minutes. Cementless and hybrid fixation rely on bone growth and may dictate partial weight bearing or non-weight bearing initially. The level of weight bearing is determined by the surgeon, typically based on the mechanical fixation of the prosthesis within the acetabulum and femur. There are advantages and disadvantages of each type of fixation, however, the primary indication for cementless fixation is a young, active individual (e.g., less than 65 years of age). Minimally invasive surgical techniques require one or two incisions, usually less than 10 centimeters in length. The benefit of minimally invasive procedures is less soft tissue trauma and an accelerated post-operative recovery. The average lifespan for a total hip arthroplasty is 15 to 20 years, and as a result, younger individuals may need one or more revision procedures in their lifetime. Complications for total hip arthroplasty include deep vein thrombosis, infection, pulmonary embolus, heterotopic ossification, femoral fractures, dislocation, and neurovascular injury.

Etiology - Total hip arthroplasty is an elective surgical procedure. Medical conditions often associated with the need for total hip arthroplasty include osteoarthritis, rheumatoid arthritis, osteomyelitis, and avascular necrosis.

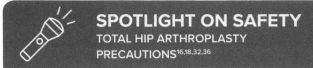

SPOTLIGHT ON SAFETY
TOTAL HIP ARTHROPLASTY PRECAUTIONS[16,18,32,36]

The specific surgical approach utilized for total hip arthroplasty is determined based on a variety of factors including patient activity level, co-morbidities, life expectancy, anticipated compliance, and surgeon familiarity. Physical therapist assistants must have an awareness of each type of approach including the structures impacted and the associated hip precautions.

Surgical approaches and associated hip precautions:

Anterolateral approach - Access to the hip occurs through the interval between the tensor fasciae latae and the gluteus medius muscle. Some portion of the hip abductors are released from the greater trochanter and the hip is dislocated anteriorly.

Hip precautions: Avoid flexion of the hip beyond 90 degrees, extension of the hip, lateral rotation, and adduction.

Direct lateral approach - This approach leaves the posterior portion of the gluteus medius attached to the greater trochanter. It requires longitudinal division of the tensor fasciae latae and vastus lateralis, along with a release of the anterior portion of the gluteus medius. Since the posterior soft tissues and capsule are left intact, the approach minimizes the probability of dislocation and may be ideal for noncompliant patients.

Hip precautions: Avoid flexion of the hip beyond 90 degrees, extension of the hip, lateral rotation, and adduction.

Posterolateral approach - Access to the hip occurs by splitting the gluteus maximus muscle in line with the muscle fibers. The short external rotators are then released and the hip abductors are retracted anteriorly. This approach maintains the integrity of the gluteus medius and vastus lateralis muscles. The femur is then dislocated posteriorly. Although it is the most commonly used approach for total hip arthroplasty, the procedure results in a high post-surgical dislocation rate.

Hip precautions: Avoid flexion of the hip beyond 90 degrees, adduction, and medial rotation.

Signs and Symptoms - Prior to surgery, there is severe pain with weight bearing, loss of mobility, gross instability or limitation in range of motion, failure of non-operative management or a previous surgical procedure.

Treatment - Initially physical therapy management focuses on decreasing inflammation and allowing tissues to heal, emphasizing adherence to hip precautions, minimizing muscle atrophy, and regaining full passive range of motion. Treatment may include ankle pumps, quadriceps and gluteal sets, active hip flexion within available range of motion, assistive device training, and progressive ambulation. As the patient progresses, treatment moves toward regaining full strength and endurance and attaining independence in the home setting.

Total Knee Arthroplasty[16,18,29,32,33,36]

Total knee arthroplasty refers to the removal of the proximal and distal joint surfaces of the knee and replacing them with an implant. The procedure is the most commonly performed surgery for advanced arthritis of the knee. Total knee arthroplasty can be classified several different ways. The first classification is based on the number of compartments replaced. Unicompartmental indicates that only the medial or lateral joint surface was replaced. Bicompartmental indicates that the entire surface of the femur and tibia were replaced, while a tricompartmental procedure includes replacement of the femur and tibia along with the patella. The implant design can be classified by the degree of constraint. An unconstrained design offers no inherent stability and relies on soft tissue integrity for stability. This type of design is used primarily with unicompartmental arthroplasty. A semiconstrained design offers some degree of stability without compromising mobility. This is the most common classification of total knee arthroplasty. A fully constrained design offers the most stability by restricting one or more planes of motion. This results in greater implant stress with a higher likelihood of implant problems (e.g., wear, failure, loosening). The average lifespan for a total knee arthroplasty is 15-20 years, and as a result, younger individuals may need one or more revision procedures in their lifetime.

Minimally invasive surgical techniques are becoming more common with total knee arthroplasty. The procedure requires only a 3-5 inch incision instead of the 8-12 inches typically required with a traditional procedure. As a result, there is less soft tissue trauma and minimal damage to the quadriceps muscle, which allows the muscle to initially produce a stronger contraction. This is extremely relevant since quadriceps weakness is correlated with an increased risk of falling. There remains a paucity of research available to determine long-term outcomes associated with the minimally invasive surgical procedure, however, preliminary data suggests positive outcomes including decreased hospital stays, improved range of motion, and improved strength.

Fixation methods include cemented, uncemented (i.e., bone ingrowth), and hybrid. The type of fixation selected is influenced by a variety of factors including patient activity level, co-morbidities, life expectancy, and tightness of fit of the femoral component achieved during surgery. Cemented remains the most common method of fixation. Potential complications of total knee arthroplasty include deep vein thrombosis, infection, pulmonary embolus, peroneal nerve palsy, restricted range of motion, periprosthetic fractures, and chronic joint effusion.

Etiology - Total knee arthroplasty is an elective surgical procedure. Medical conditions often associated with the need for total knee arthroplasty include osteoarthritis and osteomyelitis.

Signs and Symptoms - Prior to surgery there is severe pain with weight bearing, loss of mobility, gross instability or limitation in range of motion, marked deformity of the knee, failure of non-operative management or a previous surgical procedure.

Treatment - Initially, physical therapy treatment focuses on decreasing inflammation and allowing tissues to heal, emphasizing adherence to knee precautions, minimizing muscle atrophy, and regaining full passive range of motion. Knee flexion requires

CONSIDER THIS
DISCHARGE GUIDELINES FOLLOWING TOTAL HIP ARTHROPLASTY[16,18,32,36]

Patients may need to remain compliant with a strict set of discharge guidelines, typically for up to three months following total hip arthroplasty. Failure to follow the guidelines potentially jeopardizes the integrity of the surgical procedure and creates an unnecessary safety risk. The specific guidelines that are most critical for a patient upon discharge will be heavily influenced by the surgical approach and the type of fixation utilized.

General guidelines include:

- Avoid crossing the legs when in a sitting position.
- Sit in firm chairs and avoid sitting in low or soft furniture. Limit forward bending when sitting or standing up.
- Stand with the feet in a neutral position (avoid turning the toes inward).
- Use a pillow or splint between the legs when in bed.
- Avoid pulling blankets up in bed with forward bending.
- Place a nightstand on the same side of the bed as the uninvolved side.
- Use a raised toilet seat or portable commode for toileting activities.
- Use a rubber, non-skid bath mat in the shower.
- Use a long handled brush to avoid leaning forward when bathing.
- Remove all throw rugs and always walk with appropriate footwear.
- When walking, turn to the uninvolved side to avoid pivoting on the involved side.
- Walk for short periods and gradually increase the time period to improve endurance.
- When ascending stairs, step up with the uninvolved leg.
- When descending stairs, step down with the involved leg.

  *These guidelines apply to traditional total hip arthroplasty and may not be necessary with minimally invasive procedures.

a minimum of 90 degrees for activities of daily living and 105 degrees to rise comfortably from sitting. Therapeutic activities include ankle pumps, quadriceps and gluteal sets, active range of motion within available range, use of a continuous passive motion machine, assistive device training, and progressive ambulation.

As the patient progresses, treatment moves toward regaining full strength, endurance, and independence in the home setting. Advanced therapeutic activities include wall slides, controlled lunges, stationary cycling, and step ups.

Orthopedic Surgical Procedures and Considerations[18,28,29,31,32,33]

Spine

Laminectomy

Surgical considerations: A laminectomy is usually performed in the presence of a disk protrusion or spinal stenosis. A complete laminectomy involves the removal of the entire lamina, the spinous process, and the associated ligamentum flavum. A partial laminectomy involves the removal of only one lamina. In cases where a complete laminectomy is performed, the vertebral segment will be much less stable than when a partial laminectomy is performed. Both cervical and lumbar laminectomies are generally performed using a posterior approach.

Rehab considerations: There will likely be restrictions on how much weight can be lifted following surgery. The surgeon may also place restrictions on active motions, especially extension. The physical therapist assistant should emphasize the need for proper body mechanics and posture with the patient.

Spinal fusion

Surgical considerations: Spinal fusion is indicated in the presence of axial pain with unstable spinal segments, advanced arthritis, or uncontrolled peripheral pain. Bone is harvested from the patient's body (often from the iliac crest) and used to help fuse two vertebrae together. Generally the surgeon will use instrumentation (e.g., pedicle screws) to immobilize the segments while a bony callus forms between the segments. Cervical fusion typically uses an anterior approach while lumbar fusion typically uses a posterior approach. Because a fusion creates immobility at one spinal segment, it inherently leads to hypermobility at adjacent segments, which can hasten the onset of degeneration.

Rehab considerations: The surgeon will likely place restrictions on how much can be lifted following surgery. The surgeon may also place restrictions on active motion, such as bending or twisting motions. Early therapy occurs post-operatively in the hospital and involves teaching bed mobility and transfers with the patient to help them become more mobile without compromising the established precautions. Bracing (e.g., cervical collar, thoraco-lumbar-sacral orthosis) may be used to help patients comply with the movement precautions. Bracing is more likely to be used if the surgeon does not use instrumentation to stabilize the segments. Formal outpatient therapy does not usually occur until approximately 6 weeks after the surgery. If instrumentation is used, therapy will usually begin sooner and can be progressed more aggressively. Emphasis should be placed on proper body mechanics and posture, as well as core stabilization exercises.

Upper Extremity

Total shoulder arthroplasty

Surgical considerations: Shoulder arthroplasty is often performed when joint components have become arthritic, though may also be done secondary to fracture or rotator cuff arthropathy. Total shoulder arthroplasty replaces both the glenoid and humeral components, while a shoulder hemiarthroplasty replaces only one of those components. A reverse total shoulder arthroplasty is performed by reversing the concave-convex relationship of the prosthetic components and is used as the surgery of choice when the patient has a dysfunctional rotator cuff. All of these surgeries usually involve an anterior approach in which the subscapularis muscle is detached for easier access to the joint.

Rehab considerations: The patient will be immobilized in a sling for several weeks or longer if there was a repair performed on muscles/tendons (e.g., subscapularis). Protocols vary widely after these surgeries, but there likely will be some movement precautions for a short period of time (e.g., 6-8 weeks). For example, the patient often has to avoid extension and external rotation movements to help protect the healing subscapularis muscle and anterior portion of the capsule. Resisted internal rotation is also avoided for some time for this same reason. There may also be restrictions on weight bearing through the arm and limitations on lifting or carrying weight.

Subacromial decompression

Surgical considerations: This surgery is performed when cases of shoulder impingement have not responded to conservative treatment. The approach can be open (deltoid is detached), a mini-open (deltoid is only split) or arthroscopic. The procedure could involve an acromioplasty, bursectomy, removal of the distal clavicle (in cases where it is degenerated), and release of the coracoacromial ligament.

Rehab considerations: Typically patients experience a rapid recovery from this surgery. A sling will only be used for 1-2 weeks since no repair has been performed. Early rehab focuses on pain control and gentle range of motion, with strength training occurring later in rehab. If a deltoid repair was performed, passive extension is avoided initially to prevent stress on the repair site. Treatment should focus on interventions to reduce the occurrence of impingement (e.g., posture, strengthening scapular upward rotators). A full recovery is typically expected.

Rotator cuff repair

Surgical considerations: Rotator cuff tears are graded according to depth (partial vs. full) and according to width (small <1 cm, medium 1-3 cm, large 3-5 cm, massive >5 cm). Small partial-thickness tears may only require debridement; all others likely require a repair to be performed, in which the tear is reapproximated and fixated using sutures, anchors, tacks or staples. As with a subacromial decompression, the surgery is generally performed arthroscopically, though an open or mini-open approach may be necessary.

Rehab considerations: The patient will be immobilized in a sling for several weeks, and the sling may have an abduction pillow attached to it. Sling use is generally at the discretion of the surgeon and often depends on the extent of the tear/repair. Rehab protocols vary, but therapy usually consists of passive and active-assisted range of motion initially, with strengthening occurring later in the course of therapy. Precautions generally include no active range of motion, lifting, or weight bearing through the arm for several weeks. Depending on which muscle is repaired, there may be precautions set on range of motion for rotation as well. If a deltoid repair was performed, passive extension is avoided initially to prevent stress on the repair site.

Shoulder stabilization surgeries

Surgical considerations: The capsular shift procedure is performed in the presence of chronic shoulder instability. The procedure involves tightening of the joint capsule by cutting the capsule and overlapping the ends to reduce capsular redundancy. There is also an electrothermally assisted capsular shift procedure in which thermal energy is used to shrink and tighten the capsular tissue. The portion of the capsule that is tightened is dependent upon the direction of the instability. Since anterior instability is the most common form of shoulder instability, the anterior capsule is the portion that is most often tightened. In addition to the capsular shift procedure, labral repairs may also be performed since labral tears often accompany dislocation injuries. A Bankart repair involves a repair of the anterior labrum. A SLAP repair involves a repair of the superior labrum. These procedures are generally performed arthroscopically, though can also be done as an open procedure. If the procedure is open then the subscapularis muscle may need to be detached.

Rehab considerations: The type of immobilization used and the precautions will depend on the portion of the capsule that was affected. If the anterior capsule was affected, then the patient will typically utilize a normal sling. They should avoid positions of external rotation, extension, and horizontal abduction. They should also avoid resisted internal rotation if the subscapularis muscle was detached during the surgery. If the posterior capsule was affected, the patient would be immobilized in the "hand shake" position with the shoulder in neutral rotation. The patient should avoid positions of internal rotation, flexion, and horizontal adduction. Active range of motion can begin soon after the surgery. Therapists should not wait for full range of motion before beginning strengthening exercises and should not be overly aggressive in getting full motion early. If a SLAP repair has been performed, the patient should avoid contracting or stretching the biceps since the biceps is attached to the superior labrum.

Lower Extremity

Hip ORIF

Surgical considerations: Proximal hip fractures commonly occur in the femoral neck or in the intertrochanteric region. Femoral neck fractures are intracapsular and may lead to a disruption of the blood supply to the femoral head. Because of this, nonunion and osteonecrosis are more common with these fractures. Intertrochanteric hip fractures are extracapsular and therefore do not affect the blood supply. Though nonunion is less of an issue, implant failure is more of a problem with these fractures since the fixation needed is greater. Fractures can also occur in the subtrochanteric region, which is the region distal to the trochanters. There are several methods of fixation for hip fractures, and the method used depends on fracture location, amount of displacement, and the patient's activity level. Fixation usually occurs with the use of plates and screws or an intramedullary nail. For older patients with poor healing capacity, total hip arthroplasty is often considered. The surgery is always an open procedure. Depending on the approach, the tensor fasciae latae, gluteus medius, and vastus lateralis may be affected. If the fracture site is intracapsular, a capsulotomy will be performed.

Rehab considerations: New advances in this surgery have allowed for early weight bearing, though weight bearing restrictions will be based on age, the location of the fracture, and the bone quality. Early rehab consists of ambulation and range of motion. Isotonic strengthening is usually postponed until the muscles have been given a chance to heal. The muscles affected depend not only on the surgical approach, but also on the site of the fracture. For example, fractures of the greater trochanter will affect the gluteus medius, while fractures of the lesser trochanter will affect the iliopsoas. Therapists should be aware of signs of fixation failure, such as persistent thigh or groin pain, a leg length discrepancy that was not present initially, positioning the limb in external rotation, or a Trendelenburg sign that does not improve with strengthening.

Surgeries to fix articular cartilage defects

Surgical considerations: There are several different options for fixing focal cartilage defects. The microfracture procedure uses an awl to penetrate subchondral bone, which causes an ingrowth of fibrocartilage. Osteochondral autograft transplantation is a procedure in which cartilage is harvested from several non-weight bearing surfaces to form a plug that can fill the chondral defect. Autologous chondrocyte implantation is a procedure in which healthy cartilage is harvested and cultured so it will grow, then later implanted into the cartilage defect.

Rehab considerations: There will likely be weight bearing restrictions, though this is dependent upon the size and location of the lesion. Adherence to weight bearing restrictions is critical to allow healing to occur. The patient will often be in a brace that is initially locked into extension. Range of motion progression will also vary depending on the size and location of the lesion. In general, larger lesions require a slower overall progression.

Anterior cruciate ligament reconstruction

Surgical considerations: This surgery is performed on patients with an anterior cruciate ligament tear that is causing pain and/or instability. The surgery is generally performed arthroscopically.

Use of an autograft is preferred over allograft. A bone-patellar tendon-bone graft is considered the gold standard. Because it uses bone-to-bone healing, it is considered a stronger graft with good fixation. Use of the gracilis and/or semitendinosus is also common, however, the fixation is not as strong since it uses tendon-to-bone healing.

Rehab considerations: Rehab protocols will vary widely, but there generally is some period of immobilization in a hinged brace (initially locked in extension) in addition to weight bearing restrictions. The brace usually is unlocked once the patient can demonstrate good quadriceps control. Range of motion interventions should place an emphasis on achieving full knee extension early in the rehabilitative process. Strengthening exercises can occur soon after surgery and typically include isometric quadriceps strengthening, hamstrings strengthening, and closed-chain exercises. Open-chain exercises between 0-45 degrees of flexion should be avoided since they place excess stress on the graft site. Patients receiving a bone-patellar tendon-bone graft may experience anterior knee pain and should be cautious with quadriceps strengthening. Likewise, those receiving a hamstring graft should be cautious with flexion exercises. It is important for the therapist to remember that the graft tissue is most vulnerable at 6-8 weeks after surgery. As the tendon transforms into ligamentous tissue, it actually becomes weaker before it gets stronger. Failure of the graft site generally happens around that time secondary to poor compliance with the protocol. Graft maturation has been shown to be at 100% around 12-16 months post-operatively, however, most protocols allow for return to sports closer to 6 months. There are several criteria that patients wishing to return to sports must satisfy including no pain or effusion, full range of motion, no instability, quadriceps strength that is 85-90% of the opposite leg, hamstring strength that is 90-100% of the opposite leg, and functional testing (e.g., single leg hop) that is 85-90% of the opposite leg.

Posterior cruciate ligament reconstruction

Surgical considerations: Injuries to the posterior cruciate ligament (PCL) are much less common than anterior cruciate ligament (ACL) injuries. If the PCL injury occurs in isolation, surgery may not be needed. Surgery is indicated if pain and/or instability do not improve with therapy. Options for grafts are similar to those for ACL surgery.

Rehab considerations: In general, the rehab protocol is the same as with ACL surgery. However, the progression with weight bearing and with exercises tends to be more gradual. The therapist should choose exercises that will limit posterior shear forces within the knee. Repetitive knee flexion should also be avoided.

Surgeries for meniscus injuries

Surgical considerations: The surgery for a meniscus tear is generally performed arthroscopically. Meniscus tears can be dealt with surgically in two ways. The first option is a partial meniscectomy in which the torn piece of meniscus is removed. This option is usually chosen for older individuals or when the tear occurs in the inner two-thirds of the meniscus where the healing capacity is poor. The other surgical option is to perform a repair of the meniscus in which the tear is sutured back together. This option is more likely to be chosen in younger patients or when the tear is in the outer third of the meniscus.

Rehab considerations: The rehab protocol will depend on whether or not the meniscus was repaired. Following a meniscus repair, there will likely be a period of restricted weight bearing in addition to bracing. There will also likely be limitations placed on the progression of range of motion, specifically with flexion. Following a partial meniscectomy, the patient is full weight bearing without the use of a brace. There are no rehab restrictions and recovery time is significantly quicker.

Lateral ankle reconstruction

Surgical considerations: Repair of the lateral ankle ligaments is commonly performed secondary to a complete tear of the anterior talofibular ligament or calcaneofibular ligament or secondary to chronic ankle instability. There are two methods for reconstructing the ankle, both of which use an open approach. The first method involves actual repair of the torn ligaments in which they are sutured back together. The second method involves the harvesting of an autograft (usually the peroneus brevis) to replace the torn ligaments. This second option is usually performed when the original ligaments cannot be repaired due to deterioration. The surgery may also include arthroscopy or subchondral drilling since a high percentage of unstable ankles have chondral lesions within the joint.

Rehab considerations: The patient will usually be in a protective cast for a short period of time (e.g., one week), then they are placed in a walking cast or boot for several weeks, followed by a brace. Initially the patient is non-weight bearing while in the protective cast, which is progressed to partial weight bearing and full weight bearing once in the walking boot. Therapy does not usually begin immediately after surgery. Early rehab focuses on increasing the patient's range of motion while still protecting the repaired tissues. Caution should be taken when ranging the ankle into inversion since this will stress the repaired tissues. Bracing may be required long term if the patient plans to return to sports or higher level activities.

Achilles tendon repair

Surgical considerations: This surgery is performed on active patients with an Achilles tendon tear. When the repair is performed within days of the injury, it is generally done arthroscopically. The torn portion of the tendon is sutured back together. However, when the repair is delayed after the injury, the surgery may need to be performed as an open procedure. Additionally, augmentation with use of a graft (e.g., flexor hallucis longus, peroneus brevis, plantaris) may be needed for the repair instead of suturing together the original tendon.

Rehab considerations: The patient will likely be casted with the ankle in slight plantar flexion initially. Additionally, the patient may be non-weight bearing for the first several weeks. Eventually, the patient is transitioned to a cast or boot that places the ankle in neutral and they are allowed to be partial weight bearing. However, in the past few decades, there has been a push for more aggressive rehab following this surgery, in which the ankle is casted in neutral and partial weight bearing is allowed much sooner in the recovery process. Researchers have found that this leads to less restricted range of motion long term. During the healing process, the therapist should take caution with exercises that stretch the Achilles tendon or require active plantar flexion until the tendon is well healed.

Types of Fractures[31]

Avulsion fracture: A portion of a bone becomes fragmented at the site of tendon attachment due to a traumatic and sudden stretch of the tendon.

Closed fracture: A break in a bone where the skin over the site remains intact.

Comminuted fracture: A bone that breaks into fragments at the site of injury.

Compound fracture: A break in a bone that protrudes through the skin.

Greenstick fracture: A break on one side of a bone that does not damage the periosteum on the opposite side. This type of fracture is often seen in children.

Nonunion fracture: A break in a bone that has failed to unite and heal after nine to twelve months.

Stress fracture: A break in a bone due to repeated forces to a particular portion of the bone.

Spiral fracture: A break in a bone shaped like an "S" due to torsion and twisting.

Pharmacological Management of the Musculoskeletal System[37,38,39]

Disease-modifying Antirheumatic Agents

Action: Disease-modifying antirheumatic drugs (DMARD) slow or halt the progression of rheumatic disease. They are used early during the disease process to slow the progression prior to widespread damage of the affected joints. They act to induce remission by modifying the pathology and inhibiting the immune response responsible for rheumatic disease.

Indications: rheumatic disease, preferably during early treatment

Side effects: (depending on classification of DMARD) nausea, headache, joint pain and swelling, toxicity, gastrointestinal distress, sore throat, fever, liver dysfunction, hair loss, potential for sepsis, retinal damage

Implications for PT: Therapists should recognize that many of the agents have a high incidence of toxicity.

Examples: Rheumatrex, Arava

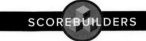

Glucocorticoid Agents (Corticosteroids)

Action: Glucocorticoids provide hormonal, anti-inflammatory, and metabolic effects including suppression of articular and systemic diseases. These agents reduce inflammation in chronic conditions that can damage healthy tissue through a series of reactions. Vasoconstriction results from stabilizing lysosomal membranes and enhancing the effects of catecholamines.

Indications: replacement therapy for endocrine dysfunction, anti-inflammatory and immunosuppressive effects; treatment of rheumatic, respiratory, and various other disorders

Side effects: muscle atrophy, gastrointestinal distress, glaucoma, adrenocortical suppression, drug-induced Cushing's syndrome, weakening with breakdown of supporting tissues (bone, ligament, tendon, skin), mood changes, hypertension

Implications for PT: A therapist must wear a mask when working with patients on glucocorticoid therapy since their immune system is weakened. A therapist must be aware of signs of toxicity including moon face, buffalo hump, and personality changes. Patients are at risk for osteoporosis and muscle wasting. Treatment of an injected joint will require special care due to ligament and tendon laxity or weakening.

Examples: Dermacort, Cordrol

Nonopioid Agents

Action: Nonopioid agents provide analgesia and pain relief, produce anti-inflammatory effects, and initiate anti-pyretic (reduces fever) properties. These drugs promote a reduction of prostaglandin formation that decreases the inflammatory process, decreases uterine contractions, lowers fever, and minimizes impulse formation of pain fibers.

Indications: mild to moderate pain of various origins, fever, headache, muscle ache, inflammation (except acetaminophen), primary dysmenorrhea, reduction of risk of myocardial infarction (aspirin only)

Side effects: nausea, vomiting, vertigo, abdominal pain, gastro-intestinal distress or bleeding, ulcer formation, potential for Reye syndrome in children (aspirin only)

Implications for PT: Patients are at increased risk for masked pain that would allow for movement beyond limitation or false understanding of their level of mobility. Complaints of stomach pain should be taken seriously with a subsequent referral to a physician.

Examples: Tylenol, Aspirin

Opioid Agents (Narcotics)

Action: Opioid agents provide analgesia for acute severe pain management. The medication stimulates opioid receptors within the CNS to prevent pain impulses from reaching their destination. Certain drugs are also used to assist with dependency and withdrawal symptoms.

Indications: moderate to severe pain of various origins, induction of conscious sedation prior to a diagnostic procedure, management of opioid dependence, relief of severe and persistent cough (codeine)

Side effects: mood swings, sedation, confusion, vertigo, dulled cognitive function, orthostatic hypotension, constipation, incoordination, physical dependence, tolerance

Implications for PT: A therapist must monitor the patient for potential side effects, especially signs of respiratory depression. Treatment that is otherwise painful should be scheduled approximately two hours after administration to maximize the analgesic benefit. A patient may not accurately report if a particular technique is painful.

Examples: Demerol, OxyContin

Musculoskeletal System Terminology[2,10,16]

Bursitis: A condition caused by acute or chronic inflammation of the bursae. Symptoms may include a limitation in active range of motion secondary to pain and swelling.

Contusion: A sudden blow to a part of the body that can result in mild to severe damage to superficial and deep structures. Treatment includes active range of motion, ice, and compression.

Edema: An increased volume of fluid in the soft tissue outside of a joint capsule.

Effusion: An increased volume of fluid within a joint capsule.

Genu valgum: A condition where the knees touch while standing with the feet separated. Genu valgum will increase compression of the lateral tibial condyle and increase stress to the medial structures. Genu valgum is also termed knock-kneed.

Genu varum: A condition where there is bowing of the legs with added space between the knees while standing with the feet together. Genu varum will increase compression of the medial tibial condyle and increase stress to the lateral structures. Genu varum is also termed bowleg.

Kyphosis: An excessive curvature of the spine in a posterior direction, usually identified in the thoracic spine. Common causes include osteoporosis, compression fractures, and poor posture secondary to paralysis.

Lordosis: An excessive curvature of the spine in an anterior direction, usually identified in the cervical or lumbar spine. Common causes include weak abdominal muscles, pregnancy, excessive weight in the abdominal area, and hip flexion contractures.

Q angle: The degree of angulation present when measuring from the midpatella to the anterior superior iliac spine and to the tibial tubercle. A normal Q angle measured in supine with the knee straight is 13 degrees for a male and 18 degrees for a female. An excessive Q angle can lead to pathology and abnormal tracking.

Sprain: An acute injury involving a ligament.

- **Grade I** – mild pain and swelling, little to no tear of the ligament
- **Grade II** – moderate pain and swelling, minimal instability of the joint, minimal to moderate tearing of the ligament, decreased range of motion
- **Grade III** – severe pain and swelling, substantial joint instability, total tear of the ligament, substantial decrease in range of motion

Strain: An injury involving the musculotendinous unit that involves a muscle, tendon or their attachments to bone.

- **Grade I** – localized pain, minimal swelling, and tenderness
- **Grade II** – localized pain, moderate swelling, tenderness, and impaired motor function
- **Grade III** – a palpable defect of the muscle, severe pain, and poor motor function

Tendonitis: A condition caused by acute or chronic inflammation of a tendon. Symptoms may include gradual onset, tenderness, swelling, and pain.

Orthotics

An orthotic is an external device that provides support or stabilization, improves function, corrects deformities, and distributes pressure from one area to another. Orthotics are made from a variety of materials including plastic, metal, leather, fabric, elastic or hybrid materials. They can be custom made or over-the-counter and are available in various prefabricated sizes. Orthotics should be lightweight, adjustable, and easy to don and doff.

Functions of orthotics include preventing deformity, maintaining proper alignment, inhibiting tone, assisting weak limbs, protecting against injury, and facilitating motion.

Factors to consider when prescribing an orthotic include static versus dynamic, temporary versus permanent, level of support required, energy efficiency, cosmesis, and cost.

Spine[36, 40, 41]

Corset

A corset is constructed of fabric and may have metal uprights within the material to provide abdominal compression and support. Corsets are utilized to provide pressure and relieve pain associated with mid and low back pathologies.

Halo Vest Orthosis

The halo vest is an invasive cervical thoracic orthosis that provides full restriction of all cervical motion. A metal ring with four posts that attach to a vest is placed on a patient and secured by inserting four pins through the ring into the skull. This orthosis is commonly used with cervical spinal cord injuries to prevent further damage or dislocation during the recovery period. A patient will wear a halo vest until the spine becomes stable.

Milwaukee Orthosis

The Milwaukee orthosis is designed to promote realignment of the spine due to scoliotic curvature. The orthosis is custom made and extends from the pelvis to the upper chest. Corrective padding is applied to the areas of severity of the curve.

Taylor Brace

The Taylor brace is a thoracolumbosacral orthosis that limits trunk flexion and extension through a three-point control design.

Thoracolumbosacral Orthosis (TLSO)

A custom molded TLSO is utilized to prevent all trunk motions and is commonly utilized as a means of post-surgical stabilization. The rigid shell is fabricated from plastics in a bivalve style using straps/Velcro to secure the orthosis.

Lower Extremity[36, 40-42]

Foot Orthosis

A semirigid or rigid insert worn inside a shoe that corrects foot alignment and improves function. May also be used to relieve pain. A foot orthosis is custom molded and is often designed for a specific level of functioning.

Ankle-foot Orthosis (AFO)

A metal ankle-foot orthosis consists of two metal uprights connected proximally to a calf band and distally to a mechanical ankle joint and shoe. The ankle joint may have the ability to be locked and not allow any motion, or set to have limited anterior/posterior capability depending on the patient's need. A plastic ankle-foot orthosis is fabricated by a cast mold of the patient's lower extremity. The use of plastic is more cosmetic, lighter, and requires that if a patient presents with edema it does not significantly fluctuate. Proper fit of a plastic ankle-foot orthosis requires that a patient be casted in a subtalar neutral position. A footplate can be incorporated into the ankle foot orthosis to assist with tone reduction. Solid ankle-foot orthoses control dorsiflexion/plantar flexion and also inversion/eversion with a trim line anterior to the malleoli. They can be fabricated to keep the ankle positioned at 90 degrees or can be fabricated with an articulating ankle joint. This articulation allows the tibia to advance over the foot during the mid to late stance phase of gait. A posterior leaf spring is a plastic AFO with a trim line posterior to the malleoli. Its primary purpose is to assist with dorsiflexion and prevent foot drop. It requires adequate medial/lateral control by the patient. Ankle-foot orthoses can also influence knee control. A floor reaction AFO assists with knee extension during stance through positioning of a calf band and/or positioning at the ankle. Ankle-foot orthoses are commonly prescribed for patients with peripheral neuropathy, nerve lesions or hemiplegia.

Knee-ankle-foot Orthosis (KAFO)

A knee-ankle-foot orthosis provides support and stability to the knee and ankle. The orthosis can be fabricated using two metal uprights extending from the foot/shoe to the thigh with calf and thigh bands. Plastic knee-ankle-foot orthoses are fabricated by a cast mold of the patient's lower extremity. A plastic thigh shell is connected to a plastic ankle-foot orthosis through metal uprights lateral and medial to the knee joint. Both types allow for a lock mechanism at the knee that provides stability. The ankle is also held in proper alignment.

Craig-Scott Knee-ankle-foot Orthosis

A knee-ankle-foot orthosis designed specifically for persons with paraplegia. This design allows a person to stand with a posterior lean of the trunk.

Hip-knee-ankle-foot Orthosis (HKAFO)

A hip-knee-ankle-foot orthosis is indicated for patients with hip, foot, knee, and ankle weakness. It consists of bilateral knee-ankle-foot orthoses with an extension to the hip joints and a pelvic band. The orthosis can control rotation at the hip and abduction/adduction. The orthosis is heavy and restricts patients to a swing-to or swing-through gait pattern.

Reciprocating Gait Orthosis (RGO)

A reciprocating gait orthosis is a derivative of the HKAFO and incorporates a cable system to assist with advancement of the lower extremities during gait. When the patient shifts weight onto a selected lower extremity, the cable system advances the opposite lower extremity. The orthoses are used primarily for patients with paraplegia.

Parapodium

A parapodium is a standing frame designed to allow a patient to sit when necessary. It is a prefabricated frame and ambulation is achieved by shifting weight and rocking the base across the floor. It is primarily used by the pediatric population.

Heel wedge: A heel wedge can be applied to the medial heel to prevent excessive hindfoot eversion or to the lateral heel to prevent excessive hindfoot inversion. Heel wedges can be used to treat symptoms associated with pes planus or pes cavus.

Heel lift: A heel lift is a rigid insert which adds extra height to the heel of a shoe. Heel lifts are commonly used to take pressure off of the Achilles tendon for patients with Achilles tendonitis or a recent repair of the tendon. Heel lifts are also used to help limit the effects of a leg length discrepancy.

Heel cushion: A heel cushion is a soft pad that is placed on the heel of the inner sole to help cushion the heel and thus decrease pain in that region. Heel cushions may be used for a patient with a calcaneal spur or plantar fasciitis.

Heel cup: A heel cup is a rigid insert that covers the plantar surface of the calcaneus and extends upwards on all three sides. A heel cup helps stabilize the calcaneus in a neutral position as well as provide some shock absorption for the heel. It is commonly used for patients with a calcaneal spur or plantar fasciitis.

Metatarsal bar/pad: A metatarsal bar or pad is a flat piece of padding that is placed just posterior to the metatarsal heads either on the outer sole (i.e., bar) or the inner sole (i.e., pad) of the shoe. The placement of the bar/pad helps relieve pressure from the metatarsal heads by transferring it to the metatarsal shafts, thus helping relieve pain for patients with metatarsalgia.

Rocker bar: A rocker bar is similar to a metatarsal bar in its placement, though it consists of a convex strip instead of a flat strip. Because of its shape and position, it assists patients who have difficulty with the terminal stance phase of gait secondary to limited mobility within the foot, especially the great toe. A rocker bar also helps relieve pressure from the metatarsal heads for patients with pain in that region.

Amputations and Prosthetics

Amputation is the surgical removal of a body part, partial or full extremity, due to disease, trauma or injury. Lower extremity amputations are significantly more common than upper extremity amputations, with peripheral vascular disease serving as the primary etiology. A commonly encountered client with limb loss is an older adult who underwent lower-limb amputation due to vascular disease. Many of these individuals have a comorbid diagnosis of diabetes. Other non-vascular causes of amputations include traumatic, cancer-related, and congenital conditions.

Amputation is considered the last course of action, but for many patients with various pathologies, it may become the only viable treatment option. Approximately 50% of all older adults with limb loss due to vascular disease will die within five years. Of the remaining individuals, 50% will experience another amputation, either on the same limb or contralaterally.

Prosthetics attempt to replace the missing body part to allow a patient improved function and cosmesis. Physical and occupational therapy are usually indicated for functional retraining with the prosthesis. Rehabilitation of an individual with limb loss requires a multidisciplinary approach typically involving a prosthetist, physical therapist, and occupational therapist.

Forequarter (scapulothoracic): Surgical removal of the upper extremity including the shoulder girdle.

Shoulder disarticulation: Surgical removal of the upper extremity through the shoulder.

Transhumeral: Surgical removal of the upper extremity proximal to the elbow joint.

Elbow disarticulation: Surgical removal of the lower arm and hand through the elbow joint.

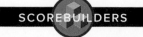

Transradial: Surgical removal of the upper extremity distal to the elbow joint.

Wrist disarticulation: Surgical removal of the hand through the wrist joint.

Partial hand: Surgical removal of a portion of the hand and/or digits at either the transcarpal, transmetacarpal or transphalangeal level.

Digital amputation: Surgical removal of a digit at either the metacarpophalangeal, proximal interphalangeal or distal interphalangeal level.

Types of Lower Extremity Amputations[40,48]

Hemicorporectomy: Surgical removal of the pelvis and both lower extremities.

Hemipelvectomy: Surgical removal of one half of the pelvis and the lower extremity.

Hip disarticulation: Surgical removal of the lower extremity from the pelvis.

Transfemoral: Surgical removal of the lower extremity above the knee joint.

Knee disarticulation: Surgical removal of the lower extremity through the knee joint.

Transtibial: Surgical removal of the lower extremity below the knee joint.

Syme's: Surgical removal of the foot at the ankle joint with removal of the malleoli.

Transverse tarsal (Chopart's): Amputation through the talonavicular and calcaneocuboid joints. The amputation preserves the plantar flexors, but sacrifices the dorsiflexors often resulting in an equinus contracture.

Tarsometatarsal (Lisfranc): Surgical removal of the metatarsals. The amputation preserves the dorsiflexors and plantar flexors.

Components of an Upper Extremity Prosthesis[40,46,48]		
	Transradial	**Transhumeral**
Socket	• Standard socket covers two-thirds of forearm • Standard socket may be shortened to allow for increased pronation/supination ability • Supracondylar sockets are self-suspending and require no additional harness apparatus	• Standard socket extends to acromion level • Modified design allows for more stability with rotational movements • Lightweight friction units may be used with passive prosthetic arms
Suspension	• Triceps cuff • Harness • Cable system	• Harness • Cable system • Suction
Elbow unit	• Attaches to either triceps cuff or upper arm pad • Flexible or rigid hinge connects socket to proximal component	• Internal or external locking elbow unit
Wrist unit	• Quick change unit • Wrist flexion unit • Ball and socket • Constant friction	• Same as transradial
Terminal device	• Voluntary opening or closing • Body-powered, externally powered, myoelectric or hybrid • Hook, mechanical hand, cosmetic glove	• Same as transradial

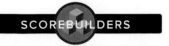

Components of a Lower Extremity Prosthesis[44,46,48]

	Transfemoral	Transtibial
Socket	• Quadrilateral socket • Ischial containment socket	• Patella tendon bearing socket (PTB) • Supracondylar patella tendon socket (PTS) • Supracondylar – suprapatellar socket (SC-SP)

Suspension	• Lanyard strap
	• Shuttle lock
	• Suction
	  – Seal-in liner suction
	  – Skin fit suction
	• Partial suction
	  – Silesian bandage
	  – Pelvic belt/band
	• Vacuum
		• Supracondylar cuff
		• Thigh corset
		• Supracondylar brim
		• "Rubber/Neoprene" sleeve suspension
		• Waist belt with fork strap
		• Suction with knee sleeve
		• Shuttle lock
		• Vacuum

Knee	• Single axis knee • Polycentric knee • Hydraulic Knee • Microprocessor knee	• Not needed
Shank	• Exoskeleton – rigid exterior • Endoskeleton – pylon covered with foam	• Same as transfemoral shank
Foot system	• Solid ankle cushion heel (SACH) • Stationary attachment flexible endoskeleton (SAFE) • Single axis • Multi-axial • Hydraulic • Powered • Dynamic response	• Same as transfemoral foot

Types of Post-Operative Dressings[40,42,43]

Rigid (Plaster of Paris)	
Advantages	**Disadvantages**
• Allows early ambulation with pylon • Promotes circulation and healing • Stimulates proprioception • Provides protection • Provides soft tissue support • Limits edema • Ability to utilize an IPOP (immediate post-operative prosthesis)	• Immediate wound inspection is not possible • Does not allow for daily dressing change • Requires professional application

Non-Weight Bearing Rigid Removable Limb Protectors	
Advantages	**Disadvantages**
• Removable • Accommodates edema fluctuation • Easily applied • Prevents contracture • Provides protection	• Not for ambulatory purposes

Semi-rigid (Unna paste, air splint)	
Advantages	**Disadvantages**
• Reduces post-operative edema • Provides soft tissue support • Allows for earlier ambulation • Provides protection • Easily changeable	• Does not protect as well as rigid dressing • Requires more changing than rigid dressing • May loosen and allow for development of edema

Soft (Ace wrap, shrinker)	
Advantages	**Disadvantages**
• Reduces post-operative edema • Provides some protection • Relatively inexpensive • Easily removed for wound inspection • Allows for active joint range of motion	• Tissue healing is interrupted by frequent dressing changes • Joint range of motion may delay the healing of the incision • Less control of residual limb pain • Cannot control the amount of tension in the bandage • Risk of a tourniquet effect • Shrinker cannot be applied until sutures/staples are removed

Influence of Prosthetic Componentry[40,44,49]

	Description	Influence
Knee	Single axis	• Difficult to reciprocate during gait • May or may not have knee extension assist and/or a weight-activated stance phase control • Constant friction mechanism
	Polycentric	• Heavier than a single axis • Reciprocal gait is more fluid • May or may not have a knee extension assist and/or a weight-activated stance phase control • Constant friction mechanism
	Hydraulic	• Variable friction for improved swing and stance phase control
	Microprocessor	• Multiple programs available to accommodate the activity level of the user • Allows for fluid management of descending stairs • Requires charging • Variable friction for improved swing and stance phase control
Foot System	SACH	• Non-articulating with a rigid keel • Inexpensive • Low maintenance • Cushioned heel for shock absorption • Lacks energy return • Cannot accommodate to uneven surfaces
	Single axis	• Allows for motion in a singular plane • Improved knee stability during weight acceptance • Lacks energy return function if not paired with a dynamic response foot
	Dynamic response	• Can be articulating or non-articulating • Keel has the capability to store and return some energy • May have a split keel to allow for improved surface accommodation
	Hydraulic/ microprocessor	• Finer control over the stability/mobility of motions • Improved shock absorption • Not appropriate for all environmental conditions and demands

Managing the Residual Limb and Prosthesis[46,48,49]

Donning and doffing a transtibial or transfemoral prosthesis requires the wearer to make sure they have all of the necessary componentry in addition to the prosthesis itself. Each suspension type has its own requirements and can vary between each individual socket system. The following is a list of the most common categories of componentry when working with individuals with limb loss.

Socket: The socket is the interface between the residual limb and the prosthesis. A properly fitting socket will disperse the pressure experienced in weight bearing throughout the limb, providing total contact with the surface. Certain areas of the residual limb are more pressure tolerant and can handle greater pressure than others (Fig. 4-70). Generally speaking, muscular areas are more tolerant than bony surfaces. Sockets can take on many shapes and sizes, however, the most common design for a transfemoral prosthesis is an ischial containment socket, while one of the more common designs for a transtibial prosthesis is a total surface bearing or patellar tendon-bearing socket.

Liner: A liner plays an important role in the comfort and health of individuals using a prosthesis. Gel liners, commonly made of silicone, are used for a variety of purposes, including cushioning the residual limb and hosting a suspension mechanism such as a pin or lanyard. Some liners are used to maintain suspension through negative pressure, such as what is seen with a transfemoral seal-in liner. Liners are, for the most part, non-breathable, which means that perspiration can buildup throughout the day. This can result in friction issues and cause irritation on the skin of the residuum. As a result, frequent doffing of the liner may be required to dry it off along with the residual limb. Liners must be carefully washed and dried to maintain a hygienic environment. Gel sheaths can be applied underneath the liner directly on the skin of the residual limb and can serve to relieve irritation when using the prosthesis.

Insert: A flexible or soft insert can be used to accommodate for space in the prosthetic socket. Soft inserts, generally made from a foam material, offer improved cushioning on the residual limb during weight bearing. Flexible inserts are usually made of plastic, and similar to a foam insert, can improve the comfort and fit of the prosthesis. Unlike a foam insert which can offer some shock absorption, the hard insert relieves pressure through a series of buildups and reliefs molded into the insert.

Sock: It is normal for an individual with limb loss to experience a decrease in residual limb volume, especially in the first year. In order to accommodate for this space, prosthetic socks are used to maintain a congruent and comfortable fit. Prosthetic socks come in various sizes and material types, including cotton, wool, and synthetic materials. Commonly encountered plys are 1, 3, and 5 ply. A general rule of thumb is that when the number of ply socks exceeds 12-15, the prosthetist should be notified as a recasting may be required. Some socks are split ply, and will have a greater/lesser ply distally than proximally. Socks must be carefully applied as to eliminate any wrinkles, otherwise the wearer may experience discomfort or breakdown in the area of increased pressure.

Self-Management Considerations[40,46,48,49]

Self-management for an individual with limb loss is a term that describes activities, knowledge, and skills that are related to living with limb loss. Therapists are instrumental in the education and indoctrination of proper self-management abilities during each phase of rehabilitation.

Hygiene: The residual limb should be carefully washed, inspected, and maintained to prevent the formation of wounds or infections. This is of particular importance for individuals with impaired vascular perfusion or a history of wounds or infection. For most patients, once the post-surgical residual limb has fully closed and no evidence of exudate is present, washing with warm water and a mild hypoallergenic soap is appropriate. If lotion use is advised, it should not be petroleum-based and it should not be applied prior to donning the prosthesis since it may inhibit suspension. The residual limb, as well as the contralateral foot, should be inspected daily for areas of breakdown. If an area of breakdown, rash, or wound is identified, it may be necessary to have the area inspected by the prosthetist and/or physician prior to donning the prosthesis.

Wear schedule: While there is no absolute rule for wearing a prosthesis, a "break-in" schedule is normally prescribed for the first few weeks of wear. This allows for careful monitoring of the limb and allows the wearer to slowly accommodate to the sensation of weight bearing through the residuum. A general rule is to start with one hour a day of total wear time, with half of the time spent ambulating. Every 30 minutes or immediately after walking, the skin should be inspected for breakdown. If the wearer is tolerating the prosthesis well and no evidence of breakdown is noted, an hour is added each day while still respecting the 50% rule of rest:use. If the skin is showing no signs of breakdown, the amount of time between inspections is gradually expanded by 15-30 minutes. Eventually, the wearer will be able to tolerate the prosthesis for extended periods of time without having to remove the prosthesis and inspect the skin.

Fit issues: The most common complaint a new prosthesis wearer makes is regarding the comfort of the socket on the residual limb. Fit issues can be potentially managed through manipulation of sock-ply, alignment of the liners in the socket, and training the patient on how to dynamically adjust the fit to accommodate fluctuations in the size of the residual limb throughout the day (Fig. 4-71). For example, if a patient complains that the prosthesis is fitting too loosely and they are using prosthetic socks to manage their fit, it would be logical to initially adjust the sock ply. If the fit of the socket is too tight, the therapist should determine if the patient has been wearing their shrinker throughout the day when not wearing their prosthesis. If they have been wearing the shrinker, a review of medications and diet may be warranted since they can adversely affect the residual limb volume.

Transtibial Residual Limb - Anterior View

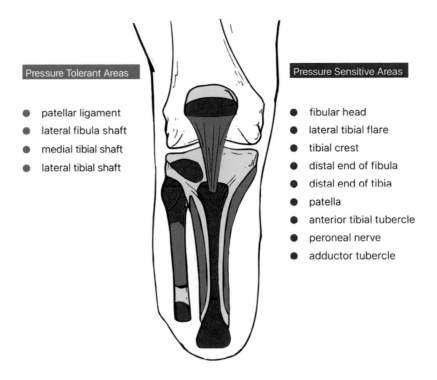

Pressure Tolerant Areas

- patellar ligament
- lateral fibula shaft
- medial tibial shaft
- lateral tibial shaft

Pressure Sensitive Areas

- fibular head
- lateral tibial flare
- tibial crest
- distal end of fibula
- distal end of tibia
- patella
- anterior tibial tubercle
- peroneal nerve
- adductor tubercle

Transfemoral Residual Limb - Anterior View

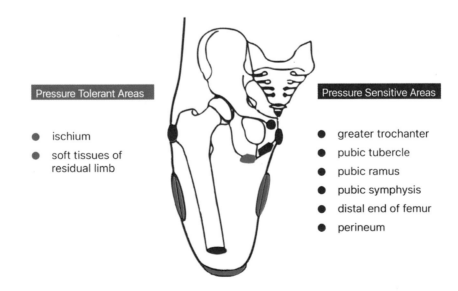

Pressure Tolerant Areas

- ischium
- soft tissues of residual limb

Pressure Sensitive Areas

- greater trochanter
- pubic tubercle
- pubic ramus
- pubic symphysis
- distal end of femur
- perineum

Fig. 4-70: Pressure Tolerant and Pressure Sensitive Areas
In a posterior view, the hamstrings' tendons are pressure sensitive and the posterior compartment is pressure tolerant.

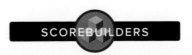

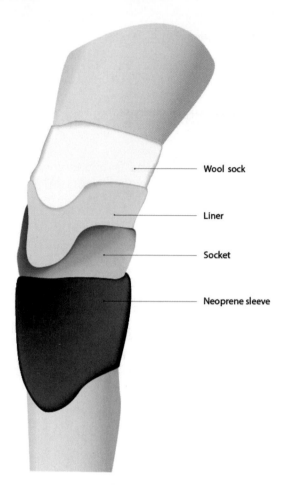

- Wool sock
- Liner
- Socket
- Neoprene sleeve

Fig. 4-71: Common components that may be worn when donning a transtibial prosthesis.

"Red flags": The patient must be educated on how to prevent, identify, and report any issues associated with their residual limb as soon as possible in order to prevent secondary complications. This includes preventing skin breakdown through daily inspections and hygiene, identifying abrasions or wounds that have formed, and discontinuing wearing the prosthesis until the limb has been examined by a physician.

Timeline: The rehabilitation of the individual with limb loss is divided into several phases. Immediately post-amputation is referred to as the pre-prosthetic phase of rehabilitation and will generally last 6 weeks in length. During this timeframe, the therapist focuses on protecting the limb, preventing contractures, developing single limb mobility skills, and preparing the patient for the prosthetic phase of rehabilitation. In some cases, a patient is fit with an immediate post-operative prosthesis (IPOP) which allows for immediate weight bearing using a temporary prosthetic device. More commonly, a patient will be evaluated for their first prosthesis once the sutures/staples have healed and the residual limb skin integrity is intact, usually between 4 and 6 weeks. A patient can begin wearing a shrinker once the sutures are removed. The patient will be sized for the shrinker by the prosthetist. Following the evaluation, the patient will receive their first prosthetic limb, known as the temporary prosthesis. This prosthetic limb is fully functional and allows the wearer to participate in the prosthetic phase of rehabilitation. Modifications may need to be made during this timeframe to improve the comfort and function of the prosthesis during weight bearing activities, which likely involve the prosthetist. After several months of working with the prosthesis, the wearer may feel the comfort and fit is appropriate, and that the residual limb volume fluctuations have stabilized. In this instance, the permanent prosthesis may be manufactured. Medicare supports a new prosthesis every five years, however, based on the activity level of the wearer, repairs/replacement may be needed prior to this period.

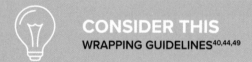

CONSIDER THIS
WRAPPING GUIDELINES[40,44,49]

- Elastic wrap should not have any wrinkles
- Diagonal and angular patterns should be used
- Do not wrap in circular patterns
- Provide pressure distally to enhance shaping
- Anchor wrap above the knee for transtibial amputations
- Anchor wrap around pelvis for transfemoral amputations
- Promote full elbow extension for transradial amputations

- Promote full knee extension for transtibial amputations
- Promote full hip extension for transfemoral amputations
- Secure the wrap with tape; do not use clips
- Use 2-4 inch wrap for upper extremity amputations
- Use 3-4 inch wrap for transtibial amputations
- Use 6 inch wrap for transfemoral amputations
- Rewrap frequently to maintain adequate pressure

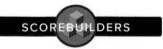

SPOTLIGHT ON SAFETY
COMPLICATIONS FOLLOWING AMPUTATION[40,43,44]

There are a multitude of potential complications patients may experience following amputation. Therapists should be aware of the potential signs and symptoms associated with these complications and, when warranted, be prepared to take immediate action.

Several of the more common complications following amputation are discussed.

Contractures
Failure to initiate full range of motion early in the post-operative phase and poor positioning of the residual limb significantly increase the likelihood of a contracture. The joint immediately proximal to the amputation site is the most susceptible. The most likely contractures based on level of amputation are: transmetatarsal and Syme's - equinus deformity; transtibial - knee flexion; transfemoral - hip flexion and abduction.

Deep Vein Thrombosis
A deep vein thrombosis is a blood clot that forms in a vein with the potential to dislodge as an embolism and travel until it blocks an artery. This is a serious medical condition since the embolus may obstruct a selected artery. Heparin is an anticoagulant commonly used to reduce the risk of deep vein thrombosis following surgery.

Hypersensitivity
Hypersensitivity of the residual limb can significantly impede or even prevent the appropriate fit and functional use of a prosthesis. Specific desensitization techniques and early fitting of a temporary prosthesis are key components in post-amputation rehabilitation. Weight bearing, massage, tapping, and residual limb wrapping are all commonly utilized interventions that facilitate desensitization.

Neuroma
A neuroma is a bundle of nerve endings that group together and can produce pain due to scar tissue, pressure from the prosthesis or tension on the residual limb.

Phantom Limb
Phantom limb refers to a painless sensation where the patient feels that the limb is still present. This is common immediately after amputation and will usually subside with desensitization and prosthetic use, however, it may continue for extended periods of time for some patients.

Phantom Pain
Phantom pain refers to the patient's perception of some form of painful stimuli as it relates to the residual limb. The pain can be continuous or intermittent, local or general, and short-term or permanent. This type of pain can disable the patient and interfere with successful rehabilitation. Treatment options include TENS, ultrasound, icing, mirror therapy, relaxation techniques, desensitization techniques, and prosthetic use.

Psychological Impact
It is extremely common for patients to experience a variety of negative thoughts and emotions following amputation. This can include denial, grief, anxiety, depression or suicidal feelings. The intensity of the thoughts and emotions may be elevated in patients following emergency amputation since the patient had insufficient time to mentally prepare for the loss.

Wound Infections
The residual limb can become infected following the surgical procedure. Antibiotics are administered at the time of surgery to reduce the risk of infection.

Considerations for Prosthetic Training[40,43,49]

Forequarter (scapulothoracic)
- Loss of all shoulder, elbow, and hand function
- Most common cause is malignancy
- Functional prosthetic use is common
- A lightweight cosmetic prosthetic is typically well-tolerated

Shoulder disarticulation
- Loss of all shoulder, elbow, and hand function
- Most commonly the result of malignancy or severe electrical injuries
- Functional prosthetic use is possible
- An external prosthetic shoulder joint is typically required

Transhumeral amputation
- Loss of all elbow and hand function
- Most commonly due to trauma
- Typically 7-10 centimeters proximal to the distal humeral condyles
- Trauma associated fracture, dislocation or peripheral nerve injury may delay prosthetic interventions
- Second most common level of upper extremity amputation

Elbow disarticulation
- Loss of all elbow and hand function
- Most commonly due to trauma
- Allows for self-suspending socket
- An external prosthetic elbow joint is typically required

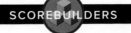

Transradial amputation

- Loss of all hand function
- Must be a minimum of five centimeters proximal to the distal radius
- Typically the result of trauma
- Trauma associated fracture, dislocation or peripheral nerve injury may delay prosthetic interventions
- Functionally preferred over wrist disarticulation or selected partial hand amputations
- Most common level of upper extremity amputation

Wrist disarticulation

- Loss of all hand function
- Relatively uncommon level of amputation
- Cosmetic and functional prosthetic disadvantages

Partial hand amputation

- Loss of a portion of digit/hand function
- Limb sparing technique utilized when functional pinch can be preserved
- Toe transfer to replace a thumb may be considered if prosthesis fails

Digit amputation

- Preserved function is highly variable depending on number of digits involved and level of amputation
- Prostheses are not typically utilized
- A long transradial amputation may be more functional if multiple digits are involved at proximal levels

Hip disarticulation/hemipelvectomy

- All functions of the hip, knee, ankle, and foot are absent
- Most common cause is malignancy
- Does not allow for activation of the prosthesis through a residual limb
- Prosthetic limb advancement initiated through pelvic motion

Transfemoral amputation

- Length of the residual limb with regard to leverage and energy expenditure
- Knee componentry will determine ability to functionally reciprocate gait
- Stance control may not activate until weight bearing occurs through the limb
- Donning can be more difficult than with a transtibial amputation
- Weight bearing through the ischium in an ischial containment socket
- Susceptible to hip flexion contracture
- Adaptation required for balance, weight of prosthesis, and energy expenditure

Knee disarticulation

- Loss of all knee, ankle, and foot function
- The residual limb can weight bear through its end
- Susceptible to hip flexion contracture
- Knee axis of the prosthesis is below the natural axis of the knee
- Gait deviations can occur secondary to the malalignment of the knee axis

Transtibial amputation

- Loss of active foot and ankle motions
- Weight bearing in the prosthesis should be distributed over the total residual limb

- Areas of primary weight bearing should be pressure tolerant
- Adaptations required for balance
- Susceptible to both knee and hip flexion contractures

Syme's amputation

- Loss of all foot functions
- Residual limb can weight bear through its end
- Residual limb is bulbous with a non-cosmetic appearance
- Dog ears must be reduced for proper prosthetic fit
- Adaptation required for the increased weight of the prosthesis
- Adaptation required due to diminished toe off during gait

Transmetatarsal and Chopart's amputation

- Loss of forefoot leverage
- Loss of balance
- Loss of weight bearing surface
- Loss of proprioception
- Tendency to develop equinus deformity

Gait Deviations[40,44,49]

Prosthetic Causes	Amputee Causes
Lateral Bending	
Prosthesis too short	Poor balance
Improperly shaped lateral wall	Abduction contracture
High medial wall	Improper training
Prosthesis aligned in abduction	Short residual limb
	Weak hip abductors on prosthetic side
	Hypersensitive and painful residual limb
Abducted Gait	
Prosthesis too long	Abduction contracture
High medial wall	Improper training
Poorly shaped lateral wall	Adductor roll
Prosthesis positioned in abduction	Weak hip flexors and adductors
Inadequate suspension	Pain over lateral residual limb
Excessive knee friction	
Circumducted Gait	
	Abduction contracture
	Improper training
	Weak hip flexors
Prosthesis too long	Lacks confidence to flex the knee
Excessive knee friction	
Socket too small	Painful anterior distal residual limb
Excessive plantar flexion	Inability to initiate prosthetic knee flexion

Prosthetic Causes	Amputee Causes
Excessive Knee Flexion During Stance	
Socket set forward in relation to foot Excessive dorsiflexion Stiff heel Prosthesis too long	Knee flexion contracture Hip flexion contracture Pain anteriorly in residual limb Decrease in quadriceps strength Poor balance
Vaulting	
Prosthesis too long Inadequate socket suspension Excessive alignment stability Excessive plantar flexion	Residual limb discomfort Improper training Fear of stubbing toe Short residual limb Painful hip/residual limb
Rotation of Forefoot at Heel Strike	
Excessive toe-out built in Loose fitting socket Inadequate suspension Rigid SACH heel cushion	Poor muscle control Improper training Weak medial rotators Short residual limb
Forward Trunk Flexion	
Socket too big Poor suspension Knee instability	Hip flexion contracture Weak hip extensors Pain with ischial weight bearing Inability to initiate prosthetic knee flexion
Medial or Lateral Whip	
Excessive rotation of the knee Tight socket fit Valgus in the prosthetic knee Improper alignment of toe break	Improper training Weak hip rotators Knee instability

Amputation and Prosthetic Terminology[40,44,49]

Acquired amputation: Refers to the surgical removal of a limb due to disease, trauma, or infection. This can be further defined as traumatic and non-traumatic amputation.

Dysvascular: Refers to the disease of the blood vessels, including peripheral vascular disease, peripheral arterial disease, and complications related to diabetes.

Endoskeletal shank: This type of shank consists of a rigid pylon covered with a material designed to simulate the contour and color of the contralateral limb.

Exoskeletal shank: This type of shank consists of a rigid external frame covered with a thin layer of tinted plastic to match the skin color distally.

Extension assist: A mechanism that assists the knee joint into extension during the swing phase of gait.

Myoelectric prosthesis: A device using electromyography signals to control movements of the prosthesis with surface electrodes or implantable wires.

Non-traumatic amputation: An amputation that is not the result of direct injury. Vascular disease and infection are types of non-traumatic amputations.

Pistoning: The translation of the prosthetic limb from the residual limb. It is the result of inadequate suspension and can result in distal residual limb skin issues.

Polycentric knee: Refers to a knee joint that has multiple axes of rotation that allows for a more natural gait cycle when compared to a single axis knee.

Prosthesis: The term refers to an artificial body part, used as a noun, not an adjective. For example, "My prosthesis is broken."

Prosthetic: The term describes an artificial body part, used as an adjective, not as a noun. For example, "The prosthetic limb is broken."

Pylon: The term used to describe a pipe-like structure used to connect the socket of the prosthesis to the foot/ankle components. The pylon assists with weight bearing and shock absorption.

Residual limb: The term used to describe the remaining extremity following an amputation. The residual limb is characterized based on its location and length.

Shrinker: An elastic sleeve that is placed over the end of the residual limb to control edema and encourage limb shaping.

Stance control (safety): A weight-activated mechanism that maintains knee extension during weight bearing even if the knee joint is not fully extended. If the knee is flexed greater than what the control mechanism is designed for, the mechanism will not engage.

Suspension: The term used to describe how the prosthetic socket is attached to the residual limb. Common types of suspension include vacuum, shuttle lock, suction, waist belt, and harness.

Traumatic amputation: An amputation performed secondary to a direct injury. A car accident or gunshot wound are potential examples of injuries resulting in traumatic amputation.

Clinical Application Templates

Clinical Application Templates* allow candidates to explore many of the elements of patient/client management for a wide variety of medical conditions. Although candidates have been exposed to a variety of medical conditions during their clinical education experiences, it is unlikely they have been exposed to the vast number of medical conditions commonly encountered on the examination. By utilizing Clinical Application Templates students can broaden their experience base and as a result be better prepared to answer examination questions.

Three specific levels of **Clinical Application Templates** (i.e., Gold, Silver, Bronze) will be presented at the conclusion of each system-based chapter.

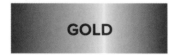

The GOLD level contains medical conditions that are commonly encountered on the NPTE-PTA. As a result, the relative breadth and depth of the template is vast due to the high return on investment.

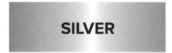

The SILVER level contains medical conditions that are occasionally encountered on the NPTE-PTA. As a result, the relative breadth and depth of the template is reduced due to the moderate return on investment.

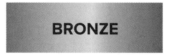

The BRONZE level contains medical conditions that are infrequently encountered on the NPTE-PTA. As a result, the relative breadth and depth of the template is minimal due to the low return on investment.

The basic assumption of this study tool is that candidates should study medical conditions proportionately to the likelihood of seeing the particular condition on the NPTE-PTA. An executive summary of selected information for each medical condition is presented at the beginning of each section (i.e., Gold, Silver, Bronze) followed by the completed Clinical Application Template.

Candidates are encouraged to review the templates and carefully reflect on the presented information. Candidates should attempt to make this activity an active learning exercise and resist the urge to simply read each of the templates. By engaging in this type of active learning exercise, candidates are able to further assess their level of preparedness for the examination. Although some candidates may be quite comfortable reviewing selected **Clinical Application Templates**, many candidates learn that they lack necessary knowledge in many others.

Candidates should not rely solely on the presented **Clinical Application Templates** and instead should utilize the template format to potentially review other medical conditions. This type of active learning is best performed by a small group of candidates with a given candidate acting as the facilitator. In this manner candidates can share their individual clinical experiences with the group and at the same time benefit from the knowledge of their classmates.

*The **Clinical Application Template** was adapted from a document by the Academy of Specialty Boards entitled "Preparing Items that Measure More than Recall." The document was originally designed to help item writers develop sample questions for the Physical Therapy Specialty Examinations.

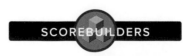

GOLD Level Clinical Application Templates

Level Clinical Application Template Executive Summary

Adhesive Capsulitis

- Occurs more in the middle-aged population with females having a greater incidence than males
- Arthrogram can assist with diagnosis by detecting decreased volume of fluid within the joint capsule
- Range of motion restriction typically in a capsular pattern (lateral rotation, abduction, medial rotation)

Ankle Sprain - Lateral - Grade II

- Typically occurs due to significant inversion and involves the lateral ligament complex, most commonly damages the anterior talofibular ligament (ATFL)
- Will likely present with significant pain or tenderness along the lateral aspect of the ankle especially at the ATFL
- Should heal fairly quickly if no other structures are involved and will return to the previous functional level within two to six weeks

Anterior Cruciate Ligament Sprain - Grade III

- Injury most commonly occurs during hyperflexion, rapid deceleration, hyperextension or landing in an unbalanced position
- Females involved in selected athletic activities have significantly higher ligament injury rates compared to males
- Approximately two-thirds of complete anterior cruciate ligament tears have an associated meniscal tear

Bicipital Tendonitis

- Increased incidence of injury is associated with selected athletic activities such as baseball pitching, swimming, rowing, gymnastics, and tennis
- Characterized by subjective reports of a deep ache directly in front and on top of the shoulder made worse with overhead activities or lifting
- Examination may reveal a positive Speed's test or Yergason's test

Lateral Epicondylitis

- Characterized by inflammation or degenerative changes at the common extensor tendon that attaches to the lateral epicondyle of the elbow
- Repeated overuse of the wrist extensors, particularly the extensor carpi radialis brevis can produce tensile stress and result in microscopic tearing and damage to the extensor tendon
- Clinical symptoms include difficulty holding or gripping objects and insufficient forearm functional strength

Level Clinical Application Template Executive Summary

Medial Collateral Ligament Sprain – Grade II

- Grade II injury is characterized by partial tearing of the ligament's fibers resulting in joint laxity when the ligament is stretched
- Mechanism of injury is usually a blow to the outside of the knee joint causing excess force to the medial side of the joint
- Return to previous functional level should occur within four to eight weeks following the injury if no other associated structures are involved

Osteoarthritis

- Degenerative process primarily involving articular cartilage resulting from excessive loading of a healthy joint or normal loading of an abnormal joint
- Typically diagnosed based on the results of a clinical examination and x-ray findings
- Prevalence is higher among women than men later in life with approximately 80-90% of individuals older than 65 years of age demonstrating evidence of osteoarthritis

Patellofemoral Syndrome

- Causes damage to the articular cartilage of the patella ranging from softening to complete cartilage destruction resulting in exposure of subchondral bone
- Etiology is unknown, however, it is extremely common during adolescence, is more prevalent in females than males, and has a direct association with activity level
- Management includes controlling edema, stretching, strengthening, improving range of motion, and activity modification

Plantar Fasciitis

- Chronic overuse condition that develops secondary to repetitive stretching of the plantar fascia through excessive foot pronation during the loading phase of gait
- Characterized by severe pain in the heel when first standing up in the morning (when the fascia is contracted, stiff, and cold)
- Intervention consists of ice massage, deep friction massage, heel insert, orthotic prescription, activity modification, and gentle stretching program of the Achilles tendon and plantar fascia

Rotator Cuff Tear

- May occur as a result of an acute traumatic incident or due to a chronic degenerative pathology such as chronic supraspinatus tendonitis
- The drop arm test and empty can test can assist in identifying supraspinatus pathology which may be indicative of a rotator cuff tear
- Failure to adequately treat a rotator cuff tear may necessitate significant activity modifications, additional surgical management, adhesive capsulitis or degenerative changes

Level Clinical Application Template Executive Summary

Rotator Cuff Tendonitis

- Caused by an inability of a weak supraspinatus muscle to adequately depress the head of the humerus in the glenoid fossa during elevation of the arm
- Participating in activities that require excessive overhead activity such as swimming, tennis, baseball, painting, and other manual labor activities increases the risk of rotator cuff tendonitis
- Patients may experience a feeling of weakness and identify the presence of a painful arc of motion most commonly occurring between 60 and 120 degrees of active abduction

Scoliosis

- Curvature is usually found in the thoracic or lumbar vertebrae and can be associated with kyphosis or lordosis
- A patient with scoliosis that ranges between 25 and 40 degrees requires a spinal orthosis and physical therapy intervention for posture, flexibility, strengthening, respiratory function, and proper utilization of the spinal orthosis
- Scoliosis does not usually progress significantly once bone growth is complete if the curvature remains below 40 degrees at the time of skeletal maturity

Spondylolisthesis - Degenerative

- Caused by the weakening of joints that allows for forward slippage of one vertebral segment on the one below due to degenerative changes
- Most common site of degenerative spondylolisthesis is the L4-L5 level
- William's flexion exercises may be indicated to strengthen the abdominals and reduce lumbar lordosis

Total Hip Arthroplasty

- Patients are typically over 55 years of age and have experienced consistent pain that is not relieved through conservative measures which serve to limit the patient's functional mobility
- Posterolateral approach allows the abductor muscles to remain intact, however, there may be a higher incidence of post-operative joint instability due to the interruption of the posterior capsule
- Cemented hip replacement usually allows for partial weight bearing initially, while a noncemented hip replacement requires toe touch weight bearing for up to six weeks

Total Knee Arthroplasty

- Primary indication for total knee arthroplasty is the destruction of articular cartilage secondary to osteoarthritis
- Post-operative care may include a knee immobilizer, elevation of the limb, cryotherapy, intermittent range of motion using a continuous passive motion (CPM) machine, and initiation of knee protocol exercises
- Patient education may include items such as avoid excessive stress to the knee, squatting, quick pivoting, using pillows under the knee while in bed, and low seating

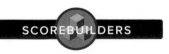

Level Clinical Application Template Executive Summary

Transfemoral Amputation due to Osteosarcoma

- A highly malignant cancer that begins in the medullary cavity of a bone and leads to the formation of a mass
- A patient status post transfemoral amputation may present with fatigue, loss of balance, phantom pain or sensation, hypersensitivity of the residual limb, and psychological issues regarding the loss of the limb
- Lying in a prone position is beneficial to decrease the incidence of a hip flexion contracture

Transtibial Amputation due to Arteriosclerosis Obliterans

- Arteriosclerosis obliterans results in ischemia and subsequent ulceration of the affected tissues
- A patient status post transtibial amputation may have a decrease in cardiovascular status depending on the frequency of intermittent claudication experienced prior to the amputation
- Preprosthetic intervention should focus on strength, range of motion, functional mobility, use of assistive devices, desensitization, and patient education for care of the residual limb

Adhesive Capsulitis

DIAGNOSIS

What condition produces a patient's symptoms?

Adhesive capsulitis (also known as "frozen shoulder") is an enigmatic shoulder disorder characterized by inflammation and fibrotic thickening of the anterior joint capsule of the shoulder. The inflamed capsule becomes adherent to the humeral head and undergoes contracture. This condition is characterized by the symptoms of limitation in glenohumeral motion and pain.

An injury was most likely sustained to which structure?

Adhesive capsulitis is classified as primary or secondary. Primary adhesive capsulitis occurs spontaneously and secondary adhesive capsulitis results from an underlying condition. Inflammation within the joint capsule causes fibrous adhesions to form and the capsule to thicken. A decrease in space within the capsule leads to a decrease of synovial fluid and further irritation to the glenohumeral joint.

INFERENCE

What is the most likely contributing factor in the development of this condition?

Primary adhesive capsulitis has no known etiology, however, it is associated with conditions such as diabetes mellitus, thyroid abnormalities, and cardiopulmonary conditions. Secondary adhesive capsulitis can result from trauma, immobilization, complex regional pain syndrome, rheumatoid arthritis, abdominal disorders, and psychogenic disorders. Orthopedic intrinsic disorders that may initiate this process include supraspinatus tendonitis, partial tear of the rotator cuff, and bicipital tendonitis. Adhesive capsulitis occurs more in the middle-aged population with females having a greater incidence than males.

CONFIRMATION

What is the most likely clinical presentation?

Data regarding the prevalence and incidence of adhesive capsulitis is lacking. According to a published study adhesive capsulitis occurs in 2% of the population within the United States and in 11% of individuals that are diagnosed with diabetes mellitus. A small percentage of patients (10-15%) develop bilateral adhesive capsulitis. Adhesive capsulitis is characterized by restricted active and passive range of motion at the glenohumeral joint. Characteristics of the acute phase include pain that radiates below the elbow and awakens the patient at night. Passive range of the shoulder is limited during this phase due to pain and guarding. During the chronic phase pain is usually localized around the lateral brachial region, the patient is not awakened by pain, and passive range is limited due to capsular stiffness. Pain is present with a loss of glenohumeral motion, restricted elevation, and lateral rotation.

What laboratory or imaging studies would confirm the diagnosis?

An arthrogram can assist with the diagnosis of adhesive capsulitis by detecting a decreased volume of fluid within the joint capsule. The glenohumeral joint normally holds approximately 16-20 ml of fluid, however, adhesive capsulitis decreases the size of the capsule so it holds only 5-10 ml of fluid. Other tests should only be performed for differential diagnosis.

What additional information should be obtained to confirm the diagnosis?

The diagnosis of adhesive capsulitis is confirmed from clinical evaluation and past medical history. The patient may present with the greatest restriction of glenohumeral motion in abduction and lateral rotation, but all planes of motion are usually affected. There is tightness within the anteroinferior joint capsule, pain with stretching, and restriction with passive and active range of motion.

EXAMINATION

What history should be documented?

Important areas to explore include past medical and surgical history, medications, family history, current symptoms, current health status, social history and habits, occupation, leisure activities, and social support system.

What tests/measures are most appropriate?

Anthropometric characteristics: circumferential measurements of bilateral upper extremities

Arousal, attention, and cognition: examine mental status, learning ability, memory, motivation

Community and work integration: analysis of community, work, and leisure activities

Cranial nerve integrity: assessment of muscle innervation by the cranial nerves, dermatome assessment

Environmental, home, and work barriers: analysis of current and potential barriers or hazards

Integumentary integrity: skin assessment, assessment of sensation

Joint integrity and mobility: assessment of hyper- and hypomobility of a joint, soft tissue swelling and inflammation

Muscle performance: strength assessment, muscle tone assessment

Pain: pain perception assessment scale, visual analogue scale, assessment of muscle soreness

Posture: analysis of resting and dynamic posture

Range of motion: active and passive range of motion

Self-care and home management: assessment of functional capacity

What additional findings are likely with this patient?

A patient with adhesive capsulitis may encounter muscle spasms around the shoulder secondary to muscle guarding. A loss of reciprocal arm swing may be seen and disuse muscle atrophy may occur over time. A thorough examination must be completed to rule out concomitant systemic, rheumatologic, inflammatory, metastatic or infectious disorders.

MANAGEMENT

What is the most effective management of this patient?

Medical management varies with adhesive capsulitis. Adhesive capsulitis is a self-limiting process that can take over 12 months in its course. Pharmacological intervention should emphasize the control of pain through acetaminophen, longer acting analgesics, NSAIDs or narcotics. A physician may inject the shoulder with corticosteroids to assist with recovery of motion. Surgical intervention to break up adhesions or release muscles adhered to the capsule is a last resort if conservative management fails. Physical therapy intervention during the acute phase includes icing or superficial heat, gentle joint mobilization, progressive strengthening, pendulum exercises, and isometric strengthening. During the chronic phase, physical therapy intervention and goals may also include ultrasound, grade III and IV mobilization, increasing the extensibility of the joint capsule, and techniques such as PNF to restore painless functional range of motion.

What home care regimen should be recommended?

A home care regimen during the acute phase should include some self-stretching, but avoid abduction secondary to the risk of damage to subacromial tissue. Once the patient enters the chronic phase, the program should emphasize self-stretching, progressive exercises, posture management, PNF and other exercises such as pendulum exercises and "wall climbing" to assist with improving range of motion.

OUTCOME

What is the likely outcome of a course of physical therapy?

Physical therapy is usually prescribed on an outpatient basis for three to five months after diagnosis. Adhesive capsulitis usually follows a nonlinear pattern of recovery. Spontaneous recovery is said to take 12-24 months in duration.

What are the long-term effects of the patient's condition?

Most patients are able to fully recover over time, but an estimated 7-14% of patients experience some permanent loss of range of motion at the shoulder joint. This loss is frequently asymptomatic and may not impair a patient's functional ability.

COMPARISON

What are the distinguishing characteristics of a similar condition?

Acute bursitis is characterized by pain that is intense and sometimes throbbing over the lateral brachial region. This condition may arise secondary to calcific tendonitis. Active and passive motion in all directions is limited by pain. Abduction greater than 60 degrees and flexion greater than 90 degrees usually produce severe pain. Acute bursitis lasts for only a few days and unlike adhesive capsulitis this condition will usually resolve itself within a few weeks.

CLINICAL SCENARIOS

Scenario One

A 29-year-old was diagnosed with primary adhesive capsulitis and referred to outpatient physical therapy. The patient is self-employed as an artist and enjoys outdoor activities. Past medical history includes diabetes mellitus since age six and a femur fracture 11 months ago. The patient noticed reduced range of motion and an increase in pain over the last few weeks.

Scenario Two

A 53-year-old female fell off her bike six months ago while cycling in a road race and sustained an injury to her shoulder complex. The patient attempted to immobilize her arm in a sling for two weeks. The patient states that she was unable to regain functional motion in her shoulder once she stopped using the sling. She saw a physician who diagnosed her with "frozen shoulder." The patient is limited to 10 degrees lateral rotation and 95 degrees of shoulder flexion.

Ankle Sprain - Lateral - Grade II

DIAGNOSIS

What condition produces a patient's symptoms?

The vast majority of ankle sprains occur due to significant inversion and involve the lateral ligament complex. This complex resists varus stress and is comprised of the anterior talofibular (ATFL), calcaneofibular (CFL), and posterior talofibular (PTFL) ligaments. The ankle is supported medially by the deltoid ligament which is the strongest of the ankle ligaments. The deltoid ligament is comprised of superficial and deep components and resists valgus stress. Since the deltoid ligament attaches in part to the medial malleolus, significant valgus stress typically causes the medial malleolus to fracture before the deltoid ligament fails mechanically.

An injury was most likely sustained to which structure?

The ATFL resists inversion of the talus and calcaneus as well as anterior translation of the talus on the tibia. The ATFL becomes taut during plantar flexion. The CFL resists inversion of the talus within the midrange of talocrural motion. The PTFL resists posterior translation of the talus and is the strongest of the lateral ligaments. The ATFL is the most likely of the three lateral ligaments to sustain damage during a lateral ankle sprain.

INFERENCE

What is the most likely contributing factor in the development of this condition?

Individuals participating in sport activities requiring high levels of agility (e.g., soccer) or jumping (e.g., basketball, volleyball) are particularly susceptible to lateral ankle sprains. Other factors such as deconditioning, poor proprioception, and obesity may also increase the risk of injury. Recurrent sprains are common and often attributed to a combination of residual ligamentous laxity and decreased proprioceptive responses.

CONFIRMATION

What is the most likely clinical presentation?

A patient with a grade II lateral ankle sprain will likely present with significant pain or tenderness along the lateral aspect of the ankle especially at the ATFL. Pain will typically limit a strength assessment, however, active range of motion should be assessed to rule out an Achilles tendon rupture. Pain will also typically contribute to an antalgic gait pattern and be elicited specifically with passive inversion and end range plantar flexion as this position maximally stretches the ATFL. There is typically discernible laxity with ligamentous testing and joint mobility. Ecchymosis and moderate to severe edema at the ankle are likely and may persist even as pain resolves and function returns.

What laboratory or imaging studies would confirm the diagnosis?

MRI is not typically utilized with suspected lateral ligament involvement without other extenuating circumstances due to the prohibitive cost.

What additional information should be obtained to confirm the diagnosis?

The anterior drawer test for the ankle specifically assesses the integrity of the ATFL during anterior translation of the talus on the tibia. The talar tilt test assesses the integrity of the CFL as the talus is moved into adduction. Though rare, neurovascular complications may accompany the ligamentous injury, therefore distal pulses and sensory integrity should also be assessed.

EXAMINATION

What history should be documented?

Important areas to explore include past medical history, medications, family history, current symptoms, current health status, social history and habits, occupation, leisure activities, and social support system.

What tests/measures are most appropriate?

Anthropometric characteristics: circumferential measurements for edema, palpation to determine ankle effusion

Arousal, attention, and cognition: examine mental status, learning ability, memory, motivation

Assistive and adaptive devices: potential utilization of crutches

Gait, locomotion, and balance: safety with/without an assistive device during gait; biomechanics of gait

Integumentary integrity: assessment of sensation

Joint integrity and mobility: special tests such as Thompson's test

Muscle performance: strength assessment, characteristics of muscle contraction

Pain: pain perception assessment scale

Range of motion: active and passive range of motion

Sensory integration: proprioception and kinesthesia

Self-care and home management: assessment of functional capacity

Ankle Sprain - Lateral - Grade II   GOLD

What additional findings are likely with this patient?

Proprioceptive deficits are common and should be addressed in the plan of care as warranted by examination findings to limit the risk of recurrent injury. Other structural injuries may also accompany a grade II lateral ankle sprain such as osteochondral or chondral injuries of the talar dome, neurovascular disruption, and Achilles tendon rupture.

MANAGEMENT

What is the most effective management of this patient?

Medical management for a grade II lateral ankle sprain usually involves conservative management including R.I.C.E. (rest, ice, compression, elevation). Pharmacological intervention is directed towards pain management through acetaminophen or NSAIDs. Surgical management is not typically indicated unless complications are identified (e.g., fracture, neurovascular disruption). The patient may utilize crutches to limit weight bearing through the involved lower extremity until full weight bearing is tolerated. Physical therapy intervention should be directed towards increasing range of motion and proprioceptive responses, decreasing edema, and beginning light resistive exercises with the involved lower extremity. Passive stretching is recommended to prevent muscle shortening. Range of motion may also be augmented with joint mobilizations if capsular restrictions are noted. Resistive exercises should include a combination of isometric, open-chain, and closed-chain exercises. Resistive exercise should include the peroneal muscles as they provide the ankle with dynamic stability. Proprioception and balance retraining should be addressed with single leg stance activities on variable surfaces. Functional activities such as gait training and stair management should be incorporated. Agility training should be based on sport-specific individual needs. Superficial modalities and electrical stimulation may be utilized to address pain, edema, inflammation, and soft tissue restrictions. Once inflammation has subsided, transverse friction massage may be applied to the healing ligament to assist in preventing the adherence of scar tissue to adjacent structures. A patient should be required to complete a functional progression prior to returning to unrestricted activity.

What home care regimen should be recommended?

The home care regimen should initially consist of R.I.C.E. Range of motion, strengthening, palliative care, and functional activities are also recommended as warranted based on the results of the patient examination. The use of crutches should continue until the patient can tolerate full weight bearing unless otherwise recommended by the referring physician.

OUTCOME

What is the likely outcome of a course of physical therapy?

A grade II lateral ankle sprain should heal fairly quickly if no other structures are involved. A patient should be able to return to their previous functional level within two to six weeks. For patients participating in recreational or competitive athletics, a period of supportive taping or bracing may be recommended to prevent the recurrence of injury.

What are the long-term effects of the patient's condition?

Proper healing time and rehabilitation should allow the patient to return to all forms of activity once the patient demonstrates full pain-free range of motion, minimal pain or tenderness with palpation, normal gait pattern, normal proprioception, and competence with agility testing. Residual laxity will increase the patient's risk of recurrence.

COMPARISON

What are the distinguishing characteristics of a similar condition?

A grade II sprain of one or more of the syndesmotic ligaments is commonly referred to as a "high ankle sprain." The syndesmotic ligaments attach to the tibia and fibula and function to stabilize the ankle mortise. Since the ligaments are deep, a great deal of force is required to cause an injury to the syndesmotic ligaments. The syndesmotic ligaments are often injured in conjunction with an ankle fracture. If the tear is unrecognized and therefore untreated, severe post-traumatic arthritis will likely result. A significant tear will require surgical repair which is not typically true for other ligamentous injuries at the ankle. Management typically is focused on the associated injuries and post-operative rehabilitation with the syndesmotic ligament requiring no specific intervention once repaired.

CLINICAL SCENARIOS

Scenario One

A 35-year-old morbidly obese female is diagnosed with a grade I lateral ligament ankle sprain. The patient was walking on a cobblestone walkway when she had an unrecoverable loss of balance and fell. The patient has enrolled in an exercise-based weight loss program. The program begins in one week and the patient does not want to postpone. The patient resides in a one story home with her mother.

Scenario Two

A 17-year-old basketball player is diagnosed with a grade III lateral ankle sprain. The patient was injured during the third week of an 11 week regular season. The patient has no significant past medical history and would like to return to her starting position before post-season playoffs begin. She is diabetic and resides with her parents in a two-story home with her bedroom on the second floor.

DIAGNOSIS

What condition produces a patient's symptoms?

The anterior cruciate ligament (ACL) extends from the anterior intercondylar region of the tibia to the medial aspect of the lateral femoral condyle in the intercondylar notch. The ligament prevents anterior translation of the tibia on the fixed femur and posterior translation of the femur on the fixed tibia. The ACL is a broad cord that has long collagen strands that permits up to 500 pounds of pressure prior to rupture. The ligament has a poor blood supply and does not have the ability to heal a complete tear. Injuries to the ACL most commonly occur during hyperflexion, rapid deceleration, hyperextension or landing in an unbalanced position.

An injury was most likely sustained to which structure?

A grade III ACL sprain refers to a complete tear of the ligament with excessive laxity. Tears of the anterior cruciate ligament most often occur in the midsubstance of the ligament and not at the ligament's attachment on the femur or tibia. Laxity rarely occurs solely in a straight plane and instead is often classified as anterolateral or anteromedial.

INFERENCE

What is the most likely contributing factor in the development of this condition?

Participation in athletic activities requiring high levels of agility (soccer, basketball, volleyball) and contact sports increases the incidence of an ACL injury. Recent studies indicate that women involved in selected athletic activities experienced significantly higher ACL injury rates than their male counterparts. There are many hypothesized reasons for this finding, but to date a definitive answer has not been identified. Causative factors for ACL disruption include body movement and positioning, muscle strength, joint laxity, Q angle, and a narrow intercondylar notch.

CONFIRMATION

What is the most likely clinical presentation?

The peak incidence of ACL injury occurs between 14 and 29 years of age. This age group corresponds to an overall higher activity level, which increases the risk of injury. A grade III ACL sprain is characterized by significant pain, effusion, and edema that significantly limits range of motion. The patient may be unable to bear weight on the involved extremity resulting in dependence on an assistive device. Ligamentous testing reveals visible laxity in the knee and may exacerbate the patient's pain level.

What laboratory or imaging studies would confirm the diagnosis?

MRI is the preferred imaging tool to identify the presence of an ACL tear and possible disruption of other soft tissue structures such as ligaments and menisci. X-rays may be used to rule out a fracture.

What additional information should be obtained to confirm the diagnosis?

Subjective reports such as hearing a loud pop or feeling as though the knee buckled is often associated with a complete tear of the ACL. Special tests such as the Lachman, anterior drawer, and pivot shift test can be used to confirm the diagnosis. It is important to perform all special tests bilaterally.

EXAMINATION

What history should be documented?

Important areas to explore include mechanism of present injury, current symptoms, past medical history, medications, living environment, social history and habits, and social support system.

What tests/measures are most appropriate?

Anthropometric characteristics: knee effusion and lower extremity circumferential measurements

Arousal, attention, and cognition: examine mental status, learning ability, memory, motivation

Assistive and adaptive devices: analysis of components and safety of a device, potential utilization of crutches

Gait, locomotion, and balance: safety during gait with an assistive device

Integumentary integrity: assessment of sensation (pain, temperature, tactile), skin assessment

Joint integrity and mobility: special tests for ligaments and menisci, Lachman and reverse Lachman test, anterior drawer test, palpation of structures, joint play, soft tissue restrictions, joint pain

Muscle performance: strength and active movement assessment, resisted isometrics, muscle contraction characteristics, muscle endurance

Orthotic, protective, and supportive devices: utilization of bracing, taping or wrapping, foot orthotic assessment

Pain: pain perception assessment scale

Range of motion: active and passive range of motion

Self-care and home management: assessment of functional capacity

Sensory integrity: proprioception and kinesthesia

Anterior Cruciate Ligament Sprain – Grade III   GOLD

What additional findings are likely with this patient?

Approximately two-thirds of the time the ACL is torn there is an accompanying meniscal tear. The collateral ligaments can also be involved although not as commonly as the menisci. When all three structures (ACL, MCL, and medial meniscus) are damaged it is referred to as the "unhappy triad."

MANAGEMENT

What is the most effective management of this patient?

Management of a patient following a grade III ACL sprain includes controlling edema, increasing range of motion, strengthening, and improving the fluidity of gait. For patients electing to have surgery, the patellar tendon is the most commonly utilized graft for intra-articular reconstruction. Patients often initially present with a knee immobilizer and crutches to protect the reconstructed ligament. Specific parameters are difficult to identify since many orthopedic surgeons utilize very specific protocols. Physical therapy management in the initial post-operative phase includes protecting the integrity of the graft, controlling edema, and improving range of motion. Specific intervention activities include pain modulation, patellar mobility, active range of motion exercises, gait activities, and quadriceps exercises. As patients progress in their rehabilitation program, treatment begins to focus on strengthening activities emphasizing closed-chain exercises and selected functional activities. Closed-chain exercises are considered more desirable than open-chain exercises since they minimize anterior translation of the tibia. Patients should be required to complete a functional progression prior to returning to unrestricted athletics. For patients opting for a conservative (non-operative) approach, it is necessary to begin an aggressive strengthening program once the acute phase of the injury has subsided.

What home care regimen should be recommended?

The home care regimen should consist of range of motion, strengthening, palliative care, and functional activities as warranted based on the results of the patient examination and course (operative versus non-operative) of treatment.

OUTCOME

What is the likely outcome of a course of physical therapy?

It is possible that with an aggressive strengthening program and/or activity modification, patients may be able to participate in light to moderate athletic activities without formal surgical reconstruction. Patients electing to have surgery can expect to return to their previous functional level in four to six months.

What are the long-term effects of the patient's condition?

Patients that sustain a complete tear of the ACL and elect not to have reconstructive surgery will likely be at increased risk for instability and subsequent deterioration of joint surfaces.

COMPARISON

What are the distinguishing characteristics of a similar condition?

A grade III posterior cruciate ligament (PCL) sprain is less common than an ACL sprain. The most common mechanism of injury for a PCL sprain is a "dashboard" injury or forced knee hyperflexion as the foot is plantar flexed. A grade III PCL injury will typically produce effusion, posterior tenderness, and a positive posterior drawer test. Knee extension is often limited due to the effusion and stretching of the posterior capsule and gastrocnemius. The rehabilitation program typically emphasizes strengthening of the quadriceps muscles. Individuals with an isolated PCL sprain may not exhibit any functional performance limitations and as a result, surgical intervention is far less common than with an ACL sprain. A PCL sprain alters the arthrokinematics of the knee joint and as a result a patient will be susceptible to degenerative changes such as arthritis.

CLINICAL SCENARIOS

Scenario One

A 16-year-old gymnast sustains a grade I ACL injury after landing awkwardly on her left leg during a vault. The patient is two days status post injury and has mild effusion in the involved knee. The patient is a competitive gymnast and needs to compete in a regional meet in slightly less than four weeks.

Scenario Two

A 35-year-old male is referred to physical therapy after injuring his knee in a softball game. The patient reports tearing the ACL ten years ago in a skiing accident. The patient is active, however, reports more recent episodes of instability. The physician notes significant arthritic changes in the involved knee including diminished joint space.

DIAGNOSIS

What condition produces a patient's symptoms?

Bicipital tendonitis is an inflammatory process of the tendon of the long head of the biceps. Impingement or an inflammatory injury can result in symptoms of shoulder pain. Repeated full abduction and lateral rotation of the humeral head can lead to irritation that produces inflammation, edema, microscopic tears within the tendon, and degeneration of the tendon itself.

An injury was most likely sustained to which structure?

Continuous or repetitive shoulder motions can cause overuse of the biceps tendon. Damaged cells within the tendon do not have time to heal, leading to tendonitis. This is common in sports or work activities that require frequent and repeated use of the upper extremities, especially when the motion is performed overhead. Athletes who throw, swim or swing a racquet or club are at greatest risk. Years of shoulder wear and tear can cause the biceps tendon to become inflamed. Degeneration in a tendon causes a loss of the normal arrangement of the collagen fibers that join together to form the tendon. Some of the individual strands of the tendon become intertwined due to the degeneration, while allowing other fibers to break and the tendon to lose strength.

INFERENCE

What is the most likely contributing factor in the development of this condition?

Bicipital tendonitis is often caused through repetitive overhead activity and motion. There is usually direct trauma to the tendon as the shoulder motion approaches excessive abduction and lateral rotation. Examples of high risk athletes include baseball pitchers, tennis players, gymnasts, rowers, and swimmers. Bicipital tendonitis can also be caused secondary to other shoulder pathology including rotator cuff disease, impingement syndrome or intra-articular pathology such as labral tears.

CONFIRMATION

What is the most likely clinical presentation?

Patients generally report the feeling of a deep ache directly in the front and on the top of the shoulder. The ache may spread down into the biceps muscle and is usually made worse with overhead activities or lifting heavy objects. Resting the shoulder typically reduces the pain. A catching or slipping sensation of the biceps muscle may indicate a tear of the transverse humeral ligament. Bicipital tendinopathy, pain to palpation over the anterior shoulder in the area of the bicipital groove, pain with the biceps resistance test (i.e., shoulder flexion against resistance with elbow extended and forearm supinated), and a positive Yergason's or Speed's test (i.e., pain with resisted supination of the forearm or with the elbow flexed at 90° and the arm adducted against the body) are positive indicators for bicipital tendonitis.

What laboratory or imaging studies would confirm the diagnosis?

There are no laboratory tests to assist with the diagnosis of bicipital tendonitis. Plain x-rays do not diagnose bicipital tendonitis, but may show calcification in the groove or subacromial spurring. Other x-rays of the neck and elbow may be indicated to rule out referred shoulder pain. MRI can view the tendon, but is expensive and not usually used unless the patient is not responding to conservative treatment.

What additional information should be obtained to confirm the diagnosis?

Testing such as the biceps resistance test, Speed's test, and Yergason's test may be performed in conjunction with a full physical examination.

EXAMINATION

What history should be documented?

Important areas to explore include past medical history, medications, current health status, nutritional status, social history and habits, occupation, living environment, and social support system.

What tests/measures are most appropriate?

Arousal, attention, and cognition: examine mental status, learning ability, memory, motivation

Community and work integration: analysis of community, work, and leisure activities

Environmental, home, and work barriers: analysis of current and potential barriers or hazards

Ergonomics and body mechanics: analysis of dexterity and coordination

Joint integrity and mobility: assessment of hyper- and hypomobility of a joint, soft tissue swelling and inflammation

Muscle performance: strength assessment, muscle tone assessment

Pain: pain perception assessment scale, visual analogue scale, assessment of muscle soreness

Posture: analysis of resting and dynamic posture

Range of motion: active and passive range of motion, Speed's test, Yergason's test

Reflex integrity: assessment of deep tendon reflexes

Self-care and home management: assessment of functional capacity

Sensory integrity: assessment of proprioception and kinesthesia

What additional findings are likely with this patient?

Patients with long-term chronic tendonitis may experience shoulder instability and subluxation secondary to biceps degeneration. Bicipital tendonitis will also frequently accompany impingement syndrome, rotator cuff tendonitis, and forms of glenohumeral instability.

MANAGEMENT

What is the most effective management of this patient?

The primary goal of medical management is to relieve pain, reduce inflammation, and regain full available range of motion. Rest and/or immobilization using a splint or a removable brace may be indicated initially for a brief period of time. Generally, the patient should avoid all overhead movement, reaching, and lifting of objects. Pharmacological intervention may include nonsteroidal anti-inflammatory medications (NSAIDs) which will reduce both pain and inflammation. Active physical therapy is not often initiated immediately, however, the patient may be referred for instruction in general education of the pathology, guidelines for restrictions, pendulum exercises, and the use of TENS. The application of heat or cold to the affected area can also assist with relief of pain. The patient may benefit from the use of iontophoresis or phonophoresis. As the patient progresses out of the acute phase, physical therapy should focus on an exercise program that stretches and strengthens the affected muscle groups. This can restore the tendon's ability to function properly, improve healing, and prevent future injury. Surgical intervention is only recommended for patients that have not progressed with conservative treatment over a six month period of time. The typical procedure includes arthroscopic decompression and acromioplasty with anterior acromionectomy.

What home care regimen should be recommended?

Patients with bicipital tendonitis are recommended to always perform warm-up activities prior to vigorous exercises, consistently perform passive selective stretching and strengthening, use proper body mechanics, and avoid any painful activity. The ongoing focus of a home program should be on strengthening and endurance surrounding the tendon. Patients will have to consistently participate in an ongoing home exercise program to prevent the risk of recurrence.

OUTCOME

What is the likely outcome of a course of physical therapy?

The goal of physical therapy is to restore full available range of motion without pain. Once the patient does not experience pain or discomfort with activity, they may slowly return to their previous level of activity. Most patients are successful with conservative treatment and are able to return to their activities after an average of six to eight weeks of physical therapy and rehabilitation.

What are the long-term effects of the patient's condition?

Although the overall prognosis depends on the level of involvement, most patients have a positive long-term outcome and are able to return to their previous level of functioning. Statistically, there are approximately 10% of patients that do not achieve a positive outcome and have further deterioration or a rupture of the tendon.

COMPARISON

What are the distinguishing characteristics of a similar condition?

The glenoid labrum is a fibrocartilage rim that surrounds the glenoid cavity, attaches to the glenoid cavity of the scapula to increase its depth, and protects the edge of the bone within the joint capsule. A labral tear is most susceptible with anterior damage or subluxation. A Bankart lesion is the name given to the avulsion of the labral ligamentous complex from the anteroinferior aspect of the glenoid. This is the most common lesion resulting in anterior joint instability. A CT scan can diagnose the tear and surgical intervention is normally successful for repair.

CLINICAL SCENARIOS

Scenario One

A 27-year-old male is referred to physical therapy by his primary care physician for "probable bicipital tendonitis." He went to see his doctor secondary to pain when performing overhead activities and lifting objects of varying weight. He works as an auto mechanic 50 hours per week. He was trying to "work through the pain," but it has worsened over the last month. He resides with his wife and twin girls in a ranch style home.

Scenario Two

A 56-year-old tennis instructor has noticed an increase in pain through a particular arc of motion at her shoulder. She was diagnosed with impingement syndrome years ago, but has not had any recurrence or discomfort again until now. She states that her goal is to return to teaching tennis.

Lateral Epicondylitis

DIAGNOSIS

What condition produces a patient's symptoms?

Lateral epicondylitis (tennis elbow) is characterized by inflammation or degenerative changes at the common extensor tendon that attaches to the lateral epicondyle of the elbow. The primary symptom of this condition is pain.

An injury was most likely sustained to which structure?

Repeated overuse of the wrist extensors, particularly the extensor carpi radialis brevis can produce tensile stress and result in microscopic tearing and damage to the extensor tendon. Other muscles that can be affected include the extensor digitorum, extensor carpi radialis longus, and extensor carpi ulnaris.

INFERENCE

What is the most likely contributing factor in the development of this condition?

The exact etiology is uncertain, however, repetitive wrist action against resistance during extension and supination appear to produce this condition. Over time inflammation of the periosteum may develop with formation of adhesions. The continued microtrauma does not allow for proper healing and will continue to injure the tissues. This pattern is best seen while hitting a backhand in tennis, however, overuse with painting, hand tools, gardening, and any repeated activity that involves forceful wrist extension can result in lateral epicondylitis. Men are more likely to develop lateral epicondylitis and it is also more common for individuals in their late 30's and 40's secondary to the normal loss of the extensibility of connective tissue with age.

CONFIRMATION

What is the most likely clinical presentation?

A typical patient with lateral epicondylitis is usually between the third and fifth decades of life and has unilateral involvement of the elbow. Lateral epicondylitis presents with pain along the lateral aspect of the elbow especially over the lateral epicondyle that sometimes radiates into the dorsum of the hand. The pain will increase with wrist flexion with elbow extension, resisted wrist extension, and resisted radial deviation. The patient may also have difficulty holding or gripping objects and insufficient forearm functional strength. Range of motion of the elbow usually remains normal, however, may be limited in severe cases. The patient will have localized tenderness over the lateral epicondyle and may present with localized swelling. The pain usually increases with activity and is noted at night.

What laboratory or imaging studies would confirm the diagnosis?

No lab or imaging studies are required to diagnose lateral epicondylitis. X-ray or MRI may be used to rule out other conditions. Electrodiagnostic tests are only beneficial if there is radial nerve involvement.

What additional information should be obtained to confirm the diagnosis?

Lateral epicondylitis is usually diagnosed based on history, physical examination of the extremity, and several manual maneuvers that specifically identify the presence of lateral epicondylitis. An increase in pain at the lateral epicondyle with resisted wrist extension implies extensor carpi radialis brevis involvement.

EXAMINATION

What history should be documented?

Important areas to explore include past medical history, medications, family history, current symptoms, current health status, social history and habits, occupation, leisure and sport activities, and social support system.

What tests/measures are most appropriate?

Anthropometric characteristics: circumferential measurements of the forearm

Arousal, attention, and cognition: examine mental status, learning ability, memory, motivation

Community and work integration: analysis of community, work, and leisure activities

Environmental, home, and work barriers: analysis of current and potential barriers or hazards

Integumentary integrity: skin assessment, assessment of sensation

Joint integrity and mobility: assessment of hypermobility and hypomobility of a joint, soft tissue swelling and inflammation, quality of movement of the elbow complex, provocative tests for lateral epicondylitis including Cozen's test, Mill's test, and lateral epicondylitis test

Muscle performance: strength assessment, muscle tone assessment, grip test dynamometer

Orthotic, protective, and supportive devices: potential utilization of bracing, splinting

Pain: pain perception assessment scale, visual analogue scale, assessment of muscle soreness

Posture: analysis of resting and dynamic posture

Range of motion: active and passive range of motion of bilateral upper extremities

Reflex integrity: assessment of deep tendon reflexes

Self-care and home management: assessment of functional capacity

What additional findings are likely with this patient?

If the patient is involved in tennis or some other potential overuse activity, there should be remediation and modification in training, technique, and equipment to minimize the chance of recurrence.

MANAGEMENT

What is the most effective management of this patient?

Medical management initially treats the pain and inflammation through protection, rest, ice, compression, and elevation. During the initial phase the patient should avoid all activities that aggravate the injury. Pharmacological intervention should include NSAIDs to alleviate pain and inflammation. Modalities may also be used such as phonophoresis with hydrocortisone or iontophoresis with dexamethasone. On occasion, resting splints may be used during the acute stage to relieve tension of the involved muscles. Physical therapy intervention should initiate stretching and strengthening to improve flexibility and increase functional activities. All exercise must remain pain free. Other modalities including electrical stimulation and cryotherapy may be beneficial. Strengthening should include elbow, wrist, and hand exercises. As a patient progresses, resistive, isokinetic, and sport-specific exercises should be introduced. Counter-force bracing in the form of a forearm band may be indicated to reduce the degree of tension in the region of the muscular attachment. A patient should wean from the brace, prior to the completion of rehabilitation so the patient does not depend on it or use it as a replacement for rehabilitation.

What home care regimen should be recommended?

A home care regimen should include the same therapeutic program the patient performs during physical therapy. Patient education should include modification of all activities that exacerbate the symptoms. It is imperative that the patient not rush or advance beyond the parameters of the home program as it will exacerbate the condition. A patient must avoid all activities that produce pain and use ice, elevation, and rest as needed.

OUTCOME

What is the likely outcome of a course of physical therapy?

Physical therapy may be indicated with goals of regaining appropriate strength, flexibility, and endurance while reducing inflammation and pain of the involved muscles. Overall outcome is favorable and a patient should be able to return to all previous functional activities without restrictions.

What are the long-term effects of the patient's condition?

Lateral epicondylitis will commonly recur, however, continued stretching and exercise will decrease the risk of future recurrence. If conservative treatment does not improve symptoms after two to three months, surgical intervention may be indicated.

COMPARISON

What are the distinguishing characteristics of a similar condition?

Medial epicondylitis (golfer's or swimmer's elbow) results from repeated microtrauma to the flexor carpi radialis and/or the humeral head of the pronator teres during pronation and wrist flexion. There is pain with resisted wrist flexion and resisted pronation and point tenderness over the medial epicondyle. Treatment is similar in protocol to lateral epicondylitis, however, is directed at the appropriate location. Complete immobilization is never recommended, however, counter-force bracing or splinting may be indicated.

CLINICAL SCENARIOS

Scenario One

A 27-year-old tennis player is seen in physical therapy diagnosed with right lateral epicondylitis. The patient plays in a competitive league and recently changed his instructor and increased the number of games played per week. He complains of pain and point tenderness over the lateral epicondyle. He is very frustrated, as this pain has had a large impact on his ability to win games.

Scenario Two

A 42-year-old female diagnosed with right lateral epicondylitis has been seen in physical therapy for four weeks. She has a past medical history that includes complex regional pain syndrome two years ago in the right upper extremity and is status post hysterectomy three months ago. She has not had any relief of pain and states that she cannot hold anything in her right hand. She enjoys gardening and works at a vegetable farm.

Medial Collateral Ligament Sprain – Grade II

DIAGNOSIS

What condition produces a patient's symptoms?

The medial collateral ligament (MCL) connects the medial epicondyle of the femur to the medial tibia and as a result resists medially directed force at the knee. The MCL is the primary stabilizer of the medial side of the knee against valgus force and lateral rotation of the tibia (especially during knee flexion). This extra-articular ligament is a thick and flat band which attaches proximally on the medial femoral condyle and extends to the medial surface of the tibia approximately six centimeters below the joint line. A common mechanism of injury is a direct blow against the lateral surface of the knee causing valgus stress and subsequent damage to the medial aspect of the knee.

An injury was most likely sustained to which structure?

A grade II injury of the MCL is characterized by partial tearing of the ligament's fibers resulting in joint laxity when the ligament is stretched. Often the medial capsular ligament is involved in a grade II sprain of the MCL.

INFERENCE

What is the most likely contributing factor in the development of this condition?

Individuals participating in contact activities requiring a high level of agility are particularly susceptible to an MCL injury. Mechanism of injury is usually a blow to the outside of the knee joint causing excess force to the medial side of the joint. The MCL can also be injured by a twisting of the knee. Muscle weakness resulting in poor dynamic stabilization may also increase the incidence of this type of injury.

CONFIRMATION

What is the most likely clinical presentation?

A patient with a grade II MCL injury will likely present with an inability to fully extend and flex the knee, pain and significant tenderness along the medial aspect of the knee, possible decrease in strength, potential loss of proprioception, and an antalgic gait. There is typically discernable laxity with valgus testing, instability of the joint, and slight to moderate swelling around the knee. More severe swelling may be indicative of meniscus or cruciate ligament involvement.

What laboratory or imaging studies would confirm the diagnosis?

MRI is a non-invasive imaging technique that can be utilized to view soft tissue structures such as ligaments. The imaging technique is extremely expensive and therefore may not be commonly employed on an individual with a suspected MCL injury without other extenuating circumstances.

What additional information should be obtained to confirm the diagnosis?

A valgus stress test is a technique designed to detect medial instability in a single plane. The examiner applies a valgus stress at the knee while stabilizing the ankle. The test is often performed initially in full extension and then in 30 degrees of flexion. A patient with a grade II MCL sprain may exhibit 5-15 degrees of laxity with valgus stress at 30 degrees of flexion.

EXAMINATION

What history should be documented?

Important areas to explore include mechanism of present injury, current symptoms, past medical history, medications, living environment, occupation, social history and habits, and social support system.

What tests/measures are most appropriate?

Anthropometric characteristics: palpation to determine knee effusion, lower extremity circumferential measurements

Arousal, attention, and cognition: examine mental status, learning ability, memory, motivation

Assistive and adaptive devices: analysis of components and safety of a device, potential utilization of crutches

Community and work integration: analysis of community, work, and leisure activities

Environmental, home, and work barriers: analysis of current and potential barriers or hazards

Gait, locomotion, and balance: safety during gait with an assistive device

Integumentary integrity: assessment of sensation (pain, temperature, tactile), skin assessment

Joint integrity and mobility: special tests for ligaments and menisci, valgus stress test, palpation of structures, joint play, soft tissue restrictions, joint pain

Muscle performance: strength assessment, assessment of active movement, resisted isometrics, muscle contraction characteristics, muscle endurance

Orthotic, protective, and supportive devices: potential utilization of bracing, taping or wrapping

Pain: pain perception assessment scale, visual analogue scale

Range of motion: active and passive range of motion

Self-care and home management: assessment of functional capacity

Sensory integrity: assessment of proprioception and kinesthesia

Medial Collateral Ligament Sprain – Grade II   GOLD

What additional findings are likely with this patient?

Anterior cruciate ligament and/or meniscal damage often accompanies a grade II MCL injury. As a result it is often prudent to perform special tests directed at these particular structures. The MCL normally has a good secondary support system with weight bearing forces compressing the medial side of the joint and adding to the overall stability of the joint. This allows the structures to be protected after injury along with use of a brace.

MANAGEMENT

What is the most effective management of this patient?

Medical management for a grade II MCL sprain usually involves conservative management including R.I.C.E. (rest, icing, compression, elevation). Pharmacological intervention is directed towards pain management through acetaminophen or NSAIDs. The patient may utilize a full-length knee immobilizer or a hinge brace and crutches to limit weight bearing through the involved lower extremity for initial rehabilitation. Physical therapy intervention should be directed towards increasing range of motion in the involved extremity and beginning light resistive exercises. Range of motion exercises may include heel slides or stationary cycling without resistance. Resistive exercises should be directed towards the quadriceps and may include isometrics and closed kinetic chain exercises. Functional activities such as gait and stair climbing should be incorporated into the treatment program. Superficial modalities and electrical stimulation may be utilized to combat pain and inflammation. Transverse friction massage may be applied to the healing ligament so it does not adhere to surrounding and adjacent structures. Care must be taken not to massage the proximal attachment of the MCL due to potential bony periosteal disruption. A patient should be required to complete a functional progression prior to returning to unrestricted activity.

What home care regimen should be recommended?

The home care regimen should consist of range of motion, strengthening, palliative care, and functional activities as warranted based on the results of the patient examination. The use of crutches should continue until the patient can adequately extend the knee joint.

OUTCOME

What is the likely outcome of a course of physical therapy?

A grade II MCL sprain should progress fairly quickly if no other structures (ACL or meniscus) are involved. A patient should be able to return to their previous functional level within four to eight weeks following the injury.

What are the long-term effects of the patient's condition?

Proper healing time and rehabilitation management should allow the patient to return to all forms of activity once the patient demonstrates full range of motion, ambulation without a limp, no visual swelling, and competence with all agility testing. If the patient has residual laxity from the injury the patient may be susceptible to reinjury.

COMPARISON

What are the distinguishing characteristics of a similar condition?

A grade II lateral collateral ligament injury differs from an MCL injury in several ways. The lateral collateral ligament attaches proximally on the lateral femoral condyle and runs distally and posteriorly to insert on the head of the fibula. Lateral collateral ligament injuries are far less common than MCL injuries. Management should focus on the same general goals (range of motion, strengthening, palliative care, functional activities) as those outlined for the MCL injury.

CLINICAL SCENARIOS

Scenario One

A 17-year-old male is diagnosed with a left grade III MCL sprain and a small tear in the medial meniscus. The patient was playing football when he was injured. The patient has no significant past medical history and plans to participate in football at the collegiate level.

Scenario Two

A 20-year-old college field hockey player complains of knee pain after being diagnosed with a grade I MCL sprain. The patient is mildly tender to palpation over the medial joint line and exhibits trace effusion. The patient has no significant past medical history and would like to return to athletic competition as soon as possible.

DIAGNOSIS

What condition produces a patient's symptoms?

Osteoarthritis (OA) is a heterogeneous group of conditions resulting in common physiological changes. The most common type of joint disease, OA is a degenerative chronic disorder resulting from the biochemical breakdown of articular cartilage in the synovial joints. Although theories indicate that OA is due to excessive wear and tear, secondary inflammatory changes may also affect the involved joints. OA has been divided into primary and secondary forms.

An injury was most likely sustained to which structure?

The progression of OA begins with degenerative alterations primarily in the articular cartilage. This degenerative process is usually a result of excessive loading of a healthy joint or normal loading of an abnormal joint. External forces create the breakdown of the chondrocytes and cause disruption of the cartilaginous matrix. Loss of cartilage results in the loss of the joint space. Through this process, reactive new bone forms, usually at the margins and subchondral areas of the joint.

INFERENCE

What is the most likely contributing factor in the development of this condition?

The etiology of primary OA is idiopathic occurring within intact joints with no history that supports the initiation of this condition. Primary OA is related to the aging process and typically occurs in older individuals. Secondary OA refers to degenerative disease of the synovial joints that results from some predisposing condition (i.e., trauma) that has adversely altered the articular cartilage and/or subchondral bone of the affected joints. Secondary OA often occurs in relatively young individuals. General risk factors include age, obesity, trauma, infection, repetitive microtrauma, genetic factors, inflammatory arthritis, neuromuscular and metabolic disorders.

CONFIRMATION

What is the most likely clinical presentation?

Potential sites for primary OA include joints of the hands specifically the distal interphalangeal joints (DIP) and inter-phalangeal joints (PIP), knees, hips, and the spine. Bilateral symmetry is often seen in cases of primary OA, particularly when the hands are affected. A patient with OA may experience a decrease in range of motion accompanied by crepitus within the affected joints. The patient will frequently complain of deep and aching joint pain exacerbated by prolonged activity and use. Heberden's nodes consist of palpable osteophytes in the DIP joints and are usually seen in women, but not men. Pain is the main reason patients seek medical attention. Initially, patients have pain during activity that is alleviated by rest and usually respond to analgesics. Morning stiffness in the affected joints usually occurs with progression of the disease, resulting in an increased pain level even at rest that may not respond to analgesics. Erythema or warmth over the joints is not usually present, but effusion may exist. Malalignment

and limitation of the joint may occur as the disease progresses in severity. The patient may also present with a deviated gait pattern, atypical movement patterns, and muscle atrophy.

What laboratory or imaging studies would confirm the diagnosis?

OA is typically diagnosed on the basis of clinical examination and x-ray findings. Laboratory tests will not diagnose OA.

What additional information should be obtained to confirm the diagnosis?

Visual inspection of the affected joints, a thorough examination, and a history of the condition will normally support the diagnosis.

EXAMINATION

What history should be documented?

Important areas to explore include past medical history, medications, current health status, nutritional status, social history and habits, occupation, living environment, and social support system.

What tests/measures are most appropriate?

Aerobic capacity and endurance: assessment of vital signs at rest and with activity, perceived exertion scale, pulse oximetry, auscultation of the lungs

Anthropometric characteristics: circumferential measurements

Arousal, attention, and cognition: mental status exam

Assistive and adaptive devices: analysis of components and safety of a device

Community and work integration: analysis of community, work, and leisure activities

Environmental, home, and work barriers: analysis of current and potential barriers or hazards

Ergonomics and body mechanics: analysis of dexterity and coordination

Gait, locomotion, and balance: static and dynamic balance in sitting and standing, safety during gait with/without an assistive device, Berg Functional Balance Scale, Functional Ambulation Profile

Integumentary integrity: assessment of sensation

Joint integrity and mobility: hypermobility and hypomobility of a joint, soft tissue swelling and inflammation

Motor function: equilibrium and righting reactions, motor assessment scales, coordination

Muscle performance: strength assessment

Pain: pain perception assessment scale, VAS

Posture: analysis of resting and dynamic posture

Range of motion: active and passive range of motion

Self-care and home management: assessment of functional capacity, Functional Independence Measure

Sensory integrity: proprioception and kinesthesia

What additional findings are likely with this patient?

In patients greater than 55 years old, the prevalence of OA is higher among women than men. DIP and PIP joint involvement resulting in Heberden's and Bouchard's nodes is also more common in women. Disease progression characteristically is slow, occurring over several years or decades. Pain is usually the initial and principal source of morbidity in OA. The patient can become progressively inactive leading to additional co-morbidities including weight gain. There is also an increased incidence of strains and sprains around joints affected with OA.

MANAGEMENT

What is the most effective management of this patient?

Medical management of a patient with OA is usually multi-faceted based on symptoms and the specific affected joints. Long-term management would include pharmacological intervention using acetaminophen or other NSAIDs to alleviate the pain. Glucocorticoid intra-articular injections may also be prescribed to improve a patient's symptoms, however, must be used sparingly due to the long-term negative effects. Nutritional education and weight reduction may be indicated to reduce the stress on the affected joints. Physical therapy may be indicated intermittently in order to preserve joint motion and flexibility. Other treatment may include posture retraining, work site evaluation, general strengthening, relaxation and endurance activities, icing or heat for pain management, hydrotherapy, modalities, patient education, aquatic therapy, and functional activities. If conservative treatment fails, a patient may be a candidate for joint replacement surgery with the goal of pain relief.

What home care regimen should be recommended?

A home care regimen for OA should include general strengthening to tolerance, AROM exercises, endurance activities, continued use of relaxation techniques, and supportive or assistive devices that would decrease pain and improve functional ability. It is very important that the patient avoid overexertion and fatigue.

OUTCOME

What is the likely outcome of a course of physical therapy?

Physical therapy can assist the patient during periods of exacerbation of the disease process, however, cannot change the ultimate outcome of the condition. OA is a progressive and chronic condition. Physical therapy can assist in minimizing the effects of the process and allow for as much independence as allowed by patient tolerance during functional activities.

What are the long-term effects of the patient's condition?

Approximately 80-90% of individuals older than 65 years have evidence of primary OA. The degree of disability also depends on the site(s) of involvement and rate of progression. Usually, the pain slowly worsens over time, but it may stabilize. OA of the knee is a leading cause of disability in elderly persons.

COMPARISON

What are the distinguishing characteristics of a similar condition?

Psoriatic arthritis is a rheumatic condition characterized by inflammatory arthritis and is often seen in combination with psoriatic skin lesions. Symptoms include silver or grey scaly spots on the scalp, elbows, knees and spine, pitting of fingernails and toenails, pain and swelling in one or more joints, and swelling of the fingers and toes. Psoriatic arthritis affects men and women of all races and usually occurs between the ages of 20 and 50, but can occur at any age. The etiology is unknown, but theories suggest a relationship to genetic inheritance, psoriasis, and environmental factors.

CLINICAL SCENARIOS

Scenario One

A 71-year-old female is referred to physical therapy with significant OA in her hands, knees, and hips. She is approximately 35 pounds overweight and has lost mobility. She rates her pain as an eight out of ten and wants to have surgery to "fix" her legs. She resides in a two-story home with her husband.

Scenario Two

A 39-year-old male has developed secondary OA as a result of a 15-year career in semi-professional football. The patient lives a very active lifestyle, however, has a significant amount of pain in both knee joints. The patient is currently married and working full-time.

Patellofemoral Syndrome

DIAGNOSIS

What condition produces a patient's symptoms?

Patellofemoral syndrome is caused by an abnormal tracking of the patella between the femoral condyles. The tracking problem places increased and misdirected forces between the patella and femur. This most commonly occurs when the patella is pulled too far laterally during knee extension.

An injury was most likely sustained to which structure?

Patellofemoral syndrome causes damage to the articular cartilage of the patella. The damage can range from softening of the cartilage to complete cartilage destruction resulting in exposure of subchondral bone.

INFERENCE

What is the most likely contributing factor in the development of this condition?

The exact etiology of patellofemoral syndrome is unknown, however, it is extremely common during adolescence, is more prevalent in females than males, and has a direct association with the activity level of the patient. In an older population patellofemoral syndrome is often associated with osteoarthritis. Additional factors associated with patellofemoral syndrome include patella alta, insufficient lateral femoral condyle, weak vastus medialis obliquus, excessive pronation, excessive knee valgus, and tightness in lower extremity muscles (iliopsoas, hamstrings, gastrocnemius, and vastus lateralis).

CONFIRMATION

What is the most likely clinical presentation?

A patient with patellofemoral syndrome often describes a gradual onset of anterior knee pain following an increase in physical activity. The pain is characteristically located behind the patella (retropatellar pain) and may be exacerbated with activities that increase patellofemoral compressive forces (stair climbing, jumping) and also with prolonged static positioning (sitting with the knee flexed at 90 degrees as in a car, plane, theatre). Point tenderness is common over the lateral border of the patella and crepitus may be elicited when the patella is manually compressed into the trochlear groove. Visible quadriceps atrophy may be noted in the involved lower extremity particularly along the vastus medialis obliquus. The patient may also complain of burning pain when sitting for prolonged periods of time or when ascending stairs.

What laboratory or imaging studies would confirm the diagnosis?

Laboratory or imaging studies are not commonly used to diagnose patellofemoral syndrome. X-rays are often used to rule out a fracture, examine the configuration of the patellofemoral joint, and identify potential osteophytes, joint space narrowing, patella alta, and arthritic changes. Arthrogram and arthroscopy can be used to examine the articular cartilage.

What additional information should be obtained to confirm the diagnosis?

Special tests such as Clarke's sign can be useful when attempting to confirm the diagnosis. The test is performed by applying pressure immediately proximal to the upper pole of the patient's patella. The physician/therapist then asks the patient to isometrically contract the quadriceps. A positive test is indicated by a failure to fully contract the quadriceps or by the presence of retropatellar pain. The test should be performed at varying degrees of flexion and extension. It is helpful to determine the patient's Q angle and examine the alignment of the patient's feet, as these factors can contribute to the causative factors.

EXAMINATION

What history should be documented?

Important areas to explore include past medical history, medications, current symptoms and health status, social history, occupation/recreational activities, living environment, and social support system.

What tests/measures are most appropriate?

Anthropometric characteristics: knee effusion, lower extremity circumferential measurements

Arousal, attention, and cognition: examine mental status, learning ability, memory, motivation

Assistive and adaptive devices: components and safety of a device, potential utilization of crutches

Environmental, home, and work barriers: analysis of current and potential barriers or hazards

Gait, locomotion, and balance: safety during gait with an assistive device

Integumentary integrity: assessment of sensation (pain, temperature, tactile), skin assessment

Joint integrity and mobility: Clarke's sign, patella grind test (active and passive), dynamic patella tracking, patella glide test, palpation of structures, joint play, soft tissue restrictions, joint pain

Muscle performance: strength assessment, assessment of active movement, resisted isometrics, muscle contraction characteristics, muscle endurance

Orthotic, protective, and supportive devices: potential utilization of bracing, taping or wrapping

Pain: pain perception assessment scale

Range of motion: active and passive range of motion

Self-care and home management: functional capacity

Sensory integrity: proprioception and kinesthesia

What additional findings are likely with this patient?

Patients diagnosed with patellofemoral syndrome often have an increased Q angle. The normal Q angle is 13 degrees in males and 18 degrees in females. The Q angle is measured using the anterior superior iliac spine, the midpoint of the patella, and the tibial tubercle. Differential diagnosis should rule out other problems such as referred pain from the hip, Osgood-Schlatter syndrome, neuroma, patellar tendonitis, plica syndrome, and infection of the knee joint.

MANAGEMENT

What is the most effective management of this patient?

Medical management of patellofemoral syndrome is usually successful with conservative measures, surgical intervention is rare. Pharmacological intervention may include acetaminophen, NSAIDs, and steroid injections into the joint. Physical therapy management includes controlling edema, stretching, strengthening, improving range of motion, and activity modification. Mobilization activities to increase medial glide can be beneficial to increase the flexibility of the lateral fascia. Strengthening activities emphasizing the vastus medialis obliquus in non-weight bearing and weight bearing positions are recommended. Biofeedback can be a useful tool in order to selectively train the muscle. Stretching activities should emphasize the hamstrings, iliotibial band, tensor fasciae latae, and rectus femoris. Strengthening activities may include quadriceps setting exercises, straight leg raising and mini-squats incorporating the hip adductors. Exercises such as deep squats should be avoided since they will tend to aggravate the patient's condition. Patellar taping to improve the position and tracking of the patella during dynamic activities can be useful to limit irritation.

What home care regimen should be recommended?

The home care regimen should consist of range of motion, strengthening, stretching, palliative care, and functional activities. An active patient must decrease their level of activities to relieve the additional stress placed on the patellofemoral joint. A patient must also comply with recommendations for proper footwear and orthotics to improve alignment and lessen aggravation of symptoms, specifically knee pain.

OUTCOME

What is the likely outcome of a course of physical therapy?

A patient with patellofemoral syndrome that undergoes conservative management may be able to return to their previous functioning within four to six weeks.

What are the long-term effects of the patient's condition?

Prognosis for a full recovery is good with successful conservative management, however, failure to adequately address the cause of the patellofemoral syndrome will likely result in a patient's condition further deteriorating. The patient may experience increased irritation of the patellofemoral joint that further impacts their ability to participate in activities of daily living. Periodic exacerbations of the condition most commonly due to an increased activity level may require further physical therapy intervention.

COMPARISON

What are the distinguishing characteristics of a similar condition?

Patellar tendonitis is an overuse condition characterized by inflammatory changes of the patellar tendon. The condition is most prevalent in athletes who participate in activities requiring repetitive jumping skills. The primary complaint is often pain over the anterior portion of the superior tibia with activities such as jumping or ascending/descending stairs. Patients may also experience pain after prolonged sitting and often exhibit point tenderness at the superior pole of the patella tendon. Management of patellar tendonitis incorporates many of the same interventions as patellofemoral syndrome such as range of motion, stretching, and palliative care.

CLINICAL SCENARIOS

Scenario One

A 14-year-old female is referred to physical therapy with patellofemoral syndrome. The patient has mild edema and is sensitive to light touch over the anterior surface of the knee. The patient reports gaining ten pounds and expresses that she is willing to do "anything" to improve her present condition.

Scenario Two

A 45-year-old male is referred to physical therapy after experiencing anterior knee pain for the last week. The patient is 19 weeks status post ACL reconstruction and has recently returned to a softball league. The patient reports an insidious onset of pain and insists that he has been faithful to his home program. A note from the referring physician confirms that the integrity of the graft is fine and he suspects patellofemoral syndrome.

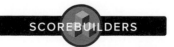

DIAGNOSIS

What condition produces a patient's symptoms?

The plantar fascia is a thin layer of tough connective tissue that supports the arch of the foot. Plantar fasciitis is an inflammatory process of the plantar fascia (or aponeurosis) at its origin on the calcaneus. Plantar fasciitis is a chronic overuse condition that develops secondary to repetitive stretching of the plantar fascia through excessive foot pronation during the loading phase of gait. This results in stress at the calcaneal origin of the plantar fascia.

An injury was most likely sustained to which structure?

Injury can occur to the plantar fascia itself and cause microtearing, inflammation, and pain. The abductor hallucis, flexor digitorum brevis, and quadratus plantae muscles share the same origin on the medial tubercle of the calcaneus and may also become inflamed and irritated.

INFERENCE

What is the most likely contributing factor in the development of this condition?

Factors that contribute to the development of plantar fasciitis include excessive pronation during gait, tightness of the foot and calf musculature, obesity, and possessing a high arch. A person participating in endurance sports such as running and dancing or a person with an occupation that requires prolonged walking or standing has an increased risk for plantar fasciitis. It is believed that development of plantar fasciitis results from a combination of predisposing factors. Although it is more common in the middle-age population, it also occurs in younger individuals, but usually in combination with calcaneal apophysitis.

CONFIRMATION

What is the most likely clinical presentation?

A patient with plantar fasciitis presents with severe pain in the heel when first standing up in the morning (when the fascia is contracted, stiff, and cold). This pain has also been reported to radiate proximally up the calf and/or distally to the toes. This is the most common symptom that relates directly to the diagnosis of plantar fasciitis and in one study was expressed in over 84% of cases. Pain typically subsides for a few hours during the day, but increases with prolonged activity or when the patient has been non-weight bearing and resumes a weight bearing posture. Pain has also been described by patients as "pain that moves around." A patient will typically experience point tenderness and pain with palpation over the calcaneal insertion of the plantar fascia. There may be bony growths in the plantar fascia near its insertion. Plantar fasciitis is usually unilateral and tightness in the Achilles tendon is found in the majority of the patients.

What laboratory or imaging studies would confirm the diagnosis?

Plantar fasciitis is initially treated based on symptoms and physical examination. If pain persists after six to eight weeks of physical therapy intervention, MRI may be used to confirm the diagnosis. Other diagnostic tools may include x-ray and bone scan to rule out a stress fracture, rheumatology workup to rule out systemic etiology, and EMG testing to rule out nerve entrapment.

What additional information should be obtained to confirm the diagnosis?

A thorough history and biomechanical assessment of the foot, observation of the fat pad, examination for Achilles tendon tightness, analysis of footwear, and gait disturbances all assist in diagnosing plantar fasciitis.

EXAMINATION

What history should be documented?

Important areas to explore include mechanism of current injury, training routine, past medical history, medications, social history and habits, occupation, living environment, and social support system.

What tests/measures are most appropriate?

Anthropometric characteristics: circumferential measurements of affected area or extremity

Arousal, attention, and cognition: examine mental status, learning ability, memory, motivation

Community and work integration: analysis of community, work, and leisure activities

Environmental, home, and work barriers: analysis of current and potential barriers or hazards

Gait, locomotion, and balance: biomechanical analysis of gait during walking and running (if appropriate), footprint analysis, dynamic plantar pressure distribution

Integumentary inspection: assessment of sensation, skin assessment

Joint integrity and mobility: assessment of swelling, inflammation, and joint restriction

Muscle performance: strength assessment, muscle endurance

Pain: pain perception scale, visual analogue scale

Orthotic, protective, and supportive devices: potential utilization of taping or use of cushions

Posture: analysis of resting and dynamic posture

Range of motion: active and passive range of motion

Sensory integrity: assessment of proprioception and kinesthesia

Self-care and home management: assessment of functional capacity

Plantar Fasciitis

What additional findings are likely with this patient?

Bony hypertrophy can occur at the origin of the plantar fascia resulting in a heel spur. Plantar fasciitis is a relative of heel spur syndrome, but is not the same condition. Heel spurs develop initially as calcium deposits that form due to the repetitive stress and inflammation in the plantar fascia.

MANAGEMENT

What is the most effective management of this patient?

Medical and pharmacological management of a patient with plantar fasciitis usually requires local corticosteroid injections or anti-inflammatory medications to reduce inflammation within the plantar fascia. Physical therapy intervention consists of ice massage, deep friction massage, shoe modification, heel insert application, foot orthotic prescription, modification of activities to include non-weight bearing endurance activities, and a gentle stretching program of the Achilles tendon and plantar fascia. Muscle strengthening exercises for the intrinsic and extrinsic muscles should be implemented once the acute symptoms have subsided. During the acute phase the patient must also modify activities and rest the affected foot. Heel cup prescription and casting may also be indicated.

What home care regimen should be recommended?

A home care regimen for a patient with plantar fasciitis should include ongoing strengthening and stretching exercises (especially stretching of the gastrocnemius and plantar fascia in the morning and prior to and after exercise), maintenance of a fitness program, the use of proper footwear, and the use of foot orthotics and heel inserts if warranted. Night tension splints may be indicated if symptoms persist.

OUTCOME

What is the likely outcome of a course of physical therapy?

Conservative physical therapy intervention on an outpatient basis in combination with a consistent home program should allow the patient to return to a more functional level within eight weeks. Total resolution of symptoms can take up to twelve months. Physical therapy, orthotic prescription, splinting, pharmacological injections, and physician follow-up are all components of the treatment program that may be required for a positive outcome.

What are the long-term effects of the patient's condition?

A patient previously diagnosed with plantar fasciitis is at an increased risk for recurrence, however, successful conservative management, compliance with a home program, and proper footwear will decrease the incidence of any negative long-term effects. If conservative management fails the patient may require surgical intervention, however, this option is relatively rare. Approximately 10% of patients can develop persistent, chronic, and disabling symptoms.

COMPARISON

What are the distinguishing characteristics of a similar condition?

The tarsal tunnel is the region where the tibial nerve passes between the medial malleolus and the calcaneus. The tibial nerve splits into the medial and lateral plantar nerves while still traversing in the tunnel along with other nerves in this region. Tarsal tunnel syndrome is characterized by pain that is experienced with weight bearing, but not with direct palpation to the plantar fascia. Characteristics of tarsal tunnel syndrome include complaints of numbness, burning pain, tingling, and paresthesias at the heel. Etiology consists of entrapment and compression of the posterior tibial nerve or plantar nerves within the tarsal tunnel due to inflammation or thickening of the flexor retinaculum.

CLINICAL SCENARIOS

Scenario One

A 19-year-old male athlete is referred to physical therapy with bilateral heel pain. The physician has ruled out systemic disorders and diagnosed bilateral mechanical plantar fasciitis. The athlete is a swimmer and began running cross-country last fall. The patient is otherwise healthy, but wants to return to athletic activities as soon as possible.

Scenario Two

A 56-year-old female is referred to physical therapy with left plantar fasciitis. The patient is mildly obese and works the night shift at a paper mill. She stands at her station throughout the shift and is required to walk between the two buildings every hour. The patient has a history of mild asthma and a cardiac murmur. She is anxious to obtain relief from her symptoms since she feels that her employment may be jeopardized.

DIAGNOSIS

What condition produces a patient's symptoms?

A rotator cuff tear may occur as a result of an acute traumatic incident or due to a chronic degenerative pathology such as chronic supraspinatus tendonitis. Tears may be classified as partial-thickness, full-thickness, acute, chronic or degenerative. Rotator cuff tears most commonly involve the supraspinatus tendon. However, with more severe or traumatic etiologies, the infraspinatus and subscapularis may also sustain damage.

An injury was most likely sustained to which structure?

The rotator cuff is comprised of the supraspinatus, infraspinatus, subscapularis, and teres minor. The muscles collectively function to provide dynamic stability to the glenohumeral (GH) joint. All four muscles originate from points on the ipsilateral scapula and insert on the proximal humerus. The muscles assist with shoulder mobility to some degree, however, support and mobility demands are greatest for the supraspinatus. This muscle assists with GH abduction and depression of the humeral head. The infraspinatus is primarily a GH lateral rotator, but also assists with GH extension. The subscapularis primarily assists with depression of the humeral head during GH mobility. The teres minor assists with GH lateral rotation.

INFERENCE

What is the most likely contributing factor in the development of this condition?

In older populations, age-related decreases in tissue elasticity and vascularity increase susceptibility to injury with the performance of everyday tasks. In younger populations, traumatic injury or repetitive high demand muscle use (e.g., professional baseball pitcher) are more typically associated with tearing.

CONFIRMATION

What is the most likely clinical presentation?

Pain and weakness are the most common complaints of a rotator cuff tear. Generalized pain exacerbated by specific movements or functional tasks is typically reported in the lateral aspect of the shoulder with radiating symptoms into the upper arm and deltoid region. Pain symptoms are likely to be more acute and specific with traumatic etiologies. Pain complaints are typically greatest with partial tearing due to increased tension on the remaining muscle fibers and associated neural tissue. A patient with a small partial-thickness tear may retain most functional abilities while a patient with a large partial-thickness or full-thickness tear will likely demonstrate significant functional deficits especially with tasks involving GH lateral rotation and abduction. Other symptoms may include complaints of shoulder instability or stiffness, a sense of GH grinding with mobility, crepitus, night pain, and discomfort when lying on the affected side.

What laboratory or imaging studies would confirm the diagnosis?

MRI is typically utilized to detect the location, size, and general characteristics of a rotator cuff tear as well as damage to adjacent structures. X-rays may also be used to assess possible bone spurs within the joint capsule.

What additional information should be obtained to confirm the diagnosis?

The drop arm test and empty can test can assist in identifying supraspinatus pathology which may be indicative of a rotator cuff tear. Pain with resisted muscle testing is likely to be greatest with a partial-thickness tear.

EXAMINATION

What history should be documented?

Important areas to explore include past medical history, medications, family history, current symptoms, current health status, social history and habits, occupation, leisure activities, and social support system.

What additional findings are likely with this patient?

Rotator cuff tears often present in association with other shoulder pathologies including chronic scapular instability, GH instability or impingement (e.g., supraspinatus tendon, long head of the biceps tendon, subacromial bursa, suprascapular nerve). In young, active individuals, the tear may be accompanied by a small avulsion fracture at the greater tuberosity of the humerus.

What tests/measures are most appropriate?

Anthropometric characteristics: circumferential measurements for upper extremity edema, palpation to determine deformity and effusion

Arousal, attention, and cognition: examine mental status, learning ability, memory, and motivation

Assistive and adaptive devices: analysis of components and safety of a device

Integumentary integrity: skin assessment, assessment of sensation

Joint integrity and mobility: soft tissue swelling and inflammation, assessment of joint play, palpation of the joint, empty can test, drop arm test

Muscle performance: strength assessment, characteristics of muscle contraction

Pain: pain perception assessment scale, visual analogue scale, assessment of muscle soreness

Posture: analysis of resting and dynamic posture

Range of motion: active and passive range of motion

Reflex integrity: assessment of deep tendon reflexes

Self-care and home management: assessment of functional capacity

Rotator Cuff Tear   GOLD

MANAGEMENT

What is the most effective management of this patient?

Medical management of a rotator cuff tear usually includes pharmacological intervention with analgesics and anti-inflammatory agents including oral NSAIDs and local cortisone injections. In older patients or chronic injuries, conservative management including physical therapy is typically attempted prior to considering surgical intervention. Surgery without conservative management may be indicated depending on the etiology, severity of symptoms, and size of the tear. Surgical interventions using an arthroscopic or open technique may include subacromial decompression, repair of the torn tendon or both. Specific parameters for post-operative protocols are difficult to identify since many orthopedic surgeons utilize very specific protocols. Patients who have undergone surgical repair are typically immobilized using a sling for a period of time to protect the repaired tissue. The acute phase of physical therapy should include cryotherapy, activity modification, range of motion, rest, and gentle isometric exercises. As surgical and non-surgical patients progress, treatment begins to focus on restoration of normal mobility with joint mobilizations, range of motion, progressive strength exercises, and palliative modalities. Activities that promote scapular stability, postural re-education, and modification of functional, work, and recreational activities are emphasized.

What home care regimen should be recommended?

A home care regimen, including the patient's adherence to post-operative mobility restrictions, is vital to a successful functional recovery. The home care regimen may vary initially for conservative versus surgically managed patients. Typical activities include palliative care, range of motion, and strengthening exercises as warranted based on the established protocol.

OUTCOME

What is the likely outcome of a course of physical therapy?

Physical therapy should begin immediately for conservatively managed patients. Depending on the surgeon's preference, patients may begin physical therapy immediately following surgical intervention or after a period of immobilization. The course of rehabilitation is variable depending on the size of the tear, treatment approach (e.g., conservative versus surgical), persistence of symptoms, patient age, patient goals, and prior level of function. In cases where the tear is especially large or complicated, repair options are often limited and patients may never fully recover shoulder function. Assuming an unremarkable recovery, a patient typically will regain functional use of the shoulder in four to six months, however, dynamic overhead activities may be restricted for as long as one year. The timeframe for a full return to sport activities may extend beyond a year.

What are the long-term effects of the patient's condition?

Failure to adequately treat a rotator cuff tear may necessitate significant activity modifications, additional surgical management, or result in the development of adhesive capsulitis or degenerative changes. Since the tendon itself does not heal, but rather forms scar tissue, there will be an increased risk of rupture or an increase in the size of the original tear. These risks are typically greater among patients who are conservatively managed.

COMPARISON

What are the distinguishing characteristics of a similar condition?

A biceps tendon rupture most commonly involves the long head of the biceps tendon (LHBT) occurring either at the bony attachment or tendon-labral junction. The injury is most prevalent among men between 40 and 60 years of age secondary to chronic inflammatory or degenerative conditions. In younger individuals, the injury is typically related to sporting activities, trauma or heavy weightlifting. Pain is a primary characteristic with some patients reporting severe pain that worsens at night and is exacerbated by overhead or repetitive activities. A palpable and often visible mass is typically noted in the upper arm where the muscle mass has retracted. A conservative or surgical treatment approach may be indicated as well as referral to physical therapy depending largely on functional deficits.

CLINICAL SCENARIOS

Scenario One

A 21-year-old male collegiate pitcher has experienced persistent supraspinatus tendonitis which has caused him to discontinue all throwing activities. He received several cortisone injections to assist with pain management. The patient is currently limited by pain with abduction and lateral rotation resistance testing and demonstrates active shoulder abduction to 60 degrees.

Scenario Two

A 73-year-old female dislocated her left shoulder during a recent fall. After four weeks of physical therapy, she continues to complain of limited functional mobility due to weakness and pain. Recent testing reveals that the drop arm test and empty can test are both positive. The patient's goal is to return to recreational swimming.

Rotator Cuff Tendonitis

DIAGNOSIS

What condition produces a patient's symptoms?

Repetitive overhead activities can produce impingement of the supraspinatus tendon immediately proximal to the greater tubercle of the humerus. The impingement is caused by an inability of a weak supraspinatus muscle to adequately depress the head of the humerus in the glenoid fossa during elevation of the arm. As a result the humerus translates superiorly due to the disproportionate action of the deltoid muscle. Primary impingement occurs from intrinsic or extrinsic factors within the subacromial space. Secondary impingement describes symptoms that occur from poor mechanics or instability at the shoulder joint.

An injury was most likely sustained to which structure?

The supraspinatus muscle has the most commonly involved tendon in rotator cuff tendonitis. The muscle originates on the supraspinatus fossa of the scapula and inserts on the greater tubercle of the humerus. Bicipital and infraspinatus tendonitis as well as bursitis may also coexist as other contributing factors.

INFERENCE

What is the most likely contributing factor in the development of this condition?

Individuals participating in activities that require excessive overhead activity such as swimming, tennis, baseball, painting, and other manual labor activities are at increased risk for rotator cuff tendonitis. Excessive use of the upper extremity following a prolonged period of inactivity also can produce this condition. Statistically, individuals from 25-40 years of age are the most likely to develop this condition.

CONFIRMATION

What is the most likely clinical presentation?

A patient with rotator cuff tendonitis often reports difficulty with overhead activities and a dull ache following periods of activity. The patient may experience a feeling of weakness and identify the presence of a painful arc of motion most commonly occurring between 60 and 120 degrees of active abduction. The patient usually presents with pain with palpation of the musculotendinous junction of the involved muscle and/or with stretching or resisted contraction of the muscle. Pain often increases at night resulting in difficulty sleeping on the affected side. The patient will often have difficulty with dressing and repetitive shoulder motions such as lifting, reaching, throwing, swinging or pushing and pulling with the involved upper extremity.

What laboratory or imaging studies would confirm the diagnosis?

Magnetic resonance imaging can be used to identify the presence of rotator cuff tendonitis, however, due to the high cost it is not commonly employed prior to the initiation of formal treatment. X-rays with the shoulder laterally rotated can be used to identify the presence of calcific deposits or other bony abnormalities.

What additional information should be obtained to confirm the diagnosis?

A number of specific special tests including the empty can test, Jobe test, Neer impingement test, and Hawkins-Kennedy impingement test can be used to confirm the presence of rotator cuff tendonitis or impingement.

EXAMINATION

What history should be documented?

Important areas to explore include past medical history, family history, medications, history of symptoms, current health status, living environment, social history and habits, occupation, and social support system.

What tests/measures are most appropriate?

Anthropometric characteristics: upper extremity circumferential measurements
Arousal, attention, and cognition: examine mental status, learning ability, memory, motivation
Assistive and adaptive devices: analysis of components and safety of a device
Community and work integration: analysis of community, work, and leisure activities
Integumentary integrity: skin assessment, assessment of sensation
Joint integrity and mobility: soft tissue swelling and inflammation, assessment of joint play, palpation of the joint, empty can test, Neer impingement test, Hawkins-Kennedy impingement test
Motor function: posture and balance
Muscle performance: strength assessment
Pain: pain perception assessment scale
Posture: analysis of resting and dynamic posture
Range of motion: active and passive range of motion
Reflex integrity: assessment of deep tendon reflexes
Self-care and home management: assessment of functional capacity

What additional findings are likely with this patient?

Rotator cuff tendonitis often presents in association with impingement syndrome. Impingement syndrome typically involves the supraspinatus tendon, glenoid labrum, long head of the biceps, and subacromial bursa. It is extremely difficult to determine through examination the exact level of involvement of each of the identified structures.

MANAGEMENT

What is the most effective management of this patient?

Medical management of acute rotator cuff tendonitis usually includes pharmacological intervention and physical therapy. Pharmacological intervention will focus on pain relief through analgesics and NSAIDs. Acute physical therapy intervention guidelines should include cryotherapy, activity modification, range of motion, and rest. As the acute phase subsides the patient is often instructed in strengthening exercises. Since the rotator cuff muscles are dependent on adequate blood supply and oxygen, it is essential that all range of motion and strengthening exercises are pain free. Range of motion exercises using a pulley system or a cane can serve as an effective intervention. Strengthening exercises are initiated with the arm at the patient's side in order to prevent the possibility of impingement. Elastic tubing or handheld weights are often the preferred equipment of choice. It is important for the entire rotator cuff to be strong prior to initiating overhead activities. Shoulder shrugs and push-ups with the arms abducted to 90 degrees can effectively be used to strengthen the upper trapezius and serratus anterior. This type of activity promotes elevation of the acromion without direct contact with the rotator cuff.

What home care regimen should be recommended?

The home care regimen should consist of range of motion, strengthening, palliative care, and functional activities as warranted based on the results of the patient examination.

OUTCOME

What is the likely outcome of a course of physical therapy?

A patient with rotator cuff tendonitis should be able to return to their previous level of functioning with conservative management within four to six weeks. Outcome can be dependent, however, on the patient's classification of stage I, II or III impingement syndrome. Stage I is usually found in the population less than 25 years of age and consists of localized inflammation, edema, and minimal bleeding around the rotator cuff. Stage II represents progressive deterioration of the tissues surrounding the rotator cuff and is common in 25 to 40-year-old patients. Stage III represents the end-stage and is usually found in patients over 40 years of age. There is usually disruption and/or rupture of numerous soft tissue structures.

What are the long-term effects of the patient's condition?

Failure to adequately treat rotator cuff tendonitis may necessitate significant activity modification or more aggressive surgical management such as subacromial decompression. Prolonged inflammation of the rotator cuff tendon may facilitate eventual tearing of the rotator cuff musculature.

COMPARISON

What are the distinguishing characteristics of a similar condition?

A rotator cuff tear is usually the result of repetitive microtrauma but can also result suddenly from a single traumatic event. Partial tears often occur in a younger population while complete tears more commonly occur in older individuals. The mechanism of injury is often a fall on an outstretched arm or a sudden strain applied to the shoulder during pushing or pulling activities. Diagnosis is made through MRI to identify the tear. Surgical repair of the rotator cuff is often required and may be done with arthroscopy or through a traditional open technique. The shoulder is usually protected by a sling and small abduction pillow for the first six weeks post surgery. Rehabilitation and return to full function can take upwards of six months, heavy lifting may be restricted for six to twelve months following surgery.

CLINICAL SCENARIOS

Scenario One

A 23-year-old female diagnosed with rotator cuff tendonitis is referred to physical therapy after experiencing pain while swimming the breaststroke in a competitive swim meet one week ago. The patient participates on a school swim team and a private club and practices four to six times per week. A few days after experiencing shoulder pain the patient was back in the pool, however, was unable to return to her previous training regimen.

Scenario Two

A 45-year-old male employed as a pipe fitter is referred to physical therapy after subacromial decompression. The patient is one week status post surgery and is anxious to "test" his involved shoulder. Prior to surgery the patient was placed on "light duty." It has been six months since the patient was able to perform his job without restrictions. The patient presently denies any pain in the involved shoulder.

DIAGNOSIS

What condition produces a patient's symptoms?

A patient with scoliosis presents with a lateral curvature of the spine. The curvature is usually found in the thoracic or lumbar vertebrae and can be associated with kyphosis or lordosis. The curvature of the spine may be towards the right or towards the left and rotation of the spine may or may not occur. Typically, the rotation will occur towards the convex side of the major curve.

An injury was most likely sustained to which structure?

The injury or deformity begins when the vertebrae of the spine deviate from the normal vertical position. The curvature disrupts normal alignment of the ribs and muscles and can create compensatory curves that attempt to keep the body in proper alignment. The vertebral column, rib cage, supporting ligaments, and muscles are all affected by a scoliosis of the spine.

INFERENCE

What is the most likely contributing factor in the development of this condition?

Idiopathic scoliosis, termed for its unknown etiology, accounts for approximately 80% of all cases. Upwards of 1:10 children are affected by some form of scoliosis with 1:4 requiring treatment for the curvature. The age of onset determines the subset of classification as infantile (0 to 3), juvenile (four to puberty), adolescent (12 for girls and 14 for boys) or adult (skeletal maturation) scoliosis. Non-structural scoliosis is a reversible curve that can change with repositioning. This type of curve is non-progressive and is usually caused by poor posture or leg length discrepancy. Structural scoliosis cannot be corrected with movement and can be caused by congenital, musculoskeletal, and neuromuscular reasons. Contributing factors of a structural curve include altered development of the spine in utero, association with neuromuscular diseases (cerebral palsy, muscular dystrophy, congenital defect of the vertebrae), and inheritance as an autosomal dominant trait. Research indicates a predisposition for scoliosis with a multifactorial etiology.

CONFIRMATION

What is the most likely clinical presentation?

A patient with a structural curve will present with asymmetries of the shoulders, scapulae, pelvis, and skinfolds. Juvenile idiopathic scoliosis is characterized by a thoracic curve with convexity towards the right. This curve may progress quickly and develop compensatory curves above and below. As the curve progresses there will be a rib hump posteriorly over the thoracic region on the convex side of the curve. The patient does not typically experience pain or other subjective symptoms until the curve has progressed. Adolescent scoliosis of greater than 30 degrees is seen more in females than males (10:1). Adult scoliosis affects approximately 500,000 adults in the United States. Curves that are less than 20 degrees rarely cause a person to experience significant problems or impairments.

What laboratory or imaging studies would confirm the diagnosis?

X-rays should be taken in an anterior and lateral view with the patient standing and with the patient bending over. A device called a scoliometer can be used to measure the angle of trunk rotation. The Cobb method can be used to determine the angle of curvature. A bone scan or MRI can be used to determine and rule out conditions such as infections, neoplasms, spondylolysis, disk herniations or compression fractures.

What additional information should be obtained to confirm the diagnosis?

Physical examination allows visual inspection of the curvature and physical asymmetries. A scoliometer can assist with measurement and the examiner can determine if the curve is non-structural or structural.

EXAMINATION

What history should be documented?

Important areas to explore include past medical history, family history, medications, current health status, living environment, school activities, and social support system.

What tests/measures are most appropriate?

Aerobic capacity and endurance: assessment of vital signs at rest and with activity, perceived exertion scale

Arousal, attention, and cognition: examine mental status, learning ability, memory, motivation

Ergonomics and body mechanics: analysis of dexterity and coordination

Integumentary integrity: skin and sensation assessment

Gait, locomotion, and balance: static and dynamic balance in sitting and standing, safety during gait with/without an assistive device, analysis of wheelchair management

Joint integrity and mobility: assessment of hypermobility and hypomobility of a joint

Muscle performance: strength assessment

Orthotic, protective, and supportive devices: analysis of components of a device, analysis of movement while wearing a device

Pain: assessment of muscle soreness

Posture: analysis of resting and dynamic posture

Range of motion: active and passive range of motion

Self-care and home management: assessment of functional capacity

What additional findings are likely with this patient?

Common postural findings with scoliosis include increased spacing between the elbow and trunk during standing, leg length discrepancy, uneven shoulder and hip heights, and prominence on one side of the pelvis or breast (due to rotation of the curve). If a progressive scoliosis is untreated, the deformity can increase to an angle in excess of 60 degrees and cause pulmonary insufficiency, significant pain, impairment in lung capacity, and degenerative changes including arthritis and disk pathology. Early screening, detection, and treatment are necessary to control the curvature and avoid surgical intervention.

MANAGEMENT

What is the most effective management of this patient?

Medical management of scoliosis is based on the type and severity of the curve, patient age, and previous management. Patients with scoliosis may utilize electrical stimulation to alleviate pain and biofeedback for education with proper posture and positioning. A patient with scoliosis that is less than 25 degrees should be monitored every three months. Breathing exercises and a strengthening program for the trunk and pelvic muscles are indicated. A patient with scoliosis that ranges between 25 and 40 degrees requires a spinal orthosis and physical therapy intervention for posture, flexibility, strengthening, respiratory function, and proper utilization of the spinal orthosis. A patient with scoliosis that is greater than 40 degrees usually requires surgical spinal stabilization. One method to surgically correct scoliosis is through posterior spinal fusion and stabilization with a Harrington rod. Physical therapy intervention after surgical fusion is indicated for breathing exercises, posture, flexibility, general strengthening, and respiratory muscle strengthening.

What home care regimen should be recommended?

A home care regimen is based on the type and severity of the curve. Exercise, stretching, posture, and flexibility are important components of an exercise program.

OUTCOME

What is the likely outcome of a course of physical therapy?

Physical therapy intervention should improve a patient's condition through patient education and therapeutic exercise. Physical therapy may be indicated for implementation of a home program, pain management, posture retraining, orthotic training or following surgical stabilization.

What are the long-term effects of the patient's condition?

Prognosis for structural scoliosis is based on the age of onset and the severity of the curve. Early intervention results in the best possible outcome. Scoliosis does not usually progress significantly once bone growth is complete if the curvature remains below 40 degrees at the time of skeletal maturity. If the curvature is over 50 degrees there likely will be ongoing progression of the curve each year of life.

COMPARISON

What are the distinguishing characteristics of a similar condition?

Torticollis is a deformity of the neck that is caused by shortened or spastic sternocleidomastoid muscles. The patient presents with a bending of the neck towards the affected side and rotation of the head towards the unaffected side. Causative factors include damage to the sternocleidomastoid muscle, malpositioning in utero, spasms secondary to central nervous system impairment or psychogenic origin. Conservative treatment for acquired torticollis includes heat, traction, massage, stretching, positioning, and bracing. Surgical intervention may be indicated if conservative management fails.

CLINICAL SCENARIOS

Scenario One

An 11-year-old female is seen in physical therapy with diagnosis of a 30-degree right thoracic scoliosis. The physician has prescribed a spinal orthosis and physical therapy. The patient denies any pain, but states that she has soreness in her back. The patient is in the marching band and plays basketball. There is no past medical history and her parents are very supportive.

Scenario Two

A seven-year-old boy is referred to physical therapy with a 12-degree right thoracic scoliosis. The physical therapy prescription requests evaluation for a home exercise program. The patient has type 1 diabetes mellitus and a low I.Q. The mother is present for the evaluation and appears to be supportive.

DIAGNOSIS

What condition produces a patient's symptoms?

Spondylolisthesis is the forward slippage of one vertebra on the vertebra below. There are several types of spondylolisthesis classified by the actual cause for the slippage. Classifications include congenital, isthmic, degenerative, post-traumatic, and pathologic spondylolisthesis. Degenerative spondylolisthesis (DS) is caused by the weakening of joints that allows for forward slippage of one vertebral segment on the one below due to degenerative changes. These changes include segmental ligamentous instability and subluxation of the hypertrophic facet joints which can result in stenosis of the spinal canal.

An injury was most likely sustained to which structure?

The most common site of DS is the L4-L5 level. The slippage causes cauda equina symptoms secondary to stenosis of the canal. It is theorized that ischemia and poor nourishment secondary to the stenosis deprives the associated spinal nerves and results in pain. The L4 nerve root is compressed in an L4-L5 spondylolisthesis. Other structures that can be irritated include the intervertebral disk, posterior and anterior longitudinal ligaments, and vertebral periosteum and bone.

INFERENCE

What is the most likely contributing factor in the development of this condition?

DS is caused by arthritis and degenerative changes in the spine. The intervertebral disk loses some of its ability to resist motion and as a result the vertebral facets increase in size and develop bone spurs to compensate. This condition can actually produce spinal stenosis and weaken the spine itself resulting in the slippage of a vertebrae. Since all structures of the spine remain intact the slippage is usually limited due to the secondary bony restraints of the spine.

CONFIRMATION

What is the most likely clinical presentation?

DS usually affects individuals over 50 years of age. It is more common with African Americans and women also have a higher incidence of occurrence than men. Back pain is a primary symptom that is said to increase with exercise, lifting overhead, prolonged standing, getting out of bed or a car, walking up stairs or an incline, and positioning in extension. The pain may be severe and radiate depending on the area of stenosis secondary to the vertebral slippage. Sensory and motor loss may be significant and follow a myotomal and/or dermatomal distribution. Most patients do not have significant neurologic deficits, however, a few do experience severe changes.

What laboratory or imaging studies would confirm the diagnosis?

Plain radiographs of the vertebral column are adequate to confirm the diagnosis of DS. CT scan or MRI may be indicated to rule out any other contributing conditions or to further assess nerve impingement.

What additional information should be obtained to confirm the diagnosis?

Physical and neurological examinations in combination with a full medical history usually provide adequate information for probable diagnosis, however, X-rays are required for definitive diagnosis of DS.

EXAMINATION

What history should be documented?

Important areas to explore include past medical history and previous testing, medications, family history, current symptoms, current health status, social history and habits, occupation, leisure activities, and social support system.

What tests/measures are most appropriate?

Arousal, attention, and cognition: examine mental status, learning ability, memory, motivation

Assistive and adaptive devices: analysis of components and safety of a device

Community and work integration: analysis of community, work, and leisure activities

Environmental, home, and work barriers: analysis of current and potential barriers or hazards

Ergonomics and body mechanics: analysis of dexterity and coordination, evaluation of proper lifting techniques

Gait, locomotion, and balance: static and dynamic balance in sitting and standing, safety during gait with/without an assistive device, Functional Ambulation Profile

Joint integrity and mobility: assessment of hyper- and hypomobility of a joint, soft tissue swelling and inflammation

Muscle performance: strength assessment

Pain: pain perception assessment scale, visual analogue scale, assessment of muscle soreness

Posture: analysis of resting and dynamic posture

Range of motion: active and passive range of motion

Self-care and home management: assessment of functional capacity

Sensory integrity: assessment of sensation

Spondylolisthesis - Degenerative

What additional findings are likely with this patient?

A patient with DS may or may not have additional slippage of the vertebra over time. If the slippage of the vertebra worsens it does not necessarily correspond to an increase in symptoms. Symptoms may increase with or without marked degenerative changes and vice versa. A patient that does experience ongoing neurological deficits will require surgical intervention regardless of the amount of slippage.

MANAGEMENT

What is the most effective management of this patient?

Medical management of a patient diagnosed with DS should initially include education, medication, activity modification, and physical therapy intervention. Pharmacological intervention should include NSAIDs to decrease acute inflammation. Corticosteroids may be indicated for severe symptoms. Epidural steroid injections and selective nerve root injections are sometimes indicated if oral medications fail. Activity modification and rest should be instituted to further allow inflammation to subside and improve overall symptoms. Long-term bed rest, however, should be avoided. Once the acute phase has subsided physical therapy should begin. William's flexion exercises should be performed to strengthen the abdominals and reduce lumbar lordosis. Back school, modalities, postural education, and other exercises that provide core stabilization and increase flexibility should be included in the patient's program. External support such as bracing or wearing of a corset may relieve intradiscal pressure. Surgical intervention is only indicated if conservative treatment fails, the pain becomes disabling or significant neurological impairment exists. Surgical intervention usually involves decompression with or without spinal fusion.

What home care regimen should be recommended?

A patient with DS should initially take NSAIDs and decrease overall activities to allow for a reduction in the acute symptoms. Once a patient is able to tolerate physical therapy the home care regimen should include prescribed exercises to improve abdominal strength and core stabilization, flexibility exercises, and proper positioning. Goals for the home program are to alleviate pain and improve function. A patient should only modify the home program per therapist instruction.

OUTCOME

What is the likely outcome of a course of physical therapy?

The majority of patients with DS are successful with conservative treatment that may include physical therapy, home program, bracing, and use of NSAIDs as needed.

What are the long-term effects of the patient's condition?

The long-term effects of DS vary based on progression and advancement of the slipped vertebrae and/or progression of symptoms. Some patients may be able to manage pain and maintain function without any further associated pathology. If symptoms continue to progress, then surgical intervention may be required.

COMPARISON

What are the distinguishing characteristics of a similar condition?

Congenital spondylolisthesis is the slippage of one vertebra on the vertebra below due to an anomaly or defect in the fusion of the neural arch. This usually occurs in the upper sacral vertebral arches or at the L5 level. The condition is usually diagnosed during the growth spurts between 12 and 16 years of age. Patients are normally pain free prior to this point and begin to express complaints of back pain, "sciatica" pain, and other symptoms. There is a strong genetic association found in this type of spondylolisthesis.

CLINICAL SCENARIOS

Scenario One

A 65-year-old female is seen in physical therapy with a diagnosis of L5 degenerative spondylolisthesis. She complains of pain in her back that can occasionally radiate down her left leg. She resides with her husband in their two-story home and works part-time at a grocery store as a clerk. She also enjoys gardening, but has been having a difficult time with all activities in the last eight weeks secondary to pain.

Scenario Two

A 74-year-old male two weeks status post spinal fusion is examined in a nursing home. The patient was diagnosed six months ago with DS, shortly after he began to exhibit neurological symptoms. The physician prescribes physical therapy daily to improve strength and functional independence.

Total Hip Arthroplasty

DIAGNOSIS

What condition produces a patient's symptoms?

A total hip arthroplasty (THA) may be warranted secondary to progressive and severe osteoarthritis or rheumatoid arthritis in the hip joint, developmental dysplasia of the hip, tumors, failed reconstruction of the hip or other hip conditions that produce incapacitating pain and disability. A THA may also be required secondary to trauma, avascular necrosis or a nonunion fracture.

An injury was most likely sustained to which structure?

Arthritis causes the hip joint to undergo a degenerative process including destruction of articular cartilage that results in bone-to-bone contact. Degenerative changes are usually apparent in both the acetabulum and the femoral head requiring a THA, however, if the acetabulum does not exhibit degenerative changes then only the femoral head will be replaced in a hemiarthroplasty procedure.

INFERENCE

What is the most likely contributing factor in the development of this condition?

Intra-articular disease or the destruction of articular cartilage may come from arthritis, repetitive microtrauma, obesity, nutritional imbalances, falls or abnormal joint mechanics. Indications for THA include osteoarthritis, rheumatoid arthritis, avascular necrosis, developmental dysplasia, osteomyelitis, failed fixation of a fracture, ankylosing spondylitis, and failed conservative management.

CONFIRMATION

What is the most likely clinical presentation?

A patient that requires a THA will present with decreased range of motion, impaired mobility skills, and persistent pain that increases with motion and weight bearing. The patient is usually over 55 years of age and has experienced consistent pain that is not relieved through conservative measures and limits the patient's functional mobility on a consistent basis.

What laboratory or imaging studies would confirm the diagnosis?

X-ray, computed tomography, and magnetic resonance imaging procedures may be used to view the integrity of the joint. These procedures are also used to rule out a fracture or a tumor.

What additional information should be obtained to confirm the diagnosis?

Patient history, current functional status, and level of pain and disability are important factors in determining the need for surgical intervention. A standardized pain assessment scale and the Arthritis Impact Measurement tool may be used to establish an objective baseline. Relative or absolute contraindications must be considered prior to the recommendation for a THA. Contraindications may include but are not limited to active infection, severe obesity, arterial insufficiency, neuromuscular disease, and certain mental illness.

EXAMINATION

What history should be documented?

Important areas to explore include past medical history, family history, medications, current symptoms, current health status, living environment, social history and habits, occupation, and social support system.

What tests/measures are most appropriate?

Aerobic capacity and endurance: assessment of vital signs at rest and with activity, perceived exertion scale

Anthropometric characteristics: hip circumferential measurements, leg length measurements

Arousal, attention, and cognition: examine mental status, learning ability, memory, motivation

Assistive and adaptive devices: analysis of components and safety of a device

Environmental, home, and work barriers: analysis of current and potential barriers or hazards

Gait, locomotion, and balance: safety during gait with/without an assistive device, Functional Ambulation Profile

Joint integrity and mobility: soft tissue swelling and inflammation

Muscle performance: strength assessment, assessment of active movement

Pain: pain perception assessment scale

Range of motion: active and passive range of motion

Self-care and home assessment: assessment of functional capacity, Barthel Index

Sensory integrity: assessment of sensation

Total Hip Arthroplasty   GOLD

What additional findings are likely with this patient?

A patient that requires a THA may also have arthritis in other areas of the body. The patient may present with low endurance and may be deconditioned secondary to inactivity from the effects of arthritis. Post-surgical complications may include nerve injury, vascular damage, dislocation, pulmonary embolism, myocardial infarction, and CVA. The prosthesis is also at risk for loosening, infection, heterotopic ossification, and fracture.

MANAGEMENT

What is the most effective management of this patient?

Medical management includes choosing a surgical approach that meets the patient's needs and level of activity. A THA that utilizes a posterolateral approach allows the abductor muscles to remain intact, however, there may be a higher incidence of post-operative joint instability due to the interruption of the posterior capsule. This type of surgical approach requires a patient to avoid excessive hip flexion greater than 90 degrees, hip adduction, and hip medial rotation. A patient with a THA that utilizes an anterolateral approach should avoid hip flexion and lateral rotation. A direct lateral approach leaves the posterior portion of the gluteus medius attached to the greater trochanter and the posterior capsule left intact. This method is preferred for patients that may be noncompliant in order to avoid posterior dislocation. Pharmacological intervention status post THA will include anticoagulant therapy and pain medication. The patient's post-operative care includes hip precautions, use of an abduction pillow (with posterolateral approach), initiation of hip protocol exercises, and physical therapy intervention. The hip protocol exercises usually include ankle pumps, quadriceps sets, gluteal sets, heel slides, and isometric abduction. Physical therapy should emphasize patient education regarding hip precautions and weight bearing status, scar management, and soft tissue mobilization. At the time of hospital discharge the patient should be able to extend the hip to neutral and flex the hip to 90 degrees. A cemented hip replacement usually allows for partial weight bearing initially and a noncemented hip replacement requires toe touch weight bearing for up to six weeks. Physical therapy encourages early ambulation training in order to avoid deconditioning and the risk of deep vein thrombosis. A patient must practice all mobility skills using the proper hip precautions. Outpatient physical therapy may be indicated to assist with progression to a cane.

What home care regimen should be recommended?

The patient should be instructed in a home care regimen that includes range of motion, strengthening, and progressive ambulation. The patient must adhere to the hip precaution guidelines for a minimum of three months or until a physician determines that the hip demonstrates adequate stability.

OUTCOME

What is the likely outcome of a course of physical therapy?

A patient status post THA will benefit from physical therapy and should attain an improved functional outcome. The patient should have diminished to no pain, increased strength and endurance, and improved mobility within six to eight weeks after surgery.

What are the long-term effects of the patient's condition?

A THA is a highly successful surgical procedure. The current lifespan of the prosthesis is less than 20 years and as a result some patients may require a subsequent replacement. Studies indicate pain relief and improved function with good to excellent results in 85-95% of the patients at 15 to 20 years post THA. Validated scoring systems such as the Harris Hip Scoring System or the Special Surgery Rating system are measures used to determine the quality of life after the THA.

COMPARISON

What are the distinguishing characteristics of a similar condition?

A hemiarthroplasty of the hip is a replacement of the femoral head due to a subcapital fracture of the femur or degeneration of the femoral head. This type of surgical intervention is sometimes used as an alternative to a THA for elderly patients that sustain a hip fracture or patients that have a shortened expected lifespan.

CLINICAL SCENARIOS

Scenario One

A patient is seen in physical therapy after THA surgery. The surgeon performed an anterolateral approach and used a noncemented prosthesis. The patient is mildly obese and has a lengthy cardiac history. The patient has osteoarthritis and had progressive pain and difficulty with mobility prior to surgery. The patient complains of soreness in the hip and is anxious to get home.

Scenario Two

A 75-year-old male is seen in physical therapy status post reduction of a dislocated right hip prosthesis. The patient had a THA three weeks ago and dislocated the hip two days ago while bending over to tie his shoes. The patient is currently using a walker for mobility and is toe touch weight bearing. The patient resides alone in a garden apartment and does not have any family in the area.

DIAGNOSIS

What condition produces a patient's symptoms?

A total knee arthroplasty (TKA) may be warranted secondary to progressive and disabling pain within the knee joint. The pain is most often due to severe degenerative osteoarthritic destruction and deformity that can occur within the knee.

An injury was most likely sustained to which structure?

Arthritis causes the knee joint to undergo a degenerative process that includes destruction of articular cartilage and resultant bone-to-bone contact within the joint. The knee presents with decreased joint space and osteophyte formation. Injury occurs to the femoral condyles, tibial articulating surface, and the dorsal side of the patella.

INFERENCE

What is the most likely contributing factor in the development of this condition?

The destruction of articular cartilage secondary to osteoarthritis is the most common indication for a TKA. A patient with a history of participation in high-impact sports or has experienced trauma to the knee is at a higher risk for arthritis and subsequent TKA. Obesity, varus/valgus deformity, previous mechanical derangement, infection, rheumatoid arthritis, hemophilia, crystal deposition diseases, avascular necrosis or bone dysplasia at the knee are some other contributing factors that may warrant a TKA.

CONFIRMATION

What is the most likely clinical presentation?

Approximately 130,000 TKAs are performed each year within the United States. A patient that requires a TKA will present with severe knee pain that worsens with motion and weight bearing, impaired range of motion, possible deformity of the knee, and impaired mobility skills. Night pain is common and may include localized or diffuse pain. Other symptoms may include stiffness, swelling, locking, and giving way of the affected knee. Patients often attempt conservative treatment measures to address the condition with only limited success.

What laboratory or imaging studies would confirm the diagnosis?

X-ray, computed tomography, and magnetic resonance imaging are used to determine the extent of deterioration and bony abnormalities within the knee joint. Radiographic images can be utilized post-operatively to ensure proper fit and obtain baseline information.

What additional information should be obtained to confirm the diagnosis?

Patient history, current functional status, and level of pain and disability are important factors in determining the need for surgical intervention. A pain assessment scale and the Arthritis Impact Measurement tool may be used to establish an objective baseline.

EXAMINATION

What history should be documented?

Important areas to explore include past medical history, family history, medications, current symptoms, living environment, social history and habits, occupation, current functional status, and social support system.

What tests/measures are most appropriate?

Aerobic capacity and endurance: assessment of vital signs at rest and with activity, perceived exertion scale

Anthropometric characteristics: knee circumferential measurements

Arousal, attention, and cognition: examine mental status, learning ability, memory, motivation

Assistive and adaptive devices: analysis of components and safety of a device

Environmental, home, and work barriers: analysis of current and potential barriers or hazards

Gait, locomotion, and balance: safety during gait/stairs with device, Functional Ambulation Profile

Joint integrity and mobility: soft tissue swelling and inflammation

Muscle performance: strength/active movement assessment

Pain: pain perception assessment scale

Range of motion: active and passive range of motion

Self-care and home assessment: assessment of functional capacity, Barthel Index

Sensory integrity: assessment of sensation

What additional findings are likely with this patient?

A patient that requires TKA may have arthritis in other joints, previous replacement surgeries or previous trauma to the knee joint. Patients with significant osteoarthritis and severe pain may exhibit sleep disorders or depression due to the disease process. Relative or absolute contraindications must be considered prior to the recommendation for a TKA. Contraindications may include but are not limited to active infection of the knee, severe obesity, significant genu recurvatum, arterial insufficiency, neuropathic joint, and certain mental illnesses. Post-surgical complications after a TKA include infection, vascular damage, patellofemoral instability, fracture surrounding the prosthesis, pulmonary embolism, nerve damage, loosening of the prosthesis, and arthrofibrosis.

MANAGEMENT

What is the most effective management of this patient?

Medical management of a patient requiring a TKA includes choosing of the appropriate surgical procedure based on the patient's symptoms and level of activity. Pharmacological intervention status post TKA will require anticoagulant therapy and pain medications. The patient's post-operative care includes a knee immobilizer, elevation of the limb, cryotherapy, intermittent range of motion using a continuous passive motion (CPM) machine, and initiation of knee protocol exercises. A cemented knee prosthesis allows for either partial weight bearing or weight bearing as tolerated post surgery based on the individual physician's discretion. A noncemented knee prosthesis requires toe touch weight bearing for up to six weeks to allow for the bone to grow and affix to the prosthesis. Physical therapy should focus on mobility training with the proper weight bearing status using an appropriate assistive device. Early ambulation training is encouraged in order to avoid deconditioning and the risk of deep vein thrombosis. Physical therapy intervention should emphasize ankle pumps, quad sets, and hamstrings sets as well as range of motion and stretching. A goal of 90 degrees of knee flexion and 0 degrees knee extension is often established prior to discharge from the hospital or rehabilitation facility. The following precautions should be used for several months after surgery to avoid excessive stress to the knee: avoid squatting, avoid quick pivoting, do not use pillows under the knee while in bed, and avoid low seating. Outpatient therapy may be recommended to progress the patient from an assistive device. Once the physician progresses the patient to weight bearing as tolerated, physical therapy intervention should include strengthening with closed-chain exercises and functional activities.

What home care regimen should be recommended?

A home care regimen would typically include range of motion, strengthening, and progressive ambulation exercises. The patient must adhere to precautions, use of an immobilizer, and proper weight bearing status until a physician determines that the knee joint demonstrates adequate stability.

OUTCOME

What is the likely outcome of a course of physical therapy?

A patient status post TKA will benefit from physical therapy and should attain an improved functional capacity. The patient should experience relief of pain that will allow for a full return to previous functional activities within eight to twelve weeks after surgery depending on a cemented or noncemented prosthesis and potential complications that were encountered.

What are the long-term effects of the patient's condition?

A TKA is a highly successful surgical procedure that should significantly reduce pain and increase function. After finishing a rehabilitation protocol, a patient may have only minor limitations in knee range of motion. A knee replacement may loosen over time and require revision, however, the life expectancy of the knee prosthesis is between 15 and 20 years.

COMPARISON

What are the distinguishing characteristics of a similar condition?

A patellectomy (surgical removal of the patella) is a surgical procedure that is indicated for a comminuted fracture of the patella that cannot be repaired with internal fixation. A patellectomy can include the entire patella or just the inferior or superior pole of the patella. The retinaculum and extensor mechanism are repaired with the surgical procedure and the patient is immobilized for six to eight weeks. Once rehabilitation is initiated the patient starts with range of motion and closed-chain exercises.

CLINICAL SCENARIOS

Scenario One

An 80-year-old female in an acute care hospital is two days status post left TKA. The patient presents with partial hearing loss and moderate dementia. The patient's past medical history includes a right CVA with no residual impairment and hypertension that is controlled by medication. The patient resides with her sister in a ranch style home with three steps to enter.

Scenario Two

A 49-year-old male is referred to outpatient physical therapy seven weeks after surgery. The patient received a noncemented knee prosthesis and has recently advanced to weight bearing as tolerated. The patient's range of motion in the involved knee is 10-85 degrees. The patient is otherwise independent with axillary crutches. No significant past medical history is noted.

DIAGNOSIS

What condition produces a patient's symptoms?

Osteosarcoma (osteogenic sarcoma) is the second most common primary bone tumor and accounts for 15-20% of bone tumors. Osteosarcoma is a highly malignant cancer that begins in the medullary cavity of a bone and leads to the formation of a mass. It usually affects bones with an active growth phase such as the femur or tibia and is often located in the metaphysis. Amputation may be necessary to remove the tumor and surrounding tissues to avoid metastatic disease.

An injury was most likely sustained to which structure?

The cancer cells are found in osteoblasts within the primitive mesenchymal cells of the medullary cavity of a bone. The cancer rapidly proliferates, replaces normal bone, and causes tissue destruction. Osteosarcoma will also metastasize to the lungs very early in the disease process.

INFERENCE

What is the most likely contributing factor in the development of this condition?

Osteosarcomas can occur as a primary or secondary cancer and the etiology remains unknown. This form of tumor primarily affects young children (especially males), adolescents, and young adults under 30 years of age. A peak time for incidence is during a growth spurt as an adolescent. Risk factors associated with secondary osteosarcoma include Paget's disease, osteoblastoma, giant cell tumor or chronic osteomyelitis. Environmental and genetic factors have been associated with the disease. In many instances amputation is required to cease the disease process.

CONFIRMATION

What is the most likely clinical presentation?

Osteosarcoma can be found most often in the long bones especially at the site of the most active epiphyseal growth plate, the distal femur, proximal tibia, proximal humerus and pelvis. The knee region accounts for approximately 50% of osteosarcomas. Patients that require amputation secondary to an osteosarcoma will present with a mass often found in the tibia or femur. The most common symptoms of osteosarcoma are pain and swelling within the extremity. Pain may worsen at night or with exercise and a lump may develop in the extremity sometime after the onset of pain. The osteosarcoma may weaken the involved extremity leading to a fracture. In some cases, a fracture may be the first sign of the osteosarcoma. Metastases appear in the lungs early in 90% of the cases.

What laboratory or imaging studies would confirm the diagnosis?

X-ray, MRI, and scintigraphy allow the physician to determine the presence, location, and size of a tumor. The "Codman's triangle" can be seen on x-ray indicating reactive bone at the site where the periosteum has been elevated by the neoplasm. Definitive diagnosis for an osteosarcoma is made through tissue biopsy of the tumor.

What additional information should be obtained to confirm the diagnosis?

Diagnosis of osteosarcoma is confirmed solely through biopsy. The course of treatment and the need for surgical amputation is determined by the size, location of the tumor, and progression of the malignancy.

EXAMINATION

What history should be documented?

Important areas to explore include past medical history, medications, family history, current symptoms and health status, social history and habits, occupation, leisure activities, and social support system.

What tests/measures are most appropriate?

Aerobic capacity and endurance: assessment of vital signs at rest and with activity, auscultation of the lungs, palpation of pulses

Anthropometric characteristics: residual limb circumferential measurements, length of limb

Arousal, attention, and cognition: examine mental status, learning ability, memory, motivation

Assistive and adaptive devices: analysis of components and safety of a device

Community and work integration: analysis of community, work, and leisure activities

Gait, locomotion, and balance: analysis of wheelchair mobility, static and dynamic balance in sitting and standing, safety during gait with an assistive device

Integumentary integrity: skin assessment, assessment of sensation, temperature of limb

Muscle performance: strength and tone assessment

Pain: phantom pain, pain perception assessment scale

Prosthetic requirements: analysis and safety of the prosthesis; alignment, efficiency, and fit of the prosthesis with the residual limb

Range of motion: active and passive range of motion

Self-care and home management: assessment of functional capacity, Barthel Index, Functional Independence Measure (FIM)

Sensory integrity: proprioception and kinesthesia

Transfemoral Amputation due to Osteosarcoma   GOLD

What additional findings are likely with this patient?

A patient status post transfemoral amputation secondary to an osteosarcoma may present with fatigue, loss of balance, phantom pain or sensation, hypersensitivity of the residual limb, and psychological issues regarding the loss of the limb. The patient may also have associated symptoms from chemotherapy that can include anemia, abnormal bleeding, infection, and kidney impairment. The presence of these findings can have a negative influence on a patient's ability to utilize a prosthesis.

MANAGEMENT

What is the most effective management of this patient?

Medical management will focus on adjunctive therapies to treat the osteosarcoma. Pharmacological intervention may include pain medication and other medication to deter effects from cancer treatment. Physical and occupational therapies should begin immediately after the transfemoral amputation. Preprosthetic intervention should focus on range of motion, positioning, strengthening, desensitization, residual limb wrapping, functional mobility, gait training, and patient education for care of the residual limb. Patients with a transfemoral amputation should lie prone for a period of time each day to prevent a hip flexion contracture. Modalities may be used to improve range of motion and decrease pain. Serial casting may be indicated if a contracture develops. Without complication, the patient should be able to return home with support and receive short-term physical therapy for prosthetic training.

What home care regimen should be recommended?

A home care regimen for a patient status post transfemoral amputation should include limb desensitization, stretching, proper positioning, and prone lying. The patient must be independent with residual limb care, skin inspection, and proper wrapping. Endurance activities, strengthening, and mobility with an assistive device are necessary as a precursor to prosthetic training.

OUTCOME

What is the likely outcome of a course of physical therapy?

Physical therapy is necessary for both preprosthetic and prosthetic training. A patient should be able to achieve the established goals and function with a prosthesis for all mobility including ambulation, balance, transfers, and stair activities. The general health, cognition, motivation, and social support system of the patient will influence the patient's functional outcome.

What are the long-term effects of the patient's condition?

The survival rate for a patient status post osteosarcoma has increased in recent years to a five-year cure rate of 70-80% with treatment that may include amputation, radiation, and chemotherapy. The transfemoral amputation should not permanently impair the patient's independence with mobility, self-care or ambulation using a prosthesis. The patient's long-term outcome is dependent on the status of the cancer.

COMPARISON

What are the distinguishing characteristics of a similar condition?

Ewing's sarcoma is a malignant nonosteogenic primary bone tumor that infiltrates the bone marrow and usually affects children and adolescents under 20 years of age. A patient will present with pain of increasing severity, swelling, and fever. This tumor is not found consistently in a specific location within the bone and is extremely malignant with a high frequency of metastases. Ewing's sarcoma requires aggressive treatment that may include amputation and adjunctive chemotherapy. The five-year survival rate is approximately 70%.

CLINICAL SCENARIOS

Scenario One

A 10-year-old female is seen in physical therapy after a right transfemoral amputation. The patient was diagnosed with osteosarcoma four months ago. The patient is in good spirits and is anxious to receive "a new leg" and begin walking. Her parents are supportive and are eager to assist her during rehabilitation.

Scenario Two

A 16-year-old male is seen for the first time in physical therapy since a left transfemoral amputation. The boy states that his leg had bothered him for a few weeks and the pain got worse each day. He also stated that he was told that the cancer was now also found in his lungs. He wants to start an exercise program so that he will be ready for his prosthesis when his residual limb heals.

DIAGNOSIS

What condition produces a patient's symptoms?

Arteriosclerosis obliterans, also known as peripheral arterial disease (PAD), is a form of peripheral vascular disease that produces thickening, hardening, and eventual narrowing and occlusion of the arteries. Arteriosclerosis obliterans results in ischemia and subsequent ulceration of the affected tissues. The affected area may become necrotic, gangrenous, and require amputation.

An injury was most likely sustained to which structure?

Injury will occur to all structures that receive blood supply from vessels that have become occluded. Prolonged ischemia results in tissue death and infection. Arteriosclerosis obliterans is the most common arterial occlusive disease and accounts for approximately 95% of the cases of vascular disease.

INFERENCE

What is the most likely contributing factor in the development of this condition?

Risk factors associated with arteriosclerosis obliterans include age, diabetes, sex, hypertension, high serum cholesterol and low-density lipid levels, smoking, impaired glucose tolerance, obesity, and sedentary lifestyle. Unsuccessful management of peripheral vascular disease may ultimately lead to uncontrolled infection, gangrene, necrosis, and amputation. Males have an overall higher incidence of arteriosclerosis than female counterparts.

CONFIRMATION

What is the most likely clinical presentation?

The patient that requires a transtibial amputation secondary to arteriosclerosis obliterans is typically an individual over 45 years that smokes (75-90%) and will present with intermittent claudication that produces cramps and pain in the affected areas. Intermittent claudication will typically present in the gastrocnemius-soleus complex, secondary to its high oxygen demand. Other characteristics include resting pain, decreased pulses, ischemia, pallor skin, and decreased skin temperature.

What laboratory or imaging studies would confirm the diagnosis?

Arteriosclerosis obliterans can be diagnosed using Doppler ultrasonography, MRI or arteriography. These diagnostic tests examine the degree of blood flow throughout the extremities. A patient with arteriosclerosis obliterans would typically demonstrate poor results including blockage, tissue damage, and tissue death.

What additional information should be obtained to confirm the diagnosis?

The physician should examine the limb for temperature, skin condition, the presence of hair, sensation, and palpable pulses when determining the need for amputation. The physician may perform a selected non-invasive test such as a claudication test that examines the presence of intermittent claudication that can occur with prolonged ambulation. The ankle-brachial index, segmental limb pressures or pulse volume recordings may also be used to assist with the diagnosis.

EXAMINATION

What history should be documented?

Important areas to explore include past medical history, medications, current health status, social history and habits, occupation, living environment, and social support system.

What tests/measures are most appropriate?

Aerobic capacity and endurance: palpation of pulses, pulse oximetry, assessment of vital signs at rest and with activity

Anthropometric characteristics: residual limb circumferential measurements, length of limb

Arousal, attention, and cognition: examine mental status, learning ability, memory, motivation

Assistive and adaptive devices: analysis of components and safety of a device

Gait, locomotion, and balance: analysis of wheelchair mobility, static and dynamic balance in sitting and standing, safety during gait with an assistive device

Integumentary integrity: examine presence of hair growth, color, temperature, assessment of sensation

Muscle performance: strength assessment, muscle tone assessment

Pain: phantom pain, pain perception assessment scale

Prosthetic requirements: (when appropriate) analysis and safety of the prosthesis; assessment of alignment, efficiency, and fit of the prosthesis; assessment of residual limb with the prosthesis

Range of motion: active and passive range of motion

Self-care and home management: assessment of functional capacity, Barthel Index, Functional Independence Measure (FIM)

Sensory integrity: assessment of proprioception and kinesthesia

Transtibial Amputation due to Arteriosclerosis Obliterans   GOLD

What additional findings are likely with this patient?

A patient status post transtibial amputation may have a decrease in cardiovascular status depending on the frequency of intermittent claudication the patient experienced prior to the amputation. The patient may initially experience diminished balance secondary to the loss of the limb. Other issues that directly affect the residual limb include phantom pain, decreased range of motion, poor skin integrity, and hypersensitivity. The presence of any of these findings can have a negative influence on a patient's ability to utilize a prosthesis.

MANAGEMENT

What is the most effective management of this patient?

A patient should be a candidate for inpatient physical therapy services immediately after the transtibial amputation. Preprosthetic intervention should focus on strength, range of motion, functional mobility, use of assistive devices, desensitization, and patient education for care of the residual limb. Intervention should focus on proper positioning in order to avoid the risk of contractures, especially a knee flexion contracture. If the patient does not experience complications they should be able to return home either independently or with support. The patient may receive continued short-term physical therapy for prosthetic intervention once the residual limb has fully healed.

What home care regimen should be recommended?

A home care regimen for a patient status post transtibial amputation should include exercises, limb desensitization, proper positioning, and stretching. Since ambulation with a prosthesis increases the energy cost, the patient should be encouraged to perform cardiovascular activities on a frequent basis. In order to be successful, the patient will need to consistently monitor the residual limb and wrap the limb to ensure proper shaping until the prosthesis is tolerated.

OUTCOME

What is the likely outcome of a course of physical therapy?

Physical therapy for both preprosthetic and prosthetic intervention is typically necessary. A patient should be able to achieve the established goals and function with a prosthesis and an assistive device if warranted. The general health, cognition, motivation, and social support system of the patient will influence the patient's functional outcome.

What are the long-term effects of the patient's condition?

Arteriosclerosis obliterans is a chronic disease that a patient should continue to manage. The current transtibial amputation should not permanently alter a patient's level of functional mobility. The patient should be able to manage all aspects of self-care and functional mobility after prosthetic training with the permanent prosthesis unless hindered by other ailments. Approximately 20% of all individuals with arteriosclerosis obliterans have a myocardial infarction or CVA at some point after diagnosis.

COMPARISON

What are the distinguishing characteristics of a similar condition?

Any amputation would be considered a similar condition, with each level of amputation possessing distinguishing characteristics. Regardless, physical therapy intervention will include desensitization, phantom pain education, proper compression and shaping, strengthening, self-care, and mobility. In most instances, patients status post amputation share the common goal of functional prosthetic use.

CLINICAL SCENARIOS

Scenario One

A two-year-old female born with congenital malformation of the ankle joint and without a foot is referred to physical therapy for a pre-operative evaluation. The child is in good health, active, and has no other past medical history. The child has become increasingly frustrated with her alternate means of mobility. Her parents are supportive and carry her for community mobility. She prefers to scoot and crawl around the house since she cannot bear weight through the affected lower extremity. She is scheduled for a Syme's amputation in one week.

Scenario Two

An 83-year-old male, status post right transtibial amputation secondary to insulin-dependent diabetes mellitus, is admitted to a skilled nursing facility for rehabilitation. The patient is obese and presents with cardiopulmonary insufficiency. The patient previously resided alone with intermittent home health care and requires two liters of oxygen with activity.

SILVER Level Clinical Application Templates

SILVER Level Clinical Application Template Executive Summary

Achilles Tendon Rupture

- Typically occurs within one to two inches above the tendinous insertion on the calcaneus
- Incidence is greatest between 30-50 years of age without history of calf or heel pain
- Patients with an Achilles tendon rupture will typically be unable to stand on their toes and tend to exhibit a positive Thompson test

Disk Herniation

- Often the result of gradual, age-related changes that cause disk degeneration
- Risk factors include being overweight and having an occupation that requires repetitive lifting, bending or twisting
- Physical therapy may consist of education on activity modification and appropriate body mechanics, soft tissue manipulation, lumbar stabilization exercises, traction, and modalities for pain relief

Glenohumeral Dislocation – Anterior

- Mechanism of injury may vary but typically involves a forceful external blow or loading force when the shoulder is in a position that combines abduction, lateral rotation and extension
- Prior to relocation of the joint, visible deformity, severe pain, and significant range of motion limitations are the most significant characteristics
- Is not life-threatening though recurrent dislocations can have a substantial impact on a patient's lifestyle

Medial Epicondylitis

- Occurs with repetitive wrist or elbow motions or gripping, and is often seen in golfers or those who play throwing or racket sports
- Initial treatment consists of rest, ice, anti-inflammatory medications, massage, stretching, and bracing to help control acute symptoms
- Home care regimen consists of stretching and strengthening exercises, especially for the wrist flexor and forearm pronator muscle groups, as well as icing to help control symptoms

Meniscal Tear

- Often involve twisting of the knee when in a semiflexed position with the foot planted on the ground
- Characterized by joint line pain and tenderness, swelling, loss of range of motion (sometimes with a mechanical block), a complaint of "catching" or "locking" within the joint, and feelings of instability
- Physical therapy focuses on interventions to reduce swelling, normalize range of motion, and improve muscular strength

Osgood-Schlatter Disease

- Refers to traction apophysitis occurring at the tibial tuberosity where symptoms are typically exacerbated by running, jumping, and squatting activities
- Characterized by localized pain and edema with point tenderness over the patella tendon's insertion on the tibial tuberosity
- Limiting symptoms may last for weeks or months before abating, however, the condition typically will resolve in time without intervention

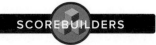

SILVER Level Clinical Application Template Executive Summary

Osteogenesis Imperfecta

- Classified into four types with a wide range of clinical presentations ranging from normal appearance with mild symptoms to severe involvement that can be fatal during infancy
- Bone densitometry may be used to measure bone mass and estimate the risk of fracture for specific sites within the body
- Children with osteogenesis imperfecta often have delayed developmental milestones secondary to ongoing fractures with immobilization, hypermobility of joints, and poorly developed muscles

Spinal Stenosis – Lumbar

- Refers to a narrowing of either the lumbar vertebral or intervertebral foramen with symptoms resulting from mechanical compression on either the spinal cord or exiting nerve roots
- Symptoms include a gradual onset and worsening of chronic pain at the midline of the lumbar region, unilateral nerve root radiculopathy, paresthesia, weakness, and diminished reflexes
- Severity of symptoms reported varies widely and directly influences expectations for long-term outcomes of physical therapy interventions

Temporomandibular Joint Dysfunction

- Females are at greater risk than males with the most common age ranging from 20-40 years of age
- Clinical presentation includes pain (persistent or recurring), muscle spasm, abnormal or limited jaw motion, headache, and tinnitus
- Intervention includes patient education, posture retraining, and modalities such as moist heat, ice, biofeedback, ultrasound, electrostimulation, TENS, and massage

Torticollis - Congenital

- Causes the neck to involuntarily contract to one side secondary to contraction of the sternocleidomastoid muscle
- The head is laterally flexed toward the contracted muscle, the chin faces the opposite direction, and there may be facial asymmetries
- Studies indicate that between 85-90% of patients with congenital torticollis respond to conservative treatment and passive stretching within the first year of life

Total Shoulder Arthroplasty

- Surgical candidates typically have irreparable damage, deterioration, and destruction to the humeral head and the glenoid fossa within the shoulder complex
- Surgical complications include mechanical loosening of the prosthesis, instability, rotator cuff tear, implant failure, heterotopic ossification, and intraoperative fracture
- Life expectancy is longer for the shoulder compared to the knee or hip since the shoulder is a non-weight bearing joint

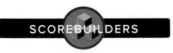

Achilles Tendon Rupture   SILVER

DIAGNOSIS

What condition produces a patient's symptoms?

Rupture of the Achilles tendon normally occurs within one to two inches above its tendinous insertion on the calcaneus. A patient will present with symptoms secondary to the rupture and discontinuity of the Achilles tendon.

An injury was most likely sustained to which structure?

The Achilles tendon is the largest and strongest tendon in the human body and is formed from the tendinous portions of the gastrocnemius and soleus muscles coalescing above the insertion on the calcaneal tuberosity. Theories suggest that an Achilles tendon rupture usually occurs in an Achilles tendon that has undergone degenerative changes. The degenerative changes will begin with hypovascularity in the Achilles tendon area. The impaired blood flow in combination with repetitive microtrauma creates degenerative changes within the tendon and as a result makes the tendon more susceptible to injury.

INFERENCE

What is the most likely contributing factor in the development of this condition?

An Achilles tendon rupture occurs most frequently when pushing off of a weight bearing extremity with an extended knee, through unexpected dorsiflexion while weight bearing or with a forceful eccentric contraction of the plantar flexors. Participation in sports that require quick-changing footwork such as softball, tennis, basketball, and football are high-risk activities. Other contributing factors include poor stretching routine, tight calf muscles, improper shoe wear during high risk activities, and altered biomechanics at the foot during activities (such as a flattened arch). The highest incidence for rupture is in individuals between 30 and 50 years of age that usually have no history of calf or heel pain and commonly participate in recreational activities.

CONFIRMATION

What is the most likely clinical presentation?

A patient with an Achilles tendon rupture will present with swelling over the distal tendon, a palpable defect in the tendon above the calcaneal tuberosity, and pain and weakness with plantar flexion. The patient may limp and will often complain that during the injury there was a snap or a pop that was associated with the severe pain. A patient will not be able to stand on their toes and in a prone position will not demonstrate any passive plantar flexion with squeezing of the affected calf muscle (the Thompson test). A complete rupture will result in a palpable gap in the tendon prior to the insertion.

What laboratory or imaging studies would confirm the diagnosis?

Confirmation of an Achilles tendon rupture should utilize x-ray to rule out an avulsion fracture or bony injury. MRI can be used to locate the presence and severity of the tear or rupture.

What additional information should be obtained to confirm the diagnosis?

Diagnosis of an Achilles tendon rupture relies on patient history of the event and a positive Thompson's test. Patient history usually reveals a popping sound and a release from the back of the ankle. Physical examination and palpation reveal a discontinuity within the tendon.

MANAGEMENT

What is the most effective management of this patient?

Medical management of a ruptured Achilles tendon incorporates immobilization through casting or a surgical approach for repair or reconstruction. Pharmacological intervention is not necessary for this condition except to relieve pain through NSAIDs, acetaminophen or narcotics depending on physician preference, and patient profile. Non-surgical treatment includes serial casting for approximately ten weeks followed by the use of a heel lift to ensure maximal healing without stress on the tendon for three to six months. Physical therapy begins when the cast is removed. If a patient requires surgical intervention then a cast or a brace is required for six to eight weeks. Physical therapy intervention is primarily the same for surgical and non-surgical patients and includes range of motion, stretching, icing, assistive device training, endurance programming, gait training, strengthening, plyometrics, and skill specific training.

What home care regimen should be recommended?

A home care regimen is vital to the success of a patient's recovery. A program must be based on a patient's post-operative impairments and follow the physician's post-surgical protocol. A home program generally incorporates icing and elevation early in the rehabilitation process. A patient is required to continue a home program throughout the six to seven months of rehabilitation. Other areas of focus include range of motion, strengthening, gait, endurance activities, and high-level skill and sport specific tasks.

OUTCOME

What is the likely outcome of a course of physical therapy?

Physical therapy should begin after surgical intervention or when the cast is removed from a non-surgical patient. Assuming an unremarkable recovery, a patient should return to their previous functional level within six to seven months.

What are the long-term effects of the patient's condition?

A patient that manages the Achilles tendon rupture without surgery and allows the tendon to heal on its own has a higher rate of rerupture (40% rerupture the tendon) compared to a patient that has surgical repair of the tendon (0-5% rerupture the tendon). An advantage to non-surgical management is a reduced risk of infection from surgery. However, it may result in an incomplete return of functional performance. A patient that has surgical intervention has a decreased risk for reinjury and a higher rate of return to athletic activities.

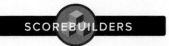

DIAGNOSIS

What condition produces a patient's symptoms?

The most common mechanism of injury for an intervertebral disk herniation is twisting and bending of the spine, often with the addition of some external load (e.g., bending over to lift a heavy object). This injury can occur acutely or gradually over time with repetitive twisting and bending movements.

An injury was most likely sustained to which structure?

The intervertebral disk is composed of two parts: an inner jelly-like material known as the nucleus pulposus and an outer cartilaginous structure known as the annulus fibrosus. A disk herniation occurs when the nucleus pulposus bulges through the exterior wall of the annulus fibrosus. Disk herniations most commonly occur on the posterolateral portion of the disk, where the disk is weakest and most likely to fissure. When the disk herniates, it often will compress nearby nerve roots and cause pain, numbness, and/or weakness into the extremities. The large majority of disk herniations occur at the L4-L5 or L5-S1 vertebral level.

INFERENCE

What is the most likely contributing factor in the development of this condition?

A disk herniation is often the result of gradual, age-related changes that cause disk degeneration. The disks lose water content over time, which makes them less flexible and increases the likelihood of tearing and rupturing of the annulus fibrosus. Risk factors for disk herniation include being overweight and having an occupation that requires repetitive lifting, bending or twisting.

CONFIRMATION

What is the most likely clinical presentation?

The clinical presentation most commonly includes low back pain followed by unilateral radicular leg pain (though bilateral leg pain is possible). Though pain is the most common symptom, the patient may also experience numbness, tingling, and weakness in the distribution of the affected nerve. Symptoms are exaggerated by sitting, walking, standing, and any increase in intra-abdominal pressure (e.g., coughing, sneezing). Though less common, disk herniations can also occur in the cervical spine.

What laboratory or imaging studies would confirm the diagnosis?

Magnetic resonance imaging is the most common imaging technique used to visualize a disk herniation. Electromyography and nerve conduction velocity testing can also be used to determine the extent of nerve damage to peripheral nerves.

What additional information should be obtained to confirm the diagnosis?

Though imaging studies are helpful, an accurate diagnosis can often be made based on a thorough medical history and physical exam. The physical exam will likely include neural provocation testing (e.g., slump test, straight leg raise test), as well as assessment of strength, sensation, and deep tendon reflexes.

MANAGEMENT

What is the most effective management of this patient?

Conservative management, consisting of avoidance of provocative positions and a course of physical therapy, is successful in the large majority of patients. Physical therapy may consist of education on activity modification and appropriate body mechanics, soft tissue manipulation, lumbar stabilization exercises, traction, and modalities for pain relief. Once tolerated, McKenzie extension exercises will likely be incorporated into the exercise program. A variety of pain medications may be administered, including NSAIDs, narcotic medications, nerve pain medications, and muscle relaxants. If conservative treatment is unsuccessful, a cortisone injection may be necessary. A small percentage of patients will eventually need surgery (i.e., microdiscectomy).

What home care regimen should be recommended?

A home care regimen will consist of activity modification and avoidance of provocative positioning, as well as lumbar stabilization exercises. Patients should use pain medications and ice or heat to help control their pain.

OUTCOME

What is the likely outcome of a course of physical therapy?

The large majority of patients will get better with conservative treatment, though complete resolution of symptoms can take months. The effectiveness of physical therapy will be dependent on the extent of disk injury, as well as the patient's age and activity level.

What are the long-term effects of the patient's condition?

The long-term effect of a patient's condition is highly dependent on the extent of the herniation. Individuals with a disk "bulge," in which the annulus fibrosus fibers are unaffected, are less likely to need surgery and more likely to experience a full recovery. Patients that have a larger herniation or rupture of the disk, in which the annulus fibrosus fibers are compromised, are more likely to experience reoccurrence of their symptoms.

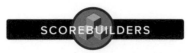

Glenohumeral Dislocation – Anterior

DIAGNOSIS

What condition produces a patient's symptoms?

An anterior glenohumeral (GH) dislocation occurs when the head of the humerus is traumatically separated from the glenoid fossa. The mechanism of injury may vary, but typically involves a forceful external blow or loading force, when the shoulder is in a position that combines abduction, lateral rotation, and extension (e.g., spiking a volleyball, throwing a ball).

An injury was most likely sustained to which structure?

Stability is primarily maintained by the GH joint capsule, ligaments, rotator cuff muscles, and glenoid labrum. Loading or other external forces applied to the joint while it is in a relatively unstable or vulnerable position may cause stretching or tearing of the stabilizing structures, allowing the joint to dislocate. Fracture may also occur.

INFERENCE

What is the most likely contributing factor in the development of this condition?

The shoulder is the most frequently dislocated joint with over 90% of shoulder dislocations occurring anteriorly. It is most common in patients engaged in sporting activities between 18 and 25 years of age. There is also a notable prevalence among the elderly with dislocation predominantly occurring secondary to a fall.

CONFIRMATION

What is the most likely clinical presentation?

Prior to relocation of the joint, visible deformity, severe pain, and significant range of motion limitations are the most significant characteristics. The affected limb will typically be positioned in slight abduction and lateral rotation with the patient unable to touch the opposite shoulder. The normal contour of the affected shoulder will be much more "square" than the unaffected side. The humeral head will typically be palpable anteriorly in the subcoracoid region. Once the dislocation has been reduced, the most severe pain symptoms typically resolve. The patient may continue to demonstrate protective or pain-limited range of motion efforts. A positive apprehension sign is likely. Diminished or absent radial pulses are suggestive of vascular injury and should be addressed immediately. Decreased sensation or motor function in the axillary, musculocutaneous, and radial nerve distributions may also be observed.

What laboratory or imaging studies would confirm the diagnosis?

X-ray imaging is typically performed both before and after the joint is reduced to assess joint position and rule out additional bony pathology. Other diagnostic procedures may also be necessary since adjacent structures may be easily damaged. MRI is typically utilized to assess suspected soft tissue injury and electromyography is utilized to assess nerve injury.

What additional information should be obtained to confirm the diagnosis?

A thorough medical history should be obtained including the mechanism of injury and any prior history of dislocation. Physical examination should include palpation as well as mobility, neurological, vascular, and pain assessments.

MANAGEMENT

What is the most effective management of this patient?

Medical management is initially focused on pharmacological pain management and joint reduction. Acutely, analgesic medications may be used to improve comfort during pre-reduction evaluative procedures and facilitate adequate relaxation of surrounding muscles prior to the reduction. After reduction, patients may require analgesics to effectively manage pain before transitioning to NSAIDs. Surgical management may be necessary if the joint cannot be conservatively reduced or if adjacent structural damage is significant (e.g., Bankart lesion, detached labrum, rotator cuff tear, fracture). Physical therapy intervention may be promptly initiated to assist with pain management and to prevent loss of function. Modalities may be used for palliative goals and to facilitate muscle retraining. Strengthening should initially emphasize isometrics, gradually progressing to resisted activities emphasizing the shoulder stabilizers. Physical therapy intervention may include range of motion, joint mobilizations, stretching, postural education, protective positioning, edema management, and activity modification.

What home care regimen should be recommended?

The home care regimen should include protective positioning, range of motion, and strengthening exercises. Pain management is typically achieved with rest, ice, and NSAIDs.

OUTCOME

What is the likely outcome of a course of physical therapy?

Typically, an aggressive strengthening program and/or activity modification will permit a return to athletic activities. The risk of re-injury is inherently greater in contact sports and is further increased depending on damage sustained to other stabilizing structures. In older or more sedentary populations, a return to prior level of function is possible. Some activity modifications emphasizing joint protection and fall prevention may be recommended.

What are the long-term effects of the patient's condition?

An anterior GH dislocation is not life-threatening though recurrent dislocations can have a substantial impact on a patient's lifestyle. Recurrent dislocations may require surgical intervention and consequently require greater restrictions or complete avoidance of participation in high-risk activities.

DIAGNOSIS

What condition produces a patient's symptoms?

Medial epicondylitis (also known as golfer's elbow) is a tendonitis that occurs at the medial epicondyle of the elbow. The condition is an overuse injury that occurs when the tendons are overworked and become inflamed, though it can also occur as the result of a traumatic event. Medial epicondylitis commonly occurs with repetitive wrist or elbow motions or gripping, and is often seen in golfers or those who play throwing or racket sports.

An injury was most likely sustained to which structure?

Medial epicondylitis affects the tendons of the muscles in the anterior forearm, which include the forearm pronators, wrist flexors, and finger flexors. The tendons of these muscles share a common tendinous sheath at their origin at the medial epicondyle of the humerus. The tendons of the flexor carpi radialis and pronator teres are most often affected. The ulnar nerve can also become irritated as it passes through the cubital tunnel in this region.

INFERENCE

What is the most likely contributing factor in the development of this condition?

This condition most often results from activities that require repetitive wrist or elbow motions or require lots of gripping. Patients who have poor flexibility, poor strength or poor endurance of the affected muscles are more prone to acquiring medial epicondylitis. Other risk factors for this condition include use of improper equipment (e.g., a racket grip that is the wrong size) or improper technique (e.g., excessive top spin in tennis).

CONFIRMATION

What is the most likely clinical presentation?

The onset of this condition is usually gradual, though it can occur suddenly after a traumatic incident. A patient with medial epicondylitis will report pain and have tenderness over the medial epicondyle. The patient will have pain with resisted wrist flexion and pronation and with gripping. There may also be weakness associated with these movements. If the ulnar nerve is affected, the patient could experience pain and paresthesias into the forearm and fourth and fifth digits.

What laboratory or imaging studies would confirm the diagnosis?

Imaging studies are generally not used in the diagnosis of medial epicondylitis. Radiographs will appear normal, though they will be necessary if the onset was traumatic. Magnetic resonance imaging can be used to identify damage to the soft tissue structures of the medial elbow, however, the diagnosis can usually be made based on the results of the physical examination alone.

What additional information should be obtained to confirm the diagnosis?

A thorough medical history and physical examination is usually enough to confirm the diagnosis of medial epicondylitis. Resisted wrist flexion or passive wrist extension can be used to elicit pain and aid in the diagnosis of medial epicondylitis. The examination should include an assessment of the ulnar collateral ligament since damage to this ligament can mimic symptoms of medial epicondylitis.

MANAGEMENT

What is the most effective management of this patient?

For the large majority of patients, the condition will improve with conservative treatment alone. Initial treatment consists of rest, ice, anti-inflammatory medications, massage, stretching, and bracing to help control acute symptoms. Bracing may involve a counterforce brace applied just distal to the elbow to help limit muscular strain at the epicondyle. Likewise, cock-up splints are sometimes used to limit repetitive movements of the wrist. Once pain subsides, strengthening exercises, especially eccentric exercises for the forearm musculature, can be initiated. A cortisone injection may be used to help alleviate symptoms. For patients who do not respond to conservative treatment, surgery may be necessary. Surgery for medial epicondylitis involves debridement of the degenerated tissue.

What home care regimen should be recommended?

The home care regimen should consist of stretching and strengthening exercises, especially for the wrist flexor and forearm pronator muscle groups, as well as icing to help control symptoms. The patient should be compliant with brace or splint use to help prevent irritation of the tissues.

OUTCOME

What is the likely outcome of a course of physical therapy?

A large majority of patients respond well to conservative treatment and are able to return to their previous functional level. Only a small percentage of patients will end up needing surgical intervention.

What are the long-term effects of the patient's condition?

While a cortisone injection can help to diminish symptoms acutely, it has no long-term effect. To prevent a recurrence of symptoms, it is important that the patient maintain good forearm flexibility and strength. Additionally, the patient should attempt to limit other risk factors by using correct technique and equipment and by limiting the volume of repetitive movements.

Meniscal Tear

SILVER

DIAGNOSIS

What condition produces a patient's symptoms?

Meniscal tears commonly occur as the result of a traumatic injury. The injury will often involve twisting of the knee when it is in a semiflexed position with the foot planted on the ground. Meniscal tears can also occur secondary to a hyperflexion injury. In older patients, meniscal tears are more likely to be caused by degeneration as opposed to acute trauma. When the meniscus has degenerated, a simple pivoting or squatting movement may be enough to cause a meniscus tear.

An injury was most likely sustained to which structure?

The menisci are C-shaped structures made of fibrocartilage that sit on each side of the tibial plateau. The menisci function to absorb shock and distribute loads within the knee joint. Because the medial meniscus is more firmly attached to the tibia, it is more commonly affected than the lateral meniscus. There are several different types of tears that can occur, including oblique, transverse, longitudinal, and complex tears. The location of the tear (e.g., inner meniscus, outer meniscus) is important in determining the most appropriate treatment. Meniscal injuries can occur in isolation or may occur in conjunction with ligamentous injuries (e.g., ACL tear).

INFERENCE

What is the most likely contributing factor in the development of this condition?

Patients who are involved in sports are more likely to experience meniscal tears, especially sports that involve quick cutting and pivoting movements. Older patients are more likely to have degenerative tears of the meniscus since, with increasing age, the cartilage thins and weakens and becomes more prone to tearing. Patients with instability of the knee, secondary to weakness or ligamentous deficiency, are also more prone to meniscal tears.

CONFIRMATION

What is the most likely clinical presentation?

Meniscal tears are characterized by joint line pain and tenderness, swelling, loss of range of motion (sometimes with a mechanical block), a complaint of "catching" or "locking" within the joint, and feelings of instability. Traumatic meniscal tears will result in a sudden onset of symptoms, whereas degenerative tears will have more of a gradual onset.

What laboratory or imaging studies would confirm the diagnosis?

While x-rays will not confirm or deny the presence of a meniscal tear, the diagnostic imaging technique is often performed to rule out other pathology (e.g., arthritis, fracture). Magnetic resonance imaging is the diagnostic test of choice for confirming the presence of a meniscal tear.

What additional information should be obtained to confirm the diagnosis?

In addition to imaging studies, a thorough medical history and physical examination should be performed on patients for whom a meniscus tear is suspected. The physical examination should include palpation, a range of motion assessment, and special tests. Common special tests for diagnosing meniscal tears include the McMurray test, the Apley's compression test, and the Thessaly test.

MANAGEMENT

What is the most effective management of this patient?

There are several considerations that must be made when determining if a patient with a meniscus tear should be treated conservatively or surgically, including the patient's age and activity level, and the location and extent of the tear. Conservative treatment for a meniscus tear involves rest including limited weight bearing, ice, use of anti-inflammatory medications, and physical therapy. Physical therapy will focus on interventions to reduce swelling, normalize range of motion, and improve muscular strength. Since some meniscus tears can heal on their own, conservative treatment is often attempted before considering surgery.

What home care regimen should be recommended?

The home care regimen will consist of rest, ice, and use of anti-inflammatory medications. The exercise program will likely consist of stretching and range of motion exercises to improve knee mobility and strengthening exercises to prevent muscular atrophy.

OUTCOME

What is the likely outcome of a course of physical therapy?

A tear in the outer one-third of the meniscus is more likely to heal spontaneously since this portion of the meniscus is vascular. Conservative treatment in these instances is often successful. If the tear is on the inner two-thirds of the meniscus, surgical intervention may be necessary.

What are the long-term effects of the patient's condition?

If the patient's condition does not respond well to conservative treatment, surgery will likely be considered. For patients who are young and whose lesion is located in the vascular portion of the meniscus, a full repair of the torn meniscus is usually performed. For older patients or for those patients who have a lesion in the avascular portion of the meniscus, a partial meniscectomy, in which the torn tissue is excised, will more likely be performed. Patients who have surgery are eventually able to return to their previous functional level without issue.

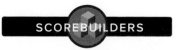

DIAGNOSIS

What condition produces a patient's symptoms?

Osgood-Schlatter disease refers to traction apophysitis occurring at the tibial tuberosity. Symptoms are typically the result of local inflammation at the tibial tuberosity and are exacerbated by running, jumping, and squatting activities.

An injury was most likely sustained to which structure?

The exact etiology is unknown though theories suggest that it may be caused by repeated microtrauma. Repeated tension at the insertion of the patella tendon can cause a small avulsion at the tuberosity thereby producing pain and edema. Over time, heterotopic bone formation may also produce a visible lump over the tibial tuberosity. The onset occurs most commonly in adolescents following a period of rapid long bone growth during which soft tissue tension may be temporarily increased before accommodating to the change in limb length.

INFERENCE

What is the most likely contributing factor in the development of this condition?

Osgood-Schlatter disease affects as many as 20% of adolescents involved in sports that require a great deal of running, jumping, swift directional changes, and repeated knee flexion (e.g., soccer, ballet). The age of onset is typically associated with periods of rapid growth during puberty. The condition is historically more prevalent among boys although the gender gap has lessened as more girls engage in competitive athletics.

CONFIRMATION

What is the most likely clinical presentation?

Osgood-Schlatter disease is characterized by localized pain and edema with point tenderness over the patella tendon's insertion on the tibial tuberosity. Pain symptoms are typically exacerbated by activities that increase traction forces at the tibial tubercle or put pressure directly on the affected area. Symptoms are typically reproducible with resisted knee extension and alleviated with rest or activity restriction. Generalized tightness in hip and knee musculature is common especially in the quadriceps. If heterotopic ossification has occurred, a firm mass will be palpable.

What laboratory or imaging studies would confirm the diagnosis?

X-ray imaging may be utilized to confirm the diagnosis and rule out other pathologies such as abnormal calcification, infection or apophyseal fracture.

What additional information should be obtained to confirm the diagnosis?

A diagnosis of Osgood-Schlatter disease is often made based entirely on symptom history and physical findings, therefore, a thorough examination is essential.

MANAGEMENT

What is the most effective management of this patient?

Medical management of Osgood-Schlatter disease is typically conservative with an emphasis on pain management. Patients should be counseled to modify or avoid pain-producing activities that increase tension on the patella tendon. The use of ice, rest, and over-the-counter medications (e.g., acetaminophen, NSAIDs) are also recommended. A knee immobilizer may be beneficial to facilitate rest during acute phases while an infrapatellar strap may assist in distributing traction forces once acuity is reduced and activity has resumed. Surgical intervention is rare though may be indicated for patients who have not responded to conservative treatment or have developed ossicles in the tendon or on the tibial tuberosity. Physical therapy intervention during an acute exacerbation may include palliative modalities, activity modification, and gentle stretching. Progressive stretching, strengthening, and cross training activities (e.g., swimming, cycling) should begin once acute symptoms have abated.

What home care regimen should be recommended?

A home care regimen should include rest, ice, and prescribed therapeutic exercise. Joint protection and cross training activities should be encouraged. Exacerbating activities should be modified or avoided until symptoms have resolved.

OUTCOME

What is the likely outcome of a course of physical therapy?

Limiting symptoms may last for weeks or months before abating. In some cases, discomfort can last for a number of years until the tibial growth plate has closed. Acute exacerbations are common until the long bones have stopped growing. Physical therapy may assist with reducing the severity of symptoms, however, the condition is typically self-limiting. Conservative treatment is successful in approximately 90% of cases.

What are the long-term effects of the patient's condition?

Osgood-Schlatter disease is a self-limiting condition that typically has an excellent prognosis. In many patients, a bony lump remains even after symptoms have resolved, though it rarely interferes with function. Complications are uncommon, but may include chronic pain, localized edema, and ossicle formation. Patients with symptoms that continue after reaching skeletal maturity may require surgical intervention.

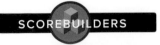

Osteogenesis Imperfecta   SILVER

DIAGNOSIS

What condition produces a patient's symptoms?

Osteogenesis imperfecta (OI) is a rare congenital disorder of collagen synthesis that affects all connective tissue in the body. The genetic defect affects collagen-producing genes and reduces production of collagen from 20-50%.

An injury was most likely sustained to which structure?

The genes for type I collagen production (COL1A1 and COL1A2) have been identified as the genes that become mutated and result in OI. Since collagen production is vital throughout the body, bones and all forms of connective tissue are compromised. OI can also compromise growth, hearing, cardiopulmonary function, and joint integrity.

INFERENCE

What is the most likely contributing factor in the development of this condition?

Most children inherit OI from parents as either an autosomal dominant or autosomal recessive trait. Twenty-five percent of the time the genetic defect occurs by spontaneous mutation of the genes. Statistics estimate that 30 to 50 thousand individuals are living with OI in the United States.

CONFIRMATION

What is the most likely clinical presentation?

OI is classified into four types and has a wide range of clinical presentations ranging from normal appearance with mild symptoms to severe involvement that is fatal during infancy. Type I is the mildest form where a child has near normal growth and appearance with frequency of fractures usually ceasing after puberty. The patient experiences mild or moderate fragility, but most times without deformity. This patient will usually present with blue sclera, easy bruising, triangular face, and possible hearing loss. Type II is the most severe form where a child dies in utero or by early childhood. This child has significant fragility of connective tissue, experiences multiple fractures with extreme deformities, and has a soft skull. Type III is severe, but these children present with greater ossification of the skull. Type III characteristics include significant growth retardation, progressive deformities, ongoing fractures, severe osteoporosis, triangular face, blue sclera, and significant limitations with functional mobility. Type IV is usually a milder course that involves mild to moderate fragility and osteoporosis (but greater than type I). The patient will experience fractures easily prior to puberty, but some children improve at that time. Type IV may or may not have a shorter stature, will have bowing of long bones, a barrel shape of their rib cage, possible hearing loss, brittle teeth, and will present with near normal sclera. These children have a near normal life expectancy.

What laboratory or imaging studies would confirm the diagnosis?

A skin biopsy is used to examine the collagen and determine what type of OI is present. X-rays and bone scans may be used for evidence of deformities and old fractures. Bone densitometry may also be used to measure bone mass and estimate the risk of fracture for specific sites within the body.

What additional information should be obtained to confirm the diagnosis?

Diagnosis should be determined based on physical examination, family and personal medical history, and formal testing.

MANAGEMENT

What is the most effective management of this patient?

Medical management is directed at controlling the symptoms of OI. General goals include maximizing independence with mobility, improving optimal bone mass and muscle strength, and prevention of fractures and deformities. Nutritional counseling and strong dental care are important in the management of OI. Lightweight orthotics may be indicated early to support the extremities, assist with ambulation, encourage weight bearing, and prevent fractures. Physical therapy intervention initially focuses on parent handling techniques, recognition of fractures, positioning, and activities that facilitate safe movement. Treatment of a child with OI should incorporate developmental activities, strengthening, positioning, weight bearing, and the use of mobility aids (scooters, riding toys or wheelchair). Swimming is also a good alternative for strengthening and exercise. All strengthening exercises should avoid rotational forces, placing weights/resistance near a joint, and using long lever arms.

What home care regimen should be recommended?

A home care regimen will be successful if parents are competent with many of the relevant aspects of care. Handling techniques, recognition of fractures, precautions and contraindications, standing program, and exercise through activities are all key components of a home program for a child with OI. A child needs to continue to move and exercise in a safe fashion in order to optimize strength and bone mass.

OUTCOME

What is the likely outcome of a course of physical therapy?

Physical therapy may be required intermittently over the course of the patient's childhood depending on the severity of OI and the secondary complications. A home program must be established for optimal therapeutic results. Physical therapy may be in an outpatient setting or through the school system. The therapist should work closely with the physician and caregivers for comprehensive care.

What are the long-term effects of the patient's condition?

A patient with OI has outcome potential based on the type of disorder, symptoms, and secondary complications encountered. A strong predictor of a child's ability to ambulate in the future also lies in the child's ability to sit by ten months of age. Some children live normal lives with minimal involvement while others use power wheelchairs for mobility and experience multiple secondary complications.

Spinal Stenosis – Lumbar

DIAGNOSIS

What condition produces a patient's symptoms?

Lumbar spinal stenosis (LSS) refers to a narrowing of either the lumbar vertebral or intervertebral foramina. Symptoms are typically produced as a result of mechanical compression on either the spinal cord or exiting nerve roots and may be further exacerbated by bony degeneration or instability. Primary spinal stenosis accounts for only a small percentage of diagnoses and is the result of a congenital malformation of spinal structures. Secondary spinal stenosis refers to narrowing due to acquired changes in the foramina.

An injury was most likely sustained to which structure?

Structural changes may include degeneration of the vertebral segments, disk herniation, osteophyte formation, and hypertrophy of structures such as the ligamentum flavum. Other etiologies include trauma, compression fracture, systemic conditions (e.g., tumor, ankylosing spondylitis), and iatrogenic factors (e.g., laminectomy, discectomy).

INFERENCE

What is the most likely contributing factor in the development of this condition?

Certain congenital conditions and defects increase the risk of primary spinal stenosis. Age is the primary risk factor for the development of secondary spinal stenosis due to the degenerative changes that are a part of the normal aging process.

CONFIRMATION

What is the most likely clinical presentation?

Typical LSS symptoms include a gradual onset and worsening of chronic pain at the midline of the lumbar region. Other complaints may include unilateral nerve root radiculopathy, paresthesia, weakness, and diminished reflexes. In rare cases, LSS may present bilaterally with bilateral weakness, paresthesia, diminished coordination, ataxic gait, balance dysfunction, bowel/bladder dysfunction, and hyperreflexia. Symptoms are typically exacerbated by activities that increase lumbar extension (e.g., standing upright, lying prone) and are alleviated by rest and activities that increase lumbar flexion (e.g., leaning on a grocery cart, sitting). Many patients adopt a stooped posture to functionally reduce their lumbar lordosis and minimize symptoms.

What laboratory or imaging studies would confirm the diagnosis?

An MRI provides the least invasive and most conclusive means of diagnosing LSS due to its ability to differentiate soft tissue pathologies such as disk damage or neural compression. A CT myelogram utilizes the injection of contrast dye into the spinal column to enhance visualization of the spinal cord, nerve roots, and areas of compression.

What additional information should be obtained to confirm the diagnosis?

A thorough medical history and physical examination should be completed to assist in ruling out similar diagnoses and determine the etiology of LSS in order to best direct treatment.

MANAGEMENT

What is the most effective management of this patient?

Medical management of LSS is typically conservative and focused on palliative pharmacological intervention. NSAIDs are often among the first medications recommended due to their dual action in providing analgesia in low doses and anti-inflammatory benefits. Muscle relaxants may be recommended to assist with sleep-related comfort. Surgical intervention such as lumbar laminectomy may be necessary if conservative measures fail and symptoms become disabling. Physical therapy intervention typically will focus on improving function and pain management. Strength, flexibility, and endurance exercises aim to improve muscular support and spinal stability. Patients who are pain-limited may also benefit from palliative modalities such as TENS to improve their tolerance for activities. Patients who are unable to assume a normal posture without exacerbation of symptoms may benefit from use of an assistive device to ease the excessive strain on postural muscles caused by a forward flexed or kyphotic posture.

What home care regimen should be recommended?

A home care regimen should include regular participation in an exercise program. Palliative home interventions may include hot or cold packs or home TENS use. Weight loss may be recommended and education should include activity modification especially for functional tasks that specifically exacerbate symptoms.

OUTCOME

What is the likely outcome of a course of physical therapy?

The severity of symptoms will vary and directly influence expectations for long-term outcomes. LSS is a progressive condition, however, for patients who are symptomatic, physical therapy can assist in minimizing the effects of the condition and maximizing independence.

What are the long-term effects of the patient's condition?

LSS is not life-threatening and in many patients is never formally diagnosed due to a relative lack of symptoms. In others, LSS can result in significant disability due to chronic pain and muscle weakness.

Temporomandibular Joint Dysfunction

SILVER

DIAGNOSIS

What condition produces a patient's symptoms?

The temporomandibular joint (TMJ) is a complex joint that is classified as a condylar, hinge, and synovial joint. The TMJ contains fibrocartilaginous surfaces and articular discs. Temporomandibular joint dysfunction (TMD) occurs due to a change in the joint structure that can cause multiple symptoms and a limitation in function. In many instances inflammation and muscle spasm surrounding the joint produces symptoms for the patient with TMD.

An injury was most likely sustained to which structure?

TMD results from injury, derangement or incongruence of the TMJ itself, intra-articular disks, and/or supporting surrounding structures. Over time the meniscus of the TMJ becomes compressed and torn allowing for the bony portion of the joint (the ball and socket) to deteriorate secondary to the grinding of bone on bone.

INFERENCE

What is the most likely contributing factor in the development of this condition?

TMD can be classified by three primary etiological factors: predisposing factors, triggering factors, and perpetuating/sustaining factors. TMD can occur secondary to multiple causative factors including injury or trauma to the joint, congenital abnormalities, internal derangement of joint structure, arthritis, dislocation, disk degeneration, metabolic conditions or stress. Risk factors include chewing on one side, eating tough food, clenching, and grinding of teeth. Habits of gum chewing and nail biting may increase the incidence of injury to the TMJ. Patients are typically between 20 to 40 years of age with a greater incidence in women. Research indicates a possible link between gender-specific hormones and the risk for TMD.

CONFIRMATION

What is the most likely clinical presentation?

The National Institute of Dental and Craniofacial Research indicates that approximately 10.8 million individuals have TMD within the United States and 90% of the individuals that are seeking treatment are women in their childbearing years. A patient with TMD will present with symptoms that include pain (persistent or recurring), muscle spasm, abnormal or limited jaw motion, headache, and tinnitus. These symptoms can be unilateral or bilateral. The patient will often complain of feeling and hearing a "clicking or popping" sound with motion at the TMJ. Clinical manifestation of symptoms relates to the actual cause of the TMD.

What laboratory or imaging studies would confirm the diagnosis?

Procedures used in diagnosing TMD and its origin may include x-ray, MRI, mandibular kinesiography, CT scan, and a dental examination.

What additional information should be obtained to confirm the diagnosis?

A physical examination, upper quarter screening, TMJ loading, condyle-meniscus relationship, review of symptoms, and past medical history are all important components in the diagnosis of TMD. An occlusion examination may be indicated to evaluate a patient's bite.

MANAGEMENT

What is the most effective management of this patient?

Medical management of TMD may include pharmacological intervention, the use of splinting, physical therapy treatment, and possible surgical intervention. Pharmacological treatment of TMD may include analgesics, NSAIDs, muscle relaxants, and antianxiety medications. A patient may also benefit from a splint to assist with realignment of the joint and a guard or bite plate to maintain proper positioning and avoid grinding of the teeth throughout the night. Specific physical therapy intervention is based on the exact etiology of the TMD. Generally, physical therapy intervention includes patient education regarding habits such as nail biting, posture retraining, the use of modalities such as moist heat, ice, biofeedback, ultrasound, electrostimulation, TENS, and massage. Soft tissue manipulation, joint mobilization, ROM, stretching, occlusal appliance prescription, and relaxation techniques are also appropriate. If conservative treatment fails or the exact etiology warrants surgical intervention (approximately 5% of cases), the patient may require a condylectomy, osteotomy, arthrotomy, arthroscopy, reduction of subluxation or joint debridement.

What home care regimen should be recommended?

A home care regimen for a patient with TMD should include relaxation techniques, self-stretching, posture retraining exercises, and progressive ROM. A patient should avoid all foods and activities (such as gum chewing) that aggravate and stress the TMJ. The patient should continue with the proper use of an occlusal appliance if indicated. In order to maintain progress the patient must have ongoing consistency with the home program.

OUTCOME

What is the likely outcome of a course of physical therapy?

Physical therapy intervention should improve a patient's condition and decrease the symptoms of the TMD. Physical therapy is usually conducted on an outpatient basis with focus on maximizing function and alleviating pain.

What are the long-term effects of the patient's condition?

A patient previously diagnosed with TMD is at an increased risk of recurrence, however, with successful management, ongoing compliance with the home program, and use of an indicated appliance, the patient may not have any long-term effects. If conservative management fails the patient may require surgical intervention for the underlying cause in order to alleviate the TMD.

DIAGNOSIS

What condition produces a patient's symptoms?

Congenital torticollis is a condition that causes the neck to involuntarily unilaterally contract to one side secondary to contraction of the sternocleidomastoid muscle. The head is laterally flexed toward the contracted muscle, the chin faces the opposite direction, and there may be facial asymmetries. The word torticollis means twisted neck. It is a disease, but also a symptom of many conditions.

An injury was most likely sustained to which structure?

Congenital torticollis is not usually seen immediately at birth. Muscle injury may be due to birth trauma, breech position in utero or other forms of intrauterine malpositioning. Infants born with torticollis appear healthy at delivery, however, over days or weeks they develop swelling over the injured sternocleidomastoid.

INFERENCE

What is the most likely contributing factor in the development of this condition?

The exact etiology of congenital torticollis is unknown, however, congenital torticollis may be caused by local trauma to the soft tissues of the neck just before or during delivery. The most common hypothesis is that birth trauma with resultant hematoma formation results in muscular contracture. Typically, children with congenital torticollis have had breech or difficult forceps delivery. The fibrosis that develops in the muscle may be due to venous occlusion and pressure on the neck in the birth canal secondary to skull and neck position. Another theory includes malpositioning in utero resulting in intrauterine compartment syndrome.

CONFIRMATION

What is the most likely clinical presentation?

The patient's head is laterally flexed towards the shortened muscle's side and the chin is pointed toward the opposite shoulder. Intermittent painful spasms of the sternocleidomastoid, trapezius, and other neck muscles may occur. The neck movements vary from jerky to smooth. The first sign may be a firm nontender enlargement of the sternocleidomastoid muscle visible at birth or within the infant's first few weeks of life. This mass, which is usually localized near the clavicular attachment of the sternocleidomastoid muscle, enlarges during the first few weeks of life, and then gradually decreases in size. Usually, the mass disappears by the sixth month of life and the only remaining clinical finding is the contracture of the sternocleidomastoid muscle that creates the torticollis posturing.

What laboratory or imaging studies would confirm the diagnosis?

Cervical spine x-rays are used to assess potential fracture or subluxation. A CT scan or MRI of the cervical spine can identify the presence of a potential neck mass. An electromyography (EMG) study may be useful in defining the degree of muscle or nerve involvement.

What additional information should be obtained to confirm the diagnosis?

The presence of the mass over the sternocleidomastoid along with the classic posturing will confirm the presence of congenital torticollis.

MANAGEMENT

What is the most effective management of this patient?

Congenital torticollis is usually treated with non-operative intervention for 12-24 months before considering surgical intervention. Pharmacological intervention may include nonsteroidal anti-inflammatory drugs (NSAIDs), benzodiazepines and other muscle relaxants, anticholinergics, and local intramuscular injections of botulinum toxin or phenol. Physical therapy includes family/caregiver education and teaching, passive stretching exercises to the sternocleidomastoid and upper trapezius muscles, massage, local heat, analgesics, sensory biofeedback, and transcutaneous electrical nerve stimulation (TENS). Active range of motion with subsequent strengthening is also indicated to correct the infant's positioning of their head. Family training is extremely beneficial if there is consistency with handling and proper positioning during feeding and sleeping in order to promote stretch and active motion of the sternocleidomastoid muscle. If conservative treatment fails, surgical intervention will consist of unipolar sternocleidomastoid release, bipolar sternocleidomastoid release or selective denervation. Physical therapy is indicated after surgery and should include manual stretching of the neck to maintain the overcorrected position. Manual stretching should be continued three times daily for 3-6 months. A cervical collar may be used for the first 6-12 weeks after surgery.

What home care regimen should be recommended?

The family must continue with the stretching program and the correct handling techniques that are recommended by the therapist. The family will need to include proper positioning for the infant's sleep and alert times in order to maximize the benefits of the intervention.

OUTCOME

What is the likely outcome of a course of physical therapy?

Studies indicate that between 85-90% of patients with congenital torticollis respond to conservative treatment and passive stretching within the first year of life. The best results for conservative management require the child to have had conservative treatment prior to the age of one. If surgical intervention is required, physical therapy will be required after surgery with an expected positive outcome for the patient..

What are the long-term effects of the patient's condition?

If a child is left untreated, congenital torticollis could have detrimental effects including the impairment of normal growth and development. The vast majority of children with congenital torticollis that receive conservative management are expected to fully recover and live a normal life.

Total Shoulder Arthroplasty   SILVER

DIAGNOSIS

What condition produces a patient's symptoms?

A patient that is a candidate for a total shoulder arthroplasty (TSA) will have severe pain and impaired shoulder motion due to deterioration of the glenohumeral joint. These candidates have undergone conservative treatment measures that have failed to improve their condition.

An injury was most likely sustained to which structure?

TSA candidates will have irreparable damage, deterioration, and destruction to the humeral head and the glenoid fossa within the shoulder complex. The joint surfaces are severely damaged or destroyed by wear and tear, inflammation, injury or previous surgery.

INFERENCE

What is the most likely contributing factor in the development of this condition?

Indications for a TSA include severe glenohumeral degenerative joint disease, pain and limited range of motion secondary to osteoarthritis, rheumatoid arthritis, avascular necrosis, fracture or rotator cuff arthropathy. Other patients that may require a TSA would include a patient with a bone tumor, Paget's disease or with recurrent dislocations. A patient will be considered for TSA if conservative treatment of the underlying cause fails.

CONFIRMATION

What is the most likely clinical presentation?

A patient will exhibit impaired range of motion at the shoulder, may lack independence with functional mobility and ADLs, and will experience severe pain. It is this unremitting pain (with failed conservative treatment) that is the primary indication for the TSA. A TSA performed secondary to arthritis is usually performed on patients between 55 and 70 years of age while TSA performed secondary to irreparable damage from dislocation or avascular necrosis is usually performed on patients between 40 and 50 years of age.

What laboratory or imaging studies would confirm the diagnosis?

X-ray will reveal the level of degeneration within the shoulder complex. MRI or CT scan will allow the physician to assess the integrity of the rotator cuff and deltoid muscles surrounding the joint as well as the overall integrity of the shoulder complex.

What additional information should be obtained to confirm the diagnosis?

A full medical history along with a physical examination is a key component that is required in determining if a patient is a candidate for a TSA. The patient must possess motivation, realistic expectations, and appropriate goals regarding outcome.

MANAGEMENT

What is the most effective management of this patient?

A patient status post TSA will remain hospitalized for an average of two to five days. Medical management of the patient will rely on a team approach including nursing, physician services, and rehabilitation therapies. The success of the TSA will rely on the style of the implant, the quality of the soft tissue and bone, and the rehabilitation program. A CPM may be prescribed by the surgeon for use during the patient's hospitalization. Pharmacological intervention includes anticoagulation and pain medications. Physical therapy is initiated the day after surgery and should follow the shoulder rehabilitation protocol designed by the surgeon. The shoulder usually remains immobilized using a sling during initial rehabilitation. The Neer shoulder protocol advocates initiating isometric shoulder exercises approximately three weeks after surgery and active shoulder exercises approximately six weeks after surgery. PROM and AAROM are indicated but AROM at the shoulder is contraindicated during the first phase of rehabilitation. Physical therapy intervention includes pain management, prevention of adhesions, functional activities, PROM/AAROM/AROM, therapeutic exercise, edema management, patient education in self-ROM and wand/pendulum exercises, and the use of modalities.

What home care regimen should be recommended?

The home care regimen should include a range of motion and therapeutic exercise program that follows the surgeon's shoulder rehabilitation protocol. During initial recovery, pendulum and wand exercises are appropriate as well as self-ROM. A patient must not perform any form of medial rotation or lateral rotation beyond 35 to 40 degrees during the first two to three weeks post surgery. Controlled motion and return to functional activity are incorporated into the home program as directed by the physician protocol. A patient must also continue to manage edema and follow other physician orders regarding precautions.

OUTCOME

What is the likely outcome of a course of physical therapy?

The goal of a TSA is to relieve pain and regain functional motion. Physical therapy should assist the patient to meet these goals unless hindered by post-surgical or other complications.

What are the long-term effects of the patient's condition?

Since the shoulder is a non-weight bearing joint there is a longer life expectancy for the prosthesis than for the knee or hip. There is a high success rate for long-term results with a TSA. Patients should avoid activities such as heavy lifting, chopping wood or contact sports since these can increase the risk of fracture, loosening of the joint replacement or rotator cuff tear.

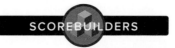

BRONZE Level Clinical Application Templates

BRONZE   Level Clinical Application Template Executive Summary

Anterior Compartment Syndrome

- Characterized by increased pressure in the lower leg secondary to swelling, which can occlude blood flow and cause ischemia and necrosis of the surrounding nerves and musculature
- Chronic cases may occur secondary to athletic exertion; acute cases are often caused by a traumatic injury and are considered a medical emergency
- Symptoms include tightness and tenderness over the muscle belly of the tibialis anterior, pain with passive stretching or active use of the muscle, and paresthesias and/or numbness in the distribution of the deep peroneal nerve

Colles' Fracture

- Frequently occurs when an individual reaches forward with their hands while attempting to break a fall; characterized by a transverse fracture of the distal radius
- Trauma related to this maneuver is commonly termed a FOOSH "fall on outstretched hand" injury
- X-ray of the wrist is the preferred method of confirming a Colles' fracture and identifying displaced fragments or damage to adjacent bony structures

De Quervain's Tenosynovitis

- Results from an inflammatory process involving the tendons and synovium of the abductor pollicis longus (APL) and extensor pollicis brevis (EPB) at the base of the thumb
- Onset is typically due to repetitive activities involving thumb abduction and extension such as racquet sports and repeated heavy lifting
- Symptom onset may be gradual or sudden depending on the mechanism of injury with report of localized pain and tenderness in the area of the anatomical snuffbox which may radiate

Myositis Ossificans

- Characterized by the calcification of muscle that is usually caused by neglecting to properly treat a muscle strain or contusion
- Development of this condition occurs within a few weeks after the initial injury and may include a noticeable hard lump in the muscle belly, an increase in pain, and a decrease in range of motion
- An x-ray is the primary imaging study used to confirm the diagnosis

Osteochondritis Dissecans

- Condition in which loss of blood flow to subchondral bone causes a piece of bone and its associated cartilage to crack and separate away from the end of the bone
- Symptoms may include pain with functional activities, joint popping or locking, weakness, swelling, and decreased range of motion
- X-ray imaging can be used to confirm the diagnosis

Osteomyelitis

- An infection that occurs within the bone, most commonly secondary to the Staphylococcus aureus microbe
- Damage to the bone from a surgical procedure, compound fracture or puncture wound that penetrates the bone may directly expose the bone to infectious microbes
- A bone biopsy is the most conclusive procedure for diagnosing osteomyelitis and determining the specific infectious microbe present

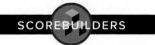

BRONZE Level Clinical Application Template Executive Summary

Piriformis Syndrome

- Characterized as the result of compression or irritation to the proximal sciatic nerve due to piriformis muscle inflammation, spasm or contracture
- Location of pain is often imprecise, though typically presents first in the area of the mid-buttock then progresses to radicular complaints in the sciatic nerve distribution
- Patients typically respond well to physical therapy interventions and are able to return to regular activities without restriction

Posterior Cruciate Ligament Sprain

- Occurs when a posteriorly directed force is applied to the tibia in relation to the femur, such as when the knee hits the dashboard in a motor vehicle accident
- Individuals participating in contact activities requiring a high level of agility are particularly susceptible to a posterior cruciate ligament injury
- A large majority of patients that experience a posterior cruciate ligament sprain are able to return to their previous level of function, including participation in athletics

Tarsal Tunnel Syndrome

- Occurs as a result of compression of the tibial nerve as it passes through the tarsal tunnel, causing neuropathy in the distribution of the nerve
- Signs and symptoms include pain, numbness, and paresthesias in the foot, muscle atrophy and weakness, diminished light touch and temperature sensation, and an antalgic gait pattern
- Tinel's sign can be used to confirm the presence of the condition, though diagnostic tests (MRI, ultrasound, EMG, NCV) may also be performed

Trochanteric Bursitis

- May occur as a result of acute or cumulative trauma to the lateral hip causing irritation to the trochanteric bursa
- Causative factors may include a true or functional leg length discrepancy, history of lateral hip surgery, and participation in sports with significant running or contact
- Patients typically respond well to conservative interventions and should be able to return fully to their prior level of function including sport activity

Ulnar Collateral Ligament Sprain – Thumb

- Occurs secondary to a traumatic event in which an excessive valgus force is applied to the metacarpophalangeal joint of the thumb
- The therapist should perform ligament stability testing of the thumb by applying a valgus force to the joint, with a movement of greater than 30-35 degrees indicating a complete tear of the ulnar collateral ligament
- X-rays should be ordered to rule out the existence of a fracture or dislocation

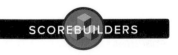

Anterior Compartment Syndrome   BRONZE

DIAGNOSIS

What condition produces a patient's symptoms?

Anterior compartment syndrome occurs when the pressure in the anterior compartment of the lower leg increases secondary to swelling. This increase in pressure results in occlusion of blood flow, which may cause ischemia and necrosis of the surrounding nerves and musculature. Acute compartment syndrome is a medical emergency, often caused by a traumatic injury, that can lead to irreversible muscle damage. Chronic compartment syndrome most often occurs secondary to athletic exertion and is typically not a medical emergency.

An injury was most likely sustained to what structure?

This condition affects the anterior compartment of the lower leg, which consists of the tibialis anterior, extensor hallucis longus, extensor digitorum longus, and peroneus tertius muscles. Because fascia does not stretch, the increase in pressure causes increased compression on the capillaries, nerves, and muscles of the anterior compartment. If not relieved, irreversible damage to the nerves and muscles may result secondary to ischemia.

CONFIRMATION

What is the most likely clinical presentation?

An increase in swelling will cause tightness and tenderness over the muscle belly of the tibialis anterior that does not decrease with elevation or pain medications. Pain increases with passive stretching or active use of the muscle. The patient will also likely experience paresthesias and/or numbness in the distribution of the deep peroneal nerve.

What laboratory or imaging studies would confirm the diagnosis?

Physicians can use compartment pressure testing, in which a needle or catheter is inserted into the affected compartment, to determine the presence of acute compartment syndrome. In the case of chronic compartment syndrome, measurements can be compared before and after exercise.

What additional information should be obtained to confirm the diagnosis?

A thorough medical history and physical examination should be completed to assist in ruling out other similar conditions such as deep venous thrombosis, fracture, and peripheral nerve injury.

Colles' Fracture   BRONZE

DIAGNOSIS

What condition produces a patient's symptoms?

A Colles' fracture frequently occurs when an individual reaches forward with their hands while attempting to break a fall. Trauma related to this maneuver is commonly termed a FOOSH (fall on outstretched hand) injury. Various types of wrist fractures can occur with a FOOSH injury due to the significant momentum and body weight that the wrist absorbs while in a hyperextended position.

An injury was most likely sustained to which structure?

A Colles' fracture is characterized by a transverse fracture of the distal radius, occurring in either an intra or extraarticular location due to direct trauma. The mechanism of injury typically causes the lunate to act as a wedge resulting in a shear force and dorsal displacement of the radius. Damage to structures on the ulnar aspect of the wrist such as the ulnar collateral ligament or styloid process are also common occurrences with a FOOSH injury.

CONFIRMATION

What is the most likely clinical presentation?

A patient with a Colles' fracture will likely present with pain and edema in close proximity to the fracture site. A "dinner fork" or "bayonet" deformity may be present with more severe Colles'

fractures as a result of dorsal displacement of the distal radius, carpals, and hand in relation to the forearm. Patients with osteoporosis are at particular risk for acquiring Colles' fractures when falling from a standing position.

What laboratory or imaging studies would confirm the diagnosis?

An x-ray of the wrist is the preferred method of confirming a Colles' fracture and identifying displaced fragments or damage to adjacent bony structures. An x-ray will commonly reveal an area of increased bone density at the fracture site with irregularities in the smooth surface line of the radius. Complete fractures will typically reveal a "dinner fork" deformity on x-ray. An MRI may be utilized if ligamentous or other significant soft tissue damage is suspected.

What additional information should be obtained to confirm the diagnosis?

The patient's subjective report of the mechanism of injury and current symptoms are extremely important when a Colles' fracture is suspected. Visual inspection, a thorough history, and careful examination will typically support the diagnosis.

De Quervain's Tenosynovitis

DIAGNOSIS

What condition produces a patient's symptoms?

De Quervain's tenosynovitis is the result of an inflammatory process involving the tendons and synovium of the abductor pollicis longus (APL) and extensor pollicis brevis (EPB) at the base of the thumb. The onset of de Quervain's tenosynovitis is typically due to repetitive activities involving thumb abduction and extension such as racquet sports and repeated heavy lifting. The associated inflammation results in pain located at the base of the thumb within the anatomical snuffbox.

An injury was most likely sustained to which structure?

The tendons of the APL and EPB are covered by a synovial sheath and pass through the anatomical tunnel that is created by the extensor retinaculum and the radial styloid process. Inflammation of the tendons and synovium results in impingement of the tendons as they move through the tunnel. Direct trauma or structural anomalies in the area can also restrict tendon mobility and cause symptoms of de Quervain's tenosynovitis.

CONFIRMATION

What is the most likely clinical presentation?

Patients will primarily report localized pain and tenderness in the area of the anatomical snuffbox which may occasionally radiate into the forearm. Symptom onset may be gradual or sudden. The degree of reported pain tends to be activity dependent and typically improves with rest and worsens with activity or resisted testing. Edema may be palpable or visible at the base of the thumb. In severe cases, edema may also cause symptoms of nerve entrapment particularly in the superficial branch of the radial nerve. De Quervain's tenosynovitis is more prevalent among women with higher risk among new mothers due to the repetitive lifting and carrying of the infant.

What laboratory or imaging studies would confirm the diagnosis?

There are no laboratory or imaging studies commonly used to assist in the diagnosis of de Quervain's tenosynovitis. A diagnosis is typically made by means of a thorough medical history and physical examination.

What additional information should be obtained to confirm the diagnosis?

Provocative testing using Finkelstein's test should be included in a physical examination to assist with the diagnosis of de Quervain's tenosynovitis. Activities of daily living and functional limitations should also be reviewed in order to identify exacerbating factors.

Myositis Ossificans

DIAGNOSIS

What condition produces a patient's symptoms?

Myositis ossificans is a condition characterized by the calcification of muscle. The condition is typically caused by neglecting to properly treat a muscle strain or contusion. Failing to apply cold therapy after an injury, applying heat after an injury or having intense therapy or massage too soon after injury are precipitating factors that disrupt healing and lead to abnormal bone growth.

An injury was most likely sustained to what structure?

The condition is characterized by bone growth in the muscle belly and often occurs in muscles prone to traumatic injury such as the muscles of the arms and legs (e.g., quadriceps). Bone will begin to grow 2-4 weeks after the injury and will mature within 3-6 months.

CONFIRMATION

What is the most likely clinical presentation?

In the initial stage post injury, the patient will present with the typical symptoms of a contusion. The patient will have pain with functional activities and stiffness and pain after prolonged rest. Swelling, tenderness, and bruising may also be present. Within a few weeks after injury, the development of further symptoms may suggest the presence of myositis ossificans. Symptoms include a noticeable hard lump in the muscle belly, an increase in pain, and a decrease in range of motion that had previously been improving.

What laboratory or imaging studies would confirm the diagnosis?

An x-ray is the primary imaging study used to confirm the diagnosis. This is performed approximately three weeks after the injury when the bone has started to grow. Magnetic resonance imaging and ultrasound imaging can also be used to assist in confirming the diagnosis.

What additional information should be obtained to confirm the diagnosis?

A thorough medical history and physical examination should be performed to assist with the diagnosis of the condition and to rule out the presence of other similar conditions (e.g., osteosarcoma).

Osteochondritis Dissecans   BRONZE

DIAGNOSIS

What condition produces a patient's symptoms?

Osteochondritis dissecans is a condition where subchondral bone and its associated cartilage crack and separate from the end of the bone. In severe cases of the condition, the bone may actually detach from the surrounding area and float freely inside the joint space. There is no definitive etiology, though it is thought the condition occurs secondary to a loss of blood flow to the affected area possibly due to repetitive microtrauma.

An injury was most likely sustained to what structure?

Loss of blood flow causes subchondral bone to die and separate from the surrounding bone. This leaves the associated articular cartilage prone to further damage. This condition primarily affects the knee joint, though is also commonly seen in the elbow and ankle.

CONFIRMATION

What is the most likely clinical presentation?

The clinical presentation varies based on the degree of subchondral bone detachment. Typical symptoms include pain with functional activities, joint popping or locking, weakness, swelling, and decreased range of motion.

What laboratory or imaging studies would confirm the diagnosis?

X-ray imaging may confirm the diagnosis of this condition, though computed tomography and magnetic resonance imaging may also be used to assist in the diagnosis and to better visualize the area of cartilage affected.

What additional information should be obtained to confirm the diagnosis?

A thorough medical history and physical examination should be performed to rule out the existence of other similar conditions (e.g., arthritis). Wilson's test can be performed to detect osteochondritis dissecans of the knee.

Osteomyelitis   BRONZE

DIAGNOSIS

What condition produces a patient's symptoms?

Osteomyelitis refers to an infection that occurs within the bone, most commonly secondary to the Staphylococcus aureus microbe. Exposure to an infectious microbe may occur through direct contamination or secondary to an infection elsewhere in the body such as the bloodstream, a wound or nearby soft tissue.

An injury was most likely sustained to which structure?

Damage to the bone (e.g., result of a surgical procedure, compound fracture or puncture wound that penetrates bone) may directly expose the bone to infectious microbes in the air or contaminating debris. In cases of secondary infection, the location of the primary injury is variable. In either circumstance, prolonged or severe cases of osteomyelitis may result in structural damage to the infected bone which could lead to amputation.

CONFIRMATION

What is the most likely clinical presentation?

Signs and symptoms of osteomyelitis are similar to those of other types of infection. Fever and chills are common systemic complaints. Localized complaints typically include pain, edema, and erythema. A conclusive diagnosis may frequently be delayed since symptoms tend to be generalized or vague. Patients who have a weakened immune system, diabetes, sickle cell disease, who are elderly or are undergoing hemodialysis are at greater risk for developing osteomyelitis. Patients who develop osteomyelitis secondary to a wound infection may show significant changes in observable wound characteristics (e.g., color, amount of exudate, type of exudate, delayed healing) as well as slow or stagnant wound healing.

What laboratory or imaging studies would confirm the diagnosis?

A bone biopsy is the most conclusive procedure for diagnosing osteomyelitis and determining the specific infectious microbe present. Blood tests, x-rays, MRI, ultrasound, CT scans, bone scans, and PET scans may provide additional information (e.g., increased white blood cell count, specific infectious microbe, bone damage), but are not considered diagnostically conclusive.

What additional information should be obtained to confirm the diagnosis?

Medical and surgical history, as well as the patient's current health status should be thoroughly reviewed. If osteomyelitis is suspected, systemic or localized signs and symptoms of infection and potential sources of exposure should be further evaluated.

BRONZE | Piriformis Syndrome

DIAGNOSIS

What condition produces a patient's symptoms?

Piriformis syndrome is the result of compression or irritation to the proximal sciatic nerve due to piriformis muscle inflammation, spasm or contracture. It is a common etiology of generalized low back pain and is sometimes referred to as "pseudosciatica" because of the similarity of symptoms.

An injury was most likely sustained to which structure?

The piriformis muscle is a flat oblique muscle that functions to abduct and externally rotate the hip. After exiting the greater sciatic foramen, the sciatic nerve passes inferior to the piriformis before continuing distally along the midline of the posterior thigh. The specific etiology of piriformis syndrome is unknown, however, trauma, mechanical dysfunction, scarring or entrapment due to soft tissue pathology are among the leading theories.

CONFIRMATION

What is the most likely clinical presentation?

The location of pain is often imprecise, though typically presents first in the area of the mid-buttock then progresses to radicular complaints in the sciatic nerve distribution. Hip, coccyx, or groin pain may also be reported. Symptoms are typically exacerbated by prolonged sitting and activities that combine medial rotation and adduction. Pain is typically reproducible on palpation and with positioning into flexion, adduction, and medial rotation. Pain and weakness are likely with resistance testing during lateral rotation with abduction. Radicular symptoms are typically exacerbated with a straight leg raise and alleviated with lower extremity traction. Often piriformis syndrome is misdiagnosed as it has a near identical symptom presentation as L5-S1 radiculopathy, which is due to either a herniated disk or stenosis.

What laboratory or imaging studies would confirm the diagnosis?

Piriformis syndrome is considered a clinical diagnosis of exclusion, therefore no specific laboratory or imaging studies are used for confirmation. X-ray, MRI, and CT scan may be used to rule out other conditions which may mimic symptoms such as disk herniation or spinal stenosis.

What additional information should be obtained to confirm the diagnosis?

A thorough medical history and examination should be obtained to assist in identifying potential etiologies and ruling out similar diagnoses such as trochanteric bursitis or myofascial pain.

BRONZE | Posterior Cruciate Ligament Sprain

DIAGNOSIS

What condition produces a patient's symptoms?

The posterior cruciate ligament (PCL) is an intracapsular ligament that attaches at the posterior tibial plateau and the lateral side of the medial femoral condyle. The PCL prevents posterior translation of the tibia on the femur and provides rotational stability to the knee. PCL injuries generally occur secondary to a traumatic event. They often occur when a posteriorly directed force is applied to the tibia in relation to the femur, such as when the knee hits the dashboard in a motor vehicle accident. Hyperflexion of the knee without a traumatic blow can also lead to a PCL sprain.

An injury was most likely sustained to which structure?

Injuries to the PCL are graded according to the normal 3-point grading scale for sprains, with a grade of 3 indicating complete rupture. Most PCL tears occur where the ligament attaches to the tibia. Isolated PCL injuries are far less common than anterior cruciate ligament (ACL) injuries, in part because the PCL is a stronger ligament. Injuries to the PCL often occur with concurrent damage to the ACL, the collateral ligaments, and/or the menisci.

CONFIRMATION

What is the most likely clinical presentation?

When a PCL injury results from acute trauma, the patient may hear an audible "pop" with an immediate onset of pain and swelling. Symptoms will vary depending on the grade of the sprain, however, this injury is generally not as debilitating as an ACL tear. Patients with a PCL sprain may complain of feelings of instability with walking and pain with descending stairs or squatting.

What laboratory or imaging studies would confirm the diagnosis?

While an x-ray will not confirm the presence of a PCL sprain, it can help rule out other pathology (e.g., fracture). An x-ray may also be used to determine if the ligament damage resulted in an associated avulsion injury. Magnetic resonance imaging is used to confirm the presence and determine the extent and location of a PCL sprain.

What additional information should be obtained to confirm the diagnosis?

A thorough medical history and physical examination should be performed. The physical examination will consist of special tests that are used to determine the presence of a PCL sprain, such as the posterior drawer test, the posterior sag sign, and the quadriceps active drawer test. An arthrometer may also be used to identify laxity in the knee and determine the extent of the damage. The examination should consist of an assessment of the other ligaments and the menisci as well since a PCL injury often occurs in conjunction with other pathology.

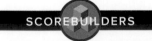

Tarsal Tunnel Syndrome   BRONZE

DIAGNOSIS

What condition produces a patient's symptoms?

The tarsal tunnel is located on the medial aspect of the ankle and is formed by the flexor retinaculum, the superior aspect of the calcaneus, the medial wall of the talus, and the medial-distal aspect of the tibia. The tibial nerve, posterior tibial artery, and tendons of the flexor hallucis longus, tibialis posterior, and flexor digitorum longus muscles pass through the tarsal tunnel. Tarsal tunnel syndrome occurs as a result of compression of the tibial nerve as it passes through the tarsal tunnel, causing neuropathy in the distribution of the nerve.

An injury was most likely sustained to which structure?

The tibial nerve is injured by compression within the tarsal tunnel causing motor and sensory disturbances. Etiologies are typically classified as either intrinsic (e.g., tumor, scar tissue), extrinsic (e.g., crush injury, severe ankle sprain) or tension factors (e.g., pes planus deformity, hindfoot valgus deformity).

CONFIRMATION

What is the most likely clinical presentation?

Symptoms include pain, numbness, and paresthesias in the foot that may be initially mistaken for plantar fasciitis. An antalgic gait pattern is common when symptoms are exacerbated. Rest typically alleviates, but does not completely resolve symptoms. Muscle atrophy may be visually observed and confirmed using manual muscle testing. Neurological signs may include a positive Tinel's sign with tibial nerve assessment posterior to the medial malleolus. Light touch and temperature sensation may be diminished in the sensory distribution of the tibial nerve and its branches. In severe or long-standing cases, trophic skin changes may also be observed.

What laboratory or imaging studies would confirm the diagnosis?

The presence of neuropathy is typically confirmed through an electromyography (EMG) or nerve conduction velocity (NCV) study. To confirm tarsal tunnel syndrome, however, the etiology of neuropathy must also be confirmed. An MRI or ultrasound may be utilized to assist in identifying compression due to a soft tissue lesion. X-ray may be utilized if bony structures are suspected to contribute to symptoms.

What additional information should be obtained to confirm the diagnosis?

A thorough medical history and physical examination should be completed to assist in ruling out alternative sources of peripheral neuropathy. A family history of neuropathy or deformities, such as hammer toes or cavus foot, may also assist in confirming the diagnosis.

Trochanteric Bursitis   BRONZE

DIAGNOSIS

What condition produces a patient's symptoms?

Trochanteric bursitis may occur from acute or cumulative trauma to the lateral hip causing irritation to the trochanteric bursa. Though symptoms typically include lateral hip pain, the pathology does not involve the actual hip joint.

An injury was most likely sustained to which structure?

The trochanteric bursa is located between the femoral trochanteric process, the gluteus medius, and the iliotibial tract. Acute trauma etiologies typically involve contusion related to direct impact occurring with activities such as falls or impact sports. Cumulative trauma etiologies are typically associated with activities such as running that produce repetitive friction between the bursa and the iliotibial band.

CONFIRMATION

What is the most likely clinical presentation?

The classic symptom of trochanteric bursitis is pain at the lateral hip which may radiate to the lateral aspect of the thigh. Point tenderness and reproduction of pain are typical with palpation. Symptoms are typically exacerbated by weight bearing activity or direct pressure on the affected area. Passive hip movement involving lateral rotation and abduction or resisted hip flexion and abduction are likely to reproduce symptoms. Patients may also complain of pain-related weakness in the affected extremity.

What laboratory or imaging studies would confirm the diagnosis?

An MRI or diagnostic ultrasound may assist in differentiating trochanteric bursitis from gluteus medius tendinitis. X-ray imaging may be utilized to rule out bony pathology or to further assess leg length discrepancies.

What additional information should be obtained to confirm the diagnosis?

A thorough medical history and physical examination should be completed to assist in ruling out similar diagnoses (e.g., sciatic pain, iliotibial band syndrome, femoral head avascular necrosis). The diagnosis is often made based on the patient's symptom history and physical examination findings.

DIAGNOSIS

What condition produces a patient's symptoms?

An ulnar collateral ligament (UCL) sprain of the thumb is the most common ligament injury in the hand. This injury occurs secondary to a traumatic event in which an excessive valgus force is applied to the metacarpophalangeal (MCP) joint of the thumb. The names "gamekeeper's thumb" and "skier's thumb" are commonly used for this injury and are derived from common mechanisms of the injury.

An injury was most likely sustained to what structure?

The UCL of the thumb is positioned on the medial side of the thumb's MCP joint and acts as an important stabilizer of the thumb. The grade of the sprain indicates the extent of injury to the ligament. With grade 1 and 2 sprains, the majority of the ligament remains intact, while a grade 3 sprain involves a complete tear of the ligament.

CONFIRMATION

What is the most likely clinical presentation?

Signs and symptoms of an UCL sprain include pain, tenderness, ecchymosis, and swelling near the thumb's MCP joint, specifically on the medial side. Other symptoms may include instability of the joint and weakness with grasping objects.

What laboratory or imaging studies would confirm the diagnosis?

X-rays should be ordered to rule out the existence of a fracture or dislocation. Ultrasound or magnetic resonance imaging may be used to determine if a ligament tear is present.

What additional information should be obtained to confirm the diagnosis?

A thorough medical history and physical examination will assist in the diagnosis. The therapist should assess the integrity of the UCL by performing ligament stability testing of the thumb. When applying a valgus force to the MCP joint, a movement of greater than 30-35 degrees indicates a complete tear of the UCL.

Musculoskeletal System Essentials

1. The body's three sources of adenosine triphosphate (ATP) include the ATP-PC (Phosphagen) System, Anaerobic Glycolysis (Lactic Acid) System, and Aerobic (Oxygen) System.

2. The ATP-PC (Phosphagen) System is used for ATP production during high intensity, short duration exercise, such as sprinting 100 meters. The system provides energy for muscle contraction for up to 15 seconds.

3. The anaerobic glycolysis system supplies ATP during high intensity, short duration exercise, such as sprinting 400 or 800 meters. The system provides energy for muscle contraction for 30-40 seconds.

4. The aerobic system supplies ATP during low intensity, long duration activities, such as running a marathon. The amount of ATP production is far greater, but requires a complicated series of chemical reactions.

5. Motion occurs in three cardinal planes of the body (frontal, sagittal, transverse) around three corresponding axes (anterior-posterior, medial-lateral, vertical).

6. Common joint receptors include free nerve endings, Golgi ligament endings, Golgi-Mazzoni corpuscles, Pacinian corpuscles, and Ruffini endings.

7. Golgi tendon organs are encapsulated sensory receptors that are sensitive to tension, especially when produced by active muscle contraction. They function to transmit information about tension or the rate of change of tension within the muscle.

8. Type I muscle fibers are described as aerobic, red, tonic, slow twitch, and slow-oxidative. Type II muscle fibers are described as anaerobic, white, phasic, fast twitch, and fast-glycolytic.

9. Muscle spindles are distributed throughout the belly of the muscle and function to send information to the nervous system about muscle length and/or the rate of change of its length.

10. The upper extremity consists of the shoulder, elbow, and wrist. The shoulder complex is formed by the glenohumeral joint, sternoclavicular joint, acromioclavicular joint, and scapulothoracic articulations. The elbow joint is formed by the radiohumeral joint, ulnohumeral joint, and proximal radioulnar joint. The wrist complex is formed by the radiocarpal and midcarpal joints.

11. The lower extremity consists of the hip, knee, ankle, and foot. The hip joint is a synovial joint formed by the head of the femur and the acetabulum. The knee joint is formed by the tibiofemoral joint and patellofemoral joint. The ankle and foot are formed by the distal tibiofibular joint, talocrural joint, subtalar joint, midtarsal joint, and forefoot.

12. The cervical spine consists of 7 vertebrae. The thoracic spine consists of 12 vertebrae, and the lumbar spine consists of 5 vertebrae.

13. An upper and lower quarter screen should, at a minimum, consist of an assessment of posture, range of motion, resistive testing, reflex testing, and dermatome testing.

14. The loose packed position of a joint is characterized by minimal stress on the joint, minimal joint congruency, and maximum ligament laxity. The close packed position of a joint is characterized by maximal stress on the joint, full joint congruency, and maximum ligament tightness.

15. End-feel refers to the type of resistance felt when passively moving a joint through the end range of motion. An end-feel classified as firm, hard or soft can be normal or abnormal depending on the joint, while an end-feel classified as empty is always abnormal.

16. Manual muscle testing grades range from zero (0/5) to normal (5/5) based on the ability to move a body segment through range with and without varying levels of resistance.

17. Active muscle insufficiency occurs when a two-joint muscle contracts across both joints simultaneously. Passive insufficiency occurs when a two-joint muscle is lengthened over both joints simultaneously.

18. Standard gait terminology includes heel strike, foot flat, midstance, heel off, toe off, acceleration, midswing, and deceleration.

Musculoskeletal System Essentials

19. Rancho Los Amigos gait terminology includes initial contact, loading response, midstance, terminal stance, pre-swing, initial swing, midswing, and terminal swing.

20. The stance phase represents approximately 60% of the gait cycle and the swing phase represents 40% of the gait cycle.

21. Step length refers to the distance measured between right heel strike and left heel strike. Stride length refers to the distance measured between right heel strike and the following right heel strike.

22. Biceps tendon pathology can be identified through Ludington's test, Speed's test, and Yergason's test.

23. Rotator cuff pathology/impairment can be identified through the drop arm test, Hawkins-Kennedy impingement test, Neer impingement test, and supraspinatus test.

24. Contractures, or tightness of the hip, can be identified through Ely's test, Ober's test, piriformis test, Thomas test, tripod sign, and 90-90 straight leg raise test.

25. An anterior cruciate ligament sprain can be identified through the anterior drawer test, Lachman test, and lateral pivot shift test.

26. Meniscal pathology of the knee can be identified through Apley's compression test, bounce home test, and McMurray test.

27. Grades I and IV mobilizations are considered small amplitude movement, while grades II and III are considered large amplitude movements.

28. Grade V manipulation is defined as small amplitude, high velocity thrust technique performed to snap adhesions at the limit of range of motion.

29. The convex/concave rule specifies that when a convex surface is moving on a concave surface, roll and slide occur in the opposite direction. When a concave surface is moving on a convex surface, roll and slide occur in the same direction.

30. Range of motion exercises are designed to improve the mobility of a single joint and may include passive, active-assisted, and active range of motion.

31. Range of motion exercises typically begin with passive range of motion, since it does not require any muscle contraction from the patient, and progress towards active range of motion.

32. Stretching exercises are used to improve muscle flexibility by increasing the extensibility of the musculotendinous unit and connective tissues.

33. Static stretching, characterized by a low intensity and long duration, is the safest form of stretching that results in the greatest gains in tissue extensibility.

34. Proprioceptive neuromuscular facilitation stretching is another stretching technique designed to improve muscle flexibility, while ballistic stretching and dynamic stretching are more often employed as a warm-up prior to initiating activity.

35. A muscle is made up of several muscle fibers and the connective tissue layers that surround and lie within the muscle.

36. Resistive training programs often employ isometric, isotonic, and isokinetic exercise.

37. Open-chain activities involve the distal segment moving freely in space, while closed-chain activities involve the body moving over a fixed distal segment.

38. Strength training parameters, such as intensity, volume, and frequency, will vary according to the desired goal of the strengthening program (e.g., strength, endurance, power).

39. Hip precautions following total hip arthroplasty using a posterolateral surgical approach include avoiding hip flexion beyond 90 degrees, adduction, and hip medial rotation.

40. Common types of fractures include avulsion, closed, comminuted, compound, greenstick, nonunion, stress, and spiral.

Musculoskeletal System Essentials

41. Common pharmacological agents used in the treatment of musculoskeletal disorders include opioid agents, nonopioid agents, glucocorticoid agents, and disease-modifying antirheumatic agents.

42. Kyphosis refers to an excessive curvature of the spine in a posterior direction usually identified in the thoracic spine. Lordosis refers to an excessive curvature of the spine in an anterior direction usually in the cervical or lumbar spine.

43. An orthotic is an external device that provides support or stabilization, improves function, corrects deformities, and distributes pressure from one area to another.

44. Lower extremity amputations are significantly more common than upper extremity amputations with peripheral vascular disease serving as the primary etiology.

45. Components of an upper extremity prosthesis include the socket, suspension, elbow unit, wrist unit, and terminal device.

46. Components of a lower extremity prosthesis include socket, suspension, knee, shank, and foot.

47. Potential complications following amputation include contractures, deep vein thrombosis, hypersensitivity, neuroma, phantom limb, phantom pain, psychological impact, and wound infections.

48. Common gait deviations with a prosthesis include lateral bending, vaulting, forward trunk flexion, medial or lateral whip, abducted gait, circumducted gait, excessive knee flexion during stance, and rotation of the forefoot at heel strike.

Musculoskeletal System Proficiencies

1. Musculoskeletal Upper Extremity Anatomy

Identify the appropriate term for each of the specified locations. Answers must be selected from the Word Bank and can be used only once.

Word Bank: brachioradialis, flexor carpi radialis, flexor carpi ulnaris, flexor digitorum superficialis, palmaris longus, pronator quadratus, pronator teres

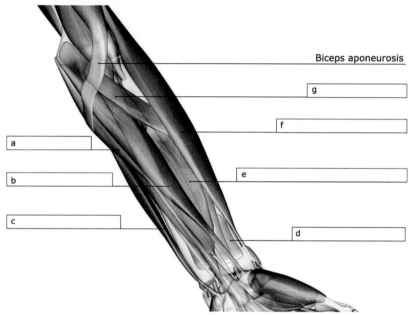

Biceps aponeurosis

g

f

a

b

e

c

d

2. Musculoskeletal Lower Extremity Anatomy I

Identify the appropriate term for each of the specified locations. Answers must be selected from the Word Bank and can be used only once.

Word Bank: gracilis, rectus femoris, sartorius, tensor fasciae latae, vastus lateralis, vastus medialis

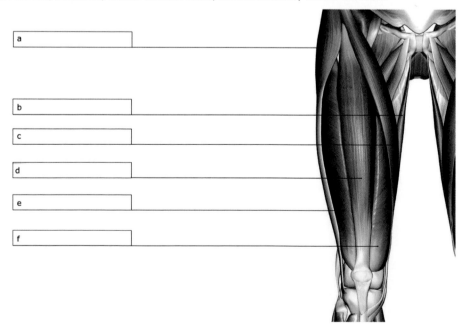

a

b

c

d

e

f

Musculoskeletal System Proficiencies

3. Musculoskeletal Lower Extremity Anatomy II

Identify the appropriate term for each of the specified locations. Answers must be selected from the Word Bank and can be used only once.

Word Bank: abductor digiti minimi, abductor hallucis, flexor digitorum brevis, flexor hallucis brevis, lumbricals, quadratus plantae

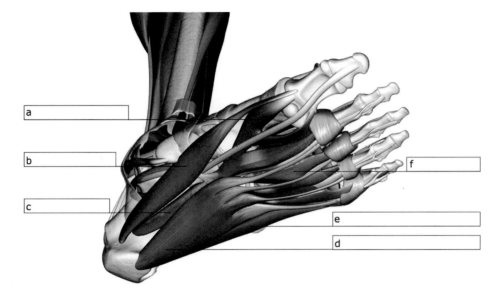

4. Muscle Function - Upper Extremity

Identify the muscle that contributes to performing each of the listed motions. Each muscle in the Word Bank must be used only once. Since a given muscle may contribute to multiple motions, it is essential for answers to be selected in a manner that allows for all muscles to be utilized.

Word Bank: anconeus, brachioradialis, coracobrachialis, extensor carpi ulnaris, flexor carpi radialis, latissimus dorsi, palmaris longus, teres major, teres minor

Shoulder	Muscle	
flexion	a	
extension	b	
lateral rotation	c	
medial rotation	d	
Elbow	**Muscle**	
flexion	e	
extension	f	
Wrist	**Muscle**	
flexion	g	
extension	h	
radial deviation	i	

Musculoskeletal System Proficiencies

5. Muscle Function - Lower Extremity

Identify the muscle that contributes to performing each of the listed motions. Each muscle in the Word Bank must be used only once. Since a given muscle may contribute to multiple motions, it is essential for answers to be selected in a manner that allows for all muscles to be utilized.

Word Bank: biceps femoris, extensor hallucis longus, gluteus medius, gracilis, iliopsoas, peroneus longus, piriformis, tibialis posterior, vastus medialis

Hip	Muscle
flexion	a
adduction	b
lateral rotation	c
medial rotation	d
Knee	**Muscle**
flexion	e
extension	f
Ankle	**Muscle**
dorsiflexion	g
inversion	h
eversion	i

6. Manual Muscle Testing

Identify the manual muscle testing grade most closely associated with the supplied description. Answers must be selected from the Word Bank and can be used only once.

Word Bank: zero, trace, poor minus, poor, poor plus, fair minus, fair, fair plus, good minus, good, good plus, normal

Grade	Description
a	The subject does not complete range of motion in a gravity-eliminated position.
b	The subject's muscle contraction can be palpated, but there is no joint movement.
c	The subject does not complete the range of motion against gravity, but does complete more than half of the range.
d	The subject completes range of motion against gravity with maximal resistance.
e	The subject completes range of motion against gravity with minimal-moderate resistance.
f	The subject completes range of motion with gravity-eliminated.
g	The subject completes range of motion against gravity with only minimal resistance.
h	The subject completes range of motion against gravity with moderate resistance.

Musculoskeletal System Proficiencies

7. Gait - Standard Terminology

Identify the sequence and phase of the gait cycle starting with heel strike and ending with deceleration. Answers must be selected from the Word Bank and can be used only once.

Word Bank: Sequence - 2nd, 3rd, 4th, 5th, 6th, 7th

Phase - acceleration, foot flat, heel off, midstance, midswing, toe off

Sequence	Phase	Description
1st	heel strike	The instant the heel touches the ground to begin stance phase.
a	b	The point in which only the toe of the stance limb remains on the ground.
c	d	The point when the swing limb is directly under the body.
e	f	The point in which the entire foot makes contact with the ground.
g	h	Begins when toe off is complete and the reference limb swings until positioned directly under the body.
i	j	The point in which the heel of the stance limb leaves the ground.
k	l	The point during the stance phase when the entire body weight is directly over the stance limb.
8th	deceleration	Begins directly after midswing as the swing limb begins to extend and ends just prior to heel strike.

8. Abnormal Gait

Identify the abnormal gait pattern most closely associated with the supplied description. Answers must be selected from the Word Bank and can be used only once.

Word Bank: antalgic, circumduction, Parkinsonian, scissor, steppage, tabetic, Trendelenburg, vaulting

Gait Pattern	Description
a	A gait pattern in which the feet and toes are lifted through hip and knee flexion to excessive heights.
b	A gait pattern characterized by the legs crossing midline upon advancement.
c	A gait pattern characterized by a circular motion to advance the leg during swing phase.
d	A protective gait pattern where the involved step length is decreased in order to avoid weight bearing on the involved side.
e	A gait pattern where the swing leg advances through a combination of elevation of the pelvis and plantar flexion of the stance leg.
f	A gait pattern characterized by excessive lateral trunk flexion and weight shifting over the stance leg due to gluteus medius weakness.
g	A gait pattern marked by quick and small steps with increased forward flexion of the trunk and knees.
h	A high stepping ataxic gait pattern in which the feet slap the ground.

Musculoskeletal System Proficiencies

9. Goniometry

Complete the blank cells with the appropriate information based on the supplied information. The number of desired responses for each cell is identified in parentheses.

Joint	Motion	Axis
shoulder	flexion	a (1)
shoulder	b (2)	olecranon process
c (1)	pronation	lateral to the ulnar styloid process
wrist	radial deviation	d (1)
hip	e (2)	anterior aspect of the patella
ankle	f (2)	lateral aspect of the lateral malleolus
g (1)	h (2)	posterior aspect of the ankle midway between the malleoli

10. Osteokinematic and Arthrokinematic Motions

Identify the concave and convex joint surface associated with the listed joints. Answers must be selected from the Word Bank and can be used more than once.

Word Bank: acetabulum, carpals, femur, fibula, glenoid, humerus, radius, talus, tibia

Joint	Concave	Convex
glenohumeral	a (1)	b (1)
radiohumeral	c (1)	d (1)
radiocarpal	e (1)	f (1)
hip	g (1)	h (1)
tibiofemoral	i (1)	j (1)
talocrural	k (2)	l (1)

Musculoskeletal System Proficiencies

11. Musculoskeletal System Basics

Mark each statement as True or False. If the statement is False correct the statement in the space provided.

True/False	Statement
a	An end-feel classified as empty can be classified as normal or abnormal depending on the joint.
Correction	
b	The loose packed position of the hip is 30 degrees flexion, 30 degrees abduction, and slight medial rotation.
Correction	
c	Stride length refers to the distance measured between right heel strike and left heel strike.
Correction	
d	The capsular pattern of the glenohumeral joint is lateral rotation, abduction, and medial rotation.
Correction	
e	According to Rancho Los Amigos gait terminology, pre-swing, midswing, and terminal swing are components of swing phase.
Correction	
f	Peak activity of the tibialis anterior occurs during the gait cycle just after heel strike.
Correction	
g	Normal elbow flexion is 0-135 degrees.
Correction	
h	The tensor fasciae latae, gluteus medius, and piriformis function as medial rotators of the hip.
Correction	
i	Muscle testing of the lower trapezius, rhomboids, and latissimus dorsi occurs with the patient positioned in prone.
Correction	
j	Sixty percent of the gait cycle occurs in the stance phase.
Correction	

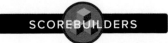

Musculoskeletal System Answer Key

1. Musculoskeletal Upper Extremity Anatomy

a. palmaris longus
b. flexor carpi radialis
c. flexor carpi ulnaris
d. pronator quadratus
e. flexor digitorum superficialis
f. brachioradialis
g. pronator teres

2. Musculoskeletal Lower Extremity Anatomy I

a. tensor fasciae latae
b. gracilis
c. sartorius
d. rectus femoris
e. vastus lateralis
f. vastus medialis

3. Musculoskeletal Lower Extremity Anatomy II

a. flexor hallucis brevis
b. abductor hallucis
c. quadratus plantae
d. flexor digitorum brevis
e. abductor digiti minimi
f. lumbricals

4. Muscle Function - Upper Extremity

a. coracobrachialis
b. latissimus dorsi or teres major
c. teres minor
d. teres major or latissimus dorsi
e. brachioradialis
f. anconeus
g. palmaris longus
h. extensor carpi ulnaris
i. flexor carpi radialis

5. Muscle Function - Lower Extremity

a. iliopsoas
b. gracilis
c. piriformis
d. gluteus medius
e. biceps femoris
f. vastus medialis
g. extensor hallucis longus
h. tibialis posterior
i. peroneus longus

6. Manual Muscle Testing

a. poor minus
b. trace
c. fair minus
d. normal
e. good minus
f. poor
g. fair plus
h. good

7. Gait - Standard Terminology

a. 5th
b. toe off
c. 7th
d. midswing
e. 2nd
f. foot flat
g. 6th
h. acceleration
i. 4th
j. heel off
k. 3rd
l. midstance

8. Abnormal Gait

a. steppage
b. scissor
c. circumduction
d. antalgic
e. vaulting
f. Trendelenburg
g. Parkinsonian
h. tabetic

9. Goniometry

a. acromial process
b. lateral rotation and medial rotation
c. forearm
d. over the middle of the dorsal aspect of the wrist over the capitate
e. lateral rotation and medial rotation
f. dorsiflexion and plantar flexion
g. subtalar
h. inversion and eversion

Musculoskeletal System Answer Key

10. Osteokinematic and Arthrokinematic Motions

a.   glenoid

b.   humerus

c.   radius

d.   humerus

e.   radius

f.   carpals

g.   acetabulum

h.   femur

i.   tibia

j.   femur

k.   tibia and fibula

l.   talus

11. Musculoskeletal System Basics*

a.   FALSE: Correction - An end-feel classified as empty is always considered abnormal due to the presence of pain.

b.   FALSE: Correction - The loose packed position of the hip is 30 degrees flexion, 30 degrees abduction, and slight lateral rotation.

c.   FALSE: Correction - Step length refers to the distance measured between right heel strike and left heel strike.

d.   TRUE

e.   FALSE: Correction - Pre-swing is a component of stance phase. Initial swing, midswing, and terminal swing are components of swing phase.

f.   TRUE

g.   FALSE: Correction - Normal elbow flexion is 0-150 degrees.

h.   FALSE: Correction - The tensor fasciae latae and gluteus medius function as medial rotators of the hip. The piriformis functions as a lateral rotator of the hip.

i.   TRUE

j.   TRUE

*The correction presented for each false statement is an example of several possible corrections.

Musculoskeletal System References

1. Guyton A. *Textbook of Medical Physiology.* W.B. Saunders Company. 1986.

2. Kendall F, McCreary E. Provance P. *Muscles: Testing and Function with Posture and Pain*. Fifth Edition. Lippincott Williams & Wilkins. 2005.

3. Norkin C, White D. *Measurement of Joint Motion: A Guide to Goniometry*. Fifth Edition. F.A. Davis Company. 2016.

4. Levangie P, Norkin C. *Joint Structure and Function: A Comprehensive Analysis*. Fifth Edition. F.A. Davis Company. 2011.

5. Tortora G, Derrickson B. *Principles of Anatomy and Physiology*. Twelfth Edition. John Wiley & Sons Inc. 2009.

6. Moore K, Dalley A. *Clinically Oriented Anatomy*. Seventh Edition. Lippincott Williams & Wilkins. 2013.

7. Patton K, Thibodeau G. *Anatomy and Physiology*. Seventh Edition. Elsevier Inc. 2010.

8. Anderson MK, Hall SJ, Martin M. *Fundamentals of Sports Injury Management*. Fourth Edition. Lippincott Williams & Wilkins. 2009.

9. Bickley L. *Bates' Guide to Physical Examination and History Taking*. Twelfth Edition. Wolters Kluwer. 2017.

10. Magee D. *Orthopedic Physical Assessment*. Sixth Edition. W.B. Saunders Company. 2014.

11. Starkey C, Ryan J. *Evaluation of Orthopedic and Athletic Injuries*. F.A. Davis Company. 2002.

12. Hoppenfeld S, Thomas H, Hutton R. *Physical Examination of the Spine and Extremities*. Prentice Hall. 1976.

13. Hertling D, Kessler R. *Management of Common Musculoskeletal Disorders*. Fourth Edition. Lippincott Williams & Wilkins. 2006.

14. Edmond S. *Joint Mobilization/Manipulation: Extremity and Spinal Techniques*. Third Edition. Mosby Inc. 2016.

15. Brody L, Hall C. *Therapeutic Exercise: Moving Toward Function*. Fourth Edition. Lippincott Williams & Wilkins. 2018.

16. Kisner C, Colby L, Borstad J. *Therapeutic Exercise Foundations and Techniques*. Seventh Edition. F.A. Davis Company. 2018.

17. Prentice W, Voight M. *Techniques in Musculoskeletal Rehabilitation*. McGraw-Hill Inc. 2008.

18. Dutton M. *Orthopaedic Examination, Evaluation, and Intervention*. Fourth Edition. McGraw-Hill Inc. 2017.

19. American College of Sports Medicine. *ACSM's Resource Manual for Guidelines for Exercise Testing and Prescription*. Seventh Edition. Lippincott Williams & Wilkins. 2014.

20. Reese N, Bandy WD. *Joint Range of Motion and Muscle Length Testing*. Second Edition. W.B. Saunders Company. 2009.

21. Hislop HJ, Avers D. *Daniels and Worthingham's Muscle Testing: Techniques of Manual Examination and Performance Testing*. Ninth Edition, W.B. Saunders Company. 2014.

22. Roy S, Wolf S, Scalzitti D. *The Rehabilitation Specialist's Handbook*. Fourth Edition. F.A. Davis Company. 2013.

23. Perry J, Burnfield J. *Gait Analysis: Normal and Pathological Function*. Second Edition. Slack Incorporated. 2010.

24. Hamill J, Knutzen K. *Biomechanical Basis of Human Movement*. Third Edition. Lippincott Williams & Wilkins. 2008.

25. Oatis C. *Kinesiology: The Mechanics and Pathomechanics of Human Movement*. Second Edition. Lippincott Williams & Wilkins. 2009.

26. Reider B. *The Orthopaedic Physical Examination*. W.B. Saunders Company. 1999.

27. Tecklin J. *Pediatric Physical Therapy*. Fifth Edition. Lippincott Williams & Wilkins. 2015.

28. Birrer R, O'Connor F. *Sports Medicine for the Primary Care Physician*. Third Edition. CRC Press. 2004.

29. Sueki D, Brechter J. *Orthopedic Rehabilitation Clinical Advisor*. Mosby Inc. 2010.

30. Palisano R, Orlin M, Shreiber J. *Campbell's Physical Therapy for Children*. Fifth Edition. Elsevier. 2017.

31. Goodman C, Fuller K. *Pathology: Implications for the Physical Therapist*. Fourth Edition. W.B. Saunders Company. 2015.

32. Brotzman SB, Wilk KE. *Clinical Orthopedic Rehabilitation*. Mosby Inc. 2003.

Musculoskeletal System References

33. Maxey L, Magnusson J. *Rehabilitation for the Postsurgical Orthopedic Patient*. Mosby Inc. 2001.

34. *Nurse's 3-Minute Clinical Reference*. Second Edition. Lippincott Williams & Wilkins. 2007.

35. Goodman C, Heick J, Lazaro R. *Differential Diagnosis for Physical Therapists – Screening for Referral*. Sixth Edition. Elsevier. 2018.

36. Cameron M, Monroe L. *Physical Rehabilitation: Evidence-Based Examination, Evaluation, and Intervention*. W. B. Saunders Company. 2007.

37. Roach S. *Pharmacology for Health Professionals*. Lippincott Williams & Wilkins. 2005.

38. Gladson B. *Pharmacology for Physical Therapists*. W. B. Saunders Company. 2006.

39. Ciccone C. *Pharmacology for Rehabilitation*. Fifth Edition. F.A. Davis Company. 2016.

40. Seymour R. *Prosthetics and Orthotics: Lower Limb and Spinal*. Lippincott Williams & Wilkins. 2002.

41. Palmer L, Toms J. *Manual for Functional Training*. Third Edition. F.A. Davis Company. 1992.

42. Radomski MV, Latham CAT. *Occupational Therapy for Physical Dysfunction*. Sixth Edition. Lippincott, Williams & Wilkins. 2008.

43. Braddom RL. *Physical Medicine and Rehabilitation*. Third Edition. Saunders. Elsevier. 2007.

44. Tan J. *Practical Manual of Physical Medicine and Rehabilitation*. Second Edition. Elsevier. 2006.

45. DeRuyter O. *Clinician's Guide to Assistive Technology*. Mosby Inc. 2002.

46. May B, Lockard M. *Prosthetics and Orthotics in Clinical Practice: A Case Study Approach*. F.A. Davis Company, 2011.

47. Means K, Kortebein P. *Geriatrics*. Demos Medical. 2013.

48. Smith D, Michael J, Bowker J. *Atlas of Amputations and Limb Deficiencies: Surgical, Prosthetic, and Rehabilitation Principles*. American Academy of Orthopaedic Surgeons. 2004.

49. Lusardi M, Milagros J, Nielsen C. *Orthotics and Prosthetics in Rehabilitation*. Third Edition. Elsevier. 2013.

5

Neuromuscular and Nervous Systems

Therese Giles

Neuromuscular and Nervous Systems represents approximately 28 - 34 questions (18.7% - 22.7%) on the NPTE-PTA.

Contributors

Scott Giles
Shawn Paquette

CHAPTER 5
Neuromuscular and Nervous Systems

Neuroanatomy: Anatomical Divisions of the Nervous System[1,2,3]

Central Nervous System (CNS)

Brain

forebrain

midbrain

hindbrain

Brainstem

midbrain, pons, medulla oblongata

- Brainstem is noted separately to acknowledge its components since it incorporates the midbrain with specific sections of the hindbrain.

Spinal Cord

- cervical, thoracic, lumbar, sacral, and coccygeal levels

Characteristics

- main centers where integration and coordination of nervous system information occur
- covered in a system of meninges and suspended in cerebrospinal fluid for protection
- surrounded by skull and vertebral column for protection
- gray matter - consists of unmyelinated neurons and contains capillaries, glial cells, cell bodies, and dendrites
- white matter - consists of myelinated axons and contains nerve fibers without dendrites
- white matter of the spinal cord is divided into three funiculi: anterior, lateral, and dorsal columns
- brain is divided into left and right cerebral hemispheres
- each hemisphere of the brain contains a frontal lobe, temporal lobe, parietal lobe, and occipital lobe

Peripheral Nervous System (PNS)

Cranial Nerves and Ganglia

- 12 pairs of cranial nerves exit the skull through the foramina

Spinal Nerves and Ganglia/Plexuses

- 31 pairs of spinal nerves exit the vertebral column through the intervertebral foramina
  - 8 cervical, 12 thoracic, 5 lumbar, 5 sacral, 1 coccygeal

Characteristics

- encased in fibrous sheaths, however, relatively unprotected
- spinal nerves each have an anterior root carrying motor information away from the CNS (efferent fibers)
- spinal nerves each have a posterior root carrying information regarding sensation to the CNS (afferent fibers)
- ganglia are clusters or swellings of cells that give rise to the peripheral and central nerve fibers

Autonomic Nervous System (ANS)

Sympathetic Division

- prepares the body for emergency response; norepinephrine neurotransmitter; generally a stimulating response

Parasympathetic Division

- conserving and restoring energy; acetylcholine neurotransmitter; generally an inhibitory response

Characteristics

- anatomically contains portions of the CNS and PNS
- concerned with innervation for involuntary processes, glands, internal organs, and smooth muscle
- emphasis on homeostasis and a person's response to stress
- impulses often do not reach our consciousness
- impulses produce largely automatic responses

CONSIDER THIS
AUTONOMIC NERVOUS SYSTEM DISORDERS[5]

- The autonomic nervous system (ANS) influences all internal organs, blood vessels, pupils and muscles of the eye, as well as sweat, salivary, and digestive glands as it relates to homeostasis. The ANS controls blood pressure, heart and breathing rates, body temperature, digestion, metabolism, electrolyte balance, production of saliva, sweat and tears, urination, defecation, sexual response, and other bodily processes.
- Disorders of the ANS can affect any body part or process. Autonomic disorders may result from outside pathology that damages autonomic nerves, such as diabetes or alcoholism, or there may be primary damage to the system. Autonomic disorders may be reversible or progressive in nature.
- Examples of ANS disorders include constipation, erectile dysfunction, Horner's syndrome, vasovagal syncope, orthostatic hypotension, and postural tachycardia syndrome.
- ANS disorders are typically treated with pharmacological intervention. These disorders may or may not have an impact on the physical therapy plan of care. Therapists need to possess an understanding of the impact of a patient's disorder and modify treatment based on their findings.

Central Nervous System

Brain

Forebrain

The brain consists of the forebrain, midbrain, and hindbrain. Each area contains different components with specific responsibilities. (Fig. 5-1).

Cerebrum

The cerebrum, which encompasses the major portion of the brain, is divided into the right and left cerebral hemispheres (Fig. 5-2). The two hemispheres are joined at the bottom by white matter, termed corpus callosum, which relays information from one side of the brain to the other. The surface of the cerebrum contains billions of neurons and glia that form the cerebral cortex. The outer surface of the cerebrum is termed gray matter and the interior is termed white matter. Sulci and fissures demark the specific lobes of the brain. Each lobe is responsible for different functions.

Fissures

- interhemispheric fissure (medial longitudinal): separates the two cerebral hemispheres
- Sylvian fissure (lateral): anterior portion separates the temporal and frontal lobes; posterior portion separates the temporal and parietal lobes

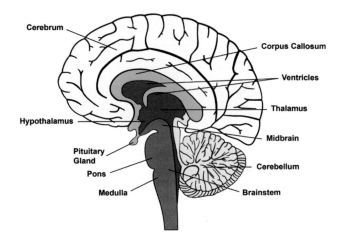

Fig. 5-1: A sagittal view of the human brain.

Sulci

- central sulcus (sulcus of Rolando): separates frontal and parietal lobes laterally
- parieto-occipital sulcus: separates the parietal and occipital lobes medially
- calcarine sulcus: separates the occipital lobe into superior and inferior halves

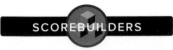

Hemisphere Specialization/Dominance[6,7]

Left

- Language
- Sequence and perform movements
- Understand language
- Produce written and spoken language
- Analytical
- Controlled
- Logical
- Rational
- Mathematical calculations
- Express positive emotions such as love and happiness
- Process verbally coded information in an organized, logical, and sequential manner

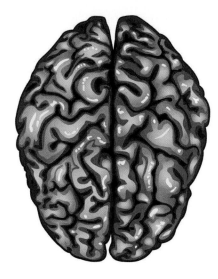

Right

- Nonverbal processing
- Process information in a holistic manner
- Artistic abilities
- General concept comprehension
- Hand-eye coordination
- Spatial relationships
- Kinesthetic awareness
- Understand music
- Understand nonverbal communication
- Mathematical reasoning
- Express negative emotions
- Body image awareness

Fig. 5-2: The two hemispheres of the brain and the corresponding characteristics of each.

Lobes of the Cerebrum[2,7,8]		
Lobe	**Function**	**Impairment**
Frontal	• voluntary movement (primary motor cortex/ precentral gyrus), intellect, orientation • Broca's area (typically located in the left hemisphere): speech, concentration • personality, temper, judgment, reasoning, behavior, self-awareness, executive functions	• contralateral weakness • perseveration, inattention • personality changes, antisocial behavior • impaired concentration, apathy • Broca's aphasia (expressive deficits) • delayed or poor initiation • emotional lability
Parietal	• associated with sensation of touch, kinesthesia, perception of vibration, and temperature • receives information from other areas of the brain regarding hearing, vision, motor, sensory, and memory • provides meaning for objects • interprets language and words • spatial and visual perception	• dominant hemisphere (typically located in the left hemisphere): agraphia, alexia, agnosia • non-dominant hemisphere (typically located in the right hemisphere): dressing apraxia, constructional apraxia, anosognosia • contralateral sensory deficits • impaired language comprehension • impaired taste
Temporal	• primary auditory processing and olfaction • Wernicke's area (typically located in the left hemisphere): ability to understand and produce meaningful speech, verbal and general memory, assists with understanding language • the rear of the temporal lobe enables humans to interpret other people's emotions and reactions	• learning deficits • Wernicke's aphasia (receptive deficits) • antisocial, aggressive behaviors • difficulty with facial recognition • difficulty with memory, memory loss • inability to categorize objects
Occipital	• main processing center for visual information • processes visual information regarding colors, light, and shapes • judgment of distance, seeing in three dimensions	• homonymous hemianopsia • impaired extraocular muscle movement and visual deficits • impaired color recognition • reading and writing impairment • cortical blindness with bilateral lobe involvement

CONSIDER THIS
TREATMENT CHALLENGES THAT RESULT FROM SPECIFIC LOBE DAMAGE[2,4]

When treating a patient with brain damage, there are predictable patterns of deficits based on the area of the brain that sustained injury. A therapist must recognize the particular concerns as it relates to the affected area(s) of the brain and integrate this into the plan of care.

- Frontal lobe lesions will produce deficits that range from paralysis and apraxia to loss of executive functions and goal-directed behaviors. Modifications to therapy may include response to perseveration, apraxia, and impaired executive functions. Patients with a frontal lobe lesion may present with apathy or may be uninhibited, distractible, and lack judgment.
- Parietal lobe lesions affect sensory awareness, interpretation, and perception. Somatosensory deficits elicit abnormal movement patterns for patients. Deficits in directional concepts hinder movement planning and require modification of therapy.
- Temporal lobe lesions will affect short and long-term memory. Damage to Wernicke's area (left hemisphere) impairs the comprehension of spoken language. Modification to therapy would include a more kinesthetic approach, relying on demonstration. New learning is available, but patients are usually unable to recall the steps that surround the new skill.
- Occipital lobe lesions produce various visual deficits that can hinder therapy. Cortical blindness occurs with damage to the occipital cortex and affects a patient's ability to receive, but not to perceive visual information. Therapy should avoid the use of diagrams, written materials, and reading. Environmental modification is required secondary to visual deficits, field cuts, and potential for visual agnosia.

Hippocampus

The hippocampus is deeply embedded within the lower temporal lobe. It is responsible for the process of forming and storing new memories of one's personal history and other declarative memory. It also possesses great importance in learning language. This "memory indexer" sends memories to appropriate areas of the cerebral hemispheres for long-term storage and retrieves memories when needed.

Basal ganglia

The basal ganglia are gray matter masses located deep within the white matter of the cerebrum and include the caudate, putamen, globus pallidus, substantia nigra, and subthalamic nuclei. The basal ganglia are collectively responsible for voluntary movement, regulation of autonomic movement, posture, muscle tone, and control of motor responses. Basal ganglia dysfunction has been associated with conditions including Parkinson's disease, Huntington's disease, Tourette's syndrome, attention-deficit disorder, obsessive-compulsive disorder, and many addictions.

Amygdala

The amygdala is a small, almond-shaped nucleus located within the temporal lobes of each hemisphere of the brain. It lies adjacent to the hippocampus and just beneath the surface of the front, medial portion of the temporal lobe. This positioning results in the bulge on the surface called the uncus. The main function of the amygdala is emotional and social processing. It is involved with fear and pleasure responses, arousal, processing of memory, and the formation of emotional memories.

Thalamus

The thalamus is a relay or processing station for the majority of information that goes to the cerebral cortex. It coordinates sensory perception and movement with other parts of the brain and spinal cord that also have a role in sensation and movement. It receives information from the cerebellum, basal ganglia, and all sensory pathways except for the olfactory tract. The thalamus then relays the information to the appropriate association cortex. Damage to the thalamus can produce thalamic pain syndrome where there is spontaneous pain on the contralateral side of the body to the thalamic lesion.

Hypothalamus

The hypothalamus receives and integrates information from the autonomic nervous system and assists in regulating hormones. The structure also controls functions such as hunger, thirst, sexual behavior, and sleeping. It regulates body temperature, the adrenal glands, the pituitary gland, and many other vital activities. Lesions can produce a variety of impairments based on the area of damage including obesity, sexual disinterest, poor temperature control, and diabetes insipidus.

Subthalamus

The subthalamus is located between the thalamus and the hypothalamus and is primarily represented by the subthalamic nucleus. It is important for regulating movements produced by skeletal muscles. It has association with the basal ganglia and substantia nigra.

Epithalamus

The epithalamus is primarily represented by the pineal gland. This gland secretes melatonin and is involved in circadian rhythms, the internal clock, selected regulation of motor pathways, and emotions.

Midbrain[9]

The midbrain is one of the three components of the brainstem and is located at the base of the brain above the spinal cord. The midbrain connects the forebrain to the hindbrain and functions as a large relay area for information passing from the cerebrum, cerebellum, and spinal cord. It is also a reflex center for visual, auditory, and tactile responses.

Hindbrain[2,3]

The hindbrain consists of the cerebellum, pons, and medulla oblongata. The pons and medulla oblongata are components of the brainstem and control the body's vital functions. The cerebellum coordinates movement and assists with maintaining balance.

Cerebellum

The cerebellum (metencephalon) is located at the posterior of the brain below the occipital lobes and is separated from the cerebrum by the tentorium. The cerebellum is responsible for fine tuning of movement and assists with maintaining posture and balance by controlling muscle tone and positioning of the extremities in space. The cerebellum controls the ability to perform rapid alternating movements. The cerebellum consists of two hemispheres of gray matter, and is divided into three lobes. Damage to one side of the cerebellum will produce ipsilateral impairment to the body. Cerebellar lesions may produce ataxia, nystagmus, tremor, hypermetria, poor coordination, and deficits in postural reflexes, balance, and equilibrium depending on the area of cerebellar lesion.

Pons

The pons (also metencephalon) is located below the midbrain and superior to the medulla oblongata. It assists with regulation of respiration rate and is associated with the orientation of the head in relation to visual and auditory stimuli. Cranial nerves V through VIII originate from the pons.

Medulla oblongata

The medulla oblongata (myelencephalon) is cone-shaped, connects to the pons superiorly, and to the spinal cord inferiorly. It's composed of white matter on the surface and gray matter within the interior. The medulla influences autonomic nervous activity and the regulation of respiration and heart rate. Reflex centers for vomiting, coughing, and sneezing are found within the medulla. Damage to motor tracts crossing within the medulla produces contralateral impairment.

Brainstem

The brainstem is a separate classification within the brain and is located in front of the cerebellum with connection to the spinal cord. It consists of three structures: the midbrain, pons, and medulla oblongata. These structures are found both within the midbrain and hindbrain. The brainstem works as a relay station, sending messages between various parts of the body and the cerebral cortex. Many of the primitive functions that are essential for survival, such as regulation of heart rate and respiratory rate, are located within the brainstem. The reticular activating system is found within the midbrain, pons, medulla, and a portion of the thalamus. Severe damage to the brainstem will often result in "brain death" secondary to the key functions that are controlled within this area. The majority of cranial nerves originate within the brainstem.

CONSIDER THIS
OCCLUSION TO A SPECIFIC ARTERY WILL PRODUCE PREDICTABLE PATTERNS OF IMPAIRMENT[2,10,11]

Blood supply is specific to particular areas within the brain. When a particular artery sustains damage via occlusion or hemorrhage, there is a specific pattern of disability that will occur. The extent of disability is determined by the extent of occlusion, the area of the brain involved, availability of collateral circulation to the affected area of the brain, and if the involved artery produces unilateral or bilateral damage. Bilateral arterial involvement will typically produce the most significant impairments.

Anterior cerebral artery
Bilateral occlusion of the anterior cerebral artery will typically produce paraplegia. Other findings include incontinence, abulic aphasia, frontal lobe symptoms such as personality changes, and potential akinetic mutism (i.e., conscious unresponsiveness).

Middle cerebral artery
Bilateral occlusion of the middle cerebral artery at the stem will produce contralateral hemiplegia and sensory impairment. Dominant hemisphere impairment includes global, Wernicke's or Broca's aphasia. Since the middle cerebral artery supplies the larger portion of the cortex, other impairments are lobe dependent.

Posterior cerebral artery
Two of the most significant impairments with posterior cerebral artery occlusion are thalamic pain syndrome and cortical blindness. Thalamic pain presents with abnormal sensation of pain, temperature, touch, and proprioception. The perceived sensation of pain can become debilitating. Cortical blindness is the loss of vision due to damage to the visual portion of the occipital cortex. Although the affected eye is physically normal, there is full or partial vision loss. The pupil continues to dilate and constrict in response to light since this occurs without influence of the brain.

Vertebral-basilar artery
There is a wide variety of clinical symptoms and syndromes based on the complex vascularity of the vertebral-basilar artery system. Severe impairment can cause locked-in syndrome, coma or vegetative state. Wallenberg syndrome secondary to lateral medullary infarct presents with a variety of symptoms including ipsilateral facial pain and temperature impairment, ipsilateral ataxia, vertigo, contralateral pain and temperature impairment of the body.

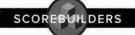

Supporting Systems of the Brain and Spinal Cord[2,7]

Meninges

Meninges consist of three layers of connective tissue covering the brain and spinal cord. The meninges provide protection from contusion and infection. There are blood vessels and cerebrospinal fluid (CSF) within the meninges.

- **dura mater:** outermost meninx; has four folds; lines the periosteum of the skull and protects the brain; subdural space separates this from the arachnoid mater

- **arachnoid mater:** the middle meninx; the arachnoid is impermeable; surrounds the brain in a loose manner; subarachnoid space separates this from the pia mater

- **pia mater:** innermost meninx; covers the contours of the brain; forms the choroid plexus in the ventricular system

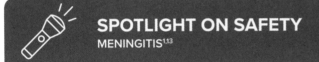

SPOTLIGHT ON SAFETY
MENINGITIS[1,13]

Meningitis is the inflammation of the meninges of the brain and spinal cord. There are various forms of meningitis with bacterial meningitis being potentially fatal within hours of onset. Acute meningitis is considered to be a medical emergency. A therapist must be aware of the signs and symptoms of meningitis including:

- fever, headache, vomiting
- complaints of a stiff and painful neck, nuchal rigidity
- pain in the lumbar area and posterior thigh
- Brudzinski's sign (flexion of the neck facilitates flexion of the hips and knees)
- Kernig's sign (pain with hip flexion combined with knee extension)
- sensitivity to light

A lumbar puncture is the gold standard for diagnosis. Early diagnosis is essential to avoid permanent neurological damage. Treatment includes antibiotic, antimicrobial, and steroid pharmacological intervention.

Dural Spaces[5,9]

- **epidural space:** an area between the skull and outer dura mater that can be abnormally occupied; also the area in the spinal cord between the dura mater and the periosteum of the vertebrae
- **subdural space:** the area between the dura and arachnoid meninges
- **subarachnoid space:** the area between the arachnoid and pia mater that contains CSF and the circulatory system for the cerebral cortex

Ventricular System[5,9]

The ventricular system is designed to protect and nourish the brain. It is comprised of four fluid-filled cavities called ventricles and multiple foramina that allow the passage of cerebrospinal fluid (CSF). Each ventricle contains specialized tissue called choroid plexus that makes CSF. An excess of CSF in the brain can cause an enlargement in the ventricles causing hydrocephalus; excess fluid within the spinal cord is termed syringomyelia.

Cerebrospinal fluid

Cerebrospinal fluid (CSF) is a clear, fluid-like substance that cushions the brain and spinal cord from injury and provides mechanical buoyancy and support. CSF provides nutrition to the central nervous system, serves as a conduit for removal of metabolites, and is constantly being absorbed and replenished within the brain and spinal cord.

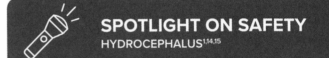

SPOTLIGHT ON SAFETY
HYDROCEPHALUS[1,14,15]

Hydrocephalus is an increase of CSF within the ventricles of the brain typically due to poor resorption, obstruction of flow or excessive production of CSF. It can be classified as congenital, acquired or idiopathic as well as communicating or non-communicating. Associated conditions and causative factors vary but may include spina bifida, choroid plexus neoplasm, cerebral palsy, tumor, meningitis or encephalocele. Successful treatment includes surgical placement of a shunt or performing an endoscopic third ventriculostomy (ETV). Often repeated neurosurgical procedures are necessary to treat hydrocephalus. Long-term health outcomes for patients with hydrocephalus remain unpredictable.

Signs of hydrocephalus or a blocked shunt include:

- enlarged head or bulging fontanelles in infants
- headache
- changes in vision
- large veins noted on scalp
- behavioral changes
- seizures
- alteration in appetite, vomiting
- "sun setting" sign or downward deviation of the eyes
- incontinence

Physical therapist assistants working with patients with hydro-cephalus or at risk for hydrocephalus must be aware of signs and symptoms of the condition as well as shunt malfunction, and when necessary, immediately notify appropriate medical personnel. There must be immediate medical intervention to alleviate the excessive fluid within the brain. Failure to act in a timely manner can result in coma and/or death.

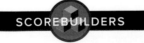

Blood-brain Barrier[5,9]

The blood-brain barrier consists of the meninges, protective glial cells, and capillary beds of the brain. It is responsible for exchange of nutrients between the central nervous system and the vascular system. The blood-brain barrier provides protection for the central nervous system by restricting certain molecules from crossing the barrier while others are able to do so freely.

Spinal Cord[6,9]

The spinal cord is a component of the central nervous system and a direct continuation of the brainstem. The spinal cord functions as a relay for information between peripheral structures and the brain in order to process information. The cord is surrounded by meninges and contained within the vertebral canal of the vertebral column (Fig. 5-4). The spinal cord contains both white and gray matter with the largest amount of gray matter found in the lumbar region. The vertebral artery forms the anterior spinal artery and two posterior spinal arteries that all surround the spinal cord. The spinal cord runs from the foramen magnum to the conus medullaris (between the 1st and 2nd lumbar vertebrae). There are 31 segments with a pair of spinal nerves arising from each segment and these nerves are components of the peripheral nervous system. Each spinal nerve contains a dorsal root (sensory) with afferent fibers and a ventral root (motor) with efferent fibers (Fig. 5-5).

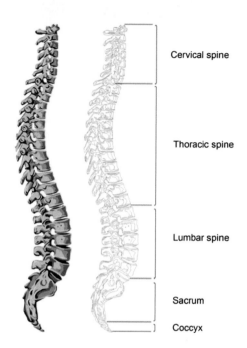

Cervical spine

Thoracic spine

Lumbar spine

Sacrum

Coccyx

Fig. 5-4: A sagittal view of the spine.

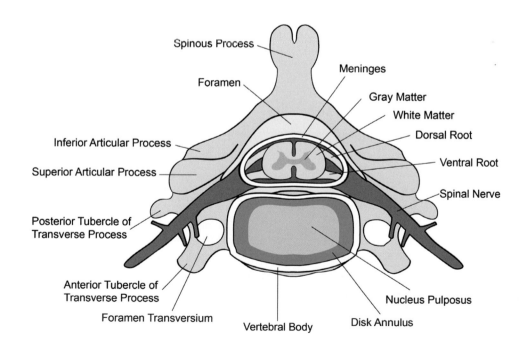

Spinous Process

Meninges

Foramen

Gray Matter

White Matter

Inferior Articular Process

Dorsal Root

Superior Articular Process

Ventral Root

Spinal Nerve

Posterior Tubercle of Transverse Process

Anterior Tubercle of Transverse Process

Foramen Transversium

Nucleus Pulposus

Vertebral Body

Disk Annulus

Fig. 5-5: A cross section of a vertebral segment.

Ascending Tracts[7,16,17]

Sensory tracts ascending in the white matter of the spinal cord arise either from cells of spinal ganglia or from intrinsic neurons within the gray matter that receive primary sensory input. Ascending tracts relay sensory feedback to the cerebrum and cerebellum. The primary afferent tracts include:

Fasciculus cuneatus (posterior or dorsal column): sensory tract for trunk, neck, and upper extremity proprioception, vibration, two-point discrimination, and graphesthesia

Fasciculus gracilis (posterior or dorsal column): sensory tract for trunk and lower extremity proprioception, two-point discrimination, vibration, and graphesthesia

Spinocerebellar tract (dorsal): sensory tract that ascends to the cerebellum for ipsilateral subconscious proprioception, tension in muscles, joint sense, and posture of the trunk and lower extremities

Spinocerebellar tract (ventral): sensory tract that ascends to the cerebellum, some fibers crossing with subsequent recrossing at the level of the pons for ipsilateral subconscious proprioception, tension in muscles, joint sense, and posture of the trunk, upper extremities, and lower extremities

Spino-olivary tract: ascends to the cerebellum and relays information from cutaneous and proprioceptive organs

Spinoreticular tract: the afferent pathway for the reticular formation that influences levels of consciousness

Spinotectal tract: sensory tract providing afferent information for spinovisual reflexes and assists with movement of eyes and head towards a stimulus

Spinothalamic tract (anterior): sensory tract for light touch and pressure

Spinothalamic tract (lateral): sensory tract for pain and temperature sensation

Descending Tracts[7,16,17]

Tracts descending to the spinal cord are involved with voluntary motor function, muscle tone, reflexes and equilibrium, visceral innervation, and modulation of ascending sensory signals. The largest, the corticospinal tract, originates in the cerebral cortex. Smaller descending tracts originate in nuclei in the midbrain, pons, and medulla oblongata. The primary efferent tracts include:

Corticospinal tract (anterior): pyramidal motor tract responsible for ipsilateral voluntary, discrete, and skilled movements

Corticospinal tract (lateral): pyramidal motor tract responsible for contralateral voluntary fine movement

- Damage to the corticospinal (pyramidal) tracts results in a positive Babinski sign, absent superficial abdominal reflexes and cremasteric reflex, and the loss of fine motor or skilled voluntary movement.

Reticulospinal tract: extrapyramidal motor tract responsible for facilitation or inhibition of voluntary and reflex activity through the influence on alpha and gamma motor neurons

Rubrospinal tract: extrapyramidal motor tract responsible for motor input of gross postural tone, facilitating activity of flexor muscles, and inhibiting the activity of extensor muscles

Tectospinal tract: extrapyramidal motor tract responsible for contralateral postural muscle tone associated with auditory/visual stimuli

Vestibulospinal tract: extrapyramidal motor tract responsible for ipsilateral gross postural adjustments subsequent to head movements, facilitating activity of the extensor muscles, and inhibiting activity of the flexor muscles

- Damage to the extrapyramidal tracts results in significant paralysis, hypertonicity, exaggerated deep tendon reflexes, and clasp-knife reaction.

CONSIDER THIS
BROWN-SEQUARD'S SYNDROME[18,19]

Afferent and efferent pathways provide consistent and predictable deficits with injury. Depending on the location of a lesion and whether or not a pathway crossed or remained on the originating side, symptoms will be noted ipsilaterally or contralaterally to the lesion. Thorough examination of a patient will allow a therapist to potentially target particular pathways that may be damaged.

As an example, Brown-Sequard's syndrome is an incomplete lesion typically caused by a stab wound, which produces hemisection of the spinal cord. There is paralysis and loss of vibratory sense and position sense on the same side as the lesion due to the damage to the corticospinal tracts and dorsal columns. There is a loss of pain and temperature sense on the opposite side of the lesion from damage to the lateral spinothalamic tract.

Peripheral Nervous System

The peripheral nervous system (PNS) contains nerves that originate within the brain and spinal cord, but end peripherally. The PNS consists of motor, sensory, and autonomic neurons that innervate end-organs that include sensory receptors, muscles, and glands. The PNS consists of 12 pairs of cranial nerves, 31 pairs of spinal nerves, and all associated ganglia and sensory receptors. Most peripheral nerves contain motor (efferent) and sensory (afferent) components (Fig. 5-6). Sensory nerves originate in the dorsal root ganglia while motor nerves originate in the anterior horn of the spinal cord. The autonomic neurons are divided into the sympathetic and parasympathetic nerves. The sympathetic nerves originate in the lateral horn of the thoracic spinal cord and the parasympathetic nerves originate from the lateral gray matter of the sacral level of the spinal cord and from the brain itself. Peripheral nerves are typically classified by axon diameter or speed of conduction.

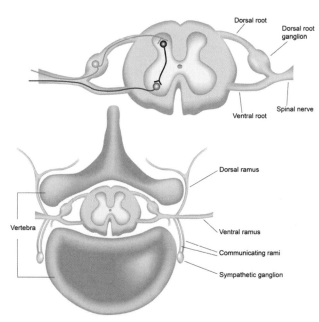

Fig. 5-6: A cross section of the spinal cord noting the spinal nerves.

Cutaneous Sensory End-organ Receptors[20]

- Thermoreceptors
- Nociceptors
- Mechanoreceptors
  - Merkel's disc
  - Ruffini's corpuscle
  - Pacinian corpuscle
  - Meissner's corpuscle
  - muscle spindle
  - free nerve ending
  - Golgi tendon organ

- Chemoreceptors
- Photoreceptors

Peripheral Nervous System Terminology[2,3,20]

Axon: a projection of a nerve away from the cell body that conducts impulses

Dendrite: an extension of the cell body that receives signals from other neurons

Motor unit: a single motor neuron and all of the muscle fibers that it innervates

Myelin: proteins and lipids that form to create a sheath around particular nerves; increases conductivity of the nerve impulse

Nerve conduction velocity: measures the speed of a nerve impulse along the axon of a nerve

Neurons: nerve cells that receive and send signals to other nerve cells; comprised of a cell body, axon, and dendrites

Nodes of Ranvier: brief gaps in myelination of an axon; serves to facilitate rapid conduction of a nerve impulse via jumping from gap node to gap node

Saltatory conduction: an action potential moving along an axon in a jumping fashion from node to node; decreases the use of sodium-potassium pumps and increases speed of conduction

Schwann cell: cells that cover the nerve fibers within the peripheral nervous system and form the myelin sheath

Classification of Peripheral Nerves[20]

A Fibers
- Large fibers
- Myelinated
- High conduction rate
- Alpha, beta, gamma, delta subsets

B Fibers
- Medium fibers
- Myelinated
- Reasonably fast conduction rate
- Preganglionic fibers of the autonomic system

C Fibers
- Small fibers
- Poorly myelinated or unmyelinated
- Slowed conduction rate
- Postganglionic fibers of the sympathetic system
- Exteroceptors for pain, temperature, and touch

Nerve Root Dermatomes, Myotomes, Reflexes, and Paresthetic Areas[21]

Nerve Root	Dermatome*	Muscle Weakness (Myotome)	Reflexes Affected	Paresthesias
C1	Vertex of skull	None	None	None
C2	Temple, forehead, occiput	Longus colli, sternocleidomastoid, rectus capitis	None	None
C3	Entire neck, posterior cheek, temporal area, prolongation forward under mandible	Trapezius, splenius capitis	None	Cheek, side of neck
C4	Shoulder area, clavicular area, upper scapular area	Trapezius, levator scapulae	None	Horizontal band along clavicle and upper scapula
C5	Deltoid area, anterior aspect of entire arm to base of thumb	Supraspinatus, infraspinatus, deltoid, biceps	Biceps, brachioradialis	None
C6	Anterior arm, radial side of hand to thumb and index finger	Biceps, supinator, wrist extensors	Biceps, brachioradialis	Thumb and index finger
C7	Lateral arm and forearm to index, long, and ring fingers	Triceps, wrist flexors (rarely, wrist extensors)	Triceps	Index, long, and ring fingers
C8	Medial arm and forearm to long, ring, and little fingers	Ulnar deviators, thumb extensors, thumb adductors (rarely, triceps)	None	Little finger alone or with two adjacent fingers; not ring or long fingers, alone or together (C7)
T1	Medial side of forearm to base of little finger	Disk lesions at upper two thoracic levels do not appear to give rise to root weakness. Weakness of intrinsic muscles of the hand is due to other pathology (e.g., thoracic outlet pressure, neoplasm of lung, ulnar nerve lesion).		
T2	Medial side of upper arm to medial elbow, pectoral and midscapular areas			
T3 – T12	T3-T6, upper thorax; T5-T7, costal margin; T8-T12, abdomen and lumbar region	Articular and dural signs and root pain are common. Root signs (cutaneous analgesia) are rare and have such indefinite area that they have little localizing value. Weakness is not detectable.		

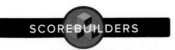

Nerve Root Dermatomes, Myotomes, Reflexes, and Paresthetic Areas[21]

Nerve Root	Dermatome*	Muscle Weakness (Myotome)	Reflexes Affected	Paresthesias
L1	Back, over trochanter and groin	None	None	Groin; after holding posture, which causes pain
L2	Back, front of thigh to knee	Psoas, hip adductors	None	Occasionally anterior thigh
L3	Back, upper buttock, anterior thigh and knee, medial lower leg	Psoas, quadriceps, thigh atrophy	Knee jerk sluggish, PKB positive, pain on full SLR	Medial knee, anterior lower leg
L4	Medial buttock, lateral thigh, medial leg, dorsum of foot, big toe	Tibialis anterior, extensor hallucis	SLR limited, neck flexion pain, weak or absent knee jerk, side flexion limited	Medial aspect of calf and ankle
L5	Buttock, posterior and lateral thigh, lateral aspect of leg, dorsum of foot, medial half of sole, first, second, and third toes	Extensor hallucis, peroneals, gluteus medius, dorsiflexors, hamstrings and calf atrophy	SLR limited one side, neck flexion painful, ankle decreased, crossed-leg raising pain	Lateral aspect of leg, medial three toes
S1	Lateral and plantar aspect of foot	Calf and hamstrings, wasting of gluteals, peroneals, plantar flexors	SLR limited, Achilles reflex weak or absent	Lateral two toes, lateral foot, lateral leg to knee, plantar aspect of foot
S2	Buttock, thigh, and posterior leg	Same as S1 except peroneals	Same as S1	Lateral leg, knee, and heel
S3	Groin, posteromedial thigh to knee	None	None	None
S4	Perineum, genitals, lower sacrum	Bladder, rectum	None	Saddle area, genitals, anus, impotence, massive posterior herniation

*In any part of which pain may be felt. PKB = prone knee bending; SLR = straight leg raising.

Adapted from Magee, DJ: Orthopedic Physical Assessment. W.B. Saunders Company, Philadelphia 2002, p.16, with permission.

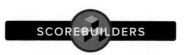

Cranial Nerves and Methods of Testing[21]

Nerve	Afferent (Sensory)	Efferent (Motor)	Test
Olfactory	Smell: Nose		Identify familiar odors (e.g., chocolate, coffee)
Optic	Sight: Eye		Test visual fields
Oculomotor		Voluntary motor: Levator of eyelid; superior, medial, and inferior recti; inferior oblique muscle of eyeball Autonomic: Smooth muscle of eyeball	Upward, downward, and medial gaze Reaction to light
Trochlear		Voluntary motor: Superior oblique muscle of eyeball	Downward and inward gaze
Trigeminal	Touch, pain: Skin of face, mucous membranes of nose, sinuses, mouth, anterior tongue	Voluntary motor: Muscles of mastication	Corneal reflex Face sensation Clench teeth; push down on chin to separate jaw
Abducens		Voluntary motor: Lateral rectus muscle of eyeball	Lateral gaze
Facial	Taste: Anterior tongue	Voluntary motor: Facial muscles Autonomic: Lacrimal, submandibular, and sublingual glands	Close eyes tight Smile and show teeth Whistle and puff cheeks Identify familiar tastes (e.g., sweet, sour)
Vestibulocochlear (acoustic nerve)	Hearing: Ear Balance: Ear		Hear watch ticking Hearing tests Balance and coordination tests
Glossopharyngeal	Touch, pain: Posterior tongue, pharynx Taste: Posterior tongue	Voluntary motor: Select muscles of pharynx Autonomic: Parotid gland	Gag reflex Ability to swallow
Vagus	Touch, pain: Pharynx, larynx, bronchi Taste: Tongue, epiglottis	Voluntary motor: Muscles of palate, pharynx, and larynx Autonomic: Thoracic and abdominal viscera	Gag reflex Ability to swallow Say "Ahhh"
Accessory		Voluntary motor: Sternocleidomastoid and trapezius muscles	Resisted shoulder shrug
Hypoglossal		Voluntary motor: Muscles of tongue	Tongue protrusion (if injured, tongue deviates toward injured side)

From Magee, DJ: Orthopedic Physical Assessment. W.B. Saunders Company, Philadelphia 2002, p.69, with permission.

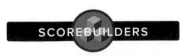

Cranial Nerve Testing Procedures[21,22]

The cranial nerves refer to twelve pairs of nerves that have their origin in the brain. Certain cranial nerves contain both sensory and motor fibers, however, many possess either sensory or motor fibers. Since lesions affecting the cranial nerves produce specific and predictable alterations, it is often prudent to perform cranial nerve testing as part of a neurological examination. The following information is a summary of some of the more common methods of testing selected cranial nerves.

Cranial Nerve I - Olfactory

The patient is positioned in sitting with the eyes closed or blindfolded. The therapist places an item with a familiar odor under the patient's nostril and the patient is asked to identify the odor. A positive test may be indicated by an inability to identify familiar odors.

Cranial Nerve II - Optic

The patient is positioned in standing a selected distance from a chart or diagram. The therapist asks the patient to identify objects or read selected items from the chart or diagram. A positive test may be indicated by an inability to identify objects at a reasonable distance.

Cranial Nerve III - Oculomotor

The patient is positioned in sitting and is asked to follow an object such as a writing utensil with their eyes as it is moved vertically, horizontally, and diagonally. The therapist should make sure the patient does not rotate their head during the testing and should inspect the patient's eyes for asymmetry or ptosis. A positive test is indicated by an identified tracking deficit, asymmetry or ptosis.

Cranial Nerve IV - Trochlear (Fig. 5-7)

The patient is positioned in sitting and asked to follow an object such as a writing utensil with their eyes as it is moved in an inferior direction. The therapist should make sure the patient does not move his head downward. A positive test is indicated by an inability to depress the eyes and/or complaints of diplopia.

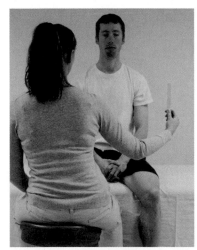

Fig. 5-7: Examination of the trochlear nerve. The patient should be able to follow the tongue depressor as it is moved in an inferior direction without moving the head.

Cranial Nerve V - Trigeminal

The patient is positioned in sitting and is asked to close their eyes. The therapist uses a piece of cotton and a safety pin to alternately touch the patient's face. The patient is asked to classify each contact with the face as "sharp" or "dull." A positive test for the sensory component may be identified by impaired or absent sensation or the inability to differentiate between "sharp" or "dull." The motor component is tested by asking the patient to perform mandibular protrusion, retrusion, and lateral deviation. A positive test may be indicated by an impaired ability to move the mandible through the specified motions.

Cranial Nerve VI - Abducens (Fig. 5-8)

The patient is positioned in sitting. The therapist asks the patient to abduct their eyes without rotating the head. A positive test is indicated by an inability to abduct the eyes.

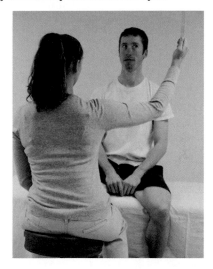

Fig. 5-8: Examination of the abducens nerve. The patient should be able to abduct the eyes without moving the head.

Cranial Nerve VII - Facial (Fig. 5-9)

The patient is positioned in sitting and is asked to distinguish between sweet and salty substances placed on the anterior portion of the tongue. A positive test for the sensory component may be identified by an inability to accurately identify sweet and salty substances. The motor component is tested by performing a manual muscle test of selected muscles involved in facial expression. A positive test for the motor component may be indicated by an inability to mimic selected facial expressions due to muscle impairment.

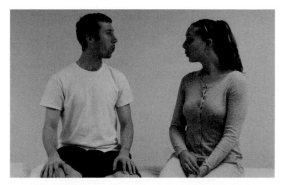

Fig. 5-9: Examination of the facial nerve. The patient should be able to mimic facial expressions. The sensory component of the nerve distinguishes between sweet and salty taste over the anterior tongue.

Cranial Nerve VIII - Vestibulocochlear

The patient is positioned in sitting in a quiet location. The therapist, positioned behind the patient and to one side, slowly brings a ticking watch toward the patient's ear. The therapist records the distance from the ear when the patient is able to identify the ticking sound. The therapist repeats the procedure on the contralateral ear and compares the measurements. A positive test is indicated by an inability to hear the ticking sound at 18-24 inches or a significant bilateral difference. Alternate tests include the Weber and Rinne tests which require a 512 Hz tuning fork.

Cranial Nerve IX - Glossopharyngeal (Fig. 5-10)

The patient is positioned in sitting. The therapist touches the pharynx with a tongue depressor. A positive test may be indicated by lack of gagging or an inability to feel the tongue depressor touch the back of the throat. The sensory component is tested by assessing the patient's ability to distinguish objects by taste after they are placed on the posterior portion of the tongue. A positive test for the sensory component may be identified by an inability to accurately identify tasted substances, especially sour and bitter substances, placed on the posterior third of the tongue.

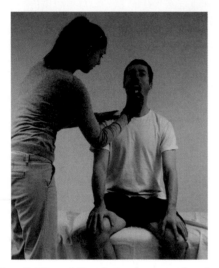

Fig. 5-10: Examination of the glossopharyngeal and vagus nerves. The tongue depressor on the tongue should produce a gag response.

Cranial Nerve X - Vagus (Fig. 5-10)

The patient is positioned in sitting. The therapist touches the pharynx with a tongue depressor. A positive test may be indicated by a lack of gagging or an inability to feel the tongue depressor touch the back of the throat (same description for Cranial Nerve IX - Glossopharyngeal). If the gag reflex is absent the therapist should carefully assess the movement of the soft palate and uvula.

Cranial Nerve XI - Accessory (Fig. 5-11)

The patient is positioned in sitting with the arms at the side. The therapist asks the patient to shrug their shoulders and maintain the position while the therapist applies resistance through the shoulders in the direction of shoulder depression. A positive test may be indicated by an inability to maintain the test position against resistance.

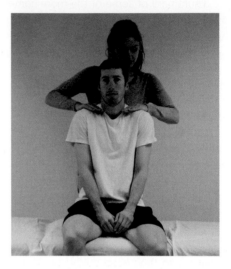

Fig. 5-11: Examination of the accessory nerve. The patient should be able to maintain a shoulder shrug against resistance.

Cranial Nerve XII - Hypoglossal (Fig. 5-12)

The patient is positioned in sitting. The therapist asks the patient to protrude the tongue. A positive test may be indicated by an inability to fully protrude the tongue or the tongue deviating to one side during protrusion.

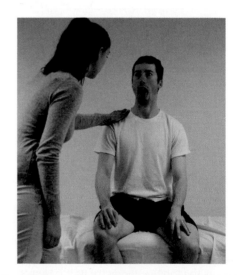

Fig. 5-12: Examination of the hypoglossal nerve. The patient should be able to protrude the tongue in a symmetrical fashion.

Nerves of the Brachial Plexus[23]

Origin	Nerves	Muscles
From the rami of the plexus	Dorsal scapular	Rhomboids, levator scapulae
	Long thoracic	Serratus anterior
From the trunks of the plexus	Nerve to subclavius	Subclavius
	Suprascapular	Infraspinatus, supraspinatus
From the lateral cord of the plexus	Lateral pectoral	Pectoralis major - clavicular head
	Musculocutaneous	Coracobrachialis, biceps brachii, brachialis
	Lateral root of the median	Flexor muscles in the forearm, except flexor carpi ulnaris, and five muscles in the hand
From the medial cord of the plexus	Medial pectoral	Pectoralis major, pectoralis minor
	Ulnar	Flexor carpi ulnaris, flexor digitorum profundus, most small muscles of the hand
	Medial root of the median	Flexor muscles in the forearm, except flexor carpi ulnaris, and five muscles of the hand
From the posterior cord of the plexus	Upper subscapular	Subscapularis
	Thoracodorsal	Latissimus dorsi
	Lower subscapular	Subscapularis, teres major
	Axillary	Deltoid, teres minor
	Radial	Brachioradialis, triceps, supinator, wrist extensors, anconeus

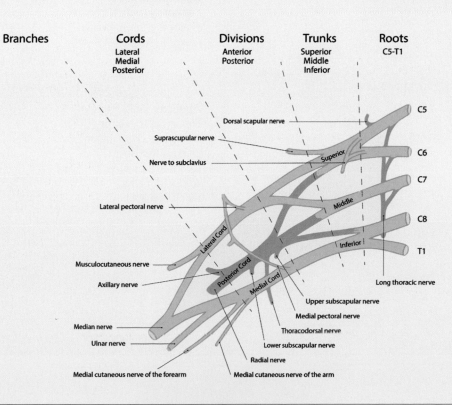

Lower Extremity Innervation[23]

Lumbar Plexus	Sciatic Nerve - Tibial Division
Psoas major Psoas minor Quadratus lumborum	Semitendinosus Semimembranosus Biceps femoris (long head)
Sacral Plexus	**Sciatic Nerve - Common Peroneal Division**
Piriformis Superior gemelli Inferior gemelli Obturator internus Quadratus femoris	Biceps femoris (short head)
Inferior Gluteal Nerve	**Deep Peroneal Nerve**
Gluteus maximus	Tibialis anterior Extensor digitorum longus Extensor hallucis longus Peroneus tertius Extensor digitorum brevis
Superior Gluteal Nerve	**Superficial Peroneal Nerve**
Gluteus medius Gluteus minimus Tensor fasciae latae	Peroneus longus Peroneus brevis
Femoral Nerve	**Medial Plantar Nerve**
Vastus lateralis Rectus femoris Vastus medialis Vastus intermedius Iliacus Sartorius Pectineus	Abductor hallucis Lumbrical I Flexor digitorum brevis Flexor hallucis brevis
Obturator Nerve	**Lateral Plantar Nerve**
Adductor longus Adductor brevis Adductor magnus Obturator externus Gracilis	Abductor digiti minimi Flexor digiti minimi Opponens digiti minimi Dorsal interossei Quadratus plantae Adductor hallucis Lumbrical II, III, IV Plantar interossei
Tibial Nerve	
Soleus Popliteus Plantaris Tibialis posterior Gastrocnemius Flexor hallucis longus Flexor digitorum longus	

Deep Tendon Reflexes[6,22,24]

Deep tendon reflexes (DTR) elicit a muscle contraction when the muscle's tendon is stimulated due to the reflex arc involving the spinal or brainstem segment that innervates the specific muscle. Hyperreflexia refers to hyperactivity or clonic reflexes. This can be indicative of a suprasegmental lesion (a lesion above the level of the spinal reflex pathways). Hyporeflexia refers to a diminished or absent response to tapping of the tendon. This can be indicative of disease that involves one or multiple components of the reflex arc itself.

Procedure Guidelines for Deep Tendon Reflex Testing[6,22]

- The patient should be relaxed and understand the testing procedure.
- Position the patient properly and symmetrically with the muscle placed on a slight stretch.
- A reflex hammer should be utilized to deliver a direct strike on the tendon with an anticipated immediate response (Fig. 5-13).
- Avoid "pecking" at the tendon with the hammer as this will not produce valid results.
- Reflexes can be graded as depressed (hypo), normal or exaggerated (hyper) on a scale of 0-4.

- If the therapist has difficulty eliciting a reflex, the Jendrassik maneuver should be employed to distract the patient, increase reflex activity, and decrease guarding. The patient can be directed to perform the Jendrassik maneuver by locking the fingers together and directly pulling against each other immediately prior to the reflex stimulus.
- The examination should provide a comparison of both sides of the body and should include all deep tendon reflexes.
- The examination should provide a comparison of "normal" areas to suspected areas of impairment.
- Examination results should assist the therapist to identify deficits within the nervous system.

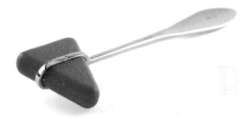

Fig. 5-13: A standard reflex hammer used to assess deep tendon reflexes.

Reflex Grading Scale[25]	
Reflex Grading	**Interpretation**
0 = no response	always abnormal
1+ = diminished/depressed response	may or may not be normal
2+ = active normal response	normal
3+ = brisk/exaggerated response	may or may not be normal
4+ = very brisk/hyperactive	always abnormal

Deep Tendon Reflex Testing[6,22,25]

Biceps tendon (Fig. 5-14)

Spinal Level: C5-C6

Procedure: support the elbow in partial flexion in sitting or supine; place the thumb firmly over the biceps tendon at the elbow and strike the hammer through the thumb

Normal Response: Contraction of the biceps muscle; flexion of the elbow

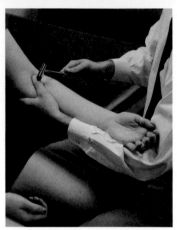

Fig. 5-14: Examination of the biceps deep tendon reflex.

Brachioradialis tendon (Fig. 5-15)

Spinal Level: C5-C6

Procedure: rest the hand on the lap in sitting with the forearm supported and in neutral; strike the radius one to two inches superior to the wrist

Normal Response: Contraction of the brachioradialis muscle; elbow flexion and/or forearm supination

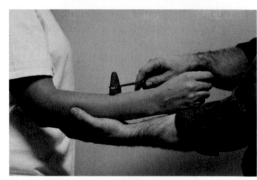

Fig. 5-15: Examination of the brachioradialis deep tendon reflex.

Triceps tendon (Fig. 5-16)

Spinal Level: C6-C7

Procedure: support the upper extremity through the humerus and allow the lower portion to hang with elbow flexion; strike the triceps tendon directly above the elbow

Normal Response: Contraction of the triceps muscle; elbow extension

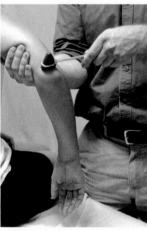

Fig. 5-16: Examination of the triceps deep tendon reflex.

Patellar tendon (Fig. 5-17)

Spinal Level: L3-L4

Procedure: supported knee flexion with the patient in sitting or supine; strike the tendon directly inferior to the patella

Normal Response: Contraction of the quadriceps; knee extension

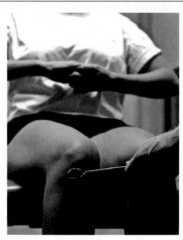

Fig. 5-17: Examination of the patellar deep tendon reflex.

Achilles tendon (Fig. 5-18)

Spinal Level: S1-S2

Procedure: in sitting, flex the foot at the ankle putting the Achilles on stretch; strike the Achilles tendon above the foot

Normal Response: Plantar flexion of the foot

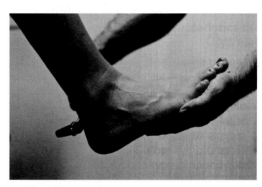

Fig. 5-18: Examination of the Achilles deep tendon reflex.

SPOTLIGHT ON SAFETY
CLINICAL RELEVANCE OF REFLEX TESTING[25]

Deep tendon reflex (DTR) testing can assist the therapist in determining the type of pathology that exists. Absent DTRs will indicate a lesion in the reflex arc itself. If absent reflexes accompany sensory loss in the distribution of the nerve that is supplying a particular reflex, the lesion is found within the afferent arc of the reflex and is located in either the nerve or dorsal horn. If an absent DTR accompanies paralysis, fasciculations or atrophy, the lesion is found within the efferent arc of the reflex and may include the efferent nerve, anterior horn cells or both.

Peripheral neuropathy is the most common etiology surrounding absent reflexes. Associated conditions can include diabetes, alcoholism, vitamin deficiencies such as pernicious anemia, certain cancers, and certain toxins (lead, arsenic, vincristine). Neuropathies will typically present with sensory, motor or mixed impairments and may affect all components of the reflex arc.

Hyperactive DTRs are found when there is interruption of the cortical supply to the lower motor neuron (secondary to upper motor neuron lesion). The interruption exists above the segment of the reflex arc, with other findings determining localization of the exact lesion. Assessment of the DTRs can provide information as to the level of lesion that exists within the central nervous system.

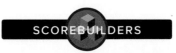

Sensation

There are several types of sensation that a physical therapist assistant will assess including superficial, deep (proprioceptive), and cortical (combined) sensations. A therapist should examine superficial and deep sensations first, followed by cortical sensations.

- **Superficial:** temperature, light touch, pain
- **Deep:** proprioception, kinesthesia, vibration
- **Cortical:** bilateral simultaneous stimulation, stereognosis, two-point discrimination, barognosis, localization of touch

Procedure Guidelines for Sensory Testing[6,22]

- The patient should be relaxed and understand the expectations of the required response.
- The examination should be conducted in an efficient manner so that the sensory system does not fatigue and allow for unreliable responses.
- The patient's vision should be obscured or the patient blindfolded so that their vision does not influence the perceived sensation.
- The pace of the examination should vary so that the patient does not expect a stimulus or respond merely to the rhythm of the test.
- The therapist should have a complete understanding of areas of the skin that have heightened or decreased sensitivity based on the type of sensation that is tested (i.e., temperature versus light touch).
- The examination should provide a comparison of both sides of the body and should include all extremities and the trunk.
- The examination should provide a comparison of "normal" areas to suspected areas of impairment.
- The examination should provide a comparison of distal versus proximal response for each tested area.
- The therapist may examine dermatomes and peripheral nerve distribution or patterns of sensation such as:
  - bilateral shoulders - C4
  - medial and lateral aspects of bilateral forearms - C6 to T1
  - thumbs and little fingers - C6 and C8
  - bilateral anterior thighs - L2 and L3
  - medial and lateral aspects of bilateral lower legs (calf)- L4 and L5
  - bilateral little toes - S1
  - saddle area - S4
- Examination results should assist the therapist to recognize the deficit as CNS, plexus or peripheral nerve pattern damage.
- Patients with sensory deficits or who are at risk for sensory impairments should be tested using Semmes Weinstein monofilaments for objective data collection regarding protective sensation (Figs. 5-19, 5-20, 5-21).

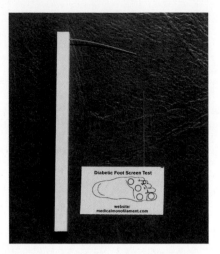

Fig. 5-19: Semmes Weinstein monofilaments.

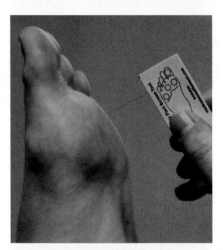

Fig. 5-20: Testing protocol requires the monofilament to be held perpendicular to the surface tested.

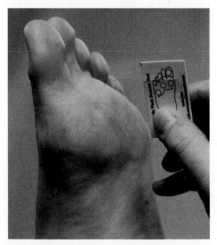

Fig. 5-21: Proper pressure has been applied when the monofilament deforms.

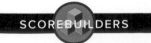

CONSIDER THIS
SCREENING OF SUPERFICIAL, DEEP, AND CORTICAL SENSATIONS[6,26]

When screening a patient's sensation, there are typical stimuli that produce an expected response that measures a patient's sensation as normal or impaired.

- **Barognosis:** perceive the weight of different objects in the hand
- **Deep pain:** squeeze the forearm or calf muscle
- **Graphesthesia:** identify a number or letter drawn on the skin without visual input
- **Kinesthesia:** identify direction and extent of movement of a joint or body part
- **Light touch:** perceive touch through light pressure or use of a cotton ball
- **Localization:** ability to identify the exact location of light touch on the body using a verbal response or gesturing
- **Proprioception:** identify a static position of an extremity or body part
- **Stereognosis:** identify an object without sight (Fig. 5-22)
- **Superficial pain:** perceive noxious stimulus using a pen cap, paper clip end or pin
- **Temperature:** perceive warm and cold test tubes
- **Two-point discrimination:** using a two-point caliper on the skin, identify one or two points without visual input (Fig. 5-23)
- **Vibration:** perceive vibration or pain through a tuning fork

Impairment found with any of the above sensations may designate lesion or pathology to a particular pathway or region of the brain. The therapist can utilize this information to enhance understanding of the neurological impairment as well as to customize the plan of care.

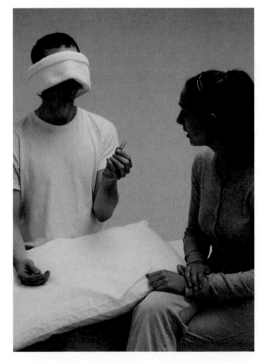

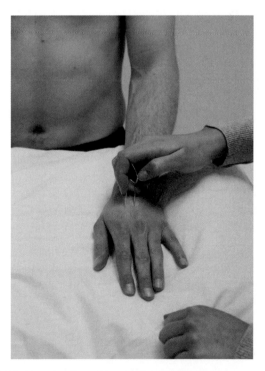

Fig. 5-22: The patient is trying to identify the paper clip without visual feedback and using only the sense of touch. This is an examination of stereognosis.

Fig. 5-23: Examination of two-point discrimination.

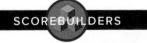

Sensory Testing[6,22,25]

Light touch (Fig. 5-24)

- instruct and demonstrate the testing procedure to the patient and ask for a response
- attempt to initiate the testing in a normal area so the patient can anticipate what to expect
- performed through touching the skin lightly or using cotton
- with eyes closed, ask patient to identify when they feel a touch
- compare sides of the body, proximal versus distal areas, and identify patterns or innervation level of impairment

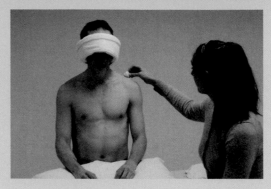

Fig. 5-24: Examination of light touch sensation using a cotton ball.

Pain

- instruct and demonstrate the testing procedure to the patient and have them note the sharp versus dull side of a pin or appropriate instrument such as a Wartenberg pinwheel (Figs. 5-25, 5-26)
- performed through touching the skin while alternating in a random fashion between the sharp and dull ends of the pin
- attempt to initiate the testing in an intact area so the patient can anticipate what to expect
- with eyes closed, ask the patient to identify if they feel a sharp or dull sensation
- allow the patient to make comparisons by asking if the stimulus is the same or different when testing different areas
- compare sides of the body, proximal versus distal areas, identify patterns or innervation level of impairment

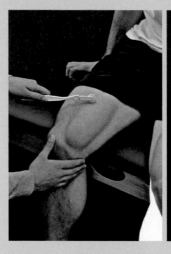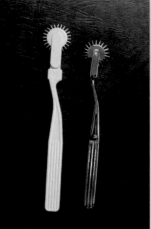

Fig. 5-25 (Left): Examination of sharp versus dull sensation using a Wartenberg pinwheel.

Fig. 5-26 (Right): Wartenberg pinwheels.

Temperature

- temperature discrimination should utilize test tubes, warm water in one and cold water in the other
- avoid extreme temperatures as this is a test of discrimination, not of a patient's tolerance to extreme temperatures
- instruct and demonstrate the testing procedure to the patient with the expectation of a response of "hot" or "cold" for each stimulus
- attempt to initiate the testing in an intact area so the patient can anticipate what to expect
- touch the skin while alternating in a random fashion between the warm and cold test tubes

- with eyes closed, ask the patient to identify if they sense a warm or cold temperature
- allow the patient to make comparisons by asking if the stimulus is the same temperature or a different temperature when testing different areas
- compare sides of the body, proximal versus distal areas, identify patterns or distribution levels of impairment
- testing for temperature discrimination will also predict pain sensation since there are sensory receptors with each modality that overlap

Sensory Testing[6,22,25]

Vibration

- instruct and demonstrate the testing procedure to the patient
- preferably performed using a 128 Hz tuning fork and alternating the testing with vibration and without vibration (Figs. 5-27, 5-28)
- initiate the test by tapping the tuning fork to produce vibration and placing it over the interphalangeal joint of a patient's finger or the interphalangeal joint of the great toe
- with eyes closed, ask patient to identify what they feel
- strike the tuning fork tines with each attempt, but stop the vibration on intermittent trials to ensure that the patient will recognize vibration versus touch or pressure
- if there is impairment, test bony prominences proximally including the wrist, elbow, spinous processes, clavicles, medial malleolus, patella, ASIS, etc.
- allow the patient to make comparisons by asking if the stimulus is the same or different when testing the different bony areas of a limb or right versus left sides of the body

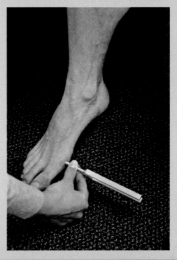

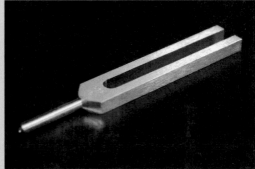

Fig. 5-27 (Above): Examination of vibration using a tuning fork.

Fig. 5-28 (Below): A tuning fork.

Pressure

- instruct and demonstrate the testing procedure to the patient and ask for a response
- attempt to initiate the testing in an intact area so the patient can anticipate what to expect
- touch the skin with a fingertip using direct pressure firm enough to stimulate the deep receptors
- with eyes closed, ask patient to identify when they feel anything
- alternate light touch and deep pressure with the patient responding "light" or "deep"
- compare sides of the body, proximal versus distal areas, identify patterns or distribution level of impairment

Peripheral Nerve Lesions[20]

A lesion of the nerve can occur through many mechanisms of injury. Possible etiologies include mechanical (compression injury), crush and percussion (fracture, compartment syndrome), laceration, penetrating trauma (stab wound), stretch (traction injury), high velocity trauma (motor vehicle accident), and cold (frostbite). This results in total loss of muscle over time with replacement by fibrous tissue.

Mononeuropathy: an isolated nerve lesion; associated conditions include trauma and entrapment

Neuroma: abnormal growth of nerve cells; associated conditions include vasculitis, AIDS, and amyloidosis

Peripheral neuropathy: impairment or dysfunction of the peripheral nerves; associated conditions include diabetic peripheral neuropathy, trauma, alcoholism

Polyneuropathy: diffuse nerve dysfunction that is symmetrical and typically secondary to pathology and not trauma; associated conditions include Guillain-Barre syndrome, peripheral neuropathy, use of neurotoxic drugs, and HIV

Classification of Acute Nerve Injuries[9,27]

Neurapraxia

- Mildest form of injury
- Conduction block usually due to myelin dysfunction
- Axonal continuity preserved
- Axons, epineurium, perineurium, and endoneurium intact
- Nerve conduction is preserved proximal and distal to the lesion
- Nerve fibers are not damaged, no evidence of nerve degeneration is noted
- Symptoms include pain, minimal muscle atrophy, numbness or greater loss of motor and sensory function, diminished proprioception
- Recovery is rapid and complete and will occur within 4-6 weeks
- Pressure injuries are the most common

CONSIDER THIS
PERIPHERAL NERVE INJURY: TYPICAL ETIOLOGIES[2,4]

Both upper and lower extremity nerves have typical etiologies that subsequently produce specific patterns of impingement or compression injuries.

In the upper extremity, brachial plexus injuries can result from trauma, penetration, traction or compression. The following lists common etiologies associated with specific nerve injuries.

Axillary: fracture of the neck of the humerus, anterior dislocation of the shoulder

Musculocutaneous: fracture of the clavicle

Radial: compression of the nerve in the radial tunnel, fracture of the humerus

Median: compression in the carpal tunnel, pronator teres entrapment

Ulnar: compression in the cubital tunnel, entrapment in Guyon's canal

In the lower extremity, many nerve injuries for women are secondary to labor, delivery or surgical procedures around the pelvis. The following lists common etiologies associated with specific nerve injuries.

Femoral: total hip arthroplasty, displaced acetabular fracture, anterior dislocation of the femur, hysterectomy, appendectomy

Sciatic: blunt force trauma to the buttocks, total hip arthroplasty, accidental injection to the nerve

Obturator: fixation of a femur fracture, total hip arthroplasty

Peroneal: femur, tibia or fibula fracture, positioning during surgical procedures

Tibial: tarsal tunnel entrapment, popliteal fossa compression

Sural: fracture of the calcaneus or lateral malleolus

Recovery is based on the degree of injury and potential for regeneration of the nerve. The majority of research indicates that children tend to have better outcomes after peripheral nerve damage than adults, although some research sees no difference between the populations. The earlier repair of a nerve yields a better outcome; the more distal the lesion, the better the outcome secondary to the nerve length that requires recovery.

Axonotmesis

- A more severe grade of injury to a peripheral nerve

- Reversible injury to damaged fibers since they maintain an anatomical relationship to each other

- Damage occurs to the axons with preservation of the endoneurium (neural connective tissue sheath), epineurium, Schwann cells, and supporting structures

- Distal Wallerian degeneration can occur

- The nerve can regenerate distal to the site of the lesion at a rate of one millimeter per day

- Recovery is spontaneous and varies from spotty to no recovery; surgery may be required for repair

- Traction, compression, and crush injuries are the most common

Neurotmesis

- The most severe grade of injury to a peripheral nerve

- Axon, myelin, connective tissue components are all damaged or transected

- Irreversible injury; no possibility of regeneration

- Flaccid paralysis and wasting of muscles occur; total loss of sensation to area supplied by the nerve

- All motor and sensory loss distal to the lesion becomes permanently impaired

- No spontaneous recovery; with surgical reattachment, potential regenerating axons may grow at one millimeter per day with proximal recovery first; sensory recovery occurs sooner than motor fibers

- Complete transection of the nerve trunk

Peripheral Nervous System Pathology[2,3,9]

Anterior Horn Cell

- Sensory component intact
- Motor weakness and atrophy
- Fasciculations
- Decreased deep tendon reflexes
- **Example:** amyotrophic lateral sclerosis (ALS), poliomyelitis

Muscle

- Sensory component intact
- Motor weakness; fasciculations are rare
- Normal or decreased deep tendon reflexes
- **Example:** muscular dystrophy

Neuromuscular Junction

- Sensory component intact
- Motor fatigue is greater than actual weakness
- Normal deep tendon reflexes
- **Example:** myasthenia gravis

Peripheral Nerve (Mononeuropathy)

- Sensory loss along the nerve route
- Motor weakness and atrophy in a peripheral distribution; may have fasciculations
- **Example:** trauma

Peripheral Polyneuropathy

- Sensory impairments; "stocking glove" distribution
- Motor weakness and atrophy; weaker distally than proximally; may have fasciculations
- Decreased deep tendon reflexes
- **Example:** diabetic peripheral polyneuropathy

Spinal Roots and Nerves

- Sensory component will have corresponding dermatomal deficits
- Motor weakness in an innervated pattern; may have fasciculations
- Decreased deep tendon reflexes
- **Example:** herniated disk

Upper Motor Neuron Disease

An upper motor neuron disease is characterized by a lesion found in descending motor tracts within the cerebral motor cortex, internal capsule, brainstem or spinal cord. Symptoms include weakness of involved muscles, hypertonicity, hyperreflexia, mild disuse atrophy, and abnormal reflexes. Damaged tracts are in the lateral white column of the spinal cord.

Examples of upper motor neuron lesions include:

- cerebral palsy
- hydrocephalus
- ALS (both upper and lower)
- CVA
- birth injuries
- multiple sclerosis
- Huntington's chorea
- traumatic brain injury
- pseudobulbar palsy
- brain tumors

Lower Motor Neuron Disease

A lower motor neuron disease is characterized by a lesion that affects nerves or their axons at or below the level of the brainstem, usually within the "final common pathway." The ventral gray column of the spinal cord may also be affected. Symptoms include flaccidity or weakness of the involved muscles, decreased tone, fasciculations, muscle atrophy, and decreased or absent reflexes.

Examples of lower motor neuron lesions include:

- poliomyelitis
- ALS (both upper and lower)
- Guillain-Barre syndrome
- tumors involving the spinal cord
- trauma
- progressive muscular atrophy
- infection
- Bell's palsy
- carpal tunnel syndrome
- muscular dystrophy
- spinal muscular atrophy

Upper versus Lower Motor Neuron Disease[1,2,3]

	UMND	LMND
Reflexes	Hyperactive	Diminished or absent
Atrophy	Mild from disuse	Present
Fasciculations	Absent	Present
Tone	Hypertonic	Hypotonic to flaccid

Involuntary Movement/Movement Disorders[1,6,22]

An involuntary movement is defined as a movement that the person does not start or stop at the person's own command or with an observer's command. Muscle fiber contractions of either central or peripheral origin can create small or large scale patterns. Common forms of hypokinesia include apraxia, rigidity, and bradykinesia. Common forms of hyperkinesia include ataxia, athetosis, chorea, tics, tremors, dysmetria, and dystonia. Select movement disorders are highlighted below.

Athetosis

Athetosis is a movement disorder that presents with slow, twisting, and writhing movements that are large in amplitude. Athetoid movement is primarily seen in the face, tongue, trunk, and extremities. When the movements are brief, they merge with chorea (choreoathetosis), and when sustained, they merge with dystonia, and it is typically associated with spasticity. Athetosis is a common finding in several forms of cerebral palsy secondary to basal ganglia pathology.

Chorea

Chorea is a form of hyperkinesia that presents with brief, irregular contractions that are rapid, but not to the degree of myoclonic jerks. Chorea is typically secondary to damage of the caudate nucleus. Chorea is often equated to "fidgeting." Ballism is a form of chorea that includes choreic jerks of large amplitude. Ballism produces flailing movements of the limbs and is typically secondary to damage of the subthalamic nucleus. Huntington's disease is an example of a pathology that presents with chorea.

Dystonia

Dystonia is a syndrome of sustained muscle contractions that frequently causes twisting, abnormal postures, and repetitive movements. All muscles can be affected and the involuntary movements are often accentuated during volitional movement and with progression, can produce overflow. Presentation varies as there are multiple types and etiologies surrounding dystonia. Etiologies range from genetic or acquired to environmental or a secondary effect from medications. Presentations can include sustained contractions of agonist and antagonist muscles; repeatedly persisting within the same muscle group; voluntary movements that create involuntary movement secondary to overflow; torsion spasms that are continual, patterned and twisting; as well as other presentations based on etiology. Common diagnoses that may include dystonia are Parkinson's disease, cerebral palsy, and encephalitis.[13]

Tics

Tics are sudden, brief, repetitive coordinated movements that will usually occur at irregular intervals. There are simple and complex tics that vary from myoclonic jerks to jumping movements that may include vocalization and repetition of other sounds. Tourette syndrome is an example of a pathology that presents with tics.

Tremors

Tremors are involuntary, rhythmic, oscillatory movements that are typically classified into three groupings:

- Resting: Tremors are observable at rest and may or may not disappear with movement; may increase with mental stress. An example is the pill-rolling tremor associated with Parkinson's disease.
- Postural: Tremors are observable during a voluntary contraction to maintain a posture. Examples include the rapid tremor associated with hyperthyroidism, fatigue or anxiety, and benign essential tremor.
- Intention (kinetic): Tremors are absent at rest, but observable with activity and typically increase as the target approaches. These tremors likely indicate a lesion of the cerebellum or its efferent pathways and are typically seen with multiple sclerosis.

Muscle/Movement Impairment Terminology[1,13,24]

Akinesia: The inability to initiate movement; commonly seen in patients with Parkinson's disease.

Asthenia: Generalized weakness, typically secondary to cerebellar pathology.

Ataxia: The inability to perform coordinated movements.

Athetosis: A condition that presents with involuntary movements combined with instability of posture. Peripheral movements occur without central stability.

Bradykinesia: Movement that is very slow.

Chorea: Movements that are sudden, random, and involuntary.

Clasp-knife response: A form of resistance seen during range of motion of a hypertonic joint where there is greatest resistance at the initiation of range that lessens with movement through the range of motion.

Clonus: A characteristic of an upper motor neuron lesion; involuntary alternating spasmodic contraction of a muscle precipitated by a quick stretch reflex.

Cogwheel rigidity: A form of rigidity where resistance to movement has a phasic quality to it; often seen with Parkinson's disease.

Dysdiadochokinesia: The inability to perform rapidly alternating movements.

Dysmetria: The inability to control the range of a movement and the force of muscular activity.

Dystonia: Closely related to athetosis, however, there is larger axial muscle involvement rather than appendicular muscles.

Fasciculation: A muscular twitch that is caused by random discharge of a lower motor neuron and its muscle fibers; suggests lower motor neuron disease, however, can be benign.

Hemiballism: An involuntary and violent movement of a large body part.

Kinesthesia: The ability to perceive the direction and extent of movement of a joint or body part.

Lead pipe rigidity: A form of rigidity where there is uniform and constant resistance to range of motion; often associated with lesions of the basal ganglia.

Rigidity: A state of severe hypertonicity where a sustained muscle contraction does not allow for any movement at a specified joint.

Tremor: Involuntary, rhythmic, oscillatory movements secondary to a basal ganglia lesion. There are various classifications secondary to specific etiology.

Balance[23,26,28]

Balance can be defined as:

- a state of physical equilibrium
- maintenance and control of the center of gravity
- achieving and maintaining an upright posture

All definitions assume integrated somatosensory, visual, and vestibular information within the central nervous system. Balance is best assessed through investigation of all three components of balance.

Somatosensory Input

Somatosensory receptors are located in the joints, muscles, ligaments, and skin to provide proprioceptive information regarding length, tension, pressure, pain, and joint position. Proprioceptive and tactile input from the ankles, knees, hips, and neck provide balance information to the brain.

- **Challenging the somatosensory system:** examination of pressure and vibration; observation of a patient when changing the surface they are standing on. Examples would be slopes, uneven surfaces, standing on foam (Figs. 5-29, 5-30).

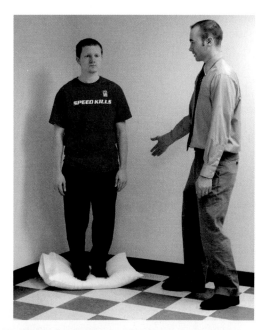

Fig. 5-29: Examination of balance while stressing the somatosensory system by using an altered surface.

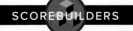

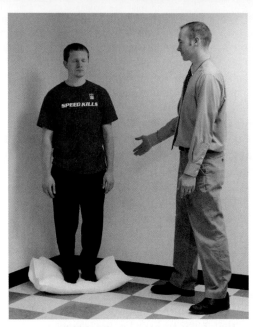

Fig. 5-30: Examination of balance by stressing the somatosensory system by using an altered surface and closing the patient's eyes. This does not allow for visual feedback regarding balance.

Visual Input

Visual receptors allow for perceptual acuity regarding verticality, motion of objects and self, environmental orientation, postural sway, and movements of the head/neck. Children rely heavily on this system for maintenance of balance.

- **Challenging the visual system:** examination of quiet standing with eyes open; observing balance strategies to maintain center of gravity with and without visual input. Assessment of potential visual field cuts, hemianopsia, pursuits, saccades, double vision, gaze control, and acuity is necessary.

Vestibular Input

The vestibular system provides the central nervous system with feedback regarding the position and movement of the head with relation to gravity. The labyrinth consists of three semicircular canals filled with endolymph and two otolith organs. Semicircular canals respond to the movement of fluid with head motion. Otoliths measure the effects of gravity and movement with regard to acceleration/deceleration.

- **Challenging the vestibular system:** examination of balance with movement of the head; testing such as Dix-Hallpike test, bithermal caloric testing, assessment for nystagmus, head thrust sign; testing of the vestibuloocular reflex.

Balance Reflexes

Vestibuloocular reflex (VOR): VOR allows for head/eye movement coordination. This reflex supports gaze stabilization through eye movement that counters movements of the head. This maintains a stable image on the retina during movement.

Vestibulospinal reflex (VSR): VSR attempts to stabilize the body and control movement. The reflex assists with stability while the head is moving as well as coordination of the trunk during upright postures.

Automatic Postural Strategies

Automatic postural strategies are automatic motor responses that are used to maintain the center of gravity over the base of support. These responses always react or respond to a particular stimulus.

Ankle strategy: The ankle strategy is the first strategy to be elicited by a small range and slow velocity perturbation when the feet are on the ground. Muscle groups contract in a distal to proximal fashion to control postural sway from the ankle joint.

Hip strategy: The hip strategy is elicited by a greater force, challenge or perturbation through the pelvis and hips. The hips will move (in the opposite direction from the head) in order to maintain balance. Muscle groups contract in a proximal to distal fashion in order to counteract the loss of balance.

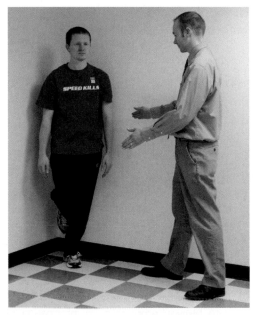

Fig. 5-31: Examination of balance with a decrease in the base of support.

Suspensory strategy: The suspensory strategy is used to lower the center of gravity during standing or ambulation in order to better control the center of gravity. Examples of this strategy include knee flexion, crouching or squatting. This strategy is often used when both mobility and stability are required during a task (such as surfing).

Stepping strategy: The stepping strategy is elicited through unexpected challenges or perturbations during static standing or when the perturbation produces such a movement that the center of gravity is beyond the base of support. The lower extremities step and/or upper extremities reach to regain a new base of support.

Balance Tests and Measures[24,29,30]

There are various tests and measures to assess the different facets of balance. Selection of the most appropriate instrument is determined based on clinical diagnosis and patient presentation. Common balance tests and measures are discussed below.

Berg Balance Scale

This is a tool designed to assess a patient's risk for falling. There are 14 tasks, each scored on an ordinal scale from 0-4. These tasks include static activities, transitional movements, and dynamic activities in sitting and standing positions. The maximum score is a 56 with a score less than 45 indicating an increased risk for falling. This tool can be used as a one-time examination or as an ongoing tool to monitor a patient who may be at risk for falls.

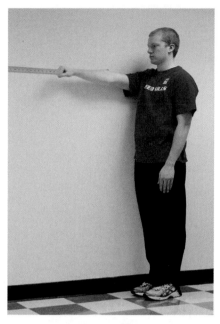

Fig. 5-32: Initial positioning for the Functional Reach Test.

Fugl-Meyer Sensorimotor Assessment of Balance Performance Battery

This tool is designed as a subset of the Fugl-Meyer Physical Performance Battery and is designed to assess balance specifically for patients with hemiplegia. Each of the seven items assessed is scored from 0-2, specific to each item with the maximum score being 14. Even though a 14 is the best score that a person can receive, the patient still may not have normal balance.

Functional Reach Test (Figs. 5-32, 5-33)

A single task screening tool used to assess standing balance and risk of falling. A person is required to stand upright with a static base of support. A yardstick is positioned to measure the forward distance that a patient can reach without moving the feet. Three trials are performed and averaged together.

The following are age-related standard measurements for functional reach:

20 - 40 years: 14.5 - 17 inches

41 - 69 years: 13.5 - 15 inches

70 - 87 years: 10.5 - 13.5 inches

A patient that falls below the age appropriate range for functional reach has an increased risk for falling. The outcome measure demonstrates high test-retest correlation and intrarater reliability.

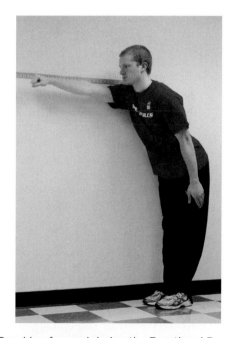

Fig. 5-33: Reaching forward during the Functional Reach Test.

Romberg Test

This is an assessment tool of balance and ataxia that initially positions the patient in unsupported standing, feet together, upper extremities folded, looking at a fixed point straight ahead with eyes open. With the eyes open, three sensory systems (visual, vestibular, somatosensory) provide input to the cerebellum to maintain standing stability. If there is a mild lesion in the vestibular or somatosensory systems, the patient will typically compensate through the visual sense.

Next the patient maintains the same standing posture, but closes the eyes (Fig. 5-34). A patient receives a grade of "normal" if they are able to maintain the position for 30 seconds. An abnormal response occurs with the inability to maintain balance when standing erect with the feet together and the eyes closed. Patients may exhibit excessive sway or begin to fall. When the visual input is removed, instability will be present if there is a larger somatosensory or vestibular deficit producing the instability. If a patient demonstrates ataxia and has a positive Romberg test, this indicates sensory ataxia and not cerebellar ataxia.

There is also a Sharpened Romberg test where the patient's balance is further assessed by performing in the same manner but with a heel-to-toe stance, typically with the non-dominant foot in front. The patient would first be tested with eyes open (Fig. 5-35) and then with eyes closed. This modification increases the challenge to the vestibular and somatosensory systems.

Timed Get Up and Go Test

This is a functional performance screening tool used to assess a person's level of mobility and balance. The person initially sits in a supported chair with a firm surface, transfers to a standing position, and walks approximately 10 feet. The patient must then turn around without external support, walk back towards the chair, and return to a sitting position. The patient is scored based on amount of postural sway, excessive movements, reaching for support, side stepping or other signs of loss of balance. The 5-point ordinal rating scale designates a score of one as normal and a score of five as severely abnormal. In an attempt to increase overall reliability the use of time was implemented. Patients who are independent can complete the multi-task process in 10 seconds or less. Patients that require over 20 seconds to complete the process are at the limit for functional independence and may be at an increased risk for falling. Patients that require 30 seconds are at a high risk for a fall.

Tinetti Performance Oriented Mobility Assessment

A tool used to screen patients and identify if there is an increased risk for falling. The first section assesses balance through sit to stand and stand to sit from an armless chair, immediate standing balance with eyes open and closed, tolerating a slight push in the standing position, and turning 360 degrees. A patient is scored from 0-2 in most categories with a maximum score of 16. The second section assesses gait at normal speed and at a rapid, but safe speed. Items scored in this section include initiation of gait, step length and height, step asymmetry and continuity, path, stance during gait, and trunk motion. A patient is scored 0-2 for each with a maximum

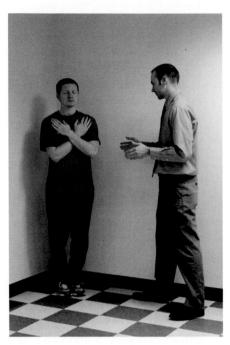

Fig. 5-34: Romberg testing for postural sway with eyes closed.

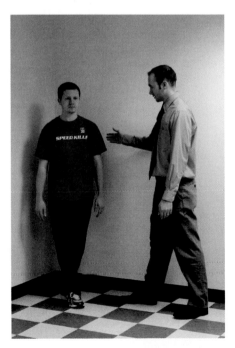

Fig. 5-35: Testing using the sharpened Romberg for postural sway with eyes open.

score of 12. The tool has a combined maximum total of 28 with the risk of falling increasing as the total score decreases. A total score less than 19 indicates a high risk for a fall.

Vestibular Rehabilitation

Vestibular rehabilitation is a therapeutic intervention that can be highly successful for patients with vestibular or central balance system disorders. Exercise protocols for vestibular retraining utilize compensation, adaptation, and plasticity to increase the brain's sensitivity, restore symmetry, improve vestibuloocular control, and subsequently increase motor control and movement.

Goals for Vestibular Rehabilitation

- Improve balance
- Improve trunk stability
- Increase strength and range of motion in order to improve musculoskeletal balance responses and strategies
- Decrease the rate and risk of falls
- Minimize dizziness

Vestibuloocular Retraining Therapeutic Guidelines

- Vestibuloocular reflex (VOR) and vestibulospinal reflex (VSR) stimulation exercises
- Ocular motor exercises
- Balance exercises
- Gait exercises
- Combination exercises (obstacle courses, functioning in a public place)
- Habituation training exercises (use only with appropriate patients)
- Individualize each program based on the patient's specific impairments (rehabilitation versus compensation training)
- Use of practice, feedback, and repetition are vital for skill refinement
- Use of gravity, varying surface conditions, visual conditions, and environmental cues should be included in therapeutic planning
- The center of gravity must be controlled at each stage of treatment
- Strategy (hip, ankle, stepping, suspense) training should be implemented during treatment so that strategies become automatic responses
- Force plate systems, electromyographic biofeedback, optokinetic visual stimulation, and videography are all technical systems that can provide feedback to motor learning during vestibular rehabilitation
- Foam, mirrors, rocker boards, BAPS boards, Swiss balls, foam rollers, trampolines, and wedges are lower "tech" treatment tools that are successfully used for vestibular rehabilitation

Communication Disorders

Aphasia[1]

Aphasia is an acquired neurological impairment of processing for receptive and/or expressive language. Aphasia is the result of brain injury, head trauma, CVA, tumor or infection. Diagnosis is based on the site of lesion in the brain and the blood vessels involved. Patients with aphasia are classified based on observation of fluent or non-fluent aphasia. Approximately 95% of right-handed persons and 66% of left-handed persons are left hemisphere dominant for language.

Prognosis is dependent on the individual patient, location, and extent of the lesion. Typically, the more sudden the onset of damage, as in the case of an acute CVA, the higher extent of aphasia can be expected. The following characteristics associated with aphasia are often associated with a poor prognosis: perseveration of speech, severe auditory comprehension impairments, unreliable yes/no answers, and the use of empty speech without recognition of impairments.

Fluent Aphasia[5,9,31]

- Lesion varies based on the type of fluent aphasia but frequently involves the temporal lobe, Wernicke's area or regions of the parietal lobe
- Word output and speech production are functional
- Prosody is acceptable, but empty speech/jargon
- Speech lacks any substance, use of paraphasias
- Use of neologisms (substitution within a word that is so severe it makes the word unrecognizable)

Non-fluent Aphasia[5,9,31]

- Lesion varies based on the type of non-fluent aphasia, but frequently the frontal lobe (anterior speech center) of the dominant hemisphere is affected
- Poor word output and dysprosodic speech (impairment in the rhythm and inflection of speech)
- Poor articulation and increased effort for speech
- Content is present, but impaired syntactical words

Types of Fluent Aphasia[5,9,31]

Wernicke's Aphasia

- Lesion: posterior region of superior temporal gyrus
- Also known as "receptive aphasia"
- Comprehension (reading/auditory) impaired
- Good articulation, use of paraphasias
- Impaired writing
- Poor naming ability
- Motor impairment not typical due to the distance from Wernicke's area to the motor cortex

Types of Non-fluent Aphasia[5,9,31]

Broca's Aphasia

- Lesion: 3rd convolution of frontal lobe
- Also known as "expressive aphasia"
- Most common form of aphasia
- Intact auditory and reading comprehension
- Impaired repetition and naming skills
- Frustration with language skill errors
- Paraphasias are common
- Motor impairment typical due to proximity of Broca's area to the motor cortex

Global Aphasia

- Lesion: frontal, temporal, parietal lobes
- Comprehension (reading/auditory) is severely impaired
- Impaired naming, writing, repetition skills
- May involuntarily verbalize, usually without correct context
- May use nonverbal skills for communication

Dysarthria[1]

Dysarthria is a motor disorder of speech that is caused by an upper motor neuron lesion that affects the muscles that are used to articulate words and sounds. Speech is often noted as "slurred" and there may also be an effect on respiratory or phonatory systems due to the weakness.

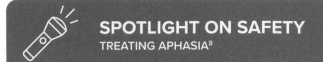

SPOTLIGHT ON SAFETY
TREATING APHASIA[8]

Treating a patient with aphasia typically requires a physical therapist and/or physical therapist assistant to alter the traditional methods of treatment in order to enhance communication and provide a safe and comfortable environment for the patient. The PT/PTA may want to co-treat or consult with the speech pathologist to establish the best means of communication with the patient. The following may be considered when treating a patient that presents with aphasia:

- Cueing strategies must avoid verbal input and use tactile and visual cues.
- Attempt to have only one person speak to the patient at a time. Extra noise and multiple voices will only confuse the patient.
- Use concise sentences and yes/no questioning for ease of understanding and response.
- Allow the patient adequate time to process and respond before progressing with treatment.
- Allow for ample time for communication during treatment. If communication is rushed, this can decrease the effectiveness of the therapy session. The patient may also become frustrated with feeling pressure to respond.
- Attempt to allow the patient to perform an activity or segment of therapy without repetitive feedback.

Medical Procedures/Testing for Neurological Dysfunction[32]

Procedure/Test	Rationale
Cerebral angiography	A cerebral angiogram is an invasive procedure that can determine the narrowing or blockage of an artery within the brain. This can be used when diagnosing a potential CVA, brain tumor, aneurysm or vascular malformation. The catheter is threaded up through the body into an artery within the neck and contrast dye is released into the bloodstream. A series of x-rays is then taken.
Computed tomography (CT scan)	Brain scan imaging is typically non-invasive and provides cross sections of the area tested with precise two dimensional views of bones, tissues, and organs. Dyes or contrast are occasionally used to provide the best view of any pathology that may exist within the tissues. A CT scan of the brain or spinal cord is required to rule out vascular malformations, tumors, cysts, herniated disks, hemorrhage, epilepsy, encephalitis, spinal stenosis, intracranial bleeding, and head injury.

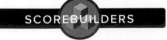

Procedure/Test	Rationale
Discography	Invasive procedure to evaluate the integrity and pathology of a spinal disk. Contrast dye is injected and CT scanning is performed in order to better assess suspected damaged areas of intervertebral disks.
Electroencephalography (EEG)	Non-invasive procedure that can continuously measure electrical activity of the brain using multiple electrodes attached to the skull. Baseline electrical activity is determined, and then various stimuli are presented and brain waves are analyzed. An EEG is used to rule out seizure disorders, brain death, brain tumors, brain damage, inflammation, alcoholism, select psychiatric disorders, and degenerative disorders that affect the brain.
Electromyography (EMG)	Invasive procedure that is used to assess nerve and muscle dysfunction or spinal cord disease. EMG records the electrical activity from the brain or spinal cord to the peripheral nerve root being tested. An EMG is used to rule out muscle pathology, nerve pathology, spinal cord disease, denervated muscle, and lower motor neuron injury.
Evoked potentials	Non-invasive procedure using two sets of electrodes that records the time it takes for an impulse to reach the brain. External stimuli (auditory, visual, proprioceptive) are used to evoke electrical potentials within the brain. This is used to rule out multiple sclerosis, brain tumor, acoustic neuroma (small tumors of the inner ear), and spinal cord injury.
Magnetic resonance imaging (MRI)	Brain scan imaging that is typically non-invasive and provides detailed images including tissues, organs, bones, and nerves. A contrast dye may be used to enhance imaging of certain tissues. The MRI is used to rule out tumors of the brain or spinal cord, multiple sclerosis, and head trauma.
Myelography	Invasive procedure of the spinal canal using contrast dye and x-ray imaging. The procedure has a high risk for headache following the spinal tap, but is used to rule out potential abnormalities surrounding the subarachnoid space, spinal nerve injury, herniated disks, fractures, back or leg pathology, and spinal tumors.
Nerve conduction velocity (NCV)	Non-invasive stimulation of a peripheral nerve to determine the nerve action potentials and the nerve's ability to send a signal. NCV rules out peripheral neuropathies, carpal tunnel syndrome, demyelination pathology, and peripheral nerve compression.
Positron emission tomography (PET)	Brain scan imaging that provides two and three-dimensional pictures of brain activity and is used to rule out cerebral circulatory pathology, metabolism dysfunction, tumors, blood flow, and brain changes following injury or drug abuse.
Spinal puncture (lumbar)	Invasive procedure that inserts a needle through lumbar puncture below the level of L1-L2 for cerebral spinal fluid sample. This procedure is most commonly performed at the L3-L4 level. A spinal puncture primarily rules out hemorrhage, inflammation, infection, meningitis, and tumor.

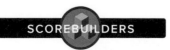

Pharmacology - Neuromuscular Management[13,33]

Antiepileptic Agents

Action: Antiepileptic agents reduce or eliminate seizure activity within the brain.

Indications: seizure activity (partial seizures, generalized seizures, unclassified seizures)

Side effects: (agent dependent) ataxia, skin issues, behavioral changes, gastrointestinal distress, headache, blurred vision, weight gain

Implications for PT: Therapists must have adequate knowledge of established protocols for responding to a seizure as well as potential side effects of antiepileptic medications. Patients with epilepsy may show greater sensitivity to environmental surroundings such as light or noise level.

Examples: Dilantin, Tegretol

Antispasticity Agents

Action: Antispasticity agents promote relaxation in a spastic muscle. Spasticity is an exaggerated stretch reflex of the muscle that can occur after injury to the CNS. Spasticity is not a primary condition, but a secondary effect from CNS damage.

Indications: increased tone, spasticity, spinal cord injury, CVA, multiple sclerosis

Side effects: drowsiness, confusion, headache, dizziness, generalized muscle weakness, hepatotoxicity potential with Dantrium, tolerance, dependence

Implications for PT: Therapists must balance the need to decrease spastic muscles with the loss of function that a patient may experience with the reduction of hypertonicity. Once spasticity is reduced, therapists should focus on therapeutic handling techniques, facilitation, and strengthening to promote overall mobility. Sedation may also alter the scheduling of therapy to allow for maximal participation.

Examples: Baclofen, Dantrium

Dopamine Replacement Agents

Action: Dopamine replacement agents assist to relieve the symptoms of Parkinson's disease secondary to the decrease in endogenous dopamine. These agents are able to cross the blood-brain barrier through active transport and transform to dopamine within the brain.

Indications: Parkinson's disease, Parkinsonism

Side effects: arrhythmias (levodopa), gastrointestinal distress, orthostatic hypotension, dyskinesias, mood and behavioral changes, tolerance

Implications for PT: Therapists and patients attain maximal benefit from scheduling therapy one hour after administration of levodopa. Therapists must understand the debilitating effects of drug holidays and should monitor the patient's blood pressure frequently due to the potential for orthostatic hypotension.

Examples: Sinemet, Madopar

Muscle Relaxant Agents

Action: Muscle relaxant agents promote relaxation in muscles that typically present with spasm that is a continuous, tonic contraction. Spasms typically occur secondary to a musculoskeletal or peripheral nerve injury rather than CNS injury.

Indications: muscle spasm

Side effects: (agent dependent) sedation, drowsiness, dizziness, nausea, vomiting, headache, tolerance, dependence

Implications for PT: Therapists must be aware of potential side effects, however, maximize the potential for relaxation through therapeutic techniques and the use of modalities during treatment. Prevention of reinjury through stretching, posture retraining, and education should assist the patient to achieve desired outcomes.

Examples: Valium, Flexeril

Neuromuscular and Nervous Systems Pathology

Alzheimer's Disease[1,6,24]

Alzheimer's disease is a progressive neurodegenerative disorder that results in deterioration and irreversible damage within the cerebral cortex and subcortical areas of the brain. Neurons that are normally involved with acetylcholine transmission deteriorate within the cerebral cortex. Development of amyloid plaques and neurofibrillary tangles result in further damage to the nervous system.

Etiology – The exact etiology of Alzheimer's disease is unknown, however, hypothesized causes include lower levels of neurotransmitters, higher levels of aluminum within brain tissue, genetic inheritance, autoimmune disease, abnormal processing of the substance amyloid, and virus. The risk of developing Alzheimer's disease increases with age and there is a higher incidence in women.

Signs and symptoms – Alzheimer's disease is initially noted by a change in higher cortical functions such as difficulty with new learning and subtle changes in memory and concentration. Progression includes a loss of orientation, word finding difficulties, depression, poor judgment, rigidity, bradykinesia, shuffling gait, and impaired ability to perform self-care skills. End-stage disease includes severe intellectual and physical destruction, incontinence, functional dependence, and an inability to speak.

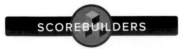

Treatment – There is no curative treatment for the disease process. Medications are administered to inhibit acetylcholinesterase, alleviate cognitive symptoms, and control behavioral changes. Physical therapy management should focus on maximizing the patient's remaining function and providing family and caregiver education. Many patients require a long-term Alzheimer's care facility secondary to personality changes, aggressive behavior, and end-stage complications.

Amyotrophic Lateral Sclerosis[1,13]

Amyotrophic lateral sclerosis (ALS) is a chronic degenerative disease that produces both upper and lower motor neuron impairments. Significant loss of anterior horn cells in the spinal cord and the motor cranial nerve nuclei in lower brainstem produces weakness and muscle atrophy. Demyelination of corticospinal and corticobulbar tracts produce the upper motor neuron symptoms. The rapid degeneration causes denervation of muscle fibers, muscle atrophy, and weakness.

Etiology – The exact etiology of ALS is unknown (90% of all cases), however, theories include genetic inheritance, virus, metabolic disturbances, and toxicity of lead and aluminum. There is a higher incidence in men and the disease typically begins between 40 to 70 years of age.

Signs and symptoms – Early clinical presentation of ALS may include both upper and lower motor neuron involvement. Lower motor neuron signs include asymmetric muscle weakness, fasciculations, cramping, and atrophy within the hands. Weakness spreads in a distal to proximal path. Upper motor neuron symptoms can include incoordination of movement, spasticity, clonus, and a positive Babinski reflex. A patient with ALS will exhibit fatigue, oral motor impairment, motor paralysis, and eventual respiratory paralysis.

Treatment – Effective management of ALS is based on supportive care and symptomatic therapy. Pharmacological intervention may include riluzole (Rilutek). Physical, occupational, speech, respiratory, and nutritional therapies may be warranted with the focus on quality of life and caregiver training.

Bell's Palsy[13]

Bell's palsy is a temporary unilateral facial paralysis secondary to trauma with demyelination and/or axonal degeneration of the facial nerve. This is a common clinical condition with the highest incidence in individuals between 15 and 45 years of age.

Etiology – The exact etiology of Bell's palsy is unclear, however, the condition may be secondary to a viral infection, specifically the herpes simplex/herpes zoster virus. Inflammation and subsequent pressure injure the nerve with varying degrees of damage. The inflammation within the auditory canal produces subsequent demyelination of the nerve and if ischemia occurs, there is axonal degeneration of the nerve.

Signs and symptoms – A patient with Bell's palsy will present with an asymmetrical facial appearance with "drooping" of the eyelid and mouth, potential for drooling, dryness of the eye, and inability to close the eyelid due to weakness.

Treatment – The sooner the person is diagnosed and treated, the better the outcome. Some patients have very mild involvement and their symptoms typically resolve within two weeks' time without formal medical intervention. In cases with greater severity, the patient may be treated with anti-viral medications along with high-dose corticosteroids. Physical therapy may be indicated for stimulation of the facial nerve, facial massage and/or exercise, depending on the degree of injury.

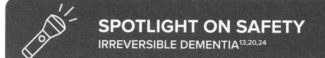

SPOTLIGHT ON SAFETY
IRREVERSIBLE DEMENTIA[13,20,24]

A therapist must be aware of each patient's medical history and level of orientation prior to treatment. This is achieved through screening of cognition, memory, and judgment regardless of the primary diagnosis. Certain pathologies can cause irreversible dementia including:

Degenerative pathology: Alzheimer's disease, Huntington's disease, multiple sclerosis

Infectious pathology: tuberculosis, AIDS

Vascular pathology: CVA, anoxia, arteriovenous malformation, multi-infarct dementia

Miscellaneous conditions at risk for dementia: head injury, hydrocephalus, toxins, alcoholism

A therapist should modify the plan of care in order to ensure that the therapeutic goals are achieved and the patient remains safe. In early stages of dementia, patients will typically attempt to conceal their shortcomings and this can significantly compromise patient safety. Thorough assessment for at-risk patients will minimize safety risks.

Carpal Tunnel Syndrome[13,20]

Carpal tunnel syndrome (CTS) is a peripheral nerve entrapment injury that occurs as a result of compression of the median nerve where it passes through the carpal tunnel. Normal tissue pressure within the tunnel is approximately 2 to 10 mm Hg, but CTS can result in pressure greater than 30 mm Hg with the wrist at rest which produces ischemia within the nerve. This results in sensory and motor disturbances in the median nerve distribution of the hand.

Etiology – The exact etiology of CTS is unclear, however, associated conditions that contribute to CTS include repetitive use, rheumatoid arthritis, pregnancy, diabetes, cumulative trauma disorders, tumor, hypothyroidism, and wrist sprain or fracture.

Signs and symptoms – A patient with CTS will initially present with sensory changes and paresthesia along the median nerve distribution in the hand. It may also radiate into the upper extremity, shoulder, and neck. Symptoms include night pain, weakness of the hand, muscle atrophy, decreased grip strength, clumsiness, and decreased wrist mobility.

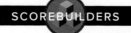

Treatment – There is no universally accepted treatment of CTS, however, typically a patient with CTS will initially receive conservative management including splinting, ergonomic measures, local corticosteroid injections, and physical therapy management. Severe cases may require surgical release of the carpal tunnel.

Cerebellar Disorders[1,13,24]

Cerebellar disorders have numerous etiologies and present differently based on etiology and location of the lesion within the cerebellum.

Etiology – Etiologies vary and include congenital malformations, hereditary ataxias, and genetic and acquired conditions.

- **Congenital malformations** manifest early in life and are non-progressive. Manifestations vary depending on the structures involved; ataxia is usually present.
- **Hereditary ataxias** may be autosomal recessive or autosomal dominant. The most common autosomal recessive ataxia is Friedreich's ataxia. Friedreich's ataxia results from a gene mutation causing abnormal repetition of the DNA sequence and ultimately, impaired mitochondrial function. Gait unsteadiness begins early in life and it is followed by upper extremity ataxia, dysarthria, and paresis. Mental function declines and slight tremors may be seen. Reflexes, vibration, and position senses are impaired.
- **Spinocerebellar ataxias** are the main autosomal dominant ataxias. Manifestations vary with many forms affecting multiple areas in the central and peripheral nervous systems. They commonly present with neuropathy, pyramidal signs, ataxia, and restless leg syndrome.
- **Acquired ataxias** may result from nonhereditary neurodegenerative systemic disorders, toxin exposure or can be idiopathic. Systemic disorders include alcoholism, hypothyroidism, and vitamin E deficiency. Toxins include carbon monoxide, heavy metals, and lithium.

Signs and symptoms – Signs and symptoms vary based on etiology, but typically include ataxia.

Treatment – Treatment is diagnosis dependent and typically supportive unless it is acquired and/or reversible. Some systemic disorders such as hypothyroidism and toxin exposure can be treated; surgical intervention may be appropriate for structural lesions (tumor, hydrocephalus), however, the majority of treatment is typically supportive.

Diabetic Neuropathy[13,34]

Diabetic neuropathy is a complication and direct effect of diabetes mellitus. Nerve ischemia results from microvascular disease combined with the direct effects of hyperglycemia on neurons resulting in the impairment of nerve function. There are many forms including cranial neuropathies, radiculopathies, and mononeuropathies. The most common include symmetric polyneuropathy and autonomic neuropathy.

Etiology – The primary etiology is the diagnosis of diabetes mellitus. Continued research attempts to understand the cause and effect of prolonged exposure to high blood glucose and its exact impact on nerve function. There are multiple factors that lead to all forms of diabetic neuropathy including metabolic factors, high blood glucose, duration of diabetes, neurovascular factors, impairment with transport of oxygen and nutrients to the nerves, autoimmune factors, inflammation in nerves, inherited traits, and the impact of environmental and lifestyle choices such as alcohol and smoking.

Signs and symptoms – Symptoms vary depending on the form of diabetic neuropathy, but typically weakness and sensory disturbances occur distally in a symmetrical pattern. Initial symptoms typically include tingling, numbness or pain, especially in the feet. Symptoms can involve the sensory, motor or autonomic systems. Additional symptoms may include wasting of muscles in the feet or hands, "stocking-glove" sensory distribution impairments, orthostatic hypotension, weakness, urinary impairments, and significant pain.

Treatment – Patients require strict monitoring of blood glucose levels to prevent further nerve pathology. Physical therapy is typically indicated to address the various symptoms including pain management, foot care, and overall fitness. Pharmacological intervention may also be warranted.

Epilepsy[13,27,34]

Epilepsy is a chronic condition where there is temporary dysfunction of the brain that results in hypersynchronous electrical discharge of cortical neurons and seizure activity that is typically unprovoked and unpredictable. A seizure is a transient event that is a symptom of interrupted brain functioning. A seizure is the hallmark sign of epilepsy, however, one seizure does not signal epilepsy.

Etiology – There are various classifications of seizures, however, many cases are idiopathic. Other associated conditions that increase risk of epilepsy include genetic influence, head trauma, dementia, CVA, cerebral palsy, Down syndrome, and autism.

Signs and symptoms – Seizure symptoms vary, depending on type and extent of the seizure. Loss of awareness or consciousness and disturbances of movement, sensation, mood or mental function may occur.

Treatment – Many patients require antiepileptic medication to manage seizures, however, there is no current medical treatment to "cure" epilepsy. Initiating antiepileptic medication is a serious decision since side effects can produce a variety of adverse effects. Surgical intervention is sometimes warranted when pharmacological management has failed and there is a high disruption of the quality of the person's life.

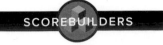

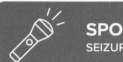

SPOTLIGHT ON SAFETY
SEIZURES: BEFORE, DURING, AND AFTER[13,27]

Epilepsy is responsible for the majority of seizures. There are various classifications of seizures including partial, generalized, and unclassified; seizures that can be simple or complex (unimpaired versus impaired consciousness), and convulsive versus nonconvulsive. Regardless of the form of seizure, a therapist should be aware of the potential course of the seizure in order to provide safe emergency treatment.

A prodromal period is rare, but can occur days or hours prior to a seizure and may include mood changes, lightheadedness, sleep disturbances, irritability, and difficulty concentrating. An aura will briefly occur within minutes before a complex partial or generalized tonic-clonic seizure. The aura is actually a simple partial seizure and produces symptoms that alert the person that something is about to happen. Symptoms vary but can include restlessness, nervousness, anxiety, heaviness, and a general feeling that something within the body is not quite right.

The therapist should consider the following when attempting to manage a person that is having a seizure:

- Stay calm and prevent injury
- Remove all objects surrounding the person to ensure that there is nothing that could harm the person during the seizure
- Maintain awareness of the length of time of the seizure
- Ensure that the person is as comfortable as possible
- Do not allow other people near the person in an effort to keep the individual isolated
- Consider your safety and do not hold the person down; there is no need for restraint if the person is thrashing during the seizure
- Avoid placing anything into the person's mouth (the person is not capable of swallowing their tongue)
- Avoid providing any water, food or medicine until the person is fully alert
- Be prepared to call 911 if the seizure lasts longer than five minutes

After the seizure is over, place the person on their left side to avoid choking in case the person vomits. The person should remain in this position until they are fully alert. The therapist should stay with the person until they have recovered which typically takes five to twenty minutes. Therapists should be aware of patients that are at-risk for seizure activity in order to avoid any unnecessary safety risks.

Guillain-Barre Syndrome[13,24]

Guillain-Barre syndrome (GBS), or acute polyneuropathy, is a temporary inflammation and demyelination of the peripheral nerves' myelin sheaths, potentially resulting in axonal degeneration. The autoantibodies of GBS attack segments of the myelin sheath of the peripheral nerves. GBS can occur at any age, however, there is a peak in frequency in the young adult population and again in adults that are between their fifth and eighth decades.

Etiology – The exact etiology of GBS is unknown, however, it is hypothesized to be an autoimmune response to a previous respiratory infection, influenza, immunization or surgery. Viral infections, Epstein-Barr syndrome, cytomegalovirus, bacterial infections, surgery, and vaccinations have been associated with the development of GBS.

Signs and symptoms – GBS results in motor weakness in a distal to proximal progression, sensory impairment, and possible respiratory paralysis. A patient with GBS will initially present with distal symmetrical motor weakness, mild distal sensory impairments, and transient paresthesias that progress towards the upper extremities and head. The level of disability usually peaks within two to four weeks after onset. Muscle and respiratory paralysis, absence of deep tendon reflexes, and the inability to speak or swallow may also occur. GBS can be life-threatening with respiratory involvement.

Treatment – Medical management of a patient with GBS typically requires hospitalization for treatment of symptoms. Pharmacological intervention often includes immunosuppressive and analgesic/narcotic medications. Cardiac monitoring, plasmapheresis, and mechanical ventilation may be required. Physical, occupational, and speech therapies are typically indicated. Physical therapy may include pulmonary rehabilitation, strengthening, mobility training, wheelchair and orthotic prescription and/or assistive device training. Intervention and rate of progression are dependent on the ultimate level of disability from GBS.

Huntington's Disease[13,20]

Huntington's disease (HD), also known as Huntington's chorea, is a neurological disorder of the CNS and is characterized by degeneration and atrophy of the basal ganglia and cerebral cortex within the brain. The neurotransmitters become deficient and are unable to modulate movement.

Etiology – HD is genetically transmitted as an autosomal dominant trait. The disease is usually perpetuated by a person that has children prior to diagnosis. The average age for developing symptoms is between 35 and 55 years, however, symptoms can develop at any age.

Signs and symptoms – HD is a movement disorder that includes affective dysfunction and cognitive impairment. The patient may present with involuntary choreic movements, mild alteration in personality, grimacing, protrusion of the tongue, and ataxia with choreoathetoid movements. Late stage HD includes mental deterioration, decrease in IQ, depression, dysphagia, incontinence, immobility, and rigidity.

Treatment – Medical management of HD requires genetic, psychological, and social counseling for the patient and family. Pharmacological management is initiated once choreiform movement impairs a patient's functional capacity. Physical therapy should maximize endurance, strength, balance, postural control, and functional mobility.

Multiple Sclerosis[13,20,24]

Multiple sclerosis (MS) produces patches of demyelination of the myelin sheaths that surround nerves within the brain and spinal cord. This decreases the efficiency of nerve impulse transmission and symptoms will vary based on the location and the extent of demyelination. There is subsequent plaque development and eventual failure of impulse transmission.

Etiology – The exact etiology of MS is unknown. Genetics, viral infections, and environment all have a role in the development of MS. It is theorized that a slow-acting virus initiates the autoimmune response in individuals that have environmental and genetic factors associated with the disease. MS can occur at any age with the highest incidence between 20-35 years of age.

Signs and symptoms – Symptoms vary based on the type of disease, location, extent of demyelination, and degree of sclerosis. Initial symptoms include visual problems, paresthesias and sensory changes, clumsiness, weakness, ataxia, balance dysfunction, and fatigue. The clinical course usually consists of periods of exacerbations and remissions, with the degree of neurologic dysfunction and subsequent recovery following typical patterns related to the specific type of MS. The frequency and intensity of exacerbations may indicate the speed/course of the disease process.

Treatment – Management of MS includes pharmacological, medical, and therapeutic interventions. The goal is to lessen the length of exacerbations and maximize the health of the patient. Pharmacological intervention is indicated along with physical, occupational, and speech therapies throughout the disease process. Nutritional and psychological counseling are also important components of medical management. Physical therapy intervention includes regulation of activity level, relaxation and energy conservation techniques, normalization of tone, balance and gait training, core stabilization, and adaptive/assistive device training.

Myasthenia Gravis[13,20,24]

Myasthenia gravis is an autoimmune disease resulting in neuromuscular junction pathology. There is a defect specifically in the transmission of nerve impulses to the muscles at the neuromuscular junction. Antibodies block or destroy the receptors that are needed for acetylcholine uptake and this prevents muscle contraction.

Etiology – This is an autoimmune disease process that also has an association with an enlarged thymus. There is also an association with diabetes, rheumatoid arthritis, lupus, and other immune disorders. There are multiple forms of myasthenia gravis that range from mild to severe involvement.

Signs and symptoms – The cardinal signs of myasthenia gravis include extreme fatiguability and skeletal muscle weakness that can fluctuate within minutes or over an extended period. The ocular muscles are typically affected first and approximately half of the patients experience ptosis and diplopia. Dysphagia, dysarthria, and cranial nerve weakness are also common findings.

Treatment – The disease process of myasthenia gravis will fluctuate and a patient will experience remissions and exacerbations. A myasthenia gravis "crisis" is a medical emergency where there is an exacerbation that includes the respiratory muscles and requires a ventilator. Anticholinesterase drug therapy, plasmapheresis, and immunosuppressive therapy may be utilized. Physical and occupational therapies are also indicated intermittently with supportive goals. Physical therapy will typically focus on obtaining a respiratory baseline and pulmonary intervention as needed. Energy conservation techniques and strengthening using isometric contractions are appropriate for most patients. Since patients typically require long-term corticosteroids, physical therapy may also focus on secondary osteoporosis.

Parkinson's Disease[13,20,24]

Parkinson's disease is a primary degenerative disorder and is characterized by a decrease in production of dopamine (neurotransmitter) within the substantia nigra of the basal ganglia. The basal ganglia store the majority of dopamine and are responsible for modulation and control of voluntary movement.

Etiology – Primary Parkinson's disease has an unknown etiology and accounts for the majority of patients with Parkinsonism. Contributing factors that can produce symptoms of Parkinson's disease include genetic defect, toxicity from carbon monoxide, excessive manganese or copper, carbon disulfide, vascular impairment of the striatum, encephalitis, and other neurodegenerative diseases such as Huntington's disease or Alzheimer's disease. The majority of patients are between 50 and 79 years of age and approximately 10% are diagnosed before 40 years.

Signs and symptoms – The majority of patients with Parkinson's disease will initially notice a resting tremor in the hands (sometimes called a pill-rolling tremor) or feet that increases with stress and disappears with movement or sleep. Early symptoms can include balance disturbances, difficulty rolling over and rising from bed, and impairment with fine manipulative movements seen in writing, bathing, and dressing. Progression of the disease process includes hypokinesia, sluggish movement, difficulty with initiating (akinesia) and stopping movement, festinating and shuffling gait, bradykinesia, poor posture, dysphagia, and "cogwheel" or "lead pipe" rigidity of skeletal muscles. Patients may also experience "freezing" during ambulation, speech, blinking, and movements of the arms. A patient with Parkinson's disease may also have a mask-like appearance with no facial expression.

Treatment – The medical management of Parkinson's disease relies heavily on pharmacological intervention. Dopamine replacement therapy is most effective in reducing movement disorders, bradykinesia, rigidity, and tremor. Physical, occupational, and speech therapies may be warranted intermittently throughout the course of the disease. Physical therapy intervention should include maximizing endurance, strength, and functional mobility. Verbal cueing and visual feedback are also effective tools to use with this population.

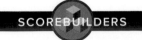

Post-polio Syndrome (PPS)[13]

Poliomyelitis is a viral infection resulting in neuropathy that includes focal and asymmetrical motor impairments. In the United States, this virus was all but eradicated in the 1960s with the development of a vaccine. Post-polio syndrome is a lower motor neuron pathology that affects the anterior horn cells of those previously affected with polio. Surviving axons were originally able to increase the size of their innervation ratio to assist denervated muscle. PPS occurs when the compensated reinnervation fails and results in ongoing muscle denervation.

Etiology – A previous diagnosis of polio is essential to diagnose PPS. Approximately 25-50% of persons with polio experience PPS decades after their initial recovery (average interval is approximately 25 years).

Signs and symptoms – Symptoms vary, however, commonly there is slow and progressive weakness, fatigue, muscle atrophy, pain, and swallowing issues.

Treatment – There is no pharmacological intervention to alter the progression of PPS. Emphasis of treatment surrounds life-style modification and symptomatic intervention. Physical therapy should emphasize supervised exercise, functional independence, adaptive equipment, and education to assist patients to maintain as much independence as possible.

Cerebrovascular Accident

A cerebrovascular accident is a specific event that results in a lack of oxygen supply to a specific area of the brain secondary to either ischemia or hemorrhage. The outcome of a CVA greatly varies and is based on etiology, extent of the CVA, the area of the brain that is affected, subsequent collateral damage, and the patient's co-morbidities and overall health status.

SPOTLIGHT ON SAFETY
RISK FACTORS FOR CEREBROVASCULAR ACCIDENT[13,20,24]

There are a number of primary and secondary risk factors that can lead to the development of a CVA. Patient education regarding risk factors and impairments secondary to CVA should be included in all treatment plans for patients that are at increased risk. Many risk factors are modifiable and can be altered to improve a patient's risk profile and overall health.

Primary	Secondary
Hypertension	Obesity
Cardiac disease or arrhythmias	High cholesterol
Diabetes mellitus	Behaviors related to hypertension (i.e., stress, excessive salt intake)
Cigarette smoking	Physical inactivity
Transient ischemic attacks	Increased alcohol consumption

Types of Cerebrovascular Accidents[13,20,24]

Transient Ischemic Attack (TIA)

A transient ischemic attack is usually linked to an atherosclerotic thrombosis which causes a temporary interruption of blood supply to an area of the brain. The effects may be similar to a CVA, but symptoms resolve quickly, typically within 24 to 48 hours. A TIA most often occurs in the carotid and vertebrobasilar arteries and may indicate future CVA.

Completed Stroke

A CVA that presents with total neurological deficits at the onset.

Stroke in Evolution

A CVA, usually caused by a thrombus that gradually progresses. Total neurological deficits are not seen for one to two days after onset.

Ischemic Stroke

Once there is a loss of perfusion to a portion of the brain (within just seconds), there is a central area of irreversible infarction surrounded by an area of potential ischemia.

- **Embolus (20% of ischemic CVAs)**

  Associated with cardiovascular disease, an embolus may be a solid, liquid or gas, and can originate in any part of the body. The embolus travels through the bloodstream to the cerebral arteries causing occlusion of a blood vessel and a resultant infarct. The middle cerebral artery is most commonly affected by an embolus from the internal carotid arteries. Due to the sudden onset of occlusion, tissues distal to the infarct can sustain higher permanent damage than those of thrombotic infarcts. An embolic CVA occurs rapidly with no warning, and often presents with a headache. Common cardiac disorders that can lead to embolism include valvular disease (i.e., rheumatic mitral stenosis), ischemic heart disease, acute myocardial infarction, arrhythmias (i.e., atrial fibrillation), patent foramen ovale, cardiac tumors, and post cardiac catheterization.

- **Thrombus**

  An atherosclerotic plaque develops in an artery and eventually occludes the artery or a branching artery causing an infarct. This type of CVA is extremely variable in onset where symptoms can appear in minutes or over several days. A thrombotic CVA usually occurs during sleep or upon awakening after a myocardial infarction or post-surgical procedure.

Hemorrhage (10 - 15% of CVAs)

Hemorrhage is an abnormal bleeding in the brain due to a rupture in blood supply. The infarct is due to disruption of oxygen to an area of the brain and compression from the accumulation of blood. Hypertension is usually a precipitating factor causing rupture of an aneurysm or arteriovenous malformation. Trauma can also precipitate hemorrhage and subsequent CVA. Characteristics include severe headache, vomiting, high blood pressure, and an abrupt onset of symptoms. Hemorrhage usually occurs during the day with symptoms evolving in relation to the speed of the bleed. Approximately 50% of deaths from hemorrhagic stroke occur within the first 48 hours.

Characteristics of a Cerebrovascular Accident[1,2,30]

Left Hemisphere	Right Hemisphere	Brainstem	Cerebellum
Weakness, paralysis of the right side	Weakness, paralysis of the left side	Unstable vital signs	Decreased balance
Increased frustration	Decreased attention span	Decreased consciousness	Ataxia
Decreased processing	Left hemianopsia	Decreased ability to swallow	Decreased coordination
Possible aphasia (expressive, receptive, global)	Decreased awareness and judgment	Weakness on both sides of the body	Nausea
Possible dysphagia	Memory deficits	Paralysis on both sides of the body	Decreased ability for postural adjustment
Possible motor apraxia (ideomotor and ideational)	Left inattention		Nystagmus
Decreased discrimination between left and right	Decreased abstract reasoning		
Right hemianopsia	Emotional lability		
	Impulsive behaviors		
	Decreased spatial orientation		

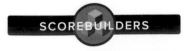

Synergy Patterns[35]

When the central nervous system is damaged as with a CVA, the higher centers of the brain are also damaged. The higher centers are responsible for both complex motor patterns and the inhibition of massive gross motor patterns. Synergy patterns result when the higher centers of the brain lose control and the uncontrolled or partially controlled stereotyped patterns of the middle and lower centers emerge.

Upper Limb

	Flexor Synergy	Extensor Synergy
Scapula	Elevation and retraction	Depression and protraction
Shoulder	Abduction and lateral rotation	Medial rotation and adduction
Elbow	Flexion	Extension
Forearm	Supination	Pronation
Wrist	Flexion	Extension
Fingers	Flexion with adduction	Flexion with adduction
Thumb	Flexion and adduction	Flexion and adduction

- The flexor synergy is seen when the patient attempts to lift up their arm or reach for an object.

Lower Limb

	Flexor Synergy	Extensor Synergy
Hip	Abduction and lateral rotation	Extension, medial rotation and adduction
Knee	Flexion	Extension
Ankle	Dorsiflexion with supination	Plantar flexion with inversion
Toes	Extension	Flexion and adduction

- The flexor synergy is characterized by great toe extension and flexion of the remaining toes secondary to spasticity.

Neurological Rehabilitation

Neurological rehabilitation may incorporate a variety of treatments based on the patient's pathology, problem list, and deficits. There are many forms of neurological rehabilitation based on each construct's beliefs regarding motor control and motor learning. A therapist must use therapeutic techniques that meet the individual patient's therapeutic objectives and goals. The following are various theories of neurological rehabilitation based on each theory's interpretation of motor control and motor learning.

Motor Control[28,30]

Motor control is the study of the nature of movement; or the ability to regulate or direct essential movement. Historically, control was thought to arise from reflex or hierarchical models where the cortex was perceived as the highest functioning component of the system and spinal level reflexes were the lowest functioning components. New models of motor control challenge these theories and believe that there is a greater distribution of control and that the cortex is not solely at the top of the hierarchy.

Motor Learning[28,36]

Motor learning is the study of the acquisition or modification of movement. Motor learning differentiates learning versus performance, provides guidelines for appropriate use of feedback, prioritizes the impact of practice as it relates to skill and movement, and also focuses on the transfer of learning across tasks and environments of practice.

Three Stage Model of Motor Learning[7,26,36]

Cognitive Stage: This is the initial stage of learning where there is a high concentration of conscious processing of information. The person will acquire information regarding the goal of the activity and begin to problem solve as to how to attain the goal. A controlled environment is ideal for learning during this stage and participation is a must for the person to progress.

Characterized by:
- large amount of errors
- inconsistent attempts
- repetition of effort allows for improvement in strategies
- inconsistent performance
- high degree of cognitive work: listening, observing, and processing feedback

Associative Stage: This is the intermediate stage of learning where a person is able to more independently distinguish correct versus incorrect performance. The person is linking the feedback that has been received with the movement that has been performed and the ultimate goal. A controlled environment is helpful but at this stage, the person can progress to a less structured or more open environment. Avoid excessive external feedback as the person should have improved internal or proprioceptive feedback for the task at hand.

Characterized by:
- decreased errors with new skill performance

- decreased need for concentration and cognition regarding the activity
- skill refinement
- increased coordination of movement
- large amount of practice yields refinement of the motor program surrounding the activity

Autonomous Stage: This is the final stage of learning or skilled learning where a person improves the efficiency of the activity without a great need for cognitive control. The person can also perform the task with interference from a variable environment.

Characterized by:
- automatic response
- mainly error-free regardless of environment
- patterns of movement are non-cognitive and automatic
- distraction does not impact the activity
- the person can simultaneously perform more than one task if needed
- extrinsic feedback should be very limited or should not be provided
- internal feedback or self-assessment should be dominant

Feedback[36]

Feedback is imperative for the progression of motor learning. A patient will rely on both intrinsic and extrinsic feedback as it relates to movement. Feedback allows for correction and adaptation within the environment. Current research supports reducing the extrinsic feedback (fading of feedback) in order to ultimately enhance learning.

Intrinsic (inherent) feedback: represents all feedback that comes to the person through sensory systems as a result of the movement including visual, vestibular, proprioceptive, and somatosensory inputs.

Extrinsic (augmented) feedback: represents the information that can be provided while a task or movement is in progress or subsequent to the movement. This is typically in the form of verbal feedback or manual contacts.

Knowledge of results: is an important form of extrinsic feedback and includes terminal feedback regarding the outcome of a movement that has been performed in relation to the movement's goals.

Knowledge of performance: is extrinsic feedback that relates to the actual movement pattern that someone used to achieve their goal of movement.

Practice[36]

Practice refers to repeated performance of an activity in order to learn or perfect a skill. Physical practice allows for direct physical experience and kinesthetic stimulation to assist with acquisition of the skill. Mental practice is the cognitive rehearsal of a task or experience without any physical movement.

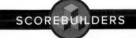

There are several commonly used terms that describe various types of practice:

Massed practice: The practice time in a trial is greater than the amount of rest between trials.

Distributed practice: The amount of rest time between trials is equal to or is greater than the amount of practice time for each trial.

Constant practice: Practice of a given task under a uniform condition.

Variable practice: Practice of a given task under differing conditions.

Random practice: Varying practice amongst different tasks.

Blocked practice: Consistent practice of a single task.

Whole training: Practice of an entire task.

Part training: Practice of an individual component or selected components of a task.

Key Terminology[28,36]

Closed system model: This is characterized by transfer of information that incorporates multiple feedback loops and larger distribution of control. In this model, the nervous system is seen as an active "participant" with the ability to enable the initiation of movement as opposed to solely "reacting" to stimuli.

Compensation: The ability to utilize alternate motor and sensory strategies due to an impairment that limits the normal completion of a task.

Habituation: The decrease in response that will occur as a result of consistent exposure to non-painful stimuli.

Learning: The process of acquiring knowledge about the world that leads to a relatively permanent change in a person's capability to perform a skilled action.

- **Non-associative:** a single repeated stimulus (habituation, sensitization)
- **Associative:** gaining understanding of the relationship between two stimuli, causal relationships or stimulus and consequence (classical conditioning, operant conditioning)
- **Procedural:** learning tasks that can be performed without attention or concentration to the task; a task is learned by forming movement habits (developing a habit through repetitive practice)
- **Declarative:** requires attention, awareness, and reflection in order to attain knowledge that can be consciously recalled (mental practice)

Motor learning: The ability to perform a movement as a result of internal processes that interact with the environment and produce a consistent strategy to generate the correct movement. It is the acquisition of, or modification of movement.

Motor program: A concept of a central motor pattern that can be activated by sensory stimuli or central processes. Motor programs are seen as containing the rules for creating spatial and temporal patterns of motor activity needed to carry out a given motor task.

Open system model: This is characterized by a single transfer of information without any feedback loop (reflexive hierarchical theory). In this theory, the nervous system is seen as awaiting stimuli in order to react.

CONSIDER THIS
MOTOR LEARNING INTERVENTION CONSTRUCTS[28,30,36]

The following are general concepts of motor learning that should be considered when evaluating, developing a plan of care, and treating patients. Many therapists will utilize therapeutic interventions from various theories of neurological rehabilitation based on the individual patient.

- Models of motor control vary based on the interpretation of brain function
- Examination determines the degree of impairment
- Intervention is designed at the level of impairment
- It is essential for a patient to relearn how to perform a functional task in order to maximize recovery and independence
- Sensory, motor, and cognitive strategies should be used to acquire postural control
- Focus is both on recovery and compensatory techniques
- Belief that sensory, motor, and perceptual input contribute to motor control
- Movement is based around a behavioral goal
- Type and amount of feedback (visual, verbal, tactile) should be determined for each individual patient
- Emphasis on postural control, alignment, and sequencing of movements is essential
- Intervention should create multiple ways to solve a movement disorder
- Belief that performance is observed, the act of learning is not
- Environmental factors must be considered with intervention, planning, and implementation

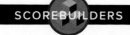

Performance: A temporary change in motor behavior seen during a particular session of practice that is a result of many variables, however, only one variable is focusing on the act of learning. Performance is not an absolute measure of learning since there are multiple variables that potentially affect performance.

Plasticity: The ability to modify or change at the synapse level either temporarily or permanently in order to perform a particular function.

Postural control: The ability of the motor and sensory systems to stabilize position and control movement.

Recovery: The ability to utilize previous strategies to return to the same level of functioning.

Sensitization: The increase in response that will occur as a result of a noxious stimulus.

Strategy: A plan used to produce a specific result or outcome that will influence the structure or system.

CONSIDER THIS
MOTOR RELEARNING INTERVENTION CONSTRUCTS[37,38]

The following are general concepts of motor relearning that should be considered when evaluating, developing a plan of care, and treating patients. Many therapists will utilize therapeutic interventions from various theories of neurological rehabilitation based on the individual patient.

- Utilizes various techniques from other treatment approaches
- Belief that treatment cannot be routine or based on diagnosis, must be individual to the patient
- Developmental sequence may not be necessary in treatment when treating adults
- Practice may include breaking the task into discrete components, followed by practice of the task as a whole
- Use of Bobath techniques for handling, facilitation, inhibitive casting, use of therapeutic ball (Figs. 5-36, 5-37)
- Use of Rood techniques of application of ice, brushing, tapping for facilitation
- Biofeedback should be utilized for decreasing hypertonicity with movement or for targeting facilitation of a muscle group
- Self-correction and self-awareness should be incorporated into treatment through the use of a mirror, verbal feedback, and biofeedback
- Intrinsic and extrinsic (augmented) feedback are important during treatment

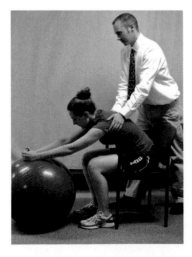

Fig. 5-36: Facilitation of movement patterns using a therapeutic ball.

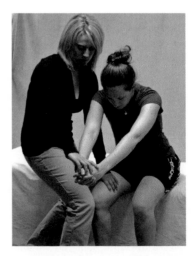

Fig. 5-37: Therapist uses handling techniques and facilitation to assist with functional activities.

Bobath: Neuro-Developmental Treatment (NDT)[30,39]

An approach developed by Karl and Berta Bobath based on the hierarchical model of neurophysiologic function. Abnormal postural reflex activity and abnormal muscle tone are caused by the loss of central nervous system control at the brainstem and spinal cord levels. The concept recognizes that interference of normal function within the brain caused by central nervous system dysfunction leads to a slowing down or cessation of motor development and the inhibition of righting reactions, equilibrium reactions, and automatic movements. The patient should learn to control movement through activities that promote normal movement patterns that integrate function.

New assumptions that have been incorporated into NDT resulting from current motor control research include:[28]

- Postural control can be learned and modified through experience
- Postural control uses both feedback and feed-forward mechanisms for execution of tasks
- Postural control is initiated from a patient's base of support
- Postural control is required for skill development
- Postural control develops by assuming progressive positions in which there is an increase in the distance between the center of gravity and base of support; the base of support should also decrease

Key Terminology

Facilitation: A technique utilized to elicit voluntary muscular contraction.

Inhibition: A technique utilized to decrease excessive tone or movement.

Key points of control: Specific handling of designated areas of the body (shoulder, pelvis, hand, and foot) will influence and facilitate posture, alignment, and control (Fig. 5-38).

Placing: The act of moving an extremity into a position that the patient must hold against gravity.

Reflex inhibiting posture: Designated static positions that Bobath found to inhibit abnormal tonal influences and reflexes.

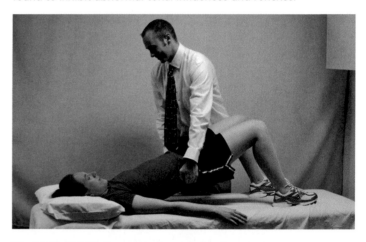

Fig. 5-38: Facilitation using key points of control.

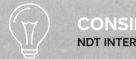

CONSIDER THIS
NDT INTERVENTION CONSTRUCTS[30,39]

The following are general concepts of NDT that should be considered when evaluating, developing a plan of care, and treating patients. Many therapists will utilize therapeutic interventions from various theories of neurological rehabilitation based on the individual patient.

- Inhibition of abnormal patterns of movement with simultaneous facilitation of normal patterns
- Alteration of abnormal tone and influencing isolated active movement
- Avoid utilization of abnormal reflexes or associated reactions during treatment
- Utilize manual contact and handling through key points of control for facilitation and inhibition (Fig. 5-39)
- Achieve a balance between muscle groups during therapeutic interventions
- Utilize the developmental sequence, dynamic reflex inhibiting patterns, and functional activities with varying levels of difficulty during therapeutic intervention
- Emphasize the use of rotation during treatment activities (Fig. 5-40)
- Provide the patient with the sensation of normal movement by inhibiting abnormal postural reflex activity
- Treatment should be active and dynamic, incorporating function
- Provide orientation to midline control by moving in and out of midline with dynamic activity (Fig. 5-41)
- Belief that compensation techniques are unnecessary and should be avoided

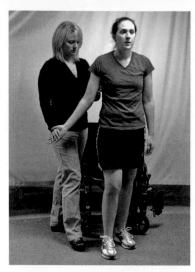

Fig. 5-39: The therapist uses an NDT technique of manual contacts and therapeutic handling to decrease tonal influence during motor output and functional activity. Key points of control can facilitate or inhibit tone based on the therapeutic goals.

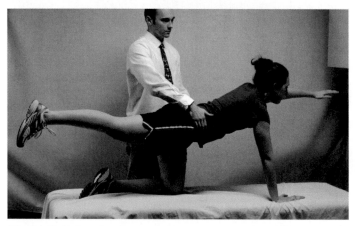

Fig. 5-41: Using developmental sequence to gain midline control. The therapist can facilitate the patient to move in and out of midline to improve dynamic mobility and control.

Brunnstrom: Movement Therapy in Hemiplegia[24,40,41]

Movement therapy in hemiplegia developed by Signe Brunnstrom is based on the hierarchical model by Hughlings Jackson. This approach created and defined the term synergy and initially encouraged the use of synergy patterns during rehabilitation. The belief was to immediately practice synergy patterns and subsequently develop combinations of movement patterns outside of the synergy. Synergies are considered primitive patterns that occur at the spinal cord level as a result of the hierarchical organization of the central nervous system. Reinforcing synergy patterns is rarely utilized now as research has indicated that reinforced synergy patterns are very difficult to change. Brunnstrom developed the seven stages of recovery, which are used for evaluation and documentation of patient progress.

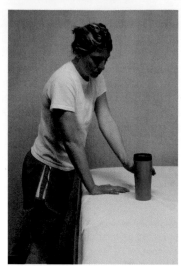

Fig. 5-40: NDT encourages the use of rotation during therapeutic activities.

Key Terminology

Associated reaction: An involuntary and automatic movement of a body part as a result of an intentional active or resistive movement in another body part.

Homolateral synkinesis: A flexion pattern of the involved upper extremity facilitates flexion of the involved lower extremity.

Limb synergies: A group of muscles that produce a predictable pattern of movement in flexion or extension patterns.

Raimiste's phenomenon: The involved lower extremity will abduct or adduct with applied resistance to the uninvolved lower extremity in the same direction.

Souques' phenomenon: Raising the involved upper extremity above 100 degrees with elbow extension will produce extension and abduction of the fingers.

Stages of recovery: Brunnstrom separates neurological recovery into seven separate stages based on progression through abnormal tone and spasticity. These seven stages of recovery describe tone, reflex activity, and volitional movement.

Seven Stages of Recovery[28]

Stage 1: No volitional movement initiated.

Stage 2: The appearance of basic limb synergies. The beginning of spasticity.

Stage 3: The synergies are performed voluntarily; spasticity increases.

Stage 4: Spasticity begins to decrease. Movement patterns are not dictated solely by limb synergies.

Stage 5: A further decrease in spasticity is noted with independence from limb synergy patterns.

Stage 6: Isolated joint movements are performed with coordination.

Stage 7: Normal motor function is restored.

CONSIDER THIS
MOVEMENT THERAPY IN HEMIPLEGIA INTERVENTION CONSTRUCTS[28,41]

The following are general concepts of movement therapy in hemiplegia that should be considered when evaluating, developing a plan of care, and treating patients. Many therapists will utilize therapeutic interventions from various theories of neurological rehabilitation based on the individual patient.

- Evaluation of strength focuses on patterns of movement rather than straight plane motion at a joint

- Sensory examination is required to assist with treating motor deficits

- Initially limb synergies are encouraged as a necessary milestone for recovery

- Encourage overflow to recruit active movement of the weak side

- Repetition of task and positive reinforcement should be emphasized during treatment activities

- A patient will follow the stages of recovery, but may experience a plateau at any point so that full recovery may not be achieved

- Movement combinations that deviate from the basic limb synergies should be introduced in stage 4 of recovery

- Treatment should incorporate only tasks that the patient can master or almost master

Kabat, Knott, and Voss: Proprioceptive Neuromuscular Facilitation (PNF)[30,40]

PNF was introduced in the early 1950's using the hierarchical model as its framework. The original goal of treatment was to establish gross motor patterns within the central nervous system. This approach is based on the premise that stronger parts of the body are utilized to stimulate and strengthen the weaker parts. Normal movement and posture is based on a balance between control of antagonist and agonist muscle groups. Development will follow the normal sequence through a component of motor learning. This theory places great emphasis on manual contacts and correct handling. Short and concise verbal commands are used along with resistance throughout the full movement pattern. The PNF approach utilizes methods that promote or hasten the response of the neuromuscular mechanism through stimulation of the proprioceptors. Movement patterns follow diagonals or spirals that each possess a flexion, extension, and rotatory component and are directed toward or away from midline.

Key Terminology

Chopping: A combination of bilateral upper extremity asymmetrical patterns performed as a closed-chain activity (Fig. 5-42).

Developmental sequence: A progression of motor skill acquisition. The stages of motor control include mobility, stability, controlled mobility, and skill.

Mass movement patterns: The hip, knee, and ankle move into flexion or extension simultaneously.

Overflow: Muscle activation of an involved extremity due to intense action of an uninvolved muscle or group of muscles.

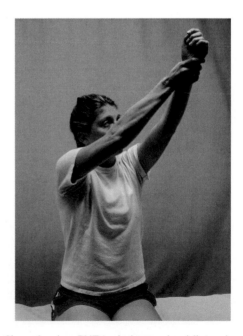

Fig. 5-42: Chopping is a PNF technique using bilateral upper extremity patterns of movement to improve strength, stability, and control.

CONSIDER THIS
PNF INTERVENTION CONSTRUCTS (KABAT, KNOTT, VOSS)[30,40]

The following are general concepts of PNF that should be considered when evaluating, developing a plan of care, and treating patients. Many therapists will utilize therapeutic interventions from various theories of neurological rehabilitation based on the individual patient.

- A patient learns diagonal patterns of movement

- Techniques must have accurate timing, specific commands, and correct hand placement

- Verbal commands must be short and concise

- Repetition of task or activity is important in motor learning

- Resistance given during the movement pattern is greater if the objective is stability (Fig. 5-43), less if the objective is mobility (Fig. 5-44)

- Techniques should utilize isometric and isotonic muscle contractions

- Treatment objectives will dictate the use of techniques through either full movement or at points within the range

- Developmental sequence is used in conjunction with PNF techniques in order to increase the balance between agonists and antagonists

- PNF techniques are implemented to progress a patient through the stages of motor control

- Functional patterns of movement are used to increase control

- Techniques should be utilized that increase strength or improve relaxation by enhancing overflow from the stronger to the weaker muscles

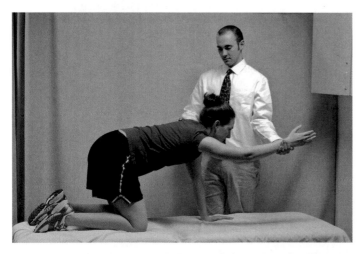

Fig. 5-43: A therapist can provide a graded amount of resistance based on therapeutic goals. This patient is working through the developmental sequence and the therapist is providing a larger amount of resistance to improve stability with a varying base of support.

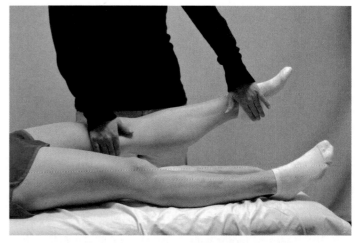

Fig. 5-44: The therapist is using minimal resistance during a lower extremity PNF pattern to improve mobility and active movement.

PNF Diagonal Patterns – Upper Extremity Responses

	D1 Flexion Pattern (Fig. 5-45)	D1 Extension Pattern	D2 Flexion Pattern	D2 Extension Pattern
Scapula	Elevation Abduction Upward rotation	Depression Adduction Downward rotation	Elevation Adduction Upward rotation	Depression Abduction Downward rotation
Shoulder	Flexion Adduction Lateral rotation	Extension Abduction Medial rotation	Flexion Abduction Lateral rotation	Extension Adduction Medial rotation
Elbow	Flexion or extension	Flexion or extension	Flexion or extension	Flexion or extension
Radioulnar	Supination	Pronation	Supination	Pronation
Wrist	Flexion Radial deviation	Extension Ulnar deviation	Extension Radial deviation	Flexion Ulnar deviation
Thumb	Adduction	Abduction	Extension	Opposition

PNF Diagonal Patterns – Lower Extremity Responses

	D1 Flexion Pattern	D1 Extension Pattern	D2 Flexion Pattern (Fig. 5-46)	D2 Extension Pattern
Pelvis	Protraction	Retraction	Elevation	Depression
Hip	Flexion Adduction Lateral rotation	Extension Abduction Medial rotation	Flexion Abduction Medial rotation	Extension Adduction Lateral rotation
Knee	Flexion or extension	Flexion or extension	Flexion or extension	Flexion or extension
Ankle and Toes	Dorsiflexion Inversion	Plantar flexion Eversion	Dorsiflexion Eversion	Plantar flexion Inversion

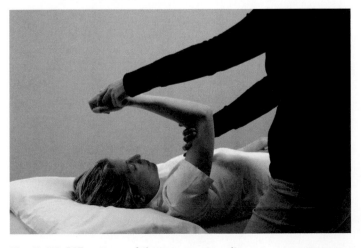

Fig. 5-45: D1F pattern of the upper extremity.

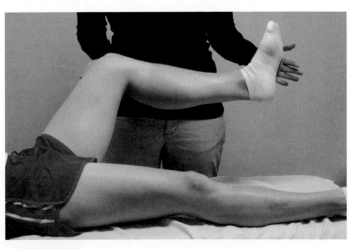

Fig. 5-46: D2F pattern of the lower extremity.

Levels of Motor Control[40]

Mobility

The ability to initiate movement through a functional range of motion.

Stability

The ability to maintain a position or posture through cocontraction and tonic holding around a joint. Unsupported sitting with midline control is an example of stability.

Controlled Mobility

The ability to move within a weight bearing position or rotate around a long axis. Activities in prone on elbows or weight shifting in quadruped are examples of controlled mobility (Fig. 5-47).

Skill

The ability to consistently perform functional tasks and manipulate the environment with normal postural reflex mechanisms and balance reactions. Skill activities include ADLs and community locomotion.

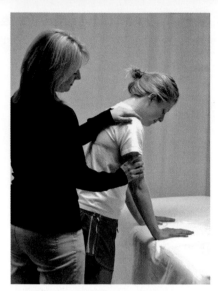

Fig. 5-47: The patient working in modified plantigrade is an example of controlled mobility.

PNF Therapeutic Exercises

Technique	Mobility		Stability	Controlled Mobility	Skill		Strength
	Increased ROM	Initiate Movement			Distal Functional Movement	Proximal Dynamic Stability	
Agonistic Reversals				X		X	
Alternating Isometrics			X				X
Contract-Relax	X						
Hold-Relax	X						
Hold-Relax Active Movement		X					
Joint Distraction	X	X					
Normal Timing					X		
Repeated Contractions		X					X
Resisted Progression						X	X
Rhythmic Initiation		X					
Rhythmical Rotation	X	X					
Rhythmic Stabilization	X		X				
Slow Reversal			X	X	X		
Slow Reversal Hold			X	X	X		
Timing for Emphasis					X		X

PNF Therapeutic Exercise Descriptions

*Blue colored terms indicate the level of developmental sequence.

Agonistic Reversals (AR)

Controlled mobility, skill: An isotonic concentric contraction performed against resistance followed by alternating concentric and eccentric contractions with resistance. AR requires use in a slow and sequential manner, and may be used in increments throughout the range to attain maximum control.

Alternating Isometrics (AI)

Stability: Isometric contractions are performed alternating from muscles on one side of the joint to the other side without rest. AI emphasizes endurance or strengthening.

Contract-Relax (CR)

Mobility: A technique used to increase range of motion. As the extremity reaches the point of limitation, the patient performs a maximal contraction of the antagonistic muscle group. The therapist resists movement for eight to ten seconds with relaxation to follow. The technique is repeated until no further gains in range of motion are noted during the session.

Hold-Relax (HR)

Mobility: An isometric contraction used to increase range of motion. The contraction is facilitated for all muscle groups at the limiting point in the range of motion. Relaxation occurs and the extremity moves through the newly acquired range to the next point of limitation until no further increases in range of motion occur. The technique is often used for patients that present with pain.

Hold-Relax Active Movement (HRAM)

Mobility: A technique to improve initiation of movement to muscle groups tested at 1/5 or less. An isometric contraction is performed once the extremity is passively placed into a shortened range within the pattern. Overflow and facilitation may be used to assist with the contraction. Upon relaxation, the extremity is immediately moved into a lengthened position of the pattern with a quick stretch. The patient is asked to return the extremity to the shortened position through an isotonic contraction.

Joint Distraction

Mobility: A proprioceptive component used to increase range of motion around a joint. Consistent manual traction is provided slowly and usually in combination with mobilization techniques. It can also be used in combination with quick stretch to initiate movement.

Normal Timing (NT)

Skill: A technique used to improve coordination of all components of a task. NT is performed in a distal to proximal sequence. Proximal components are restricted until the distal components are activated and initiate movement. Repetition of the pattern produces a coordinated movement of all components.

Repeated Contractions (RC)

Mobility: A technique used to initiate movement and sustain a contraction through the range of motion. RC is used to initiate a movement pattern, throughout a weak movement pattern or at a point of weakness within a movement pattern. The therapist provides a quick stretch followed by isometric or isotonic contractions.

Resisted Progression (RP)

Skill: A technique used to emphasize coordination of proximal components during gait. Resistance is applied to an area such as the pelvis, hips or extremity during the gait cycle in order to enhance coordination, strength or endurance.

Rhythmic Initiation (RI)

Mobility: A technique used to assist in initiating movement when hypertonia exists. Movement progresses from passive ("let me move you"), to active assistive ("help me move you"), to slightly resistive ("move against the resistance"). Movements must be slow and rhythmical to reduce the hypertonia and allow for full range of motion.

Rhythmic Stabilization (RS)

Mobility, stability: A technique used to increase range of motion and coordinate isometric contractions. The technique requires isometric contractions of all muscles around a joint against progressive resistance. The patient should relax and move into the newly acquired range and repeat the technique. If stability is the goal, RS should be applied as a progression from AI in order to stabilize all muscle groups simultaneously around the specific body part.

Rhythmical Rotation (RR)

Mobility: A passive technique used to decrease hypertonia by slowly rotating an extremity around the longitudinal axis. Relaxation of the extremity will increase range of motion.

Slow Reversal (SR)

Stability, controlled mobility, skill: A technique of slow and resisted concentric contractions of agonists and antagonists around a joint without rest between reversals. This technique is used to improve control of movement and posture.

Slow Reversal Hold (SRH)

Stability, controlled mobility, skill: Using slow reversal with the addition of an isometric contraction that is performed at the end of each movement in order to gain stability.

Timing for Emphasis (TE)

Skill: Used to strengthen the weak component of a motor pattern. Isotonic and isometric contractions produce overflow to weak muscles.

Rood[28,30]

This theory is based on Sherrington and the reflex stimulus model. Rood believed that all motor output was the result of both past and present sensory input. Treatment is based on sensorimotor learning. It takes into account the autonomic nervous system and emotional factors as well as motor ability. Rood used a developmental sequence, which was seen as "key patterns" in the enhancement of motor control. A goal of this approach is to obtain homeostasis in motor output and to activate muscles to perform a task independent of a stimulus. Exercise is seen as a treatment technique only if the response is correct and if it provides sensory feedback that enhances the motor learning of that response. Once a response is obtained during treatment, the stimulus should be withdrawn. Rood introduced the use of sensory stimulation to facilitate or inhibit responses such as icing and brushing in order to elicit desired reflex motor responses.

Sensory Stimulation Techniques

Facilitation	Inhibition
• Approximation (Fig. 5-48) • Joint compression • Icing • Light touch • Quick stretch • Resistance • Tapping • Traction	• Deep pressure • Prolonged stretch • Warmth • Prolonged cold

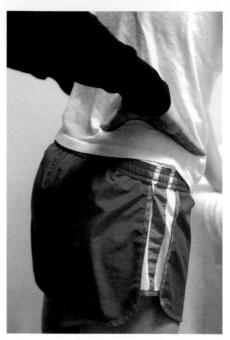

Fig. 5-48: The therapist is providing approximation to the hips while the patient is in standing in order to improve cocontraction around the joint and subsequent stability.

Key Terminology

Heavy work: A method used to develop stability by performing an activity (work) against gravity or resistance. Heavy work focuses on the strengthening of postural muscles.

Light work: A method used to develop controlled movement and skilled function by performing an activity (work) without resistance. Light work focuses on the extremities.

Key patterns: A developmental sequence designed by Rood that directs patients' mobility recovery from synergy patterns through controlled motion.

CONSIDER THIS
ROOD SENSORY INTERVENTION CONSTRUCTS[28,30]

The following are general concepts of Rood that should be considered when evaluating, developing a plan of care, and treating patients. Many therapists will utilize therapeutic interventions from various theories of neurological rehabilitation based on the individual patient.

- Utilization of sensory stimulation to achieve motor output during treatment
- Movement is considered autonomic and noncognitive
- Homeostasis of all systems is essential
- Techniques such as neutral warmth, maintained pressure, and slow rhythmical stroking can be used to calm a patient
- Tactile stimulation is used to facilitate normal movement
- The environment can influence the effects of therapeutic intervention
- Exercise must provide proper sensory feedback in order to be therapeutic
- Belief in techniques used to stimulate the proprioceptive, exteroceptive, and vestibular channels of the central nervous system

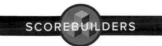

Neuromuscular and Nervous Systems Terminology[1,2,3,27]

Agnosia: The inability to interpret information.

Agraphesthesia: The inability to recognize symbols, letters or numbers traced on the skin.

Agraphia: The inability to write due to a lesion within the brain and is typically found in combination with aphasia.

Anosognosia: The denial or unawareness of one's illness; often associated with unilateral neglect.

Aphasia: The inability to communicate or comprehend due to damage to specific areas of the brain.

Apraxia: The inability to perform purposeful learned movements or activities even though there is no sensory or motor impairment that would hinder completion of the task.

Astereognosis: The inability to recognize objects by sense of touch.

Body schema: Having an understanding of the body as a whole and the relationship of its parts to the whole.

Constructional apraxia: The inability to reproduce geometric figures and designs. A person is often unable to visually analyze how to perform a task.

Decerebrate rigidity: A characteristic of a corticospinal lesion at the level of the brainstem that results in extension of the trunk and all extremities (Fig. 5-49).

Decorticate rigidity: A characteristic of a corticospinal lesion at the level of the diencephalon where the trunk and lower extremities are positioned in extension and the upper extremities are positioned in flexion (Fig. 5-50).

Diplopia: Double vision.

Dysarthria: Slurred and impaired speech due to a motor deficit of the tongue or other muscles essential for speech.

Dysphagia: The inability to properly swallow.

Dysprosody: Impairment in the rhythm and inflection of speech.

Emotional lability: A characteristic of a right hemisphere infarct where there is an inability to control emotions and outbursts of laughing or crying that are inconsistent with the situation.

Fluent aphasia: Characteristic of receptive aphasia where speech produces functional output regarding articulation, but lacks content and is typically dysprosodic using neologistic jargon.

Hemiparesis: A condition of weakness on one side of the body.

Hemiplegia: A condition of paralysis on one side of the body.

Homonymous hemianopsia: The loss of the right or left half of the field of vision in both eyes.

Ideational apraxia: The inability to formulate an initial motor plan and sequence tasks where the proprioceptive input necessary for movement is impaired.

Ideomotor apraxia: A condition where a person plans a movement or task, but cannot volitionally perform it. Automatic movement may occur, however, a person cannot impose additional movement on command.

Non-fluent aphasia: Characteristic of expressive aphasia where speech is non-functional, effortful, and contains paraphasias. Writing is also impaired.

Nystagmus: An abnormal eye movement that entails nonvolitional, rhythmic oscillation of the eyes. The speed of movement is typically faster in one direction and its origins is congenital or acquired.

Perseveration: The state of repeatedly performing the same segment of a task or repeatedly saying the same word/phrase without purpose.

Synergy: Mass movement patterns that are primitive in nature and coupled with spasticity due to brain damage.

Unilateral neglect: The inability to interpret stimuli and events on the contralateral side of a hemispheric lesion. Left-sided neglect is most common with a lesion to the right inferior parietal or superior temporal lobes.

Vertigo: The sensation of movement and rotation of oneself or the surrounding environment. Vertigo may have a peripheral or central origin.

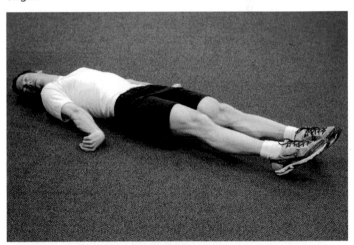

Fig. 5-49: Decerebrate positioning.

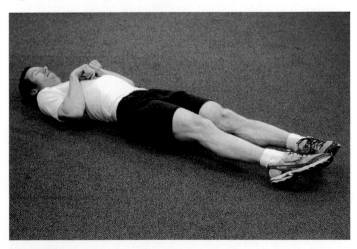

Fig. 5-50: Decorticate positioning.

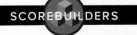

Spinal Cord Injury (SCI)

When there is sufficient force exerted on the spinal cord, there can be permanent damage with extensive neurological deficits. There are approximately 250,000 people in the United States today with traumatic spinal cord injuries. Motor vehicle accidents are the largest cause of traumatic SCI. Other etiologies include stabbing, falls, sports injuries, and high-risk behaviors. The mechanism of injury often dictates the predicted pattern of deficits. Flexion injuries occur most often at the C5-C6 level of the spine while extension injuries occur most at the C4-C5 level. Axial loading and rotatory injuries are other mechanisms for spinal cord damage. A spinal cord injury will have an area of primary damage followed by an area of secondary damage that can extend multiple spinal segments beyond the initial segment of injury.

Types of Spinal Cord Injury[18,19,24]

Complete lesion: A lesion to the spinal cord where there is no preserved motor or sensory function below the level of the lesion.

Incomplete lesion: A lesion to the spinal cord with incomplete damage to the cord. There may be scattered motor function, sensory function or both below the level of the lesion.

Specific Incomplete Lesions[18,19,24]

Anterior Cord Syndrome

An incomplete lesion that results from compression and damage to the anterior part of the spinal cord or anterior spinal artery. The mechanism of injury is usually cervical flexion. There is loss of motor function and pain and temperature sense below the lesion due to damage of the corticospinal and spinothalamic tracts.

Brown-Sequard's Syndrome

An incomplete lesion usually caused by a stab wound, which produces hemisection of the spinal cord. There is paralysis and loss of vibratory and position sense on the same side as the lesion due to the damage to the corticospinal tract and dorsal columns. There is a loss of pain and temperature sense on the opposite side of the lesion from damage to the lateral spinothalamic tract. Pure Brown-Sequard's syndrome is rare since most spinal cord lesions are atypical.

Cauda Equina Injuries

An injury that occurs below the L1 spinal level where the long nerve roots transcend. Cauda equina injuries can be complete, however, they are frequently incomplete due to the large number of nerve roots in the area. A cauda equina injury is considered a peripheral nerve injury. Characteristics include flaccidity, areflexia, and impairment of bowel and bladder function. Full recovery is not typical due to the distance needed for axonal regeneration.

Central Cord Syndrome

An incomplete lesion that results from compression and damage to the central portion of the spinal cord. The mechanism of injury is usually cervical hyperextension that damages the spinothalamic tract, corticospinal tract, and dorsal columns. The upper extremities present with greater involvement than the lower extremities and greater motor deficits exist as compared to sensory deficits.

Posterior Cord Syndrome

A relatively rare syndrome that is caused by compression of the posterior spinal artery and is characterized by loss of proprioception, two-point discrimination, and stereognosis. Motor function is preserved.

Spinal Cord Injury Tests and Measures

ASIA Impairment Scale (American Spinal Injury Association)[42]

A =	**Complete:** No sensory or motor function is preserved in sacral segments S4-S5.
B =	**Sensory Incomplete:** Sensory but not motor function is preserved below the neurologic level and extends through sacral segments S4-S5.
C =	**Motor Incomplete:** Motor function is preserved below the neurologic level, and most key muscles below the neurologic level have a muscle grade less than 3.
D =	**Motor Incomplete:** Motor function is preserved below the neurologic level, and most key muscles below the neurologic level have a muscle grade greater than or equal to 3.
E =	**Normal:** Sensory and motor functions are normal.

Classification of Level of Injury

Motor level: The motor level is determined by the most caudal key muscles that have muscle strength of 3 or greater with the superior segment tested as normal or 5.

Motor index scoring: Testing each key muscle using the 0-5 scoring, with total points of 25 per extremity for the total possible score of 100.

Sensory level: The sensory level is determined by the most caudal dermatome with a normal score of 2/2 for pinprick and light touch.

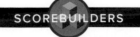

Key Muscles Tested

C5	Elbow flexors (biceps, brachialis)
C6	Wrist extensors (extensor carpi radialis longus and brevis)
C7	Elbow extensors (triceps)
C8	Finger flexors (flexor digitorum profundus) to the middle finger
T1	Small finger abductors (abductor digiti minimi)
L2	Hip flexors (iliopsoas)
L3	Knee extensors (quadriceps)
L4	Ankle dorsiflexors (tibialis anterior)
L5	Long toe extensors (extensor hallucis longus)
S1	Ankle plantar flexors (gastrocnemius, soleus)

Potential Complications of Spinal Cord Injury[18,19,24]

Deep Vein Thrombosis (DVT)

Deep vein thrombosis results from the formation of a blood clot that becomes dislodged and is termed an embolus. This is considered a serious medical condition since the embolus may obstruct a selected artery. A patient with a spinal cord injury has a greater risk of developing a DVT due to the absence or decrease in the normal pumping action by active contractions of muscles in the lower extremities. Homans' sign is a special test designed to confirm the presence of a DVT. Prevention of a DVT should include prophylactic anticoagulant therapy, maintaining a positioning schedule, range of motion, proper positioning to avoid excessive venous stasis, and use of elastic stockings.

Symptoms: Swelling of the lower extremity, pain, sensitivity over the area of the clot, and warmth in the area are cardinal symptoms of DVT.

Treatment: Once a DVT is suspected, there should be no active or passive movement performed to the involved lower extremity. Bed rest and anticoagulant pharmacological intervention are usually indicated. Surgical procedures can be performed if necessary.

Sensory Testing for Light Touch and Pinprick

0=Absent, 1=Impaired/hyperesthesia, 2=Intact

Level	Site for Sensory Testing
C2	Occipital protuberance
C3	Supraclavicular fossa
C4	Top of the acromioclavicular joint
C5	Lateral side of antecubital fossa
C6	Thumb
C7	Middle finger
C8	Little finger
T1	Medial side of antecubital fossa
T2	Apex of axilla
T3	Third intercostal space (IS)
T4	Fourth IS at the nipple line
T5	Fifth IS (midway between T4 and T6)
T6	Sixth IS at the level of the xiphisternum
T7	Seventh IS (midway between T6 and T8)
T8	Eighth IS (midway between T6 and T10)
T9	Ninth IS (midway between T8 and T10)
T10	10th IS or umbilicus
T11	11th IS (midway between T10 and T12)
T12	Midpoint of inguinal ligament
L1	Half the distance between T12 and L2
L2	Midanterior thigh
L3	Medial femoral condyle
L4	Medial malleolus
L5	Dorsum of the foot at third metatarsophalangeal joint
S1	Lateral heel
S2	Popliteal fossa in the midline
S3	Ischial tuberosity
S4-5	Perianal area (taken as 1 level)

SPOTLIGHT ON SAFETY
AUTONOMIC DYSREFLEXIA: A MEDICAL EMERGENCY[18,43]

Autonomic dysreflexia is perhaps the most dangerous complication of spinal cord injury and can occur in patients with lesions at or above T6. A noxious stimulus below the level of the lesion triggers the autonomic nervous system causing a sudden elevation in blood pressure. Common causes include distended or full bladder, kink or blockage in the catheter, bladder infections, pressure ulcers, extreme temperature changes, tight clothing or even an ingrown toenail. If not treated, this condition can lead to convulsions, hemorrhage, and death.

Symptoms: High blood pressure, severe headache, blurred vision, stuffy nose, profuse sweating, goose bumps below the level of the lesion, and vasodilation (flushing) above the level of injury.

Treatment: The therapist should immediately check the catheter for blockage while having the patient assume or remain in a sitting position. Lying a patient down is contraindicated and will only assist to further elevate blood pressure. The patient should be examined for any other irritating stimuli and potentially checked for bowel impaction. If the cause remains unknown, the patient should receive immediate medical intervention.

Ectopic Bone

Ectopic bone or heterotopic ossification refers to the spontaneous formation of bone in the soft tissue. It typically occurs adjacent to larger joints such as the knees or the hips. Theories regarding etiology range from tissue hypoxia to abnormal calcium metabolism.

Symptoms: Early symptoms include edema, decreased range of motion, and increased temperature of the involved joint.

Treatment: Pharmacological intervention usually involves diphosphates that inhibit ectopic bone formation. Physical therapy and surgery are often incorporated into treatment. Physical therapy should focus on maintaining functional range of motion and allowing the patient the most independent functional outcome possible.

Orthostatic Hypotension

Orthostatic hypotension or postural hypotension occurs due to a loss of sympathetic control of vasoconstriction in combination with absent or severely reduced muscle tone. Venous pooling is fairly common during the early stages of rehabilitation. A decrease in systolic blood pressure greater than 20 mm Hg after moving from a supine position to a sitting position or a decrease in diastolic blood pressure greater than 10 mm Hg is typically indicative of orthostatic hypotension.

Symptoms: Complaints of dizziness, lightheadedness, nausea, and "blacking out" when going from a horizontal to a vertical position are primary symptoms of this condition.

Treatment: Monitoring vital signs assists with minimizing the effects of orthostatic hypotension. The use of elastic stockings, Ace wraps to the lower extremities, and abdominal binders are common. Gradual progression to a vertical position using a tilt table is often indicated. Pharmacological intervention may be indicated in order to increase blood pressure.

Pressure Ulcers

A pressure ulcer is caused by sustained pressure, friction, and/or shearing to a surface. The most common areas susceptible to pressure ulcers are the coccyx, sacrum, ischium, trochanters, elbows, buttocks, malleoli, scapulae, and prominent vertebrae. Pressure ulcers require immediate medical intervention and often can significantly delay the rehabilitation process.

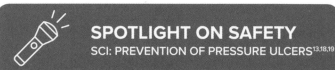

SPOTLIGHT ON SAFETY
SCI: PREVENTION OF PRESSURE ULCERS[13,18,19]

Recent data shows that between 60-80% of people with SCI develop a pressure ulcer within their lifetime. Patients with spinal cord injury potentially experience many of the risk factors associated with the development of a pressure ulcer including:

* immobility
* decreased or absent sensation
* prolonged pressure to an area
* shearing forces
* poor positioning
* poor nutrition

Prevention should include:

Proper positioning while sitting and in bed: protecting all bony prominences, equal distribution of weight, use of equipment such as specialized cushions, mattress pads, and other pressure relief devices

Proper skin care: full cleansing and drying of skin, consistently inspect all skin and monitor any red areas closely; use of skin care products that are recommended by health care professionals

Proper changing of position: consistently change position every two hours; need to weight shift in sitting at a minimum of every 15-20 minutes

Proper nutrition: attain adequate nutrition and calories each day, drink the recommended amount of water, limit empty calories and alcohol intake

Clothing: wear clothing that is not high risk for skin breakdown (e.g., zippers), avoid tight clothing; clothing should be breathable with a comfortable fit

Mobility: daily activity is recommended and should include a cardiovascular component; however, avoid activities with a high shear or drag component

Symptoms: Primarily there is a reddened area that persists or an open area of the skin.

Treatment: Prevention is of greatest importance. A patient should change position frequently, maintain proper skin care, sit on an appropriate cushion, consistently weight shift, and maintain proper nutrition and hydration. Surgical intervention is often necessary with advanced pressure ulcers.

Spasticity

Spasticity can occasionally be useful to a patient with a spinal cord injury, however, more often serves to interfere with functional activities. Spasticity can be enhanced by both internal and external

sources such as stress, decubiti, urinary tract infections, bowel or bladder obstruction, temperature changes or touch.

Symptoms: Increased involuntary contraction of muscle groups, increased tonic stretch reflexes, and exaggerated DTRs.

Treatment: Medications are usually administered in an attempt to reduce the degree of spasticity (Dantrium, Baclofen, Lioresal). Aggressive treatment includes phenol blocks, rhizotomies, myelotomies, and other surgical interventions. Physical therapy intervention includes positioning, aquatic therapy, weight bearing, functional electrical stimulation, range of motion, resting splints, and inhibitive casting.

Functional Outcomes for Complete Lesions[24]

Functional Skills	Level of Assistance Required (by SCI level groups)			
	High Tetraplegia (C1-C5)	Mid-level Tetraplegia (C6)	Low Tetraplegia (C7-C8)	Paraplegia
Bed Mobility • Rolling side to side • Rolling supine/prone • Supine/sitting • Scooting all directions	− Dependent (C1-C4) − Moderate to maximal assistance (C5) − Verbally direct	− Minimal assistance to modified independent with equipment − Verbally direct	− Independent with all	− Independent
Transfers • Bed • Car • Toilet • Bath equipment • Floor • Upright wheelchair	− Dependent (C1-C4) − Maximal assistance with level sliding board transfers (C5) − Verbally direct	− Minimal assistance to modified independent for sliding board transfers − Dependent with wheelchair loading in car − Dependent with floor transfers and uprighting wheelchair − Verbally direct	− Modified independent to independent with level surface transfer (sliding board) − Moderate assistance to modified independent with car transfer − Maximal to moderate assistance with floor transfers and uprighting wheelchair − Verbally direct	− Independent with level surface and car transfers (depression) − Minimal assistance to independent with floor transfers and uprighting wheelchair − Verbally direct
Weight Shifts • Pressure relief • Repositioning in wheelchair	− Setup to modified independent with power recline/tilt weight shift − Dependent with manual recline/tilt/lean weight shift − Verbally direct	− Modified independent with power recline/tilt weight shift − Minimal assistance to modified independent with side to side/forward lean weight shift − Verbally direct	− Modified independent with side to side/forward lean, or depression weight shift	− Modified independent with depression weight shift
Wheelchair Management • Wheel locks • Armrests • Footrests/legrests • Safety strap(s) • Cushion adjustment • Anti-tip levers • Wheelchair maintenance	− Dependent with all − Able to verbally direct	− Some assistance required − Able to verbally direct	− May require assistance with cushion adjustment, anti-tip levers, and wheelchair maintenance − Able to verbally direct	− Independent with all

Functional Outcomes for Complete Lesions[24]

Functional Skills	Level of Assistance Required (by SCI level groups)			
	High Tetraplegia (C1-C5)	Mid-level Tetraplegia (C6)	Low Tetraplegia (C7-C8)	Paraplegia
Wheelchair Mobility • Smooth surfaces • Up/down ramps • Up/down curbs • Rough terrain • Up/down steps (manual wheelchair only)	– Supervision/ setup to modified independent on smooth, ramp, and rough terrain with power wheelchair – Modified independent with manual wheelchair on smooth surface in forward direction (C5) – Maximal assistance to dependent with manual wheelchair in all other situations (C5) – Able to verbally direct	– Modified independent in smooth, ramp, and rough terrain with power wheelchair – Dependent to maximal assistance up/down curb with power wheelchair – Modified independent on smooth surfaces with manual wheelchair – Moderate to minimal assistance on ramps and rough terrain with manual wheelchair – Maximal to moderate assistance up/down curbs with manual wheelchair – Able to verbally direct	– Modified independent on smooth, ramp, and rough terrain with power wheelchair – Dependent to maximal assistance up/down curb with power wheelchair – Modified independent on smooth surfaces and up/down ramps with manual wheelchair – Minimal assistance to modified independent on rough terrain – Moderate to minimal assistance up/down curbs with manual wheelchair – Dependent to maximal assistance up/down steps with manual wheelchair – Can verbally direct	– Minimal assistance to modified independent up/down 6" curbs with manual wheelchair – Modified independent with descending steps with manual wheelchair – Maximal to minimal assistance to ascend steps with manual wheelchair – Able to verbally direct
Gait • Don/doff orthoses • Sit/stand • Smooth surfaces • Up/down ramps • Up/down curbs • Up/down steps • Rough terrain • Safe falling	– Not applicable	– Not applicable	– Not applicable	Abilities range from: – exercise only with KAFOs* – household gait with KAFOs – limited community gait with KAFOs or AFOs* – functional community ambulation with or without orthoses
ROM/Positioning • PROM to trunk, legs, and arms • Pad/position in bed	– Dependent – Able to verbally direct	– Moderate assistance to modified independent with all – Able to verbally direct	– Minimal assistance to modified independent with all – Able to verbally direct	– Independent
Feeding • Drinking • Finger feeding • Utensil feeding	– Dependent (C1-C4) – Minimal assistance with adaptive equipment (C5) – Able to verbally direct	– Modified independent with adaptive equipment	– Modified independent with adaptive equipment (C7)	– Independent

Functional Outcomes for Complete Lesions[24]

Functional Skills	Level of Assistance Required (by SCI level groups)			
	High Tetraplegia (C1-C5)	Mid-level Tetraplegia (C6)	Low Tetraplegia (C7-C8)	Paraplegia
Grooming • Face • Teeth • Hair • Makeup • Shaving face	– Dependent (C1-C4) – Minimal assistance with adaptive equipment for face, teeth, makeup/shaving (C5) – Maximal/moderate assistance for hair grooming (C5) – Able to verbally direct	– Modified independent with adaptive equipment	– Modified independent	– Independent
Dressing • Dressing and undressing (in bed or wheelchair) • Upper body/lower body (in bed or wheelchair)	– Dependent – Able to verbally direct	– Modified independent for upper body in bed or wheelchair – Minimal assistance with lower body dressing in bed – Moderate assistance with lower body undressing in bed – Able to verbally direct	– Modified independent for upper/lower body dressing in bed – Minimal assistance with lower body dressing/undressing in wheelchair (C7) – Modified independent for upper/lower body dressing/undressing in wheelchair (C8) – Able to verbally direct	– Modified independent
Bathing • Bathing and drying off • Upper body and lower body	– Dependent – Able to verbally direct	– Minimal assistance for upper body bathing and drying – Moderate assistance for lower body bathing and drying – Use of shower or tub chair – Able to verbally direct	– Modified independent with all using shower or tub chair	– Modified independent with all on tub bench or tub bottom cushion
Bowel/Bladder Problems • Intermittent catheterization • Leg bag care • Condom application • Clean up • In bed/wheelchair (bladder) • Feminine hygiene • Bowel program	– Dependent – Able to verbally direct	**Bladder:** – Minimal assistance for male in bed or wheelchair – Moderate assistance for female in bed **Bowel:** – Moderate assistance with use of equipment – Able to verbally direct	**Bladder:** – Modified independent for male in bed or wheelchair – Modified independent for female in bed; moderate assistance for female in wheelchair **Bowel:** – Minimal assistance to modified independent with use of equipment – Able to verbally direct	**Bladder:** – Modified independent for male and female **Bowel:** – Modified independent for male and female

*KAFO = knee-ankle-foot orthosis; AFO = ankle-foot orthosis
From Umphred DA: Neurological Rehabilitation. Mosby-Year Book, Inc. 1995, p. 502-505, with permission.

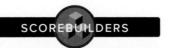

Spinal Cord Injury Terminology[18,19,24]

Cauda equina injury: A term used to describe injuries that occur below the L1 level of the spine. A cauda equina injury is considered to be a lower motor neuron lesion.

Dermatome: Designated sensory areas based on spinal segment innervation.

Myelotomy: A surgical procedure that severs certain tracts within the spinal cord in order to decrease spasticity and improve function.

Myotome: Designated motor areas based on spinal segment innervation.

Neurectomy: A surgical removal of a segment of a nerve in order to decrease spasticity and improve function.

Neurogenic nonreflexive bladder: The bladder is flaccid as a result of a cauda equina or conus medullaris lesion. The sacral reflex arc is damaged.

Neurogenic reflexive bladder: The bladder empties reflexively for a patient with an injury above the level of T12. The sacral reflex arc remains intact.

Neurologic level: The lowest segment (most caudal) of the spinal cord with intact strength and sensation. Muscle groups at this level must receive a grade of fair.

Paradoxical breathing: A form of abnormal breathing that is common in tetraplegia where the abdomen rises and the chest is pulled inward during inspiration. On expiration the abdomen falls and the chest expands.

Paraplegia: A term used to describe injuries that occur at the level of the thoracic, lumbar or sacral spine.

Rhizotomy: A surgical resection of the sensory component of a spinal nerve in order to decrease spasticity and improve function.

Sacral sparing: An incomplete lesion where some of the innermost tracts remain innervated. Characteristics include sensation of the saddle area, movement of the toe flexors, and rectal sphincter contraction.

Spinal shock: A physiologic response that occurs between 30 and 60 minutes after trauma to the spinal cord and can last up to several weeks. Spinal shock presents with total flaccid paralysis and loss of all reflexes below the level of injury.

Tenodesis: Patients with tetraplegia that do not possess motor control for grasp can utilize the tight finger flexors in combination with wrist extension to produce a form of grasp.

Tenotomy: A surgical release of a tendon in order to decrease spasticity and improve function.

Tetraplegia (quadriplegia): A term adopted by the American Spinal Injury Association to describe injuries that occur at the level of the cervical spine.

Zone of preservation: A term used to describe poor or trace motor or sensory function for up to three levels below the neurologic level of injury.

CONSIDER THIS
SPINAL CORD INJURY INTERVENTION CONSTRUCTS[13,20,24]

Patients with spinal cord injury will likely have a unique course of rehabilitation based on their primary diagnosis, secondary complications, co-morbidities, and level of impairment. The following guidelines, however, reflect areas that should be incorporated into the plan of care for patients with spinal cord injury.

- Positioning
- Prevention of pressure ulcers
- Pressure relief techniques and equipment
- Range of motion
- Family/caregiver teaching
- Bowel and bladder programming
- Respiratory training/airway clearance

  - Assisted cough and secretion clearance
  - Breathing exercises
  - Abdominal binders
  - Mechanical ventilation
  - Glossopharyngeal breathing (GPB)

- Wheelchair, cushion (Figs. 5-51, 5-52), and orthotic prescriptions
- Wheelchair mobility
- Balance and center of gravity retraining
- Motor function retraining (transitioning between positions, seated scooting) (Figs. 5-53, 5-54)
- Mobility training including floor transfers if appropriate (Figs. 5-55, 5-56, 5-57)
- Pain management
- Use of FES, biofeedback, TENS if appropriate
- Self-care skills
- Gait training (T9 or lower)

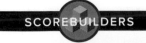

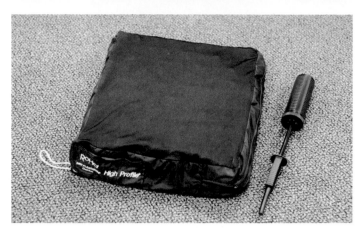

Fig. 5-51: Roho high profile specialized cushion with cover.

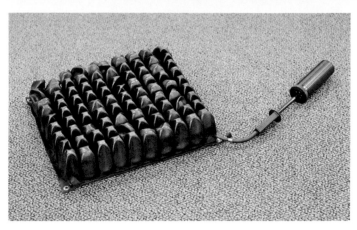

Fig. 5-52: Roho high profile specialized cushion for wheelchair seating.

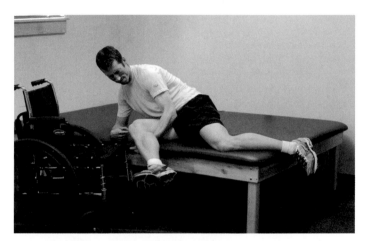

Fig. 5-53: Functional retraining of a patient with spinal cord injury, specifically transfers from the wheelchair to the mat surface.

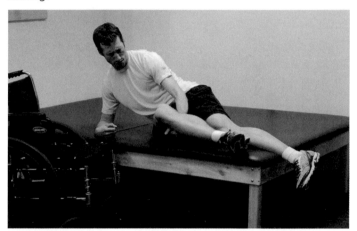

Fig. 5-54: The patient must compensate by looping the upper extremity under the lower extremity in combination with momentum in order to swing the lower extremity onto the mat surface.

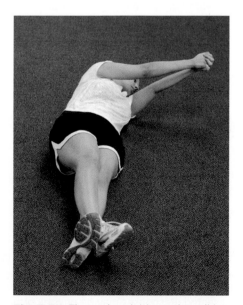

Fig. 5-55: The patient initiates the roll by manually crossing legs, using the upper extremities to create movement and momentum.

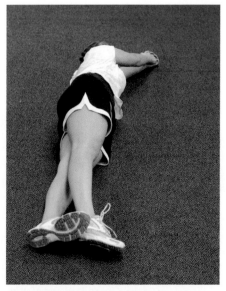

Fig. 5-56: The patient begins to roll using momentum and gravity.

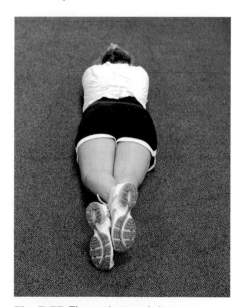

Fig. 5-57: The patient ends in prone position as anticipated.

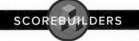

Traumatic Brain Injury

According to the Centers for Disease Control and Prevention, more than 1.7 million people annually sustain a traumatic brain injury. Approximately 52,000 die from the trauma and an additional 80,000 experience long-term impairment and disability on an annual basis. The leading risk factor for TBI is a motor vehicle accident, followed by falls, high risk behaviors, and gunshot wounds. Brain injury is classified as open versus closed with primary and secondary brain damage. Secondary damage within the brain can be significant due to the widespread areas that are affected.

Types of Brain Injury[20,44]

Open Injury

An injury of direct penetration through the skull to the brain. Location, depth of penetration, and pathway determine the extent of brain damage. Examples include gunshot wound, knife or sharp object penetration, skull fragments, and direct trauma.

Closed Injury

An injury to the brain without penetration through the skull. Examples include concussion, contusion, hematoma, injury to extracranial blood vessels, hypoxia, drug overdose, near drowning, and acceleration or deceleration injuries.

Primary Injury

Initial injury to the brain sustained by impact. Examples include skull penetration, skull fractures, and contusions to gray and white matter.

Coup lesion: A direct lesion of the brain under the point of impact. Local brain damage is sustained.

Contrecoup lesion: An injury that results on the opposite side of the brain. The lesion is due to the rebound effect of the brain after impact.

Secondary Injury

Brain damage that occurs as a response to the initial injury. Examples include hematoma, hypoxia, ischemia, increased intracranial pressure, and post-traumatic epilepsy.

Epidural hematoma: A hemorrhage that forms between the skull and dura mater.

Subdural hematoma: A hemorrhage that forms due to venous rupture between the dura and arachnoid.

Levels of Consciousness[20,44]

Coma: A state of unconsciousness and a level of unresponsiveness to all internal and external stimuli.

Stupor: A state of general unresponsiveness with arousal occurring from repeated stimuli.

Obtundity: A state of consciousness that is characterized by a state of sleep, reduced alertness to arousal, and delayed responses to stimuli.

Delirium: A state of consciousness that is characterized by disorientation, confusion, agitation, and loudness.

Clouding of consciousness: A state of consciousness that is characterized by quiet behavior, confusion, poor attention, and delayed responses.

Consciousness: A state of alertness, awareness, orientation, and memory.

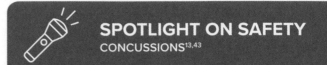

SPOTLIGHT ON SAFETY
CONCUSSIONS[13,43]

A concussion can occur as a result of injury, specifically a blow to the head. This may or may not produce a temporary loss of consciousness. There is damage to the reticular activating system that allows for immediate changes in vital signs. Concussions occur frequently secondary to acute trauma such as motor vehicle accidents or through athletics.

The American Academy of Neurology classifies concussions as:

Grade 1 – A concussion that results from head injury where there was no loss of consciousness but typically some transient confusion by the patient. Symptoms will typically resolve within 15 minutes of the event. The patient may exhibit full memory of the event. An athlete should be removed from the competition and return only if symptom free after one week of rest.

Grade 2 – A concussion that results from a moderate head injury with transient confusion that will last longer than 15 minutes. The patient may exhibit poor concentration, and retrograde and anterograde amnesia. An athlete should be removed immediately from the competition and receive a medical evaluation. CT scan is indicated if symptoms worsen and return to play should be deferred until the athlete is asymptomatic for two weeks at rest and with exertion.

Grade 3 – A concussion that results from head injury with any form of loss of consciousness. A patient should require transport to the emergency room for full neurological evaluation. Hospitalization is warranted if altered consciousness or mental status persists. An athlete should be withheld from competition after a grade 3 concussion once symptom free for a minimum of one month. This form of concussion is secondary to diffuse axonal injury and, if severe, can result in coma.

Traumatic Brain Injury Tests and Measures

Rancho Los Amigos Levels of Cognitive Functioning[24]

I. NO RESPONSE

Patient appears to be in a deep sleep and is completely unresponsive to any stimuli.

II. GENERALIZED RESPONSE

Patient reacts inconsistently and non-purposefully to stimuli in a nonspecific manner. Responses are limited and often the same regardless of stimulus presented. Responses may be physiological changes, gross body movements, and/or vocalization.

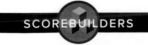

III. LOCALIZED RESPONSE

Patient reacts specifically, but inconsistently to stimuli. Responses are directly related to the type of stimulus presented. May follow simple commands such as closing the eyes or squeezing the hand in an inconsistent, delayed manner.

IV. CONFUSED-AGITATED

Patient is in a heightened state of activity. Behavior is bizarre and non-purposeful relative to the immediate environment. Does not discriminate among persons or objects; is unable to cooperate directly with treatment efforts. Verbalizations frequently are incoherent and/or inappropriate to the environment; confabulation may be present. Gross attention to environment is very brief; selective attention is often nonexistent. Patient lacks short and long-term recall.

V. CONFUSED-INAPPROPRIATE

Patient is able to respond to simple commands fairly consistently. However, with increased complexity of commands or lack of any external structure, responses are non-purposeful, random, or fragmented. Demonstrates gross attention to the environment, but is highly distractible and lacks the ability to focus attention on a specific task. With structure, may be able to converse on a social automatic level for short periods of time. Verbalization is often inappropriate and confabulatory. Memory is severely impaired; often shows inappropriate use of objects; may perform previously learned tasks with structure, but is unable to learn new information.

VI. CONFUSED-APPROPRIATE

Patient shows goal-directed behavior, but is dependent on external input or direction. Follows simple directions consistently and shows carryover for relearned tasks such as self-care. Responses may be incorrect due to memory problems, but they are appropriate to the situation. Past memories show more depth and detail than recent memory.

VII. AUTOMATIC-APPROPRIATE

Patient appears appropriate and oriented within the hospital and home setting. Goes through daily routine automatically, but frequently robot-like. Patient shows minimal to no confusion and has shallow recall of activities. Shows carryover for new learning, but at a decreased rate. With structure is able to initiate social or recreational activities; judgment remains impaired.

VIII. PURPOSEFUL-APPROPRIATE

Patient is able to recall and integrate past and recent events and is aware of and responsive to environment. Shows carryover for new learning and needs no supervision once activities are learned. May continue to show a decreased ability relative to premorbid abilities, abstract reasoning, tolerance for stress, and judgment in emergencies or unusual circumstances.

From Professional Staff Association, Rancho Los Amigos Hospital, p.87-88, with permission

Glasgow Coma Scale[24]

A neurological assessment tool used initially after injury to determine arousal and cerebral cortex function. A total score of eight or less correlates to severe brain injury and coma in 90% of patients. Scores of 9 to 12 indicate moderate brain injuries and scores from 13 to 15 indicate mild brain injuries.

Glasgow Coma Scale

Eye Opening	E
Spontaneous	4
To speech	3
To pain	2
Nil	1
Best Motor Response	**M**
Obeys commands	6
Localizes pain	5
Withdraws	4
Abnormal flexion	3
Extensor response	2
Nil	1
Verbal Response	**V**
Oriented	5
Confused conversation	4
Inappropriate words	3
Incomprehensible sounds	2
Nil	1
Coma Score (E+M+V) = 3 to 15	

From Management of Head Injuries by Bryan Jennett and Graham Teasdale, Copyright-1981 by Oxford University Press, Inc. Used by permission of Oxford University Press, Inc.

Memory Impairments

Anterograde amnesia: The inability to create new memory. Anterograde memory is usually the last to recover after a comatose state. Contributing factors include poor attention, distractibility, and impaired perception of stimuli.

Post-traumatic amnesia: The time between the injury and when the patient is able to recall recent events. The patient does not recall the injury or events up until this point of recovery. Post-traumatic amnesia is used as an indicator of the extent of damage.

Retrograde amnesia: An inability to remember events prior to the injury. Retrograde amnesia may progressively decrease with recovery.

CONSIDER THIS
TRAUMATIC BRAIN INJURY INTERVENTION CONSTRUCTS[20,24,44]

Patients with brain injury will likely have a unique course of rehabilitation based on their primary diagnosis, secondary complications, co-morbidities, and level of impairment. The following guidelines, however, reflect areas that should be incorporated into the plan of care for patients with a brain injury.

- Emphasis on motivation
- Promote independence
- Therapy should be goal-directed and functional
- Focus on orientation and behavior modification activities
- Repetition is typically helpful
- Educate patient in compensatory strategies for success
- Structure is essential depending on the level of the patient
- Avoid overstimulation during therapy using a calm voice and simple commands
- Perform activities that are both familiar and enjoyable for the patient
- Family education and support can enhance and assist the rehabilitation process
- Flexibility in treatment is needed based on patient's immediate needs and state of mind

- Intervention should include:
  - Cognitive and orientation training
  - Therapeutic exercise
  - Positioning
  - Sensory integration
  - Balance and vestibular training
  - Range of motion
  - Motor function training
  - Wheelchair and adaptive equipment prescription
  - Splinting and serial casting
  - Mobility training

Pediatrics and Development

Apgar Score

Apgar Sign	0	1	2
Appearance (skin color)	Blue; pale	Normal body color, except blue hands and feet	Normal color "pink"
Pulse	Absent	Below 100 beats per minute	Above 100 beats per minute
Grimace (reflex irritability)	No response to stimulation	Minimal response to stimulation	Pulls away, sneeze or cough
Activity (muscle tone)	No movement, "floppy"	Flexing of the arms and legs	Active movement
Respiration	Absent	Slow, irregular	Vigorous cry

The Apgar score is a method for objectively reporting the health of a newborn shortly after it is delivered. The score is determined by rating five different criteria: **A**ppearance (skin color), **P**ulse rate, **G**rimace (reflex irritability), **A**ctivity, and **R**espiration. Each criterion is graded on a scale from 0-2, with a score of 2 indicating a normal response.

Total scores are calculated at one minute and at five minutes following birth. A newborn is considered to be in good condition if they have a score of 7-10. A score of 3 or below is considered to be low and is an indicator that the newborn requires immediate medical attention.

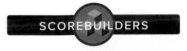

Concepts of Development[45,46]

Cephalic to Caudal: A person develops head and upper extremity control prior to trunk and lower extremity control. There is a general skill acquisition from the direction of head to toe.

Gross to Fine: A general trend for large muscle movement acquisition with progression to small muscle skill acquisition.

Mass to Specific: A general trend for a person to acquire simple movements and progress towards complex movements.

Proximal to Distal: A concept that uses the midline of the body as the reference point. Trunk control (midline stability) is acquired first with subsequent gain in distal control (extremities).

Infant Reflexes and Possible Effects if Reflex Persists Abnormally[47]

Primitive Reflex	Possible Negative Effect on Movement with Abnormal Persistence of Reflex
Asymmetrical Tonic Neck Reflex (ATNR)	
Stimulus: Head position, turned to one side **Response:** Arm and leg on face side are extended, arm and leg on scalp side are flexed, spine curved with convexity toward face side **Normal age of response:** Birth to 6 months	Interferes with: • Feeding • Visual tracking • Midline use of hands • Bilateral hand use • Rolling • Development of crawling • Can lead to skeletal deformities (e.g., scoliosis, hip subluxation, hip dislocation)
Symmetrical Tonic Neck Reflex (STNR)	
Stimulus: Head position, flexion or extension **Response:** When head is in flexion, arms are flexed, legs extended. When head is in extension, arms are extended, legs are flexed **Normal age of response:** 6 to 8 months	Interferes with: • Ability to prop on arms in prone position • Attaining and maintaining hands-and-knees position • Crawling reciprocally • Sitting balance when looking around • Use of hands when looking at object in hands in sitting position
Tonic Labyrinthine Reflex (TLR)	
Stimulus: Position of labyrinth in inner ear - reflected in head position **Response:** In the supine position, body and extremities are held in extension; in the prone position, body and extremities are held in flexion **Normal age of response:** Birth to 6 months	Interferes with: • Ability to initiate rolling • Ability to prop on elbows with extended hips when prone • Ability to flex trunk and hips to come to sitting position from supine position • Often causes full body extension, which interferes with balance in sitting or standing
Galant Reflex	
Stimulus: Touch to skin along spine from shoulder to hip **Response:** Lateral flexion of trunk to side of stimulus **Normal age of response:** 30 weeks of gestation to 2 months	Interferes with: • Development of sitting balance • Can lead to scoliosis

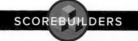

Infant Reflexes and Possible Effects if Reflex Persists Abnormally[47]

Primitive Reflex	Possible Negative Effect on Movement with Abnormal Persistence of Reflex
Palmar Grasp Reflex	
Stimulus: Pressure in palm on ulnar side of hand **Response:** Flexion of fingers causing strong grip **Normal age of response:** Birth to 4 months	Interferes with: • Ability to grasp and release objects voluntarily • Weight bearing on open hand for propping, crawling, protective responses
Plantar Grasp Reflex	
Stimulus: Pressure to base of toes **Response:** Toe flexion **Normal age of response:** 28 weeks of gestation to 9 months	Interferes with: • Ability to stand with feet flat on surface • Balance reactions and weight shifting in standing
Rooting Reflex	
Stimulus: Touch on cheek **Response:** Turning head to same side with mouth open **Normal age of response:** 28 weeks of gestation to 3 months	Interferes with: • Oral-motor development • Development of midline control of head • Optical righting, visual tracking, and social interaction
Moro Reflex	
Stimulus: Head dropping into extension suddenly for a few inches **Response:** Arms abduct with fingers open, then cross trunk into adduction; cry **Normal age of response:** 28 weeks of gestation to 5 months	Interferes with: • Balance reactions in sitting • Protective responses in sitting • Eye-hand coordination, visual tracking
Startle Reflex	
Stimulus: Loud, sudden noise **Response:** Similar to Moro response, but elbows remain flexed and hands closed **Normal age of response:** 28 weeks of gestation to 5 months	Interferes with: • Sitting balance • Protective responses in sitting • Eye-hand coordination, visual tracking • Social interaction, attention
Positive Support Reflex	
Stimulus: Weight placed on balls of feet when upright **Response:** Stiffening of legs and trunk into extension **Normal age of response:** 35 weeks of gestation to 2 months	Interferes with: • Standing and walking • Balance reactions and weight shift in standing • Can lead to contractures of ankles into plantar flexion
Walking (Stepping) Reflex	
Stimulus: Supported upright position with soles of feet on firm surface **Response:** Reciprocal flexion/extension of legs **Normal age of response:** 38 weeks of gestation to 2 months	Interferes with: • Standing and walking • Balance reactions and weight shifting in standing • Development of smooth, coordinated reciprocal movements of lower extremities

From Ratliffe KT: Clinical Pediatric Physical Therapy: A Guide for the Physical Therapy Team. Mosby Inc., Philadelphia 1998, p.266, with permission.

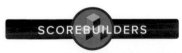

Developmental Gross and Fine Motor Skills[47]

Gross Motor Skills	Fine Motor Skills
Newborn to 1 Month	
Prone Physiological flexion Lifts head briefly Head to side **Supine** Physiological flexion Rolls partly to side **Sitting** Head lag in pull to sit **Standing** Reflex standing and walking	Regards objects in direct line of sight Follows moving object to midline Hands fisted Arm movements jerky Movements may be purposeful or random
2 to 3 Months	
Prone Lifts head 90 degrees briefly Chest up in prone position with some weight through forearms Rolls prone to supine **Supine** Asymmetrical tonic neck reflex (ATNR) influence is strong Legs kick reciprocally Prefers head to side **Sitting** Head upright, but bobbing Variable head lag in pull to sitting position Needs full support to sit **Standing** Poor weight bearing Hips in flexion, behind shoulders	Can see farther distances Hands open more Visually follows through 180 degrees Grasp is reflexive Uses palmar grasp

Gross Motor Skills	Fine Motor Skills
4 to 5 Months	
Prone Bears weight on extended arms Pivots in prone to reach toys **Supine** Rolls from supine to side position Plays with feet to mouth **Sitting** Head steady in supported sitting position Turns head in sitting position Sits alone for brief periods **Standing** Bears all weight through legs in supported standing	Grasps and releases toys Uses ulnar-palmar grasp
6 to 7 Months	
Prone Rolls from supine to prone position Holds weight on one hand to reach for toy **Supine** Lifts head **Sitting** Lifts head and helps when pulled to sitting position Gets to sitting position without assistance Sits independently **Mobility** May crawl backward	Approaches objects with one hand Arm in neutral when approaching toy Radial-palmar grasp "Rakes" with fingers to pick up small objects Voluntary release to transfer objects between hands

Developmental Gross and Fine Motor Skills (continued)[47]

Gross Motor Skills	Fine Motor Skills
8 to 9 Months	

Gross Motor Skills	Fine Motor Skills
Prone	Develops active supination
Gets into hands-knees position	Radial-digital grasp develops
Supine	Uses inferior pincer grasp
Does not tolerate supine position	Extends wrist actively
Sitting	Points with index finger
Moves from sitting to prone position	Pokes with index finger
Sits without hand support for longer periods	Release of objects is more refined
Pivots in sitting position	Takes objects out of container
Standing	
Stands at furniture	
Pulls to stand at furniture	
Lowers to sitting position from supported stand	
Mobility	
Crawls forward	
Walks along furniture (cruising)	

10 to 11 Months	
Standing	Fine pincer grasp developed
Stands without support briefly	Puts objects into container
Pulls to stand using half-kneel intermediate position	Grasps crayon adaptively
Picks up object from floor from standing with support	
Mobility	
Walks with both hands held	
Walks with one hand held	
Creeps on hands and feet (bear walk)	

Gross Motor Skills	Fine Motor Skills
12 to 15 Months	
Walks without support	Marks paper with crayon
Fast walking	Builds tower using two cubes
Walks sideways	Turns over small container to obtain contents
Bends over to look between legs	
Creeps or hitches upstairs	
Throws ball in sitting	

16 to 24 Months	
Squats in play	Folds paper
Walks backward	Strings beads
Walking upstairs and downstairs with one hand held using both feet on step	Stacks six cubes
Propels ride-on toys	Imitates vertical and horizontal strokes with crayon on paper
Kicks ball	Holds crayon with thumb and fingers
Throws ball	
Throws ball forward	
Picks up toy from floor without falling	

2 Years	
Rides tricycle	Turns knob
Walks on tiptoe	Opens and closes jar
Runs on toes	Able to button large buttons
Walks downstairs alternating feet	Uses child-size scissors with help
Catches large ball	Does 12 to 15 piece puzzles
Hops on one foot	Folds paper or clothes

Developmental Gross and Fine Motor Skills (continued)[47]

Gross Motor Skills	Fine Motor Skills
Preschool Age (3 to 4 Years)	
Throws ball 10 feet	Controls crayons more effectively
Walks on a line 10 feet	Copies a circle or cross
Hops 2-10 times on one foot	Matches colors
Jumps distances of up to two feet	Cuts with scissors
Jumps over obstacles up to 12 inches	Draws recognizable human figures with head and two extremities
Throws and catches small ball	Draws squares
Runs fast and avoids obstacles	May demonstrate hand preference
Early School Age (5 to 8 Years)	
Skips on alternate feet	Hand preference is evident
Gallops	Prints well, starting to learn cursive writing
Can play hopscotch, balance on one foot, controlled hopping, and squatting on one leg	Able to button small buttons
Jumps with rhythm, control (jump rope)	
Bounces large ball	
Kicks ball with greater control	
Limbs growing faster than trunk allowing greater speed, leverage	

Gross Motor Skills	Fine Motor Skills
Later School Age (9 to 12 Years)	
Mature patterns of movement in throwing, jumping, running	Develops greater control in hand usage
Competition increases, enjoys competitive games	Learns to draw
Improved balance, coordination, endurance, attention span	Handwriting is developed
Boys may develop preadolescent fat spurt	
Girls may develop prepubescent and pubescent changes in body shape (hips, breasts)	
Adolescence (13 Years+)	
Rapid growth in size and strength, boys more than girls	Develops greater dexterity in fingers for fine tasks (knitting, sewing, art, crafts)
Puberty leads to changes in body proportions, center of gravity rises toward shoulders for boys, lowers to hips for girls	
Balance and coordination skills, eye-hand coordination, endurance may plateau during growth spurt	

From Ratliffe KT: Clinical Pediatric Physical Therapy: A Guide for the Physical Therapy Team. Mosby Company Inc., Philadelphia 1998, p.45-47, with permission.

Pediatric Therapeutic Positioning

Proper positioning is essential to obtain maximum function for the pediatric population. Positioning is used for many purposes including facilitation of desired patterns of movement, inhibition of abnormal reflexes, normalization of tone, midline orientation, enhancement of respiratory capacity, pulmonary hygiene, maintaining skin integrity, and prevention of contractures.

Ideal Positioning[47]

	Supine	Prone	Sidelying	Sitting
Pelvis and Hips	Pelvis in line with trunk. Hips in 30 to 90 degrees of flexion. Neutral rotation of pelvis. Hips symmetrically abducted 10 to 20 degrees.	Pelvis in line with trunk. Hips in extension. Neutral rotation of pelvis. Hips symmetrically abducted 10 to 20 degrees.	Pelvis in line with trunk. Hips in flexion. Neutral rotation. Hips in 10 to 20 degrees abduction.	Pelvis in line with trunk. Hips at 90 degrees flexion. Neutral rotation of pelvis. Hips symmetrically abducted 10 to 20 degrees.
Trunk	Straight. Shoulders in line with hips. Neutral rotation of trunk.	Straight. Shoulders in line with hips. Neutral rotation.	Straight. Shoulders in line with hips. Slight sidebending okay.	Straight. Shoulders over hips. Not rotated.
Head and Neck	Head in neutral position. Facing forward. Slight cervical flexion.	Head in neutral position. Facing to one side. Slight cervical flexion.	Head in neutral position. Facing forward. Slight cervical flexion.	Head in neutral position. Facing forward. Head evenly on shoulders.
Shoulders and Arms	Arms fully supported. Arms forward of trunk. Forearms rest on trunk or pillow.	Arms fully supported. Arms forward of trunk. Flexion at shoulders. Flexion at elbows.	Both arms supported. Lower arm forward, not lying on point of shoulders. Lower arm neutral rotation. Upper arm may have 0 to 40 degrees medial rotation.	Arms fully supported. Elbows in flexion. 0 to 45 degrees internally rotated shoulders.
Legs and Feet	Knees supported in flexion. Feet positioned at 90 degrees.	Knees extended. Feet positioned at 90 degrees.	Knees in flexion. Feet positioned at 90 degrees. Pillow between knees.	Knees at 90 degrees. Ankles at 90 degrees. Feet fully supported. Thighs fully supported.

From Ratliffe KT: Clinical Pediatric Physical Therapy: A Guide for the Physical Therapy Team. Mosby Inc., Philadelphia 1998, p.266, with permission.

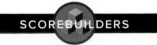

Neuromuscular and Nervous Systems Pediatric Pathology

Arthrogryposis Multiplex Congenita (AMC)[45,46,47]

Arthrogryposis multiplex congenita is a non-progressive neuromuscular disorder that is estimated to occur during the first trimester in utero. The restriction in utero allows for fibrosis of muscles and structures within the joints.

Etiology – An exact etiology of AMC is unknown, however, causative factors include poor movement during early development due to myopathic, neuropathic or joint abnormalities. The causative factor for a small percentage of children with this condition is genetic inheritance as an autosomal dominant trait.

Signs and symptoms – AMC characteristics include cylinder-like extremities with minimal definition, significant and multiple contractures, dislocation of joints, and muscle atrophy.

Treatment – The goal of treatment is to attain the maximum level of developmental skills through positioning, stretching, strengthening, splinting, and use of adaptive equipment. Significant family involvement is required for the home program. Surgical intervention may be indicated.

Autism Spectrum Disorder[13,46]

Autism spectrum disorder (ASD) is a group of complex brain development disorders that are characterized by difficulties with social interaction, communication, and repetitive behaviors. Children with ASD can vary widely in their functional level since ASD is an umbrella term that includes four previously isolated disorders: autistic disorder, childhood disintegrative disorder, pervasive development disorder (not otherwise specified), and Asperger syndrome.

Etiology – The etiology for ASD is not well understood, but it is thought to have a multifactorial cause that includes genetic and environmental influences.

Signs and Symptoms – Initial signs and symptoms generally become apparent around the age of two or three. These often include nonpurposeful speech or the complete absence of speech, diminished facial expressions, an inability to understand nonverbal cues, limited interest or awkwardness in social interactions, a lack of empathy, defensiveness or indifference towards sensory stimulation, repetitive self-stimulating behaviors, perseverations, preoccupation with routines and rituals, and decreased coordination. Children that have more severe forms of ASD may be significantly limited in their ability to participate in expected social roles, while children with mild ASD (e.g., Asperger syndrome) may have relatively few limitations and only be recognized as being socially awkward. Many children with ASD have exceptional talents in music, art, and academic skills.

Treatment – Generally multidisciplinary and may focus on improving social communication and decreasing nonpurposeful movements and vocalizations. Sensory integration therapy may also be used to help those patients that have difficulty with sensory processing. The prognosis for patients with ASD is directly related to the severity of the condition.

Cerebral Palsy (CP)[13,45,46,47]

Cerebral palsy is an umbrella term used to describe movement disorders due to brain damage that are non-progressive and are acquired in utero, during birth or infancy. The brain damage decreases the brain's ability to monitor and control nerve and voluntary muscle activity.

Etiology – CP can occur before or during birth secondary to a lack of oxygen, maternal infections, drug or alcohol abuse, placental abnormalities, toxemia, prolonged labor, prematurity, and Rh incompatibility. The etiology of acquired cerebral palsy includes meningitis, CVA, seizures, and brain injury.

Signs and symptoms – Characteristics vary from mild and undetectable to severe loss of control accompanied by profound intellectual disability. All types of cerebral palsy demonstrate abnormal muscle tone, impaired modulation of movement, presence of abnormal reflexes, and impaired mobility.

Cerebral Palsy Primary Motor Patterns (mixed motor patterns exist)

- **Spastic** - indicating a lesion in the motor cortex of the cerebrum; upper motor neuron damage
- **Athetoid** - indicating a lesion involving the basal ganglia

Distribution of Involvement

- **Monoplegia** - one extremity
- **Diplegia** - bilateral lower extremity involvement, however, upper extremities may be affected
- **Hemiplegia** - unilateral involvement of the upper and lower extremities
- **Quadriplegia** - involvement of the entire body

Treatment – Treatment of cerebral palsy is a lifelong process. Intervention includes ongoing family and caregiver education, normalization of tone, stretching, strengthening, motor learning and developmental milestones, positioning, weight bearing activities, and mobility skills. Splinting, assistive devices, and specialized seating may be indicated. Surgical intervention may be required for orthopedic management or reduction of spasticity.

Down Syndrome[45,46,47]

Down syndrome is a genetic abnormality consisting of an extra twenty-first chromosome, termed trisomy 21.

Etiology – The etiology of Down syndrome includes incomplete cell division of the 21st pair of chromosomes due to nondisjunction, translocation or mosaic classification. Advanced maternal age increases the risk of genetic imbalance.

Signs and symptoms – Signs and symptoms of this syndrome include intellectual disability, hypotonia, joint hypermobility, flattened nasal bridge, narrow eyelids with epicanthal folds, small mouth, feeding impairments, flat feet, scoliosis, congenital heart disease, and visual and hearing loss.

Treatment – Treatment should emphasize exercise and fitness, stability, maximizing respiratory function, and education for caregivers. Surgical intervention may be indicated for cardiac abnormalities.

Duchenne Muscular Dystrophy[13,45,46,47]

Duchenne muscular dystrophy is a progressive disorder caused by the absence of the gene required to produce the muscle proteins dystrophin and nebulin. Without dystrophin and nebulin, cell membranes weaken, myofibrils are destroyed, and muscle contractility is lost. Fat and connective tissue eventually replace muscle, and death usually occurs from cardiopulmonary failure prior to age 25, usually in the teenage years.

Etiology – The causative factor is inheritance as an X-linked recessive trait. The child's mother is a silent carrier and only male offspring will manifest the disease.

Signs and symptoms – Characteristics usually manifest between two and five years of age. Progressive weakness, disinterest in running, falling, toe walking, excessive lordosis, and pseudohypertrophy of muscle groups are common symptoms. Progressive impairment with ADLs and mobility begins around age five and the inability to ambulate follows.

Treatment – Intervention focuses on family and caregiver education, respiratory function, submaximal exercise, mobility skills, splinting, orthotics, and adaptive equipment. Medical management includes the use of immunosuppressants, steroids, and surgical intervention for orthopedic impairments.

Prader-Willi Syndrome[45,46,47]

Prader-Willi syndrome is a genetic condition that is diagnosed by physical attributes and patterns of behavior rather than genetic testing.

Etiology – The causative factor is a partial deletion of chromosome 15.

Signs and symptoms – Characteristics include physical and behavioral attributes such as small hands, feet, and sex organs, hypotonia, almond-shaped eyes, obesity, and a constant desire for food. This child will present with coordination impairments and intellectual disability.

Treatment – Physical therapy includes postural control, exercise and fitness, and gross and fine motor skills training.

Spina Bifida[13,45,46,47]

Spina bifida is a developmental abnormality due to insufficient closure of the neural tube by the 28th day of gestation. This defect usually occurs in the low thoracic, lumbar or sacral regions and affects the central nervous, musculoskeletal, and urinary systems.

Etiology – A single etiology has not been identified, however, causative factors include genetic predisposition, environmental influence, low levels of maternal folic acid, maternal hyperthermia, and certain classifications of drugs. Classifications of spina bifida include:

- **Spina Bifida Occulta** - An impairment and non-fusion of the spinous processes of a vertebra, however, the spinal cord and meninges remain intact. There is usually no associated disability.
- **Spina Bifida Cystica** - Presents with a cyst-like protrusion through the non-fused vertebrae, which results in impairment.

  Meningocele - Herniation of meninges and cerebrospinal fluid into a sac that protrudes through the vertebral defect. The spinal cord remains within the canal.

  Myelomeningocele - A severe form characterized by herniation of meninges, cerebrospinal fluid, and the spinal cord extending through the defect in the vertebrae. The cyst may or may not be covered by skin.

Signs and symptoms – Characteristics and associated impairments of myelomeningocele include motor loss below the level of the defect in the spinal cord, sensory deficits, hydrocephalus, Arnold-Chiari Type II malformation, osteoporosis, clubfoot, scoliosis, tethered cord syndrome, latex allergy, bowel and bladder dysfunction, and learning disabilities.

Treatment – Physical therapy treatment emphasizes significant family teaching regarding positioning, handling, range of motion, and therapeutic exercise. Additional therapeutic activities include facilitation of developmental milestones, skin care, strengthening, balance and mobility training, adaptive equipment, splinting, orthotic prescription, and wheelchair prescription. Physical therapy is ongoing through adolescence and is based on the severity of impairments and needs of the child.

Spinal Muscular Atrophy (SMA)[13,45,46,47]

Spinal muscular atrophy is characterized by progressive degeneration of the anterior horn cell.

Etiology – The causative factor of spinal muscular atrophy is an autosomal recessive genetic inheritance. Certain types of this disease involve a mutation on chromosome 5.

Signs and symptoms – Characteristics for all categories of the disease are the same, and vary in onset and speed of progression. Characteristics include progressive muscle weakness and atrophy, diminished or absent deep tendon reflexes, normal intelligence, intact sensation, and end-stage respiratory compromise.

Treatment – Treatment includes positioning, vestibular and visual stimulation, and access to play. Treatment for the slower progressing categories is primarily supportive including educating caregivers, mobility training, and use of assistive devices and adaptive equipment.

Legislation Acts and Amendments for the Education of Children with Disabilities[48]

Over the last 25 years, there have been various forms of legislation that were enacted in order to improve health care, medical benefits, and education specifically for children. The largest reforms are listed below.

Education for All Handicapped Children Act (enacted 1975)

The groundbreaking law was intended to support states and localities in protecting the rights of, meeting the individual needs of, and improving the results for infants, toddlers, children, and youths with disabilities and their families. This is the origin of the Individuals with Disabilities Education Improvement Act (IDEA).

Carl D. Perkins Vocational Education Act of 1984

Each state was required to meet the special needs of individuals with handicaps or adults that are disadvantaged, adults in need of training and retraining, single parents or homemakers, programs designed to eliminate sex bias/stereotyping, and criminal offenders.

Perkins Vocational and Applied Technology Act (enacted 1990)

Reauthorization and modification of the Education for All Handicapped Children Act (EHA). Provides free, appropriate education in the least restrictive environment for individuals with disabilities from age 3-21.

IDEA (Individuals with Disabilities Education Improvement Act) Amendments (enacted 1991)

Reauthorized early intervention; established Federal Interagency Coordination Council.

Rehabilitation Act Amendments (enacted 1992)

Transition planning at high school graduation includes coordination of assistive technology services and the rehabilitation system.

IDEA Amendments (enacted 1997)

Restructuring of IDEA into four distinct and individual parts. It defines the responsibilities of school districts in providing services to ensure that children with certain specified disabilities receive free, appropriate education. School districts must prepare an Individualized Education Program (IEP) for each eligible child. Related services most commonly include speech, physical, and occupational therapies, and child counseling.

No Child Left Behind Act (enacted 2002)

The most sweeping reform of the Elementary and Secondary Education Act since its enactment in 1965. This act redefines the federal role in K-12 education. It requires accountability for all children, including student groups based on poverty, race and ethnicity, disability, and limited English proficiency (LEP). Its goal is to close the achievement gap between disadvantaged, disabled, and minority students and their peers.

Before the IDEA

- One in five children with disabilities was educated.
- Over 1 million children with disabilities were excluded from the education system.
- 3.5 million children with disabilities did not receive appropriate services.

Impact of the IDEA

- Currently 6.5 million children with disabilities are served.
- 96% of students with disabilities are now served in a regular school setting.
- There is an increase in the number of children from birth to three that receive services.

MOTIVATIONAL MOMENT

See Page 990

GOLD Level Clinical Application Templates

Level Clinical Application Template Executive Summary

Alzheimer's Disease

- Progressive neurological disorder that results in deterioration and irreversible damage within the cerebral cortex and subcortical areas of the brain
- Disease is initially noted by a change in higher cortical functions characterized by subtle changes in memory, impaired concentration, and difficulty with new learning
- Typical course of the disease averages between 7-11 years with death resulting from infection or dehydration

Amyotrophic Lateral Sclerosis

- Risk is higher in males than females and usually occurs between 40-70 years of age
- Clinical presentation may include both upper and lower motor neuron involvement with weakness occurring in a distal to proximal progression
- Average course of the diagnosis is two to five years with 20-30% of patients surviving longer than five years

Carpal Tunnel Syndrome

- Incidence is higher in females than males with the most common age being from 35-55 years of age
- Muscle atrophy is often noted in the abductor pollicis brevis muscle and later in the thenar muscles
- Electromyography studies, Tinel's sign, and Phalen's test can be used to assist with confirming the diagnosis

Cerebral Palsy

- Spastic cerebral palsy involves upper motor neuron damage; athetoid cerebral palsy involves damage to the basal ganglia
- Clinical presentation includes motor delays, abnormal muscle tone and motor control, reflex abnormalities, poor postural control, and balance impairments
- Intellectual disability and epilepsy are present in 50-60% of children diagnosed with cerebral palsy

Cerebrovascular Accident

- Types of CVA include ischemic stroke (thrombus, embolus, lacunar) and hemorrhagic stroke (intracerebral, subdural, subarachnoid)
- Left CVA may present with weakness or paralysis to the right side, impaired processing, heightened frustration, aphasia, dysphagia, and motor apraxia
- Right CVA may present with weakness or paralysis to the left side, poor attention span, impaired awareness and judgment, spatial deficits, memory deficits, emotional lability, and impulsive behavior

Down Syndrome

- Clinical manifestations include hypotonia, flattened nasal bridge, Simian line (palmar crease), epicanthal folds, enlargement of the tongue, and developmental delay
- Detection occurs in approximately 60-70% of women tested that are carrying a baby with Down syndrome
- Exercise is essential for a child with Down syndrome in order to avoid inactivity and obesity

Level Clinical Application Template Executive Summary

Duchenne Muscular Dystrophy

- X-linked recessive trait manifesting in only male offspring while female offspring become carriers
- Clinical presentation includes waddling gait, proximal muscle weakness, toe walking, pseudohypertrophy of the calf, and difficulty climbing stairs
- There is usually rapid progression of this disease with the inability to ambulate by ten to twelve years of age with death occurring as a teenager or less frequently in the 20's

Guillain-Barre Syndrome

- Results in motor weakness in a distal to proximal progression, sensory impairment, and possible respiratory paralysis
- Etiology of the disease is unknown, however, it is hypothesized to be an autoimmune response to a previous respiratory infection, influenza, immunization or surgery
- Majority of patients experience full recovery, 20% have remaining neurologic deficits, and 3-5% of patients die from respiratory complications

Multiple Sclerosis

- Characterized by demyelination of the myelin sheaths that surround nerves within the brain and spinal cord resulting in plaque development, decreased nerve conduction velocity, and eventual failure of impulse transmission
- Clinical symptoms may include visual problems, paresthesias, sensory changes, clumsiness, weakness, ataxia, balance dysfunction, and fatigue
- Intervention includes regulation of activity level, relaxation and energy conservation techniques, normalization of tone, balance activities, gait training, and core stabilization

Parkinson's Disease

- Degenerative disorder characterized by a decrease in production of dopamine (neurotransmitter) within the substantia nigra of the basal ganglia
- Clinical presentation may include hypokinesia, difficulty initiating and stopping movement, festinating and shuffling gait, bradykinesia, poor posture, and "cogwheel" or "lead pipe" rigidity
- Medical management includes dopamine replacement therapy (Levodopa, Sinemet, Madopar) which is designed to minimize bradykinesia, rigidity, and tremor

Sciatica Secondary to a Herniated Disk

- The sciatic nerve experiences an inflammatory response and subsequent damage secondary to compression from the herniated disk
- Sciatica is characterized by low back and gluteal pain that typically radiates down the back of the thigh along the sciatic nerve distribution
- Pain will increase in a sitting position or when lifting, forward bending or twisting

Level Clinical Application Template Executive Summary

Spinal Cord Injury – Complete C7 Tetraplegia

- Clinical presentation includes impaired cough and ability to clear secretions, altered breathing pattern, and poor endurance
- Outcomes at this level include independence with feeding, grooming, dressing, self-range of motion, independent manual wheelchair mobility, independent transfers, and independent driving with an adapted automobile
- The triceps, extensor pollicis longus and brevis, extrinsic finger extensors, and flexor carpi radialis will remain the lowest innervated muscles

Spinal Cord Injury – Complete L3 Paraplegia

- Patients possess at least partial innervation of the gracilis, iliopsoas, quadratus lumborum, rectus femoris, and sartorius with full upper extremity use
- Additional findings that can exist include sexual dysfunction, a nonreflexive bladder, the need for a bowel program, urinary tract infections, muscle contractures, and pressure sores
- Patients with L3 paraplegia should be able to live independently with education regarding the management of their disability

Thoracic Outlet Syndrome

- Results from compression and damage to the brachial plexus nerve trunks, subclavian vascular supply, and/or the axillary artery
- Contributing factors in the development of the condition include the presence of a cervical rib, an abnormal first rib, postural deviations, hypertrophy or spasms of the scalene muscles, and an elongated cervical transverse process
- Females are at two to three times greater risk than males, with the most common age ranging from 30-40 years of age

Traumatic Brain Injury

- Occurs due to an open head injury where there is penetration through the skull or closed head injury where the brain makes contact with the skull secondary to a sudden, violent acceleration or deceleration
- Brain injury may include swelling, axonal injury, hypoxia, hematoma, hemorrhage, and changes in intracranial pressure
- High risk groups include ages 0-4, 15-19, and greater than 65 (males are at greater risk in each category)

DIAGNOSIS

What condition produces a patient's symptoms?

Alzheimer's disease is a progressive neurological disorder that results in deterioration and irreversible damage within the cerebral cortex and subcortical areas of the brain. The loss of neurons results from the breakdown of several processes that would normally sustain the brain cells.

An injury was most likely sustained to which structure?

Neurons that are normally involved with acetylcholine transmission deteriorate within the cerebral cortex of the brain. Postmortem biopsy reveals neurofibrillary tangles within cytoplasm, amyloid plaques, and cerebral atrophy. Amyloid plaques contain fragmented axons, altered glial cells, and cellular waste that result in an inflammatory response that causes further damage to the nervous system. Amyloid can also cause atrophy of the smooth muscle of the arteries of the brain, predisposing them to rupture.

INFERENCE

What is the most likely contributing factor in the development of this condition?

The exact etiology of Alzheimer's disease is unknown, however, hypothesized causes include lower levels of neurotransmitters, higher levels of aluminum within brain tissue, genetic inheritance, autoimmune disease, abnormal processing of the substance amyloid, and virus. Approximately 4.5 million individuals are living with Alzheimer's disease in the United States. The risk of developing Alzheimer's disease increases with age and there is a higher incidence in women. The prevalence of Alzheimer's disease is 6% of individuals over 65 and 20% of individuals over 80 years of age.

CONFIRMATION

What is the most likely clinical presentation?

Alzheimer's disease is initially noted by a change in higher cortical functions characterized by subtle changes in memory, impaired concentration, and difficulty with new learning. These symptoms progress in the early stages and there is a loss of orientation, word finding difficulties, emotional lability, depression, poor judgment, and impaired ability to perform self-care skills. During the middle stages of Alzheimer's disease the patient will develop behavioral and motor problems characterized by neurological symptoms such as aphasia, apraxia, perseveration, agitation, and violent or socially unacceptable behavior that can include wandering. Eventually all ability to learn is lost and long-term memory also disappears. End-stage Alzheimer's disease is characterized by severe intellectual and physical destruction. Patients in this stage will present with vegetative symptoms including incontinence, functional dependence, the inability to speak, and seizure activity.

What laboratory or imaging studies would confirm the diagnosis?

Alzheimer's disease presently cannot be confirmed until a postmortem biopsy reveals the neurofibrillary tangles and amyloid plaques. MRI can be used to assess any abnormalities or signs of atrophy within the brain that is associated with Alzheimer's disease or to rule out other medical conditions. Single photon emission computed tomography (SPECT) may be used to determine brain activity and predict potential for Alzheimer's disease. Blood work, urine, and spinal fluid may be required to rule out other diseases that may cause signs of dementia.

What additional information should be obtained to confirm the diagnosis?

A physical examination, neurological examination, and neuropsychological testing are required for diagnosis of probable Alzheimer's disease. The patient must demonstrate at least two deficits of cognition, memory, and related cognitive functioning with the absence of all other brain disease or disturbances in consciousness that may contribute to the identified deficits. Family history and symptoms may provide insight into the expected speed of progression of the disease.

EXAMINATION

What history should be documented?

Important areas to explore include past medical history, family history, history of current symptoms, current health status, living environment, social history and habits, occupation, and social support system.

What tests/measures are most appropriate?

Aerobic capacity and endurance: assessment of vital signs at rest and with activity

Arousal, attention, and cognition: examine mental status, learning ability, memory, motivation, Mini-Mental State Examination, level of consciousness

Assistive and adaptive devices: analysis of components and safety of a device

Environmental, home, and work barriers: analysis of current and potential barriers or hazards

Gait, locomotion, and balance: static and dynamic balance in sitting and standing, safety during gait with/without an assistive device, Functional Ambulation Profile, Berg Balance Scale

Motor function: equilibrium and righting reactions, coordination, physical performance scales

Muscle performance: strength assessment

Posture: analysis of resting and dynamic posture

Range of motion: active and passive range of motion

Reflex integrity: assessment of deep tendon and pathological reflexes (e.g., Babinski, ATNR)

Self-care and home management: assessment of functional capacity, Functional Independence Measure (FIM), Barthel Index

Alzheimer's Disease   GOLD

What additional findings are likely with this patient?

A patient with end-stage Alzheimer's disease is at high risk for infection and pneumonia. These patients may experience complications from a persistent vegetative state such as contractures, decubiti, fracture, and pulmonary compromise.

MANAGEMENT

What is the most effective management of this patient?

Medical management of Alzheimer's disease may include pharmacological intervention during the early stages of the disease process. Medications are administered to inhibit acetylcholinesterase, alleviate cognitive symptoms, and control behavioral changes. Drug therapies are usually short-term in effect lasting six to nine months. Tacrine (Cognex), donepezil (Aricept), and rivastigmine (Exelon) are common pharmacological agents used to treat Alzheimer's disease, however, the side effects can be substantial. Physical therapy management should focus on maximizing the patient's remaining function and providing family and caregiver education. The therapist should attempt to create an emotional and physical environment that provides the patient with the opportunity to experience success. Modifying the layout of the patient's living space in order for the patient to easily find items is one example of creating an environment that encourages success. Safety with functional mobility and gait training may be indicated in the early stages of the disease. Later stages may require ongoing caregiver education regarding assistance with mobility, range of motion, and positioning. Many patients require a long-term care facility that specializes in Alzheimer's disease secondary to personality changes, aggressive behavior, and end-stage complications.

What home care regimen should be recommended?

During the early stages of Alzheimer's disease a patient should continue with activity as tolerated and utilize a memory book or other compensatory strategies at home. As the disease progresses, a patient will rely on caregiver support to assist with a daily exercise program. The patient should be encouraged to exercise, ambulate, and participate in everyday activities such as folding laundry, making beds, and assisting with dinner in order to avoid restlessness and wandering.

OUTCOME

What is the likely outcome of a course of physical therapy?

Physical therapy may be indicated intermittently throughout the course of the disease, however, the therapy will not alter or cease the progression of the disease process.

What are the long-term effects of the patient's condition?

Alzheimer's disease is a chronic and progressive disorder and is the fourth leading cause of death in adults. The typical course of the disease averages between seven and eleven years. The leading cause of death of a patient with Alzheimer's disease is infection or dehydration.

COMPARISON

What are the distinguishing characteristics of a similar condition?

Multi-infarct dementia produces symptoms in a step-like manner secondary to ongoing cerebral infarcts. This form of dementia is usually found in patients that are over 70 years of age and is more common in males. Hypertension is a primary risk factor and depression is common. A patient may also experience neurological deficits such as hemiplegia and emotional lability.

CLINICAL SCENARIOS

Scenario One

A 65-year-old female is referred to physical therapy for gait disturbances. The patient resides alone and drives on a regular basis. During the examination the patient reveals that she is sometimes confused when driving. The patient complains that she has difficulty managing her time around the house and requires an extended amount of time to get ready in the morning.

Scenario Two

A 79-year-old male is seen by a therapist in an Alzheimer's residential facility. The physician recommends gait training with a walker. The patient enjoys walking around the unit, however, has fallen several times within the last month.

Amyotrophic Lateral Sclerosis

DIAGNOSIS

What condition produces a patient's symptoms?

Amyotrophic lateral sclerosis (ALS) is a chronic degenerative disease that produces both upper and lower motor neuron impairments. Demyelination, axonal swelling, and atrophy within the cerebral cortex, premotor areas, sensory cortex, and temporal cortex cause the symptoms of ALS.

An injury was most likely sustained to which structure?

Rapid degeneration and demyelination occur in the giant pyramidal cells of the cerebral cortex and affect areas of the corticospinal tracts, cell bodies of the lower motor neurons in the gray matter, anterior horn cells, and areas within the precentral gyrus of the cortex. The rapid degeneration causes denervation of muscle fibers, muscle atrophy, and weakness.

INFERENCE

What is the most likely contributing factor in the development of this condition?

The exact etiology of ALS is unknown (90% of all cases), however, there are multiple theories of causative factors that include genetic inheritance as an autosomal dominant trait, a slow acting virus, metabolic disturbances, and theories of toxicity of lead and aluminum. Familial ALS occurs in 5-10% of all cases. Risk for ALS is higher in men and usually occurs between 40 to 70 years of age.

CONFIRMATION

What is the most likely clinical presentation?

Early clinical presentation of ALS may include both upper and lower motor neuron involvement. Early lower motor neuron signs include asymmetric muscle weakness, cramping, and atrophy that are usually found within the hands. Muscle weakness due to denervation eventually causes significant fasciculations, atrophy and wasting of the muscles. The weakness spreads throughout the body over the course of the disease and generally follows a distal to proximal path. Upper motor neuron symptoms occur due to the loss of inhibition of the muscle. Incoordination of movement, spasticity, clonus, and a positive Babinski reflex are some of the indicators of upper motor neuron involvement. Bulbar involvement is characterized by dysarthria, dysphagia, and emotional lability. Initially a person may have either upper or lower motor neuron involvement, but eventually both categories are affected. A patient with ALS will exhibit fatigue, oral motor impairment, fasciculations, spasticity, motor paralysis, and eventual respiratory paralysis.

What laboratory or imaging studies would confirm the diagnosis?

There are multiple tests used to assist with diagnosing ALS. Electromyography assesses fibrillation and muscle fasciculations. Muscle biopsy verifies lower motor neuron involvement rather than muscle disease and a spinal tap may reveal a higher protein content in some patients with ALS. CT scan will appear normal until late in the disease process.

What additional information should be obtained to confirm the diagnosis?

Diagnosis relies heavily on symptoms that determine both upper and lower motor neuron involvement. A patient that presents with motor impairment without sensory impairment is a primary indicator of ALS. Definitive diagnosis also first requires a physician to rule out other neurological conditions such as multiple sclerosis, spinal cord tumors, progressive muscular dystrophy, Lyme disease, and syringomyelia.

EXAMINATION

What history should be documented?

Important areas include past medical history, family history, history of current symptoms, current health status, living environment, social history and habits, occupation, and social support system.

What tests/measures are most appropriate?

Aerobic capacity and endurance: assessment of vital signs at rest and with activity, perceived exertion scale

Anthropometric characteristics: weight and height

Arousal, attention, and cognition: examines mental status, learning ability, memory, motivation

Assistive and adaptive devices: analysis of components and safety of a device

Environmental, home, and work barriers: analysis of current and potential barriers or hazards

Gait, locomotion, and balance: static and dynamic balance in sitting and standing, safety during gait with/without an assistive device

Motor function: motor assessment scales, coordination, equilibrium and righting reactions

Muscle Performance: strength assessment, muscle endurance, muscle tone assessment, muscle atrophy

Neuromotor development and sensory integration: analysis of reflex movement patterns, assessment of involuntary movements, sensory integration tests, gross and fine motor skills

Posture: analysis of resting and dynamic posture

Range of motion: active and passive range of motion

Reflex integrity: assessment of deep tendon and pathological reflexes (e.g., Babinski, ATNR)

Self-care and home management: Barthel Index

Ventilation, respiration, and circulation: respiratory muscle strength, accessory muscle utilization, assessment of cough

What additional findings are likely with this patient?

During the initial stages of ALS there are various effects on the body. Progression of the disease allows for significant deterioration within the brain and spinal cord and a patient may exhibit paralysis of vocal cords, swallowing impairment, contractures, decubiti, and breathing difficulty that requires ventilatory support. Throughout the course of ALS, however, sensation, eye movement, and bowel and bladder function remain preserved.

MANAGEMENT

What is the most effective management of this patient?

Effective management of ALS is based on supportive care and symptomatic therapy. Pharmacological intervention may include riluzole (Rilutek). This drug appears to have an effect on the progression of the disease process, however, its long-term effects are unknown. Symptomatic therapy may include anticholinergic, antispasticity, and antidepressant medications. Physical, occupational, speech, respiratory, and nutritional therapies may be warranted. Physical therapy intervention should focus on the quality of life and should include a low-level exercise program, range of motion, mobility training, assistive/adaptive devices, wheelchair prescription, bronchial hygiene, and energy conservation techniques. Patient, family, and caregiver training are important as the disease continues to progress.

What home-care regimen should be recommended?

A home care regimen for a patient with ALS must consider the rate of disease progression and level of respiratory involvement. Goals should focus on maximizing the patient's functional capacity. A low-level exercise program may be indicated as long as the patient does not exercise to fatigue and promote further weakness. Family involvement is encouraged to support the patient through the course of the disease and assist with mobility, pacing skills, energy conservation techniques, and overall safety. During the latter part of the disease the family and caregivers must be competent with positioning, bronchial hygiene, range of motion, and assistance with mobility.

OUTCOME

What is the likely outcome of a course of physical therapy?

Physical therapy intervention may assist with current issues, however, therapy does not hinder progression of ALS. Therapeutic goals will consider disease progression and focus on teaching for the patient and caregivers.

What are the long-term effects of the patient's condition?

ALS is usually a rapidly progressing neurological disease with an average course of two to five years with 20-30% of patients surviving longer than five years. Research indicates that although there is no structured course of this disease process, if a patient is diagnosed before 50 years of age the disease is usually longer in course. Death usually occurs from respiratory failure.

COMPARISON

What are the distinguishing characteristics of a similar condition?

Muscular dystrophy (MD) is the term for a group of inherited disorders that are progressive and exhibit degeneration of muscles without sensory or neural impairment. Progressive weakness occurs to the muscle fibers secondary to the absence of dystrophin within the skeletal muscles. This group of disorders presents early in life and usually shortens life expectancy. Disuse atrophy, muscle deterioration, contractures, and cardiac and respiratory weakness are common characteristics of this disease process. A patient with MD usually dies from respiratory/cardiac complications secondary to the primary disease process.

CLINICAL SCENARIOS

Scenario One

A 56-year-old male is diagnosed with ALS and presents with mild atrophy of the hand. The patient owns his own business as a painter and wants to continue working for as long as he can. The patient is referred to physical therapy for a home exercise program.

Scenario Two

A 60-year-old female is referred to physical therapy secondary to a left CVA. The patient was also diagnosed with ALS two years ago, requires the use of a wheelchair for mobility, and occasionally chokes while eating. The patient has assistance at home from her husband who is in good health.

Carpal Tunnel Syndrome

DIAGNOSIS

What condition produces a patient's symptoms?

The carpal tunnel is created by the transverse carpal ligament, the scaphoid tuberosity and trapezium, the hook of the hamate and pisiform, and the volar radiocarpal ligament and volar ligamentous extensions between the carpal bones. The median nerve, four flexor digitorum profundus tendons, four flexor digitorum superficialis tendons, and the flexor pollicis longus tendon pass through the carpal tunnel. Carpal tunnel syndrome (CTS) occurs as a result of compression of the median nerve where it passes through the carpal tunnel.

An injury was most likely sustained to which structure?

The median nerve is injured by compression within the carpal tunnel at the wrist. Normal tissue pressure within the tunnel is 2 to 10 mm Hg, but CTS can result in pressure above 30 mm Hg, which further increases with flexion and extension of the wrist. The increase in pressure produces ischemia in the nerve. This results in sensory and motor disturbances in the median nerve distribution of the hand.

INFERENCE

What is the most likely contributing factor in the development of this condition?

Any condition such as edema, inflammation, tumor or fibrosis may cause compression of the median nerve within the carpal tunnel and result in ischemia. The exact etiology of CTS is unclear, however, conditions that produce inflammation of the carpal tunnel that can contribute to CTS include repetitive use, rheumatoid arthritis, pregnancy, diabetes, trauma, tumor, hypothyroidism, and wrist sprain or fracture. Other etiologies include a congenital narrowing of the tunnel and vitamin B6 deficiency.

CONFIRMATION

What is the most likely clinical presentation?

Approximately five million individuals in the United States are diagnosed with CTS. Most patients are diagnosed between 35 and 55 years of age with greater prevalence in women. A patient with CTS will initially present with sensory changes and paresthesia along the median nerve distribution in the hand. It may also radiate into the upper extremity, shoulder, and neck. Symptoms include night pain, weakness of the hand, muscle atrophy, decreased grip strength, clumsiness, and decreased wrist mobility. Initially, muscle atrophy is often noted in the abductor pollicis brevis muscle and progresses to the thenar muscles.

What laboratory or imaging studies would confirm the diagnosis?

Electromyography and electroneurographic studies can be used to diagnose a motor conduction delay along the median nerve within the carpal tunnel. MRI is sometimes used to identify inflammation of the median nerve, altered tendon or nerve positioning within the tunnel or thickening of the tendon sheath.

What additional information should be obtained to confirm the diagnosis?

Physical examination, history, and review of symptoms are extremely important when diagnosing CTS. Provocation testing such as a positive Tinel's sign, a positive Phalen's test, and a positive tethered median nerve stress test along with the other symptoms will assist to confirm the diagnosis.

EXAMINATION

What history should be documented?

Important areas to explore include past medical history, medications, history of symptoms, current health status, occupation, living environment, social history and habits, leisure activities, and social support system.

What tests/measures are most appropriate?

Anthropometric characteristics: wrist and hand circumferential measurements

Arousal, attention, and cognition: examine mental status, learning ability, memory, motivation

Community and work integration: analysis of community, work, and leisure activities

Environmental, home, and work barriers: analysis of current and potential barriers or hazards

Ergonomics and body mechanics: analysis of dexterity and coordination

Integumentary integrity: skin and nailbed assessment, assessment of sensation

Joint integrity and mobility: assessment of hypomobility of a joint, assessment of soft tissue swelling/inflammation, Tinel's sign, Phalen's test, tethered median nerve stress test

Muscle performance: strength assessment including hand musculature

Orthotic, protective, and supportive devices: potential utilization of bracing or splinting

Pain: pain perception assessment scale

Range of motion: active and passive range of motion

Self-care and home management: assessment of functional capacity

Carpal Tunnel Syndrome

What additional findings are likely with this patient?

Advanced CTS can present with muscle atrophy of the hand, radiating pain in the forearm and shoulder, and nerve damage with motor and sensory loss. Unrelieved compression creates initial neurapraxia with some demyelination of the axons. This results in eventual axonotmesis and Wallerian degeneration within the nerve distribution. The patient may present with ape hand deformity caused by atrophy of the thenar musculature and first two lumbricals. Research indicates that approximately 50% of cases include bilateral involvement.

MANAGEMENT

What is the most effective management of this patient?

A patient with CTS will initially receive conservative management including local corticosteroid injections, splinting, and physical therapy management. Recent pharmacological intervention has included Methylprednisolone injected proximally to the tunnel. Physical therapy is one aspect of conservative management and includes splinting, carpal mobilization, and gentle stretching. Biomechanical analysis and adaptation of a patient's occupation, work place, leisure activities, and living environment may be necessary.

If conservative treatment fails the patient may require surgery to release the carpal ligament and decompress the median nerve. Newer surgical techniques allow for smaller incisions, less manipulation of the nerve, and are highly successful for long-term relief of symptoms. Post-surgical physical therapy intervention should include the use of moist heat with electrical stimulation, iontophoresis, cryotherapy, gentle massage, desensitization of the scar, tendon gliding exercises, and active range of motion. A patient should initially avoid wrist flexion and a forceful grasp. After four weeks, a patient can progress with active wrist flexion, gentle stretching, putty exercises, light progressive resistive exercise, and continued modification of body mechanics. Radial deviation against resistance should be avoided due to the tendency for irritation and inflammation. Post-surgical rehabilitation usually lasts six to eight weeks.

What home care regimen should be recommended?

A home care regimen should consist of continued stretching and strengthening exercises. The patient must be competent and compliant regarding the use of a splint and follow all work and leisure modifications.

OUTCOME

What is the likely outcome of a course of physical therapy?

Physical therapy intervention should improve a patient's condition and decrease symptoms of CTS within four to six weeks. If conservative treatment fails and the patient requires surgical intervention, rehabilitation may last six to eight weeks.

What are the long-term effects of the patient's condition?

CTS can have minor effects on some patients while having debilitating effects on others. The overall long-term effects are dependent on the degree of involvement, the amount of permanent damage, and the level of success with conservative or surgical management. It is possible to have no long-term effects from this condition if the patient responds positively to physical therapy and the rehabilitation process. Other patients may be left with permanent motor and sensory impairments along the median nerve distribution.

COMPARISON

What are the distinguishing characteristics of a similar condition?

Compression in the tunnel of Guyon occurs with inflammation to the ulnar nerve between the hook of the hamate and the pisiform. This condition occurs from tasks such as leaning during extended handwriting, leaning on bike handles while riding, repetitive gripping activities or trauma. The patient will present with paresthesias along the ulnar distribution, weakness and atrophy of the hypothenar musculature, decreased mobility of the pisiform, and impaired grip strength. This condition can be treated with conservative management or surgical intervention.

CLINICAL SCENARIOS

Scenario One

A 26-year-old female is seen in physical therapy with a diagnosis of bilateral CTS. The patient has not been treated previously for this syndrome and is employed as a telephone sales specialist. The patient complains of pain in her hands, numbness when sleeping and while performing at work, and muscle soreness in both hands.

Scenario Two

A 45-year-old male with CTS is referred to physical therapy ten days after surgical decompression. The patient's post-operative routine includes resting the hand, using a splint, icing, and elevation. Minimal edema is noted at the wrist. The patient is anxious to return to work.

DIAGNOSIS

What condition produces a patient's symptoms?

Cerebral palsy (CP) is an umbrella term used to describe a group of non-progressive movement disorders that result from brain damage. CP is the most common cause of permanent disability in children.

An injury was most likely sustained to which structure?

There is a wide variety of neurological damage that can occur with injury. Autopsy reports have indicated lesions that include hemorrhage below the lining of the ventricles, damage to the central nervous system that caused neuropathy and anoxia, and hypoxia that caused encephalopathy. Hypoxic and ischemic injuries disrupt normal metabolism that results in global damage to the developing fetus. CP is classified by neurological dysfunction and extremity involvement. Spastic CP involves upper motor neuron damage; athetoid CP involves damage to the basal ganglia.

INFERENCE

What is the most likely contributing factor in the development of this condition?

The etiology may be multifactorial and is sometimes unknown. Risk factors are categorized as prenatal (80%) or perinatal and postnatal (20%) cases. Prenatal risk factors include Rh incompatibility, maternal malnutrition, hypothyroidism, infection, diabetes, and chromosome abnormalities. Perinatal factors include multiple or premature births, breech delivery, low birth weight, prolapsed cord, placenta abruption, and asphyxia. Postnatal factors include CVA, head trauma, neonatal infection, and brain tumor. The most common causative factor of CP is prenatal cerebral hypoxia.

CONFIRMATION

What is the most likely clinical presentation?

CP is the second most common neurological impairment seen in children (following intellectual disability). CP is a neuromuscular disorder of posture and controlled movement, however, clinical presentation is highly variable based on the area and extent of CNS damage. A child may present with high tone, low tone or athetoid movement. CP is classified as monoplegia (one involved extremity), hemiplegia (unilateral involvement of the upper and lower extremities), and quadriplegia (involvement of all extremities). CP is also classified as mild, moderate, and severe. General characteristics include motor delays, abnormal muscle tone and motor control, reflex abnormalities, poor postural control, high risk for hip dislocations, and balance impairments. Intellect, vision, hearing, and perceptual skills are usually altered in conjunction with CP. All other characteristics of CP are classification dependent.

What laboratory or imaging studies would confirm the diagnosis?

If CP is suspected through clinical findings, including seizures, an electroencephalography (EEG) may be performed. X-ray of the hip may rule out hip dislocation; blood and urine tests can be used to investigate a metabolic cause of CP. Observation usually will diagnose CP secondary to the observed outward characteristics.

What additional information should be obtained to confirm the diagnosis?

Diagnosis of CP is regularly confirmed through an extensive neurological evaluation, patient observation, and patient history including developmental progress, and the presence of pathological reflexes. Differential diagnosis is performed to rule out other potential disorders.

EXAMINATION

What history should be documented?

Important areas to explore include past medical history, risk factors, maternal course of pregnancy, medications, family history, current characteristics, social history, and social support system.

What tests/measures are most appropriate?

Aerobic capacity and endurance: assessment of vital signs at rest and with activity, auscultation of the lungs

Arousal, attention, and cognition: examine mental status, learning ability, memory, motivation

Assistive and adaptive devices: analysis of components and safety of a device

Environmental, home, and work barriers: analysis of current and potential barriers or hazards

Gait, locomotion, and balance: static/dynamic balance

Integumentary integrity: skin assessment, assessment of sensation

Joint integrity and mobility: assessment of hyper- and hypomobility of a joint

Motor function: equilibrium and righting reactions, coordination, posture and balance, sensorimotor integration, Barthel Index, Bayley Scale of Infant Development, Bruininks-Oseretsky Test of Motor Proficiency, Alberta Infant Motor Scale, Pediatric Evaluation of Disability Inventory

Muscle performance: muscle tone assessment, strength assessment if appropriate

Neuromotor development and sensory integration: analysis of reflex movement patterns, assessment of involuntary movements, sensory integration tests, gross and fine motor skills, developmental milestones

Orthotic, protective, and supportive devices: analysis of components of a device

Pain: adapted pain scale

Posture: analysis of resting and dynamic posture

Range of motion: active and passive range of motion, assessment of contractures

Reflex integrity: assessment of deep tendon and pathological reflexes (e.g., Babinski, ATNR, Moro)

Sensory integrity: proprioception and kinesthesia

Ventilation, respiration, and circulation: breathing patterns, respiratory strength, accessory muscle utilization

Cerebral Palsy

What additional findings are likely with this patient?

Specific additional findings are dependent on the classification and extent of CP. Generally, complications can include aspiration, pneumonia, contractures, scoliosis, and constipation. Intellectual disability and epilepsy are present in 50-60% of children diagnosed with CP. Common co-morbidities include learning disabilities, seizure disorders, vision and hearing impairments, bowel and bladder dysfunction, microcephalus, and hydrocephalus. Secondary impairments may include psychosocial issues for the patient and family members.

MANAGEMENT

What is the most effective management of this patient?

Effective medical management of CP requires a life-long team approach. Pharmacological intervention may require antianxiety, antispasticity, and anticonvulsant medications. Physical therapy for CP often uses neurodevelopmental treatment and sensory integration techniques. Treatment should include normalization of tone, patient and caregiver education, motor learning, developmental milestones, positioning, stretching, strengthening, balance, and mobility skills. Adaptive equipment, specialized wheelchair seating, and orthotic prescription may be indicated. Surgical management may be required and include hip correction, contracture release, motor point block, dorsal rhizotomy or correction of scoliosis.

What home care regimen should be recommended?

A home care regimen for a patient with CP is also a life-long process that will require ongoing modification to meet the progression of goals. Family and caregiver involvement are vital for patients with moderate to severe CP. A home program may include patient and caregiver education, exercise, positioning, stretching, mobility training, and strengthening.

OUTCOME

What is the likely outcome of a course of physical therapy?

Physical therapy will attempt to maximize a patient's level of current function and prevent secondary loss. If a patient is going to ambulate, this will usually occur by the age of eight. The ability or inability to ambulate will have a large impact on the direction and goals of therapeutic intervention.

What are the long-term effects of the patient's condition?

CP is a non-progressive, but permanent condition. The long-term effects and overall functional outcome depend on the extent of injury, associated impairments, and caregiver support. Prognosis for mild to moderate CP is a near normal lifespan. Fifty percent of children with severe CP die by the age of ten.

COMPARISON

What are the distinguishing characteristics of a similar condition?

Arthrogryposis multiplex congenita (AMC) occurs in utero and is also considered to be non-progressive. AMC is a neuromuscular syndrome classified into three forms. The infant is born with multiple contractures and may have fibrous bands that developed in place of muscle. A patient with AMC should have a normal life expectancy and is typically of normal intelligence. It is usually difficult for these individuals to live independently due to their level of physical disability.

CLINICAL SCENARIOS

Scenario One

A two-year-old female diagnosed with moderate spastic quadriplegia is seen in physical therapy. She is delayed in developmental milestones and beginning to acquire contractures. The parents are very supportive and the child appears happy and cooperative. The child's chart indicates normal intelligence.

Scenario Two

A nine-year-old male is seen in physical therapy at the request of his parents. The patient is diagnosed with moderate low tone quadriplegia, has minimal impairments with intelligence, and has acquired a 30-degree left thoracic scoliosis. The parents requested the evaluation since the child remains nonambulatory.

DIAGNOSIS

What condition produces a patient's symptoms?

Cerebrovascular accident (CVA) occurs when there is an interruption of cerebral circulation that results in cerebral insufficiency, destruction of surrounding brain tissue, and subsequent neurological deficit. The ischemia occurs from either a stroke in evolution (the infarct slowly progresses over one to two days) or as a completed stroke (an abrupt infarct with immediate neurological deficits).

An injury was most likely sustained to which structure?

CVA results from prolonged ischemia to an artery within the brain. This condition can cause subsequent neurological damage relative to the size and location of the infarct. Disruption of blood flow to a certain artery will lead to damage of a specific area of the brain and its functions. There are different types of CVA that include ischemic stroke (thrombus, embolus, lacunar) and hemorrhagic stroke (intracerebral, subdural, subarachnoid).

INFERENCE

What is the most likely contributing factor in the development of this condition?

The primary risk factors for CVA are classified as modifiable and non-modifiable. Modifiable factors include hypertension, atherosclerosis, heart disease, diabetes, elevated cholesterol, smoking, and obesity. Hypertension is the most prevalent modifiable cause of CVA. Non-modifiable risk factors include age, race, family history, and sex. Age constitutes the greatest risk for CVA, in fact 73% of patients sustaining a stroke are greater than 65 years of age.

CONFIRMATION

What is the most likely clinical presentation?

It is estimated there are four million stroke survivors living today. The clinical presentation of a CVA is determined by the location and extent of the infarct. Typical characteristics can include hemiplegia or hemiparesis, sensory, visual, and perceptual impairments, balance abnormalities, dysphagia, aphasia, cognitive deficits, incontinence, and emotional lability.

What laboratory or imaging studies would confirm the diagnosis?

Computed tomography can confirm an area of infarct in the brain and its vascular origin, however, it can present as negative for up to a few days after the event. MRI allows for the diagnosis of ischemia within the brain almost immediately after onset. Positron emission tomography (PET) can provide information regarding cerebral perfusion and cell function. Ultrasonography identifies areas of diminished blood flow in vessels and angiography may identify a clot and determine if surgical intervention is necessary.

What additional information should be obtained to confirm the diagnosis?

A chest x-ray may be warranted to rule out lung disease, while an electrocardiogram is used to examine potential cardiac abnormalities. Diagnosis is usually based upon patient history, physical and neurological examinations, symptoms, and diagnostic testing.

EXAMINATION

What history should be documented?

Important areas to explore include past medical history, medications, risk factor profile, current health status, social history and habits, occupation, living environment, and social support system.

What tests/measures are most appropriate?

Arousal, attention, and cognition: examine mental status, learning ability, memory, motivation, Mini-Mental State Exam, Boston Diagnostic Aphasia Examination

Assistive and adaptive devices: analysis of components and safety of a device

Gait, locomotion, and balance: static and dynamic balance in sitting and standing, safety during gait with an assistive device, Berg Balance Scale, Tinetti Performance Oriented Mobility Assessment, Functional Ambulation Profile

Integumentary integrity: skin and sensation assessment

Motor function: equilibrium and righting reactions, coordination, motor assessment scales

Muscle performance: muscle tone assessment, assessment of active movement, Stroke Rehabilitation Assessment of Movement (STREAM)

Neuromotor development and sensory integration: assess involuntary movements, sensory integration, gross and fine motor skills, reflex movement patterns

Orthotic, protective, and supportive devices: analysis of components of a device, analysis of movement while wearing a device

Posture: analysis of resting and dynamic posture

Pain: pain perception assessment scale

Range of motion: active and passive range of motion

Reflexes: assessment of pathological reflexes (e.g., Babinski, ATNR)

Self-care and home management: assessment of functional capacity, Rankin Scale, NIH Stroke Scale, Functional Independence Measure (FIM)

Sensory integrity: proprioception and kinesthesia

What additional findings are likely with this patient?

A patient with a left CVA may present with weakness or paralysis to the right side, impaired processing, heightened frustration, aphasia, dysphagia, motor apraxia, and right hemianopsia. A patient with a right CVA may present with weakness or paralysis to the left side, poor attention span, impaired awareness and judgment, spatial deficits, memory deficits, left inattention, emotional lability, impulsive behavior, and left hemianopsia. Coma and death are the most severe consequences of a CVA. It is common for patients post CVA to have residual complications and deficits that persist.

MANAGEMENT

What is the most effective management of this patient?

Medical management will initially include medically stabilizing the patient through medication and surgical intervention. Pharmacological intervention can include thrombolytic agents, anticoagulants (contraindicated for hemorrhagic CVA), diuretics, antihypertensives, and potential long-term use of aspirin. Respiratory care must also be a priority during acute rehabilitation. Physical therapy during the acute phase focuses on positioning, pressure relief, sensory awareness and integration, ROM, weight bearing, facilitation, muscle re-education, balance, and postural control. The therapist is responsible for implementing the most appropriate therapeutic strategies based on the degree of impairment. There are many approaches to neurological rehabilitation that include, but are not limited to Bobath's Neuro-Developmental Treatment (NDT), motor control, Brunnstrom's Movement Therapy in Hemiplegia, Rood, and Kabat, Knott, and Voss' Proprioceptive Neuromuscular Facilitation (PNF). Many therapists integrate facets from multiple approaches based on the patient's response to selected interventions.

What home care regimen should be recommended?

Approximately 75% of patients that have experienced a CVA return home at various levels of functional mobility. The majority of patients require ongoing therapy services as part of their home care regimen. A therapeutic program should be designed for a patient to continue at home independently or with the required level of assistance. Fall prevention, control of spasticity, endurance training, and optimizing functional mobility are important components of a successful home program.

OUTCOME

What is the likely outcome of a course of physical therapy?

A patient that experiences neurological deficits due to a CVA may require physical therapy to assist with motor re-education, sensory stimulation, and functional mobility. The outcome is dependent on the patient's overall health, level of cognition and motivation, motor recovery, residual deficits, and family support.

What are the long-term effects of the patient's condition?

The effects of a CVA can be quite diverse ranging from spontaneous recovery to permanent disability requiring compensatory strategies and techniques in order to function. The first three months of recovery typically reveals the most measurable neurologic recovery and is usually a good indicator of the long-term outcome. Long-term outcome is based on several factors including the site and extent of CVA, premorbid status, age, potential for plasticity of the nervous system, and motivation. Research indicates that a patient can continue to improve the control of movement and show progress for an average of two to three years post CVA.

COMPARISON

What are the distinguishing characteristics of a similar condition?

A transient ischemic attack (TIA) is also characterized by diminished blood supply to the brain, however, It is transient. Although the patient may present with similar symptoms of a CVA, the symptoms last for only a brief period of time. Unlike a CVA, the TIA does not cause permanent residual neurological deficits. A TIA is an indication, however, of future risk for a CVA.

CLINICAL SCENARIOS

Scenario One

A 43-year-old male is diagnosed with a left hemorrhagic CVA due to an aneurysm of the middle cerebral artery. The patient resides with his wife and two teenage sons.

Scenario Two

A 79-year-old female is diagnosed with a right CVA involving the anterior cerebral artery. The patient was unconscious for two days and is functioning at a very low-level. The patient was residing in an independent living facility where she had meals provided for her in the dining area.

DIAGNOSIS

What condition produces a patient's symptoms?

Down syndrome (trisomy 21) occurs when there is an error in cell division either through nondisjunction (95%), translocation (4%) or mosaicism (1%) and the cell nucleus results in 47 chromosomes. Nondisjunction occurs when faulty cell division results in three specific chromosomes instead of two and extra chromosomes are then replicated for every cell. Translocation occurs when part of a chromosome breaks off during cell division and attaches to another chromosome. The total number of chromosomes remains 46, but Down syndrome exists. Mosaicism occurs right after fertilization when nondisjunction occurs in the initial cell divisions. This results in a mixture of cells with 46 and 47 chromosomes.

An injury was most likely sustained to which structure?

The pair of 21st chromosomes is responsible for Down syndrome when nondisjunction, translocation or mosaicism occurs during cell division.

INFERENCE

What is the most likely contributing factor in the development of this condition?

The exact etiology of Down syndrome is currently unknown. Some theories suggest that an increase in maternal age (and age of the oocyte) may cause predisposition to errors in meiosis. Environmental factors such as virus, paternal age, medical exposure, reproductive medications, and intrinsic predispositions have been associated with Down syndrome.

CONFIRMATION

What is the most likely clinical presentation?

Down syndrome occurs once in every 800-1,000 live births. In the United States there are approximately 350,000 individuals living with Down syndrome. Down syndrome is the most common cause of intellectual disability. Other clinical manifestations include hypotonia, flattened nasal bridge, almond-shaped eyes, abnormally shaped ears, Simian line (palmar crease), epicanthal folds, enlargement of the tongue, congenital heart disease, developmental delay, and a variety of musculoskeletal disorders.

What laboratory or imaging studies would confirm the diagnosis?

During pregnancy a female can be tested for Alpha-fetoprotein, human chorionic gonadotropin, and unconjugated estrogen levels (the triple screen). Three diagnostic studies include chorionic villus sampling, amniocentesis or percutaneous umbilical blood sampling. Detection of Down syndrome occurs in approximately 60-70% of the women tested that are carrying a baby with Down syndrome. After birth a chromosome analysis called a karyotype can be performed to confirm the suspected diagnosis.

What additional information should be obtained to confirm the diagnosis?

In most cases, diagnosis of Down syndrome is made through the physical attributes that are present at birth. Chromosomal testing is used to determine the exact chromosomal pathogenesis.

EXAMINATION

What history should be documented?

Important areas to explore include past medical history including cardiac status, family history, history of seizures, current health status, physical attributes, developmental delay, and social support system.

What tests/measures are most appropriate?

Arousal, attention, and cognition: mental status, learning ability, memory, intelligence testing

Environmental, home, and work barriers: analysis of current and potential barriers or hazards

Ergonomics and body mechanics: analysis of dexterity and coordination

Gait, locomotion, and balance: static and dynamic balance in sitting and standing, safety during gait with/without an assistive device

Integumentary integrity: skin and sensation assessment

Joint integrity and mobility: assessment of hypermobility and hypomobility of a joint, ligamentous laxity

Motor function: equilibrium and righting reactions, motor assessment scales, coordination, posture and balance in sitting, assessment of sensorimotor integration, Peabody Developmental Motor Scales

Muscle performance: strength and tone assessment

Neuromotor development and sensory integration: analysis of reflex movement patterns, assessment of involuntary movements, sensory integration tests, gross and fine motor skills, Bayley Scales of Infant Development

Posture: analysis of resting and dynamic posture

Range of motion: active and passive range of motion

Reflex integrity: assessment of deep tendon and pathological reflexes (e.g., Babinski, ATNR)

Self-care and home management: assessment of functional capacity, WEE-FIM

Ventilation, respiration, and circulation: assessment of cough and clearance of secretions, breathing patterns, respiratory muscle strength, accessory muscle utilization and vital capacity, perceived exertion scale, pulse oximetry, palpation of pulses, pulmonary function testing, auscultation of the lungs and heart

Down Syndrome

What additional findings are likely with this patient?

There are many associated impairments that a child with Down syndrome may inherit. Potential manifestations and secondary complications that are associated with Down syndrome include atlantoaxial instability, sensory, hearing, and visual impairments, umbilical hernia, respiratory compromise, and Alzheimer's disease. Persons with Down syndrome also have an increased incidence of celiac disease, epilepsy, constipation, as well as blood, dermatologic, and musculoskeletal disorders.

MANAGEMENT

What is the most effective management of this patient?

Medical management of Down syndrome is a team approach that requires lifelong intervention and should be directed toward the specific medical and developmental goals. The overall goal of treatment is to achieve maximum potential and level of function. Pharmacological intervention is based on a particular characteristic or complication such as leukemia or a seizure disorder. Physical therapy intervention plays an important role in the treatment of Down syndrome. Developmental delay, hypotonia, laxity of the ligaments, and poor strength are key areas for the focus of physical therapy treatment. A child with Down syndrome will also require learning strategies based on his or her level of intellectual disability. Children with Down syndrome regularly have significant verbal-motor impairments when they verbally respond to a stimulus. Physical therapy will not accelerate developmental milestones, but will help the patient avoid compensatory patterns with static positioning and mobility.

What home care regimen should be recommended?

A home care regimen should be multifaceted with caregivers being proficient with all aspects of care. A routine of exercise is highly important for a child with Down syndrome in order to avoid inactivity and obesity. Positioning and handling are key components in order to maximize proper alignment and to minimize pathological reflexes, malalignment, and instability.

OUTCOME

What is the likely outcome of a course of physical therapy?

Physical therapy will assist a child by teaching optimal movement patterns during developmental activities and by improving strength. Physical therapy will be indicated on an intermittent basis based on level of function and secondary complications. Strengthening and endurance activities should be encouraged within a home program.

What are the long-term effects of the patient's condition?

Individuals with Down syndrome today have a longer life expectancy secondary to advances in medical care, however, it is still less than standard life expectancy. Higher mortality results from issues such as congenital heart defects and gastrointestinal anomalies. Immune system dysfunction, repeated respiratory infections, onset of leukemia, pulmonary hypertension, and complications from Alzheimer's disease all contribute to a higher overall mortality rate compared to the general population. Approximately 80% of patients with Down syndrome reach the age of 55.

COMPARISON

What are the distinguishing characteristics of a similar condition?

Prader-Willi syndrome is a genetic disorder that occurs when there is a partial deletion of chromosome 15. Characteristics include hypotonia, difficulties with feeding during infancy, short stature, excessive appetite, and obesity through childhood. Learning disabilities also exist.

CLINICAL SCENARIOS

Scenario One

A six-month-old boy with Down syndrome is evaluated for outpatient physical therapy. Moderate hypotonia exists and the child does not roll or sit with support. The child's chart indicates atlantoaxial instability with minimal subluxation between C1 and C2. The boy's parents are supportive but both work full-time and are concerned about the competence of the daycare provider.

Scenario Two

A 12-year-old-girl with Down syndrome is seen in physical therapy two times per week at her school. The child is status post right femur fracture and the cast was taken off two weeks ago. The physician orders strengthening and cardiovascular endurance activities. The child has mild scoliosis and minimal learning deficits. The child is moderately obese and complains of pain consistently during treatment.

Duchenne Muscular Dystrophy

DIAGNOSIS

What condition produces a patient's symptoms?

Duchenne muscular dystrophy (DMD) is a progressive neuromuscular degenerative disorder that manifests symptoms once fat and connective tissue begin to replace muscle that has been destroyed by the disease process. The mutation of the dystrophin gene causes the symptoms of DMD.

An injury was most likely sustained to which structure?

A patient with DMD is born with a mutation in the dystrophin gene Xp21 that normally codes for the muscle membrane protein dystrophin. This gene is found on the X-chromosome and since it is a recessive trait, only males are affected while females are carriers. The lack of dystrophin allows for damage within the sarcolemma with contraction of the muscle. The mutated gene causes weakening of cell membranes, destruction of myofibrils, and loss of muscle contractility. The destroyed muscle cells are replaced with fatty deposits.

INFERENCE

What is the most likely contributing factor in the development of this condition?

The etiology of DMD is inheritance as an X-linked recessive trait. The mother is the silent carrier of this disorder. Since it is a recessive trait, only male offspring will manifest the disorder while female offspring become carriers.

CONFIRMATION

What is the most likely clinical presentation?

The incidence of DMD in the United States is 20-35:100,000 live male births. Diagnosis of DMD usually occurs between two and five years of age. The first symptoms include a waddling gait, proximal muscle weakness, clumsiness, toe walking, excessive lordosis, pseudohypertrophy of the calf and other muscle groups, and difficulty climbing stairs. DMD primarily affects the shoulder girdle musculature, pectorals, deltoids, rectus abdominis, gluteals, hamstrings, and calf muscles, and is initially identified when a child begins to have difficulty getting off the floor, needing to use the Gowers' maneuver. During this technique a patient uses his hands to stabilize and walk up his legs in order to attain an upright posture. Approximately one-third of patients have some form of learning disability secondary to the dystrophin abnormalities. The disabilities usually present as subtle cognitive and/or behavioral deficits. There is usually rapid progression of this disease with the inability to ambulate by ten to twelve years of age.

What laboratory or imaging studies would confirm the diagnosis?

Electromyography is used to examine the electrical activity within the muscles. A muscle biopsy can be performed to determine the absence of dystrophin and evaluate the muscle fiber size. DNA analysis and high serum creatinine kinase levels in the blood also assist with confirming the diagnosis.

What additional information should be obtained to confirm the diagnosis?

Clinical examination, current symptoms, and family history are used to assist in the diagnosis, the type, and progression of the disease. Definitive diagnosis is made from clinical findings along with EMG and muscle biopsy results.

EXAMINATION

What history should be documented?

Important areas to explore include past medical history, family history, medications, current symptoms, current health status, living and school environment, and social support system.

What tests/measures are most appropriate?

Anthropometric characteristics: circumferential measurements to monitor muscle atrophy

Aerobic capacity and endurance: assessment of vital signs at rest and with activity

Arousal, attention, and cognition: examine mental status, learning ability, memory, motivation

Assistive and adaptive devices: analysis of components and safety of a device

Environmental, home, and work barriers: analysis of current and potential barriers or hazards

Gait, locomotion, and balance: static and dynamic balance in sitting and standing, safety during gait with/without an assistive device

Joint integrity: assessment of hypermobility and hypomobility of a joint, assessment of deformity

Muscle performance: assessment of active movement

Orthotic, protective, and supportive devices: analysis of components of a device, analysis of movement while wearing a device

Pain: pain perception assessment scale

Posture: analysis of resting and dynamic posture

Range of motion: active and passive range of motion, contracture assessment

Ventilation, respiration, and circulation: breathing patterns, respiratory muscle strength, accessory muscle utilization, pulmonary function testing

Duchenne Muscular Dystrophy

What additional findings are likely with this patient?

Additional findings occur with progression of the disease. Disuse atrophy, contractures, scoliosis, inability to ambulate, weight gain/obesity, cardiac and respiratory impairments, musculoskeletal deformity, and gastrointestinal dysfunction are the most common findings. Respiratory problems and scoliosis progress once the child is utilizing a wheelchair.

MANAGEMENT

What is the most effective management of this patient?

Medical management of DMD focuses on maintaining function of the unaffected musculature for as long as possible. Pharmacological intervention may include glucocorticoids and immunosuppressant medications. Physical therapy intervention is initially indicated to assist a young child with progression through the developmental milestones. Once a child presents with impairments, physical therapy should focus on maintaining available strength, encouraging mobility, adapting to the loss of function, and promoting family involvement in a home program. Manual muscle testing and range of motion should be evaluated on a consistent basis to determine the pattern and rate of disability. Orthotic prescription, adaptive devices, and wheelchair prescription are areas that will require attention during the course of the disease. Respiratory care will also become a vital part of the plan of care as the patient weakens and strength diminishes. As DMD progresses, treatment will include range of motion, prevention of contracture/deformity, positioning, pain management, breathing exercises and postural drainage, and the use of a wheelchair or adaptive equipment. Ongoing emotional support for the child/family is necessary.

What home care regimen should be recommended?

A home care regimen relies on family involvement for a successful home program. Proper positioning, range of motion, submaximal exercise, and breathing exercises are all important aspects that assist a child to maintain function for as long as possible.

OUTCOME

What is the likely outcome of a course of physical therapy?

Physical therapy is an important aspect in the care of a child with DMD, however, it will not alter the degenerative process of the disease. The goals of physical therapy throughout the course of the disease are to maintain present function, adapt to the progressive loss of mobility skills, and educate the patient and family. It is the role of the therapist to ensure that full and proper training has been completed on all aspects of a patient's care to ensure the highest level of function.

What are the long-term effects of the patient's condition?

DMD is a progressive disorder that occurs early in childhood and progresses rapidly. DMD usually affects cardiac muscle in the later stages of the disease. Death occurs primarily from cardiopulmonary complications due to cardiac muscle involvement or respiratory muscle dysfunction. Death usually takes place by the time a patient is a teenager or less frequently into their 20's.

COMPARISON

What are the distinguishing characteristics of a similar condition?

Facioscapulohumeral dystrophy (FSHD), also known as Landouzy-Dejerine dystrophy, is a form of muscular dystrophy that is also inherited, but the exact genetic origin is unclear. This disease presents later in a child's life, usually between seven and twenty years of age. Characteristics include facial and shoulder girdle weakness, weakness lifting the arms over the head, and difficulty closing the eyes. This disease is more common in males than females. Females tend to be carriers of the disorder. Lifespan remains normal.

CLINICAL SCENARIOS

Scenario One

A three-year-old male was recently diagnosed with DMD. The mother reports that the child can ambulate, but prefers to be carried. The child crawls up the stairs and has been falling more frequently. The patient has two sisters at home and resides in a two-story home. At present, both parents work full-time and the child is enrolled in a home daycare.

Scenario Two

A 12-year-old male diagnosed with DMD is referred to physical therapy secondary to increased weakness and frequent falls. The patient is currently ambulating with bilateral Lofstrand crutches. There is evidence of pseudohypertrophy and a mild plantar flexion contracture. The patient's mother is concerned that he is at risk for serious injury while ambulating at school.

DIAGNOSIS

What condition produces a patient's symptoms?

Guillain-Barre syndrome (GBS) or acute polyneuropathy is a temporary inflammation and demyelination of the peripheral nerves' myelin sheaths, potentially resulting in axonal degeneration. GBS results in motor weakness in a distal to proximal progression, sensory impairment, and possible respiratory paralysis.

An injury was most likely sustained to which structure?

The autoantibodies of GBS attack segments of the myelin sheath of the peripheral nerves. The infecting organism is of similar structure to molecules found on the surface of myelin sheaths. The antibodies produced attack both the organism of infection as well as the Schwann cells due to the similar structure. This decreases nerve conduction velocity and results in weakness or paralysis of the involved muscles. The demyelination that is initiated at Ranvier's nodes occurs secondary to macrophage response and inflammation, and as a result, destruction of the myelin. The body responds to this process and attempts to repair the damage through Schwann cell division and myelinization of the damaged nerves. Motor fibers are predominantly affected.

INFERENCE

What is the most likely contributing factor in the development of this condition?

The exact etiology of GBS is unknown, however, it is hypothesized to be an autoimmune response to a previous respiratory infection, influenza, immunization or surgery. Viral infections, Epstein-Barr syndrome, cytomegalovirus, bacterial infections, surgery, and vaccinations have been associated with the development of GBS.

CONFIRMATION

What is the most likely clinical presentation?

GBS can occur at any age, however, there is a peak in frequency in the young adult population and again in adults that are between their fifth and eighth decades. Incidence is slightly greater in males than females and in Caucasians than African Americans. A patient with GBS will initially present with distal symmetrical motor weakness and will likely experience mild distal sensory impairments and transient paresthesias. The weakness will progress towards the upper extremities and head. The level of disability usually peaks within two to four weeks after onset. Muscle and respiratory paralysis, absence of deep tendon reflexes, and the inability to speak or swallow may also occur. GBS can be life threatening if there is respiratory involvement. There are multiple subtypes of GBS, but the classic type involves acute onset of symptoms with peak impairment within four weeks, followed by a two to four week static period and gradual recovery that can take months to years.

What laboratory or imaging studies would confirm the diagnosis?

GBS can be diagnosed through a cerebrospinal fluid sample that contains high protein levels and little to no lymphocytes. Electromyography will result in abnormal and slowed nerve conduction.

What additional information should be obtained to confirm the diagnosis?

A physical and neurological examination, strength testing, and a review of relevant medical history are all important in the diagnosis of GBS. The National Institute of Neurologic and Communicative Disorders and Stroke has established criteria to assist with the diagnosis of GBS.

EXAMINATION

What history should be documented?

Important areas to explore include past medical, family, and surgical history, recent illness, medications, immunizations, current symptoms and health status, social history and habits, occupation, living environment, and social support system.

What tests/measures are most appropriate?

Aerobic capacity and endurance: vital signs at rest/activity, responses to positional changes

Arousal, attention, and cognition: examine mental status, learning ability, memory, motivation

Assistive and adaptive devices: analysis of components and safety of a device

Cranial nerve integrity: assessment of muscles innervated by the cranial nerves, dermatome assessment

Community and work integration: analysis of community, work, and leisure activities

Gait, locomotion, and balance: static and dynamic balance in sitting and standing, safety during gait with/without an assistive device, Berg Balance Scale, Tinetti Performance Oriented Mobility Assessment, analysis of wheelchair management

Integumentary integrity: skin and sensation assessment

Motor function: equilibrium and righting reactions, coordination, motor assessment scales

Muscle performance: strength and tone assessment

Orthotic, protective, and supportive devices: potential utilization of bracing

Pain: pain perception assessment scale

Range of motion: active and passive range of motion

Reflex integrity: assessment of deep tendon and pathological reflexes

Self-care and home management: assessment of functional capacity

Ventilation, respiration and circulation: pulmonary function tests, assessment of cough and secretions

Guillain-Barre Syndrome
GOLD

What additional findings are likely with this patient?

The extent of impairment for each patient depends on the clinical course of the GBS. The patient may also experience pelvic floor muscle weakness, deep muscle pain, and autonomic nervous system involvement including arrhythmia, tachycardia, postural hypotension, heart block, and absent reflexes. Up to 30% of patients require mechanical ventilation during the acute stage. Respiratory assistance can last as long as 50-60 days.

MANAGEMENT

What is the most effective management of this patient?

Medical management of a patient with GBS may require hospitalization for treatment of symptoms. Pharmacological intervention often includes immunosuppressive and analgesic/narcotic medications. Corticosteroids are controversial and usually contraindicated. Cardiac monitoring, plasma exchange (through plasmapheresis), and mechanical ventilation may be required. A tracheostomy may be performed for ventilation. Physical, occupational, and speech therapies are indicated to facilitate neurological rehabilitation. Physical therapy should be initiated upon admission to the hospital with focus on passive range of motion, positioning, and light exercise. During the acute stage a therapist must limit overexertion and fatigue to avoid exacerbation of symptoms. As the patient progresses, intervention may include orthotic, wheelchair or assistive device prescription, exercise and endurance activities, family teaching, functional mobility and gait training, and progressive respiratory therapy. The therapeutic pool may be indicated to initiate movement without the effects of gravity.

What home-care regimen should be recommended?

A home care regimen should include breathing exercises and incentive spirometry for respiratory involvement. A patient, along with the caregiver, must continue with therapeutic exercise, ongoing functional mobility training, and endurance activities as tolerated.

OUTCOME

What is the likely outcome of a course of physical therapy?

Physical therapy may assist with recovery, but it cannot alter the course of the disease. Physical therapy intervention may be required on an ongoing basis to assist with recovery that can last from 3-12 months.

What are the long-term effects of the patient's condition?

GBS is an autoimmune response that varies in severity from person to person. Recovery is slow and can last up to two years after onset. Although most patients experience full recovery, statistics indicate that 20% have remaining neurologic deficits, and 3-5% of patients die from respiratory complications.

COMPARISON

What are the distinguishing characteristics of a similar condition?

Polyneuropathy is a progressive condition that affects the nerves. The most common etiology is metabolic conditions such as diabetes mellitus. Polyneuropathy develops slowly, bilaterally, and symmetrically. The first symptom is often sensory impairment of the distal lower extremities. Pain, diminished deep tendon reflexes, and motor loss are other symptoms of this condition that is marked by exacerbations and remissions. Medical management will focus on stabilizing the underlying metabolic condition.

CLINICAL SCENARIOS

Scenario One

A 25-year-old female has been hospitalized for one week with a diagnosis of GBS. The patient's strength assessment reports 3-/5 bilateral hip strength, 2+/5 bilateral knee strength, and 2-/5 bilateral ankle strength. The patient is anxious to improve and is eager to begin physical therapy. The patient resides alone in a second floor apartment and works as a bank teller.

Scenario Two

A 43-year-old male was admitted to the hospital one month ago with GBS. The patient had significant paralysis and was ventilator dependent. The patient began to improve two weeks ago and was taken off the ventilator. The patient was in good health prior to admission and worked as an independent international sales representative. The patient is diabetic and has a history of alcoholism. He is divorced with no children.

DIAGNOSIS

What condition produces a patient's symptoms?

Multiple sclerosis (MS) produces patches of demyelination that decreases the efficiency of nerve impulse transmission. Symptoms vary based on the location and the extent of demyelination.

An injury was most likely sustained to which structure?

Multiple sclerosis is characterized by demyelination of the myelin sheaths that surround the nerves within the brain and spinal cord. Myelin breakdown results in plaque development, decreased nerve conduction velocity, and eventual failure of impulse transmission. Lesions are scattered throughout the central nervous system and do not follow a particular pattern.

INFERENCE

What is the most likely contributing factor in the development of this condition?

The exact etiology of MS is unknown. Genetics, viral infections, and environment all have a role in the development of MS. It is theorized that a slow acting virus initiates the autoimmune response in individuals that have environmental and genetic factors for the disease. The incidence of MS is higher in Caucasians between the ages of 20 and 35 years and is nearly twice as common in women as in men. There is also a higher incidence of MS in temperate climates.

CONFIRMATION

What is the most likely clinical presentation?

The prevalence of MS differs by geographic area, sex, and race. In the United States the prevalence is 340-360:100,000 with over 800,000 current cases. The highest incidence is 20-35 years of age, however, MS can occur at any age. MS can be classified as relapsing-remitting MS (85%), secondary-progressive MS, primary-progressive MS or progressive-relapsing MS. The clinical presentation varies based on the type of disease, the location, extent of demyelination, and degree of sclerosis. Initial symptoms can include visual problems, paresthesias and sensory changes, clumsiness, weakness, ataxia, balance dysfunction, and fatigue. The clinical course usually consists of periods of exacerbations and remissions, however, the degree of neurologic dysfunction and subsequent recovery will follow typical patterns of the specific type of MS. The frequency and intensity of exacerbations may indicate the speed/course of the disease process.

What laboratory or imaging studies would confirm the diagnosis?

There is not a single testing procedure to diagnose MS early in the disease. MRI may assist with observation and establishing a baseline for lesions, evoked potentials may demonstrate slowed nerve conduction, and cerebrospinal fluid can be analyzed for an elevated concentration of gamma globulin and protein levels.

What additional information should be obtained to confirm the diagnosis?

Clinical presentation and reliable patient history of symptoms are vital in the diagnosis of MS. Guidelines indicate that a clinically definitive diagnosis of MS can be made if a person experiences two separate attacks and shows evidence of two separate lesions. Other diagnoses (having specific criteria) include laboratory-supported definite MS, clinically probable MS, and laboratory-supported probable MS.

EXAMINATION

What history should be documented?

Important areas to explore include past medical history, history of symptoms, medications, current health status, social history, occupation, living environment, and social support system.

What tests/measures are most appropriate?

Aerobic capacity and endurance: assessment of vital signs at rest and with activity

Arousal, attention and cognition: examine mental status, learning ability, memory, and motivation, Mini-Mental State Examination

Assistive and adaptive devices: analysis of components and safety of a device

Community and work integration: analysis of community, work, and leisure activities

Gait, locomotion, and balance: static/dynamic balance in sitting/standing, Tinetti Performance Oriented Mobility Assessment, Berg Balance Scale

Motor function: assessment of dexterity and coordination; assessment of postural, equilibrium, and righting reactions; gross and fine motor skills

Muscle performance: strength and tone assessment, tremor assessment, muscle endurance, Modified Fatigue Impact Scale

Neuromotor development and sensory integration: analysis of reflex movement patterns

Pain: pain perception assessment scale

Posture: resting/dynamic posture, potential contracture

Range of motion: active and passive range of motion

Self-care and home management: Barthel Index, assessment of functional capacity and safety, Kurtzke Expanded Disability Status Scale

Multiple Sclerosis

What additional findings are likely with this patient?

A low percentage of patients experience benign MS and have little to no long-term disability. The majority experience progressive degeneration through periods of exacerbations and remissions. As the disease advances exacerbations leave greater ongoing disability and the length of remissions decrease. Ongoing symptoms can include emotional lability, depression, dementia, psychological problems, spasticity, tremor, weakness, paralysis, sexual dysfunction, and loss of bowel and bladder control.

MANAGEMENT

What is the most effective management of this patient?

Management of MS includes pharmacological, medical, and therapeutic intervention. The goal of medical treatment of MS is to lessen the length of exacerbations and maximize the health of the patient. Pharmacological intervention is quite complex and can include ABC drugs (approved in the treatment of MS) that are classified as immunomodulatory medications. Physical, occupational, and speech therapies are indicated throughout the clinical course of the disease and well as nutritional and psychological counseling. Physical therapy intervention includes regulation of activity level, relaxation and energy conservation techniques, normalization of tone, balance activities, gait training, core stabilization and control, and adaptive/assistive device training. Patient and caregiver education regarding safety, energy conservation, patterns of fatigue, and the use of adaptive devices is vital to the quality of life.

What home care regimen should be recommended?

A home care regimen should include a submaximal exercise/endurance program. Exercise in the morning when the patient is rested is advisable to avoid fatigue. The patient may need frequent rest periods throughout the day and may benefit from breaking a task into smaller steps to avoid fatigue. Ongoing ambulation and mobility activities are important to maintain endurance and prevent disuse atrophy. Aquatic therapy may also be beneficial to this population.

OUTCOME

What is the likely outcome of a course of physical therapy?

Physical therapy is indicated intermittently throughout the clinical course of MS with the goal of maximizing functional capacity and the quality of life. Physical therapy will not alter the progression of the disease process, but rather treat the current symptoms and assist the patient to attain the highest level of function. Factors that influence exacerbations include heat, stress, infection, trauma, and pregnancy.

What are the long-term effects of the patient's condition?

MS is generally a progressive degenerative disease process that creates permanent damage and disability. Factors that influence exacerbations include heat, stress, and trauma. Most patients live with MS for many years and die from secondary complications such as disuse atrophy, pressure sores, contractures, pathological fractures, renal infection, and pneumonia. If left untreated 50% of patients will require a wheelchair within 15 years post diagnosis. Overall mortality rate and long-term outcome correlates to age at diagnosis, number of attacks and exacerbations, frequency and duration of remissions, and type of MS. Suicide is also seven times greater when compared to the same age control group without MS.

COMPARISON

What are the distinguishing characteristics of a similar condition?

Dystonia is a neurologic syndrome that presents with involuntary and sustained muscle contractions that cause repetitive movements. Idiopathic dystonia has a genetic basis and accounts for two-thirds of all cases. Secondary dystonia usually results from brain damage or CNS damage. There are no definitive tests to diagnose dystonia. Treatment is based on current symptoms and includes pharmacological intervention, physical therapy, and occasional surgical intervention. Prognosis is based on age of onset and spontaneous remission occurs in 25-30% of the cases.

CLINICAL SCENARIOS

Scenario One

A 28-year-old female has recently had visual difficulty, urinary urgency, tingling, and upper extremity weakness on two separate occasions. The patient has an aunt with MS, however, has no other significant medical history. The patient was referred to physical therapy by her primary physician.

Scenario Two

A 42-year-old male with MS is referred to physical therapy. The patient has experienced several exacerbations and remissions with full recovery in the past. The patient presently appears to have an exacerbation of symptoms including excessive fatigue. He lives alone and works in a library.

DIAGNOSIS

What condition produces a patient's symptoms?

Parkinsonism syndrome is used to describe a group of disorders within subcortical gray matter of the basal ganglia that produces a similar disturbance of balance and voluntary movements. This syndrome occurs as a secondary effect or disorder from another disease process. Parkinson's disease is a primary degenerative disorder and is characterized by a decrease in production of dopamine (neurotransmitter) within the substantia nigra portion of the basal ganglia. The degeneration of the dopaminergic pathways creates an imbalance between dopamine and acetylcholine. This process produces the symptoms of Parkinson's disease.

An injury was most likely sustained to which structure?

Injury occurs to the subcortical gray matter within the basal ganglia, specifically the substantia nigra and the corpus striatum. The basal ganglia store the majority of dopamine and are responsible for modulation and control of voluntary movement. A patient with Parkinson's disease exhibits degeneration of dopaminergic neurons that results in depletion of dopamine production within the basal ganglia. Change in the neurochemical production damages the complex loop between the basal ganglia and the cerebrum.

INFERENCE

What is the most likely contributing factor in the development of this condition?

Primary Parkinson's disease has an unknown etiology and accounts for the majority of patients with Parkinsonism. Contributing factors that can produce symptoms of Parkinson's disease include genetic defect, toxicity from carbon monoxide, excessive manganese or copper, carbon disulfide, vascular impairment of the striatum, encephalitis, and other neurodegenerative diseases such as Huntington's disease or Alzheimer's disease.

CONFIRMATION

What is the most likely clinical presentation?

There are approximately 500,000 individuals affected by Parkinsonism and about 42% of these are diagnosed specifically with Parkinson's disease. The risk for developing Parkinson's disease increases with age and 1:100 are affected over the age of 75. The majority of patients are between 50 and 79 years of age and approximately 10% are diagnosed before 40 years. The majority of patients with Parkinson's disease will initially notice a resting tremor in the hands (sometimes called a pill-rolling tremor) or feet that increases with stress and disappears with movement or sleep. Early in the disease process a patient may attribute symptoms to "old age" such as balance disturbances, difficulty rolling over and rising from bed, and impairment with fine manipulative movements seen in writing, bathing and dressing. A patient's symptoms slowly progress and often include hypokinesia, sluggish movement, difficulty with initiating (akinesia) and stopping movement, festinating and shuffling gait, bradykinesia, poor posture, dysphagia, and "cogwheel" or "lead pipe" rigidity of skeletal muscles. Patients may also experience "freezing" during ambulation, speech, blinking, and movements of the arms. A patient with Parkinson's disease will also have a mask-like appearance with no facial expression.

What laboratory or imaging studies would confirm the diagnosis?

There are no laboratory or imaging studies that initially diagnose Parkinson's disease. CT scan or MRI may be used to rule out other neurodegenerative diseases and obtain a baseline for future comparison.

What additional information should be obtained to confirm the diagnosis?

Definitive diagnosis is difficult during the early stages of the disease. Parkinson's disease is believed to progress slowly over 25 to 30 years prior to the onset of pharmacological intervention. Diagnosis is made from patient history, history of symptoms, and differential diagnosis to rule out other potential disorders. There are evaluation tools that are utilized to classify a patient by stage of the disease process.

EXAMINATION

What history should be documented?

Important areas to explore include past medical history, medications, current symptoms, current health status, social history and habits, occupation, living environment, and social support system.

What tests/measures are most appropriate?

Aerobic capacity and endurance: assessment of vital signs at rest and with activity

Arousal, attention, and cognition: examine mental status, learning ability, memory, motivation, and Mini-Mental State Examination

Environmental, home, and work barriers: analysis of current and potential barriers or hazards

Gait, locomotion, and balance: static and dynamic balance in sitting and standing, Functional Reach Test, Tinetti Performance Oriented Mobility Assessment, Berg Balance Scale, outcome measurement tools, safety with/without an assistive device during gait

Joint integrity and mobility: analysis of quality of movement, examine joint hypermobility and hypomobility

Motor function: assessment of dexterity, coordination and agility, assessment of postural, equilibrium, and righting reactions

Muscle performance: strength assessment, muscle tone assessment, and tremor assessment

Posture: analysis of resting and dynamic posture

Range of motion: active and passive range of motion

Parkinson's Disease

Self-care and home management: functional capacity, Barthel Index, safety assessments, Parkinson's disease Questionnaire (PDQ-39)

Sensory integration: assessment of combined sensation, assessment of proprioception and kinesthesia

Ventilation, respiratory, and circulation: assessment of chest wall mobility, expansion, and excursion

What additional findings are likely with this patient?

Since Parkinson's disease is a progressive condition there are ongoing physical and cognitive impairments. A patient may develop a stooped posture and an increased risk for falling. Progression of the disease may result in dysphagia, difficulty with speech, and pulmonary impairment. Greater attention is required for skin care once nutrition and mobility are further compromised. Many patients with Parkinson's disease die from complications of bronchopneumonia.

MANAGEMENT

What is the most effective management of this patient?

The medical management of Parkinson's disease relies heavily on pharmacological intervention. Dopamine replacement therapy, (levodopa, Sinemet, Madopar) is the most effective treatment in reducing the symptoms of Parkinson's disease such as movement disorders, bradykinesia, rigidity, and tremor. Antihistamines, anticholinergics, and antidepressants are also utilized. Physical, occupational, and speech therapies may be warranted intermittently throughout the course of the disease. Physical therapy intervention should include maximizing endurance, strength, and functional mobility. Verbal cueing and oral/visual feedback are effective tools to use with this population. Family teaching, balance activities, gait training, stretching, trunk rotation activities, assistive device training, relaxation techniques, and respiratory therapy are all important components in the treatment of Parkinson's disease. Psychological and nutritional counseling are recommended.

What home care regimen should be recommended?

A home care regimen should include an exercise routine, functional mobility skills, the use of relaxation techniques, range of motion and stretching exercises, and endurance activities. A competent caretaker is vital to the success of the home program and must continuously motivate the patient to continue with mobility and endurance activities in order to avoid deleterious effects of the disease process.

OUTCOME

What is the likely outcome of a course of physical therapy?

Physical therapy is recommended on an intermittent basis throughout the course of the disease and will focus on current symptoms that arise. Physical therapy will not prevent further degeneration or cure the movement disorder, however, it will assist the patient to maximize their level of function and quality of life.

What are the long-term effects of the patient's condition?

Parkinson's disease does not significantly alter a patient's lifespan if the patient is diagnosed with a generalized form between 50 and 60 years of age. As the disease progresses, however, there will be an exacerbation of all symptoms and significant loss of mobility. The inactivity and deconditioning allow for complications and eventual death.

COMPARISON

What are the distinguishing characteristics of a similar condition?

Wilson's disease is inherited as an autosomal recessive trait and causes a defect in the metabolism of copper. The accumulation of copper within the erythrocytes, liver, brain, and kidneys produces the associated degenerative changes. The patient presents with hepatic insufficiency, tremor, choreoathetoid movements, dysarthria, and progressive rigidity.

CLINICAL SCENARIOS

Scenario One

A 35-year-old female is sent to physical therapy shortly after being diagnosed with Parkinson's disease. She is presently having difficulty maintaining a grasp on items from an assembly line at work and complains of frequently tripping.

Scenario Two

A 42-year-old male was diagnosed with Parkinson's disease four years ago. The patient requires physical therapy to reassess gait and prescribe an assistive device. The son states that the patient sits a great deal at home and lacks motivation to engage in exercise.

GOLD   **Sciatica Secondary to a Herniated Disk**

DIAGNOSIS

What condition produces a patient's symptoms?

A herniated disk is an intervertebral disk that bulges and protrudes posterolaterally against a nerve root. Sciatica is the diagnosis of compression of the sciatic nerve (L4, L5, S1, S2, S3) secondary to a herniated disk causing a patient's symptoms. Other causes for sciatica include tumor, infection, spondylolisthesis, narrowing of the canal, and blood clots.

An injury was most likely sustained to which structure?

As a patient gets older there are natural and significant alterations in the composition of the intervertebral disks and supporting structures. In a herniated disk the nucleus pulposus has bulged posterolaterally secondary to a weakening of the outer annulus fibrosis and posterior longitudinal ligament. The sciatic nerve experiences an inflammatory response and subsequent damage secondary to the compression from the herniated disk.

INFERENCE

What is the most likely contributing factor in the development of this condition?

The most common contributing factor for this condition is the natural aging process. Each decade the composition of the annulus fibrosus and nucleus pulposus is altered and decreases in overall stability. Once there is adequate structural breakdown within the disk, a patient becomes a high risk for injury. A "normal mechanical load on a normal disk" is now an "excessive load on a compromised disk." As expected, sciatica secondary to a herniated disk is most often seen in patients between 40 and 60 years of age.

CONFIRMATION

What is the most likely clinical presentation?

Sciatica is characterized by low back and gluteal pain that typically radiates down the back of the thigh along the sciatic nerve distribution. Sciatic pain occurs from nerve root compression and can be dull, aching or sharp. Pain may have a sudden onset or develop gradually over time. Early sciatica may involve discomfort or pain limited to the low back and gluteal region. Leg pain can become greater than the back pain and can radiate the entire length of the nerve to the toes. The patient may also experience intermittent numbness and tingling localized to the dermatomal distribution, limited thoracolumbar range of motion in all planes, tenderness to palpation at the segment of herniation, and muscle guarding.

What laboratory or imaging studies would confirm the diagnosis?

Radiologic testing of the spine and electrophysiologic studies are initially performed to assist with diagnosis. Other imaging may include myelogram, discography, CT scan or MRI. Blood work may assist with differential diagnosis.

What additional information should be obtained to confirm the diagnosis?

A full examination should be performed that includes history (trauma, osteoporosis, corticosteroid use), functional assessment, inspection, palpation, and special tests. The straight leg raise test will reproduce symptoms in the case of a herniated disk. The exam should also include testing for non-organic back pain to rule out psychological factors.

EXAMINATION

What history should be documented?

Important areas to explore include past medical history and treatment, history of trauma and accidents, medications, family history, current symptoms, current health status, social history and habits, occupation, leisure activities, and social support system.

What tests/measures are most appropriate?

Arousal, attention, and cognition: examine mental status, learning ability, memory, motivation

Assistive and adaptive devices: analysis of components and safety of a device

Community and work integration: analysis of community, work, and leisure activities

Environmental, home, and work barriers: analysis of current and potential barriers or hazards

Ergonomics and body mechanics: analysis of dexterity and coordination

Gait, locomotion, and balance: static and dynamic balance in sitting and standing, Functional Ambulation Profile

Integumentary integrity: skin assessment, assessment of sensation, dermatome testing of the lower extremities

Joint integrity and mobility: assessment of hypermobility and hypomobility of a joint, soft tissue swelling and inflammation

Muscle performance: strength assessment, resisted isometrics, straight leg raise testing

Pain: Oswestry Function Test, McGill Pain Questionnaire, visual analogue scale

Posture: analysis of resting and dynamic posture

Range of motion: active and passive movement of the spine, combined movements, segmental mobility testing

Reflex integrity: assessment of deep tendon and pathological reflexes (clonus)

Self-care and home management: assessment of functional capacity, Functional Independence Measure

Sciatica Secondary to a Herniated Disk   GOLD

What additional findings are likely with this patient?

Sciatica will produce pain that increases with certain positions due to an increase in intradiskal pressure. Pain will increase in a sitting position or when lifting, forward bending or twisting. Sneezing and coughing can also exacerbate the pain. Although a patient may want to stop all activity to relieve pain, prolonged bed rest is contraindicated and will not relieve pain on a long-term basis.

MANAGEMENT

What is the most effective management of this patient?

Medical management of sciatica due to a herniated disk includes short-term bed rest, overall reduction of intradiskal pressure, patient education, physical therapy, medications, and in rare instances surgical intervention. Pharmacological intervention will incorporate NSAIDs initially to relieve pain followed by epidural injections of cortisone and local anesthetics that may be indicated for temporary relief, however, do not alter the root of the problem. Physical therapy intervention should include patient education on positioning and biomechanics, pain management, traction, heat, lumbar stabilization exercises, McKenzie exercises, stretching, and endurance activities. Swimming, stationary bicycling and walking are indicated within tolerance. Lifting, squatting, and climbing are contraindicated due to the significant increase in intradiskal pressure. Most herniations will spontaneously decrease in size with conservative treatment. Research indicates that the majority of patients improve with two to four months of conservative treatment, however, approximately 2% of patients undergo surgery. Common surgical intervention may include laminectomy, discectomy, chemonucleolysis, laser discectomy or laminotomy.

What home care regimen should be recommended?

A home care regimen should include ongoing caution regarding positioning and constant effort to decrease intradiskal pressure. A home exercise program including stabilization exercises is indicated as well as other aerobic/endurance activities to tolerance.

OUTCOME

What is the likely outcome of a course of physical therapy?

Most patients improve with conservative treatment over a two to four month period. Physical therapy intervention combined with a consistent home program will provide the patient with the necessary tools to relieve pain and improve function.

What are the long-term effects of the patient's condition?

Sciatica secondary to a herniated disk can be corrected through rest and physical therapy intervention. Healing of the disk can also occur and scarring can reinforce the posterior aspect and annular fibers so that it is protected from further protrusion. Restoration of functional mobility is plausible, however, surgical intervention may be required if neurological symptoms increase or no progress is made with conservative measures.

COMPARISON

What are the distinguishing characteristics of a similar condition?

Spinal stenosis is another condition that can be a causative factor of sciatica. Symptoms that would indicate spinal stenosis include lower extremity weakness with or without sciatica, back and leg pain after ambulating a short distance, increasing symptoms with continued ambulation, and relief of symptoms through flexion. Radiologic results reveal disk narrowing and degenerative spondylolisthesis. Surgery is only recommended as a last resort when conservative treatment fails.

CLINICAL SCENARIOS

Scenario One

A 42-year-old female is referred to physical therapy with an L5 herniated disk and sciatica. The patient injured her back skiing three months ago. She presently works 50 hours per week at a daycare facility. Current symptoms include radiating pain down the left leg, a "feeling of weakness," and an inability to sleep at night due to pain.

Scenario Two

A 65-year-old male has been seen in physical therapy for three months with sciatica secondary to a L4 herniated disk. The patient states that he experiences constant pain. The therapist questions the patient's overall compliance with his established home exercise program. The physician orders are prescribed as physical therapy three times per week.

DIAGNOSIS

What condition produces a patient's symptoms?

The majority of traumatic spinal cord injuries result from compression, flexion or extension of the spine with or without rotation. Spinal cord injuries are classified as a concussion, contusion or laceration, and injury results in primary and secondary neural destruction. Traumatic injury to the spinal cord produces a physiological and biochemical chain of events that results in vascular impairment and permanent tissue and nerve damage.

An injury was most likely sustained to which structure?

A patient sustains primary damage to the spinal cord and surrounding tissues at the C7 level through disruption of the membrane, displacement or compression of the spinal cord, and subsequent hemorrhage and vascular damage. Secondary damage occurs beyond the level of injury due to biochemicals that are released as a result of the initial damage. This process destroys adjacent cells and neural tracts due to the acute inflammation and can last for days or even weeks. After injury, C7 is the most distal segment of the spinal cord that both the motor and sensory components remain intact.

INFERENCE

What is the most likely contributing factor in the development of this condition?

There is an estimated 250,000 persons living with SCI within the United States. Statistics from the National Spinal Cord Injury Database (NSCID) indicate that motor vehicle accidents, violence, and falls are the top causes of traumatic spinal cord injury. Statistics also indicate a higher ratio of injury in men (approximately 80%) and Caucasians. The highest incidence of age of injury (over 50%) occurs between 15 to 30 years of age.

CONFIRMATION

What is the most likely clinical presentation?

Spinal shock, which is the total depression of all nervous system function below the level of lesion, occurs immediately following injury and may last for days. Presentation includes total flaccid paralysis and loss of all reflexes and sensation. Surgical intervention may be required after injury in order to stabilize the spinal cord through decompression and fusion at the site of injury. A Halo device is commonly used with cervical injuries to stabilize the spine. As spinal shock subsides, a patient will experience an increase in muscle tone below the level of lesion and neurologic reflexes reappear. Spasticity will evolve and may become problematic. Autonomic dysreflexia and loss of thermoregulation are other impairments that occur secondary to autonomic nervous system dysfunction. A patient with C7 tetraplegia will also present with impaired cough and ability to clear secretions, altered breathing pattern, and poor endurance. The patient is at high risk for contractures and impaired skin integrity.

What laboratory or imaging studies would confirm the diagnosis?

X-rays of the cervical spine observe the positioning and damage of the involved vertebrae. The results of imaging determine subsequent medical intervention including stabilization of the spine. A myelogram or tomogram may be useful to confirm the extent of surrounding damage at the level of the injury.

What additional information should be obtained to confirm the diagnosis?

Other information commonly obtained in order to support the diagnosis includes physician conducted interviews regarding the mechanism of injury as well as a full neurological examination.

EXAMINATION

What history should be documented?

Important areas to explore include past medical history, medications, mechanism of injury, precautions, current health status, social history and habits, occupation or school responsibilities, living environment, and social support system.

What tests/measures are most appropriate?

Aerobic capacity and endurance: autonomic responses to positional changes, vital signs at rest/activity

Arousal, attention, and cognition: examine mental status, learning ability, memory, motivation

Assistive and adaptive devices: analysis of components and safety of a device, wheelchair prescription, adaptive devices, environmental controls

Integumentary integrity: skin assessment, American Spinal Injury Association (ASIA) - Standard Neurological Classification of Spinal Cord Injury Sensory Examination

Motor function: posture and balance in sitting

Muscle performance: ASIA - Standard Neurological Classification of Spinal Cord Injury Motor Examination, muscle tone assessment

Neuromotor development and sensory integration: analysis of reflex movement patterns

Pain: dysesthetic pain (deafferentation pain), nerve root pain, musculoskeletal pain

Posture: positioning, resting and dynamic posture

Range of motion: active and passive range of motion

Reflex integrity: assessment of deep tendon reflexes and pathological reflexes

Sensory integrity: proprioception and kinesthesia

Ventilation, respiration, and circulation: assessment of cough and clearance of secretions, breathing patterns, respiratory muscle strength, accessory muscle utilization, pulmonary function tests

What additional findings are likely with this patient?

There are many additional findings that can exist with a C7 injury, but the most common complications include orthostatic hypotension, pressure sores, spasticity, heterotopic ossification, and autonomic dysreflexia. Autonomic dysreflexia is considered a medical emergency and requires immediate attention to remove the noxious stimuli and lower the blood pressure or the patient will be at risk for subarachnoid hemorrhage. Other findings that require management include sexual dysfunction, respiratory complications, and pain management (neurogenic, central cord, peripheral nerve or musculoskeletal pain).

MANAGEMENT

What is the most effective management of this patient?

Medical management of a SCI injury has both an acute and rehabilitation phase. The acute phase begins at injury and includes medically stabilizing the patient. Pharmacological intervention is started immediately using methylprednisolone (corticosteroid), lipid peroxidation inhibitors, and drugs that block opiate receptors. These drugs appear to control the amount of secondary damage and improve neurological outcome. Once a patient is medically stable, inpatient rehabilitation, which is typically six to eight weeks, should initially focus on range of motion, positioning in bed, and respiratory management such as cough, clearance of secretions, postural drainage, and incentive spirometry. Compensatory techniques, strengthening, muscle substitution, the use of momentum, and the head-hips relationship should be utilized during all activities. Ongoing intervention should include mat and endurance activities, pressure relief training, wheelchair skills, self-range of motion, transfer skills, and community reintegration.

What home care regimen should be recommended?

A home care regimen should include breathing exercises, incentive spirometry, stretching, and mobility skills. Physical therapy intervention may be indicated for continuation of community skills and furthering the patient's independence within the boundaries of the physical limitations.

OUTCOME

What is the likely outcome of a course of physical therapy?

A patient diagnosed with C7 tetraplegia will require extensive physical therapy with projected outcomes based upon the C7 level of motor and sensory innervation. Typical outcomes at this level include independence with feeding, grooming, and dressing, self-range of motion, independent manual wheelchair mobility, independent transfers, and independent driving with an adapted automobile. Independent living with adaptive equipment is possible.

What are the long-term effects of the patient's condition?

At this time there is no cure for a complete spinal cord injury, therefore a patient with a complete C7 injury will not regain innervation below this level. The triceps, extensor pollicis longus and brevis, extrinsic finger extensors, and flexor carpi radialis will remain the lowest innervated muscles. There will be ongoing musculoskeletal and cardiopulmonary deficits that can increase the risk for other health issues. The latest research suggests, however, that approximately 40% of the spinal cord injured population have a life expectancy over 45 years of age.

COMPARISON

What are the distinguishing characteristics of a similar condition?

Brown-Sequard's syndrome is a condition that results from injury to one side of the spinal cord. Motor function, proprioception, and vibration are lost ipsilateral to the lesion and vibration, pain, and temperature are absent contralateral to the lesion.

CLINICAL SCENARIOS

Scenario One

A patient is diagnosed with T12 paraplegia after a motor vehicle accident. Neurological examination reveals no active movement or sensation below T12. The patient is a chemistry teacher and coaches basketball. He is otherwise in good health.

Scenario Two

A 25-year-old male was injured when he was hit from behind. The blow produced cervical hyperextension and bleeding within the central gray matter of the spinal cord. The patient was diagnosed with central cord syndrome and referred to physical therapy. The patient resides alone in a second floor apartment and is a full-time graduate student.

DIAGNOSIS

What condition produces a patient's symptoms?

The majority of traumatic spinal cord injuries result from compression, flexion or extension of the spine with or without rotation. Spinal cord injuries are classified as a concussion, contusion or laceration, and injury results in primary and secondary neural destruction. Traumatic injury to the spinal cord produces a physiological and biochemical chain of events that results in vascular impairment and permanent tissue and nerve damage.

An injury was most likely sustained to which structure?

The forces responsible for spinal fractures are compression, flexion, extension, rotation, shear or distraction forces or a combination of these. A patient sustains primary damage to the spinal cord and surrounding tissues at the L3 level through the disruption of the membrane, displacement or compression of the spinal cord, and subsequent hemorrhage and vascular damage. Secondary damage occurs beyond the level of injury due to biochemicals that are released as a result of the initial damage. This process destroys adjacent cells and neural tracts due to the acute inflammation that can last for days or even weeks. After a complete injury at this level, L3 is the most distal segment of the spinal cord that both the motor and sensory components remain intact.

INFERENCE

What is the most likely contributing factor in the development of this condition?

Statistics from the National Spinal Cord Injury Database (NSCID) indicate that motor vehicle accidents, violence, and falls are the top causes of traumatic spinal cord injury. Statistics also indicate a higher ratio of injury in men (approximately 80%) and Caucasians. The highest incidence of age of injury (over 50%) occurs between 15 to 30 years of age.

CONFIRMATION

What is the most likely clinical presentation?

Spinal shock occurs immediately after the injury and can last for days. Surgical intervention may be required for stabilization of the spine. The patient is usually required to wear a spinal orthosis to maintain stability. As spinal shock subsides, a patient will experience an increase in muscle tone below the level of lesion and neurologic reflexes reappear. Spasticity will evolve and may become problematic. Patients specifically with a complete lesion at the L3 level typically have at least partial innervation of the gracilis, iliopsoas, quadratus lumborum, rectus femoris, and sartorius. Patients have full use of their upper extremities and have hip flexion, adduction, and knee extension.

What laboratory or imaging studies would confirm the diagnosis?

The evaluation of a patient with an acute lumbar spine fracture should include routine laboratory tests, such as CBC, and electrolytes. X-rays, CT scan, and MRI allows for bony and ligamentous injury diagnosis.

What additional information should be obtained to confirm the diagnosis?

A detailed neurological evaluation should include evaluation of sensory level, posterior column function, normal and abnormal reflexes, and examination of rectal tone and perianal sensation. The cutaneous abdominal reflex, bulbocavernosus reflex, and the presence of the Babinski sign also should be examined.

EXAMINATION

What history should be documented?

Important areas to explore include past medical history, medications, mechanism of injury, precautions, current health status, nutritional status, social history, living environment occupation, and social support system.

What tests/measures are most appropriate?

Aerobic capacity and endurance: autonomic responses to positional changes, vital signs at rest/activity

Arousal, attention, and cognition: examine mental status, memory, motivation, level of consciousness

Assistive and adaptive devices: analysis of components and safety of a device, wheelchair prescription, adaptive devices, environmental controls

Community and work integration: analysis of community, work, and leisure activities

Environmental, home, and work barriers: analysis of current and potential barriers or hazards

Gait, locomotion, and balance: static and dynamic balance in sitting, analysis of wheelchair management

Integumentary integrity: skin assessment, American Spinal Injury Association (ASIA) – Standard Neurological Classification of Spinal Cord Injury Sensory Examination

Motor function: equilibrium and righting reactions, posture and balance in sitting

Muscle performance: ASIA – Standard Neurological Classification of Spinal Cord Injury Motor Examination, muscle tone assessment

Neuromotor development and sensory integration: analysis of reflex movement patterns

Orthotic, protective, and supportive devices: analysis of components of a device and movement with a device

Pain: dysesthetic pain (deafferentation pain), nerve root pain, musculoskeletal pain

Range of motion: active and passive range of motion

Reflex integrity: assessment of deep tendon and pathological reflexes

Self-care and home management: assessment of functional capacity, Functional Independence Measure

Sensory integrity: proprioception and kinesthesia

Spinal Cord Injury – Complete L3 Paraplegia   GOLD

What additional findings are likely with this patient?

There are many additional findings that can exist with a L3 injury including sexual dysfunction, a nonreflexive bladder, and the need for a bowel program. These patients usually present with flaccid paralysis below the level of lesion and are at risk for pain, urinary tract infections, muscle contractures, and pressure sores.

MANAGEMENT

What is the most effective management of this patient?

Medical emergency management of a patient with a L3 SCI is initiated by stabilization of the patient's airway in order to secure adequate oxygenation. As soon as the patient is stabilized all patients with spinal cord injuries should immediately receive intravenous methylprednisolone since it has proven to control the amount of secondary damage and improve the neurological outcome. The patient may be placed in a thoracolumbar orthosis (TLSO) with restriction of activities or undergo stabilization surgery followed by the use of a TLSO. Once the patient's spine is stable, rehabilitation should be initiated on an inpatient basis for approximately four to eight weeks. Rehabilitation management may include physical, occupational, vocational therapies, physiatry, nutritional consult, counseling services, and case management. Physical therapy should initially focus on mobility including transfers, bed mobility, and wheelchair mobility. Range of motion and selective strengthening programs, endurance activities, and balance activities should be performed on an ongoing basis in order to optimize functional outcomes. Orthotic prescription (KAFOs or AFOs) is recommended once the patient has gained strength to assist with ambulation using crutches. Community reintegration must be a component of the overall rehabilitation program.

What home care regimen should be recommended?

A home care regimen for a patient with L3 SCI should include continued selective strengthening, selective stretching, endurance activities, balance and postural control training, and continued use of all orthotics and assistive/adaptive devices. The patient must continue with a home program in order to attain and maintain the highest level of functioning and endurance.

OUTCOME

What is the likely outcome of a course of physical therapy?

A patient with L3 SCI will usually participate in four to eight weeks of inpatient rehabilitation immediately after injury and stabilization. The patient should be able to function independently from a wheelchair level and ambulation level. Outcome is based on the degree of injury, the patient's mental capacity, outside support, emotional stability, motivation, and co-morbidities.

What are the long-term effects of the patient's condition?

There are approximately 12,000 persons that sustain a spinal cord injury each year and nearly 5,000 of these cases are diagnosed with paraplegia. Patients with SCI are always at a greater risk for osteoporosis, pressure ulcers, hypertension, and heterotopic ossification. The leading cause of death at present is pneumonia, followed by nonischemic heart disease and sepsis. Patients with L3 paraplegia should be able to live independently with education regarding the management of their disability.

COMPARISON

What are the distinguishing characteristics of a similar condition?

There are various outcomes from spinal cord injuries that occur in the lumbosacral region. Fractures of the thoracolumbar junction can produce a mixture of cord and root syndromes caused by lesions of the conus medullaris and lumbar nerve roots. Complete damage of the conus medullaris presents with no motor function or sensation below L1. Patients with complete damage to the sacral portion of the cord have no control of bowel and bladder function and sacral motor paralysis.

CLINICAL SCENARIOS

Scenario One

A 16-year-old male involved in an MVA sustained a complete L4 injury that required surgery to stabilize his spine. He has just been transferred to rehabilitation and has a TLSO for support. His parents are divorced and he lives between their two homes.

Scenario Two

A 23-year-old male sustained a conus medullaris injury in an MVA. He was admitted to the acute care hospital and has been having complications regulating his blood glucose level. The patient was diagnosed with type 1 diabetes mellitus when he was seven years old. The patient resides in a two-story condominium.

DIAGNOSIS

What condition produces a patient's symptoms?

Thoracic outlet syndrome is a term used to describe a group of disorders that presents with symptoms secondary to neurovascular compression of fibers of the brachial plexus. This usually occurs between the points of the interscalene triangle and the inferior border of the axilla. Compression of the nerves and blood supply can also occur as they pass over the first rib.

An injury was most likely sustained to which structure?

Thoracic outlet syndrome results from compression and damage to the brachial plexus nerve trunks, subclavian vascular supply, and/or the axillary artery. Nerve injury can result in neurapraxia with segmental degeneration and progress to axonotmesis due to continued and unrelieved compression.

INFERENCE

What is the most likely contributing factor in the development of this condition?

Contributing factors in the development of thoracic outlet syndrome include the presence of a cervical rib, an abnormal first rib, postural deviations or changes, body composition, chronic hyperabduction of the arm, hypertrophy or spasms of the scalene muscles, degenerative disorders, and an elongated cervical transverse process.

CONFIRMATION

What is the most likely clinical presentation?

A patient with thoracic outlet syndrome will present with symptoms based on nerve and/or vascular compression. Typical symptoms include diffuse pain in the arm most often at night, paresthesias in the fingers and through the upper extremities, weakness and muscle wasting, poor posture, edema, and discoloration. If the upper plexus is involved, pain will be reported in the neck that may radiate to the face and may follow the lateral aspect of the forearm into the hand. If the lower plexus is involved, pain is reported in the back of the neck and shoulder, which will radiate over the ulnar distribution to the hand. A patient's symptoms are usually enhanced with behaviors that aggravate the symptoms such as poor posture, lifting activities, and movements overhead.

What laboratory or imaging studies would confirm the diagnosis?

X-ray will confirm the presence of a cervical rib or other bony abnormality. Nerve conduction velocity testing may be valuable if a neuropathy exists. Otherwise, diagnosis relies solely on a thorough history of patient symptoms, provocative testing, and a physical examination. Other testing should be used for differential diagnosis to rule out cervical radiculopathy, RSD, myofascial pain syndrome, tumor, carpal tunnel syndrome, brachial plexus injury, ulnar nerve compression, and angina.

What additional information should be obtained to confirm the diagnosis?

A patient can be diagnosed with thoracic outlet syndrome following a thorough history of symptoms, physical examination, and provocative testing that includes Adson maneuver, Wright test, Roos' test, Halstead maneuver, Allen test, and the costoclavicular and hyperabduction tests.

EXAMINATION

What history should be documented?

Important areas to explore include past medical history, family history, medications, history of symptoms, current health status, living environment, social history and habits, occupation, and social support system.

What tests/measures are most appropriate?

Anthropometric characteristics: upper extremity circumferential measurements

Arousal, attention, and cognition: examine mental status, learning ability, memory, motivation

Community and work integration: analysis of community, work, and leisure activities

Cranial nerve integrity: assessment of muscles innervation by the cranial nerves, dermatome assessment

Environmental, home, and work barriers: analysis of current and potential barriers or hazards

Ergonomics and body mechanics: analysis of dexterity and coordination

Integumentary integrity: skin assessment, assessment of sensation

Joint integrity and mobility: soft tissue swelling and inflammation, assessment of joint play, palpation of the joint

Motor function: posture and balance; upper quarter screening

Muscle performance: strength assessment

Pain: pain perception assessment scale, assessment of interscalene triangle point tenderness

Posture: analysis of resting and dynamic posture

Range of motion: active and passive range of motion

Reflex integrity: assessment of deep tendon and pathological reflexes (e.g., Babinski, ATNR)

Self-care and home management: assessment of functional capacity

Thoracic Outlet Syndrome   GOLD

What additional findings are likely with this patient?

A patient with thoracic outlet syndrome may have difficulty sleeping due to excessive pillows or malpositioning of the arm. The patient may have difficulty at work with carrying items on the affected side or with driving a car. Thoracic outlet most commonly affects the population between 30 and 40 years of age with women being affected two to three times more than men.

MANAGEMENT

What is the most effective management of this patient?

Initial medical management of thoracic outlet syndrome takes a conservative approach. If conservative management fails, it is followed by surgical intervention. A patient with thoracic outlet syndrome requires physical therapy intervention to assist with modification of posture, breathing patterns, positioning in bed and at the work site, and gentle stretching. Physical therapy should focus on pain management, strengthening (especially the trapezius, levator scapulae, and rhomboids), joint mobilization, body mechanics, flexibility, and postural awareness. A therapist may utilize modalities such as transcutaneous nerve stimulation, ultrasound, and biofeedback to attain goals. Work site analysis and subsequent activity modification may be necessary to relieve the pain and other symptoms. A patient may benefit from anti-inflammatory agents in combination with physical therapy. If physical therapy management fails, the patient may require surgical decompression of bony or fibrotic abnormalities. The exact type of surgical intervention and approach is chosen by the surgeon based on symptoms and current damage.

What home care regimen should be recommended?

A home care regimen for a patient with thoracic outlet syndrome should include stretching, strengthening, and postural awareness. The patient should utilize these strategies on an ongoing basis at work and with recreational activities in order to promote pain free movement and limit undesirable symptoms associated with the condition.

OUTCOME

What is the likely outcome of a course of physical therapy?

Most patients with thoracic outlet syndrome have positive results from physical therapy intervention and are able to return to their previous level of function within four to eight weeks.

What are the long-term effects of the patient's condition?

If a patient has positive results from physical therapy intervention, there will not be any long-term impairments, however, if the patient's symptoms persist for three to four months, surgical intervention may be warranted. Approximately 75% of patients post surgery have a positive response, however, complications from surgery can include winging of the scapula, pneumothorax, and nerve compression. Research indicates no significant long-term difference between surgical resection of the first rib and successful conservative management.

COMPARISON

What are the distinguishing characteristics of a similar condition?

A radial nerve lesion may be caused by direct trauma, excessive traction, entrapment or compression. A patient presents with an inability to extend the wrist, thumb, and fingers. The patient will also present with impaired grip strength and coordination. Splinting is recommended to maintain proper positioning. Passive range of motion is necessary to prevent secondary impairments such as contractures within the hand.

CLINICAL SCENARIOS

Scenario One

A 35-year-old female is seen in physical therapy secondary to pain and paresthesias throughout the left upper extremity. The patient's work history reveals that she is employed as a telemarketer and is required to hold the phone between her ear and shoulder throughout her shift. The patient carries a five-pound brief case with a shoulder strap as she walks one-half mile to work. The patient has a one-year-old child.

Scenario Two

A 45-year-old female is referred to physical therapy secondary to pain when reaching overhead and carrying objects. The patient recently complains of waking up during the night with pain and paresthesias in the involved arm. The patient is very anxious and concerned because she is required to carry items and place them above her head as part of her job at a local production mill.

DIAGNOSIS

What condition produces a patient's symptoms?

Traumatic brain injury (TBI) occurs due to an open head injury where there is penetration through the skull or closed head injury where the brain makes contact with the skull secondary to a sudden, violent acceleration or deceleration impact. Traumatic brain injury can also occur secondary to anoxia as with cardiac arrest or near drowning.

An injury was most likely sustained to which structure?

Any structure within the brain is vulnerable to injury; however, primary damage will occur at the site of impact. Secondary damage occurs as a result of metabolic and physiologic reactions to the trauma. Brain injury may include swelling, axonal injury, hypoxia, hematoma, hemorrhage and changes in intracranial pressure (ICP).

INFERENCE

What is the most likely contributing factor in the development of this condition?

Statistics from the Centers for Disease Control indicate that falls (32.5%) and motor vehicle accidents (17.3%) are the two leading causes of TBI. Pediatric TBI occurs 50% of the time as a result of a fall. Motor vehicle accidents account for 31.8% of deaths from TBI. High risk groups include ages 0-4, 15-19, and greater than 65 years of age. Males are at greater risk in each demographic category.

CONFIRMATION

What is the most likely clinical presentation?

The incidence of head injury is close to two million individuals per year with an estimated five million individuals living with a brain injury. The clinical presentation of a TBI varies due to the type, area, extent of injury, and secondary damage within the brain. Characteristics of a TBI may include altered consciousness (coma, obtundity, delirium), cognitive and behavioral deficits, changes in personality, motor impairments, alterations in tone, and speech and swallowing issues.

What laboratory or imaging studies would confirm the diagnosis?

Diagnostic imaging such as CT scan or MRI should be performed immediately in order to rule out hemorrhage, infarction, and swelling. X-rays taken of the cervical spine can be used to rule out fracture and potential for subluxation. An electroencephalogram (EEG), positron emission tomography (PFT), and cerebral blood flow mapping (CBF) may also be utilized for diagnosis and baseline data.

What additional information should be obtained to confirm the diagnosis?

A full neurological evaluation by a physician should include a mental examination, cranial nerve assessment, tonal assessment and pupillary reactivity assessment. The physician will classify the patient using the Glasgow Coma Scale and indicate severe (coma), moderate or mild brain injury. The Rancho Los Amigos Levels of Cognitive Functioning can also be used to classify injury and assist with developing an appropriate plan of care.

EXAMINATION

What history should be documented?

Important areas to explore include past medical history, medications, family history, current symptoms, level of cognitive functioning, social history and habits, occupation, leisure activities, and social support system.

What tests/measures are most appropriate?

Aerobic capacity and endurance: vital signs at rest/activity, pulse oximetry, auscultation of lungs

Arousal, attention, and cognition: using Rancho Los Amigos Levels of Cognitive Functioning

Assistive and adaptive devices: analysis of components and safety of a device

Cranial nerve integrity: muscle innervation by the cranial nerves, dermatome assessment

Environmental, home, and work barriers: analysis of current and potential barriers or hazards

Gait, locomotion, and balance: static and dynamic balance in sitting and standing, safety during gait with/without an assistive device, Berg Balance Scale, Tinetti Performance Oriented Mobility Assessment, analysis of wheelchair management

Integumentary integrity: skin and sensation assessment

Joint integrity and mobility: assessment of hypermobility and hypomobility of a joint

Motor function: equilibrium and righting reactions, motor assessment scales, coordination, posture and balance in sitting, assessment of sensorimotor integration, physical performance scales

Muscle performance: strength assessment, muscle tone assessment

Neuromotor development and sensory integration: analysis of reflex movement patterns, assessment of involuntary movements, sensory integration tests, gross and fine motor skills

Orthotic, protective, and supportive devices: analysis of components and movement while wearing a device

Pain: pain perception assessment scale, visual analogue scale, assessment of muscle soreness

Posture: analysis of resting and dynamic posture

Range of motion: active and passive range of motion

Reflex integrity: assessment of deep tendon and pathological reflexes (e.g., Babinski, ATNR)

Self-care and home management: assessment of functional capacity, Functional Independence Measure (FIM), Barthel Index, Rankin Scale, Rivermead Motor Assessment

What additional findings are likely with this patient?

There are multiple impairments that can develop secondary to TBI. Intracranial pressure must be monitored initially since it is at risk to increase or develop hemorrhage. A patient can develop heterotopic ossification, contractures, skin breakdown, seizures, and deep vein thrombosis. A patient with a severe TBI may remain in a persistent vegetative state.

MANAGEMENT

What is the most effective management of this patient?

Medical management is initiated at the site of injury or in the emergency room for life preserving measures. The initial goal is to stabilize the patient, control intracranial pressure, and prevent secondary complications. Surgical intervention may be required in attempt to regain homeostasis within the brain secondary to hemorrhage or fracture. Once a patient is medically stable, physical therapy rehabilitation is initiated. Treatment of a patient with TBI usually includes a team approach with goals based on the patient's level of injury. Pharmacological intervention may include cerebral vasoconstrictive agents, psychotropic agents, hypertensive agents, antispasticity agents, and medication to assist with cognition and attention. Physical therapy will focus on sensory stimulation and PROM for a comatose patient or pathfinding and high-level balance activities for a patient with a mild injury. Physical therapy may include functional mobility training, behavior modification, serial casting, compensatory strategies, vestibular rehabilitation, task specific activities, wheelchair seating, and pulmonary intervention.

What home care regimen should be recommended?

A home care regimen should include ongoing therapeutic activities that focus on goals associated with the patient's current Rancho Los Amigos level. Consistency is vital to the success of a home program. The patient may also participate in a community re-entry based program for the TBI population if warranted by their level of current function.

OUTCOME

What is the likely outcome of a course of physical therapy?

A patient diagnosed with TBI does not have a specific projected outcome. Outcome is based on the degree of primary and secondary damage and the extent of cognitive and behavioral impairments. Physical therapy should continue in all settings until the patient has attained all realistic goals.

What are the long-term effects of the patient's condition?

TBI affects approximately 1.7 million Americans each year. Approximately 52,000 individuals die each year as a result of TBI. Long-term effects are determined by the extent of injury and impairments resulting from the TBI. Many patients experience lifelong deficits that do not allow them to return to their pre-injury lifestyle.

COMPARISON

What are the distinguishing characteristics of a similar condition?

Meningitis is a bacterial or viral infection that spreads through the cerebrospinal fluid to the brain. The meninges of the brain become inflamed as well as the meningeal membranes. The patient will have a headache and may complain of stiffness in the neck. The patient may also show symptoms of confusion, fatigue, and irritability. As the virus progresses the patient may experience seizures and may progress into a coma. Medical treatment varies based on the causative strain of the virus/bacteria. Mortality ranges from 5-25% and approximately 30% have some degree of permanent neurological impairment.

CLINICAL SCENARIOS

Scenario One

A 22-year-old male with TBI is admitted to an inpatient rehabilitation hospital. The patient is presently classified as Rancho Los Amigos Level IV. The patient required surgical decompression after the TBI. The patient's parents are with the patient almost constantly.

Scenario Two

A 42-year-old female sustained a severe TBI in a motor vehicle accident and is presently classified as Rancho Los Amigos Level II. The accident was two weeks ago. Prior to admission the patient was healthy and worked full-time. She has a supportive husband.

SILVER Level Clinical Application Templates

SILVER Level Clinical Application Template Executive Summary

Anterior Cord Syndrome

- An incomplete spinal cord lesion in which the anterior two-thirds of the spinal cord is damaged
- Occurs through a traumatic incident that causes compression or damage to the anterior spinal artery, most often associated with fracture or dislocation
- Typically presents with complete loss of motor function and loss of pain and temperature sensation bilaterally below the level of the lesion due to the damage to the corticospinal and spinothalamic tracts

Cauda Equina Syndrome

- Considered to be a peripheral nerve injury and results from damage and loss of function involving two or more nerves of the cauda equina
- May result from compression on the cauda equina nerve roots, including spinal structure pathology, trauma, infectious conditions, tumor or iatrogenic factors
- Is a self-limiting condition, however, the longer a patient is symptomatic prior to intervention, the less likely the patient is to achieve a complete recovery

Central Cord Syndrome

- An incomplete spinal cord lesion that most often results from a cervical hyperextension injury
- Clinical presentation involves motor loss that is greater in the upper extremities than the lower extremities
- Most common incomplete spinal cord lesion accounting for approximately 30% of all incomplete forms of tetraplegia

Erb's Palsy

- Muscles affected are supplied by cervical roots C5 and C6 which result in a loss of function of the rotator cuff, deltoid, brachialis, coracobrachialis, and biceps brachii
- Brachial plexus injury in a newborn usually occurs during a difficult delivery, due to a large baby, a breech presentation with a prolonged labor or with the use of forceps
- Results in flaccid paralysis nicknamed the "waiter's tip deformity" (characterized by a loss of shoulder function, loss of elbow flexion, loss of forearm supination, and the hand positioned in a pinch grip manner)

Huntington's Disease

- Chronic progressive genetic disorder that is fatal within 15 to 20 years after clinical manifestation
- Characterized by degeneration and atrophy of the basal ganglia (specifically the striatum) and cerebral cortex within the brain
- Clinical presentation includes enlarged ventricles secondary to atrophy of the basal ganglia, mental deterioration, speech disturbances, and ataxic gait

Myasthenia Gravis

- An autoimmune disorder that affects the transmission of neuromuscular signals
- Primary feature is muscle weakness within the skeletal muscles, with other neurologic findings being normal (e.g., reflexes, sensation)
- Muscles affected commonly include the ocular muscles and limb musculature (proximal greater than distal)

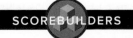

SILVER   Level Clinical Application Template Executive Summary

Post-Polio Syndrome
- 25-50% of patients with poliomyelitis will eventually develop post-polio syndrome.
- Symptoms of post-polio syndrome include muscle weakness, atrophy, fatigue, and sometimes muscular or joint pain
- Treatment is generally multidisciplinary and aimed at controlling symptoms and improving daily function

Spina Bifida – Myelomeningocele
- Classifications include occulta (incomplete fusion of the posterior vertebral arch with no neural tissue protruding), meningocele (incomplete fusion of the posterior vertebral arch with neural tissue/meninges protruding outside the neural arch), and myelomeningocele (incomplete fusion of the posterior vertebral arch with both meninges and spinal cord protruding outside the neural arch)
- Approximately 75% of vertebral defects are found in the lumbar/sacral region most often at L5-S1
- Prenatal testing of alpha-fetoprotein (AFP) in the blood will show an elevation in levels that indicate a probable neural tube defect at approximately week 16 of gestation

Vestibular Disorders
- Occurs when there is a disruption of the sensory information processed by the inner ear and brain with respect to the body's control of balance and eye movements
- Classified as either peripheral or central, with the majority of cases diagnosed as peripheral
- Effects can be quite diverse ranging from spontaneous recovery to permanent disability

Anterior Cord Syndrome
SILVER

DIAGNOSIS:

What condition produces a patient's symptoms?

Anterior cord syndrome is an incomplete spinal cord lesion in which the anterior two-thirds of the spinal cord is damaged. Since the dorsal columns are not affected, it is considered an incomplete spinal cord injury or syndrome. The mechanism of injury is typically a cervical flexion injury or through infarction of the anterior spinal artery.

An injury was most likely sustained to which structure?

A flexion injury to the cervical spine can result in the anterior structures becoming compressed and damaged, specifically the anterior spinal artery. The anterior spinal artery supplies blood to the anterior two-thirds of the spinal cord. Damage to this artery results in decreased perfusion to the spinal tracts that it supplies, including the anterior and lateral corticospinal tracts and spinothalamic tracts. The corticospinal tracts are responsible for motor function while the spinothalamic tracts are responsible for the sensations of pain and temperature.

INFERENCE:

What is the most likely contributing factor in the development of this condition?

Anterior cord syndrome can occur through a traumatic incident that causes compression or damage to the anterior spinal artery, most often associated with fracture or dislocation. However, decreased perfusion and vascular insufficiencies can also occur through non-traumatic etiologies. Atherosclerosis, external compression such as a disk protrusion or mass, and aortic pathology have caused anterior cord syndrome.

CONFIRMATION:

What is the most likely clinical presentation?

The patient will typically present with complete loss of motor function and loss of pain and temperature sensation bilaterally below the level of the lesion due to the damage to the corticospinal and spinothalamic tracts. Sensations controlled through the dorsal columns (e.g., proprioception, vibration) remain intact. Autonomic dysfunction such as loss of bowel and bladder function and sexual function are both likely, though this is dependent on the level of the lesion. Respiratory function may also be affected.

What laboratory or imaging studies would confirm the diagnosis?

MRI is used to determine the location and extent of the injury. X-rays may be used to determine if there is a fracture or dislocation of a vertebral segment. CT scan may also be used as it is more sensitive than x-ray in detecting injuries to the spine and spinal canal.

What additional information should be obtained to confirm the diagnosis?

Though imaging studies will be used to confirm the presence of anterior cord syndrome, a thorough neurological examination should be performed. Special attention should be given to sensory and motor testing. The ASIA impairment scale can be used to determine the extent of the patient's spinal cord injury.

MANAGEMENT:

What is the most effective management of this patient?

Medical management of a SCI has both an acute and rehabilitation phase. Initial management will consist of medical immobilization and stabilization of the patient. Pharmacological management is immediate and includes methylprednisolone administered in high doses to limit swelling and secondary damage and improve potential neurological outcome. An orthosis (e.g., halo, Minerva) may be used for continued immobilization if a cervical fracture has occurred. Acute physical therapy intervention should include range of motion, respiratory management, pressure relief, skin care education and management, and functional mobility. During the rehabilitation phase, physical therapy consists of strengthening, transfer training, adaptive device training, and ambulation and/or wheelchair management. Compensatory techniques, muscle substitution, the use of momentum, and the head-hips relationship should be utilized during all activities. Most patients with anterior cord syndrome will need to be trained to utilize a wheelchair.

What home care regimen should be recommended?

A home care regimen should consist of exercise such as range of motion and strengthening, functional mobility, and skin care management. Community skill training may be appropriate and participation in an outpatient physical therapy program may be warranted.

OUTCOME:

What is the likely outcome of a course of physical therapy?

A patient with anterior cord syndrome will require extensive physical therapy with projected outcomes based on the actual level of injury. Physical therapy can assist patients to compensate for the injury, however, only minor improvement in motor function is anticipated. Significant neurological recovery following spinal cord infarct is unusual.

What are the long-term effects of the patient's condition?

Currently, there is no cure for a spinal cord injury, though there can be some level of recovery that occurs for 1-2 years after the initial injury. The prognosis for anterior cord syndrome is best when recovery is noted within the first 24 hours after the injury. Otherwise, the prognosis is poor compared to other spinal cord injury syndromes. It is associated with high mortality and poor functional outcomes.

Cauda Equina Syndrome

DIAGNOSIS

What condition produces a patient's symptoms?

Cauda equina syndrome (CES) is considered to be a peripheral nerve injury and results from damage and loss of function involving two or more nerves of the cauda equina. CES is associated with numerous mechanisms of injury and typically presents as a complex of symptoms.

An injury was most likely sustained to which structure?

The spinal cord typically extends to L1, terminating with the conus medullaris. Paired lower lumbar, sacral, and coccygeal nerve roots extend beyond the conus medullaris and are termed the cauda equina. The cauda equina provides sensory innervation to the "saddle area" of the lower extremities, lower extremity motor innervation, parasympathetic innervation to the bowel and bladder, and voluntary control over the associated sphincters. The nerves of the cauda equina are more susceptible to damage than most other nerve root pairs due to a poorly developed protective epineurium and the tendency to form edema even with mild injury.

INFERENCE

What is the most likely contributing factor in the development of this condition?

CES may result from any source of compression on the cauda equina nerve roots, including spinal structure pathology (e.g., ruptured disk, fracture, stenosis), trauma (e.g., fall, gunshot wound), infectious conditions (e.g., abscess or tuberculosis), tumor or iatrogenic factors.

CONFIRMATION

What is the most likely clinical presentation?

CES may develop slowly or rapidly depending on the underlying pathology. For patients with gradual onset, diagnosis may be difficult since early symptoms may be poorly defined or mimic other conditions. Altered reflexes, pain, and decreased strength and sensation are common symptoms. Other symptoms can include severe back pain, functional impairment, diminished sensation in the saddle distribution, bowel and bladder dysfunction (e.g., retention or incontinence), and sexual dysfunction. The incidence of CES is higher in adults, however, children with spinal birth defects may also be at an increased risk.

What laboratory or imaging studies would confirm the diagnosis?

MRI studies are able to identify the widest range of potential etiologies as they are able to best delineate soft tissue structures and pathology (e.g., tumor, abscess). Compression due to bony abnormalities, such as narrowed disk spaces, altered bony alignment or arthritic changes are more readily identified with x-ray imaging or a CT scan.

What additional information should be obtained to confirm the diagnosis?

A thorough medical history should be obtained and a physical examination performed if CES is suspected. The physical examination should include an assessment of lower extremity muscle strength, sensation, and deep tendon reflexes. Perineal sensation, reflexes, and rectal tone should also be assessed.

MANAGEMENT

What is the most effective management of this patient?

Surgical and medical interventions are typically directed toward nerve root decompression. Though CES is not fatal, it can signal a surgical emergency since delayed intervention may limit long-term outcomes. Medical management may include radiation therapy or chemotherapeutic agents for tumor-related compression. Other pharmaceutical agents may also be used for compression (e.g., anti-inflammatory, antibiotic agents). Physical therapy interventions should emphasize maximal functional return and accommodation for residual deficits. Therapeutic exercise, functional mobility training, coordination activities, sensory stimulation, orthotics, and adaptive equipment training are typical components of the plan of care. Physical therapist assistants may also provide education related to bowel and bladder retraining. Modalities such as biofeedback and neuromuscular electrical stimulation may assist in targeted muscle retraining.

What home care regimen should be recommended?

A home care regimen should be consistent with physical therapy interventions, including therapeutic exercise and activities that emphasize functional independence with adaptive equipment.

OUTCOME

What is the likely outcome of a course of physical therapy?

A patient with CES does not have a specific projected outcome. Outcomes are based on the degree of primary and secondary damage and the extent of motor and sensory impairments. Physical therapy should continue until the patient has attained realistic goals.

What are the long-term effects of the patient's condition?

Long-term effects are determined by the extent of injury and the resulting impairments. CES is a self-limiting condition, however, the longer a patient is symptomatic prior to intervention, the less likely the patient is to achieve a complete recovery. Morbidity is typically associated with long-term effects including weakness and bowel or bladder dysfunction. Other complications may include the development of decubitus ulcers or thrombus formation.

Central Cord Syndrome SILVER

DIAGNOSIS

What condition produces a patient's symptoms?

Central cord syndrome (CCS) is an incomplete spinal cord lesion that most often results from a cervical hyperextension injury. Symptoms are secondary to damage to the central aspect of the spinal cord. CCS usually occurs from a fall but can occur from other forms of trauma such as a motor vehicle accident.

An injury was most likely sustained to which structure?

The spinal cord sustains bleeding into the central gray matter that causes damage to the centrally located cervical tracts. Injury is caused by a ligamentum flavum (hyperextension) injury or otherwise from anterior compression of the cord due to osteophyte formation. Studies often reveal axonal disruption in the lateral columns at the level of injury with preservation of the gray matter.

INFERENCE

What is the most likely contributing factor in the development of this condition?

The most common mechanism of injury for CCS is a hyperextension injury of the cervical spine. Other potential contributing factors in the development of CCS include cervical spondylosis, narrowing or congenital defect of the spinal canal, tumor, rheumatoid arthritis or syringomyelia. CCS predominantly affects the population over 50 years of age with a greater incidence in men.

CONFIRMATION

What is the most likely clinical presentation?

CCS presents with motor loss that is greater in the upper extremities than the lower extremities and is most severe distally in the upper extremities. This presentation is due to the damage that occurs within the central location of the spinal cord. Sensory loss found below the level of the lesion is usually limited, but can be variable. Lumbar, thoracic, and cervical components proceed medially in order towards the center of the spinal cord. Sacral segments are usually unaffected since they are located laterally within the spinal cord. Bowel and bladder functions resolve in 55-85% of patients with CCS after six months.

What laboratory or imaging studies would confirm the diagnosis?

MRI is used to assess spinal cord impingement from bone or disk. CT scan of the spine will assess spinal canal compromise and the degree of impingement. X-rays can be utilized to assess potential fractures, dislocations, and degree of spondylotic deterioration.

What additional information should be obtained to confirm the diagnosis?

Diagnosis is made using results of MRI, CT scan, and x-ray findings. Information may be obtained from past medical history and mechanism of injury that usually supports the diagnosis of CCS.

MANAGEMENT

What is the most effective management of this patient?

Rehabilitation services are initiated once the patient is medically stable. Medical management should include physiatry, physical therapy, occupational therapy, vocational counseling, and social services. Methylprednisolone should be administered within eight hours of injury to assist with neurologic recovery. Other pharmacological intervention may include blood pressure medication to combat autonomic dysreflexia, antispasticity medication for treatment of spasticity, anticonvulsants for treatment of neurogenic pain, prophylactic anticoagulants, and antidepressants if warranted. Physical therapy intervention should include patient and caregiver education, range of motion, strengthening, endurance activities, balance retraining, proximal stabilization exercises, and functional mobility based on the patient's current functional status. Adaptive devices may be required to assist with overall mobility. If a patient ambulates, a platform attachment walker may initially be indicated since hand function is usually poor for grasp. Surgical intervention is rare, but may be indicated if compression within the spinal cord persists or progress ceases without cause.

What home care regimen should be recommended?

A home care regimen should include a continuation of exercise, endurance, and functional mobility training based on the patient's current functional abilities. Outpatient physical therapy may be warranted and should modify the home program as necessary.

OUTCOME

What is the likely outcome of a course of physical therapy?

Physical therapy can assist a patient with CCS to attain maximum functional outcome based on level and extent of injury. Overall outcome, however, is based on age, motivation, compliance, and extent of injury.

What are the long-term effects of the patient's condition?

CCS is the most common incomplete spinal cord lesion and accounts for approximately 30% of overall incomplete tetraplegia. Statistics indicate 77% of patients with CCS will ambulate, 53% will gain bowel and bladder control, and 42% regain some hand function. Older patients do not tend to recover as well as younger ones. Favorable long-term prognostic factors for a good outcome include early hand function, improvement of strength in all extremities during the inpatient stay, and little to no lower extremity involvement.

Erb's Palsy

DIAGNOSIS

What condition produces a patient's symptoms?

Erb's palsy is a term used to denote an upper brachial plexus injury or palsy that usually results from a difficult birth. This type of injury is the most common palsy related to the brachial plexus. It primarily affects the muscles of the shoulder and elbow.

An injury was most likely sustained to which structure?

The brachial plexus is damaged with the most common avulsion located at Erb's point (which is an area in the anterolateral neck). This damages the nerves supplying the ipsilateral upper limb and shoulder. The muscles affected are those supplied by cervical roots C5 and C6: axillary, lateral pectoral, upper and lower subscapular, suprascapular and partial paralysis of the long thoracic and the musculocutaneous nerves. The result is loss of rotator cuff, deltoid, brachialis, coracobrachialis, and biceps brachii function.

INFERENCE

What is the most likely contributing factor in the development of this condition?

A brachial plexus injury in a newborn usually occurs during a difficult delivery, due to a large baby, with a breech presentation, with a prolonged labor or with the use of forceps. One side of the baby's neck is stretched which damages the nerves. If the upper nerves are affected the condition is termed Erb's palsy. One theory suggests that congenital chicken pox or amniotic bands may also produce this condition. When it occurs in adults, the cause typically is an injury that has caused stretching, tearing or other trauma to the upper brachial plexus network.

CONFIRMATION

What is the most likely clinical presentation?

There are four types of brachial plexus injuries: avulsion, rupture, neuroma, and neurapraxia. The clinical presentation is a flaccid paralysis that is nicknamed the "waiter's tip deformity," characterized by a loss of shoulder function, loss of elbow flexion, loss of forearm supination, and the hand positioned in a pinch grip manner.

What laboratory or imaging studies would confirm the diagnosis?

An x-ray or magnetic resonance imaging (MRI) may be performed to see if there is any damage to the bones and joints of the neck and shoulder. The physician may also use an electromyogram (EMG) or nerve conduction studies (NCS) to see if any nerve signals are present in the upper extremity muscles. In complete injuries, motor and sensory nerve conduction studies of median, ulnar, and radial nerves may be conducted.

What additional information should be obtained to confirm the diagnosis?

A complete history from the patient or parent should be taken regarding upper extremity weakness. Other testing that may assist with diagnosis includes the active movement scale, Gilbert Shoulder Classification, and the Pediatric Outcomes Data Collection Instrument.

MANAGEMENT

What is the most effective management of this patient?

Physical therapy is recommended for a patient with Erb's palsy with the goal of developing a program that focuses on increasing active and passive movement and promoting use of the weak upper extremity for functional activities. Occupational and physical therapies are usually indicated immediately when the patient is diagnosed. The length of treatment will depend on the patient's recovery of active movements. If a patient has spontaneous recovery (full active movements) within three to four months, the caregivers are usually given a home program. However, if spontaneous recovery does not occur within that timeframe, the patient may continue in therapy with close monitoring of progress. If conservative management fails, surgery may be indicated. Surgery will not restore normal function. After surgery, the infant will wear a splint for approximately three to four weeks. Caregiver education is very important regarding positioning to avoid any further traction during the child's daily activities. Other treatment techniques may include adaptation of developmental milestones, weight bearing activities, and other sensory techniques.

What home care regimen should be recommended?

The patient's caregivers must be competent with all aspects of the home program and must perform the program in a consistent fashion. The program should include AROM, PROM, general strengthening, functional activities and integration of the weakened upper extremity into all functional activities.

OUTCOME

What is the likely outcome of a course of physical therapy?

The therapeutic management of a patient with Erb's palsy must begin in infancy (or immediately) in order to achieve optimal functional return. Nerve regeneration remains at a constant speed, however, physical therapy intervention can assist with overall strength and function during recovery.

What are the long-term effects of the patient's condition?

Approximately nine out of ten infants with brachial plexus palsy can recover with conservative treatment. The final functional outcome will depend on the degree of damage to the nerves and the caregiver's ability to maintain their motion and their level of interest towards the affected upper extremity during the initial first few months of life. Since nerves grow at a rate of one inch per month, it may take several months or even years for nerves repaired at the cervical spine to reach the muscles of the hand.

Huntington's Disease   SILVER

DIAGNOSIS

What condition produces a patient's symptoms?

Huntington's disease (HD), also known as Huntington's chorea, is a neurological disorder of the CNS and is characterized by degeneration and atrophy of the basal ganglia (specifically the striatum) and cerebral cortex within the brain.

An injury was most likely sustained to which structure?

HD affects the basal ganglia and cerebral cortex of the brain. The ventricles of the brain become enlarged secondary to atrophy of the basal ganglia and there is extensive loss of small and medium sized neurons. There appears to be an overall decrease in the quantity and activity of gamma-aminobutyric acid (GABA) and acetylcholine neurons that are produced in these areas. The identified neurotransmitters become deficient and are unable to modulate movement. Loss of neurons creates dysfunction in inhibition that results in the symptoms of chorea, bradykinesia, and rigidity.

INFERENCE

What is the most likely contributing factor in the development of this condition?

HD is genetically transmitted as an autosomal dominant trait with the defect linked to chromosome four and to the gene identified as IT-15. The disease is usually perpetuated by a person that has children prior to the normal onset of symptoms and without knowledge that he/she possesses the defective gene. Genetic testing is able to identify the defective gene for HD prior to the onset of symptoms.

CONFIRMATION

What is the most likely clinical presentation?

The average age for developing symptoms of HD ranges between 35 and 55 years, however, symptoms can develop at any age. HD is a disease that produces a movement disorder, affective dysfunction, and cognitive impairment. The patient will initially present with involuntary choreic movements and a mild alteration in personality. Unintentional facial expressions such as a grimace, protrusion of the tongue, and elevation of the eyebrows are common. As the disease progresses gait will become ataxic and a patient experiences choreoathetoid movement of the extremities and the trunk. Speech disturbances and mental deterioration are common. Late stage HD is characterized by a decrease in IQ, dementia, depression, dysphagia, incontinence, inability to ambulate or transfer, and progression from choreiform movements to rigidity.

What laboratory or imaging studies would confirm the diagnosis?

Magnetic resonance imaging (MRI) or computed tomography (CT scan) may indicate atrophy or abnormalities within the cerebral cortex as well as the basal ganglia. Positron emission tomography (PET) may be used to augment other testing and obtain information regarding blood flow, oxygen uptake, and metabolism of the brain. A DNA marker study may be administered to determine if the autosomal dominant trait is present for HD.

What additional information should be obtained to confirm the diagnosis?

A physical examination, review of symptoms, and family history are important components in the diagnosis of HD.

MANAGEMENT

What is the most effective management of this patient?

Education regarding disease process, coping strategies, and genetic consequences should be initiated immediately following diagnosis. Medical treatment will focus on symptoms and pharmacological management. Drug classes such as anticonvulsants and antipsychotics may assist as these block dopamine transmission, however, have very serious side effects. Physical, occupational, and speech therapy interventions may be warranted intermittently throughout the course of the disease and should focus on current problems with mobility and self-care skills. Physical therapy should maximize endurance, strength, balance, postural control, and functional mobility. Intervention should focus on motor control and utilize techniques including coactivation of muscles, trunk stabilization, the use of biofeedback, and relaxation in an attempt to maintain a patient's functional status. Patient education should include prone lying, stretching, prevention of deformity and contracture, and safety with mobility. As the disease progresses, the degree of dementia will influence treatment and goals. The therapist must continue to emphasize family involvement and caregiver teaching. As the patient continues to lose function the caregiver will require education regarding posture, seating, assistance with transfers, mobility, and the use of adaptive equipment.

What home care regimen should be recommended?

A home care regimen should include an exercise routine, functional mobility skills, relaxation techniques, range of motion, stretching exercises, and endurance activities. Participation in a home care regimen can assist to maintain the optimal quality of life during the progression of the disease process.

OUTCOME

What is the likely outcome of a course of physical therapy?

Physical therapy is recommended on an intermittent basis throughout the course of the disease. Physical therapy will not prevent further degeneration, however, it will maximize the patient's functional potential and safety. The goal of physical therapy is to attain an optimal functional outcome within the limitations of the disease process.

What are the long-term effects of the patient's condition?

HD is a chronic progressive genetic disorder that is fatal within 15 to 20 years after clinical manifestation. Late stages of the disease result in total physical and mental incapacitation. The patient usually requires an extended care facility due to the burden of care and physical, cognitive, and emotional dysfunction.

SILVER   **Myasthenia Gravis**

DIAGNOSIS

What condition produces a patient's symptoms?

Myasthenia gravis is an autoimmune disorder that affects the transmission of neuromuscular signals. The immune system produces antibodies that attack nerve receptors. Because neuromuscular function is decreased, patients with myasthenia gravis have symptoms of weakness and fatigue.

An injury was most likely sustained to which structure?

The pathology associated with myasthenia gravis occurs at the neuromuscular junction. Normally, there are receptors on the motor end plate that accept acetylcholine, which results in the transmission of an action potential. In patients with myasthenia gravis there are fewer receptors on the motor end plate, secondary to the immune system attacking these receptors, which results in an inefficient nerve transmission process.

INFERENCE

What is the most likely contributing factor in the development of this condition?

Though there is no known cause for myasthenia gravis, abnormalities with thymus function likely plays a role. The majority of patients with myasthenia gravis have abnormalities of the thymus (e.g., tumor, hyperplasia), and it is thought that dysfunction of this gland may cause an autoimmune reaction within the body. Women tend to develop the condition in their twenties and thirties while men develop it in their fifties and sixties. In general, women are more likely to be affected by this condition.

CONFIRMATION

What is the most likely clinical presentation?

The primary feature of myasthenia gravis is muscle weakness within the skeletal muscles, with other neurologic findings being normal (e.g., reflexes, sensation). The muscles fatigue rapidly with activity, however, rest quickly improves muscle function. Muscles affected commonly include the ocular muscles and limb musculature (proximal greater than distal). Because the ocular muscles are commonly affected, the patient can experience diplopia and ptosis. Myasthenia gravis can also affect the muscles involved in facial expression, chewing, swallowing, and speech. Triggers that may make a patient's symptoms worse include activity, heat, stress, illness, certain medications, menstruation, and pregnancy. A myasthenic crisis refers to an episode in which the respiratory muscles experience paralysis and the patient needs ventilation to assist with respiration.

What laboratory or imaging studies would confirm the diagnosis?

There are several tests that can be performed to confirm the presence of myasthenia gravis. Laboratory testing of the blood can be used to identify the presence of the antibodies that attack the acetylcholine receptors. Electromyography can be used to identify the characteristic symptom of myasthenia gravis, rapid fatigue with repeated muscle stimulation. Edrophonium chloride, a drug that blocks the degradation of acetylcholine, can be administered to determine if symptoms temporarily improve secondary to increased acetylcholine uptake. Imaging studies (e.g., x-ray, CT scan, MRI) may be performed if the presence of a thymus tumor is suspected.

What additional information should be obtained to confirm the diagnosis?

A thorough medical history and physical examination should be performed to identify the characteristic symptoms of myasthenia gravis and differentiate this condition from other similar conditions, such as hyperthyroidism or botulism. The physical examination will likely consist of an assessment of the ocular and facial muscles, as well as other neurologic testing including sensory, strength, and reflex testing. The examination may also include pulmonary function testing to determine if the respiratory muscles have been affected.

MANAGEMENT

What is the most effective management of this patient?

Patients with myasthenia gravis are often administered a medication that helps to inhibit acetylcholinesterase, the enzyme that breaks down acetylcholine. This allows acetylcholine to build up at the neuromuscular junction, which diminishes the symptoms of weakness and fatigue. Though this medication helps to improve symptoms, it only does so temporarily. Other medications, such as corticosteroids, can help suppress the immune system, thereby improving symptoms. Surgical intervention to remove the thymus gland is another possible treatment to reduce symptoms, especially for those patients who have a thymus tumor. In serious cases with acute worsening of symptoms, plasmapheresis can be performed to remove the antibodies from the blood. Physical therapy should focus on strength and endurance training with caution to avoid overexertion. Therapy may also involve training in breathing techniques to improve respiratory function.

What home care regimen should be recommended?

The home care regimen should consist of a general exercise program to help improve strength and endurance. The patient should follow energy conservation techniques to avoid overexertion.

OUTCOME

What is the likely outcome of a course of physical therapy?

Physical therapy will not be the primary intervention for patients with myasthenia gravis, though a course of physical therapy can help patients to improve muscular strength and endurance and improve functioning with daily activities. Patients will also be instructed in energy conservation techniques.

What are the long-term effects of the patient's condition?

With appropriate treatment, the prognosis for myasthenia gravis is fairly good. Symptoms are generally most severe within the first few years of diagnosis. Afterwards, symptoms either plateau or improve. Though complete remission is rare, symptoms can be well controlled and patients can experience a high quality of life. Removal of the thymus can result in complete remission of symptoms in some patients. Overall, mortality rates are very low.

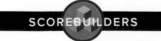

Post-Polio Syndrome   SILVER

DIAGNOSIS

What condition produces a patient's symptoms?

Poliomyelitis is a neurologic condition characterized by asymmetric weakness and/or paralysis caused by a viral infection. Vaccines for the virus were created in the 1950s resulting in eradication of the disease in developing countries. However, for patients who had poliomyelitis and recovered, new neuromuscular symptoms can appear years after their recovery. This new onset of weakness is termed post-polio syndrome.

An injury was most likely sustained to which structure?

The original condition involved a viral attack on the nervous system, specifically on the anterior horn cells within the spinal cord. With the death of anterior horn cells, the motor nerves degrade and the muscles experience atrophy. Recovery of strength in these patients was thought to occur secondary to collateral sprouting to help reinnervate denervated muscles (i.e., a single nerve innervates a larger proportion of muscle fibers). Though the collateral sprouting allows for a period of recovery, the increased demands placed on the remaining nerves leads to deterioration of these nerves over time, leading to a new onset of weakness.

INFERENCE

What is the most likely contributing factor in the development of this condition?

Post-polio syndrome only occurs in individuals previously diagnosed with poliomyelitis. It is estimated that 25-50% of patients with poliomyelitis will eventually develop post-polio syndrome. It is thought that patients who have a more serious initial onset of poliomyelitis (i.e., greater motor involvement) are more likely to develop post-polio syndrome. Women are also more likely to develop post-polio syndrome.

CONFIRMATION

What is the most likely clinical presentation?

The main symptoms of post-polio syndrome include muscle weakness, atrophy, fatigue, and sometimes muscular or joint pain. Weakness can also affect axial musculature and result in difficulties with breathing or swallowing. Post-polio syndrome tends to primarily affect the muscles that were affected during the initial poliomyelitis attack, though it can affect previously unaffected muscles. Pain and weakness generally increase with physical activity and with exposure to cold. The patient will experience decades of recovery after their initial acute poliomyelitis attack before the symptoms of post-polio syndrome begin. With the onset of post-polio syndrome, weakness progresses slowly over the course of years and is interspersed with periods of stability where there is no progression of symptoms.

What laboratory or imaging studies would confirm the diagnosis?

Laboratory and imaging studies are used to exclude the presence of other similar conditions that may be causing neuromuscular symptoms. Electromyography can be performed to determine if muscles have become newly denervated. Muscle biopsy may be utilized for this same reason.

What additional information should be obtained to confirm the diagnosis?

The diagnosis of post-polio syndrome is a clinical diagnosis confirmed primarily through the exclusion of other similar diseases. Because the diagnosis is made clinically, a thorough medical history and physical examination are very important. Patients diagnosed with post-polio syndrome must have a previous history of poliomyelitis that was followed by years of recovery and then a gradual onset of new symptoms.

MANAGEMENT

What is the most effective management of this patient?

There is no cure for post-polio syndrome, therefore treatment is generally multidisciplinary and aimed at controlling symptoms and improving daily function. Medications to combat fatigue (e.g., anticholinesterases, intravenous immunoglobulin) may be prescribed, however, these medications have only shown moderate success in patients with post-polio syndrome. Physical therapy interventions focus on improving overall conditioning. Intense exercise that leads to fatigue or exhaustion should be avoided since this can result in worsening of symptoms. Patients with post-polio syndrome should be taught energy conservation techniques to allow for improved function. Training in the use of assistive devices or orthoses may also be necessary.

What home care regimen should be recommended?

The patient's home care regimen should focus on aerobic exercises as well as strengthening exercises to help improve overall strength and endurance. Exercise is typically performed every other day to allow for adequate rest and recovery.

OUTCOME

What is the likely outcome of a course of physical therapy?

Physical therapy has been shown to help patients with post-polio syndrome improve their levels of strength and endurance, leading to greater daily function and quality of life. Additionally, patients who engage in physical activity demonstrate better gait quality than those who do not.

What are the long-term effects of the patient's condition?

Post-polio syndrome is generally not a life-threatening disease, though this may not be true for those patients who have respiratory involvement. Despite the fact that the majority of patients have a normal lifespan, the disease can still greatly affect a patient's quality of life. Symptoms generally slowly progress over a long period of time, though periods of progression are usually interspersed with periods of stability, which can last years without any progression of symptoms.

Spina Bifida – Myelomeningocele

DIAGNOSIS

What condition produces a patient's symptoms?

Spina bifida is a congenital neural tube defect that generally occurs in the lumbar spine but can also occur at the sacral, cervical, and thoracic levels. Spina bifida has three classifications that include spina bifida - occulta (incomplete fusion of the posterior vertebral arch with no neural tissue protruding), spina bifida - meningocele (incomplete fusion of the posterior vertebral arch with neural tissue/meninges protruding outside the neural arch), and spina bifida - myelomeningocele (incomplete fusion of the posterior vertebral arch with both meninges and spinal cord protruding outside the neural arch).

An injury was most likely sustained to which structure?

Spina bifida - myelomeningocele is characterized by a sac or cyst that protrudes outside the spine and contains a herniation of meninges, cerebrospinal fluid, and the spinal cord through the defect in the vertebrae. The cyst may or may not be covered by skin. Spina bifida results from failure of neural tube closure by day 28 of gestation when the spinal cord is expected to form. Approximately 75% of vertebral defects are found in the lumbar/sacral region, typically L5-S1 with injury to the structures at that level and below.

INFERENCE

What is the most likely contributing factor in the development of this condition?

The incidence of neural tube defects varies by socioeconomic status, geographic area, and ethnic background. The overall incidence is declining due to improved prenatal care. The exact etiology for spina bifida - myelomeningocele has not been identified, however, causative and risk factors include genetic predisposition, environmental influence (certain solvents, lead, herbicides, glycol ethers), insulin-dependent diabetes, low levels of maternal folic acid, alcohol, maternal hyperthermia, and certain classifications of drugs (teratogenic exposure and vitamin A toxicity). Prenatal care including recommended amounts of folic acid, especially in the first six weeks of pregnancy, appears to be the most effective way to prevent neural tube defects.

CONFIRMATION

What is the most likely clinical presentation?

Myelomeningocele is a severe condition that is characterized by a sac that is seen on an infant's back protruding from a specific area of the spinal cord. Impairments associated with myelomeningocele include motor and sensory loss below the vertebral defect, hydrocephalus, Arnold-Chiari type II malformation, clubfoot, scoliosis, bowel and bladder dysfunction, and learning disabilities. The higher the neural lesion the worse the prognosis is for survival. The infant will require surgical intervention to close the lesion and in 90% of the cases a shunt is required for hydrocephalus. Approximately two-thirds of children with myelomeningocele and shunted hydrocephalus have normal intelligence and the other third demonstrate only mild retardation. Regardless of intelligence, children with myelomeningocele exhibit difficulties with perceptual abilities, attention, problem solving, and memory.

What laboratory or imaging studies would confirm the diagnosis?

Prior to birth a fetal ultrasound may identify the myelomeningocele defect in the spine. Prenatal testing of alpha-fetoprotein (AFP) in the blood will show an elevation in levels that indicate a probable neural tube defect at approximately week 16 of gestation. At birth an obvious sac will be present over the spinal defect.

What additional information should be obtained to confirm the diagnosis?

Diagnosis is confirmed through prenatal testing or upon visual observation at birth. Past medical history of the mother, history of the pregnancy, and family history of neural tube defects may be noted.

MANAGEMENT

What is the most effective management of this patient?

Medical management of a patient with myelomeningocele begins with immediate surgical intervention to repair and close the defect and for placement of a shunt to alleviate hydrocephalus. Orthopedic surgical intervention may be warranted throughout a patient's life to correct deformities such as clubfoot, hip dysplasia, and scoliosis. Physical and occupational therapies are important components in the management of myelomeningocele. Physical therapy is initiated immediately and focuses on family education regarding positioning, handling techniques, range of motion, and therapeutic play. Long-term physical therapy attempts to maximize functional capacity and may include range of motion, facilitation of developmental milestones, therapeutic exercise, skin care, strengthening, balance, and mobility training. Physical therapy will also assist with wheelchair prescription, assistive and adaptive device selection, and the use of orthotics and splinting.

What home care regimen should be recommended?

A home care regimen should include a formal exercise program, range of motion, and mobility training. Family and caregiver involvement are important in assisting a patient through their exercise program. The home program will require modification as the child matures and goals change.

OUTCOME

What is the likely outcome of a course of physical therapy?

Physical therapy initially evaluates and documents the baseline information regarding the patient's motor and sensory function and level of ability. Physical therapy is ongoing through adolescence and is based on the severity of impairments and the needs of the child. Physical therapy is usually initiated based on symptoms, functional problems, and disability.

What are the long-term effects of the patient's condition?

A patient with myelomeningocele has a near normal life expectancy as long as the patient receives consistent and thorough health care. Functional outcome of the patient depends on the level of injury, the amount of associated impairments, and the caregiver support that is provided.

Vestibular Disorders

SILVER

DIAGNOSIS

What condition produces a patient's symptoms?

A vestibular disorder occurs when there is a disruption of the sensory information processed by the inner ear and brain with respect to the body's control of balance and eye movements. Typically, disease or injury to these processing areas will result in a vestibular disorder, however, genetic, environmental, and idiopathic etiologies have been recognized as well.

An injury was most likely sustained to which structure?

A vestibular disorder may encompass numerous specific diagnoses including Meniere's disease, benign paroxysmal positional vertigo (BPPV), labyrinthitis, ototoxicity, and acoustic neuroma. Vestibular disorders are classified as either peripheral (e.g., dysfunction of the auditory or vestibular structures in the inner ear) or central (e.g., dysfunction of the nervous system in processing spatial and balance information) with the majority of cases diagnosed as peripheral.

INFERENCE

What is the most likely contributing factor in the development of this condition?

Ear infection, whiplash injury, and head injury are among the most common causes of vestibular disorders in younger individuals. In many individuals, especially those over 50 years of age, the onset of symptoms is idiopathic.

CONFIRMATION

What is the most likely clinical presentation?

The clinical presentation of a vestibular disorder may vary greatly. Symptoms may be intermittent or persistent presenting as either a single attack or repeatedly over time. In many cases, symptoms will diminish or resolve without intervention as the body either heals or compensates for deficits. Typical characteristics can include vertigo, dizziness, nausea, altered balance, auditory changes, and difficulties with cognition, memory or coordination.

What laboratory or imaging studies would confirm the diagnosis?

A vestibular disorder is typically diagnosed based on a patient's past medical history and a clinical examination. MRI may be utilized to rule out soft tissue abnormalities such as tumor, acoustic neuroma or CVA. Depending on the patient's presentation, laboratory blood and allergy testing may also assist in ruling out differential diagnoses.

What additional information should be obtained to confirm the diagnosis?

Various auditory and vestibular tests may assist in the confirmation of a vestibular disorder. Vestibular testing typically emphasizes assessment of the vestibuloocular reflex (e.g., Dix-Hallpike test, electronystagmography, videonystagmography) and an assessment of balance reactions (e.g., gait on varied surfaces, postural sway with eyes closed). Auditory testing is typically performed formally by an audiologist.

MANAGEMENT

What is the most effective management of this patient?

Medical management may include pharmacological intervention, nutritional counseling, psychological counseling, and surgical intervention depending on the etiology and severity of the patient's symptoms. Pharmacological intervention emphasizes symptom management and is typically only recommended either with the initial onset of symptoms, once differential diagnoses have been ruled out or during an acute exacerbation of symptoms. Long-term suppression of symptoms is not typically recommended since the body must experience symptoms in order to develop compensatory strategies. For specific etiologies, antibiotic or antiviral medications may also be prescribed. Nutritional counseling typically emphasizes regulation of the body's fluid balance to stabilize the volume and electrolyte concentrations of the inner ear's endolymph fluid. This may include altering the intake of substances such as sodium and sugar, managing fluid intake, eliminating caffeine and alcohol, and avoiding substances likely to trigger symptoms (e.g., nicotine, aspirin, NSAIDs). For patients who have been unsuccessful in conservatively managing symptoms, surgical options do exist, however, they may be limited depending on the specific etiology. Vestibular rehabilitation includes specific physical therapy interventions designed to assist the patient to habituate (e.g., become less sensitive) to symptoms through adaptation, substitution, cognitive, and symptom prediction strategies. Activities to retrain balance reactions, proprioception, and the vestibuloocular reflex are typically key components of a treatment plan. Examples include gaze stabilization with head movements, single leg stance on variable surfaces, gait with head movement, and maintaining balance with eyes closed. Goals typically include improved static and dynamic balance, decreased reports of dizziness, decreased symptom-related anxiety, and reduced dependence on visual and somatosensory information.

What home care regimen should be recommended?

The home care regimen should include activities which facilitate symptom accommodation and habituation. Activities should be assigned as warranted based on the results of the patient examination with the physical therapist and physical therapist assistant ensuring that each task can be performed safely and without debilitating symptom exacerbation.

OUTCOME

What is the likely outcome of a course of physical therapy?

Vestibular rehabilitation is typically recommended if a patient's symptoms have not resolved within an extended timeframe. However, the risk of falling and incidence of falls may be reduced when therapy interventions are initiated closer to the onset. Though largely dependent on the location and severity of damage, vestibular exercises have been shown to be effective in most patients.

What are the long-term effects of the patient's condition?

The effects of vestibular disorders can be quite diverse ranging from spontaneous recovery to permanent disability.

BRONZE Level Clinical Application Templates

BRONZE Level Clinical Application Template Executive Summary

Bell's Palsy

- Refers to an acute onset of sensory and motor deficits in structures supplied by the facial nerve
- Primarily affects the muscles associated with facial expression, however, it can also impact saliva and tear production
- Is a self-limiting condition that is not life-threatening with majority of patients experiencing a spontaneous recovery that occurs within weeks to months

Epilepsy

- Injury to the brain can cause abnormal activity of the brain's nerve cells in which the electrical discharge of the neurons becomes hypersynchronous, resulting in epileptic seizures
- Symptoms vary widely depending on the type of seizure (e.g., tonic, clonic) and may include mood disturbances, staring, loss of consciousness, uncontrollable jerking of the arms and legs, stiffening of muscles, and loss of muscle control
- An electroencephalogram measures electrical activity of the brain and is the most common test used to confirm the diagnosis of epilepsy

Polyneuropathy

- Characterized by damage or disease that affects multiple peripheral nerves, which is most commonly caused by diabetes mellitus
- Polyneuropathy often starts in the distal lower extremities, generally symmetrically, and may progress to include the hands and more proximal portions of the limbs
- Electromyography and nerve conduction testing are often used to determine the location and extent of nerve damage

Trigeminal Neuralgia

- Typically the result of abnormal pressure on or irritation of the trigeminal nerve
- Symptoms are typically unilateral and may be either episodic or constant; sudden pain described as sharp, jolting, stabbing or shock-like or persistent aching or burning sensations
- Diagnostic testing is often inconclusive with a diagnosis typically made based on the patient's reported symptoms

Bell's Palsy

DIAGNOSIS

What condition produces a patient's symptoms?

Bell's palsy refers to an acute onset of sensory and motor deficits in structures supplied by the facial nerve. Bell's palsy is typically the result of abnormal pressure on the facial nerve, commonly associated with edema or inflammation. It primarily affects the muscles associated with facial expression, however, it can also impact saliva and tear production.

An injury was most likely sustained to which structure?

The facial nerve (cranial nerve VII) is sometimes referred to as the "nerve of facial expression." It is associated with taste sensation on the anterior aspect of the tongue and voluntary motor control of most facial muscles. The nerve originates in the brainstem, traveling with the vestibulocochlear nerve (cranial nerve VIII) around middle ear structures before exiting through the stylomastoid foramen and passing through the parotid gland where it divides into five major branches.

CONFIRMATION

What is the most likely clinical presentation?

The onset of Bell's palsy may occur suddenly or progress over a few days. Symptoms typically affect only one side of the face and often begin with a feeling of generalized stiffness or tightness. A facial droop is the most recognizable characteristic of the condition. Other symptoms include difficulties with motor skills that may interfere with eye and mouth closure, eating, and facial expressions (e.g., one-sided smile). Decreased taste sensation, altered tear and saliva production, and increased auditory sensitivity may also be reported.

What laboratory or imaging studies would confirm the diagnosis?

An MRI or CT scan may assist in identifying the presence of an infection or structural abnormality (e.g., tumor, fracture) which may be the cause of pressure on the facial nerve. Blood tests and imaging may be used to rule out conditions which may mimic Bell's palsy, such as Lyme disease and CVA.

What additional information should be obtained to confirm the diagnosis?

A thorough medical history should be obtained to assist in ruling out similar diagnoses and identifying conditions associated with an increased incidence of Bell's palsy. Electromyogram (EMG) may be utilized to evaluate the extent and severity of nerve damage. The preliminary diagnosis is typically made based on a functional assessment of facial muscle performance and symmetry with activities such as smiling, frowning, closing the eyes, baring the teeth, and raising the eyebrows.

Epilepsy

DIAGNOSIS

What condition produces a patient's symptoms?

Epilepsy is a chronic central nervous system disorder characterized by epileptic seizures due to abnormal neuronal activity within the brain. Epilepsy has no identifiable etiology in approximately half of the population with the condition. Known conditions that can cause epilepsy include brain injury (e.g., head trauma, stroke, tumor), infectious disease (e.g., AIDS, meningitis), genetic influence, and developmental disorders (e.g., cerebral palsy).

An injury was most likely sustained to what structure?

Injury to the brain can cause abnormal activity of the brain's nerve cells in which the electrical discharge of the neurons becomes hypersynchronous. This abnormal neuronal activity precipitates the patient's seizure symptoms.

CONFIRMATION

What is the most likely clinical presentation?

Seizures are often unpredictable and unprovoked and vary widely in their presentation depending on the type of seizure (e.g., simple focal, absence, tonic, clonic). Symptoms may include mood disturbances, staring, loss of consciousness, uncontrollable jerking of the arms and legs, stiffening of muscles, and loss of muscle control. A seizure is the hallmark sign of epilepsy, though one seizure does not signify that a patient has epilepsy.

What laboratory or imaging studies would confirm the diagnosis?

An electroencephalogram measures electrical activity of the brain and is the most common test used to confirm the diagnosis of epilepsy. It is common for patients to have abnormal brain wave patterns even when they are not experiencing a seizure. Other imaging and laboratory studies, such as magnetic resonance imaging, computed tomography, and blood tests, may be used to identify the cause of the seizures.

What additional information should be obtained to confirm the diagnosis?

A thorough medical history, physical examination, and neurological examination may assist in the diagnosis of epilepsy and rule out other similar conditions (e.g., syncope, metabolic conditions, movement disorders, migraine).

Polyneuropathy
BRONZE

DIAGNOSIS:

What condition produces a patient's symptoms?

Polyneuropathy is a condition characterized by damage or disease that affects multiple peripheral nerves. The most common etiology of polyneuropathy is diabetes mellitus (both type 1 and type 2). Other causes include advanced age, certain drugs (e.g., chemotherapy), alcohol abuse, AIDS, environmental toxins, and inherited neurological conditions.

An injury was most likely sustained to what structure?

Polyneuropathy typically affects peripheral nerves, especially distally in the extremities, though it can also affect cranial nerves and nerves of the autonomic nervous system. Polyneuropathy can affect solely the sensory nerves, solely the motor nerves, or both. Neuropathy may involve damage to the axon, the myelin sheath or the nerve's cell body depending on the cause of the neuropathy.

CONFIRMATION

What is the most likely clinical presentation?

Polyneuropathy often starts in the distal lower extremities, typically symmetrically, and may progress to include the hands and more proximal portions of the limbs. Symptoms include numbness, tingling, and pain in a "stocking" and "glove" pattern. Additional symptoms include loss of position and vibration sense as well as ataxia. If motor nerves are affected, the condition will involve muscle weakness, and possibly atrophy. Autonomic symptoms include constipation, loss of bowel and bladder control, and orthostatic hypotension.

What laboratory or imaging studies would confirm the diagnosis?

Electromyography and nerve conduction testing are often used to determine the location and extent of nerve damage. Other laboratory testing (e.g., blood tests) may be performed to determine the cause of the neuropathy.

What additional information should be obtained to confirm the diagnosis?

The physician can often diagnose the condition based on a thorough medical history and a neurological examination. The examination consists of assessments of sensation (superficial and deep), strength, deep tendon reflexes, and coordination.

Trigeminal Neuralgia
BRONZE

DIAGNOSIS

What condition produces a patient's symptoms?

Trigeminal neuralgia is typically the result of abnormal pressure on or irritation of the trigeminal nerve. Common etiologies for abnormal pressure include tumor or a swollen blood vessel. Irritation of the nerve is more commonly associated with conditions that cause demyelination such as multiple sclerosis. In some cases, the continuous pulsations and consequent friction of a blood vessel in contact with the nerve can cause demyelination and subsequent symptoms over time.

An injury was most likely sustained to which structure?

The trigeminal nerve (cranial nerve V) is a mixed sensory and motor nerve that originates in the brainstem and branches into the ophthalmic, mandibular, and maxillary nerves. Pressure or demyelination injury produces a chronic pain condition which may impact the entire nerve distribution depending on the specific location and severity of the pathology. The most common location of injury is in the narrow space where the nerve exits the brainstem.

CONFIRMATION

What is the most likely clinical presentation?

Symptoms of trigeminal neuralgia are typically unilateral and may be either episodic or constant. Episodic symptoms most commonly present as a sudden onset of pain described as sharp, jolting, stabbing or shock-like. Spasms or tics may also occur. Episodic symptoms may be triggered by touch or sound with attacks that often result from activities of daily living such as shaving, chewing or oral care. Chronic symptoms are more commonly described as persistent aching or burning sensations which may be exacerbated by the same type of daily activities that trigger an episodic attack. Symptoms of either form can be progressive and in severe cases, may be debilitating. Trigeminal neuralgia is more common among women and individuals over the age of 50.

What laboratory or imaging studies would confirm the diagnosis?

Magnetic resonance angiography utilizes a colored dye to visualize blood flow near the brainstem and identify vessel pathology that may be causing compression of the trigeminal nerve.

What additional information should be obtained to confirm the diagnosis?

A thorough medical history should be obtained to identify potential sources of trigeminal nerve trauma (e.g., recent sinus or oral surgery, stroke, facial trauma). Diagnostic testing is often inconclusive with a diagnosis typically made based on the patient's reported symptoms.

Neuromuscular and Nervous Systems Essentials

1. The nervous system is composed of specialized cells that function to receive, integrate, control, and transmit information throughout the body. Components of the nervous system include the central nervous system (CNS), peripheral nervous system (PNS), autonomic nervous system (ANS), somatic nervous system (SNS), and limbic system.

2. The central nervous system anatomically consists of the brain and the spinal cord. There are two hemispheres of the brain and each hemisphere includes a frontal, temporal, parietal, and occipital lobe. The brain can also be divided into the forebrain, midbrain, and hindbrain. Each area is responsible for interpretation and control of certain biological processes and movement.

3. The peripheral nervous system consists of 12 pairs of cranial nerves and 31 pairs of spinal nerves. These nerves all have afferent and efferent fibers for communication between the body and the central nervous system.

4. The autonomic nervous system (ANS) consists of two divisions: the sympathetic division (generally a stimulating response) and the parasympathetic division (generally an inhibitory response). Anatomically, the ANS contains portions of the CNS and PNS. Impulses to the ANS typically do not reach the level of consciousness and instead produce automatic responses.

5. The somatic nervous system (SNS) regulates body movement through sensory and motor neurons that transmit information from the brain to muscle fibers throughout the body. The SNS controls voluntary movement, influences the five senses, and is responsible for reflex arcs such as deep tendon reflexes.

6. The limbic system is found within the brain and is involved with control and expression of mood, processing, memory, appetite, and olfaction. Lesions to this area can produce aggression, fearlessness, alterations in motivation, and other behaviors.

7. The forebrain consists of the telencephalon (cerebral cortex, hippocampus, basal ganglia, amygdala) and the diencephalon (thalamus, hypothalamus, subthalamus, epithalamus).

8. The cerebrum consists of gray matter on the surface and white matter interiorly, while sulci and fissures demark the specific lobes.

9. The left hemisphere has specific responsibilities including the ability to understand language, sequencing of movements, producing written and spoken language, expression of positive emotions, and the ability to be analytical, controlled, and logical. The right hemisphere has specific responsibilities including nonverbal processing, artistic expression, comprehension of general concepts, spatial relationships, kinesthetic awareness, mathematical reasoning, and body image awareness.

10. Each lobe of the brain has specific responsibilities: Frontal: intellect, orientation, voluntary movement, Broca's area, executive functions; Parietal: receives information associated with touch, kinesthesia, vibration; Temporal: auditory processing, Wernicke's area, production of meaningful speech; Occipital: visual processing, judgment of distance, vision in three dimensions.

11. The midbrain is located at the base of the brain above the spinal cord. It consists of the tectum and tegmentum and serves as a relay area, connecting the forebrain to the hindbrain. It is also a reflex center for visual, auditory, and tactile responses.

12. The hindbrain consists of the cerebellum, pons, and medulla oblongata. The cerebellum coordinates movement and assists with maintenance of balance. The pons and medulla assist with control of the body's vital functions.

13. From the Circle of Willis, the anterior cerebral artery, middle cerebral artery, posterior cerebral artery, and vertebral-basilar artery perfuse different regions of the brain and will produce impairments with vascular pathology specific to each artery.

14. The meninges are three layers of connective tissue that provide covering and protection for the brain and spinal cord. The dura mater is the outermost layer, followed by the arachnoid, and the pia mater (innermost layer). Dural spaces are areas normally surrounding meninges that may contain cerebrospinal fluid.

Neuromuscular and Nervous Systems Essentials

15. Cerebrospinal fluid is a clear fluid-like substance that cushions the brain and spinal cord and provides nutrition to the CNS. The ventricular system assists to produce and circulate CSF.

16. The spinal cord is a component of the CNS and a direct continuation of the brainstem. It serves as a relay for information between the brain and peripheral structures. Spinal nerves each possess afferent and efferent fibers for transmission of information through ascending and descending tracts of the spinal cord.

17. The peripheral nervous system contains nerves that have sensory, motor, and autonomic responsibilities. Cutaneous sensory end organs include thermoreceptors, nociceptors, mechanoreceptors, chemoreceptors, and photoreceptors that provide feedback through different channels of stimulation.

18. Peripheral nerve fibers may be classified as A, B or C fibers. A fibers are large and myelinated with a high conduction speed. B fibers are medium and myelinated with a moderate speed. C fibers are small and unmyelinated or poorly myelinated with a slow speed.

19. Nerve roots from C1 through S4 each innervate a particular region for sensation (dermatome), and for motor innervation (myotome), and provide a pattern of anticipated weakness with impairment.

20. The cranial nerves include olfactory, optic, oculomotor, trochlear, trigeminal, abducens, facial, vestibulocochlear, glossopharyngeal, vagus, accessory, and hypoglossal nerves. Each has a specific testing protocol to ensure accuracy of results.

21. The brachial plexus innervates the muscles of the upper extremity while the lower extremity is innervated by the lumbar plexus and sacral plexus.

22. Superficial reflexes are a response to stimulation of the receptors within the skin. The sensory signal must reach the spinal cord and ascend to the brain for processing. Common superficial reflexes include the abdominal, corneal, cremasteric, gag, and plantar reflexes. The Babinski reflex is an abnormal plantar reflex.

23. Deep tendon reflexes (DTR) elicit a muscle contraction through stimulation of the muscle's tendon through a reflex arc. DTRs are graded from 0 to 4+ and results of testing may be indicative of a lesion to the reflex arc or a suprasegmental lesion.

24. Superficial sensations include light touch, temperature, and pain. Deep sensations include kinesthesia, proprioception, and vibration. Cortical sensations include localization of touch, bilateral simultaneous stimulation, two-point discrimination, stereognosis, and barognosis.

25. Acute injury to a peripheral nerve will produce neurapraxia (the mildest form of injury with axons preserved and recovery rapid and complete), axonotmesis (more severe injury with reversible damage, potential for spontaneous recovery), and neurotmesis (most severe damage, axon and myelin are damaged, irreversible injury, no spontaneous recovery, surgery may allow for some recovery).

26. Upper motor neuron lesions are found within the motor cortex, internal capsule, brainstem or spinal cord. Hyperactive reflexes, mild atrophy, and increased tone are characteristic findings with this form of pathology.

27. Lower motor neuron lesions are found in nerves or their axons at or below the level of the brainstem. Hypoactive or absent reflexes, atrophy, fasciculations, and decreased tone are characteristic findings with this form of pathology.

28. Tremors, tics, chorea, dystonia, and athetosis are all forms of movement disorders that present with involuntary movements.

29. Balance is the state of physical equilibrium with maintenance and control of the center of gravity. There are somatosensory, visual, and vestibular systems that provide feedback to the CNS regarding balance.

30. The vestibuloocular reflex (VOR) supports gaze stabilization through eye movement that counters movements of the head. The vestibulospinal reflex (VSR) attempts to stabilize the body while the head is moving in order to manage upright posture.

Neuromuscular and Nervous Systems Essentials

31. Vestibular rehabilitation is targeted for patients with central or peripheral balance disorders and can include VOR and VSR exercises, ocular motor exercises, habituation training, balance training, center of gravity control, varying environments, visual conditions, and use of gravity to challenge the balance system.

32. Communication disorders can include all forms of aphasia, verbal apraxia, and dysarthria. Aphasia is typically classified as receptive, expressive or global. Treatment will be modified based on the patient's ability to communicate or understand alternative forms of communication.

33. Common pharmacological agents used in the treatment of neurological disorders include antiepileptic agents, antispasticity agents, cholinergic agents, dopamine replacement agents, and muscle relaxant agents.

34. A cerebrovascular accident (CVA) is a specific event that results in a lack of oxygen to a specific area of the brain secondary to ischemia or hemorrhage. CVAs are typically termed a completed stroke, stroke in evolution, transient ischemic attack, ischemic stroke or hemorrhage.

35. A patient presents with predictable patterns of impairment when ischemia occurs secondary to a CVA in the left hemisphere, right hemisphere, brainstem or cerebellum.

36. The flexor synergy for the upper extremity includes scapular elevation and retraction; shoulder abduction and lateral rotation; elbow flexion; forearm supination; wrist flexion; and finger and thumb flexion with adduction. The extensor synergy for the upper extremity includes scapular depression and protraction; shoulder adduction and medial rotation; elbow extension; forearm pronation; wrist extension; and finger and thumb flexion with adduction.

37. The flexor synergy for the lower extremity includes hip abduction and lateral rotation; knee flexion; ankle dorsiflexion with supination; and toe extension. The extensor synergy for the lower extremity includes hip extension, medial rotation, and adduction; knee extension; ankle plantar flexion with inversion; and toe flexion and adduction.

38. Neurological rehabilitation may incorporate a variety of treatments based on the patient's pathology and goals. The variety of constructs base each of the theories of rehabilitation on their particular interpretation of motor control and motor learning.

39. Motor control is the study of the nature of movement and the ability to direct essential movement. Motor learning is the study of the acquisition or modification of movement. Stages of motor learning include the cognitive stage, associative stage, and autonomous stage. Feedback is imperative for the progression of motor learning.

40. Practice is integral to motor learning. Various types of practice include massed and distributed practice; constant and variable practice; random and blocked practice; and whole training and part training.

41. Bobath developed Neuro-Developmental Treatment based on the hierarchical model of neurophysiologic function. This approach includes facilitation and inhibition of tone, reflex inhibiting postures, key points of control, proximal control, and the use of rotation during treatment.

42. Brunnstrom's Movement Therapy in Hemiplegia utilizes synergy patterns to assist with developing movement combinations outside of synergy patterns. Raimiste's phenomenon and Souques' phenomenon are used in treatment along with associated reactions, stages of recovery, overflow, and limb synergies.

43. Proprioceptive Neuromuscular Facilitation (PNF) is based on establishing gross motor patterns within the CNS, allowing for stronger parts to stimulate and strengthen the weaker parts. Treatment emphasizes developmental sequence, mass movement patterns, and diagonal patterns.

44. Rood's theory of neurological rehabilitation is based on the reflex stimulus model where motor output is the result of past and present sensory input. The goal of homeostasis is achieved using key patterns to enhance motor control. Treatment includes sensory stimulation to facilitate or inhibit a response.

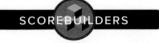

Neuromuscular and Nervous Systems Essentials

45. Spinal cord injury (SCI) refers to permanent damage that can occur to the spinal cord after a sufficient force has been exerted on the spinal cord itself. Motor vehicle accidents have the highest incidence for SCI. There are complete and incomplete lesions with regard to motor and sensory function.

46. Incomplete lesions can include anterior cord syndrome, Brown-Sequard's syndrome, central cord syndrome, posterior cord syndrome, and cauda equina injuries.

47. The ASIA Impairment Scale is widely used for assessment of a patient with a SCI. This tool classifies complete versus incomplete lesions along with key muscles to test.

48. Autonomic dysreflexia is a common complication of a SCI and is considered a medical emergency. An excessive and uncontrolled increase in blood pressure places the patient at risk. A kinked catheter is the most typical stimulus for this condition.

49. Functional outcomes are anticipated for each level of spinal cord injury. A physical therapist assistant must be able to recognize a patient's potential based on expected functional outcomes.

50. Traumatic brain injury is classified as either open or closed with primary and secondary brain damage. Primary injuries typically consist of coup and contrecoup lesions with secondary injury typically due to an epidural or subdural hematoma.

51. The Glasgow Coma Scale is used to assess patients with suspected head injury in order to classify the injury from mild to severe.

52. Rancho Los Amigos Levels of Cognitive Functioning Scale will also assist to classify the level of injury based on where the patient best meets the criteria of each level. The levels include: no response; generalized response; localized response; confused-agitated; confused-inappropriate; confused-appropriate; automatic-appropriate; and purposeful-appropriate.

53. The concepts of development include cephalic to caudal; gross to fine; mass to specific; and proximal to distal.

54. Primitive reflexes are elicited with a predictable stimulus that causes a predictable response until the time when the primitive reflex is integrated. When reflexes do not integrate, there is typically interference with progressing through the developmental milestones.

55. Developmental milestones for gross and fine motor skills follow a tentative schedule that children will follow through the teenage years. Developmental delay and other pediatric pathology may cause the child to experience difficulty progressing through the milestones.

56. Therapeutic positioning is essential to obtain maximum function for the pediatric population and is used to facilitate desired movement, inhibit unwanted tonal influences, normalize tone, prevent contractures, enhance midline orientation, and improve respiratory capacity.

57. Legislation such as the Individuals with Disabilities Education Improvement Act (IDEA), Rehabilitation Act, and No Child Left Behind Act have provided improved services and benefits for children with disabilities. These laws have been updated and amended to improve services for children with disabilities.

Neuromuscular and Nervous Systems Proficiencies

1. Brain Anatomy

Identify the appropriate term for each of the specified locations. Answers must be selected from the Word Bank and can be used only once.

Word Bank: cerebellum, corpus callosum, hypothalamus, medulla oblongata, midbrain, pituitary gland, thalamus

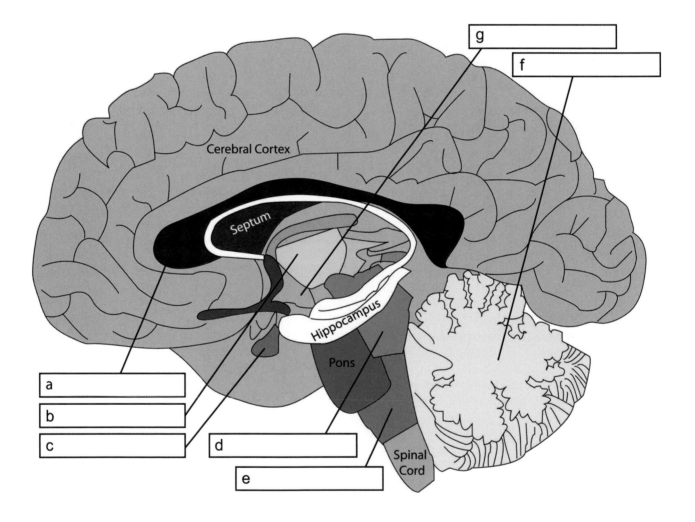

Neuromuscular and Nervous Systems Proficiencies

2. Cranial Nerve Function

Indicate "yes" or "no" in each cell based on the presence or absence of a sensory (afferent) and/or motor (efferent) component for each cranial nerve.

Cranial Nerve	Sensory	Motor
Olfactory	a	b
Optic	c	d
Oculomotor	e	f
Trochlear	g	h
Trigeminal	i	j
Abducens	k	l
Facial	m	n
Vestibulocochlear	o	p
Glossopharyngeal	q	r
Vagus	s	t
Accessory	u	v
Hypoglossal	w	x

3. Cranial Nerve Testing

Identify the most appropriate method of testing for each of the cranial nerves. Answers must be selected from the Word Bank and can be used more than once if indicated.

Word Bank: downward and inward gaze; face sensation; familiar odors; familiar tastes; gag reflex (2); hearing test; lateral gaze; resisted shoulder shrug; tongue protrusion; upward, downward, and medial gaze; visual fields

Cranial Nerve	Cranial Nerve Test
Olfactory	a
Optic	b
Oculomotor	c
Trochlear	d
Trigeminal	e
Abducens	f
Facial	g
Vestibulocochlear	h
Glossopharyngeal	i
Vagus	j
Accessory	k
Hypoglossal	l

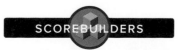

Neuromuscular and Nervous Systems Proficiencies

4. Hemispheric Specialization

Identify the specific hemisphere most closely associated with each described function. Answers must be selected from the Word Bank and can be used more than once.

Word Bank: left, right

Hemisphere	Function
a	logical and rational
b	understand nonverbal communication
c	understand and express language
d	spatial relationships
e	artistic abilities
f	mathematical calculations
g	body image awareness
h	express positive emotions
i	express negative emotions

5. Innervation Levels

Identify the primary innervation level most closely associated with the described myotome, dermatome or reflex. Answers must be selected from the Word Bank and can be used more than once.

Word Bank: C4, C5, C6, C7, C8, L4, L5, S1, S3

Myotome	Innervation Level
trapezius	a
triceps	b
extensor hallucis longus	c
gastrocnemius-soleus	d

Dermatome	Innervation Level
deltoid area	e
radial side of hand to thumb and index finger	f
medial arm and forearm to long, ring, and little fingers	g
groin, medial thigh to knee	h

Reflex	Innervation Level
biceps	i
triceps	j
patellar	k
Achilles	l

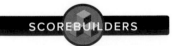

Neuromuscular and Nervous Systems Proficiencies

6. Sensory Testing

Identify the type of sensory testing most closely associated with the supplied description. Answers must be selected from the Word Bank and can be used only once.

Word Bank: deep pain, graphesthesia, kinesthesia, light touch, proprioception, temperature, two-point discrimination, stereognosis, superficial pain, vibration

Sensation	Description
a	squeeze the forearm or calf muscle
b	use a tuning fork
c	identify a static position of an extremity
d	use a cotton ball applied to the skin
e	identify direction and extent of movement of a body part
f	use hot and cold test tubes
g	draw a letter on the skin with a finger
h	identify one or two points without sight
i	identify an object without sight
j	use a paper clip end or a pen cap

7. Upper versus Lower Motor Neuron Lesions

Indicate whether each pathology is an upper motor neuron or lower motor neuron lesion. Answers must be selected from the Word Bank and can be used more than once.

Word Bank: upper motor neuron, lower motor neuron

Pathology	Type of Lesion
multiple sclerosis	a
traumatic brain injury	b
Bell's palsy	c
Guillain-Barre syndrome	d
Huntington's chorea	e
muscular dystrophy	f
poliomyelitis	g
cerebral palsy	h
CVA	i

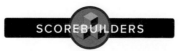

Neuromuscular and Nervous Systems Proficiencies

8. Brunnstrom's Stages of Recovery

Identify the appropriate sequence of Brunnstrom's Stages of Recovery based on the supplied description. Answers must be selected from the Word Bank and can be used only once.

Word Bank: Sequence - 1, 2, 3, 4, 5, 6, 7

Sequence	Description
a	The synergies are performed voluntarily; spasticity increases.
b	Normal motor function is restored.
c	The appearance of basic limb synergies. The beginning of spasticity.
d	Spasticity begins to decrease. Movement patterns are not dictated solely by limb synergies.
e	No volitional movement initiated.
f	A further decrease in spasticity is noted with independence from limb synergy patterns.
g	Isolated joint movements are performed with coordination.

9. Sensory Stimulation Techniques

Identify whether the sensory stimulation technique is used for facilitation or inhibition. Answers must be selected from the Word Bank and can be used more than once.

Word Bank: facilitation, inhibition

Technique	Use
icing	a
deep pressure	b
warmth	c
joint compression	d
prolonged stretch	e
quick stretch	f
tapping	g
light touch	h

Neuromuscular and Nervous Systems Proficiencies

10. Pediatric Reflexes I

Identify the type of pediatric reflex associated with the supplied stimulus. Answers must be selected from the Word Bank and can be used only once.

Word Bank: asymmetrical tonic neck reflex, Galant reflex, Moro reflex, palmar grasp reflex, plantar grasp reflex, positive support reflex, rooting reflex, startle reflex, symmetrical tonic neck reflex, walking (stepping) reflex

Reflex	Stimulus
a	touch on the cheek
b	head position, turned to one side
c	loud, sudden noise
d	head position, flexion or extension
e	head dropping into extension suddenly for a few inches
f	touch to the skin along the spine from the shoulder to the hip
g	weight placed on the balls of the feet when upright
h	pressure to the base of the toes
i	pressure in the palm on the ulnar side of the hand
j	supported upright position with the soles of the feet on a firm surface

11. Pediatric Reflexes II

Identify the type of pediatric reflex associated with the described response. Answers must be selected from the Word Bank and can be used only once.

Word Bank: asymmetrical tonic neck reflex, Galant reflex, Moro reflex, palmar grasp reflex, plantar grasp reflex, positive support reflex, rooting reflex, symmetrical tonic neck reflex, tonic labyrinthine reflex, walking (stepping) reflex

Reflex	Response
a	arms abduct with fingers open, then cross trunk into adduction; cry
b	arm and leg on the face side are extended; arm and leg on the scalp side are flexed
c	when the head is in flexion, the arms are flexed and the legs are extended
d	when in a supine position, the body and the extremities are held in extension
e	flexion of the fingers causing a strong grip
f	lateral flexion of the trunk to the side of the stimulus
g	toe flexion
h	reciprocal flexion and extension of the legs
i	turning the head to the same side with the mouth open
j	stiffening of the legs and the trunk into extension

Neuromuscular and Nervous Systems Proficiencies

12. Neuromuscular and Nervous Systems Terminology

Identify the neuromuscular term most closely associated with the supplied description. Answers must be selected from the Word Bank and can be used only once.

Word Bank: agraphia, aphasia, constructional apraxia, emotional lability, hemiparesis, homonymous hemianopsia, ideomotor apraxia, perseveration, unilateral neglect

Terminology	Description
a	The state of repeatedly performing the same segment of a task or repeatedly saying the same word/phrase without purpose.
b	The inability to write due to a lesion within the brain.
c	The inability to control emotion with outbursts of laughing or crying that are inconsistent with the situation.
d	The loss of the right or left half of the field of vision in both eyes.
e	The inability to interpret stimuli and events on the contralateral side of a hemispheric lesion.
f	A condition where a person plans a movement or task, but cannot volitionally perform it.
g	The inability to communicate or comprehend due to damage to specific areas of the brain.
h	A condition of weakness on one side of the body.
i	The inability to reproduce geometric figures and designs.

13. Neuromuscular and Nervous Systems Basics

Mark each statement as True or False. If the statement is False, correct the statement in the space provided.

True/False	Statement
a	The occipital lobe of the cerebrum contains the primary motor cortex and Broca's area.
Correction	
b	The meninges consist of three distinct layers termed the dura mater, arachnoid, and pia mater.
Correction	

Neuromuscular and Nervous Systems Proficiencies

True/False	Statement
c	The fasciculus gracilis is a motor tract responsible for voluntary, discrete, and skilled movement.
Correction	
d	The axillary and radial nerves originate from the posterior cord of the brachial plexus.
Correction	
e	The plantar reflex is assessed by stroking the lateral aspect of the sole of the foot to the ball of the foot toward the base of the great toe.
Correction	
f	A reflex grade of 1+ is indicative of a brisk or exaggerated response.
Correction	
g	Elbow flexion and/or forearm supination is a normal response when eliciting the brachioradialis deep tendon reflex.
Correction	
h	Graphesthesia refers to the ability to perceive the weight of different objects placed in the hand.
Correction	
i	Slopes, uneven surfaces, and standing on foam could be used to challenge the somatosensory system during a balance assessment.
Correction	

Neuromuscular and Nervous Systems Proficiencies

True/False	Statement
j	Crouching or squatting is an example of the suspensory postural strategy.
Correction	
k	The Berg Balance Scale consists of fourteen tasks, each scored on an ordinal five point scale.
Correction	
l	Patients with Brown-Sequard's syndrome present with a loss of pain and temperature sense on the ipsilateral side of the lesion.
Correction	
m	Guillain-Barre syndrome results in motor weakness in a proximal to distal progression.
Correction	
n	The Glasgow Coma Scale has a minimum score of 0 and a maximum score of 15.
Correction	

Neuromuscular and Nervous Systems Answer Key

1. Brain Anatomy

a. corpus callosum
b. thalamus
c. pituitary gland
d. midbrain
e. medulla oblongata
f. cerebellum
g. hypothalamus

2. Cranial Nerve Function

a. yes
b. no
c. yes
d. no
e. no
f. yes
g. no
h. yes
i. yes
j. yes
k. no
l. yes
m. yes
n. yes
o. yes
p. no
q. yes
r. yes
s. yes
t. yes
u. no
v. yes
w. no
x. yes

3. Cranial Nerve Testing

a. familiar odors
b. visual fields
c. upward, downward, and medial gaze
d. downward and inward gaze
e. face sensation
f. lateral gaze
g. familiar tastes
h. hearing test
i. gag reflex
j. gag reflex
k. resisted shoulder shrug
l. tongue protrusion

4. Hemispheric Specialization

a. left
b. right
c. left
d. right
e. right
f. left
g. right
h. left
i. right

5. Innervation Levels

a. C4
b. C7
c. L5
d. S1
e. C5
f. C6
g. C8
h. S3
i. C5
j. C7
k. L4
l. S1

6. Sensory Testing

a. deep pain
b. vibration
c. proprioception
d. light touch
e. kinesthesia
f. temperature
g. graphesthesia
h. two-point discrimination
i. stereognosis
j. superficial pain

Neuromuscular and Nervous Systems Answer Key

7. Upper versus Lower Motor Neuron Lesions

a. upper motor neuron
b. upper motor neuron
c. lower motor neuron
d. lower motor neuron
e. upper motor neuron
f. lower motor neuron
g. lower motor neuron
h. upper motor neuron
i. upper motor neuron

8. Brunnstrom's Stages of Recovery

a. 3
b. 7
c. 2
d. 4
e. 1
f. 5
g. 6

9. Sensory Stimulation Techniques

a. facilitation
b. inhibition
c. inhibition
d. facilitation
e. inhibition
f. facilitation
g. facilitation
h. facilitation

10. Pediatric Reflexes I

a. rooting reflex
b. asymmetrical tonic neck reflex
c. startle reflex
d. symmetrical tonic neck reflex
e. Moro reflex
f. Galant reflex
g. positive support reflex
h. plantar grasp reflex
i. palmar grasp reflex
j. walking (stepping) reflex

11. Pediatric Reflexes II

a. Moro reflex
b. asymmetrical tonic neck reflex
c. symmetrical tonic neck reflex
d. tonic labyrinthine reflex
e. palmar grasp reflex
f. Galant reflex
g. plantar grasp reflex
h. walking (stepping) reflex
i. rooting reflex
j. positive support reflex

12. Neuromuscular and Nervous Systems Terminology

a. perseveration
b. agraphia
c. emotional lability
d. homonymous hemianopsia
e. unilateral neglect
f. ideomotor apraxia
g. aphasia
h. hemiparesis
i. constructional apraxia

13. Neuromuscular and Nervous Systems Basics*

a. FALSE: Correction - The frontal lobe of the cerebrum contains the primary motor cortex and Broca's area.
b. TRUE
c. FALSE: Correction - The corticospinal tract is a motor tract responsible for voluntary, discrete, and skilled movement.
d. TRUE
e. TRUE
f. FALSE: Correction - A reflex grade of 1+ is indicative of a diminished or depressed response.
g. TRUE
h. FALSE: Correction - Barognosis refers to the ability to perceive the weight of different objects placed in the hand.
i. TRUE
j. TRUE
k. TRUE
l. FALSE: Correction - Patients with Brown-Sequard's syndrome present with a loss of pain and temperature sense on the contralateral side of the lesion.

Neuromuscular and Nervous Systems Answer Key

m. FALSE: Correction - Guillain-Barre syndrome results in motor weakness in a distal to proximal progression.

n. FALSE: Correction - The Glasgow Coma Scale has a minimum score of 3 and a maximum score of 15.

   *The correction presented for each false statement is an example of several possible corrections.

Neuromuscular and Nervous Systems References

1.   Rowland LP, Pedley TA. *Merritt's Neurology*. 12th Edition. Lippincott Williams & Wilkins. 2009.

2.   Snell RS. *Clinical Neuroanatomy*. 7th Edition. Philadelphia, PA: Lippincott Williams & Wilkins. 2009.

3.   Lundy-Ekman L. *Neuroscience: Fundamentals for Rehabilitation*. Fifth Edition. Elsevier. 2018.

4.   McCaffrey P. The Corpus Striatum, Rhinencephalon, Connecting Fibers, and Diencephalon. www.csuchico.edu/~pmccaffrey/syllabi/CMSD%20320/362unit5.html Neuroscience on the Web Series. November, 2010. Accessed March, 2011.

5.   Cohen H. *Neuroscience for Rehabilitation*. JB Lippincott Company. 1999.

6.   DeMyer W. *Technique of the Neurologic Examination*. Fifth Edition. McGraw-Hill Companies. 2004.

7.   Bertoti, DB. *Functional Neurorehabilitation Through the Life Span*. F.A. Davis. 2004.

8.   Gillen G, Burkhardt A. *Stroke Rehabilitation: A Functional Approach*. Mosby. 1998.

9.   Conn PM. *Neuroscience in Medicine*. JB Lippincott Company. 2008.

10. Freemon FR. Akinetic Mutism and Bilateral Anterior Cerebral Artery Occlusion. http://www.ncbi.nlm.nih.gov/pmc/articles/PMC1083504/ Journal of Neurology, Neurosurgery, and Psychiatry. Accessed March, 2011.

11. Dawson VL, Hsu CY, Liu TH, Dawson TM, Wamsley JK. Receptor alterations in subcortical structures after bilateral middle cerebral artery infarction of the cerebral cortex. http://www.ncbi.nlm.nih.gov/pubmed/8070526. Accessed April, 2011.

12. Slater D, Curtin S, Johns J. Middle cerebral artery stroke. http://emedicine.medscape.com/article/323120-overview. Accessed March 2011.

13. Goodman C, Fuller K. *Pathology: Implications for the Physical Therapist*. Fourth Edition. W.B. Saunders Company. 2015.

14. Palisano R, Orlin M, Shreiber J. *Campbell's Physical Therapy for Children*. Fifth Edition. Elsevier. 2017.

15. Campbell S. *Decision Making in Pediatric Neurologic Physical Therapy*. Churchill Livingstone. 1999.

16. Human Nervous System. Encyclopedia Britannica Online, http://www.britannica.com/EBchecked/topic/409709/human-nervous-system. Updated 2010. Retrieved November 29, 2010.

17. Gutman S. *Quick Reference Neuroscience for Rehabilitation Professionals*. Second Edition. Slack Inc. 2008.

18. Field-Fote E. *Spinal Cord Injury Rehabilitation*. F.A. Davis Company. 2009.

19. Sisto SA, Druin E, Macht-Sliwinski M. *Spinal Cord Injuries Management and Rehabilitation*. Mosby Elsevier. 2009.

20. Cameron M, Monroe L. *Physical Rehabilitation: Evidence-Based Examination, Evaluation, and Intervention*. W. B. Saunders Company. 2007.

21. Magee DJ. *Orthopedic Physical Assessment*. Sixth Edition. W. B. Saunders Company. 2014.

22. Bickley L. *Bates' Guide to Physical Examination and History Taking*. Twelfth Edition. Wolters Kluwer. 2017.

23. Kendall F, McCreary E, Provance, P. *Muscles Testing and Function with Posture and Pain*. Fifth Edition. Lippincott Williams & Wilkins. 2005.

24. Umphred D. *Neurological Rehabilitation*. Sixth Edition. Mosby Inc. 2013.

25. Walker HK, Hall WD, Hurst JW. *Clinical Methods: The History, Physical, and Laboratory Examinations*. Third Edition. Butterworths. 1990.

Neuromuscular and Nervous Systems References

26. O'Sullivan S, Schmitz T, Fulk G. *Physical Rehabilitation: Assessment and Treatment*. Sixth Edition. F.A. Davis Company. 2014.

27. Roy S, Wolf S, Scalzitti D. *The Rehabilitation Specialist's Handbook*. Fourth Edition. F.A .Davis Company. 2013.

28. Montgomery PC, Connolly BH. *Clinical Applications for Motor Control*. Slack, Incorporated. 2003.

29. *Physical Therapist's Clinical Companion*, Springhouse Corporation. 2000.

30. Bennett S, Karnes J. *Neurological Disabilities: Assessment and Treatment*. Lippincott-Raven Publishers. 1998.

31. Barnes M, Dobkin B, Bogousslavsky J. *Recovery after Stroke*. Cambridge University Press. 2005.

32. Neurological Diagnostic Tests and Procedures. National Institute of Neurological Disorders and Stroke, National Institutes of Health. http://www.ninds.nih.gov/disorders/misc/diagnostic_tests.htm. Accessed June 2011.

33. Ciccone C. *Pharmacology in Rehabilitation*. Fifth Edition. F.A.Davis Company. 2016.

34. *Miller-Keane: Encyclopedia and Dictionary of Medicine, Nursing, and Allied Health*. Seventh Edition. W.B. Saunders Company. 2003.

35. Davies PM. *Steps to Follow: The Comprehensive Treatment of Patients with Hemiplegia*. Springer-Verlag. 2004.

36. Shumway-Cook A, Woollacott M. *Motor Control: Translating Research into Clinical Practice*. Fourth Edition. Lippincott Williams & Wilkins. 2011.

37. Carr J, Shepherd R. *Neurologic Rehabilitation: Optimizing Motor Performance*. Churchill Livingstone. 2010.

38. Carr J, Shepard R. *Stroke Rehabilitation: Guidelines for Exercise and Training to Optimize Motor Skill*. Elsevier Science Limited. 2003.

39. Bobath B. *Adult Hemiplegia: Evaluation and Treatment*. Third Edition. Butterworth-Heinemann. 1990.

40. Sullivan P, Markos P. *Clinical Decision Making in Therapeutic Exercise*. Appleton & Lange. 1995.

41. Brunnstrom S. *Movement Therapy in Hemiplegia*. Harper and Row Publishers Inc. 1992.

42. Mesulam MM. Motor Exam Guide and Key Sensory Points. National Institute of Health http://www.asia-spinalinjury.org/# American Spinal Injury Association (ASIA). Accessed June 2011.

43. Goodman C, Heick J, Lazaro R. *Differential Diagnosis for Physical Therapists – Screening for Referral*. Sixth Edition. Elsevier. 2018.

44. Campbell M. *Rehabilitation for Traumatic Brain Injury: Physical Therapy Practice in Context*. Churchill Livingstone. 2000.

45. Long T, Toscano K. *Handbook of Pediatric Physical Therapy*. Second Edition. Lippincott Williams & Wilkins. 2002.

46. Tecklin J. *Pediatric Physical Therapy*. Fifth Edition. Lippincott Williams & Wilkins. 2015.

47. Ratliffe KT. *Clinical Pediatric Physical Therapy: A Guide for the Physical Therapy Team*. Mosby Inc. 1998.

48. Special Education and Rehabilitative Services. ehttp://www2.ed.gov/policy/speced/leg/edpicks.jhtml?src=ln. The US Department of Education. Accessed June 2011.

6

Cardiovascular and Pulmonary Systems

Michael Fillyaw

Cardiovascular and Pulmonary Systems represents approximately 21 - 26 questions (14% - 17.3%) on the NPTE-PTA.

Contributors

Scott Giles
Shawn Paquette

CHAPTER 6
Cardiovascular and Pulmonary Systems

Anatomy and Physiology of the Cardiovascular System

Heart

Topology of the Heart

Apex: The lowest part of the heart formed by the inferolateral part of the left ventricle. It projects anteriorly and to the left at the level of the 5th intercostal space and the left midclavicular line.

Base: The upper border of the heart involving the left atrium, part of the right atrium, and the proximal portions of the great vessels. It lies approximately below the second rib at the level of the second intercostal space.

Endocardium: The endothelial tissue that lines the interior of the heart chambers and valves.

Epicardium: The serous layer of the pericardium. The epicardium contains the epicardial coronary arteries and veins, autonomic nerves, and lymphatics.

Myocardium: The thick contractile middle layer of muscle cells that forms the bulk of the heart wall.

Pericardium: A double-walled connective tissue sac that surrounds the outside of the heart and great vessels.

Great Vessels of the Heart

Aorta: The body's largest artery and the central conduit of blood from the heart to the body. The aorta begins at the upper part of the left ventricle, and after ascending for a short distance arches backward and to the left (arch of the aorta). It then descends within the thorax (thoracic aorta) and passes into the abdominal cavity (abdominal aorta).

Inferior vena cava: The vein that returns venous blood from the lower body and viscera to the right atrium.

Pulmonary arteries: The arteries that carry deoxygenated blood from the right ventricle to the left and right lungs.

Pulmonary veins: The veins that carry oxygenated blood from the right and left lungs to the left atrium.

Superior vena cava: The vein that returns venous blood from the head, neck, and arms to the right atrium.

Heart Chambers and Valves

The superior chambers of the heart are the right atrium (RA) and left atrium (LA). The wall between the atria is the atrial septum. The two inferior chambers of the heart are the right ventricle (RV) and left ventricle (LV). The wall between the ventricles is the ventricular septum. The right chambers collect blood from the body and pump it to the lungs. The left chambers collect blood from the lungs and pump it to the rest of the body.

The heart has four valves that function to maintain unidirectional blood flow (Fig. 6.1). The atrioventricular valves (AV) are between the atria and ventricles and are named by the number of leaflets or cusps. The right AV valve, or tricuspid valve, has three leaflets. It controls blood flow between the RA and RV. The left AV valve, or mitral valve, has two leaflets. It controls blood flow between the LA and LV. The aortic valve is between the LV and aorta; the pulmonary valve is between the RV and pulmonary artery.

Venous blood from the superior and inferior vena cava enters the RA and is pumped through the tricuspid valve into the RV. The tricuspid valve closes while the RV contracts to pump blood through the pulmonary valve and into the pulmonary trunk, which divides into right and left pulmonary arteries serving the right and left lungs, respectively. After picking up oxygen and releasing carbon dioxide in the pulmonary capillaries, oxygenated blood returns via the pulmonary veins to the LA. Contraction of the LA forces blood through the mitral valve into the LV. The mitral valve closes when the LV contracts to pump blood through the aortic valve into the aorta where it is distributed into the coronary circulation and systemic circulation (Fig. 6-1).

Coronary Arteries

The coronary arteries are a network of progressively smaller vessels that carry oxygenated blood to the myocardium. The right and left coronary arteries arise from the ascending aorta just beyond where the aorta leaves the left ventricle. These arteries and their branches supply all parts of the myocardium (Fig. 6-2).

HEART
Chambers of the Heart

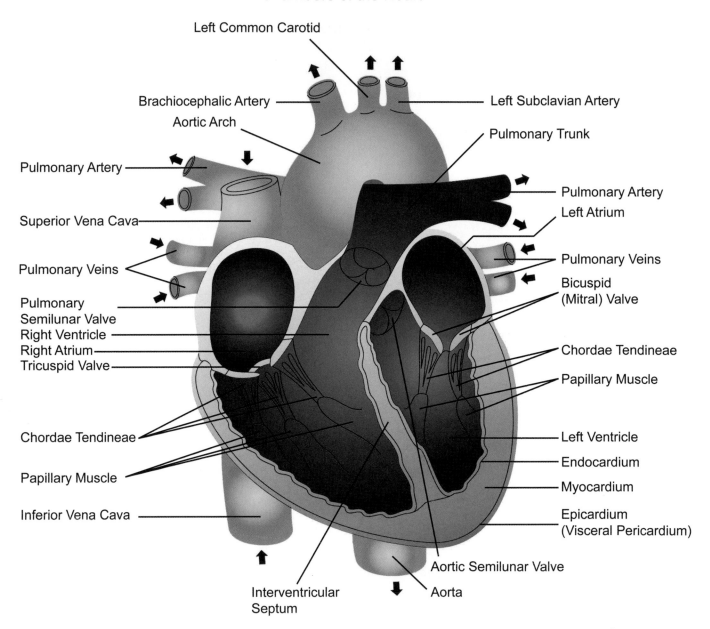

Left Common Carotid

Brachiocephalic Artery

Aortic Arch

Left Subclavian Artery

Pulmonary Trunk

Pulmonary Artery

Superior Vena Cava

Pulmonary Artery

Left Atrium

Pulmonary Veins

Pulmonary Veins

Pulmonary Semilunar Valve

Bicuspid (Mitral) Valve

Right Ventricle

Right Atrium

Tricuspid Valve

Chordae Tendineae

Papillary Muscle

Chordae Tendineae

Papillary Muscle

Left Ventricle

Endocardium

Myocardium

Inferior Vena Cava

Epicardium (Visceral Pericardium)

Aortic Semilunar Valve

Interventricular Septum

Aorta

Anterior View

Fig. 6-1: Cross section of the anterior of the heart showing the chambers and valves.

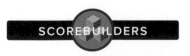

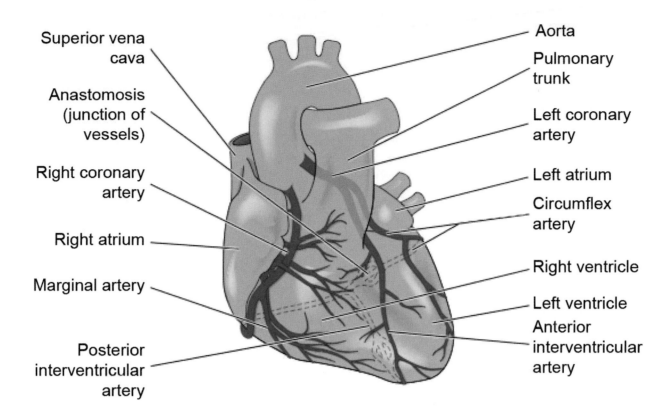

Fig. 6-2: Anterior surface of the heart showing the great vessels and coronary arteries.

Coronary Veins

The coronary venous circulation includes the coronary sinus, cardiac veins, and thebesian veins. The great cardiac vein, along with the small and middle cardiac veins, drain into the coronary sinus, emptying into the right atrium. The thebesian veins arise in the myocardium and drain into all chambers of the heart, but primarily into the right atrium and right ventricle.

Cardiac Conduction System

The cardiac conduction system includes the sinoatrial (SA) node and the atrioventricular (AV) node. Each cardiac myocyte has an intrinsic ability to depolarize and propagate electrical impulses from cell to cell without nerve stimulation.

The SA node is the normal pacemaker of the heart. Specialized conduction tracts conduct the cardiac impulse between the SA node and AV node and to the atrial musculature.

Innervation of the Heart

Although cardiac automaticity is intrinsic to the SA node; heart rate, rhythm, and contractility are also influenced by the autonomic nervous system. The vagus and sympathetic cardiac nerves converge to form the cardiac plexus at the base of the heart.

- The sympathetic influence is achieved by release of epinephrine and norepinephrine. Sympathetic nerves stimulate the chambers to beat faster (chronotropic effect) and with greater force of contraction (inotropic effect).

- The parasympathetic influence is achieved via acetylcholine release from the vagus nerve. Parasympathetic nerves slow the heart rate (chronotropic effect) primarily through their influence on the SA node.

Neural Reflexes and Circulatory Control

The balance between the sympathetic and parasympathetic components of the autonomic nervous system determines cardiovascular responses.

Baroreceptor reflex: Baroreceptors are mechanoreceptors that detect changes in pressure. The reflexes by which blood pressure is maintained are collectively known as the baroreflex, which includes arterial baroreceptors (high pressure receptors located in the carotid sinus, aortic arch, and origin of the right subclavian artery) and cardiopulmonary receptors (low pressure receptors). Sympathetic activation leads to increased cardiac contractility, increased heart rate, venoconstriction, and arterial vasoconstriction, ultimately leading to increased blood pressure via elevation of total peripheral resistance and cardiac output. Parasympathetic activation leads to a decrease in heart rate and a small decrease in contractility, resulting in a decrease in blood pressure.

Bainbridge reflex: An increase in venous return stretches receptors in the wall of the right atrium which sends vagal afferent signals to the cardiovascular center within the medulla. The signals inhibit parasympathetic activity, resulting in an increased heart rate.

Chemoreceptor reflex: Chemosensitive cells located in the carotid bodies and the aortic body respond to changes in pH status and blood oxygen tension.

Valsalva maneuver: Forced expiration against a closed glottis produces increased intrathoracic pressure, increased central venous pressure, and decreased venous return. The resultant decrease in cardiac output and blood pressure is sensed by baroreceptors, which reflexively increase heart rate and myocardial contractility through sympathetic stimulation.

Cardiac Cycle

The cardiac cycle refers to the sequence of events that occur when the heart beats.

Atrial systole: The contraction of the right and left atria pushing blood into the ventricles.

Atrial diastole: The period between atrial contractions when the atria are repolarizing.

Ventricular systole: Contraction of the right and left ventricles pushing blood into the pulmonary arteries and aorta.

Ventricular diastole: The period between ventricular contractions when the ventricles are repolarizing.

Preload: Refers to the tension in the ventricular wall at the end of diastole. It reflects the venous filling pressure that fills the left ventricle during diastole.

Afterload: Refers to the forces that impede the flow of blood out of the heart, primarily the pressure in the peripheral vasculature, the compliance of the aorta, and the mass and viscosity of blood.

Stroke volume (SV): Refers to the volume of blood ejected by each contraction of the left ventricle. Normal SV ranges from 60 to 80 ml depending on age, sex, and activity.

Cardiac output (CO): The amount of blood pumped from the left or right ventricle per minute. It is equal to the product of stroke volume and heart rate. Normal CO for an adult male at rest is 4.5 to 5.0 L/min with women producing slightly less. CO can increase up to 25 L/min during exercise.

Venous return: The amount of blood that returns to the right atrium each minute. This is similar in volume to the CO. Because the cardiovascular system is a closed loop, venous return must equal CO when averaged over time.

Systemic Circulation

The systemic arterial circulation carries oxygenated blood from the left ventricle through the aorta, arteries, and arterioles to the capillaries in the tissues of the body. From the capillaries, deoxygenated blood returns through a series of venules and veins.

Blood and Components of Blood[1]

Blood transports oxygen and nutrients to the cells of the body and returns waste products from these cells. Normal blood volume of an adult is between 4.5 and 5.0 L, with women's volume being slightly less than men.

Plasma

Plasma is the liquid component of blood, in which the blood cells and platelets are suspended. Plasma consists of water, electrolytes, and proteins, and accounts for more than half of the total blood volume. Plasma is important in regulating blood pressure and temperature.

Red blood cells

Red blood cells (i.e., erythrocytes) make up approximately 40% of blood volume. Red blood cells contain hemoglobin, a protein that gives blood its red color and enables it to bind with oxygen. When the number of red blood cells is too low (anemia), the blood carries less oxygen, resulting in fatigue and weakness. If the number of red blood cells is too high (polycythemia), the blood is too thick, increasing the risk of stroke or heart attack.

Blood platelets

Blood platelets (i.e., thrombocytes) assist in blood clotting by clumping together at a bleeding site and forming a plug that helps to seal the blood vessel. A low number of platelets (thrombocytopenia) increases the risk for bruising and abnormal bleeding. A high number of platelets (thrombocythemia) increases the risk of thrombosis, which may result in a stroke or heart attack.

White blood cells

White blood cells (i.e., leukocytes) protect against infection. A low number of white blood cells (leukopenia) increases the risk of infection. An abnormally high number of white blood cells (leukocytosis) can indicate an infection or leukemia. There are five main types of white blood cells (Fig. 6-3):

Neutrophils: help protect the body against infections by ingesting bacteria and debris.

Lymphocytes: consist of three main types - T lymphocytes and natural killer cells, which help protect against viral infections and can detect and destroy some cancer cells, and B lymphocytes, which develop into cells that produce antibodies.

Monocytes: ingest dead or damaged cells and help defend against infectious organisms.

Eosinophils: kill parasites, destroy cancer cells, and are involved in allergic responses.

Basophils: participate in allergic responses.

Erythrocytes   Thrombocytes

Fig. 6-3: Blood cells. Left to right: top row - erythrocytes and thrombocytes; bottom row – monocyte, basophil, eosinophil, neutrophil, lymphocyte.

Anatomy and Physiology of the Respiratory System

Thorax

The bony thorax encloses and protects the heart, lungs and other organs and provides attachment sites for ventilatory muscles and other muscles. The thorax is bounded posteriorly by the 12 thoracic vertebrae, intervertebral disks, and ribs; anteriorly by the sternum, costal cartilages, and ribs; and laterally by the ribs. Although not considered part of the thorax, the clavicles and scapulae provide attachment sites for the accessory muscles of inspiration.

Sternum

The sternum consists of three parts – manubrium, body, and xiphoid process. The manubrium, the superior portion, articulates with the right and left clavicles at the clavicular notch. The manubrium articulates with the body of the sternum forming the sternal angle (angle of Louis). A notch at the junction of the manubrium and body provides for the articulation of the second rib. The xiphoid process is the inferior portion of the sternum.

Ribs

Most of the bony thorax is formed by the 12 pairs of ribs. Anteriorly, ribs 1 through 7 (true ribs) attach to the sternum by costal cartilage. The costal cartilages of ribs 8 through 10 (false ribs) attach to the cartilage of the rib above and do not reach the sternum. The ventral ends of ribs 11 and 12 (floating ribs) have no skeletal attachment.

Thoracic vertebrae

Except for ribs 1, 10, 11, and 12, which articulate only with one vertebra, the head of each rib has both a superior and inferior facet for articulation with the bodies of two adjacent thoracic vertebrae. The inferior facet articulates with the superior costal facet of the vertebra of the same number. The superior facet articulates with the inferior costal facet of the vertebra numbered one lower. The transverse process of each vertebra has a transverse costal facet

that articulates with the facet on the tubercle of the rib forming the costotransverse joints.

Muscles of Inspiration

The diaphragm and external intercostals are considered the principal muscles of inspiration. The diaphragm is a dome-shaped muscle that separates the thoracic cavity from the abdominal cavity. Contraction of the diaphragm causes the chest to expand longitudinally and the lower ribs to elevate to allow for inspiration.

The intercostal muscles occupy the spaces between the ribs. External intercostal muscles are oriented obliquely upward and backward from the upper border of one rib to the lower border of the rib above. Internal intercostal muscles are oriented obliquely upward and forward from the upper border of one rib to the lower border of the rib above. Contraction of the external and internal intercostal muscles elevates the ribs. Upward movement of the upper ribs increases the anterior-posterior (A-P) diameter of the chest; elevation of the lower ribs increases the transverse diameter.

Other muscles that attach to the sternum and ribs and ordinarily contribute to movement of the chest wall only during high levels of ventilation are considered accessory muscles of inspiration. These include the sternocleidomastoid, scalenes, pectoralis major (sternocostal portion), pectoralis minor, and serratus anterior.

Muscles of Exhalation

During quiet breathing, exhalation results from passive recoil of the lungs and rib cage. During forceful breathing, the rectus abdominis, external oblique, internal oblique, and transverse abdominis depress the lower ribs and compress the abdominal contents, thus pushing up the diaphragm and assisting with active exhalation.

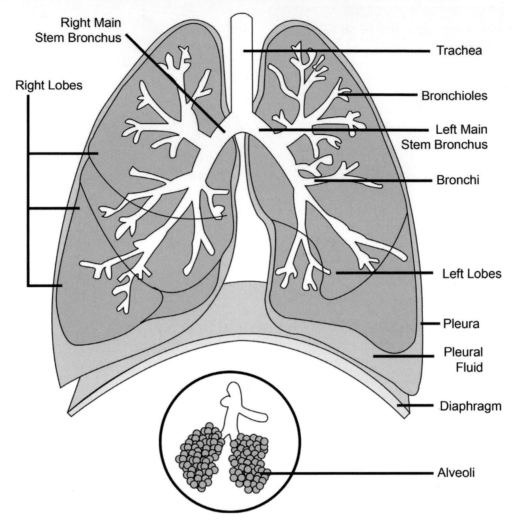

Right Main Stem Bronchus

Right Lobes

Trachea

Bronchioles

Left Main Stem Bronchus

Bronchi

Left Lobes

Pleura

Pleural Fluid

Diaphragm

Alveoli

Fig. 6-4: Diagram of the human lungs.

Upper Respiratory Tract

The upper respiratory tract includes the nasal cavity, pharynx (nasopharynx, oropharynx, laryngopharynx), and larynx. In addition to serving as gas conduits, these passages humidify, cool or warm inspired air, and filter foreign matter before it can reach the alveoli. The hairs in the nostrils filter out many particles while the remaining particles settle on mucous membranes in the nose or near the tonsils and adenoids.

Lower Respiratory Tract

The lower respiratory tract extends from the larynx to the alveoli in the lungs and consists of the conducting airways and the terminal respiratory units. Between the trachea and the alveoli, the airways divide approximately 23 times.

Trachea

Beginning at the larynx (approximately at the base of the neck) and ending at the carina (at the level of the fourth thoracic vertebra and the sternal angle) the trachea consists of a series of horseshoe-shaped rings of cartilage which support the anterior and lateral walls.

Lung Lobes and Segments

The lungs are located on either side of the mediastinum, each within its own pleural cavity. The right lung has three lobes (upper, middle, and lower) and the left lung has two lobes (upper and lower). The lingula of the left upper lobe is analogous to the right middle lobe (Fig. 6-4).

Bronchopulmonary segments

The bronchopulmonary segments are the topographic units of the lungs. There are ten bronchopulmonary segments in the right lung and eight bronchopulmonary segments in the left lung.

Right lung

The right main bronchus gives rise to the superior, middle, and inferior lobar bronchi.

Left lung

The left main bronchus divides into the superior and inferior lobar bronchi, which correspond to the upper and lower lobes, respectively.

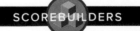

Lung Volumes and Capacities

Anatomic dead space volume (VD)	The volume of air that occupies the non-respiratory conducting airways.
Expiratory reserve volume (ERV)	The maximal volume of air that can be exhaled after a normal tidal exhalation. ERV is approximately 15% of total lung volume.
Forced expiratory volume (FEV)	The maximal volume of air exhaled in a specified period of time: usually the 1st, 2nd, and 3rd second of a forced vital capacity maneuver.
Forced vital capacity (FVC)	The volume of air expired during a forced maximal expiration after a forced maximal inspiration.
Functional residual capacity (FRC)	The volume of air in the lungs after normal exhalation. FRC = ERV + RV. FRC is approximately 40% of total lung volume.
Inspiratory capacity (IC)	The maximal volume of air that can be inspired after a normal tidal exhalation. IC = TV + IRV. IC is approximately 60% of total lung volume.
Inspiratory reserve volume (IRV)	The maximal volume of air that can be inspired after normal tidal volume inspiration. IRV is approximately 50% of total lung volume.
Minute volume ventilation (VE)	The volume of air expired in one minute. VE = TV x respiratory rate.
Peak expiratory flow (PEF)	The maximum flow of air during the beginning of a forced expiratory maneuver.
Residual volume (RV)	The volume of gas remaining in the lungs at the end of a maximal expiration. RV is approximately 25% of total lung volume.
Tidal volume (TV)	Total volume inspired and expired with each breath during quiet breathing. TV is approximately 10% of total lung volume.
Total lung capacity (TLC)	The volume of air in the lungs after a maximal inspiration; the sum of all lung volumes. TLC = RV + VC or TLC = FRC + IC.
Vital capacity (VC)	The volume change that occurs between maximal inspiration and maximal expiration. VC = TV + IRV + ERV. VC is approximately 75% of total lung volume.

Alveolar–capillary units

The bronchi branch many times before terminating in the acinus or respiratory unit of the lung. Oxygen diffuses across the alveolar-capillary septum into the red blood cells in the lung capillaries where it combines with hemoglobin to be transported back to the heart. Carbon dioxide diffuses in the opposite direction.

Pleurae

A membranous serous sac called visceral pleura covers each lung. The pleura covering the surface of the lungs is called the visceral pleura. The pleural tissue covering the inner surfaces of the chest wall, ribs, vertebrae, diaphragm, and mediastinum is called parietal pleura. Normally, the two pleurae remain in contact throughout the respiratory cycle, separated only by serous fluid. Under abnormal circumstances, the pleural space may contain air (pneumothorax), blood (hemothorax), pus or increased amounts of serous fluid, which compress the lung and cause respiratory distress.

Pulmonary Circulation

The portion of the circulatory system that carries deoxygenated blood from the heart to the lungs via the pulmonary arterial trunk, right and left pulmonary arteries, lobar arteries, arterioles, and capillaries. The pulmonary circulation returns oxygenated blood from the lungs to the left atrium via the pulmonary veins.

Bronchial Circulation

The portion of the circulatory system that supplies oxygenated blood to the bronchi and connective tissue of the lungs via the bronchial arteries, which drain directly into the bronchial veins.

Control of Breathing[2]

Although spontaneous breathing is largely an involuntary process, also it is under voluntary control. Breathing control is achieved by integrated activity of the central respiratory center in the brainstem and peripheral receptors in the lungs, airways, chest wall, and blood vessels. The respiratory center integrates the information transmitted from the central and peripheral chemoreceptors and mechanoreceptors in the chest wall to stimulate motor neurons that innervate the respiratory muscles.

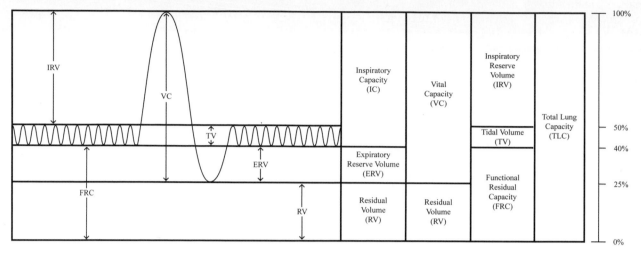

ERV = ~15% total volume   RV = ~25% total volume
IRV = ~50% total volume   IC = ~60% total volume
FRC = ~40% total volume   TV = ~10% total volume
VC = ~75% total volume   TLC = 100% volume

Fig. 6-5: Spirogram showing lung volumes and capacities.

Oxygen and Carbon Dioxide Transport

Oxygen is physically dissolved in the blood plasma and chemically combined with hemoglobin in red blood cells. Much more oxygen is combined with hemoglobin than is dissolved in the plasma.

Carbon dioxide is physically dissolved in the blood, chemically combined with the amino acids of hemoglobin as carbamino compounds, and as bicarbonate ions. About 5-10% of the total carbon dioxide transported by the blood is dissolved in physical solution. A similar percentage is in the form of carbamino compounds. The remaining 80-90% of the carbon dioxide is transported by the blood as bicarbonate ions.

Pathology of the Heart and Blood Vessels

Aneurysm[3]

A localized abnormal dilation of a blood vessel, usually an artery. Common sites include the thoracic and abdominal aorta and vessels within the brain.

Etiology – Congenital defect; weakness in the wall of the vessel often due to chronic hypertension; connective tissue disease (e.g., Marfan syndrome); trauma; infection.

Signs and symptoms – Variable based on the site. Aortic aneurysms are usually asymptomatic, but may include generalized abdominal or low back pain. Abdominal aortic aneurysms may cause pulsations near the navel. A cerebral aneurysm can cause a sudden and severe headache, nausea and vomiting, stiff neck, seizure, loss of consciousness, and double vision.

Treatment – Antihypertensive medications may be recommended for hypertension. Surgery is recommended to repair large aortic aneurysms and consists of replacing the aneurysm with a synthetic fabric graft.

Angina Pectoris[3]

A transient precordial sensation of pressure or discomfort resulting from myocardial ischemia. Common types of angina pectoris are:

- **Stable angina** - Occurs at a predictable level of exertion, exercise or stress and responds to rest or nitroglycerin.

- **Unstable angina** - Usually is more intense, lasts longer, is precipitated by less exertion, occurs spontaneously at rest, is progressive, or any combination of these features.

- **Prinzmetal (variant) angina** - Occurs due to coronary artery spasm most often associated with coronary artery disease.

Etiology – Inadequate blood flow and oxygenation of the heart muscle mostly due to coronary artery disease.

Signs and symptoms – Usually described as pressure, heaviness, fullness, squeezing, burning or aching behind the sternum, but may also be felt in the neck and back, jaw, shoulders, and arms. The sensation may be associated with difficulty breathing, nausea or vomiting, sweating, anxiety or fear (anginal equivalents). It is typically triggered by exertion or strong emotion and subsides with rest.

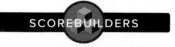

Treatment – Treatments for acute angina include supplemental oxygen, nitroglycerin, and rest. Chronic or recurring angina pectoris is treated with long-acting nitrates, beta blockers, and calcium channel blockers. Angioplasty with stenting of the coronary arteries or coronary artery bypass surgery may be performed when medications are not effective.

Atherosclerosis[3]

A slow progressive accumulation of fatty plaques on the inner walls of arteries. Over time the plaque can restrict blood flow, causing a blood clot.

Etiology – Although the exact cause is unknown, the process may begin with damage or injury to the inner wall of the artery from hypertension, high cholesterol, smoking or diabetes. Over time, fatty plaques made of cholesterol and other cellular waste products build up at the site of the injury and harden, narrowing the artery and impeding blood flow (Fig. 6-6).

Signs and symptoms – Varies based on the severity of disease and the artery affected. When the coronary arteries are affected, angina pectoris may result. When cerebral arteries are affected, numbness or weakness of the arms or legs, difficulty speaking or slurred speech, or drooping face muscles may result. When peripheral arteries are affected, intermittent claudication may result.

Treatment – Lifestyle changes, medications, and surgery may be recommended. Lifestyle changes include smoking cessation, regular exercise, healthy diet, and stress management. Medications may include antihypertensive, antiplatelet, and antilipidemic agents. Surgical procedures may include: angioplasty, endarterectomy, and bypass surgery.

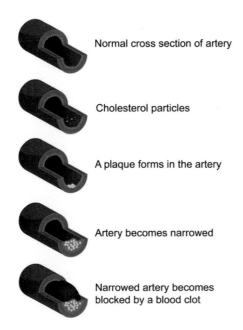

Normal cross section of artery

Cholesterol particles

A plaque forms in the artery

Artery becomes narrowed

Narrowed artery becomes blocked by a blood clot

Fig. 6-6: Changes in an artery due to atherosclerosis.

Chronic Venous Insufficiency (CVI)[3]

A condition in which the veins and valves in the lower extremity are damaged and cannot keep blood flowing toward the heart. This causes the veins to remain filled with blood.

Etiology – Weak or damaged valves inside the veins. Risk factors include age, female gender, obesity, pregnancy, and prolonged sitting or standing.

Signs and symptoms – Leg swelling, varicose veins, aching, heaviness or cramping, itching, redness or skin ulcers of the legs and ankles.

Treatment – Compression stockings and elevation of the legs help decrease chronic swelling. Varicose vein stripping may be performed for cases with persistent leg pain or skin ulcers due to poor circulation.

Cor Pulmonale[4]

Cor pulmonale, also known as pulmonary heart disease, refers to hypertrophy of the right ventricle caused by altered structure or function of the lungs.

Etiology – Pulmonary hypertension from chronically increased resistance in the pulmonary circulation.

Signs and symptoms – The cardinal symptom is progressive shortness of breath, especially with exertion. Other signs and symptoms are fatigue, palpitations, atypical chest pain, swelling of the lower extremities, dizziness, and syncope.

Treatment – Supplemental oxygen sufficient to maintain $SaO_2 >$ 90% and/or $PaO_2 > 60$ mm Hg. General measures include diuretics and anticoagulation.

Coronary Artery Disease (CAD)[3]

CAD is the narrowing or blockage of the coronary arteries due to atheromatous plaques resulting in diminished blood flow.

Etiology – CAD is thought to begin with damage or injury to the inner layer of a coronary artery. Once the inner wall is damaged, fatty plaques made of cholesterol and other cellular waste products tend to accumulate at the site of injury. If a plaque ruptures, platelets will clump at the site to try to repair the artery. This clump can block the artery, leading to a heart attack. Risk factors for CAD are the same as those for atherosclerosis: high blood levels of LDL cholesterol, low blood levels of HDL cholesterol, type 2 diabetes mellitus, smoking, obesity, and physical inactivity. Genetic factors, hypertension, and hypothyroidism also contribute to risk.

Signs and symptoms – The degree of stenosis required to produce signs and symptoms varies with the oxygen demand. The diminished blood flow may cause angina, shortness of breath or other symptoms, which may not be felt until >70% of the lumen is occluded. A complete blockage can cause a heart attack.

Treatment – Aggressive modification of atherosclerosis risk factors to slow progression and induce regression of existing plaques and restore or improve coronary blood flow. This includes smoking cessation; weight loss; a heart-healthy diet low in saturated fat, cholesterol and sodium; regular exercise; modification of serum lipids; and control of hypertension and diabetes. Drug therapy includes: antiplatelet agents (e.g., aspirin, Clopidogrel), ACE inhibitors, angiotensin II receptor blockers, and statins. Percutaneous angioplasty and coronary artery bypass graft surgery are considered for patients at high risk of mortality.

Deep Vein Thrombosis (DVT)[3]

A condition in which a blood clot forms in one or more of the deep veins, usually in the lower extremities. DVT is a serious condition because the clot can break loose and travel to the lungs, resulting in a pulmonary embolism.

Etiology – Any condition that impairs normal circulation or normal blood clotting. Many factors increase the risk of a DVT including prolonged sitting or bed rest, inherited blood clotting disorders, injury or surgery of the veins, pregnancy, cancer, birth control or hormone replacement therapy, being overweight, obesity, and smoking.

Signs and symptoms – About 50% of DVT cases are asymptomatic. When signs and symptoms occur they can include swelling, pain, redness, and warmth in the affected leg.

Treatment – The goal of treatment is to prevent the blood clot from getting bigger and to prevent it from breaking loose and causing a pulmonary embolism. Medications include anticoagulant and thrombolytic agents. "Filters" may be surgically inserted into the vena cava to prevent clots from reaching the lungs. Compression stockings may be recommended to reduce blood pooling.

Heart Failure[5]

Also known as congestive heart failure, heart failure is a progressive condition in which the heart cannot maintain a normal cardiac output to meet the body's demands for blood and oxygen. Heart failure often develops after other conditions have damaged or weakened the heart. The ventricles weaken and dilate to the point that the heart can't pump efficiently. It can affect the right side, left side or both sides of the heart, but typically begins with the left ventricle. The term "congestive heart failure" comes from blood backing up into the liver, abdomen, lower extremities, and lungs. The condition can be acute or chronic.

Etiology – Coronary artery disease, hypertension, diabetes mellitus, myocardial infarction, abnormal heart valves, and cardiomyopathy.

Signs and symptoms – Shortness of breath; fatigue and weakness; swelling in the legs, feet and abdomen; rapid or irregular heartbeat with S3 or S4 heart sound; persistent cough or wheezing; and weight gain from fluid retention.

Treatment – Sometimes treating the underlying cause can correct heart failure (e.g., repairing a damaged heart valve or controlling an abnormal heart rhythm). In most cases, treatment is a balance of medications, devices, and lifestyle changes to help the heart contract normally. Medications include anticoagulants, antihypertensives, and digitalis to increase the strength of contraction. In severe cases, surgery and medical devices may be needed to correct the underlying cause of the heart failure. These include coronary artery bypass graft, heart valve repair, implantable cardioverter-defibrillator (ICD), biventricular pacemaker, left ventricular assist device, and heart transplant. Lifestyle changes include smoking cessation, restricting sodium intake, maintaining healthy weight, limiting alcohol and fluids, stress reduction, and moderate exercise.

Hypertension[6]

Normal blood pressure is defined as systolic blood pressure less than 120 mm Hg and diastolic blood pressure less than 80 mm Hg. Levels of hypertension include Elevated, Stage 1, and Stage 2.

Etiology – Primary or essential hypertension has no known cause. Hypertension with an identified cause (usually renal disease) is called secondary hypertension.

Signs and symptoms – Hypertension is often asymptomatic until complications develop in the organs. An S4 heart sound is an early sign. Severe hypertension (DBP > 120 mm Hg) can cause significant CNS symptoms (e.g., confusion, cortical blindness, hemiparesis, seizures), cardiovascular symptoms (e.g., chest pain, dyspnea), and renal involvement.

Treatment – Recommendations include lifestyle modifications (aerobic physical activity at least 30 min/day most days of the week; weight loss to a body mass index of 18.5 to 24.9; smoking cessation; reduced intake of dietary sodium and alcohol; increased consumption of fruits, vegetables, and low-fat dairy products with reduced saturated and total fat content); and medications. Classes of medications for hypertension include diuretics, beta blockers, calcium channel blockers, ACE inhibitors, angiotensin II receptor blockers, and direct vasodilators.

Classification of Hypertension in Adults		
BP Classification	SBP mm Hg	DBP mm Hg
Normal	<120 (and)	<80
Elevated	120–129 (and)	<80
Stage 1	130–139 (or)	80–89
Stage 2	at least 140 (or)	at least 90

Blood pressure guidelines update – November 2017. American Heart Association and American College of Cardiology.

Myocardial Infarction (MI)[8]

Also known as a heart attack, a MI occurs when the blood flow through one or more of the coronary arteries is severely reduced or cut off completely. This causes irreversible necrosis to the portion of myocardium supplied by the blocked artery.

Etiology – Most heart attacks occur when a ruptured atherosclerotic plaque or blood clot blocks the flow of blood through a coronary artery. An uncommon cause is a spasm of a coronary artery.

Signs and symptoms – Chest discomfort with pressure, squeezing or pain; shortness of breath; discomfort in the upper body including the arms, shoulder, neck or back; nausea, vomiting, dizziness, sweating, and palpitations.

Treatment – Treatment of a MI varies from medication to surgery, or both, depending on the severity and the amount of heart damage. Medications used to treat the acute MI include anticoagulants and thrombolytic agents, pain relievers, antihypertensives, and cholesterol-lowering medications. Surgical procedures may include coronary angioplasty with stenting or coronary artery bypass surgery. Recommended lifestyle changes include smoking cessation, moderate exercise, maintaining a healthy diet and weight, stress reduction, and consuming alcohol only in moderation.

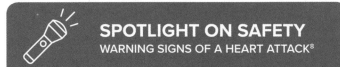

SPOTLIGHT ON SAFETY
WARNING SIGNS OF A HEART ATTACK[8]

Heart attack symptoms vary. Not all people who have heart attacks experience the same symptoms or experience them to the same degree. Some heart attacks are sudden and intense, but most start slowly, with mild pain or discomfort. Signs that can indicate a heart attack include:

- Discomfort in the center of the chest that lasts more than a few minutes, or that goes away and comes back. It can feel like uncomfortable pressure, squeezing, fullness or pain.
- Pain or discomfort in one or both upper extremities, the back, neck, jaw or stomach.
- Shortness of breath with or without chest discomfort.
- Breaking out in a cold sweat, nausea or lightheadedness.

The most common heart attack symptom is chest pain or discomfort in both men and women. Women are somewhat more likely than men to experience shortness of breath, nausea/vomiting, and back or jaw pain.

Often people affected aren't sure what's wrong and wait too long before getting help. Even if a patient or therapist is not sure it's a heart attack, they should have it checked by a doctor. Patients should not wait more than five minutes to call 911 or an emergency response number. It is best to call Emergency Medical Services (EMS) for rapid transport to an emergency room. EMS staff can begin treatment when they arrive and can revive someone whose heart has stopped.

Peripheral Arterial Disease[9]

Stenotic, occlusive, and aneurysmal diseases of the aorta and peripheral arteries.

Etiology – Caused primarily by atherosclerosis and thromboembolic processes that alter the structure and function of the aorta and its branches.

Signs and symptoms – Fatigue, aching, numbness, or pain primarily in the buttock, thigh, calf, or foot at rest or when walking; poorly healing wounds of the legs or feet; distal hair loss, trophic skin changes, and hypertrophic nails.

Treatment – For patients with asymptomatic disease, treatment consists of smoking cessation, lipid lowering medications, and control of diabetes and hypertension (with beta blockers). For patients with disabling intermittent claudication, treatment consists of revascularization procedures (e.g., angioplasty, stent, lasers, atherectomy devices) and surgery (e.g., aortobifemoral bypass, aortoiliac bypass, aortofemoral bypass, iliofemoral bypass) may be recommended. Supervised exercise training should be performed for a minimum of 30 to 45 minutes, at least three times per week, for a minimum of 12 weeks.

Valvular Heart Disease[10]

Damage to one or more of the heart's valves results in regurgitation or stenosis of blood flow. In regurgitation, also known as insufficiency or incompetence, the blood leaks backward through the damaged valve. Stenosis happens when the leaflets thicken, stiffen or fuse together and do not open wide enough to allow adequate blood flow through the valve.

Etiology – Congenital defects, calcific degeneration, infective endocarditis, coronary artery disease, myocardial infarction, and rheumatic fever.

Signs and symptoms – Varies based on the type and severity of valve disease, but may include heart palpitations, shortness of breath, chest pain, coughing, ankle swelling, and fatigue.

Treatment – Patients with minimal symptoms may not require treatment. Treatment for moderate cases includes medications to reduce the workload of the heart, regulate the heart rhythm, and prevent clotting. These medications may include digitalis, diuretics, antiplatelet and anticoagulant agents, beta blockers, and calcium channel blockers. Severe cases may require balloon valvuloplasty or surgery to repair or replace the affected valve.

Pathology of the Airways and Lungs

Asthma[11]

Asthma is a chronic inflammation of the airways caused by an increased airway hypersensitivity to various stimuli.

Etiology – Factors that trigger asthma include respiratory infections; allergens such as pollen, mold, animal dander, feathers, dust, food, and cockroaches; exposure to cold air or sudden temperature change; cigarette smoke; excitement/stress; and exercise.

Signs and symptoms – Range from mild to severe depending on the level of airway restriction. A mild attack presents with wheezing, chest tightness, and slight shortness of breath. A severe attack presents with dyspnea, flaring nostrils, diminished wheezing, anxiety, cyanosis, and the inability to speak. A severe attack can result in respiratory failure if left untreated.

Treatment – Reducing exposure to known triggers is a critical step toward controlling asthma. Two classes of medications are used to treat asthma: anti-inflammatory agents and bronchodilators. Anti-inflammatory agents interrupt bronchial inflammation and have a preventive action. These agents include inhaled corticosteroids, cromolyn sodium, and leukotriene modifiers. Bronchodilators dilate the airways by relaxing bronchial smooth muscle. They include beta-adrenergic agonists, methylxanthines, and anticholinergics. Physical therapy management includes caregiver education, airway clearance, breathing exercises, relaxation, and endurance and strength training.

Bronchitis[3]

Bronchitis is an inflammation of the bronchi characterized by hypertrophy of the mucus secreting glands, increased mucus secretions, and insufficient oxygenation due to mucus blockage. Chronic bronchitis is characterized by a productive cough for three months over the course of two consecutive years.

Etiology – Acute bronchitis may be caused by cold viruses and exposure to smoke and other air pollutants. Cigarette smoking is the primary cause of chronic bronchitis, but exposure to air pollutants, dust, or toxic gases in the environment or workplace can also contribute.

Signs and symptoms – Persistent cough with production of thick sputum, increased use of accessory muscles of breathing, wheezing, dyspnea, cyanosis, and increased pulmonary artery pressure. Patients with chronic bronchitis present with a cough that is worse in the morning and in damp weather and may experience frequent respiratory infections.

Treatment – Focuses on relieving symptoms and improving breathing. For acute bronchitis, treatment includes rest, fluids, breathing warm and moist air, cough suppressants, and acetaminophen or aspirin. For chronic bronchitis, treatments include antibiotics, anti-inflammatory agents, and bronchodilators. Recommended lifestyle changes include smoking cessation, avoiding respiratory irritants, using an air humidifier, using a cold-air face mask if cold air aggravates cough and promotes shortness of breath, and pulmonary rehabilitation (airway clearance, breathing exercises, and endurance and strength training).

Chronic Obstructive Pulmonary Disease (COPD)[3]

COPD refers to a group of lung diseases that block airflow due to narrowing of the bronchial tree. Emphysema and chronic bronchitis are the two main conditions that make up COPD. COPD can also refer to damage caused by chronic asthmatic bronchitis. Progression of the disease includes alveolar destruction and subsequent air trapping. Patients have an increased total lung capacity with a significant increase in residual volume.

Etiology – In the majority of cases, COPD is caused by long-term smoking or exposure to secondhand smoke. Other irritants can cause COPD, including air pollution and certain occupational fumes. In rare cases, COPD results from a genetic disorder that causes low levels of the protein alpha-1-antitrypsin.

Signs and symptoms – Excessive mucus production, chronic productive cough, wheezing, shortness of breath, fatigue, and reduced exercise capacity.

Treatment – Medications include bronchodilators, inhaled steroids, supplemental oxygen, and antibiotics (if a bacterial infection is present). Surgery may include lung volume reduction surgery, bullectomy, and lung transplantation. Lifestyle modifications include smoking cessation, influenza shots, avoiding respiratory irritants, maintaining good nutrition, and pulmonary rehabilitation (airway clearance, breathing exercises, and endurance and strength training).

Cystic Fibrosis (CF)[13]

CF is an autosomal recessive genetic disease of the exocrine glands that primarily affects the lungs, pancreas, liver, intestines, sinuses, and sex organs. People who have CF inherit two faulty CF genes, one from each parent.

Etiology – The causative factor is a mutation of the cystic fibrosis transmembrane conductance regulator on chromosome 7. A defective gene and its protein product cause the body to produce unusually thick, sticky mucus that leads to life-threatening lung infections, obstructs the pancreas, and inhibits normal digestion and absorption of food.

Signs and symptoms – Symptoms vary with the progression of the disease and may include salty tasting skin, persistent and productive coughing, frequent lung infections, wheezing, shortness of breath, poor growth/weight gain in spite of a good appetite, and frequent greasy, bulky stools.

Treatment – Medications include antibiotics, nutritional supplements, pancreatic enzyme replacements, mucolytics, and bronchodilators. Physical therapy includes airway clearance, breathing techniques, assisted cough, and ventilatory muscle training. General exercise is indicated to improve overall strength and endurance, except with severe lung disease.

Emphysema[3]

In emphysema, the alveolar walls are gradually destroyed and the alveoli are turned into large, irregular pockets with gaping holes in the walls. In addition, the elastic fibers that hold open the bronchioles are destroyed, so that they collapse during exhalation, not letting air escape from the lungs. The alveoli are permanently overinflated and dead space increases within the lungs.

Etiology – Smoking is the leading cause of emphysema. One to two percent of individuals with emphysema have a genetic disorder that causes low levels of the protein alpha-1-antitrypsin, which protects the elastic structures in the lungs. Without this protein, enzymes can cause progressive lung damage, eventually resulting in emphysema.

Signs and symptoms – Shortness of breath, wheezing, chronic coughing, orthopnea, barrel chest, increased use of accessory muscles, increased respiration rate, fatigue, and reduced exercise capacity.

Treatment – Medications include bronchodilators, inhaled steroids, supplemental oxygen, and antibiotics (if a bacterial infection is present). Surgery may include lung volume reduction surgery, bullectomy, and lung transplantation. Lifestyle modifications include smoking cessation, annual influenza inoculation, avoiding respiratory irritants, maintaining good nutrition, and pulmonary rehabilitation (airway clearance, breathing exercises, and endurance and strength training).

Pneumonia[3]

Pneumonia refers to inflammation of the lungs (Fig. 6-7).

Etiology – Usually caused by bacterial, viral, fungal, or parasitic infection.

Signs and symptoms – Symptoms are variable depending on the cause of the infection. Common signs and symptoms include fever, cough, shortness of breath, sweating, shaking chills, chest pain that fluctuates with breathing, headache, muscle pain, and fatigue.

Treatment – Variable depending on the severity of the symptoms and the type of pneumonia. Antibiotics are used for bacterial and mycoplasma pneumonias. Antiviral agents are used to treat a few forms of viral pneumonia. Antifungal agents are used to treat fungal pneumonia. Lifestyle remedies include rest and drinking plenty of liquids.

Pulmonary Edema[3]

Pulmonary edema occurs when fluid collects in the alveoli within the lungs, making it difficult to breathe. Acute pulmonary edema is a medical emergency.

Etiology – In most cases, pulmonary edema occurs when the left ventricle is unable to pump blood adequately (e.g., left-sided heart failure). As a result, pressure increases inside the left atrium and then in the pulmonary veins and capillaries, causing fluid to be pushed through the capillary walls into the alveoli. In noncardiac pulmonary edema, fluid leaks from the capillaries within the alveoli since the capillaries themselves become more permeable. This may result from pneumonia, exposure to certain toxins and medications, smoke inhalation, respiratory distress syndrome, and living at high elevations.

Signs and symptoms – Depending on the cause, symptoms can develop suddenly or slowly. Signs and symptoms that come on suddenly may include extreme shortness of breath and difficulty breathing; a feeling of suffocating or drowning; wheezing or gasping for breath; anxiety; restlessness; a sense of apprehension; coughing; frothy, blood-tinged sputum; chest pain (if a cardiac cause); and a rapid, irregular pulse.

Treatment – Variable depending on the underlying cause, but often includes supplemental oxygen and medications.

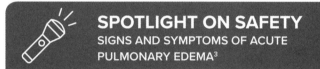

SPOTLIGHT ON SAFETY
SIGNS AND SYMPTOMS OF ACUTE PULMONARY EDEMA[3]

Acute pulmonary edema is life-threatening. Call 911 or emergency medical services immediately if any of the following signs or symptoms develop:

- Extreme shortness of breath or difficulty breathing with profuse sweating

- A bubbly, wheezing or gasping sound during breathing

- A cough that produces frothy sputum that may be tinged with blood

- Cyanotic skin color

- A rapid, irregular pulse

- A severe drop in blood pressure

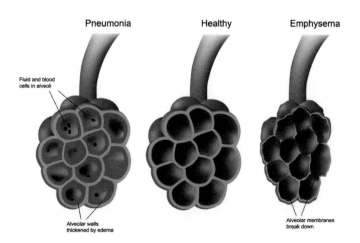

Pneumonia   Healthy   Emphysema

Fluid and blood cells in alveoli

Alveolar walls thickened by edema

Alveolar membranes break down

Fig. 6-7: Changes in alveoli with pneumonia and emphysema.

Pulmonary Embolism (PE)[3]

PE is a condition where one or more arteries in the lungs become blocked. PE can be life-threatening, but prompt treatment with anti-clotting medications can greatly reduce the risk of death.

Etiology – In most cases, PE is caused by blood clots from the lower extremities.

Signs and Symptoms – Symptoms can vary greatly, depending on how much of the lung is involved, the size of the clot, and overall health of the patient (especially the presence or absence of underlying lung disease or heart disease). Common signs and symptoms include sudden onset of shortness of breath; chest pain that becomes worse with deep breathing, coughing, eating or bending; and coughing up bloody or blood-streaked sputum. Other signs and symptoms include wheezing, lower extremity swelling, excessive sweating, rapid or irregular pulse, and lightheadedness or fainting.

Treatment – Pulmonary embolism can be life-threatening, but prompt treatment with anticoagulants and thrombolytic agents greatly reduces the risk of death. Surgery may be done to remove the clot or insert a filter into the inferior vena cava. Preventing clot formation in the deep leg veins reduces the risk of PE. Prevention includes compression stockings, pneumatic compression, physical activity, and drinking fluids.

Restrictive Lung Dysfunction (RLD)[14]

RLD is an abnormal reduction in lung expansion and pulmonary ventilation.

Etiology - RLD is caused by abnormal lung parenchyma (e.g., atelectasis, pneumonia, pulmonary fibrosis, pulmonary edema, acute respiratory distress syndrome), abnormal pleura (e.g., pleural effusion, pleural fibrosis, pneumothorax, hemothorax), and disorders affecting ventilatory pump function (e.g., decrease in respiratory drive, neurologic and neuromuscular diseases, muscle disease or weakness, thoracic deformity or trauma, connective tissue disorders affecting the thoracic joints, pregnancy, obesity, and ascites).

Signs and Symptoms – Dyspnea on exertion, a persistent non-productive cough, increased respiratory rate, hypoxemia, decreased vital capacity, abnormal breath sounds, and reduced exercise tolerance.

Treatment – Variable depending on the etiology (e.g., antibiotics for pneumonia, treatment of edema, reversal of CNS depression). Additional supportive measures include mechanical ventilation, supplemental oxygen, nutrition support, and pulmonary rehabilitation (airway clearance, breathing exercise, respiratory muscle training, endurance and strength training).

Common Laboratory Tests

Arterial Blood Gas (ABG)

Arterial blood gases are collected to evaluate acid–base status (pH), ventilation ($PaCO_2$), and oxygenation of arterial blood (PaO_2). The partial pressure of oxygen in arterial blood (PaO_2) and the percent oxygen saturation of hemoglobin (SaO_2) provide information about how well the lungs are functioning to oxygenate the blood. The partial pressure of carbon dioxide in arterial blood ($PaCO_2$) provides information on how well the lungs are able to remove carbon dioxide. Changes in $PaCO_2$ directly affect the balance of pH in the body. Blood pH is tightly regulated, as an imbalance in either direction can affect the nervous system and can cause convulsions or coma. Bicarbonate (HCO_3^-) is an important component of the chemical buffering system that keeps the blood from becoming too acidic or basic and is often part of an ABG test.

Mean (range) of adult normal ABG values:

pH: 7.4 (7.35 - 7.45)

$PaCO_2$: 40 mm Hg at sea level breathing ambient air (35 - 45 mm Hg)

PaO_2: 97 mm Hg at sea level breathing ambient air (80 - 100 mm Hg)

HCO_3^-: 24 mEq/L (22 – 26 mEq/L)

SaO_2: 95 - 98%

By convention, ABG results are written or spoken in the following order: pH→$PaCO_2$→PaO_2→HCO_3^- (e.g., 7.4/40/97/24)

Acidemia: elevated acidity of blood (pH < 7.35)

Alkalemia: decreased acidity of blood (pH > 7.45)

Eucapnia: normal level of CO_2 in arterial blood ($PaCO_2$ 35 - 45 mm Hg)

Hypercapnia: elevated level of CO_2 in arterial blood ($PaCO_2$ > 45 mm Hg)

Hypocapnia: low level of CO_2 in arterial blood ($PaCO_2$ < 35 mm Hg)

Hypoxemia: low level of O_2 in arterial blood (PaO_2 < 80 mm Hg)

Hypoxia: low level of O_2 in the tissue despite adequate perfusion of the tissue

Reference Values in Hematology

	Conventional Units	SI Units
Erythrocytes		
Adult males	4.3 – 5.6 x 10^6/ml	4.3 – 5.6 x 10^{12}/L
Adult females	4.0 – 5.2 x 10^6/ml	4.0 – 5.2 x 10^{12}/L
Leukocytes		
Total	3.54 – 9.06 x 10^3/mm^3	3.54 – 9.06 x 10^9/L
Differential Blood Count		
Neutrophils	0.40 – 0.70	40 – 70%
Lymphocytes	0.20 – 0.50	20 – 50%
Monocytes	0.04 – 0.08	4 – 8%
Eosinophils	0.00 – 0.06	0 – 6%
Basophils	0.00 – 0.02	0 – 2%
Platelet Count	165 – 415 x 10^3/mm^3	165 – 415 x 10^9/L
Partial Thromboplastin Time (PTT)	26.3 – 39.4 sec	26.3 – 39.4 sec
Hematocrit		
Adult males	0.388 – 0.464	38.8 – 46.4%
Adult females	0.354 – 0.444	35.4 – 44.4%
Hemoglobin		
Adult males	13.3 – 16.2 gm/dL	13.3 – 16.2 g/dL
Adult females	12.0 – 15.8 gm/dL	12.0 – 15.8 g/dL

Reference Values in Clinical Chemistry

	Conventional Units		SI Units
Serum Cholesterol			
Total	< 200 mg/dL	Desirable	< 5.17 mmol/L
	200 – 239 mg/dL	Borderline	5.17 – 6.20 mmol/L
	> 240 mg/dL	High	≥ 6.21 mmol/L
LDL cholesterol	< 100 mg/dL	Optimal	< 2.59 mmol/L
	100 – 129 mg/dL	Near optimal	2.59 – 3.35 mmol/L
	130 – 159 mg/dL	Borderline	3.36 – 4.12 mmol/L
	160 – 189 mg/dL	High	4.13 – 4.90 mmol/L
	≥ 190 mg/dL	Very high	≥ 4.91 mmol/L
HDL cholesterol	< 40 mg/dL	Low	< 1.03 mmol/L
	≥ 60 mg/dL	High	≥ 1.55 mmol/L
Triglyceride	< 150 mg/dL	Desirable	< 1.70 mmol/L
	150 – 199 mg/dL	Borderline	1.70 – 2.25 mmol/L
	200 – 499 mg/dL	High	2.26 – 5.63 mmol/L
	≥ 500 mg/dL	Very high	> 5.64 mmol/L

The values are for illustrative purposes. Each clinical laboratory establishes its own reference values.

Adapted from: Kratz A, Pesce MA, Fink DJ. Reference Values for Laboratory Tests. In: Fauci A, Braunwald E, Kasper D, Hauser, Longo D, Jameson J, Loscalzo J. Harrison's Manual of Medicine, 17th ed. New York, NY: McGraw-Hill Medical; 2009.

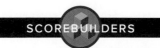

Cholesterol Test[15]

Also called a lipid panel or lipid profile, a cholesterol test measures the amount of cholesterol and triglycerides in the blood in order to determine the risk of atherosclerosis. Cholesterol is carried in the circulation in association with lipoproteins. A complete lipid profile includes the measurement of four types of lipids in the blood: total cholesterol, high-density lipoprotein (HDL) cholesterol, low-density lipoprotein (LDL) cholesterol, and triglycerides. HDL cholesterol is referred to as the "good" cholesterol because it helps carry away LDL cholesterol and is protective against atherogenesis. LDL cholesterol is referred to as the "bad" cholesterol since it is associated with the buildup of fatty plaques within the arteries which reduce blood flow. The body converts any calories it does not need to use right away into triglycerides, which are stored in adipose tissue. High levels of triglycerides are seen in overweight people, in those consuming too many sweets or too much alcohol, and in people with diabetes who have elevated blood sugar levels.

Complete Blood Count (CBC)[15]

A CBC measures red blood cell count, total white blood cell count, white blood cell differential, platelets, hemoglobin, and hematocrit.

Common Diagnostic Procedures

Ambulatory Electrocardiography[5]

Also known as Holter monitoring, ECG electrodes are placed on the chest and attached to a small battery-operated recording monitor carried in a pocket or in a small pouch around the neck (Fig. 6-8). The ECG is recorded for 24 to 48 hours or longer to evaluate cardiac rhythm, the efficacy of medications, and pacemaker function. It is then correlated with a diary of the patient's symptoms and activities.

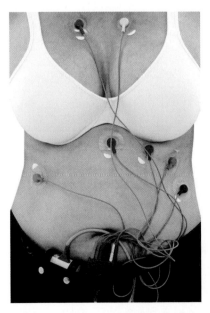

Fig. 6-8: Woman wearing a Holter monitor.

A CBC is performed to assess health, to diagnose and monitor a medical condition, and to monitor the effects of medical treatment.

Hematocrit (HCT)[15]

Hematocrit is the percentage of red blood cells in total blood volume. A low hematocrit may indicate anemia, blood loss, and vitamin or mineral deficiencies. A high hematocrit may indicate dehydration or polycythemia vera, a condition that causes an overproduction of red blood cells.

Partial Thromboplastin Time (PTT) and Prothrombin Time (PT)[15]

PTT and PT tests measure how quickly the blood clots. The tests are commonly used to monitor oral anticoagulant therapy or to screen for selected bleeding disorders. The tests examine all of the clotting factors of the intrinsic pathway with the exception of platelets. Partial thromboplastin time is more sensitive than prothrombin time in detecting minor deficiencies.

Angiography[15]

A radiologic examination that injects a contrast medium into the blood vessels. Coronary angiograms are part of the group of procedures known as cardiac catheterization. An angiogram can show the location of plaques in the coronary arteries and the extent of occlusion.

Bronchoscopy[15]

A procedure for direct visualization of the bronchial tree performed for diagnostic and therapeutic purposes. A bronchoscope is a fiber optic instrument that transmits an image to an eyepiece or video camera and can identify tumors, bronchitis, foreign bodies, and bleeding. Tissue specimens may be removed from the lungs by biopsy or bronchoalveolar lavage.

Cardiac Catheterization[5]

A thin catheter inserted into an artery in the leg or arm is advanced to the coronary arteries where a contrast dye is injected. The test can evaluate narrowing or occlusion of the coronary arteries and measure blood pressure in the heart and oxygen in the blood. Some treatments, such as coronary angioplasty, are performed using cardiac catheterization.

Chest Radiograph[5]

Chest radiographs are used to visualize the location, size, and shape of the heart, lungs, blood vessels, ribs, and bones of the spine. Chest radiographs can also reveal fluid in the lungs or pleural space, pneumonia, emphysema, cancer, and other conditions.

Computed Tomography (CT scan)[5]

A CT scan is a diagnostic test that uses an x-ray machine that rotates around a patient lying on a table. A computer processes the information from the scanner and creates a picture of the organ and surrounding structures. The pictures are slices of the body called tomograms and each picture is called a computed tomograph. The newest models of CT scanners allow pictures of the coronary arteries to be taken without the need, in some cases, for catheterization.

Echocardiography[5]

An echocardiogram uses high frequency sound waves non-invasively to evaluate the functioning of the heart via real time images. An echocardiogram can provide information on the size and function of the ventricles, thickness of the septums, and function of the walls, valves, and chambers of the heart.

Fluoroscopy[5]

A continuous x-ray procedure that shows the heart and lungs. Because fluoroscopy involves a relatively high dose of radiation, it has been largely replaced by echocardiography and other diagnostic tests. It is still a component of cardiac catheterization and electrophysiological testing.

Invasive Hemodynamic Monitoring[14]

Continuous monitoring of cardiovascular status is performed by intra-arterial catheters and intravenous lines that measure pressure, volume, and temperature. A balloon catheter, also known as a Swan-Ganz catheter, is placed in the pulmonary artery to obtain the pulmonary artery wedge pressure and left atrial pressure. A thermodilution catheter can be used to measure cardiac output. A central venous pressure (CVP) line measures pressure in the vena cava or right atrium.

Magnetic Resonance Imaging (MRI)[15]

MRI uses a magnetic field and radio waves to create 3-D images of the heart and blood vessels to assess the size and function of the chambers, thickness and movement of the walls, extent of damage caused by myocardial infarction or heart disease, structural problems in the aorta (e.g., aneurysms, dissections), and the presence of plaques and blockages in blood vessels. MRI is also used to image masses located in the mediastinum, but is of limited value for imaging the lungs.

Myocardial Perfusion Imaging (MPI)[16]

Also known as radionuclide stress test and nuclear stress test, the test shows how well the heart muscle is perfused at rest and under exercise stress. A radionuclide agent is injected into the blood at rest and at a maximum level of exercise. Images of the heart reveal areas that have reduced blood supply due to narrowing of one or more coronary arteries.

Pharmacological Management of Heart and Vascular Diseases

Alpha Adrenergic Antagonist Agents[18,19]

Action: Alpha adrenergic antagonist agents reduce peripheral vascular tone by blocking alpha-1-adrenergic receptors. This action causes dilation of arterioles and veins and decreases blood pressure.

Indications: hypertension, benign prostatic hyperplasia

Side effects: dizziness, palpitations, orthostatic hypotension, drowsiness

Implications for PT: Use caution when rising from a sitting or lying position due to the risk of dizziness and/or orthostatic hypotension. Closely monitor patient during exercise.

Examples: Cardura, Minipress

Angiotensin-Converting Enzyme (ACE) Inhibitor Agents[18,19]

Action: ACE inhibitor agents decrease blood pressure and afterload by suppressing the enzyme that converts angiotensin I to angiotensin II.

Indications: hypertension, congestive heart failure

Side effects: hypotension, dizziness, dry cough, hyperkalemia, hyponatremia

Implications for PT: Avoid sudden changes in posture due to the risk of dizziness and fainting from hypotension. Patients with heart failure should avoid rapid increases in physical activity.

Examples: Capoten, Vasotec

Anticoagulant Agents[18,19]

Action: Anticoagulant agents inhibit platelet aggregation and thrombus formation.

Indications: post percutaneous transluminal coronary angioplasty and coronary artery bypass graft surgery, prevention of venous thromboembolism and cardioembolic events in patients with atrial fibrillation and prosthetic heart valves

Side effects: hemorrhage, increased risk of bleeding, gastrointestinal distress with oral medication

Implications for PT: A therapist must be careful to avoid injury secondary to the risk of excessive bleeding or bruising. Patient education regarding common side effects is also indicated to protect the patient.

Examples: Heparin, Coumadin

Antihyperlipidemia Agents[18,19]

Action: There are five categories of lipid-modifying agents. The most commonly used drugs, the statins, inhibit enzyme action in cholesterol synthesis, break down low density lipoproteins, decrease triglyceride levels, and increase HDL levels. The other categories are bile acid sequestrants, nicotinic acid, cholesterol absorption inhibitors, and fibric acid derivatives.

Indications: hyperlipidemia, atherosclerosis, prevent coronary events in patients with existing coronary disease, diabetes or peripheral vascular disease

Side effects: headache, gastrointestinal distress, myalgia, rash

Implications for PT: Aerobic exercise can increase high density lipoproteins and maximize the effects of drug therapy.

Examples: Lipitor, Zocor

Antithrombotic (Antiplatelet) Agents[18,19]

Action: Antithrombotic agents inhibit platelet aggregation and clot formation.

Indications: post-myocardial infarction, atrial fibrillation, prevent arterial thrombus formation

Side effects: hemorrhage, thrombocytopenia, potential liver toxicity with the use of aspirin, gastrointestinal distress

Implications for PT: A therapist must be careful to avoid injury secondary to the risk of excessive bleeding. Patient education regarding common side effects is also indicated to protect the patient.

Examples: Bayer, Plavix

Beta Blocker Agents (Beta-Adrenergic Blocking Agents)[18,19]

Action: Beta blocker agents decrease the myocardial oxygen demand by decreasing heart rate and contractility by blocking ß-adrenergic receptors.

Indications: hypertension, angina, arrhythmias, heart failure, migraines, essential tremor

Side effects: bradycardia, cardiac arrhythmias, fatigue, depression, dizziness, weakness, blurred vision

Implications for PT: Heart rate and blood pressure response to exercise will be diminished. Rate of perceived exertion may be used to monitor exercise intensity. Closely monitor patients during positional changes due to an increased risk for orthostatic hypotension.

Examples: Tenormin, Lopressor

Calcium Channel Blocker Agents[18,19]

Action: Calcium channel blocker agents decrease the entry of calcium into vascular smooth muscle cells resulting in diminished myocardial contraction, vasodilation, and decreased oxygen demand of the heart.

Indications: hypertension, angina pectoris, arrhythmias, congestive heart failure

Side effects: dizziness, headache, hypotension, peripheral edema

Implications for PT: Heart rate and blood pressure response to exercise will be diminished. Monitor patient closely when moving to an upright position secondary to dizziness and/or orthostatic hypotension. Observe the patient for signs and symptoms of congestive heart failure such as worsening peripheral edema, dyspnea or weight gain.

Examples: Procardia, Cardizem

Diuretic Agents[18,19]

Action: Diuretic agents increase the excretion of sodium and urine. This causes a reduction in plasma volume which decreases blood pressure. Classifications include thiazide, loop, and potassium sparing agents.

Indications: hypertension, edema associated with heart failure, pulmonary edema, glaucoma

Side effects: dehydration, hypotension, electrolyte imbalance, polyuria, increased low-density lipoproteins, arrhythmias

Implications for PT: Positioning changes can increase the risk of dizziness and falls due to decreased blood pressure. Monitor patients closely for signs and symptoms of electrolyte imbalance and muscle weakness or cramping.

Examples: Diuril, Lasix

Nitrate Agents[18,19]

Action: Nitrate agents decrease ischemia through smooth muscle relaxation and dilation of peripheral vessels.

Indications: angina pectoris

Side effects: headache, dizziness, orthostatic hypotension, reflex tachycardia, nausea, vomiting

Implications for PT: Patients must be educated to come to a standing position slowly to minimize the risk of orthostatic hypotension. Sublingual administration of nitroglycerin is the preferred method to treat an acute angina attack.

Examples: Nitrostat

Positive Inotropic Agents[18,19]

Action: Positive inotropic agents increase the force and velocity of myocardial contraction, slow the heart rate, decrease conduction velocity through the AV node, and decrease the degree of activation of the sympathetic nervous system.

Indications: heart failure, atrial fibrillation

Side effects: cardiac arrhythmias, gastrointestinal distress, dizziness, blurred vision

Implications for PT: Therapists should monitor heart rate during activity, teach the patient and family to take the patient's pulse, and seek health care provider's advice for rates less than 60 beats/minute or more than 100 beats/minute

Examples: Lanoxin

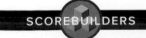

Thrombolytic Agents[18,19]

Action: Thrombolytic agents facilitate clot dissolution through conversion of plasminogen to plasmin. Plasmin breaks down clots and allows occluded vessels to reopen to maintain blood flow.

Indications: acute myocardial infarction, pulmonary embolism, ischemic stroke, arterial or venous thrombosis

Side effects: hemorrhage (specifically intracranial in certain populations), allergic reaction, cardiac arrhythmia

Implications for PT: Therapists must be careful to avoid situations that may cause trauma due to altered clotting activity.

Examples: Kinlytic, Activase

Medical Procedures for Heart and Vascular Diseases

Balloon Angioplasty[15]

Angioplasty involves temporarily inserting a small balloon-tipped catheter into a stenotic artery and expanding the balloon at the site of blockage to help widen a narrowed artery (Fig. 6-9). Angioplasty is usually combined with implantation of a small metal coil called a stent in the narrowed artery to help prop it open and decrease the chance of restenosis.

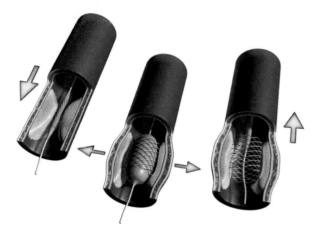

Fig. 6-9: Balloon angioplasty.

Coronary Artery Bypass Graft Surgery (CABG)[15]

CABG surgery is performed to treat coronary arteries that are narrowed or occluded in an attempt to revascularize the myocardium. In this procedure, blood is rerouted around the affected artery joining the patient's own saphenous vein, internal thoracic/mammary artery, or radial artery to connect the affected artery above and below the occlusion.

Heart Transplant[15]

A surgical procedure in which a failing, diseased heart is replaced with a healthier donor heart. A heart transplant is reserved for patients with end-stage heart failure for whom other treatments have not been successful (e.g., patients with cardiomyopathy, coronary artery disease, valvular disease, and congenital heart disease).

Ventricular Assist Devices (VAD)[15]

A VAD is a miniature pump that is implanted in the chest to provide mechanical support to the ventricle. A right ventricular device (RVAD) attaches to the right atrium and pulmonary artery, bypassing the right ventricle. A left ventricular device (LVAD) attaches to the left atrium, bypassing the left ventricle. With a biventricular device (BiVAD), both ventricles are bypassed. VADs are commonly used as a temporary treatment for people waiting for a heart transplant and increasingly as a permanent treatment for heart failure.

Cardiac Pacemaker[14]

A pacemaker is a surgically implanted battery-powered device placed under the skin, usually in the left anterior chest wall. Pacemakers are a standard treatment for conditions affecting the electrical conduction system including a slow heart rate and arrhythmias. By preventing a slow heart rate, pacemakers can treat fatigue, lightheadedness, and fainting.

Pharmacological Management of Airway and Lung Diseases

Antihistamine Agents[18,19]

Action: Antihistamine agents block the effects of histamine resulting in a decrease in nasal congestion, mucosal irritation, and symptoms of the common cold, sinusitis, conjunctivitis, and allergies.

Indications: respiratory seasonal allergies, rhinitis and sneezing from the common cold, allergic conjunctivitis, motion sickness, and Parkinson's disease

Side effects: arrhythmias, postural hypotension, gastrointestinal distress, dizziness, drowsiness, headache, blurred vision, fatigue, nausea, thickening of bronchial secretions

Implications for PT: Increase guarding when rising from a sitting or lying position due to the risk of orthostatic hypotension. Closely monitor patient during exercise.

Examples: Benadryl, Allegra, Claritin

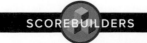

Anti-Inflammatory Agents[18,19]

Action: Inhaled corticosteroids, leukotriene modifiers, and mast-cell stabilizers help prevent inflammatory-mediated bronchoconstriction by inhibiting production of inflammatory cells, suppressing release of inflammatory mediators (cytokines, prostaglandins, leukotrienes), and reversing capillary permeability, in turn reducing airway edema.

Indications: bronchospasm, asthma

Side effects: Corticosteroid: systemic side effects are decreased with the inhaled form of corticosteroids, but may include damage of supporting tissues, skin breakdown, osteoporosis, decreased bone density, glaucoma, and delayed growth. Local effects include nasal irritation and dryness, sneezing, and bloody mucus; Leukotriene modifier: liver dysfunction; Mast-cell stabilizer: bronchospasm, throat and nasal irritation, cough, gastrointestinal distress.

Implications for PT: Instruct the patient in the correct use of the inhaler and to rinse their mouth with water after use to avoid irritation of local mucosa. Advise the patients that these agents are not bronchodilators and should not be used to treat acute episodes of asthma. Inform patients to contact their health care provider immediately if they experience signs and/or symptoms of liver dysfunction (e.g., fatigue, flu-like symptoms, jaundice, lethargy).

Examples: Pulmicort, AeroBid

Bronchodilator Agents[18,19]

Action: Bronchodilator agents relieve bronchospasm by stimulating the receptors that cause bronchial smooth muscle relaxation or by blocking the receptors that trigger bronchoconstriction. Primary classifications of bronchodilators include anticholinergic, sympathomimetics, and xanthine derivatives.

Indications: bronchospasm, wheezing, and shortness of breath in asthma and COPD

Side effects: (depending on class of drug) paradoxical broncho-spasm, dry mouth, gastrointestinal distress, chest pain, palpitations, tremor, nervousness. Long-acting sympathomimetics, including salmeterol, increase the risk of asthma-related death.

Implications for PT: Therapists should advise patients to take their bronchodilator medication as prescribed before therapy and to bring their short acting sympathomimetics (rescue medications) with them. Cardiac or vision abnormalities may indicate toxicity, and the physician should be notified immediately.

Examples: Atrovent, Ventolin, Serevent

Expectorant Agents[18,19]

Action: Expectorant agents increase respiratory secretions which help to loosen mucus. Reducing the viscosity of secretions and increasing sputum volume improves the efficiency of the cough reflex and of ciliary action in removing accumulated secretions.

Indications: cough associated with respiratory tract infections and related conditions such as sinusitis, pharyngitis, bronchitis, and asthma, when complicated by tenacious mucus or mucus plugs and congestion

Side effects: gastrointestinal distress, drowsiness

Implications for PT: Therapists can exploit the effects of expectorant agents by performing airway clearance interventions within one hour after drug administration. Therapists should encourage the patient to take the medication with a glass of water.

Examples: Mucinex

Mucolytic Agents[18,19]

Action: Mucolytic agents decrease the viscosity of mucus secretions by altering their composition and consistency, making them easier to expectorate. They are administered by a nebulizer.

Indications: viscous mucus secretions due to pneumonia, emphysema, chronic bronchitis, and cystic fibrosis

Side effects: pharyngitis, oral mucosa inflammation, rhinitis, chest pain

Implications for PT: Therapists can exploit the effects of mucolytic agents by performing airway clearance interventions within one hour after drug administration. Patients should be instructed in the proper use and maintenance of the nebulizer and compressor system used in its delivery.

Examples: Pulmozyme, Mucomyst

Medical Procedures for Airway and Lung Diseases

Airway Adjuncts[14]

A variety of devices are used to maintain or protect the airway, to provide mechanical ventilation or to promote airway clearance.

Oral pharyngeal airway: A plastic tube shaped to fit the curvature of the soft palate and tongue that holds the tongue away from the back of the throat and maintains the patency of the airway.

Nasal pharyngeal airway: A latex or rubber tube inserted through the nose to allow for nasotracheal suctioning.

Endotracheal tube: A plastic tube inserted in the trachea from the mouth or nose to provide an airway and to allow for mechanical ventilation.

Tracheostomy tube: An artificial airway inserted into the trachea from an incision in the neck below the vocal cords used in patients needing prolonged mechanical ventilation.

Airway Suctioning[14]

Suctioning is the mechanical aspiration of secretions from the nasopharynx, oropharynx, and trachea using a suction catheter. Endotracheal suctioning refers to the mechanical aspiration of pulmonary secretions from a patient with an artificial airway in place. Nasotracheal suctioning refers to the insertion of a suction catheter through the nasal passage and pharynx into the trachea without a tracheal tube or tracheostomy to aspirate accumulated secretions or foreign material. Indications for suctioning include increased or thickened secretions and inadequate cough. The frequency of suctioning is dependent on the amount of secretion produced.

Lung Transplant[3]

A surgical procedure to replace one or both diseased or failing lungs with healthy donor lungs. A lung transplant is reserved for patients with end-stage COPD, interstitial pulmonary fibrosis, cystic fibrosis, and other serious lung diseases, but who do not have serious comorbidities.

Mechanical Ventilation[14]

Patients with severe pulmonary dysfunction may need assistance to breathe from a positive pressure mechanical ventilator or breathing machine. The positive pressure from the ventilator provides the force that delivers air into the lungs by increasing intrathoracic pressure. Mechanical ventilation involves an automatic cycling ventilator connected to a tracheostomy tube or mask to assist or breathe for the patient.

Oxygen Therapy[14]

Liquid or gaseous oxygen is indicated for the treatment of acute and chronic hypoxemia in patients with a $PaO_2 \leq 55$ mm Hg, or an oxygen saturation $\leq 88\%$ while seated at rest, or a PaO_2 of 56 to 59 mm Hg, or oxygen saturation of 89% in the presence of cor pulmonale or polycythemia. A number of devices are available to

deliver the supplemental oxygen to the patient including nasal cannula, simple face mask, partial rebreathing mask, nonrebreathing mask, aerosol face mask, Venturi mask, and transtracheal catheter.

Thoracotomy[20]

A surgical incision cutting the chest wall to access the heart, great vessels, lungs, esophagus, and diaphragm for diagnostic and therapeutic purposes. The incision may be made under the arm (axillary thoracotomy), through the sternum (median sternotomy), from the back to the side (posterolateral thoracotomy) or under the breast (anterolateral thoracotomy).

Tracheostomy[15]

A surgically created hole through the neck into the trachea below the level of the vocal cords. The term for the surgical procedure to create the opening is tracheotomy. There are two primary indications for tracheostomy: airway obstruction at or above the level of the larynx and respiratory failure requiring prolonged mechanical ventilation. The tracheostomy can be surgically closed when it is no longer needed.

Physical Therapy Tests and Measures

Angina Pain Scales

A number of pain scales are used to grade the severity of angina pectoris.[21,22] One of the more commonly used angina scales rates angina pain from one to four.

Rating	Description
1	Mild, barely noticeable
2	Moderate, bothersome
3	Moderately severe, very uncomfortable
4	Most severe or intense pain ever experienced

Ankle-Brachial Index (ABI)[15]

Also known as the ankle-arm index, the ABI compares systolic blood pressures at the ankle and arm to check for peripheral artery disease.

Procedure

- Systolic blood pressures are measured in both brachial arteries and both tibialis posterior arteries with a sphygmomanometer and a handheld Doppler ultrasound device.

- The ABI is calculated by dividing the higher of the two blood pressure measurements in the ankles by the higher of the two systolic blood pressure measurements at the arms.

Interpretation

> 1.30	Indicates rigid arteries and the need for an ultrasound test to check for peripheral artery disease
1.0 – 1.30	Normal; no blockage
0.8 – 0.99	Mild blockage; beginnings of peripheral artery disease
0.4 – 0.79	Moderate blockage; may be associated with intermittent claudication during exercise
< 0.4	Severe blockage suggesting severe peripheral artery disease; may have claudication pain at rest

Arterial Blood Pressure[6]

Noninvasive measurement of arterial blood pressure (BP) with a pneumatic cuff and sphygmomanometer is considered one of the "vital signs" and an important indicator of health (Fig. 6-10). Deviations from normal pressure provide important information regarding a variety of cardiovascular conditions.

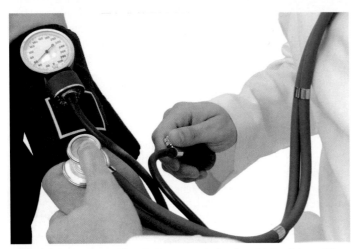

Fig. 6-10: Checking blood pressure at the brachial artery with a sphygmomanometer and stethoscope.

Procedure

- Use the appropriate sphygmomanometer cuff for the size of the body part. The bladder inside the cuff should encircle 80% of the arm in adults and 100% of the arm in children younger than 13 years old. If the bladder is too small, false high readings may result. If in doubt, use a larger cuff.

- The brachial artery is occluded by a sphygmomanometer cuff wrapped snugly around the upper arm and inflated to above the anticipated systolic pressure.

- As the cuff is slowly deflated (no more than 2-3 mm Hg per second), pulsatile blood flow is re-established and accompanied by sounds that can be detected by a stethoscope held over the artery.

- The sounds, known as Korotkoff sounds, originate from a combination of turbulent blood flow and oscillations of the arterial wall. As the pressure is reduced, the sounds change in quality and intensity.

    Phase I - first appearance of clear tapping sounds corresponding to the appearance of a palpable pulse; Phase I corresponds to systolic blood pressure (SBP)

    Phase II - sounds become softer and longer

    Phase III - sounds become crisper and louder

    Phase IV - sounds become muffled and softer

    Phase V - sounds disappear completely; the diastolic pressure (DBP) is the pressure at the last audible sound

Interpretation

In November of 2017, the American Heart Association and the American College of Cardiology released new guidelines that lowered the standards for high blood pressure. The result is that high blood pressure will now be treated earlier with lifestyle changes and in some cases medication. The new guidelines represent the first significant change in blood pressure guidelines since 2003.

- **In adults:**

    Normal BP: < 120 mm Hg SBP and < 80 mm Hg DBP

    Elevated: 120 – 129 mm Hg SBP and < 80 mm Hg DBP

    Stage 1 Hypertension: 130 – 139 mm Hg SBP or 80-89 mm Hg DBP

    Stage 2 Hypertension: at least 140 mm Hg SBP or at least 90 mm Hg DBP

    Hypertensive Crisis: greater than 180 mm Hg SBP and/ or greater than 120 mm Hg DBP

Auscultation of Heart Sounds[23]

Listening to the intensity and quality of heart sounds over the surface of the chest can provide useful information about the condition and function of the heart. Although considered an advanced skill, with supervised practice, the therapist should be able to differentiate normal heart sounds from blatantly abnormal sounds such as loud murmurs and gallops.

Procedure

The bell or diaphragm of the stethoscope is held directly on the patient's bare skin with enough pressure to provide a skin seal while the patient breathes quietly through the nose.

- Listen over four designated auscultatory areas (Fig. 6-11):

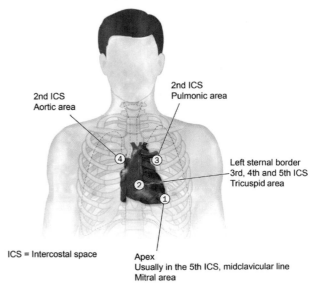

Fig. 6-11: Four areas to auscultate for heart sounds generated from the aortic, pulmonic, tricuspid, and mitral valves.

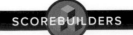

Aortic area – 2nd intercostal space at the right sternal border

Pulmonic area – 2nd intercostal space at the left sternal border

Mitral area – 5th intercostal space, medial to the left midclavicular line

Tricuspid area – 4th intercostal space at the left sternal border

- Listen to the overall rate and rhythm of the heart sounds.
- Listen separately to each sound and each pause in the cardiac cycle for as many beats as necessary to evaluate the sounds in one area before moving to the next area.
- Listen for extra sounds or murmurs while concentrating on systole and diastole.

Interpretation

S1 (lub)

- 1st heart sound - closure of the mitral and tricuspid (atrioventricular) valves at the onset of ventricular systole.
- High frequency sound with lower pitch and longer duration than S2.

S2 (dub)

- 2nd heart sound - closure of the aortic and pulmonic (semilunar) valves at the onset of ventricular diastole.
- High frequency sound with higher pitch and shorter duration than S1 (Fig. 6-12).

S3

- 3rd heart sound - vibrations of the distended ventricle walls due to passive flow of blood from the atria during the rapid filling phase of diastole.
- Normal in healthy young children; termed "physiologic" 3rd heart sound.
- Abnormal in adults; may be associated with heart failure; often called "ventricular gallop."

S4

- 4th heart sound - pathological sound of vibration of the ventricular wall with ventricular filling and atrial contraction.
- May be associated with hypertension, stenosis, hypertensive heart disease or myocardial infarction; often called an "atrial gallop".

Murmurs

- Heart murmurs are vibrations of longer duration than the heart sounds and are often due to disruption of blood flow past a stenotic or regurgitant valve; the sounds are variably described as soft, blowing or swishing.
- When the leaflets of the heart valves are thickened, the forward flow of blood is restricted; when the leaflets lose competency and fail to close tightly, blood can flow backwards (regurgitation).

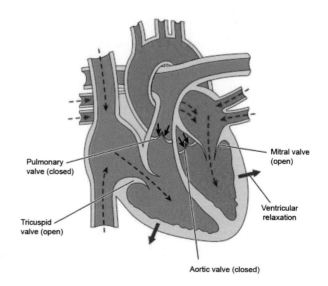

The first heart sound (S1), is caused by the closure of the mitral and tricuspid valves at the beginning of ventricular contraction (systole).

The second heart sound (S2), is caused by the closure of the aortic and pulmonary valves at the end of ventricular systole.

Fig. 6-12: Origin of the first and second heart sounds, S1 and S2, respectively.

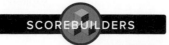

Auscultation of Lung Sounds[24]

Movement of air in the tracheobronchial tree produces sounds that can be heard with a stethoscope. Auscultation of lung sounds and voice sounds is performed to assist in diagnosis and to evaluate the effects of treatment. Lung or breath sounds are characterized by pitch, intensity, quality, and the duration of the inspiratory and expiratory phases.

Procedure

- Place the diaphragm of the stethoscope in firm contact with the patient's unclothed chest wall (Fig. 6-13).

- Start at the apices and work downward, comparing symmetrical points sequentially (Figs. 6-14, 6-15).

- Have the patient breathe in and out through the mouth, a little deeper than normal.

- Listen to at least one cycle of inspiration and expiration in each pulmonary segment.

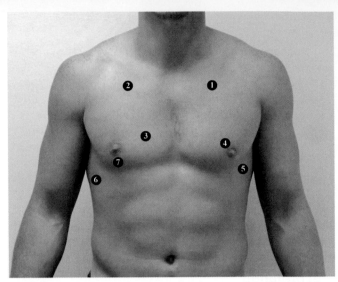

Fig. 6-14: Areas to auscultate for lung or breath sounds on the anterior thorax. Listen to at least one breath sound in each bronchopulmonary segment comparing the sounds from the left and right sides.

Interpretation

Normal breath sounds

These are sounds that are heard in their normal location or phase of respiration.

- Tracheal and bronchial sounds
  - Loud, tubular sounds normally heard over the trachea.
  - Inspiratory phase is shorter than the expiratory phase and there is a slight pause between them.

    Note: Bronchial sounds heard over distal airways are abnormal and represent consolidation or compression of lung tissue that facilitates transmission of sound.

- Vesicular breath sounds
  - High pitched, breezy sounds normally heard over the distal airways in healthy lung tissue.
  - Inspiratory phase is longer than expiratory phase and there is no pause between them.

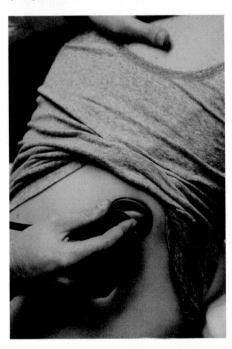

Fig. 6-13: Auscultation of lung sounds from the posterior thorax.

If abnormal sounds are suspected:

- Compare the intensity, pitch, and quality of the sounds heard on one side with sounds heard in the same location on the other side.

- Identify the breath sounds as vesicular, bronchovesicular bronchial or absent by the duration of inspiration and expiration, and by the quality and pitch.

- Note the presence or absence of adventitious (extra) sounds.

Abnormal breath sounds

These are sounds that are heard outside of their normal location or phase of respiration.

Adventitious breath sounds

Abnormal breath sounds heard with inspiration and/or expiration that can be continuous or discontinuous.

Crackle (formerly rales)

- An abnormal, discontinuous, high-pitched popping sound heard more often during inspiration. May be associated with restrictive or obstructive respiratory disorders.

Pleural friction rub

- Dry, crackling sound heard during both inspiration and expiration.

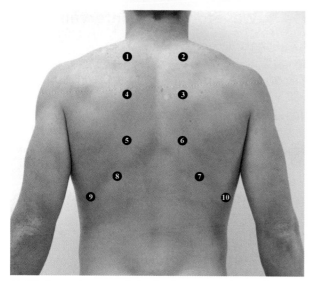

Fig. 6-15: Areas to auscultate for lung sounds on the posterior thorax.

Rhonchi

- Continuous low-pitched sounds described as having a "snoring" or "gurgling" quality that may be heard during both inspiration and expiration.

Stridor

- Continuous high-pitched wheeze heard with inspiration or expiration.

Wheeze

- Continuous "musical" or whistling sound composed of a variety of pitches heard during both inspiration and/or expiration, but variable from minute to minute and area to area.

Body Mass Index (BMI)[25]

BMI describes relative weight for height and is a measurement used to identify increased risk for mortality and morbidity due to excess weight and obesity. It can also monitor changes in body weight from treatment. Although BMI can be used for most men and women, it may overestimate body fat in athletes and others who have a muscular build and underestimate body fat in older persons and others who have lost muscle.

Procedure

- Measure the subject's standing height and body weight.
- BMI = weight [kg] ÷ height [m²] OR BMI = weight [lb] ÷ height [in²] x 703

Interpretation

Adult BMI	Classification
< 18.5	Underweight
18.5 – 24.9	Normal
25.0 – 29.9	Overweight
30.0 – 34.9	Obesity (Class 1)
35.0 – 39.9	Obesity (Class 2)
≥ 40.0	Extreme obesity (Class 3)

Classifications do not apply to children and adolescents as BMI changes with age and sex:

- BMI between the 85th and 95th percentile for age and sex is considered at risk for becoming overweight.
- BMI ≥ the 95th percentile is considered overweight or obese.

Capillary Refill Time[23]

The time it takes the capillary bed to refill after it is occluded by pressure is an indicator of impaired perfusion to the extremities.

Procedure

- Apply firm pressure over a nail bed or bony prominence (e.g., chin, forehead, or sternum) until the nail or skin blanches.
- Release the pressure.
- Observe the time for the nail or skin to regain its full color.

Interpretation

- Normal – Full color returns in < 2 seconds
- Abnormal – Refill time is > 2 seconds; indicates capillary blood flow is compromised (e.g., arterial occlusion, hypovolemic shock, hypothermia)

Dyspnea Scales

Dyspnea is an uncomfortable awareness of breathing that may result from decreased oxygenation, hypoventilation, hyperventilation, or increased work of breathing due to changes in respiratory mechanics or anxiety. A number of scales are available to rate dyspnea.[21, 29-31]

Borg Dyspnea Scale[29]	
0	No breathlessness at all
0.5	Very, very slight
1	Very slight
2	Slight breathlessness
3	Moderate
4	Somewhat severe
5	Severe breathlessness
6	
7	Very severe breathlessness
8	
9	Very, very severe breathlessness
10	Maximal

Electrocardiogram (ECG)[32]

The ECG is a graphic representation of the heart's electrical activity recorded from electrodes on the surface of the body. The ECG provides insight into the electrical behavior of the heart and its modification by physiologic, pharmacologic, and pathologic events. A 12-lead ECG provides 12 views of the heart. It is used to assess cardiac rhythm, to diagnose the location, extent, and acuteness of myocardial ischemia and infarction, and to evaluate changes with activity (Fig. 6-16).

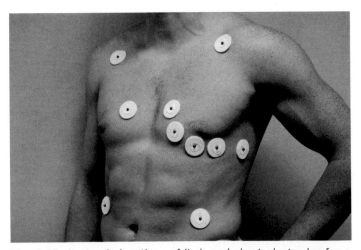

Fig. 6-16: Anatomic locations of limb and chest electrodes for a 12-lead ECG recording.

Waveforms and Intervals

- **P wave:** Atrial depolarization
- **PR interval:** Time for atrial depolarization and conduction from the SA node to the AV node. Normal duration is 0.12 to 0.20 seconds
- **QRS complex:** Ventricular depolarization and atrial repolarization. Normal duration is 0.06 to 0.10 seconds
- **QT interval:** Time for both ventricular depolarization and repolarization. Normally ranges from 0.20 to 0.40 seconds, depending on heart rate
- **ST segment:** Isoelectric period following QRS when the ventricles are depolarized
- **T wave:** Ventricular repolarization

Sinus Node Rhythms

- **Normal sinus rhythm:** Atrial depolarization begins in the SA node and spreads normally throughout the electrical conduction system with a heart rate between 60 and 100 beats/minute
- **Sinus bradycardia:** Sinus rhythm with a heart rate less than 60 beats/minute (in adults)
- **Sinus tachycardia:** Sinus rhythm with a heart rate more than 100 beats/minute (in adults)
- **Sinus arrhythmia:** A sinus rhythm, but with quickening and slowing of impulse formation in the SA node resulting in a slight beat-to-beat variation of the rate
- **Sinus arrest:** A sinus rhythm, except with intermittent failure of either SA node impulse formation or AV node conduction that results in the occasional complete absence of P or QRS waves

Exercise Stress Testing[21]

Exercise stress tests are used to assess the patient's ability to tolerate increasing intensity of exercise while ECG, BP, HR, and symptoms are monitored for evidence of myocardial ischemia, abnormal electrical conduction, or other abnormal signs and symptoms of exertion. They may be used to evaluate disease severity and prognosis and to determine functional capacity, especially for exercise prescription and counseling. A number of exercise protocols are available using a treadmill, cycle ergometer or upper extremity ergometer.

Procedure

- Generally, the patient is required to exercise at progressively greater increments of work, by varying the speed and grade of the treadmill, or the speed and resistance to pedaling an upper extremity or cycle ergometer.
- HR, BP, ECG, RPE, and signs and symptoms are monitored before, during, and after the test
- Absolute indications for terminating an exercise test:
  - Drop in SBP > 10 mm Hg from baseline despite increase in workload with other evidence of ischemia

– Moderately severe angina (three on a scale of four)

– Increasing nervous system symptoms (e.g., ataxia, dizziness)

– Signs of poor perfusion (cyanosis, pallor)

– Sustained ventricular tachycardia

– 1.0 mm ST elevation in leads without diagnostic Q waves

• Relative indications for terminating an exercise test:

– Drop in SBP > 10 mm Hg from baseline despite increase in workload without other evidence of ischemia

– > 2 mm ST segment depression

– Arrhythmias other than sustained ventricular tachycardia, including multifocal PVCs, supraventricular tachycardia, heart block or bradyarrhythmias

– Fatigue, shortness of breath, wheezing, leg cramps, and claudication

– Development of bundle branch block or intraventricular conduction delay

– Increasing chest pain

– Hypertensive response (SBP > 250 mm Hg and/or DBP > 115 mm Hg)

Interpretation

A negative test indicates a low probability of coronary artery disease; a positive test indicates a high probability of coronary artery disease.

Prognosis can be assessed using various multivariate indices (e.g., Duke Treadmill Test score and Veteran's Administration Score).

An aerobic exercise prescription can be determined from performance on the exercise test (see also Physical Therapy Procedural Interventions - Cardiac Rehabilitation).

Homans' Sign for Deep Vein Thrombosis[33]

Homans' sign is a test to detect deep vein thrombosis (DVT) in the lower leg.

Procedure

Passively dorsiflex the foot at the ankle with the knee straight.

Interpretation

Homans' sign is positive for DVT if the maneuver produces pain in the calf or popliteal space.

Clinical findings alone are insensitive and nonspecific and cannot be relied on to confirm or exclude the diagnosis of DVT.

Despite the lack of specificity, a positive Homans' sign warrants further evaluation.

Palpation of Peripheral Arterial Pulses

The peripheral pulse is a periodic fluctuation in the flow of blood through a peripheral artery caused by the ejection of blood with each heartbeat. Normal pulses are strong and regular. The pulse will be irregular with a cardiac arrhythmia and weak and difficult to palpate in peripheral artery disease. A higher intensity pulse will be present when stroke volume is increased (e.g., exercise, fever).

Procedure

• Heart rate and rhythm, as well as blood flow in the extremity, are assessed by palpating over the artery with the tip of the index or middle finger with enough pressure to feel the pulse, but without obstructing blood flow.

• Common arteries used include brachial, carotid, dorsal pedal, femoral, popliteal, posterior tibial, radial, and temporal.

• Note the time between pulsations.

• For regular rhythms (i.e., time between pulsations is approximately equal), count the pulses in 15 seconds and multiply by four.

• For irregular rhythms (i.e., time between pulsations is not equal), count the pulses in 60 seconds.

• Note the volume and quality of the pulse and any differences between the pulses in the two limbs.

Pulse Points of Selected Peripheral Arteries	
Artery	**Pulse Point**
Carotid	The medial aspect of the sternocleidomastoid muscle in the lower half of the neck (Fig. 6-17)
Brachial	Medial to the biceps tendon and lateral to the medial epicondyle of the humerus
Radial	At the wrist, lateral to the flexor carpi radialis tendon (Fig. 6-18)
Ulnar	At the wrist, between the flexor digitorum superficialis and the flexor carpi ulnaris tendons
Femoral	In the upper thigh, one-third of the distance from the pubis to the anterior superior iliac spine
Popliteal	In the popliteal space of the posterior knee
Posterior tibial	In the space between the medial malleolus and the Achilles tendon, above the calcaneus
Dorsalis pedis	Near the center of the long axis of the foot, between the first and second metatarsal bones (Fig. 6-19)

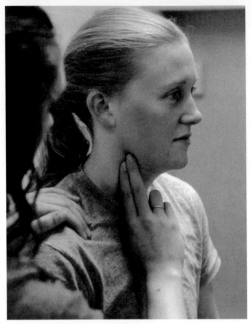

Fig. 6-17: Palpating the carotid artery.

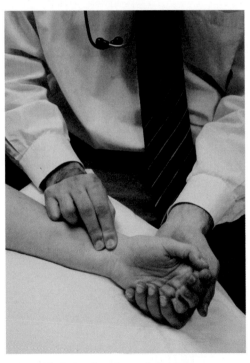

Fig. 6-18: Palpating the radial artery.

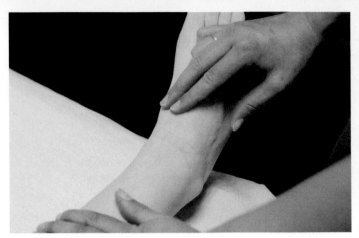

Fig. 6-19: Palpating the dorsalis pedis artery.

Interpretation

Characterize the heart rate	
Normal infant	100 to 130 beats/minute
Normal child	80 to 100 beats/minute
Normal adult	60 to 100 beats/minute
Bradycardia	< 60 beats/minute
Tachycardia	> 100 beats/minute
Characterize the volume or amplitude of the pulse[34]	
3+	= large or bounding pulsation
2+	= normal or average pulsation
1	= small or reduced pulsation
0	= absence of pulsation

Pulmonary Function Testing (PFT)[35]

Pulmonary function testing measures the volume or flow of air during inhalation and exhalation (Fig. 6-20). The measurements include, but are not limited to, forced vital capacity (FVC), and other forced expiratory flow measurements such as peak expiratory flow (PEF), the forced expiratory volume in the first second (FEV_1), and the mid-expiratory flow (FEF 25-75%).

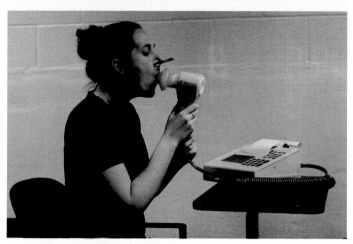

Fig. 6-20: Performing a pulmonary function test with a bedside digital spirometer.

Procedure

- While maintaining an upright posture, the subject exhales into the spirometer mouthpiece as hard and as fast as possible for six seconds until no more air can be expelled.

- An adequate FVC test requires three acceptable maneuvers.

- Modern spirometers calculate "predicted normal" values, (i.e., the test value the patient should normally attain based on age, sex, height, weight, and race).

Interpretation[36]

Obstructive ventilatory impairment

- Characterized by decreased expiratory flows.

- Airway narrowing during exhalation causes a disproportionate reduction of maximal air flow compared to the maximal volume displaced from the lungs.

- $FEV_1/FVC < 70\%$ is the primary indicator of an obstructive impairment.

- Pathologies include asthma, emphysema, and chronic bronchitis

Restrictive ventilatory impairment

- Characterized by reduced lung volumes (total lung capacity, FVC, FEV_1) and relatively normal expiratory flow rates.

- Inferred from spirometry when FVC is reduced and FEV_1/FVC is normal or $> 80\%$.

- Pathologies include interstitial lung disease, pleural diseases, chest wall deformities, obesity, pregnancy, neuromuscular disease, and tumor.

Pulse Oximetry[37]

A pulse oximeter estimates the percent of arterial oxygen saturation of hemoglobin by placing a sensor on the finger or earlobe (Fig. 6-21). The sensor measures the differential absorption of light by oxygenated and nonoxygenated hemoglobin. This estimate is denoted as SpO_2, which is an indication of the partial pressure of oxygen in arterial blood.

Procedure

- Apply the sensor to the earlobe or fingertip.

- Assess the strength of the waveform or pulse amplitude to assure that the oximeter is detecting adequate arterial blood flow.

- Holding the finger dependent and motionless and covering the finger sensor to occlude ambient light improves the quality of readings.

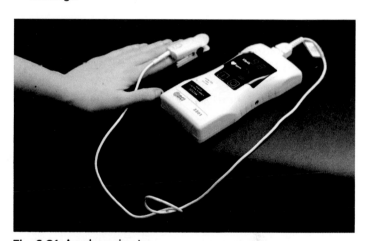

Fig. 6-21: A pulse oximeter.

Interpretation

SpO_2 is only an estimate of the arterial O_2 saturation; actual arterial oxygen saturation is $\pm 4\%$ of SpO_2. A number of factors limit the accuracy of oximeter readings:

- Motion artifact
- Abnormal hemoglobin
- Intravascular dyes
- Exposure of probe to ambient light during measurement
- Poor cutaneous perfusion at the measurement site due to hypotension, hypothermia, low cardiac output or vasoconstrictor medications
- Skin pigmentation
- Nail polish or nail coverings (with finger probe)

If $SpO_2 < 90\%$ in acutely ill patients or $< 85\%$ in patients with chronic lung disease, activity should be stopped and a discussion with the physician should take place to consider adding or increasing supplemental oxygen.

Rate Pressure Product (RPP)[14]

RPP, or double-product, is an index of myocardial oxygen consumption and coronary blood flow. RPP provides an easy to measure physiologic correlate to the onset of angina pectoris or the development of ECG abnormalities in patients with heart disease. These signs and symptoms of myocardial ischemia generally occur at a reproducible RPP value.

Procedure

- Measure SBP and heart rate (HR) during the same exercise workload
- RPP = HR x SBP
- RPP is usually reported as a two digit number x 10^3 (e.g., if HR = 150 and SBP = 170, RPP = $25.5 \cdot 10^3$).

Interpretation

In patients with fixed-threshold angina:

- A relatively constant level of activity will precipitate angina.
- RPP obtained during an exercise test may be used to guide the exercise prescription.
- Keeping the intensity of exercise below the RPP value will reduce the risk of developing angina.

Rating of Perceived Exertion (RPE)[38]

The RPE is used to quantify the subject's overall sense of effort during activity. The reported RPE provides the therapist with an idea of the amount of strain or level of exertion the patient is experiencing.

Procedure

- There are two RPE scales that are widely used: the original 6 – 20 scale and the revised 0 – 10 scale. These scales are often referred to as the Borg Scale.
- Recommended instructions for administering the RPE scale:[29]

"While doing physical activity, we want you to rate your perception of exertion. This feeling should reflect how heavy and strenuous the exercise feels to you, combining all sensations and feelings of physical stress, effort, and fatigue. Do not concern yourself with any one factor such as leg pain or shortness of breath, but try to focus on your total feeling of exertion."

"Choose the number that best describes your level of exertion. This will give you a good idea of the intensity level of your activity. Try to appraise your feeling of exertion as honestly as possible, without thinking about what the actual physical load is. Your own feeling of effort and exertion is important, not how it compares to other people's."

Interpretation

RPE of 13 - 14 represents about 70% of maximum heart rate during exercise on a treadmill or cycle ergometer. RPE of 11 - 13 corresponds to the upper limit of prescribed training heart rates early in cardiac rehabilitation.[39] RPE can substitute for HR in prescribing the intensity of exercise when:

- Ability to monitor HR is compromised (e.g., sensory deficits)
- Patients begin an exercise-based rehabilitation program without a preliminary exercise test
- The HR response to exercise is altered (e.g., cardiac transplant)
- Physical activities other than cardiorespiratory endurance activity are assessed
- Clinical status or medical therapy changes

Ratings can be influenced by psychological state, environmental conditions, mode of exercise, and age.

Original RPE Scale		Revised RPE Scale	
6		0	Nothing at all
7	Very, very light	0.5	Very, very weak
8		1	Very weak
9	Very light	2	Weak
10		3	Moderate
11	Fairly light	4	Somewhat strong
12		5	Strong
13	Somewhat hard	6	
14		7	Very strong
15	Hard	8	
16		9	
17	Very hard	10	Very, very strong
18		• Maximal	
19	Very, very hard		
20			

Respiratory Rate, Rhythm, and Pattern

A complete assessment of respiration considers four parameters: rate, rhythm, depth, and character. Respiratory rate is the number of breaths per minute. Rhythm refers to the regularity of inspirations and expirations. Depth of respiration refers to the volume of air exchanged with each breath. The character of respirations refers to the effort and sound produced during breathing.

Procedure

- Observe the patient's breathing at rest for 60 seconds (an alternate method is to place your hand over the patient's upper thorax or abdomen and observe and feel movement with each respiration).

- Document the rate, rhythm, depth, and character of respiration.

Interpretation

Resting respiratory rates for healthy individuals[40]

- **Newborn:** 33 - 45 breaths/minute
- **1 year:** 25 - 35 breaths/minute
- **10 years:** 15 - 20 breaths/minute
- **Adult:** 12 - 20 breaths/minute

Respiratory rhythm

- **Normal:** Inspiration (I) is half as long as expiration (E); I:E ratio is 1:2
- **COPD:** I:E ratio reflects a longer expiration phase; 1:3 or 1:4

Depth of respiration

- Characterized as deeper or shallower than normal tidal volume

Character of respiration

- Normal breathing is quiet and effortless
- Labored breathing is evident by the use of accessory muscles of respiration
- Wheezes and crackles are abnormal sounds produced by changes in the airways

Common Breathing Patterns[23]	
Apnea	absence of spontaneous breathing
Biot's	irregular breathing; breaths vary in depth and rate with periods of apnea; often associated with increased intracranial pressure or damage to the medulla
Bradypnea	slower than normal respiratory rate; < 12 breaths/minute in adults; may be associated with neurologic or electrolyte disturbance, infection or high level of cardiorespiratory fitness
Cheyne-Stokes (periodic)	decreasing rate and depth of breathing with periods of apnea; can occur due to central nervous system damage
Eupnea	normal rate and depth of breathing
Hyperpnea	increased rate and depth of breathing
Hypopnea	decreased rate and depth of breathing
Tachypnea	faster than normal respiratory rate; > 20 breaths/minute in adults

Six-Minute Walk Test (6MWT)[41]

The 6MWT is used to measure functional status and to document treatment outcomes in patients with heart and lung disease as well as healthy and older adults.

Procedure

- Walk on a measured "track" at least 100 feet (30 meters) in length.
- Subjects may self-administer any medications ordinarily taken before activity, may use supplemental O_2 at their prescribed flow rate for exercise, and may use any assistive device for walking.
- Three walks are recommended with at least 15 minutes of rest between each walk.
- BP, HR, RR, RPE, and O_2 saturation may be measured before and immediately after the test.

- Standard instructions are given:

  "The purpose of this test is to find out how far you can walk in six minutes. You will start from this point and follow the hallway to the marker at the end, then turn around and walk back. You will go back and forth as many times as you can in the six-minute period. You may stop and rest, if you need to, just remain where you are until you can go on again. The most important thing is that you cover as much ground as you possibly can during the six minutes. I will tell you the time, and I will let you know when the six minutes are up. When I say 'stop', stand right where you are."

- Standard words of encouragement are provided at regular intervals (e.g., "you're doing well," "keep up the good work," "you have three minutes to go").

Interpretation

The therapist should record the distance walked and the number of rest stops.

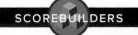

Physical Therapy Procedural Interventions

Aerobic Exercise Prescription[21,39]

Aerobic exercise, or cardiorespiratory endurance exercise, refers to submaximal, rhythmic repetitive exercise of large muscle groups during which adenosine triphosphate is synthesized primarily by the long-term energy system and the utilization of inspired oxygen.

Indications

- Reduced cardiorespiratory endurance
- Primary and secondary prevention of cardiovascular disease

Precautions/Contraindications

- Appropriate screening or health appraisal should be performed prior to beginning exercise training to identify known diseases, risk factors for coronary artery disease, and other factors that will optimize adherence, minimize risk, and maximize benefits.
- Avoid Valsalva maneuver

Procedure

Effective aerobic exercise training and improvement in VO_{2max} is directly related to the intensity, frequency, and duration of aerobic activity interacting with the two major principles of exercise training: overload and specificity. The overload principle states that to improve its function, a tissue or organ must be exposed to a stress or load greater than that which it normally encounters. The principle of specificity states that the long-term adaptations to the metabolic and physiologic systems derived from exercise are specific to the exercises performed and the muscles involved.

Mode

- Rhythmic activities that use large muscle groups and can be performed continuously and safely (e.g., walking, hiking, running, jogging, bicycling, cross-country skiing, aerobic dance/calisthenics, rope skipping, rowing, skating, stair climbing, swimming, and various endurance game activities).

Intensity

- A target heart rate (THR) zone is established from lower and upper heart rate limits calculated using different percentage training intensities depending on the individual's age, fitness level, health status, and goals.
- **Method 1:** Percent of maximum heart rate (HRmax)

    Lower THR = HRmax x 55%

    Upper THR = HRmax x 90%
- **Method 2:** Heart rate reserve (HRR) or Karvonen formula

    Lower THR = [(HRmax – HRrest) x 40%] + HRrest

    Upper THR = [(HRmax – HRrest) x 85%] + HRrest

    – HRmax = maximum heart rate measured during a graded exercise test or estimated by 220 - age

    – HRrest = resting heart rate

Duration

- Duration is dependent on the intensity of the activity.
- 20 – 60 minutes of continuous or intermittent activity (minimum of 10-minute bouts accumulated throughout the day).
- Lower intensity activity should be performed over a longer period of time ($\geq$ 30 minutes).
- Higher intensity activity should be performed for 20 minutes or longer.
- Moderate intensity activity of longer duration is recommended for adults not training for athletic competition due to the potential hazards and adherence problems associated with high-intensity activity.

Frequency

- 3 – 5 days per week

Expected Outcomes

The therapist should be aware of the normal cardiorespiratory responses to aerobic exercise as well as the chronic adaptations that occur from a successful long-term aerobic exercise training program.

Normal Cardiorespiratory Response to Acute Aerobic Exercise

- Increased oxygen consumption due to increased cardiac output, increased blood flow, and oxygen utilization in the exercising skeletal muscles.
- Linear increase in SBP with increasing workload (8 to 12 mm Hg per MET)
- No change or moderate decrease in DBP
- Increased respiratory rate and tidal volume

Chronic Adaptations to Aerobic Exercise

- VO_{2max}: increased at maximal exercise
- HR: no change or decrease at maximal exercise; decreased at submaximal exercise
- Arteriovenous oxygen difference: increased at maximal exercise; no change at submaximal exercise
- SBP and DBP: no change or slight increase at maximal exercise; no change or slight decrease at submaximal exercise
- Blood lactate: increased at maximal exercise; decreased at submaximal exercise
- Oxidative capacity of muscle: increase in mitochondrial number and size, capillary density, and oxidative enzymes
- Maximal voluntary ventilation: increased at maximal exercise
- Plasma volume: increased
- Skeletal muscle blood flow: increase at maximum exercise; no change at submaximal exercise

- Reduced body mass and body fat and increase in fat free body mass
- Improved body heat transfer due to larger plasma volume and more responsive thermoregulatory mechanisms
- Psychological benefits: reduced anxiety, stress, and depression; improved mood, and self-esteem

Airway Clearance Techniques

Airway clearance techniques are intended to manage or prevent the consequences of impaired mucociliary transport or the inability to protect the airway (e.g., impaired cough). The techniques may include breathing strategies, manual and mechanical techniques, and postural drainage.

Indications for airway clearance[42]

- Retained secretions in the central airways
- Prophylaxis against postoperative pulmonary complications
- Obtain sputum for diagnostic analysis
- Difficulty clearing secretions
- Atelectasis caused by or suspected of being caused by mucus plugging

Active cycle of breathing

The active cycle of breathing (ACB) technique was developed under the name "forced expiratory technique" to assist secretion clearance in patients with asthma. The name of the technique was changed to "active cycle of breathing" to emphasize that ACB always couples breathing exercise with the huff cough. It includes three phases: breathing control, thoracic expansion exercises, and forced expiratory technique.[43]

Procedure

- Breathing control:
  - Gentle, relaxed breathing (may be diaphragmatic breathing at patient's tidal volume and resting respiratory rate for 5 – 10 seconds, or as long as the patient needs in order to prepare for the next phase).
- Thoracic expansion exercise:
  - Three to four deep, slow, relaxed inhalations to inspiratory reserve with passive exhalation
  - Chest percussion, vibration or shaking may be combined with exhalation
- Forced expiratory technique:
  - One or two huffs at mid to low lung volumes with the glottis open into the expiratory reserve volume
  - A brisk adduction of the upper arms may be added to self-compress the thorax

Precautions/Contraindications

- Splinting postoperative incisions to achieve adequate expiratory force
- Bronchospasm or hyperreactive airways

Autogenic drainage (AD)

AD uses controlled breathing to mobilize secretions by varying expiratory airflow without using postural drainage positions or coughing. The theory is to improve airflow in small airways to facilitate the movement of mucus. AD requires patience to learn, so this may not be suitable for young children and patients who are not motivated or easily distracted. Because AD does not require the assistance of another person or equipment, it can be performed anywhere and during activities of daily living.[43]

Procedure

- The patient is sitting upright in a chair with back support.
- Controlled breathing at three lung volumes
  - "Unsticking phase": slowly breathe in through the nose at low-lung volumes followed by a two to three second breath-hold to allow collateral ventilation to get air behind the secretions, then exhale down into the expiratory reserve volume
  - "Collecting phase": breathe at tidal volume, interspersed by two to three second breath-holds
  - "Evacuating phase": deeper inspirations from low-to-mid inspiratory reserve volume, with breath holding followed by a huff
- Exhalation through pursed-lips may be used to control expiratory flow rate.
- An average treatment is 30 to 45 minutes.

Precautions/Contraindications

- Requires motivation and concentration to learn

Directed cough and huffing[44]

A directed cough tries to compensate for the patient's physical limitations to elicit a maximum forced exhalation.

Huffing is a forced expiratory maneuver performed with the glottis open. The maneuver is similar to fogging a pair of glasses with your breath. Although a huff does not produce the same airflow velocity as a cough, the potential for airway collapse is less. Huffing may be reinforced by a quick adduction of the arms to self-compress the chest wall.

Procedure

Cough

- Inhale maximally, close the glottis and hold breath for two to three seconds.
- Contract the expiratory muscles to produce increased intra-thoracic pressure against the closed glottis.
- Cough sharply two to three times through a slightly open mouth.
- Post-surgical patients may need to splint the chest or abdomen by applying pressure over the incision with a pillow or blanket roll.

Huff

- Inhale deeply through an open mouth.
- Contract the abdominal muscles during a rapid exhalation with the glottis open, saying, "Ha, ha, ha."

Precautions/Contraindications

- Inability to control possible transmission of infection from patients suspected or known to have pathogens transmittable by droplets
- Elevated intracranial pressure or known intracranial aneurysm
- Reduced coronary artery perfusion (e.g., acute myocardial infarction)
- Acute unstable head, neck or spine injury
- Potential for regurgitation/aspiration
- Acute abdominal pathology, abdominal aortic aneurysm, hiatal hernia or pregnancy
- Untreated pneumothorax
- Osteoporosis
- Flail chest

Postural drainage, percussion, and vibration[42]

Postural drainage consists of positioning the patient so that gravity will help drain bronchial secretions from specific lung segments toward the central airways where they can be removed by cough or mechanical aspiration.

Percussion, also known as cupping and clapping, is the rhythmic clapping or striking of the thorax with a cupped hand or mechanical percussor directly over the lung segment being drained. This rhythmic sequence should last for several minutes and should not be painful.

Vibration is the application of a fine, tremulous action on the chest wall over the lung segment being drained in the direction the ribs move during exhalation. It may be performed manually or with a mechanical vibrator. Vibration should be performed during exhalation.

Procedure for postural drainage

- The patient assumes the appropriate position for the affected lung segment (Figs. 6-22, A-J).
- Standard positions may be modified as the patient's condition and tolerance warrant.
- Maintain each position for two to three minutes.

Precautions/Contraindications

All positions are contraindicated for:

- Intracranial pressure > 20 mm Hg
- Head and neck injury until stabilized
- Active hemorrhage with hemodynamic instability
- Recent spinal surgery (e.g., laminectomy) or acute spinal injury
- Active hemoptysis
- Empyema

- Bronchopleural fistula
- Pulmonary edema associated with congestive heart failure
- Large pleural effusion
- Pulmonary embolism
- Confused or anxious patients who do not tolerate position changes
- Rib fracture, with or without flail chest
- Surgical wound or healing tissue

Trendelenburg position is contraindicated for:

- Uncontrolled hypertension
- Distended abdomen
- Esophageal surgery
- Recent gross hemoptysis related to lung carcinoma treated surgically or with radiation therapy
- Uncontrolled airway at risk for aspiration (e.g., tube feeding or recent meal)

Procedure for percussion and vibration

- Place the patient in the appropriate postural drainage position.
- Cover the skin overlying the affected segment with a thin material (towel, t-shirt, hospital gown).
- Therapist rhythmically strikes the chest with a cupped hand for two to three minutes per lung segment (Fig. 6-23).
- Therapist places one hand on top of the other over affected area or one hand on each side of the rib cage.
- Vibrate the chest wall as the patient exhales by tensing the muscles of the hands and arms while applying moderate pressure downward.
- The maneuver is performed in the direction in which the ribs move on expiration.
- Encourage the patient to cough or huff after two or three vibrations.

Precautions/Contraindications

- All contraindications listed for postural drainage
- Subcutaneous emphysema
- Recent epidural spinal infusion or spinal anesthesia
- Recent skin grafts, or flaps, on the thorax
- Burns, open wounds, and skin infections of the thorax
- Recently placed transvenous or subcutaneous pacemaker
- Suspected pulmonary tuberculosis
- Lung contusion
- Bronchospasm
- Osteomyelitis of the ribs
- Osteoporosis
- Complaint of chest wall pain

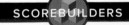

Postural Drainage Positioning

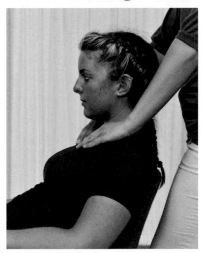

Fig. 6-22A: Apical segments right and left upper lobes: The patient is in a sitting position, leaning back 30-40 degrees. Percussion and vibration are performed above the clavicles.

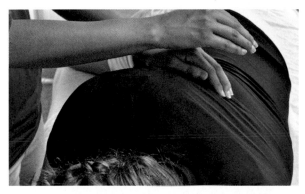

Fig. 6-22B: Posterior segment right upper lobe: The patient is turned ¼ from prone on the left side with the bed horizontal and the head and shoulders raised on a pillow. Percussion and vibration are performed around the medial border of the right scapula.

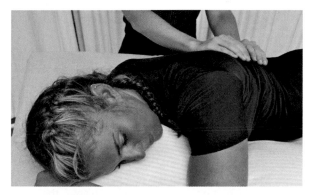

Fig. 6-22C: Posterior segment left upper lobe: The patient is turned ¼ from prone on the right side with the head of the bed elevated 45 degrees and the head and shoulders raised on a pillow. Percussion and vibration are performed around the medial border of the left scapula.

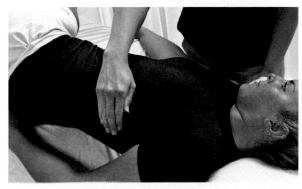

Fig. 6-22D: Lingula left upper lobe: The patient is turned ¼ from supine on the right side with the foot of the bed elevated 12 inches. Percussion and vibration are performed over the left chest between the axilla and the left nipple.

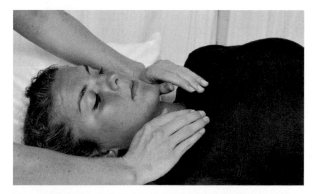

Fig. 6-22E: Anterior segments right and left upper lobes: The patient is in supine with the bed horizontal. Percussion and vibration are performed below the clavicles.

Postural Drainage Positioning (continued)

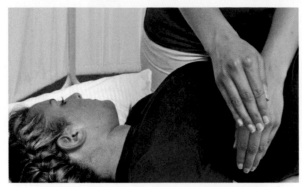

Fig. 6-22F: Right middle lobe: The patient is turned ¼ from supine on the left side with the foot of the bed elevated 12 inches. Percussion and vibration are performed over the right chest between the axilla and the right nipple.

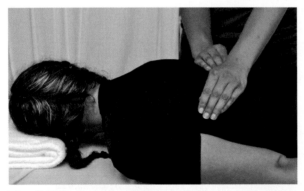

Fig. 6-22G: Superior segments left and right lower lobes: The patient is prone with the bed horizontal. Percussion and vibration are performed below the inferior border of the left and right scapulae.

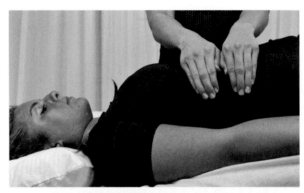

Fig. 6-22H: Anterior basal segments left and right lower lobes: The patient is in supine with the foot of the bed elevated 18 inches. Percussion and vibration are performed over the lower ribs on the left and right side.

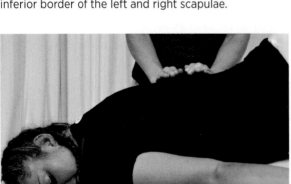

Fig. 6-22I: Posterior basal segments left and right lower lobes: The patient is in prone with the foot of the bed elevated 18 inches. Percussion and vibration are performed over the lower ribs on the left and right side of the chest.

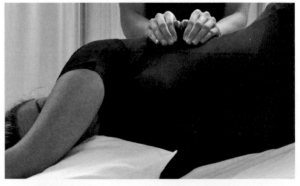

Fig. 6-22J: Lateral basal segments lower lobes: The patient is in sidelying with the foot of the bed elevated 18 inches. Percussion and vibration performed over the lower ribs. The image shows the position for the lateral segment of the left lower lobe with the patient lying on the right side. For the lateral segment of the right lower lobe, the patient lies on the left side.

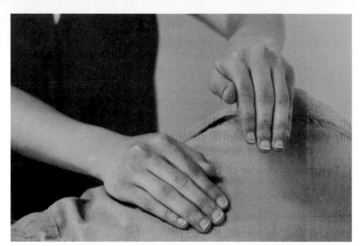

Fig. 6-23: Percussion of the thorax during postural drainage.

Expected outcomes of airway clearance

- Easier clearance of secretions and increased volume of secretions during and after treatments
- Improved breath sounds in the lungs being treated
- Increase in sputum production
- Change in vital signs - moderate changes in respiratory rate and/or pulse rate are expected
- Resolution or improvement of atelectasis and localized infiltrates observed with chest x-ray
- Improvement in arterial blood gas values or oxygen saturation

Breathing Exercises

Diaphragmatic breathing (DB)[45,46]

DB involves breathing predominantly with the diaphragm while minimizing the action of accessory muscles and motion of the upper rib cage during inspiration (Fig. 6-24).

Indications

- Post-surgical patient with pain in the chest wall or abdomen, or restricted mobility
- Patient learning active cycle of breathing or autogenic drainage airway clearance techniques
- Dyspnea at rest or with minimal activity
- Inability to perform ADLs due to dyspnea or inefficient breathing pattern

Precautions/Contraindications

- Moderate to severe COPD and marked hyperinflation of the lungs without diaphragmatic movement
- Patients with paradoxical breathing patterns, or who demonstrate increased inspiratory muscle effort, and increased dyspnea during DB

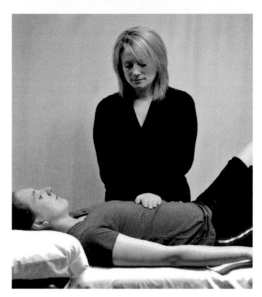

Fig. 6-24: A physical therapist assistant teaches diaphragmatic breathing.

Procedure

- Semi-Fowler's position is a good starting position.
- Sniffing can be used to facilitate contraction of the diaphragm.
- Have the patient place one hand on the upper chest and the other just below the rib cage.
- Instruct the patient to:

"Breathe in slowly through your nose so that your stomach moves out against your hand. The hand on your chest should remain as still as possible. Feel your abdomen gently rise into your hand. Exhale through pursed lips, let the hand on your abdomen descend, while the hand on your upper chest remains still."

Expected Outcomes

- Decrease respiratory rate
- Decrease use of accessory muscles of inspiration
- Increase tidal volume
- Decrease respiratory flow rate
- Subjective improvement of dyspnea
- Improve tolerance for activity

Inspiratory muscle training (IMT)[45,47,48]

IMT attempts to strengthen the diaphragm and intercostal muscles. Two different IMT devices provide different modes of training: flow resistive breathing and threshold breathing. During flow resistive breathing, the patient inspires through a mouthpiece and adapter with an adjustable diameter. Decreasing the diameter increases the resistance to breathing, provided that breathing rate, tidal volume, and inspiratory time are kept constant. Threshold loading requires a buildup of negative pressure before flow occurs through a valve that opens at a critical pressure. Threshold breathing provides consistent and specific pressure for IMT, regardless of how quickly or slowly patients breathe.

Indications

- Impaired inspiratory muscle strength and/or a ventilatory limitation to exercise performance

Precautions/Contraindications

- Clinical signs of inspiratory muscle fatigue (in characteristic order of appearance)
  - Tachypnea
  - Reduced tidal volume
  - Increased $PaCO_2$
  - Bradypnea and decreased minute ventilation

Procedure

- Measure the patient's maximum inspiratory pressure (MIP) with a manometer. Use the measured MIP to calculate the training load.

Expected Outcomes

- Increase inspiratory muscle strength and endurance
- Decrease dyspnea at rest and during exercise
- Increase functional exercise capacity

Paced breathing and exhale with effort[45]

Paced breathing is a strategy to decrease the work of breathing and prevent dyspnea during activity. It allows anyone who experiences shortness of breath to become less fearful of activity and exercise.

Exhale with effort is a breathing strategy employed during activity to prevent a patient from holding their breath. The technique breaks any activity into one or more breaths with inhalation during the resting or less active phase of the activity and exhalation during the movement or more active phase of the activity.

Indications

- Patients with dyspnea at rest or with minimal activity
- Inability to perform activity due to pulmonary limitation
- Inefficient breathing pattern during activity

Precautions/Contraindications

- Avoid Valsalva maneuver during activity

Procedure

- Perform activity at a tempo that does not exceed the patient's breathing limitations.
- Find a comfortable inspiration to expiration (I:E) time to synchronize with the exertion phase of activity.
- Synchronize breathing with components of the activity:
  - inhale before or during the easier component of the activity
  - exhale during the more vigorous component of the activity
- Do not hold breath or rush through the activity.

Walking:

- Inhale through the nose while walking two steps and then pause; exhale through pursed lips while walking four steps

Climbing stairs:

- Inhale through the nose while standing
- Exhale through pursed lips while stepping up (or down) one or two stairs
- Remain on the step until breathing control is restored

Lifting:

- Inhale through the nose while standing or sitting; exhale through pursed lips while bending to reach the object
- Pause
- Inhale through the nose while grabbing the object; exhale through pursed lips while standing up

Expected Outcomes

- Complete activity without dyspnea
- Decrease patient's fear of becoming short of breath during activity

Pursed-lip breathing (PLB)[49]

PLB is a simple technique to reduce respiratory rate, reduce dyspnea, and maintain a small positive pressure in the bronchioles, which may help prevent airway collapse in patients with emphysema. Any patient who is short of breath may use this technique.

Indications

- Tachypnea
- Dyspnea

Precautions/Contraindications

- Forcing exhalation

Procedure

- Semi-Fowler's is a good position to initiate the breathing technique.
- Instruct the patient to:

"Breathe in slowly through your nose with the mouth closed for two counts. Pucker, or purse your lips as if you were going to whistle, then gently breathe out through pursed lips, as if trying to make a candle flame flicker, for a four count. Do not blow with force."

Expected Outcomes

- Decrease respiratory rate
- Relieve dyspnea
- Reduce arterial partial pressure of carbon dioxide ($PaCO_2$)
- Improve tidal volume
- Improve oxygen saturation
- Prevent airway collapse in patients with emphysema
- Increase activity tolerance

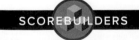

Segmental breathing[45,50]

Segmental breathing, also known as localized breathing or thoracic expansion exercise, is intended to improve regional ventilation and prevent and treat pulmonary complications after surgery. It is based on the presumption that asymmetrical chest wall motion may coincide with underlying pathology (e.g., pneumonia, pleuritic chest wall pain, retained secretions) and that inspired air can be directed to a particular area by facilitation or inhibition of chest wall movement through proper hand placements, verbal cues or coordination of breathing.

Indications

- Decreased intrathoracic lung volume
- Decreased chest wall lung compliance
- Increased flow resistance from decreased lung volume
- Ventilation:perfusion (V:Q) mismatch

Precautions/Contraindications

- None

Procedure

- Position the patient:
  - Sitting position for basal atelectasis
  - Sidelying with affected lung uppermost
  - Postural drainage positions with affected lung uppermost to assist with secretion removal
- Therapist applies firm pressure at the end of exhalation to the patient's chest wall overlying the area to be expanded.
- Patient inhales deeply and slowly expands the rib cage under the therapist's hands.
- Therapist reduces hand pressure during the patient's inhalation.

Expected Outcomes

- Increase chest wall mobility
- Expand collapsed alveoli via airflow through collateral ventilation channels
- Assist with secretion removal

Sustained maximal inhalation with incentive spirometer[51]

In a sustained maximal inspiration (SMI), a maximal inspiratory effort is held for three or more seconds at the point of maximum inspiration before exhalation. Many airway clearance techniques include SMI to compensate for asynchronous ventilation, to promote air passage past mucus obstructions in airways, and to maximize alveolar expansion. SMI is also called incentive spirometry when using a device that provides visual or other feedback to encourage the patient to take long, slow, deep inhalations (Fig. 6-25).

Indications

- Decreased intrathoracic lung volume
- Decreased chest wall lung compliance
- Increased flow resistance from decreased lung volume
- Ventilation:perfusion (V:Q) mismatch

- Atelectasis or risk of atelectasis due to thoracic and upper abdominal surgery
- Restrictive lung defect associated with quadriplegia and/or dysfunctional diaphragm

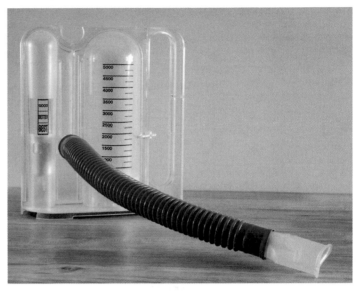

Fig. 6-25: Incentive spirometer.

Precautions/Contraindications

- Patient is not cooperative or is unable to understand or demonstrate proper use of the incentive spirometer.
- Patient is unable to deep breathe effectively (e.g., with vital capacity less than 10 mL/kg or inspiratory capacity less than one-third of predicted).
- Patients with moderate to severe COPD with increased respiratory rate and hyperinflation.

Procedure

- Hold the incentive spirometer in a vertical position.
- Have the patient exhale completely, then seal his lips around the mouthpiece.
- Breathe in slowly and deeply through the mouth, raising the ball or piston of the spirometer.
- Encourage the patient to move the diaphragm and expand the lower chest, not the upper chest.
- Hold the breath for at least three seconds and note the highest level the piston reaches.
- Perform SMI independently five to ten breaths per hour when awake.

Expected Outcomes

- Absence of or improvement in signs of atelectasis
- Decreased respiratory rate
- Resolution of fever
- Normal pulse rate

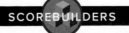

- Normal chest x-ray
- Improved PaO_2
- Increased forced vital capacity and peak expiratory flows

Positions to Relieve Dyspnea

A number of positions may be used to provide relief from dyspnea. The choice of position will depend on the circumstances at the time. The forward leaning position often provides relief of dyspnea to patients with lung disease.

Forward leaning with arm support optimizes the length-tension relationship of the diaphragm and allows the pectoralis minor and pectoralis major muscles to assist in elevating the rib cage during inspiration. The positions may be combined with other breathing techniques.

Reverse Trendelenburg position

The opposite of the Trendelenburg position, the reverse Trendelenburg position places a person in supine with their head above their trunk and lower extremities, decreasing the weight of the abdominal contents on the diaphragm and reducing the resistance to movement during breathing.

Semi-Fowler's position

The semi-Fowler's position places a patient in supine with the head of the bed elevated to 45 degrees and pillows under the knees for support and maintenance of a proper lumbar curve. This position is used often for patients with congestive heart failure or other cardiac conditions.

CONSIDER THIS
MET VALUES OF COMMON PHYSICAL ACTIVITIES[14]

Once the appropriate MET levels for exercise are determined for the patient, activities with the desired aerobic requirement can be selected from a published table of MET values.

Light	Moderate	Vigorous
Walking, Jogging, Running		
Walking slowly at home or office = 2.0	Walking 3 mph = 3.0 – 4.0	Walking 4.5 mph = 6.3
	Walking 4 mph = 4.5 – 7.0	Jogging 5 mph = 8.0
		Running 7 mph = 11.5
Self-care, Household, and Occupation		
Toileting = 1.0 – 2.0	Washing windows or car = 3.0	Shoveling = 7.0
Driving a car = 1.0 – 2.0	Sweeping, vacuuming = 3.0 – 3.5	Carrying heavy loads = 7.5
Working at a computer or desk = 1.5	Light gardening = 3.0 – 4.0	Heavy farm work = 8.0
Making bed, washing dishes = 2.0	Carrying, stacking wood = 5.5	Digging ditches = 9.5
Bathing = 2.0 – 3.0	Power lawn mowing = 5.5	
Cooking = 2.0 – 3.0		
Leisure Time and Sports		
Playing cards, arts, and crafts = 1.5	Slow dancing = 3.0	Backpacking = 5.0 – 11.0
Playing musical instrument = 2.0 – 2.5	Table tennis = 4.0	Basketball game = 8.0
Fishing (sitting) = 2.5	Fast dancing = 4.5	Bicycling (flat) 12 – 14 mph = 8.0
	Basketball shooting around = 4.5	Bicycling (flat) 14 – 16 mph = 10.0
	Sexual intercourse = 4.0 – 5.0	
	Golf (walking) = 4.0 – 7.0	
	Swimming = 4.0 – 8.0	
	Tennis doubles = 5.0	
	Bicycling (flat) 10 – 12 mph = 6.0	

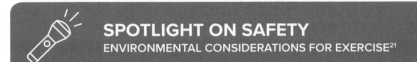

SPOTLIGHT ON SAFETY
ENVIRONMENTAL CONSIDERATIONS FOR EXERCISE[21]

Physical therapist assistants should be aware of the special problems encountered during exercise in hot and cold environments and at high altitudes.

Exercise in Hot Environments

Activity in hot environments should be modified to include access to fluids, increased frequency/duration of rest breaks, and shorter exercise time.

Moderate dehydration (loss of ≥ 6% of body weight) contributes to a drop in exercise performance and increases the risk of heat illness. To maintain hydration, measure body weight before and after exercise and drink at least one pint of fluid for each pound of body weight lost.

Wear clothing with a high wicking capacity to assist in evaporative heat loss. Remove clothing and equipment to permit heat loss, especially head gear.

Signs and symptoms of heat-related illnesses:

Heat stroke: disorientation, dizziness, apathy, headache, nausea, vomiting, hyperventilation, dry skin

Heat exhaustion: low blood pressure, elevated heart rate and respiratory rate, wet and pale skin, weakness, dizziness

Heat syncope: decreased heart rate and respiratory rate, pale skin, weakness, vertigo, nausea

Heat cramps: localized muscle spasms progressing to debilitating muscle cramps

Exercise in Cold Environments

Exercise in the cold may lower the angina threshold and increase the risk of death or injury in individuals with heart disease. Inhalation of cold air may exacerbate asthma.

Signs and symptoms of cold-related illnesses:

Frostbite: Loss of feeling and a white or pale appearance in fingers, toes, ear lobes, and the tip of the nose

Hypothermia: Body temperature < 97° Fahrenheit, shivering, confusion, disorientation, incoherence, poor coordination, slurred speech

Hypothermia develops when heat loss exceeds heat production. Factors that increase the risk of developing hypothermia include water immersion, rain, wet clothing, low body fat, age ≥ 60 years, and hypoglycemia.

Clothing should be adjusted during activity to minimize sweating and reduce sweat accumulation.

Exercise in High-Altitude Environments

The decreased atmospheric pressure at ≥ 5000 feet reduces the partial pressure of oxygen in the air, resulting in decreased arterial oxygen levels. The immediate compensatory responses include increases in ventilation and heart rate and a decrease in performance.

Acclimatization to altitude is the best prevention and treatment for altitude-related illness. Staging, or living at a moderate elevation for as long as one week before ascending to the final elevation, minimizing activity, and maintaining hydration and food intake reduce risk and facilitate recovery. If severe signs and symptoms persist, descending to a lower altitude is effective.

Signs and symptoms of altitude-related illnesses:

Acute mountain sickness: headache, nausea, fatigue, poor appetite and sleep, mild swelling in hands, feet or face

High altitude pulmonary edema: crackles/rales in the lungs, cyanosis of lips and nail beds

GOLD Level Clinical Application Templates

Level Clinical Application Template Executive Summary

Congestive Heart Failure

- Common etiologies contributing to CHF include arrhythmia, pulmonary embolism, hypertension, valvular heart disease, myocarditis, unstable angina, renal failure, and severe anemia
- Left-sided heart failure is generally associated with signs of pulmonary venous congestion; right-sided heart failure is associated with signs of systemic venous congestion
- Diminished cardiac output causes compensatory changes including an increase in blood volume, cardiac filling pressure, heart rate, and cardiac muscle mass

Cystic Fibrosis

- Causes the exocrine glands to overproduce thick mucus which causes subsequent obstruction
- Autosomal recessive genetic disorder (both parents are carriers of the defective gene) located on the long arm of chromosome seven
- The most common cause of death is respiratory failure

Emphysema

- Results from a long history of chronic bronchitis, recurrent alveolar inflammation or from genetic predisposition of a congenital alpha 1-antitrypsin deficiency
- Clinical presentation may include barrel chest appearance, increased subcostal angle, rounded shoulders secondary to tight pectorals, and rosy skin coloring
- Symptoms of emphysema worsen with the progression of the disease and include a persistent cough, wheezing, difficulty breathing especially with expiration, and an increased respiration rate

Myocardial Infarction

- Myocardial infarction occurs when there is poor coronary artery perfusion, ischemia, and subsequent necrosis of the cardiac tissue usually due to thrombus, arterial blockage or atherosclerosis
- Risk factors include patient or family history of heart disease, smoking, physical inactivity, stress, hypertension, elevated cholesterol, diabetes mellitus, and obesity
- Clinical presentation may include deep pain or pressure in the substernal area with or without pain radiating to the jaw or into the left arm or the back

Peripheral Vascular Disease

- Characterized by narrowing of the lumen of blood vessels causing a reduction in circulation usually secondary to atherosclerosis
- Risk factors include phlebitis, injury or surgery, autoimmune disease, diabetes mellitus, smoking, hyperlipidemia, inactivity, hypertension, positive family history, increased age, and obesity
- Patient education is paramount regarding the disease process, limb protection, foot and skin care, and risk factor reduction (smoking cessation, avoid cold exposure)

DIAGNOSIS

What condition produces a patient's symptoms?

Congestive heart failure (CHF) occurs when the heart can no longer meet the metabolic demands of the body. The heart's inability to pump a sufficient amount of blood occurs when there is insufficient or defective cardiac filling and/or impaired contraction and emptying of the heart. The impairment in cardiac output causes the body to compensate for this deficit and this results in an increase in blood volume, cardiac filling pressure, heart rate, and cardiac muscle mass.

An injury was most likely sustained to which structure?

CHF is not an independent disease process but rather a symptom of pathology within the heart muscle itself or in the cardiac valves. Injury within the heart can be left-sided, right-sided or both. The abnormal retention of fluids and diminished blood flow causes further stress and injury to the cardiac system.

INFERENCE

What is the most likely contributing factor in the development of this condition?

There are many pathologies (reversible and irreversible) that can contribute to CHF. Common etiologies shown to contribute to CHF include arrhythmia (e.g., atrial fibrillation), pulmonary embolism, hypertension, valvular heart disease, myocarditis, unstable angina, renal failure, medication-induced problems, high salt intake, and severe anemia. CHF occurs when there is a decrease in cardiac output, abnormalities in skeletal muscle metabolism, impaired left ventricular function or all of the above.

CONFIRMATION

What is the most likely clinical presentation?

A patient with CHF will initially show signs of tachycardia. Other signs include venous congestion, high catecholamine levels, and finally impaired cardiac output. As the severity of CHF increases, signs of venous congestion usually become apparent. Left-sided heart failure is generally associated with signs of pulmonary venous congestion; right-sided heart failure is associated with signs of systemic venous congestion. Impairment to either ventricle can affect the other, leading to both systemic and pulmonary venous congestion. A patient may present with pulmonary edema, nocturnal dyspnea, orthopnea, S3 gallop, dry cough, exertional dyspnea with low level exercise, sudden weight gain, possible cyanotic extremities, cardiac hypertrophy, and shortness of breath.

What laboratory or imaging studies would confirm the diagnosis?

Lab tests including urinalysis and a CBC count that includes electrolyte, thyroid stimulating hormone, blood urea nitrogen (BUN), and serum creatinine levels should be performed. A chest x-ray, electrocardiogram, and echocardiogram are also recommended. A Doppler echocardiogram can determine systolic and diastolic performance, the cardiac output (ejection fraction), and pulmonary artery and ventricular filling pressures.

What additional information should be obtained to confirm the diagnosis?

A patient history and administration of cardiac questionnaires will assist with diagnosis of CHF. In the Framingham classification system, the diagnosis of CHF requires that either two major criteria or one major and two minor criteria be present concurrently. The New York Heart Association Functional Capacity Classification also classifies heart disease based on symptomology as it relates to physical activity.

EXAMINATION

What history should be documented?

Important areas to explore include past medical history, medications, current health status, nutritional status, social history and habits, occupation, living environment, and social support system.

What tests/measures are most appropriate?

Aerobic capacity and endurance: assessment of vital signs at rest and with activity, perceived exertion scale, pulse oximetry, auscultation of the lungs

Anthropometric characteristics: circumferential measurements

Arousal, attention, and cognition: examine mental status, learning ability, memory, motivation

Community and work integration: analysis of community, work, and leisure activities

Environmental, home, and work barriers: analysis of current and potential barriers or hazards

Gait, locomotion, and balance: static and dynamic balance in sitting and standing, safety during gait with/without an assistive device

Integumentary integrity: skin assessment

Muscle performance: strength assessment

Pain: pain perception assessment scale, VAS

Range of motion: active and passive range of motion

Self-care and home management: assessment of functional capacity, Functional Independence Measure

Sensory integrity: proprioception and kinesthesia

Ventilation, respiration, and circulation: assessment of cough and clearance of secretions, breathing patterns, vital capacity, perceived exertion scale, pulse oximetry, palpation of pulses, auscultation of the lungs and heart

What additional findings are likely with this patient?

Diagnoses such as left ventricular infarction, aortic or mitral valve disease, and hypertension create pulmonary congestion that may result in left-sided CHF. Over time, however, fluid accumulation spreads and ankle edema, congestive hepatomegaly, ascites, and pleural effusion occur. This leads the patient to develop right-sided CHF as well. Later stages of CHF are characterized by symptoms of low cardiac output.

MANAGEMENT

What is the most effective management of this patient?

A patient with CHF will be treated based on the root cause of the heart failure. Medical management includes the use of diuretics, nitrates, analgesics, and angiotensin-converting enzyme inhibitor agents. Medications play a vital role in the optimal management of this disease process. Therapists must be aware of the potential side effects such as digitalis toxicity when treating this population. The patient may be referred to physical therapy for generalized conditioning and mobility. Primary goals include improving exercise tolerance and increasing knowledge of the disease process. Therapeutic intervention has to be individualized by each patient since the etiology, current medications, and overall health play a role in the plan of care. Walking is commonly used to initiate an exercise program with cardiac patients. Patients can progress their overall endurance following their own heart rate and perceived exertion guidelines. Caregiver education and instruction may also be appropriate. Psychosocial support, nutritional counseling (no salt diet and no alcohol), and caretaker education are also important components of the plan of care.

What home care regimen should be recommended?

A patient will usually follow a similar program at home once they are discharged from the hospital or in addition to their outpatient therapy. The patient should continue energy conservation and pacing techniques with all activities. The family and patient must be fully educated as to the signs and symptoms of concern as well as potential medication toxicity.

OUTCOME

What is the likely outcome of a course in physical therapy?

A patient can live with CHF and should benefit from physical therapy in order to improve endurance and strength after a decline in function from hospitalization or bed rest. Physical therapy will improve skeletal muscle function, blood flow, metabolic capacity, and overall exercise tolerance. Physical therapy, however, will not cure CHF or its cause.

What are the long-term effects of the patient's condition?

CHF is a common disorder. Approximately 4.6 million Americans are being treated for CHF, and over 500,000 new cases are diagnosed each year. The prevalence of CHF increases significantly with age, occurring in 1-2% of persons aged 50-59 years and in up to 10% of persons older than 75 years. Despite the heart's compensatory mechanisms, the ability of the heart to contract and relax progressively worsens and eventually fails. Thirty-year data from the Framingham heart study demonstrated a median survival of 3.2 years for males and 5.4 years for females after diagnosis.

COMPARISON

What are the distinguishing characteristics of a similar condition?

Cor pulmonale is a form of right-sided heart failure but is normally seen as a consequence of chronic obstructive pulmonary disease. Sustained hypoxia produces an increase in pulmonary artery pressure that leads to right ventricular hypertrophy and finally, right-sided heart failure. When the right side fails, the left side does not receive adequate amounts of blood and then cannot sustain a normal cardiac output. This is not congestive in nature, however, as there is no fluid buildup within the lungs. The right-sided heart failure also does not present with an audible S3 gallop.

CLINICAL SCENARIOS

Scenario One

A 69-year-old male has been hospitalized for five days with congestive heart failure. He was diagnosed last year with the condition and has been doing well on medication. He started having shortness of breath and noted a six pound weight gain. His medications have been adjusted and he is motivated to get home to his wife. The physician requests a physical therapy consult for baseline data and a home exercise program.

Scenario Two

An 82-year-old female resides in a nursing home since her husband who cared for her passed away last summer. She was diagnosed with a left CVA three years ago that resulted in moderate weakness of her right upper extremity and as a result she requires assistance for ADLs. She requires a quad cane and supervision for ambulation. She has been in bed for the last month due to pneumonia and she currently has been diagnosed with CHF.

DIAGNOSIS

What condition produces a patient's symptoms?

Cystic fibrosis (CF) is an inherited disease that affects the ion transport of the exocrine glands resulting in impairment of the hepatic, digestive, respiratory, and reproductive systems. The disease causes the exocrine glands to overproduce thick mucus (that causes subsequent obstruction), overproduce normal secretions or overproduce sodium and chloride.

An injury was most likely sustained to which structure?

CF affects multi-systems within the body, however, the respiratory and gastrointestinal systems are usually the most involved in the disease process. There is an underlying impermeability of epithelial cells to chloride that results in viscosity of mucous gland secretions within the lungs, sweat glands, pancreas, and intestines. CF creates an elevation of sodium chloride and pancreatic enzyme insufficiency.

INFERENCE

What is the most likely contributing factor in the development of this condition?

CF is an autosomal recessive genetic disorder (both parents are carriers of the defective gene) and is located on the long arm of chromosome seven. This disorder creates an abnormality in the CF transmembrane conductance regulator (CFTR) protein. CFTR normally is involved with the process that allows for chloride to pass through the plasma membrane of epithelial cells. It is estimated that 5% of the population carry a recessive gene for CF.

CONFIRMATION

What is the most likely clinical presentation?

CF is the most common lethal genetic disorder affecting Caucasian children in the United States. Incidence is estimated at 1:2,500 births for Caucasians compared to 1:17,000 births for African Americans. CF can be diagnosed shortly after birth, however, it is sometimes not diagnosed for years. The most consistent symptom is the finding of high concentrations of sodium and chloride in the sweat. Parents will notice a salty taste when kissing their child. Other symptoms vary depending on the systems that are affected by the disease and the course of progression. These systems include pulmonary, gastrointestinal, digestive (liver, intestinal, pancreatic), genitourinary, and musculoskeletal impairments. Early symptoms may include a persistent cough, salty skin, sputum production, wheezing, poor weight gain, and recurrent infections.

What laboratory or imaging studies would confirm the diagnosis?

Neonates' meconium can be tested as a screening tool for increased albumin. The quantitative pilocarpine iontophoresis sweat test is the sole diagnostic tool in determining the presence of CF. Sodium and chloride amounts greater than 60 mEq/l (standard value is 40 mEq/l) is a positive diagnosis for CF. The sweat test should be performed twice to ensure accuracy.

What additional information should be obtained to confirm the diagnosis?

Additional information in the diagnosis of CF is found through a positive family history, genetic screening of the parents, a previous diagnosis of failure to thrive, and in the manifestation of symptoms.

EXAMINATION

What history should be documented?

Important areas to explore include past medical history (if diagnosed after birth), medications, current health status, developmental milestones, living environment, and social support system.

What tests/measures are most appropriate?

Aerobic capacity and endurance: assessment of vital signs at rest and with activity, perceived exertion scale

Arousal, attention, and cognition: examine mental status, learning ability, memory, motivation

Assistive and adaptive devices: analysis of components and safety of a device

Integumentary integrity: skin assessment, sweat test findings, clubbing of the digits

Muscle performance: active motion, strength assessment

Posture: analysis of resting and dynamic posture, especially thorax and shoulder girdle

Range of motion: active and passive range of motion, chest wall mobility

Self-care and home management: functional capacity

Ventilation, respiration, and circulation: assess cough and clearance of secretions, pulmonary function testing (FEV_1 and FVC), pulse oximetry, auscultation of the lungs, accessory muscle utilization and vital capacity

Cystic Fibrosis

GOLD

What additional findings are likely with this patient?

The most common complication of CF is an exacerbation of obstructive pulmonary disease. Pulmonary function testing results in a decreased forced expiratory volume (FEV_1) and forced vital capacity (FVC). The functional residual capacity (FRC) and residual volume (RV) become increased. Hypoxemia and hypercapnia develop due to the alteration in perfusion. Chronic pulmonary infections and poor absorption often lead to barrel chest, pectus carinatum, and kyphosis deformities. Approximately 90% of patients have pancreatic enzyme deficiency, degeneration, and eventual progressive fibrosis of the pancreas. This process interferes with digestion and absorption of nutrients. Airway obstruction can cause pulmonary hypertension, atelectasis, pneumonia, and lung abscess. Severe complications can include cirrhosis, diabetes mellitus, pneumothorax, cardiac pathology, pancreatitis, cor pulmonale, and intestinal obstruction.

MANAGEMENT

What is the most effective management of this patient?

Medical management of CF is a multidisciplinary approach that should focus on the quality of life, providing emotional and psychosocial support, and controlling symptoms. Nutritional support is necessary throughout the patient's life to ensure adequate nutrition. Pharmacological intervention is required to treat infections, thin mucus secretions, replace pancreatic enzymes, reduce inflammation, and assist with breathing. Psychological counseling is indicated as needed. Gene therapy is experimental and attempts to correct the defect in CF cells. Physical therapy intervention is essential for management of the disease. Chest physical therapy should be performed several times per day and includes postural drainage, percussion, vibration, breathing and assistive cough techniques, and ventilatory muscle training. Posture training, mobilization of the thorax, and breathing exercises must be incorporated into the overall program. A patient may also be trained to use autogenic drainage, a positive expiratory pressure (PEP) device or Flutter valve therapy to assist with independent postural drainage. General exercise and stretching are indicated to optimize overall function. Family and patient education are vital to the survival of the patient.

What home care regimen should be recommended?

A home care regimen for a patient with CF requires an ongoing routine performing postural drainage and chest physical therapy several times each day. Family members are trained to provide this ongoing support at home. Mechanical percussors may be used to ease the time and energy spent on manual percussion by the care provider. Mechanical percussors also offer the patient control and independence with treatment. Physical conditioning including exercise and endurance training are indicated except with severe lung disease. Exercise programs may improve pulmonary function, increase maximal work capacity, improve mucus expectoration, and increase self-esteem.

OUTCOME

What is the likely outcome of a course in physical therapy?

A patient with CF will require intermittent physical therapy throughout his or her life. The goals of physical therapy are to maximize secretion clearance from the lungs, optimize pulmonary function, and maximize the patient's quality of life.

What are the long-term effects of the patient's condition?

CF is a terminal disease, however, the median age of death has increased to 35 years of age due to early detection and comprehensive management. The most common cause of death for patients with CF remains respiratory failure. A child that initially presents with gastrointestinal symptoms generally has a good clinical course whereas a child that initially presents with pulmonary symptoms is more likely to clinically deteriorate at a faster pace. Males generally have a better prognosis than females.

COMPARISON

What are the distinguishing characteristics of a similar condition?

There is no other respiratory disease that is similar to the etiology of CF, however, chronic obstructive pulmonary disease (COPD) has similar lung characteristics. COPD is characterized by altered pulmonary function tests, difficulty with expiration, cough, sputum production, and physical damage to specific portions of the lungs. Chest physical therapy and pharmacological intervention are indicated for moderate to advanced COPD.

CLINICAL SCENARIOS

Scenario One

A four-week-old infant is referred to physical therapy after being diagnosed with CF. The infant has a pleasant disposition and does not have any observable discomfort, however, the parents are very anxious. The patient has three siblings that do not have CF.

Scenario Two

A 26-year-old female with CF is referred to physical therapy with a severe respiratory infection. The patient recently moved into an apartment with her boyfriend and works 30 hours per week in a hair salon. Prior to the infection the patient was living at home and was able to manage the disease with occasional assistance from family members. The physical therapy referral is for chest physical therapy.

DIAGNOSIS

What condition produces a patient's symptoms?

Emphysema refers to a pathologic accumulation of air in the lungs found with chronic obstructive pulmonary disease (COPD). There are three classifications of emphysema that include centrilobular emphysema, panlobular emphysema, and paraseptal emphysema. Emphysema results from a long history of chronic bronchitis, recurrent alveolar inflammation or from genetic predisposition of a congenital alpha 1-antitrypsin deficiency.

An injury was most likely sustained to which structure?

Emphysema results from a non-reversible injury and destruction of elastin protein within the alveolar walls. This process causes permanent enlargement of the air spaces distal to the terminal bronchioles within the lungs. Anatomical changes include loss of elastic recoil, excessive airway collapse during exhalation, and chronic obstruction of airflow. Progression of the disease includes further destruction of the alveolar walls, collapse of the peripheral bronchioles, and impaired gas exchange. Emphysema causes pockets of air to form between the alveolar spaces, (known as blebs), and within the lung parenchyma (known as bullae). This results in an increase in dead space within the lungs that diminishes gas exchange.

INFERENCE

What is the most likely contributing factor in the development of this condition?

The primary risk factors for the development of emphysema include chronic bronchitis, lower respiratory infections, cigarette smoking, and genetic predisposition. Environmental influence includes air pollution and other airborne toxins. The risk of acquiring emphysema increases with age.

CONFIRMATION

What is the most likely clinical presentation?

COPD is the second leading cause of disability in individuals under 65 years of age worldwide. There are two million individuals in the United States diagnosed with emphysema (and another 14 million with some form of COPD). Emphysema can be asymptomatic until middle age and is most often diagnosed between 55 and 60 years of age. Centrilobular emphysema usually destroys the bronchioles in the upper lungs while the alveolar sacs usually remain intact. Panlobular emphysema destroys the air spaces of the acinus and is usually found in the lower lungs. Paraseptal emphysema destroys the alveoli in the lower lobes resulting in blebs along the lung periphery. Symptoms of emphysema worsen with the progression of the disease and include a persistent cough, wheezing, difficulty breathing especially with expiration, and an increased respiration rate. Advanced disease symptoms include increased use of accessory muscles, severe dyspnea, cor pulmonale, and cyanosis.

What laboratory or imaging studies would confirm the diagnosis?

X-ray is utilized to visually evaluate the shape and spacing of the lungs. Other imaging studies include a planogram to detect bullae and a bronchogram to evaluate mucus ducts and detect possible enlargement of the bronchi. Arterial blood gases may indicate a decreased PaO_2.

What additional information should be obtained to confirm the diagnosis?

A physical examination, thorough patient history (including cigarette smoking), and pulmonary function tests are required for diagnosis. Pulmonary function testing will result in impaired forced expiratory volume (FEV_1), vital capacity (VC), and forced vital capacity (FVC). Total lung capacity (TLC), residual volume (RV), and functional residual capacity (FRC) will be increased.

EXAMINATION

What history should be documented?

Important areas to explore include past medical history, history of smoking, medications, current health status, social history and habits, occupation, living environment, and social support system.

What tests/measures are most appropriate?

Aerobic capacity and endurance: assessment of vital signs at rest and with activity, perceived exertion scale, Six-Minute Walk Test, Three-Minute Step Test

Arousal, attention, and cognition: examine mental status, learning ability, memory, motivation

Assistive and adaptive devices: analysis of components and safety of a device

Environmental, home, and work: analysis of current and potential barriers or hazards

Gait, locomotion, and balance: static and dynamic balance in sitting and standing, safety during gait with/without an assistive device

Muscle performance: strength assessment, assessment of active movement, and muscle endurance

Posture: analysis of resting and dynamic posture

Self-care and home management: functional capacity

Ventilation, respiration, and circulation: assessment of thoracoabdominal movement, auscultation of vesicular sounds/potential rhonchi, pulse oximetry, pulmonary function testing, accessory muscle utilization

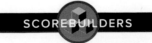

Emphysema

What additional findings are likely with this patient?

A patient with emphysema may present with a barrel chest appearance, an increased subcostal angle, rounded shoulders secondary to tight pectorals, rosy skin coloring, and may utilize pursed-lip breathing to assist with ventilation. Patients will also have high rates of anxiety associated with difficulty breathing and may present with claustrophobia, insomnia, and depression. Complications such as the formation and rupture of bullae and blebs can lead to pneumothorax. Cor pulmonale is a serious complication that can occur with advanced emphysema.

MANAGEMENT

What is the most effective management of this patient?

Medical management of a patient with emphysema includes pharmacological intervention, oxygen therapy, and physical therapy. Pharmacological intervention promotes bronchodilation, improved oxygenation, and ventilation. Drugs such as oral/inhaled bronchodilators, anti-inflammatory agents, mucolytic expectorants, mast cell membrane stabilizers, and antihistamines may be used in the treatment of emphysema. Preventative immunizations against influenza and pneumonia are also recommended. Physical therapy intervention is based on the severity of the disease process and can include general exercise and endurance training, breathing exercises including pursed-lip breathing, ventilatory muscle strengthening, chest wall exercises, and patient education on posture, airway secretion clearance, and energy conservation techniques. Pulse oximetry should be used to monitor a patient's oxygen saturation during activities and exercise. This will assist with patient education and deter the effects of hypoxemia. Chest physical therapy is required during advanced stages of emphysema.

What home care regimen should be recommended?

The home care regimen should include breathing strategies and exercises, energy conservation, pacing techniques, and general strength and endurance training.

OUTCOME

What is the likely outcome of a course in physical therapy?

A patient with emphysema may require physical therapy intermittently as the disease progresses. The goals of physical therapy are to maximize the patient's functional abilities and optimize pulmonary function.

What are the long-term effects of the patient's condition?

Emphysema is a chronic progressive disease process. Patients require ongoing medical care and intermittent physical therapy intervention. Life expectancy decreases to less than five years with severe expiratory slowing measured at a rate of <1L of air during forced expiratory volume (FEV_1).

COMPARISON

What are the distinguishing characteristics of a similar condition?

Bronchiectasis is inherited or acquired and is characterized by chronic inflammation and dilation of bronchi and destruction of the bronchial walls. This disease is associated with chronic bacterial infections and is an extreme form of bronchitis. Incidence within the United States is low. Bronchiectasis has a higher risk for development in patients with cystic fibrosis, sinusitis, Kartagener's syndrome, and endobronchial tumors. Characteristics include a chronic cough with sputum, hemoptysis, wheezing, dyspnea, and recurrent respiratory infections. Primary treatment includes physical therapy, bronchodilators, and antibiotics.

CLINICAL SCENARIOS

Scenario One

A 65-year-old male is referred to physical therapy after recently being diagnosed with emphysema. The patient works in an oil refinery part-time and manages a small dairy farm. The patient's past medical history is negative for smoking and consists of recurrent respiratory infections and chronic cough. The patient complains of shortness of breath with exertion, however, pulmonary function testing indicates only minimal impairment in lung volumes.

Scenario Two

A 75-year-old female requires physical therapy for management of emphysema. The patient has a history of smoking cigarettes for over 40 years and continues to smoke approximately one pack per day. The patient has an oxygen saturation rate of 94% at rest and requires two liters of oxygen with exertion. The patient has moderate impairment in pulmonary function testing and a persistent cough. The patient presently resides in a two-story home and assists with the care of her disabled husband.

DIAGNOSIS

What condition produces a patient's symptoms?

Myocardial infarction (MI) occurs when there is poor coronary artery perfusion, ischemia, and subsequent necrosis of the cardiac tissue usually due to thrombus, arterial blockage or atherosclerosis. The location and severity of the infarct will determine symptoms and the overall acute clinical picture.

An injury was most likely sustained to which structure?

A MI produces ischemia and subsequent necrosis to a portion of the myocardium. The extent of the damage to the myocardium is dependent on the duration of ischemia and on the thickness of the tissue involved. A transmural MI involves the full-thickness of the myocardium while a nontransmural MI involves the subendocardial area (inner third of the myocardium). The myocardium has three zones that form concentric circles around the point of infarct termed zone of infarct, zone of hypoxic injury, and zone of ischemia. Thrombosis of the anterior descending branch of the left coronary artery is the most common location of infarct and affects the left ventricle. A right coronary artery thrombosis can result in an infarct of the posteroinferior portion of the left ventricle and can potentially affect the right ventricular myocardium.

INFERENCE

What is the most likely contributing factor in the development of this condition?

The primary risk factors for MI include patient or family history of heart disease, smoking, physical inactivity, stress, hypertension, elevated cholesterol, diabetes mellitus, and obesity. The use of cocaine and aortic stenosis may also cause a MI. It has been documented that a MI will occur more frequently in the morning hours and during the November to December holiday season.

CONFIRMATION

What is the most likely clinical presentation?

MI occurs in 1.5 million individuals each year within the United States with a mortality rate of 500,000 deaths annually. Approximately two-thirds of patients experience prodromal symptoms days to weeks before the event, including unstable angina, shortness of breath, and fatigue. A patient that is experiencing a MI will initially present with deep pain or pressure in the substernal area. The pain may or may not radiate to the jaw and down the left arm or to the back. The patient cannot alleviate the pain with rest or nitroglycerin and the pain may last for hours. The patient is usually anxious, pale, sweating, fatigued, and may present with nausea and vomiting. Symptoms of a MI frequently do not follow a typical pattern, especially in females. There are also instances of a silent MI where no symptoms are noted.

What laboratory or imaging studies would confirm the diagnosis?

The primarily tool to detect a MI is a 12-lead electrocardiogram. An inverted T wave indicates myocardial ischemia, elevated ST segment indicates acute infarction, and a depressed ST segment indicates a pending subendocardial or transmural infarction. A blood serum analysis can be utilized to determine the level of selected cardiac enzymes. The level of selected enzymes such as creatine phosphokinase (CPK), aspartate transferase (AST), and lactic dehydrogenase (LDH) can be dramatically altered during and after a MI. A complete blood count (CBC), chest radiograph, radionuclide imaging, and amylase level may be ordered to assist with the diagnosis.

What additional information should be obtained to confirm the diagnosis?

Additional information in the diagnosis of a MI is found through the manifestation of symptoms and clinical examination including a thorough past medical history and history of current symptoms.

EXAMINATION

What history should be documented?

Important areas to explore include past medical history, family history, medications, current health status, living environment, social history and habits, occupation, and social support system.

What tests/measures are most appropriate?

Aerobic capacity and endurance: vital signs at rest and during activity, palpation of pulses, perceived exertion scale, electrocardiogram analysis, auscultation of the heart and lungs, pulse oximetry

Arousal, attention, and cognition: examine mental status, learning ability, memory, motivation

Assistive and adaptive devices: analysis of components and safety of a device

Environmental, home, and work: analysis of current and potential barriers or hazards

Gait, locomotion, and balance: assessment of static and dynamic balance in sitting and standing, safety during gait with/without an assistive device

Muscle performance: strength assessment through active movement only (no manual muscle testing)

Pain: pain perception scale, visual analogue scale

Posture: analysis of resting and dynamic posture

Self-care and home management: assessment of functional capacity, Barthel Index

Ventilation, respiration, and circulation: ventilation, respiration, and circulation; assessment of pulses

Myocardial Infarction   GOLD

What additional findings are likely with this patient?

A patient status post MI is at risk for complications that include arrhythmias, hypotension, pericarditis, impaired cardiac output, pulmonary edema, congestive heart failure, cardiogenic shock, recurrent infarction, and sudden death. Arrhythmias occur in 90% of patients post MI and are caused by ischemia, ANS impairment, electrolyte imbalances, conduction defects, and other chemical imbalances.

MANAGEMENT

What is the most effective management of this patient?

Initial medical management of a MI is to stabilize the patient and initiate pharmacological intervention to hinder the evolution of the MI. Anticoagulants, beta-blockers, thrombolytic agents, angiotensin-converting enzyme inhibitors, vasodilators, and estrogen (in women) may be used. Once stable, the patient is managed through a cardiac rehabilitation program. Surgical intervention including angioplasty, stenting, endarterectomy, and bypass grafting may be indicated based on the underlying cause of the MI. Exercise testing is performed within three days of the MI in order to establish baseline guidelines for patients that are cleared to exercise and do not exhibit any arrhythmias or angina. Physical therapy intervention usually follows a multi-phase cardiac rehabilitation program and continues in an outpatient setting once the patient is discharged from the hospital. Low-level therapeutic exercise, functional activities, relaxation, breathing techniques, endurance training, and continuous monitoring of vital signs are key components of this program. Patient education regarding reduction of risk factors, return to activity, and commitment to fitness and health are also important to the success of physical therapy intervention.

What home care regimen should be recommended?

A home care regimen should follow the guidelines indicated for each phase of cardiac rehabilitation. A patient must continue with safe exercise and integration of risk factor reduction. Symptom recognition and nutritional strategies are also important in a daily routine.

OUTCOME

What is the likely outcome of a course in physical therapy?

Cardiac rehabilitation is recommended status post MI. The patient should start in the coronary care unit (CCU) and progress through each of the phases of cardiac rehabilitation. The goal is successful completion of a cardiac rehabilitation program allowing the patient to resume all activities of daily living and recreational pursuits. Upon completion, the patient should possess self-management skills associated with symptoms/risk factors of heart disease.

What are the long-term effects of the patient's condition?

A patient that has experienced a MI may be able to return to all previous activities after successful completion of a cardiac rehabilitation program. A patient must continue to reduce the modifiable risk factors and maintain an appropriate level of exercise in order to limit a possible subsequent MI. Long-term outcome is dependent on prior functional ability, the extent and damage to the heart, and factors that negatively affect prognosis such as age, cardiovascular disease, hypotension, the presence of co-morbidities, and an abnormal treadmill exercise test.

COMPARISON

What are the distinguishing characteristics of a similar condition?

Angina pectoris is a myocardial ischemic disorder that occurs when there is an oxygen deficit to the coronary arteries. Coronary artery disease accounts for 90% of all cases of angina. Angina is classified as stable, post-infarction, Prinzmetal's, resting, unstable, nocturnal or variant. Symptoms often occur during exertion and include chest pain that may radiate. Rest or nitroglycerin normally provides relief of the symptoms. Treatment of the underlying cause is essential to prevent further damage to the heart.

CLINICAL SCENARIOS

Scenario One

A 51-year-old male is referred to a phase I cardiac rehabilitation program after a transmural MI two days ago. The patient has hypertension, high cholesterol, smokes, and is obese. The patient currently supervises a local automobile dealership. The patient is divorced and lives in a two-story home.

Scenario Two

A 78-year-old female is status post nontransmural MI. The patient is very active and plays golf. The patient's past medical history includes treatment for a cardiac arrhythmia, obesity, and diabetes mellitus. The physician referred the patient for cardiac rehabilitation.

Peripheral Vascular Disease

DIAGNOSIS

What condition produces a patient's symptoms?

Peripheral vascular disease (PVD) is a condition where there has been narrowing of the lumen of blood vessels causing a reduction in circulation usually secondary to atherosclerosis. This can be compounded by either emboli or thrombi.

An injury was most likely sustained to which structure?

PVD, also known as arteriosclerosis obliterans, is primarily the result of atherosclerosis. Damage can occur to the walls of both arteries and veins from fatty plaque buildup that creates hard and narrow vessels. The atherosclerotic process will gradually progress to significant or complete occlusion of medium and large arteries.

INFERENCE

What is the most likely contributing factor in the development of this condition?

The primary factor for developing PVD is atherosclerosis. Other etiologies and risk factors that have been associated with the development of PVD may include phlebitis, injury or surgery, autoimmune disease, diabetes mellitus, smoking, hyperlipidemia, inactivity, hypertension, positive family history, increased age, and obesity.

CONFIRMATION

What is the most likely clinical presentation?

Symptoms and clinical presentation will differ depending on which vessel or blood flow has been compromised. During the early stages of PVD intermittent claudication may be the only manifestation. Symptoms are precipitated by walking a predictable distance and are normally relieved by rest. Claudication also may present as buckling or "giving out" of the lower extremity after a certain period of exertion and may not demonstrate the typical symptom of pain on exertion. Other symptoms may include tingling and numbness of the affected extremities, pain at rest and during sleep, slowed healing, changes in skin coloring, a decrease in skin temperature, absence of hair on the extremity, and a weak or absent pulse.

What laboratory or imaging studies would confirm the diagnosis?

Routine blood tests generally are indicated and include CBC, BUN, creatinine, and electrolytes studies. Doppler ultrasound studies are used to determine flow status. MRI, angiogram or arteriogram can also be used to assist with the diagnosis.

What additional information should be obtained to confirm the diagnosis?

The ankle-brachial index (ABI) can be used to provide a ratio of systolic blood pressure of the lower extremity compared to the upper extremity. A rubor of dependency test, transcutaneous oximetry, and treadmill exercise test may also assist with baseline information and diagnosis of insufficiency.

EXAMINATION

What history should be documented?

Important areas to explore include past medical history, medications, current health status, nutritional status, social history and habits, occupation, living environment, and social support system.

What tests/measures are most appropriate?

Aerobic capacity and endurance: assessment of vital signs at rest and with activity, perceived exertion scale, pulse oximetry, auscultation of the lungs

Arousal, attention, and cognition: examine mental status, memory, motivation

Assistive and adaptive devices: analysis of components and safety of a device

Community and work integration: analysis of community, work, and leisure activities

Environmental, home, and work barriers: analysis of current and potential barriers or hazards

Gait, locomotion, and balance: static and dynamic balance in sitting and standing, safety during gait with/without an assistive device, Functional Ambulation Profile

Integumentary integrity: skin assessment, assessment of sensation

Muscle performance: strength assessment

Pain: pain perception assessment scale, visual analogue scale, assessment of muscle soreness

Posture: analysis of resting and dynamic posture

Range of motion: active and passive range of motion

Self-care and home management: assessment of functional capacity, Functional Independence Measure

Sensory integrity: proprioception and kinesthesia

Ventilation, respiration, and circulation: palpation of pulses, pulse oximetry, ABI, capillary refilling test

Peripheral Vascular Disease   GOLD

What additional findings are likely with this patient?

Ischemic rest pain can occur from the combination of PVD and inadequate perfusion. It is fairly common for a patient with PVD to be diagnosed with coronary artery disease or diabetes mellitus. There is a higher risk for complications such as deep vein thrombosis, insufficiency ulcers, gangrene, and amputation.

MANAGEMENT

What is the most effective management of this patient?

The medical management of a patient with PVD should include a physician, psychiatrist or psychologist, nurse, nutritionist, occupational therapist, physical therapist, vocational therapist, and case manager. Pharmacological intervention may be utilized to reduce morbidity and prevent complications. Anticoagulants such as heparin, antiplatelet agents and thrombolytics may be indicated. Patient education is paramount regarding the disease process, limb protection, foot and skin care, and risk factor reduction (smoking cessation, avoid cold exposure). Physical therapy is an important component in the treatment of PVD. A walking program will initially have the patient walk until near maximal pain and then rest until the pain is relieved. The goal is to have the patient achieve longer walking periods with less rest, eventually walking for 30 minutes continuously. Non-weight bearing exercises such as swimming or stationary cycling can supplement the program. After 4-6 weeks of therapy including isometric and active range exercises, the patient should tolerate the implementation of resistive exercise. Physical rehabilitation, involving dynamic aerobic exercise and resistance training improves cardiovascular endurance and demonstrates a positive impact on patient function and independence. In more severe cases, surgical intervention may be required. Common procedures include balloon angioplasty, endarterectomy, stent implantation or bypass surgery.

What home care regimen should be recommended?

A patient must continue with their walking program and a generalized exercise program to tolerance. They should perform skin and foot inspections daily and continue with smoking cessation and a low cholesterol diet. For patients with pain at rest, particularly at night, the head of the bed should be elevated 4-6 inches, which should improve lower extremity perfusion by the effects of gravity on blood flow.

OUTCOME

What is the likely outcome of a course in physical therapy?

Physical therapy can be instrumental in managing PVD through education of the disease process, implementing a walking program that allows for the development of collateral circulation, and designing an exercise program that allows the patient to gain strength and endurance for activities. The patient must have the desire, discipline, and motivation to continue with habit modification and maintain their exercise regimen in order to be successful.

What are the long-term effects of the patient's condition?

PVD can be controllable with pharmacological treatment, risk factor reduction, and in some cases, surgical intervention. Patients with PVD are at a higher risk overall for complications such as permanent numbness, tingling or weakness in lower extremities and/or feet, permanent sensory changes such as burning or aching pain, gangrene, and amputation of the affected body part. Patients with PVD are also at higher risk of heart attack and stroke. Symptomatic PVD has at least a 30% risk of death within five years and approximately 50% in ten years, secondary to MI or cerebrovascular disease.

COMPARISON

What are the distinguishing characteristics of a similar condition?

Coronary artery disease (CAD) is the narrowing or blockage due to fatty build up (cholesterol) within the artery walls reducing the overall blood flow to the cardiac muscle. Patient symptoms will vary based on the location and severity of blockage. Patients range from asymptomatic to symptoms at rest. These symptoms can include nausea, vomiting, heartburn, shortness of breath, and profuse sweating. Risk factors include hypertension, smoking, obesity, stress, elevated cholesterol, and sedentary lifestyle. Electrocardiograms and angiograms are typically used to diagnose CAD.

CLINICAL SCENARIOS

Scenario One

A 66-year-old male is seen in physical therapy with a new diagnosis of PVD. The patient's past medical history consists of L5 disc herniation with surgical stabilization and type 2 diabetes mellitus. The patient complains of increasing lower extremity pain with ambulation while at his job as a surveyor. The patient lives alone and has two dogs.

Scenario Two

An 82-year-old female is seen in physical therapy in an acute care hospital with orders for whirlpool secondary to an ulcer on her right lower extremity. The patient has moderate to severe PVD affecting both lower extremities. She presents with sensory loss and significant pain with ambulation greater than 20 feet. She also complains of pain at night. She resides with her husband in a first floor apartment.

SILVER   Level Clinical Application Templates

SILVER **Level Clinical Application Template Executive Summary**

Angina Pectoris

- Results from diminished myocardial perfusion, most commonly caused by narrowing of one or more of the coronary arteries (e.g., due to embolism, atherosclerosis, inflammation)
- Described as an uncomfortable or painful feeling of tightness, pressure, fullness or squeezing in the center of the chest
- Medical management varies greatly with symptom severity and type (i.e., stable versus unstable), focusing primarily on the underlying pathology

Coronary Artery Disease

- Occurs as a result of atherosclerotic plaque buildup within the coronary arteries; develops slowly, often going unnoticed for years before producing symptoms
- Risk factors include hypertension, diabetes, obesity, chronic kidney disease, elevated cholesterol and triglyceride levels, and a family history of the condition
- Cardiac rehabilitation is recommended and upon completion, the patient should possess self-management skills associated with symptom recognition and reduction of risk factors

Hypertension

- A condition in which blood pressure is persistently elevated; Stage 1 hypertension: 130–139 mm Hg systolic blood pressure or 80–89 mm Hg diastolic blood pressure; Stage 2 hypertension: at least 140 mm Hg systolic blood pressure or at least 90 mm Hg diastolic blood pressure
- Symptoms may not be recognized until blood pressure becomes dangerously high producing a headache, confusion, visual changes, fatigue, arrhythmia or tinnitus
- Medical management is largely focused on risk reduction through modifiable risk factors and pharmacological intervention

Restrictive Lung Disease

- Classification of disorders caused by a pulmonary or extrapulmonary restriction that produces impairment in lung expansion and an abnormal reduction in pulmonary ventilation
- Pulmonary restriction of the lungs can be caused by tumor, interstitial pulmonary fibrosis, scarring within the lungs, pleural effusion, chest wall stiffness, structural abnormality, and respiratory muscle weakness
- Pathogenesis includes a decrease in lung and chest wall compliance, decrease in lung volumes, and an increase in the work of breathing

Angina Pectoris

DIAGNOSIS

What condition produces a patient's symptoms?

Angina pectoris results from diminished myocardial perfusion, most commonly caused by narrowing of one or more of the coronary arteries (e.g., due to embolism, atherosclerosis, inflammation). When the tissue's oxygen demand is greater than that provided by the coronary arteries, myocardial ischemia results producing characteristic chest pain. This specific type of pain is termed angina pectoris and is most commonly associated with underlying coronary artery disease (CAD).

An injury was most likely sustained to which structure?

Angina pectoris is not an independent disease process, but rather a symptom of myocardial ischemia. Damage to the myocardial tissue is dependent on the location, extent, and duration of the ischemia. Certain etiologies may also result in localized vessel damage, as well as narrowing or blockages that can produce angina.

INFERENCE

What is the most likely contributing factor in the development of this condition?

Risk factors for angina pectoris are consistent with those of CAD and include a family history of heart disease, smoking, physical inactivity, stress, hypertension, elevated cholesterol, diabetes mellitus, and obesity.

CONFIRMATION

What is the most likely clinical presentation?

Angina pectoris is typically described as an uncomfortable or painful feeling of tightness, pressure, fullness or squeezing in the center of the chest. Symptoms will typically present on the left side of the body in the back, arm, shoulder, neck or jaw when accompanied by radiating pain. Shortness of breath and unexplained fatigue are also frequently reported. Angina pectoris may be classified as either stable or unstable. Stable angina occurs predictably in response to activities that increase the oxygen demands of myocardial tissue (e.g., exercise, stress, cold weather, large meals). Stable angina symptoms typically do not last longer than 15 minutes and are relieved with rest or nitroglycerin. Unstable angina is typically considered to be more serious since it occurs without cause and is often unresponsive to nitroglycerin.

What laboratory or imaging studies would confirm the diagnosis?

A 12-lead electrocardiogram (ECG) is most commonly used to diagnose angina pectoris with an inverted T wave indicating myocardial ischemia. In patients with normal resting ECG readings, a more provocative exercise ECG or stress test may be required. A diagnosis of angina pectoris is most often confirmed by first diagnosing the underlying pathology causing the ischemia.

What additional information should be obtained to confirm the diagnosis?

A thorough medical history should be completed to assist in identifying cardiac risk factors. The patient's history of symptoms should include detail regarding exacerbating and alleviating factors. A thorough clinical examination should also be performed in order to rule out similar diagnoses.

MANAGEMENT

What is the most effective management of this patient?

The medical management of angina pectoris varies greatly with symptom severity and type (i.e., stable versus unstable), focusing primarily on the underlying pathology. Pharmacological intervention may target vessel relaxation, heart rate, the blood's clotting ability or cholesterol levels. Aspirin, nitrates, beta-blockers, statins, calcium channel blockers, and ACE inhibitors may be used in the treatment of angina. The goal of surgical intervention is typically to widen a coronary artery in order to improve blood flow. Angioplasty, stent placement, endarterectomy, and coronary artery bypass graft are common surgical procedures. Lifestyle changes such as smoking cessation, weight management, increased activity level, and stress management are recommended. Physical therapy intervention usually follows a multi-phase cardiac rehabilitation program for patients with stable angina.

What home care regimen should be recommended?

A home care regimen should follow the guidelines indicated for each phase of cardiac rehabilitation. Patients should continue to safely exercise and incorporate the reduction of modifiable risk factors. Symptom recognition and nutritional management are also important in a daily routine.

OUTCOME

What is the likely outcome of a course of physical therapy?

Cardiac rehabilitation is recommended for patients with angina pectoris. Patients with stable angina that are managed with lifestyle changes and medication may initiate cardiac rehabilitation in an outpatient setting. The goal is successful completion of the cardiac rehabilitation program, allowing the patient to resume all activities of daily living and recreational pursuits.

What are the long-term effects of the patient's condition?

Patients with angina pectoris typically have some degree of pre-existing cardiac pathology. These patients are at an increased risk for developing cardiac arrhythmias or experiencing a myocardial infarction or cardiac arrest. The severity of risk is linked to the severity of the underlying disease process as well as prior cardiac history and the patient's response to pharmaceutical management.

Coronary Artery Disease   SILVER

DIAGNOSIS

What condition produces a patient's symptoms?

Coronary artery disease (CAD) occurs as a result of atherosclerotic plaque buildup within the coronary arteries. The plaque is primarily comprised of fatty deposits containing cholesterol and other blood products that accumulate over time. CAD typically develops slowly and often goes unnoticed for years before producing symptoms.

An injury was most likely sustained to which structure?

The right and left coronary arteries are branches of the ascending aorta. The right coronary artery primarily supplies the right atrium and ventricle and the left coronary artery primarily supplies the left atrium and ventricle. As plaques develop, the arteries harden and narrow, decreasing the volume of blood available to perfuse cardiac tissue when demand is increased. Diminished perfusion significantly increases the risk of myocardial ischemia and permanent cardiac damage.

INFERENCE

What is the most likely contributing factor in the development of this condition?

The risk factors for CAD include hypertension, diabetes, obesity, chronic kidney disease, elevated cholesterol and triglyceride levels, and family history. Modifiable risk factors include smoking, inactivity, alcohol abuse, and stress.

CONFIRMATION

What is the most likely clinical presentation?

Certain patients with CAD never develop symptoms or complications from the disease. In others, symptoms typically develop when arteries are no longer able to adequately perfuse cardiac tissue resulting in ischemia. The severity of symptoms varies with the exacerbating activity and degree of occlusion. A partial occlusion may cause exertion-related shortness of breath, weakness or angina pectoris and is often the initial indicator of underlying pathology. In some cases, however, the first symptom of CAD may be as severe as a myocardial infarction secondary to plaques that have completely occluded an artery.

What laboratory or imaging studies would confirm the diagnosis?

Cardiac catheterization with coronary angiography introduces contrast dye via small catheters into the coronary arteries for x-ray imaging. This invasive diagnostic procedure provides the most accurate information regarding both the location and severity of CAD. CT scan and magnetic resonance coronary angiograms provide a less invasive means of visualizing the coronary arteries with contrast dye introduced either intravenously or via injection.

What additional information should be obtained to confirm the diagnosis?

A thorough medical history should be completed to assist in identifying cardiac risk factors. The patient's history should include details of symptoms including alleviating and exacerbating factors, frequency, and duration. A thorough clinical examination should also be performed in order to rule out similar diagnoses.

MANAGEMENT

What is the most effective management of this patient?

The medical management of CAD is largely focused on risk reduction and pharmacological intervention. Lifestyle changes are typically recommended to address modifiable risk factors. Pharmacological agents facilitate vessel relaxation, modify heart rate or reduce the blood's clotting ability or cholesterol levels. Aspirin, nitrates, beta-blockers, statins, calcium channel blockers, and ACE inhibitors may be used alone or in combination. Surgical intervention is typically performed to widen one or more of the coronary arteries in order to improve blood flow. Angioplasty, stent placement, endarterectomy, and coronary artery bypass are common surgical procedures. Physical therapy intervention is typically provided through a formal multi-phase cardiac rehabilitation program. Patients who have undergone surgical intervention will begin during their inpatient stay. Others may begin cardiac rehabilitation on an outpatient basis. Patients should be educated regarding target heart rate zones and self-monitoring of cardiac status during exercise.

What home care regimen should be recommended?

A home care regimen should follow the guidelines indicated for each phase of cardiac rehabilitation. Patients should continue to safely exercise and incorporate healthy habits. Nutritional management and the ability to recognize symptoms of cardiac distress are also important in a daily routine.

OUTCOME

What is the likely outcome of a course of physical therapy?

Cardiac rehabilitation is recommended for patients diagnosed with CAD. At the conclusion of physical therapy, the patient should possess self-management skills associated with symptom recognition and the reduction of cardiac risk factors.

What are the long-term effects of the patient's condition?

Patients diagnosed with CAD are at increased risk of developing angina pectoris, heart failure, cardiac arrhythmias, and cardiac arrest. The severity of risk is linked to the severity of disease. The patient's response to pharmacological and lifestyle interventions can also influence the overall risk of complications.

Hypertension

DIAGNOSIS

What condition produces a patient's symptoms?

Hypertension (HTN) is a condition in which blood pressure is persistently elevated. Primary HTN occurs without an identifiable cause and typically develops slowly over time. Secondary HTN occurs as a result of underlying pathology (e.g., pre-eclampsia, kidney disease, congenital vessel defects, atherosclerosis, stress) or as a side effect of certain medications.

An injury was most likely sustained to which structure?

Blood pressure measures represent the force of blood against interior arterial walls. The systolic component represents the maximum pressure exerted as the heart contracts. The diastolic component represents the minimum pressure exerted when the heart is at rest. In patients with primary HTN, increased forces may cause damage to the arteries, increasing the risk of more serious comorbidities such as CVA or MI. For patients with secondary HTN, structural injuries may also be linked to the specific underlying pathology.

INFERENCE

What is the most likely contributing factor in the development of this condition?

Patients of African descent, men, post-menopausal women, and those with a family history of HTN have a higher risk of developing HTN. Risk increases further with age. Certain conditions (e.g., pregnancy, diabetes, sleep apnea) and modifiable risk factors (e.g., obesity, sedentary lifestyle, stress, tobacco use, excessive alcohol use, excess dietary sodium) are also associated with HTN.

CONFIRMATION

What is the most likely clinical presentation?

Hypertension is classified based on the degree of elevation. Classifications include Stage 1 hypertension, Stage 2 hypertension, and hypertensive crisis. Both systolic and diastolic values are relevant, however, many patients over 50 years of age demonstrate significantly elevated systolic measures with normal diastolic findings. This is referred to as isolated systolic hypertension (ISH). Patients do not typically report symptoms due to the slow onset of primary HTN. Secondary HTN may present with or without symptoms depending on the specific etiology and how quickly the condition progresses. Symptoms may not be recognized until blood pressure becomes dangerously high producing a headache, confusion, visual changes, fatigue, arrhythmia or tinnitus.

What laboratory or imaging studies would confirm the diagnosis?

There are no specific laboratory or imaging studies used to diagnose HTN. Specific testing (e.g., electrocardiogram, urinalysis, blood cholesterol) may be used to identify underlying pathologies so that medical management may be specifically targeted.

What additional information should be obtained to confirm the diagnosis?

A thorough medical history and physical examination should be completed to assist in identifying risk factors associated with the development of HTN. This is typically diagnosed by assessing blood pressure at least twice to determine if hypertension exists. Some patients may be asked to monitor their blood pressure at home if a medical office is felt to be stressful and contributing to elevated readings.

MANAGEMENT

What is the most effective management of this patient?

The medical management of HTN is largely focused on risk reduction through modifiable risk factors and pharmacological intervention. Lifestyle changes are recommended to address modifiable risk factors associated with HTN. Pharmacological agents may be used to decrease preload, dilate peripheral vessels or alter heart rate. Diuretics, beta-blockers, calcium channel blockers, and angiotensin-converting enzyme inhibitors may be used alone or in combination, depending on the pathology. Physical therapy intervention is typically focused on risk factor modification through progressive exercise and education. A patient may also qualify for a formal cardiac rehabilitation program depending on the degree of hypertension and existence of other comorbidities.

What home care regimen should be recommended?

A home care regimen should include progressive exercise and a comprehensive plan emphasizing risk reduction through lifestyle modification.

OUTCOME

What is the likely outcome of a course of physical therapy?

Patient compliance in a home care regimen is essential in reducing hypertension and associated risk factors. With appropriate management and controlled hypertension, most patients are able to participate in functional and recreational activities without limitation.

What are the long-term effects of the patient's condition?

Most patients are able to effectively manage HTN through risk factor modification and medication management. For patients with secondary HTN, further intervention may be necessary to treat the underlying pathology. Morbidity and mortality are typically associated with poorly controlled HTN which increases the risk for metabolic syndrome, myocardial infarction, heart failure, cerebrovascular accident, aneurysm, cognitive changes, kidney dysfunction, and visual impairment.

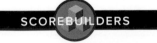

Restrictive Lung Disease   SILVER

DIAGNOSIS

What condition produces a patient's symptoms?

Restrictive lung disease (RLD) is a classification of disorders caused by a pulmonary or extrapulmonary restriction that produces impairment in lung expansion and an abnormal reduction in pulmonary ventilation. There are multiple conditions that can cause restrictive lung disease. Many symptoms are common regardless of the underlying etiology and other symptoms are disease-specific.

An injury was most likely sustained to which structure?

Pulmonary restriction of the lungs can be caused by tumor, interstitial pulmonary fibrosis, scarring within the lungs, and pneumonia. Extrapulmonary restrictions of the lungs include pleural effusion, chest wall stiffness, structural abnormality, postural deformity, respiratory muscle weakness, and central nervous system injury.

INFERENCE

What is the most likely contributing factor in the development of this condition?

There are varying etiologies for the group of disorders that cause restrictive lung disease. Musculoskeletal etiology includes scoliosis, pectus excavatum or other chest wall deformity, rib fractures, ankylosing spondylitis, and kyphosis. Pulmonary etiology includes idiopathic pulmonary fibrosis, pneumonia, pleural effusion, sarcoidosis, hyaline membrane disease, and tumor within the lungs. Other etiologies include inhalation of toxic fumes, drug therapy, asbestos, rheumatoid arthritis, systemic lupus erythematosus, muscular dystrophy, spinal cord injury, obesity, and other neurologic and neuromuscular diseases.

CONFIRMATION

What is the most likely clinical presentation?

The clinical presentation varies based on the underlying cause or disease process. The pathogenesis of RLD includes a decrease in lung and chest wall compliance, decrease in lung volumes and an increase in the work of breathing. Generally, restrictive lung disease is characterized by a reduction of lung volumes (total lung capacity, vital capacity, inspiratory reserve volume, tidal volume, expiratory reserve volume, and inspiratory capacity) due to impaired lung expansion. A patient with restrictive lung disease will present with decreased chest mobility, decreased breath sounds, shortness of breath, hypoxemia, a rapid and shallow respiratory pattern (tachypnea), respiratory muscle weakness, ineffective cough, and increased use of accessory muscles.

What laboratory or imaging studies would confirm the diagnosis?

A chest radiograph is utilized to evaluate lung structure and evidence of fibrosis, infiltrates, tumor, and deformity. Arterial blood gas analysis may indicate a decrease in PaO_2.

What additional information should be obtained to confirm the diagnosis?

Pulmonary function testing will result in impaired vital capacity (VC), forced vital capacity (FVC), and total lung capacity (TLC). The patient will usually present with normal residual volume (RV) and expiration flow rates. Expiratory reserve volume (ERV) and functional residual capacity (FRC) are often decreased. Arterial blood gas analysis examines the presence of hypoxemia and hypocapnia.

MANAGEMENT

What is the most effective management of this patient?

Medical management of restrictive lung disease includes treatment of the underlying cause through pharmacological intervention, physical therapy, and potential surgical intervention. Physical therapy intervention is based on the severity of the condition, but is consistently oriented toward the goals of maximizing gas exchange and obtaining maximal functional capacity. Physical therapy intervention may include body mechanics, posture training, diaphragm and ventilatory muscle strengthening, relaxation and energy conservation techniques, and the use of these techniques during functional mobility. Breathing exercises, coughing techniques, and airway secretion clearance are often components of a comprehensive care plan.

What home care regimen should be recommended?

A home care regimen should include breathing strategies and exercises, proper positioning, energy conservation and pacing techniques, general strengthening and endurance activities, and postural awareness with mobility. Low-level general strengthening and endurance training are indicated as tolerated.

OUTCOME

What is the likely outcome of a course in physical therapy?

Physical therapy intervention is specific to the underlying cause of the restrictive lung disease. Outcome is based on the etiology of the restrictive lung disease and patient response to physical therapy intervention. Treatment goals should include improving oxygenation and obtaining the maximal level of functioning.

What are the long-term effects of the patient's condition?

Long-term effects from restrictive lung disease are also specific to the underlying cause. Some disorders require surgical intervention that alleviates the condition while other conditions are progressive and irreversible. Some patients with end-stage disease may be candidates for lung transplantation, however, most eventually progress to ventilatory failure. Idiopathic pulmonary fibrosis is a restrictive lung disease that has a high mortality rate within four to six years of diagnosis whereas many conditions that cause restrictive lung disease are alleviated through appropriate management.

BRONZE **Level Clinical Application Templates**

BRONZE | Level Clinical Application Template Executive Summary

Aneurysm

- Abnormal balloon-like bulge in the wall of a blood vessel (most often the aorta) that occurs when the blood vessel becomes weakened and can no longer handle the pressure of the blood
- Symptoms will differ based on the site of the aneurysm (e.g., thoracic versus abdominal aorta) and whether the aneurysm has ruptured or not
- Symptoms include low back, abdominal or groin pain, nausea and vomiting, lightheadedness, and a rapid heart rate; symptoms of a thoracic aortic aneurysm include jaw, neck, back or chest pain, coughing or hoarseness, and shortness of breath

Chronic Venous Insufficiency

- Typically affects the distal lower extremities and is characterized by venous incompetence and resultant venous hypertension
- Symptoms include edema, feelings of heaviness, tingling sensations, and dull, aching pain in the distal lower extremities
- Symptoms generally improve and may resolve fully with elevation, however, reappear once dependent positioning is resumed

Pneumothorax

- Occurs when air accumulates in the pleural cavity and causes a collapsed lung
- Symptoms vary widely depending on the type and size of the pneumothorax, but may include chest pain, shortness of breath, hypoxemia, cyanosis, and hypotension
- Tension pneumothorax is a specific type of pneumothorax that results in large increases in pressure in the pleural cavity and is considered a medical emergency

Pulmonary Edema

- Characterized by excess fluid in the lungs that often occurs when the left ventricle is unable to adequately pump blood to the systemic circulation
- Acute pulmonary edema is considered a medical emergency and is characterized by extreme shortness of breath, wheezing or gasping, anxiety, a cough that produces frothy sputum, chest pain, and palpitations
- A chest x-ray is the primary imaging study to confirm the presence of fluid in the lungs

Pulmonary Embolism

- Occurs most commonly as a result of venous thrombi that have detached and traveled from elsewhere in the body before lodging in a pulmonary artery
- Symptoms include a sudden onset of dyspnea, coughing, hypoxia, and chest pain which may mimic myocardial infarction
- Pulmonary angiogram is the most conclusive means of identifying a pulmonary embolism, however, complication risks are high and so it is used only when other diagnostic methods are inconclusive

BRONZE Level Clinical Application Template Executive Summary

Respiratory Acidosis

- Refers to a state in which the pH of body fluids is abnormally low indicating acidemia
- Hypoventilation prevents adequate removal of CO_2 from the body causing hypercapnia and as a result, bicarbonate (HCO_3^-) levels decrease altering the body's acid-base balance
- Initial symptoms are often vague and more closely related to the underlying pathology; as the condition worsens, symptoms include lethargy, confusion, altered mental status, and cyanosis

Respiratory Alkalosis

- Refers to a state in which the pH of body fluids is abnormally high indicating alkalemia
- Hyperventilation removes more CO_2 from the body than can be produced causing hypocapnia and as a result, hydrogen ($H+$) levels decrease altering the body's acid-base balance
- Initial symptoms are often vague and more closely related to the underlying pathology, however, tachypnea, tachycardia, hyperventilation, and dizziness are commonly observed

Tuberculosis

- Highly contagious infectious disease spread via airborne transmission primarily caused by the Mycobacterium tuberculosis bacteria
- Active TB typically presents with generalized symptoms of infection including fever, chills, fatigue, weight loss, decreased appetite, and night sweats; left untreated can be fatal
- Diagnosed based on a skin test where a small amount of the substance tuberculin is injected at a forearm site with the skin's reaction then assessed 48 to 72 hours later

Venous Thrombosis

- The formation of a blood clot within a vein, most commonly occurring in the deep veins of the lower extremities
- Signs and symptoms include swelling, redness, warmth, and pain in the affected leg, though it can occur without any noticeable symptoms
- Ultrasound imaging is most commonly used to identify the presence of a venous thrombus

Aneurysm   BRONZE

DIAGNOSIS

What condition produces a patient's symptoms?

An aneurysm is an abnormal balloon-like bulge in the wall of a blood vessel. An aneurysm occurs when the wall of the blood vessel becomes weakened and can no longer tolerate the pressure of the blood, thus leading to bulging of the wall. There are many factors which may lead to damage or weakening of the blood vessel walls, including smoking, high blood pressure, atherosclerosis, infections, genetic conditions (e.g., Marfan syndrome), trauma, and advanced age.

An injury was most likely sustained to what structure?

This condition involves injury to the wall of a blood vessel, typically an artery. Most aneurysms occur in the aorta, and are labeled thoracic aortic aneurysms (TAA) or abdominal aortic aneurysms (AAA) based on the portion of the aorta affected. Aneurysms also occur in the brain, specifically in the Circle of Willis circulation, or in any peripheral artery.

CONFIRMATION

What is the most likely clinical presentation?

Symptoms will differ based on the site of the aneurysm and whether the aneurysm has ruptured or not. Symptoms of a ruptured AAA include low back, abdominal or groin pain, nausea and vomiting, lightheadedness, and a rapid heart rate. The internal bleeding from a ruptured AAA will typically lead to hypovolemic shock and is fatal in the large majority of cases. Symptoms of a TAA include jaw, neck, back or chest pain, coughing or hoarseness, and shortness of breath. A brain aneurysm may cause fatigue, loss of balance, and speech and vision problems. A ruptured brain aneurysm will result in a subarachnoid hemorrhage. Symptoms may include severe headache, loss of vision or double vision, loss of consciousness, vomiting, change in mental status, and seizure. This is a medical emergency.

What laboratory or imaging studies would confirm the diagnosis?

The imaging studies that may be performed to detect an aneurysm include ultrasound, computed tomography, magnetic resonance imaging, echocardiography, and angiography.

What additional information should be obtained to confirm the diagnosis?

A thorough medical history and physical examination should be performed to rule out other similar conditions. With a large AAA, palpation may reveal a throbbing mass in the abdominal area. If a ruptured brain aneurysm is suspected, a lumbar puncture may be performed to detect blood within the cerebrospinal fluid.

Chronic Venous Insufficiency   BRONZE

DIAGNOSIS

What condition produces a patient's symptoms?

Chronic venous insufficiency (CVI) typically affects the distal lower extremities and is characterized by venous incompetence and resultant venous hypertension. CVI increases fluid volume within interstitial spaces, eventually overloading the lymphatic system resulting in edema. The accumulation of protein-rich fluid causes local inflammation, hypoxia, and fibrotic changes within the tissues. These changes are significant factors in the development of venous stasis ulcers and delayed healing.

An injury was most likely sustained to which structure?

Typically, the bicuspid valves prevent the back flow within vessels returning blood from the periphery to the heart. Malfunctioning valves create venous incompetence and allow blood to pool within the vessels causing venous hypertension. At the capillary level, venous hypertension alters the pressure gradient between the capillaries and interstitium, impeding reabsorption and blood flow.

CONFIRMATION

What is the most likely clinical presentation?

Patients typically report symptoms more closely associated with resultant venous hypertension and stasis than the CVI itself. Symptoms include edema, feelings of heaviness, and dull, aching pain in the distal lower extremities. Symptoms generally improve and may resolve fully with elevation, however, they reappear once dependent positioning is resumed. Untreated venous hypertension and stasis related symptoms will cause a brawny skin discoloration and hyperkeratosis. Chronic inflammation can lead to poor wound healing and fibrotic changes in the subcutaneous tissue.

What laboratory or imaging studies would confirm the diagnosis?

Diagnosis will often include bidirectional or color-flow studies using venous ultrasonography to visualize structures and flow patterns and to identify reflux. A medical history and a thorough physical examination are also indicated.

What additional information should be obtained to confirm the diagnosis?

A complete medical history and description of daily activities is important. Patients who are obese, have vessel damage or who are pregnant are at greater risk for developing CVI due to structural or tissue impedance of venous structures. Patients who spend extended periods in sitting or standing are also at increased risk.

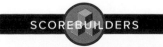

BRONZE   Pneumothorax

DIAGNOSIS

What condition produces a patient's symptoms?

A pneumothorax is an accumulation of air in the pleural cavity that results in a collapsed lung. A primary pneumothorax is one that occurs without a known etiology, while a secondary pneumothorax occurs in the presence of existing lung pathology. Causes of secondary pneumothorax include trauma, airway disease (e.g., cystic fibrosis, emphysema), lung infections (e.g., pneumonia, tuberculosis), lung disease (e.g., sarcoidosis, pulmonary fibrosis), connective tissue disease (e.g., rheumatoid arthritis, systemic sclerosis), and cancer.

An injury was most likely sustained to what structure?

A pneumothorax occurs when air leaks into the pleural cavity. The pleural cavity refers to the space between the lungs and chest wall. The increase in pressure in the pleural space causes partial collapse of the lung, which results in impaired gas exchange and decreased oxygenation of the blood. If the pneumothorax is large, it can cause a shift in position of the mediastinum.

CONFIRMATION

What is the most likely clinical presentation?

The presentation varies widely, from asymptomatic to life-threatening, depending on the type and size of the pneumothorax. Symptoms include chest pain, shortness of breath, hypoxemia, cyanosis, and hypotension. A tension pneumothorax occurs when damaged tissue causes a one-way valve into the chest and results in large increases in pressure. A tension pneumothorax is a medical emergency that leads to significant impairment of respiration and circulation and requires immediate medical attention.

What laboratory or imaging studies would confirm the diagnosis?

A chest x-ray is typically the first imaging study performed to confirm the diagnosis of pneumothorax. Computed tomography and ultrasound imaging can also be useful in providing more detailed information regarding the condition.

What additional information should be obtained to confirm the diagnosis?

A thorough medical history and physical examination should be performed to rule out the existence of other similar conditions (e.g., pulmonary embolism, acute respiratory distress syndrome). Auscultation of the lungs typically reveals decreased breath sounds and decreased fremitus.

BRONZE   Pulmonary Edema

DIAGNOSIS

What condition produces a patient's symptoms?

Pulmonary edema is a condition characterized by excess fluid within the lungs. This often occurs when the left ventricle is unable to adequately pump blood to the systemic circulation (e.g., left-sided heart failure). This causes fluid to back up into the pulmonary circulation and the lungs. Other causes of fluid buildup within the lungs include living at high elevations, respiratory distress syndrome, pulmonary embolism, adverse drug reactions, viral infections, smoke inhalation, and exposure to toxins. Acute pulmonary edema is considered a medical emergency.

An injury was most likely sustained to what structure?

When the left ventricle is unable to adequately pump blood to the systemic circulation, fluid backs up into the left atrium and then into the pulmonary circulation. As the pressure in the pulmonary circulation increases, the fluid moves from the lung capillaries into the alveoli, which makes breathing more difficult. In noncardiogenic pulmonary edema, the fluid buildup in the alveoli is not caused by an increase in pressure in the pulmonary circulation, but rather an increase in permeability of the capillaries themselves.

CONFIRMATION

What is the most likely clinical presentation?

Depending on the etiology, symptoms can develop slowly or suddenly. Acute pulmonary edema is characterized by extreme shortness of breath (especially when lying down), wheezing or gasping, anxiety, a cough that produces frothy sputum (may be tinged with blood), chest pain, and palpitations. Chronic pulmonary edema is characterized by shortness of breath that worsens when lying down or during physical activity, wheezing, weight gain, lower extremity swelling, and fatigue.

What laboratory or imaging studies would confirm the diagnosis?

A chest x-ray is the primary imaging study used to confirm the presence of fluid within the lungs. Other tests may be ordered to determine the cause of the pulmonary edema, including blood tests, electrocardiogram, and echocardiogram.

What additional information should be obtained to confirm the diagnosis?

A thorough medical history and physical examination should be performed to rule out other similar conditions that may cause shortness of breath (e.g., asthma, chronic obstructive pulmonary disease, pulmonary embolism).

Pulmonary Embolism
BRONZE

DIAGNOSIS

What condition produces a patient's symptoms?

An embolism that blocks a pulmonary artery is referred to as a pulmonary embolism (PE). A PE occurs as a result of venous thrombi that have detached and traveled from elsewhere in the body before lodging in a pulmonary artery. In most cases, multiple thrombi must be present to create a blockage large enough to produce PE symptoms.

An injury was most likely sustained to which structure?

A PE will cause decreased perfusion in the lung tissue supplied by the blocked vessel. As a result, the tissue becomes ischemic and fails to provide adequate oxygen for the body. Localized damage to venous structures associated with the initial thrombus formation may also occur.

CONFIRMATION

What is the most likely clinical presentation?

Signs and symptoms of PE include a sudden onset of dyspnea, coughing, hypoxia, and chest pain which may mimic myocardial infarction. Dyspnea presents both at rest and with activity. Complaints of chest pain typically worsen with coughing, eating, deep breathing or bending activities. Coughing may produce blood tinged sputum. Other signs and symptoms may include unilateral lower extremity edema, cyanosis, wheezing, diaphoresis, fainting, and a rapid or weak pulse.

What laboratory or imaging studies would confirm the diagnosis?

A ventilation-perfusion scan (V-Q scan) uses nuclear imaging of inhaled and injected radioactive substances to visualize air and blood flow through the lungs and identify blockages. The 3-D images produced by a spiral CT scan may be used to confirm the presence and location of a PE. MRI or diagnostic ultrasound may also be ordered to rule out the presence of additional thrombi, especially in the lower extremities. A pulmonary angiogram is the most conclusive and accurate means of identifying a PE, however, complication risks are high and so it is typically used only when other diagnostic methods are inconclusive.

What additional information should be obtained to confirm the diagnosis?

A complete medical and surgical history should be obtained in order to identify PE risk factors. Patients who are elderly or have certain inherited blood abnormalities (e.g., fibrinogen anomalies, antithrombin III deficiency) are at increased risk for developing a PE. Acquired risk factors are typically identified through the patient's history. These include extended periods of immobility, recent surgery, pregnancy, estrogen replacement use, smoking, and heart disease.

Respiratory Acidosis
BRONZE

DIAGNOSIS

What condition produces a patient's symptoms?

Respiratory acidosis refers to a state in which the pH is abnormally low indicating acidemia. Hypoventilation prevents adequate removal of CO_2 from the body causing hypercapnia. As a result, bicarbonate (HCO_3-) levels decrease altering the body's acid-base balance. Common etiologies include pulmonary disease, medications that suppress breathing, structural factors that limit effective lung expansion (e.g., severe scoliosis, morbid obesity), and conditions that cause respiratory muscle weakness (e.g., Guillain-Barre syndrome, amyotrophic lateral sclerosis).

An injury was most likely sustained to which structure?

Respiratory acidosis is not an independent disease process, but rather a symptom of some other underlying condition or disease. Injuries sustained vary with the etiology of the altered respiratory state and associated acidosis.

CONFIRMATION

What is the most likely clinical presentation?

Initial signs and symptoms of respiratory acidosis are often vague and more closely related to the underlying pathology. As the condition worsens, patients may present with lethargy, confusion, altered mental status, and cyanosis. Respiratory acidosis may present as a chronic or acute condition. Patients with chronic respiratory acidosis are likely to become stable if renal function is normal and HCO_3- excretion can be modulated to compensate for respiratory-induced acidemia. This renal compensation will be reflected in laboratory values that typically show a near normal pH and partial pressure of CO_2 ($PaCO_2$) measures toward the upper limits of normal. Acute respiratory acidosis is considered an emergent condition due to the rapid buildup of CO_2. This results in acidemia and $PaCO_2$ levels above the normal reference range.

What laboratory or imaging studies would confirm the diagnosis?

Laboratory analysis of arterial blood gases (e.g., serum CO_2 and O_2 levels), metabolic panel blood analysis (e.g., serum electrolytes), and urine pH are used to identify abnormal acidity and differentiate between respiratory and metabolic acidosis.

What additional information should be obtained to confirm the diagnosis?

A thorough medical history is necessary to assist in identifying conditions or medications which may contribute to alveolar hypoventilation and respiratory acidosis. Physical examination should include assessments of posture and respiratory muscle strength as well as mechanics.

Respiratory Alkalosis

DIAGNOSIS

What condition produces a patient's symptoms?

Respiratory alkalosis refers to a state in which the pH is abnormally high indicating alkalemia. Hyperventilation removes more CO_2 from the body than can be produced causing hypocapnia. As a result, hydrogen (H+) levels decrease altering the body's acid-base balance. Numerous conditions (e.g., pulmonary embolism, hyperthyroidism, sepsis), medications (e.g., catecholamines, nicotine), external influences (e.g., high altitude), and internal influences (e.g., CNS response to trauma, pain, anxiety, fever) can induce hyperventilation and subsequent alkalosis.

An injury was most likely sustained to which structure?

Respiratory alkalosis is not an independent disease process, but rather a symptom of some other underlying condition or disease. Injuries sustained vary with the etiology of the altered respiratory state and associated alkalosis.

CONFIRMATION

What is the most likely clinical presentation?

Initial signs and symptoms of respiratory alkalosis may be vague and are often closely related to the underlying pathology. Tachypnea, tachycardia, hyperventilation, and dizziness are commonly observed. In severe cases, a patient may develop seizures. If the patient is also hypoxic, cyanosis may be observed. Respiratory alkalosis may present as either a chronic or acute condition. As a chronic condition, lab values will reflect a partial pressure of CO_2 ($PaCO_2$) measure below normal reference values and serum pH alkalemia. Acute respiratory alkalosis will also reflect a $PaCO_2$ measure below normal reference values while serum pH will be normal or near normal.

What laboratory or imaging studies would confirm the diagnosis?

Laboratory analysis of arterial blood gases (e.g., serum CO_2 and O_2 levels), metabolic panel blood analysis (e.g., serum electrolytes), and urine pH are used to identify abnormal alkalinity and differentiate between respiratory and metabolic alkalosis.

What additional information should be obtained to confirm the diagnosis?

A thorough medical history is necessary to assist in identifying conditions or medications which may contribute to alveolar hyperventilation and respiratory alkalosis. Additional diagnostic testing may be required to identify a patient's underlying etiology so that respiratory alkalosis treatment interventions may be specifically targeted.

Tuberculosis

DIAGNOSIS

What condition produces a patient's symptoms?

Tuberculosis (TB) is a highly contagious infectious disease spread via airborne transmission. The infection is primarily caused by the Mycobacterium tuberculosis bacteria. Multiple antibiotic-resistant strains of the bacteria have been identified. Patients with latent TB are infected, however, it is not contagious and produces no symptoms. Active TB will produce symptoms and may develop from the latent bacteria or from a recent exposure to a contagious individual.

An injury was most likely sustained to which structure?

TB typically affects the lungs. Less common infection sites include the brain, spine, and kidneys with each producing different clinical symptoms. Patients with a weakened immune system are most likely to contract TB.

CONFIRMATION

What is the most likely clinical presentation?

Patients with active TB in the lungs typically present with symptoms including fever, chills, and fatigue. Weight loss, decreased appetite, and night sweats are also common. Complaints of a persistent cough for greater than three weeks, bloody sputum, and chest pain associated with deep breathing or coughing may be present. Physical examination will reveal abnormal lung sounds suggestive of pleural effusion and enlarged lymph nodes which may be tender with palpation. Clubbing of the digits may also be observed in patients with advanced TB. Patients who have been on an appropriate pharmacological regimen for at least two weeks are no longer considered contagious. Most recover from TB without long-term effects, however, untreated TB can spread to other areas of the body and become fatal.

What laboratory or imaging studies would confirm the diagnosis?

TB is typically diagnosed based on the results of a skin test. A small amount of the substance tuberculin is injected at a forearm site and the skin's reaction is then assessed 48 to 72 hours later. This diagnostic tool is, however, known to produce false results especially in patients who have previously had a TB vaccination or have recently been infected.

What additional information should be obtained to confirm the diagnosis?

A thorough medical history should be obtained to assist in identifying risk factors and ruling out similar diagnoses. Social history may also be significant if the patient has a high risk of occupational exposure or has ever visited or lived abroad.

Venous Thrombosis   BRONZE

DIAGNOSIS

What condition produces a patient's symptoms?

Venous thrombosis is a condition characterized by the formation of a blood clot (thrombus) within a vein. Any condition which slows or changes the flow of blood within a vein can increase the risk for thrombus formation. These risk factors include prolonged immobility, recent surgery, pregnancy, obesity, cigarette smoking, medications (e.g., birth control, hormone replacement), blood conditions characterized by "thick" blood (e.g., polycythemia), blood-clotting disorders, cancer, and certain autoimmune disorders.

An injury was most likely sustained to what structure?

Venous thrombosis most commonly affects the deep veins of the lower extremities. A thrombus can break off from its site of origin and travel within the bloodstream (i.e., embolus) to the brain, lungs or heart and cause severe damage.

CONFIRMATION

What is the most likely clinical presentation?

Signs and symptoms include swelling, redness, warmth, and pain in the affected leg, most commonly in the calf, though the condition can occur without any noticeable symptoms.

What laboratory or imaging studies would confirm the diagnosis?

Ultrasound imaging is most commonly used to identify the presence of a venous thrombus. Blood tests will also be ordered to detect elevated levels of clot-dissolving substances. Other imaging studies less often used include magnetic resonance imaging, computed tomography, and venography.

What additional information should be obtained to confirm the diagnosis?

A thorough medical history and physical examination should be performed to help diagnose the presence of a venous thrombus. Homans' sign may be performed as part of the physical examination, though further evaluation should be performed due to the poor diagnostic value of this test.

Cardiovascular and Pulmonary Systems Essentials

1. The components of the cardiac conduction system include the sinoatrial (SA) node, internodal tracts, atrioventricular (AV) node, common AV bundle or bundle of His, right and left bundle branches, and Purkinje fibers.

2. Sympathetic nerves stimulate the heart to beat faster (chronotropic effect) and with greater force of contraction (inotropic effect). Parasympathetic nerves slow the heart rate (chronotropic effect) primarily through their influence on the SA node.

3. The Valsalva maneuver produces increased intrathoracic pressure, increased central venous pressure, and decreased venous return and should be avoided, especially by patients with heart, blood vessel or lung disease.

4. Ventricular systole denotes contraction of the ventricles; ventricular diastole denotes the relaxation phase.

5. Cardiac output is the product of heart rate and stroke volume. It is approximately 5.0 – 5.5 L/min in resting adults, but can increase fivefold during exercise.

6. The components of blood are plasma, red blood cells, white blood cells, and platelets.

7. Oxygen is both dissolved in the blood plasma and chemically combined to hemoglobin in red blood cells. Only about 0.3 mL O_2 is dissolved in 100 mL of arterial blood; the rest is attached to hemoglobin.

8. The diaphragm is the primary muscle of inspiration. Secondary muscles of inspiration are the internal and external intercostals, sternocleidomastoids, and scalenes.

9. The bronchopulmonary segments are the topographic units of the lungs. There are ten bronchopulmonary segments in the right lung and eight in the left lung.

10. The most common sign of a heart attack in both men and women is chest pain or discomfort.

11. Blood pressure classifications include normal, elevated, Stage 1 hypertension, Stage 2 hypertension, and hypertensive crisis.

12. Pulmonary edema can be fatal if not treated. Seek immediate emergency medical assistance if the signs or symptoms of acute pulmonary edema develop including extreme shortness of breath or difficulty breathing, a feeling of suffocating or drowning, wheezing or gasping for breath, anxiety, restlessness or a sense of apprehension or a cough that produces frothy sputum tinged with blood.

13. Arterial blood gases evaluate acid–base status (pH), ventilation ($PaCO_2$), and oxygenation (PaO_2). Mean arterial blood gas values in adults at sea level are: pH = 7.4; $PaCO_2$ = 40 mm Hg; PaO_2 = 97 mm Hg; HCO_3- = 24 mEq/L.

14. A complete blood count (CBC) measures red blood cell count, total white blood cell count, white blood cell differential, platelets, hemoglobin, and hematocrit.

15. Antihypertensive medications include diuretics, calcium channel blockers, ACE inhibitors, angiotensin II blockers, ß-adrenergic blockers, and alpha adrenergic antagonists.

16. Bronchodilator agents work to relieve bronchospasm by stimulating the receptors that cause bronchial smooth muscle relaxation or by blocking the receptors that trigger bronchoconstriction. Primary classifications of bronchodilators include anticholinergic, sympathomimetics, and xanthine derivatives.

17. BMI describes relative weight for height and is a useful measurement for identifying adults at increased risk for mortality and morbidity due to being overweight and obese. BMI = weight [kg] ÷ height [m^2].

18. Normal heart sounds are S1 (closing of the mitral and tricuspid valves) and S2 (closing of the aortic and pulmonic valves).

19. ST segment depression on the ECG may indicate ischemia of the myocardium.

20. Adventitious inspiratory or expiratory breath sounds include crackles, pleural friction rub, rhonchi, stridor, and wheeze.

Cardiovascular and Pulmonary Systems Essentials

21. Pulmonary function tests help to differentiate obstructive and restrictive forms of lung dysfunction. Obstructive defects are characterized by decreased expiratory flows ($FEV_1/FVC < 70\%$). Restrictive defects are characterized by reduced lung volumes and relatively normal expiratory flow rates (FVC is reduced and FEV_1/FVC is normal or increased).

22. If the percent of arterial oxygen saturation of hemoglobin falls below 90% in acutely ill patients or below 85% in patients with chronic lung disease, activity should be stopped and a discussion with the physician should take place to consider adding or increasing supplemental oxygen.

23. The rate pressure product (RPP), the product of heart rate and systolic blood pressure, is a clinical index of myocardial oxygen consumption that provides an easy to measure physiologic correlate to the onset of angina pectoris or the development of ECG abnormalities in patients with previous heart disease.

24. Active cycle of breathing and autogenic drainage are breathing techniques that patients can perform independently to assist with airway clearance.

25. Huffing is a forced expiratory maneuver performed with the glottis open that can be used instead of a cough.

26. Pursed-lip breathing helps to reduce respiratory rate, reduce dyspnea, and prevent airway collapse in patients with emphysema. Any patient who is short of breath may use this technique.

27. An incentive spirometer provides visual or other feedback to encourage the patient to take long, slow, deep inhalations, which is especially important after thoracic and abdominal surgery.

28. Intensity of aerobic exercise can be regulated by heart rate, MET level, and RPE.

29. One MET is the energy expended while sitting quietly (3.5 mLO_2/kg/min or 1kcal/kg/h).

30. RPE of 11 - 13 corresponds to the upper limit of prescribed training heart rates for patients in the early phase of outpatient cardiac rehabilitation.

31. There is no optimal exercise intensity for the aerobic exercise training of patients in pulmonary rehabilitation. Intensity is determined primarily by patient tolerance and safety.

Cardiovascular and Pulmonary Systems Proficiencies

1. Heart Anatomy

Identify the appropriate term for each of the specified locations. Answers must be selected from the Word Bank and can be used only once.

Word Bank: inferior vena cava, left ventricle, left atrium, left pulmonary veins, left pulmonary arteries, left subclavian artery, left cardiac vein, left common carotid artery, right pulmonary veins, right atrium, right coronary artery, superior vena cava

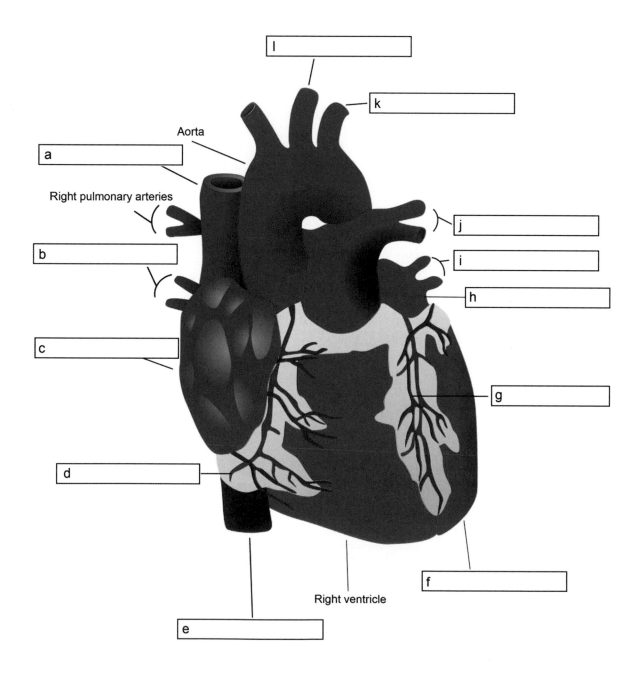

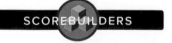

Cardiovascular and Pulmonary Systems Proficiencies

2. Heart Circulation

Identify the appropriate term for each of the specified locations. Answers must be selected from the Word Bank and can be used only once.

Word Bank: aortic valve, deoxygenated blood from body, deoxygenated blood to left lung, deoxygenated blood to right lung, left atrium, left ventricle, mitral valve, oxygenated blood from left lung, oxygenated blood to body, pulmonary valve, right atrium, right ventricle, tricuspid valve

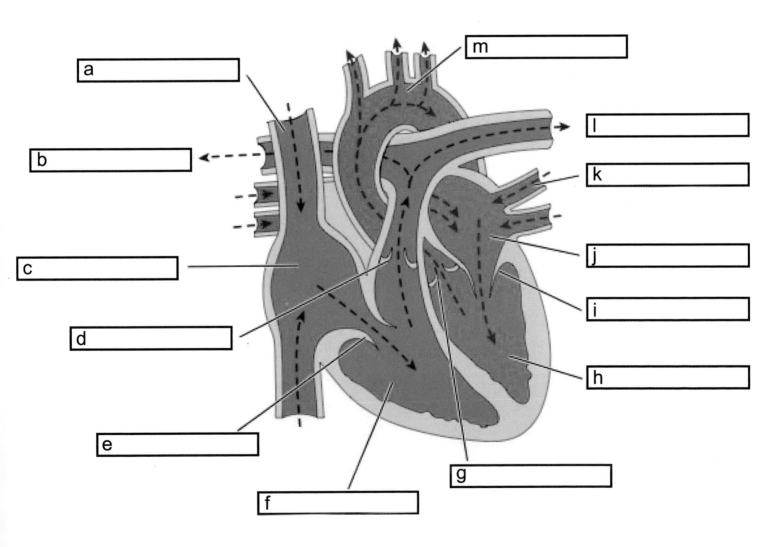

Cardiovascular and Pulmonary Systems Proficiencies

3. Vessels of the Heart

Identify the appropriate vessel of the heart based on the described function. Answers must be selected from the Word Bank and can each be used only once.

Word Bank: aorta, inferior vena cava, pulmonary arteries, pulmonary veins, superior vena cava

Great Vessel	Description
a	returns blood to the right atrium from the head, neck and arms
b	takes blood away from the right ventricle to the left and right lungs
c	returns blood from the left and right lungs to the left atrium
d	takes blood away from the left ventricle
e	returns blood to the right atrium from the lower body and viscera

4. Heart Valves

Identify the areas associated with each valve. Answers must be selected from the Word Bank. Answers can be used more than once.

Word Bank: aorta, left atrium, left ventricle, pulmonary artery, right atrium, right ventricle

a. The tricuspid valve controls blood flow between the _____ and the _____.

b. The pulmonary valve controls blood flow between the _____ and the _____.

c. The aortic valve controls blood flow between the _____ and the _____.

d. The mitral valve controls blood flow between the _____ and the _____.

5. Lung Capacities

Identify the components of each of the listed lung capacities. The sum of the identified components must equal the stated capacity. A list of possible components is provided in the Word Bank. The components can be used more than once.

Word Bank: Expiratory Reserve Volume (ERV), Functional Residual Capacity (FRC), Inspiratory Capacity (IC), Inspiratory Reserve Volume (IRV), Residual Volume (RV), Tidal Volume (TV), Vital Capacity (VC)

Measure	Components
functional residual capacity	a
inspiratory capacity	b
total lung capacity	c
vital capacity	d

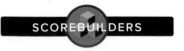

Cardiovascular and Pulmonary Systems Proficiencies

6. Lung Volumes and Capacities

Identify the volumes and capacities most closely associated with the supplied descriptions. Answers must be selected from the Word Bank and can each be used only once.

Word Bank: anatomic dead space volume, expiratory reserve volume, forced vital capacity, functional residual capacity, inspiratory capacity, inspiratory reserve volume, residual volume, tidal volume, total lung capacity, vital capacity

Volumes and Capacities	Description
a	The maximal volume of air that can be inspired after a normal tidal exhalation.
b	The volume of air in the lungs after normal exhalation.
c	The maximal volume of air that can be exhaled after a normal tidal exhalation.
d	The volume change that occurs between maximal inspiration and maximal expiration.
e	The volume of air in the lungs after a maximal inspiration; the sum of all lung volumes.
f	The volume of gas remaining in the lungs at the end of a maximal expiration.
g	The volume of air expired during a forced maximal expiration after a forced maximal inspiration.
h	Total volume inspired and expired with each breath during quiet breathing.
i	The volume of air that occupies the non-respiratory conducting airways.
j	The maximal volume of air inspired after normal tidal volume inspiration.

7. Pathology of the Cardiovascular and Pulmonary Systems

Identify the appropriate medical condition based on the supplied descriptions. Answers must be selected from the Word Bank and can each be used only once.

Word Bank: angina pectoris, asthma, atherosclerosis, bronchitis, cor pulmonale, cystic fibrosis, pulmonary edema

Pathology	Description
a	hypertrophy of the right ventricle caused by altered structure or function of the lungs
b	inflammation of the bronchi characterized by hypertrophy of the mucus secreting glands
c	fluid collects in the alveoli in the lungs making it difficult to breathe
d	a transient precordial sensation of pressure or discomfort resulting from myocardial ischemia
e	a slow progressive accumulation of fatty plaques on the inner walls of arteries
f	chronic inflammation of the airways caused by increased airway sensitivity to various stimuli
g	an autosomal recessive genetic disease of the exocrine glands

Cardiovascular and Pulmonary Systems Proficiencies

8. Arterial Blood Gas Values

Identify the appropriate arterial blood gas measure for each of the supplied values. Answers must be selected from the Word Bank and can each be used only once.

Word Bank: HCO_3^-, $PaCO_2$, PaO_2, pH, SaO_2

Measure	Value
a	7.35 - 7.45
b	40 mm Hg
c	97 mm Hg
d	24 mEq/L
e	95-98%

9. Pharmacology of the Cardiovascular and Pulmonary Systems

Identify the appropriate medication based on the supplied descriptions. Answers must be selected from the Word Bank and can each be used only once.

Word Bank: alpha adrenergic antagonist agents, angiotensin-converting enzyme inhibitor agents, anticoagulant agents, anti-inflammatory agents, beta blocker agents, calcium channel blockers, diuretics, expectorant agents, nitrates, positive inotropic agents

Drug	Action
a	decrease the entry of calcium into vascular smooth muscle cells
b	increase the excretion of sodium and urine
c	decrease blood pressure and afterload by suppressing a specific enzyme
d	decrease ischemia through smooth muscle relaxation and dilation of peripheral vessels
e	reduce peripheral vascular tone causing dilation of arterioles and veins resulting in decreased blood pressure
f	decrease myocardial oxygen demand by decreasing heart rate and contractility
g	increase respiratory secretions which help to loosen mucus
h	inhibit platelet aggregation and thrombus formation
i	prevent inflammatory-mediated bronchoconstriction
j	increase the force and velocity of myocardial contraction, slow the heart rate, and decrease conduction through the AV node

Cardiovascular and Pulmonary Systems Proficiencies

10. Hypertension

Next to each value state whether the BP is normal, elevated, stage 1 hypertension, or stage 2 hypertension. Classification should be made based on the November 2017 Blood Pressure Guidelines. Answers must be selected from the Word Bank and can each be used more than once.

Word Bank: normal, elevated, stage 1 hypertension, stage 2 hypertension

Blood Pressure Value	Classification
125/89 mm Hg	a
170/105 mm Hg	b
155/95 mm Hg	c
110/75 mm Hg	d
142/105 mm Hg	e
135/82 mm Hg	f

11. Heart Sounds

Identify the appropriate heart sounds for each of the supplied descriptions. Answers must be selected from the Word Bank and can each be used only once.

Word Bank: S1, S2, S3, S4, murmur

Heart Sound	Definition
a	closure of the aortic and pulmonary valves at the onset of diastole
b	closure of the mitral and tricuspid valves at the onset of systole
c	pathological sound of vibration of the ventricle walls with ventricular filling and atrial contraction
d	vibrations of the distended ventricle walls due to passive flow of blood from the atria during diastole
e	vibrations of longer duration than the heart sounds due to disrupted blood flow past a stenotic or regurgitant valve

12. Abnormal Breath Sounds

Identify the appropriate abnormal breath sound for each of the supplied descriptions. Answers must be selected from the Word Bank and can each be used only once.

Word Bank: crackle, pleural friction rub, rhonchi, stridor, wheeze

Breath Sound	Definition
a	dry, crackling sound heard during inspiration and expiration
b	continuous low-pitched sounds resembling snoring or gurgling during inspiration and expiration
c	continuous high-pitched wheeze heard with inspiration or expiration
d	discontinuous high-pitched popping sound heard during inspiration
e	continuous musical or whistling sound composed of a variety of pitches

Cardiovascular and Pulmonary Systems Proficiencies

13. Peripheral Pulses

Identify the appropriate artery based on the supplied descriptions. Answers must be selected from the Word Bank and can each be used only once.

Word Bank: brachial, carotid, dorsalis pedis, femoral, popliteal, posterior tibial, radial, ulnar

Artery	Pulse Location
a	the medial aspect of the sternocleidomastoid muscle in the lower half of the neck
b	at the wrist, lateral to the flexor carpi radialis tendon
c	in the upper thigh, one-third of the distance from the pubis to the anterior superior iliac spine
d	in the space between the medial malleolus and the Achilles tendon, above the calcaneus
e	medial to the biceps tendon and lateral to the medial epicondyle of the humerus
f	at the wrist, between the flexor digitorum superficialis and the flexor carpi ulnaris tendons
g	in the popliteal space of the posterior knee
h	near the center of the long axis of the foot, between the first and second metatarsal bones

14. Cardiovascular and Pulmonary Systems Basics

Mark each statement as True or False. If the statement is False correct the statement in the space provided.

True/False	Statement
a	Cardiac output refers to the volume of blood ejected by each contraction of the left ventricle.
Correction:	
b	Preload refers to the tension in the ventricular wall at the end of diastole.
Correction:	
c	The radial artery is assessed at the wrist, medial to the flexor carpi radialis tendon.
Correction:	

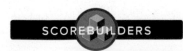

Cardiovascular and Pulmonary Systems Proficiencies

True/False	Statement
d	The dorsalis pedis artery is assessed near the center of the long axis of the foot, between the second and third metatarsals.
Correction:	
e	White blood cells, also known as leukocytes, protect the body from infection by ingesting bacteria and debris.
Correction:	
f	Minute volume ventilation is calculated by multiplying total lung capacity and respiratory rate.
Correction:	
g	The pulmonic area of the heart is auscultated by placing the diaphragm of the stethoscope over the fourth intercostal space at the left sternal border.
Correction:	
h	A body mass index of 27.5 would be classified as normal.
Correction:	
i	When observing an electrocardiogram, the P wave represents atrial depolarization.
Correction:	
j	A rating of 14 on a rate of perceived exertion scale represents approximately 50% of the maximum heart rate during exercise on a treadmill.
Correction:	

Cardiovascular and Pulmonary Systems Proficiencies

True/False	Statement
k	Eupnea refers to the absence of spontaneous breathing.
Correction:	
l	When performing pursed lip breathing, the inspiratory phase is twice as long in duration as the expiratory phase.
Correction:	
m	Activities requiring 3-6 metabolic equivalents would be considered moderate level activity.
Correction:	
n	A compression rate of greater than or equal to 100 compressions per minute should be used when performing cardiopulmonary resuscitation on an adult.
Correction:	

Cardiovascular and Pulmonary Systems Answer Key

1. Heart Anatomy

a. superior vena cava
b. right pulmonary veins
c. right atrium
d. right coronary artery
e. inferior vena cava
f. left ventricle
g. left cardiac vein
h. left atrium
i. left pulmonary veins
j. left pulmonary arteries
k. left subclavian artery
l. left common carotid artery

2. Heart Circulation

a. deoxygenated blood from body
b. deoxygenated blood to right lung
c. right atrium
d. pulmonary valve
e. tricuspid valve
f. right ventricle
g. aortic valve
h. left ventricle
i. mitral valve
j. left atrium
k. oxygenated blood from left lung
l. deoxygenated blood to left lung
m. oxygenated blood to body

3. Vessels of the Heart

a. superior vena cava
b. pulmonary arteries
c. pulmonary veins
d. aorta
e. inferior vena cava

4. Heart Valves

a. The tricuspid valve controls blood flow between the right atrium and the right ventricle.
b. The pulmonary valve controls blood flow between the right ventricle and the pulmonary artery.
c. The aortic valve controls blood flow between the left ventricle and the aorta.
d. The mitral valve controls blood flow between the left atrium and the left ventricle.

5. Lung Capacities

a. FRC = ERV + RV
b. IC = TV + IRV
c. TLC = RV + VC or TLC = FRC + IC
d. VC = TV + IRV + ERV

6. Lung Volumes and Capacities

a. inspiratory capacity
b. functional residual capacity
c. expiratory reserve volume
d. vital capacity
e. total lung capacity
f. residual volume
g. forced vital capacity
h. tidal volume
i. anatomic dead space volume
j. inspiratory reserve volume

7. Pathology of the Cardiovascular and Pulmonary Systems

a. cor pulmonale
b. bronchitis
c. pulmonary edema
d. angina pectoris
e. atherosclerosis
f. asthma
g. cystic fibrosis

Cardiovascular and Pulmonary Systems Answer Key

8. Arterial Blood Gas Values

a. pH
b. $PaCO_2$
c. PaO_2
d. HCO_3-
e. SaO_2

9. Pharmacology of the Cardiovascular and Pulmonary Systems

a. calcium channel blockers
b. diuretics
c. angiotensin-converting enzyme inhibitor agents
d. nitrates
e. alpha adrenergic antagonist agents
f. beta blocker agents
g. expectorant agents
h. anticoagulant agents
i. anti-inflammatory agents
j. positive inotropic agents

10. Hypertension

a. stage 1 hypertension
b. stage 2 hypertension
c. stage 2 hypertension
d. normal
e. stage 2 hypertension
f. stage 1 hypertension

11. Heart Sounds

a. S2
b. S1
c. S4
d. S3
e. murmur

12. Abnormal Breath Sounds

a. pleural friction rub
b. rhonchi
c. stridor
d. crackle
e. wheeze

13. Peripheral Pulses

a. carotid
b. radial
c. femoral
d. posterior tibial
e. brachial
f. ulnar
g. popliteal
h. dorsalis pedis

14. Cardiovascular and Pulmonary Systems Basics*

a. FALSE: Correction - Stroke volume refers to the volume of blood ejected by each contraction of the left ventricle.
b. TRUE
c. FALSE: Correction - The radial artery is assessed at the wrist, lateral to the flexor carpi radialis tendon.
d. FALSE: Correction - The dorsalis pedis artery is assessed near the center of the long axis of the foot, between the first and second metatarsal.
e. TRUE
f. FALSE: Correction - Minute volume ventilation is calculated by multiplying tidal volume and respiratory rate.
g. FALSE: Correction - The tricuspid area of the heart is auscultated by placing the diaphragm of the stethoscope over the fourth intercostal space at the left sternal border.
h. FALSE: Correction - A body mass index of 18.5 - 24.9 would be considered normal.
i. TRUE
j. FALSE: Correction - A rating of 14 on a rate of perceived exertion scale represents approximately 70% of the maximum heart rate during exercise on a treadmill.
k. FALSE: Correction - Apnea refers to the absence of spontaneous breathing. Eupnea refers to the normal rate and depth of breathing.

Cardiovascular and Pulmonary Systems Answer Key

l.   FALSE: Correction - When performing pursed lip breathing, the expiratory phase is twice as long in duration as the inspiratory phase.

m. TRUE

n.   TRUE

*The correction presented for each false statement is an example of several possible corrections.

Cardiovascular and Pulmonary Systems References

1. Components of Blood. The Merck Manuals Online Medical Library. http://www.merckmanuals.com/home/sec14/ch169/ch169b. html#sec14-ch169-ch169b-4. Updated August 2006. Accessed January 3, 2011.

2. DePalo VA, McCool F D. Pulmonary Anatomy & Physiology. In: Hanley ME, Welsh CH, eds. *CURRENT Diagnosis & Treatment in Pulmonary Medicine*. New York, NY: McGraw-Hill; 2003. http://0-www.accessmedicine.com.lilac.une.edu/content. aspx?aID=575000. Accessed January 3, 2011.

3. Diseases and Conditions. Mayo Clinic Web site. http://www. mayoclinic.com/health/DiseasesIndex/DiseasesIndex. Accessed January 3, 2011.

4. Lawrence EC, Brigham KL. Chronic Cor Pulmonale. In: Fuster V, O'Rourke RA, Walsh RA, Poole-Wilson P, eds. *Hurst's the Heart*, 12th ed. New York, NY: McGraw-Hill; 2008. http://0-www. accessmedicine.com.lilac.une.edu/content.aspx?aID=3070848. Accessed January 13, 2011.

5. Diagnostic tests and procedures. American Heart Association Web site. http://www.heart.org/HEARTORG/Conditions/ HeartAttack/SymptomsDiagnosisofHeartAttack/Diagnostic-Tests-Procedures_UCM_303929_Article.jsp. Updated November 3, 2010. Accessed January 2, 2011.

6. Chobanian AV, Bakris GL, Black HR, et al. Seventh report of the joint national committee on prevention, detection, evaluation, and treatment of high blood pressure: the JNC 7 complete report. *Hypertension*. 2003; 42: 1206–1252.

7. The Seventh Report of the Joint National Committee on Prevention, Detection, Evaluation, and Treatment of High Blood Pressure (JNC 7). National Heart Lung and Blood Institute Web site. http://www.nhlbi.nih.gov/guidelines/hypertension/jnc7full. pdf. Accessed January 3, 2011.

8. Cardiac procedures and surgeries. American Heart Association Web site. http://www.heart.org/HEARTORG/Conditions/ HeartAttack/PreventionTreatmentofHeartAttack/Cardiac-Procedures-and-Surgeries_UCM_303939_Article.jsp. Updated November 3, 2010. Accessed January 2, 2011.

9. ACC/AHA 2005 Practice guidelines for the management of patients with peripheral arterial disease (lower extremity, renal, mesenteric, and abdominal aortic) *Circulation* 2006; 113:1474-1547.

10. Valve disease. Texas Heart Institute Web site. http://www. texasheartinstitute.org/HIC/Topics/Cond/valvedis.cfm Updated July 2010. Accessed January 3, 2011.

11. Asthma. American Lung Association website. http://www.lungusa. org/lung-disease/asthma/. Accessed January 3, 2011.

12. Diseases and conditions index. National Heart Lung and Blood Institute Web site. http://www.nhlbi.nih.gov/health/dci/index.html. Updated June 2010. Accessed January 3, 2010.

13. About cystic fibrosis. Cystic Fibrosis Foundation Web site. http://www.cff.org/AboutCF/. Accessed January 3, 2011.

14. Watchie J. *Cardiovascular and Pulmonary Physical Therapy. A Clinical Manual.* 2nd ed. St. Louis, MO: Saunders Elsevier; 2010.

15. Tests and procedures. Mayo Clinic Web site. http://www. mayoclinic.com/health/tests-and-procedures/Test Procedure Index. Accessed January 3, 2011.

16. Fuster V, O'Rourke RA, Walsh RA, Poole-Wilson P. Nuclear Cardiology. In: Fuster V, O'Rourke RA, Walsh RA, Poole-Wilson P, eds. Hurst's The Heart, 12th ed. New York, NY: McGraw-Hill; 2008. http://0-www.accessmedicine.com.lilac.une.edu/content. aspx?aID=3059284. Accessed January 13, 2011.

17. Chang AM, Maisel AS, Hollander JE. Diagnosis of heart failure. *Heart Failure Clinics*. 2009; 5:25-35.DOI: 10.1016/j.hfc.2008.08.013.

18. Drug Facts and Comparison. Facts and Comparisons Web site. http:www.factsandcomparisons.com. Accessed January 3, 2011.

19. Monographs A-Z. Clinical Pharmacology Web site. http://www. clinicalpharmacology.com/?epm=2_1. Accessed January 3, 2011.

20. Nason KS, Maddaus MA, Luketich JD. Chest Wall, Lung, Mediastinum, and Pleura. In: Brunicardi FC, Andersen DK, Billiar TR, Dunn DL, Hunter JG, Matthews JB, Pollock RE, eds. *Schwartz's Principles of Surgery*, 9th ed. New York, NY: McGraw-Hill; 2010. http://0-www.accessmedicine.com.lilac.une.edu/content. aspx?aID=5016069. Accessed January 3, 2010.

21. American College of Sports Medicine. *ACSM's Resource Manual for Guidelines for Exercise Testing and Prescription*. Seventh Edition. Lippincott Williams & Wilkins. 2014.

22. Campeau L. The Canadian Cardiovascular Society grading of angina pectoris revisited 30 years later. *Can J Cardiol*. 2002:18:371-9.

23. Seidel HM, Ball JW, Dains JE, Benedict GW. *Mosby's Guide to Physical Examination*. Fifth Edition. St. Louis, MO: Mosby; 2003.

24. LeBlond RF, DeGowin RL, Brown DD. Cardiovascular and Respiratory Signs. DeGowin's Diagnostic Examination. 9th ed. New York: McGraw-Hill Medical; 2009. http://0-www. accessmedicine.com.lilac.une.edu/content.aspx?aID=3661627. Accessed January 3, 2011.

25. Assessing your weight and health risk. National Heart Lung and Blood Institute website. http://www.nhlbi.nih.gov/health/public/ heart/obesity/lose_wt/risk.htm. Accessed January 3, 2011.

26. Zuther JE. Lymphedema Management. *The Comprehensive Guide for Practitioners*. New York, NY: Thieme; 2005

27. *Guide to Physical Therapist Practice*. 2nd ed. Phys Ther. 2001; 81:583.

Cardiovascular and Pulmonary Systems References

28. Wullink M, Stoffers HE, Kuipers H. A primary care walking exercise program for patients with intermittent claudication. *Med Sci Sports Exerc*. 2001; 33:1629-1634.

29. Borg G. Borg's Perceived Exertion and Pain Scales. Champaign IL: Human Kinetics; 1998.

30. Prasad SA, Randall SD, Balfour-Lynn IM. Fifteen-count breathlessness score: an objective measure for children. *Pediatr Pulmonol*. 2000 30(1):56-62.

31. American Thoracic Society. Dyspnea. Mechanisms, assessment, and management: A consensus statement. *Am J Respir Crit Care Med*. 1999; 159:3321-340.

32. Goldberger AL. *Clinical Electrocardiography: A Simplified Approach*. 7th ed. Philadelphia, PA: Mosby Elsevier; 2006.

33. American Thoracic Society. The diagnostic approach to acute venous thromboembolism. Clinical practice guideline. *Am J Respir Crit Care Med*. 1999; 160:1043-1066.

34. O'Rourke RA, Shaver JA, Silverman ME. The History, Physical Examination, and Cardiac Auscultation. In: Fuster V, O'Rourke RA, Walsh RA, Poole-Wilson P, eds. *Hurst's The Heart*, 12th ed. New York, NY: McGraw-Hill; 2008. http://0-www.accessmedicine.com. lilac.une.edu/content.aspx?aID=3057120. Accessed January 3, 2011.

35. Miller MR, Hankinson J, Brusasco V, Burgos R, et al. Standardisation of spirometry. *Eur Respir J*. 2005; 26: 319-338.

36. American Thoracic Society. Lung function testing: Selection of reference values and interpretative strategies. *Am Rev Respir Dis*. 1991; 144:1202-1218.

37. AARC Clinical Practice Guideline: Exercise testing for evaluation of hypoxemia and/or desaturation. *Respir Care*. 1992; 37: 907-912.

38. Borg GAV: Psychophysical bases of perceived exertion. *Med Sci Sports Exerc*. 1982;14:377.

39. Wallace J. Principles of cardiorespiratory endurance programming. In: *ACSM's Resource Manual for Guidelines for Exercise Testing and Prescription*. Philadelphia, PA: Lippincott Williams & Wilkins; 2006; 336-349.

40. Krider SJ. Vital Signs. In: Wilkins RL, Krider SJ, Sheldon RL, eds. *Clinical Assessment in Respiratory Care*, 4th ed. St. Louis, MO: Mosby; 2000.

41. ATS statement: Guidelines for the six-minute walk test. *Am J Respir Crit Care Med*. 2002; 166:111-117.

42. AARC Clinical Practice Guideline. Postural drainage therapy. *Respir Care*. 1991; 36:1418-1426

43. Hardy KA. A review of airway clearance: new techniques, indications and recommendations. *Respir Care*. 1994; 39:440.

44. AARC Clinical Practice Guideline. Directed cough. *Respir Care*. 1993; 38:495-499

45. Levenson CR. Breathing exercises. In: *Pulmonary Management in Physical Therapy*. In: Zadai CC. Ed. New York, NY; 1992: 135-155.

46. Cahalin LP, Braga M, Matsuo Y, Hernandez ED. Efficacy of diaphragmatic breathing in persons with chronic obstructive pulmonary disease: a review of the literature. *J Cardiopulm Rehabil*. 2002; 22:7-21.

47. Shekleton M, Berry JK, Covey MK. Respiratory muscle weakness and training. In: Frownfelter D, Dean E, eds. *Principles and Practice of Cardiopulmonary Physical Therapy*. Fifth ed. St. Louis, Mo: Mosby; 2012: 443-452.

48. Lotters F, van Tol B, Kwakkel G, Gosselink R. Effects of controlled inspiratory muscle training in patients with COPD: a meta-analysis. *Eur Respir*. 2002; 20:570-576.

49. Gosselink R. Controlled breathing and dyspnea in patients with chronic obstructive pulmonary disease (COPD) *J Rehabil Res Dev*. 2003;40(5): Suppl 2:25-33.

50. Humberstone N, Tecklin JS. Respiratory treatment. In: Irwin S, Tecklin JS, eds. *Cardiopulmonary Physical Therapy*. 3rd ed. St. Louis, Mo: Mosby; 1995; 356-374.

51. AARC Clinical Practice Guideline. Incentive spirometry. *Respir Care*. 1991; 36:1402-1405.

52. American Association of Cardiovascular & Pulmonary Rehabilitation. *Guidelines for Cardiac Rehabilitation and Secondary Prevention Programs*. 4th ed. Champaign,IL: Human Kinetics; 2004.

53. Balady GJ, Ades PA, Comoss P, Limacher M, et al. Core components of cardiac rehabilitation/secondary prevention programs: A statement for healthcare professionals from the American Heart Association and the American Association of Cardiovascular and Pulmonary Rehabilitation. *Circulation*. 2000;102:1069-1073.

54. Keteyian SJ, Brawner CA. Cardiopulmonary Adaptations to Exercise. In: Kaminsky LA, ed. ACSM's *Resource Manual for Guidelines for Exercise Testing and Prescription*. 5th ed. Baltimore, MD: Williams & Wilkins; 2006.

55. AARC Clinical Practice Guideline Pulmonary Rehabilitation. *Respir Care* 2002; 47:617-625.

56. American Association of Cardiovascular & Pulmonary Rehabilitation. *Guidelines for Pulmonary Rehabilitation Programs*. 3rd ed. Champaign, IL: Human Kinetics; 2004.

57. Troosters T, Casaburi R, Gosselink R, Decramer M. Pulmonary rehabilitation in chronic obstructive pulmonary disease. Am J Respir Crit Care Med 2005:172:19-38.

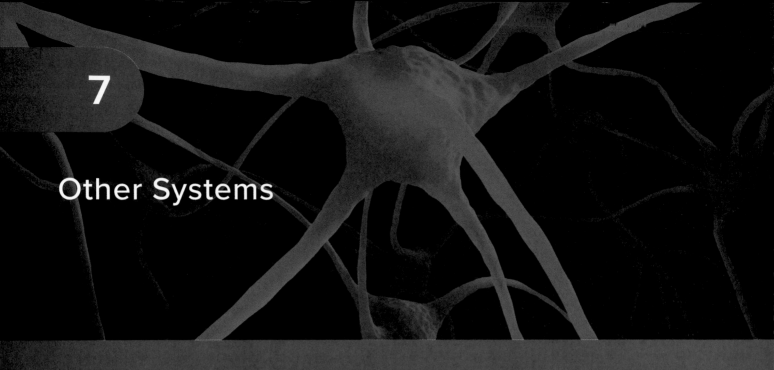

7

Other Systems

Therese Giles
Scott Giles

Other Systems represents approximately 18 - 38 questions (12% - 25.3%) on the NPTE-PTA.

Contributors

Shawn Paquette
Daniel Lee
Danielle Cowan
Ryan Bailey

CHAPTER 7
Other Systems

Integumentary System

Foundational Science: Integumentary System

The integumentary system (or skin) is the body's largest organ consisting of stratified dermal and epidermal layers, hair follicles, nails, sebaceous glands, and sweat glands. The avascular epidermis is the most superficial layer of skin. The dermis, known as the true skin, is well vascularized, and is characterized as elastic, flexible, and tough (Fig. 7-1).[1]

Key Functions of the Integumentary System

- Protection

- Sensation

- Thermoregulation

- Excretion of sweat

- Vitamin D synthesis

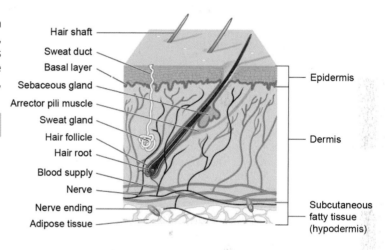

Fig. 7-1: Anatomy of the skin.

Phases of Normal Wound Healing[1,2]

Normal wound healing occurs as damaged tissues move through distinct yet overlapping phases of repair. In chronic wounds, this progression is either interrupted or delayed causing the wound to become "stuck" in a particular phase of healing.

Inflammatory Phase (1 to 10 days)[3,4]

Inflammation is the immune system's initial response to a wound. Temporary repair mechanisms rapidly re-establish hemostasis through platelet activation and the clotting cascade. Debris and necrotic tissue are removed and bacteria are killed by mast cells, neutrophils, and leukocytes. Processes occurring in the inflammatory phase establish a clean wound bed which signals tissue restoration and permanent repair processes to begin. Re-epithelialization typically begins within 24 hours at the wound borders, though visible signs are usually not observed earlier than three days after injury.

Proliferative Phase (3 to 21 days)[3,4]

The formation of new tissue signals the beginning of the proliferative phase. Capillary buds and granulation tissue begin to fill the wound bed creating a support structure for the migration of epithelial cells. Keratinocytes, endothelial cells, and fibroblasts are active and the collagen matrix is formed. Skin integrity is restored in the proliferative phase with wound closure occurring through epithelialization and wound contraction.

Maturation Phase (7 days to 2 years)[3,4]

The maturation, or remodeling phase is initiated when granulation tissue and epithelial differentiation begin to appear in the wound bed. As the maturation phase progresses, mechanisms of fiber reorganization and contraction shrink and thin the scar. An immature scar will appear red, raised, and rigid while a mature scar will appear pale, flat, and pliable. Scar tissue is remodeled and strengthened through the processes of collagen lysis and synthesis. Newly repaired tissues have approximately 15% of pre-injury tensile integrity and should be protected to prevent re-injury. Over time, tensile integrity may increase to as much as 80% of the pre-injury strength. Hypertrophic scarring, especially in relation to burn injuries, can significantly impact maturation phase progression. A burn without hypertrophic scarring will typically mature within four to eight weeks; burns with hypertrophic scarring, however, may require up to two years to reach maturity.

CONSIDER THIS
THE INFLAMMATORY PHASE AND CHRONIC WOUNDS[2]

An abnormal inflammatory response (e.g., chronic or delayed) is believed to be the most significant factor in delayed wound healing and chronicity. Re-injury, infection, poor tissue perfusion or the body's failure to initiate appropriate responses may prolong the inflammatory phase. Inflammation that persists chronically for weeks or months interferes with the initiation of proliferative phase processes and increases the risk of infection.

Anti-inflammatory or immunosuppressive medications, arterial insufficiency or conditions that alter immune responses (e.g., diabetes mellitus, alcoholism, AIDS) can limit the body's response to a wound. This can occur to the extent that the healing process is never truly initiated, resulting in a chronic wound. Differing from chronically inflamed wounds, chronic wounds show little if any of the usual inflammatory phase characteristics and fail to progress.

Healing by Intention[2,4]

Primary Intention

Healing by primary intention most commonly occurs in acute wounds with minimal tissue loss. Smooth clean edges are reapproximated and closed with sutures, staples or adhesives to facilitate re-epithelialization. Superficial partial-thickness wounds, such as abrasions or blisters, also heal by primary intention with epithelial migration over the wound bed frequently completed within 72 hours. Wounds healing by primary intention typically have minimal scarring and heal quickly in an uncomplicated and orderly progression (e.g., surgical incision, laceration, puncture, and superficial and partial-thickness wounds).

Secondary Intention

Healing by secondary intention permits wounds to close on their own without superficial closure. Wounds with characteristics such as significant tissue loss or necrosis, irregular or nonviable wound margins that cannot be reapproximated, infection or debris contamination typically heal by secondary intention. These wounds are often associated with pathology such as diabetes, ischemic conditions, pressure damage or inflammatory disease. A layer of granulation tissue will gradually fill the wound bed to the level of the surrounding skin, with closure occurring by wound contraction and scar formation. Wounds healing by secondary intention require ongoing wound care and have significantly larger scars than those healing by primary intention (e.g., neuropathic, arterial, venous or pressure ulcers, most full-thickness wounds, and chronically inflamed wounds).

Tertiary Intention

Healing by tertiary intention may also be referred to as delayed primary intention healing. Wounds at risk for developing complications, such as sepsis or dehiscence, may be temporarily left open. Once risk factors have been alleviated (e.g., wounds with significant edema, contamination from debris, at high risk for infection or with questionable vascular integrity) the wound is closed by the usual primary intention methods.

Factors Influencing Wound Healing

There are a variety of factors, not inherent to the wound itself, which can significantly impact the rate and degree of wound healing. Physical therapist assistants should encourage patients to make positive changes with modifiable factors and assist them in compensating for unmodifiable factors.

Age: The epidermis thins and flattens as part of the aging process, making it more fragile and susceptible to injury from friction and shear. Decreased metabolism in older adults is also correlated with a decrease in the overall rate of wound healing.[2,4]

Co-morbidities: Medical co-morbidities such as cardio-pulmonary disease, vascular conditions, and diabetes mellitus can significantly delay wound healing. This is often attributed to poor tissue perfusion which limits the wound's ability to sustain cellular activity. Co-morbidities which suppress or compromise the immune system can result in altered inflammatory responses and increased risk of infection.[1,2]

Edema: Some degree of edema is considered a normal part of the body's inflammatory response to a wound. However, increased tissue pressure from excessive edema, such as with venous insufficiency or lymphedema, can negatively impact both tissue perfusion and the removal of cellular waste. This alteration in hemodynamics decreases the availability of oxygen and nutrients thus delaying healing and increasing the risk of infection.[1,2]

Harsh or Inappropriate Wound Care: Failure to use appropriate technique or best-practice interventions in wound care can contribute to wound healing delays. Vigorous wound irrigation, aggressive debridement, prolonged whirlpool exposure or the use of harsh cleansing techniques and agents can impair healing by further damaging peripheral and granulating tissues.[4]

Infection: Wound infection negatively impacts the restorative processes necessary for wound healing. Immune responses become overwhelmed as infectious bacteria compete with the body's own cells for available nutrients. Infectious bacteria can also release toxins into the wound causing further tissue damage and increasing the rate of cellular necrosis.[1,2]

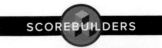

Lifestyle: Regular physical activity and good nutrition facilitate wound healing by enhancing tissue perfusion and the availability of nutrients needed to sustain cellular activity. In contrast, smoking dramatically impedes wound healing by limiting the blood's oxygen carrying capacity. The resulting wound hypoxia slows healing and creates an ideal environment for anaerobic bacteria growth, thereby increasing the risk of wound infection.[1,2]

Medication: Medications from a variety of pharmacological classes can negatively impact wound healing. Common classes include anti-inflammatory, immunosuppressive, anti-coagulant, anti-neoplastic, steroid, and oral contraceptive agents. Undesirable physiologic effects may include a poor or prolonged inflammatory response, reduced blood supply, delayed collagen synthesis, and decreased tensile strength of repaired tissues.[1,2]

Obesity: Obesity is associated with numerous medical co-morbidities in addition to various inherent factors that may negatively impact wound healing. Poor periwound skin quality is susceptible to fissuring which increases the risk of wound infection. Increased skin tension heightens the risk of skin tears and limits options for reapproximation. Large skin folds create moist, warm environments contributing to skin maceration and bacterial growth which may lead to both the onset and perpetuation of wounds in skin crevasses.[2,5]

CONSIDER THIS
CONTAMINATED, COLONIZED OR INFECTED?[4]

Contamination: The presence of non-replicating bacteria on a wound surface that causes no additional tissue injury and does not stimulate an inflammatory immune response.

Colonization: The presence of replicating bacteria on a wound surface that does not invade or further injure tissues and does not stimulate an inflammatory immune response. Colonization can delay wound healing, however, colonized bacteria occasionally benefit wound healing by preventing more virulent organisms from proliferating in the wound bed.

Infection: The presence of replicating bacteria that invades viable tissue beyond the wound surface causing a visible inflammatory immune response. Infection will significantly delay wound healing and, if untreated, can progress to sepsis, osteomyelitis, and gangrene.

Wound Types

Acute Wounds[2]

Abrasion: An abrasion is a wound caused by a combination of friction and shear forces, typically over a rough surface, resulting in the scraping away of the skin's superficial layers.

Avulsion: A soft tissue avulsion, sometimes referred to as degloving, is a serious wound resulting from tension that causes skin to become detached from underlying structures.

Incisional wound: An incisional wound is most often associated with surgery and is created intentionally by means of a sharp object such as a scalpel or scissors.

Laceration: A laceration is a wound or irregular tear of tissues often associated with trauma. Lacerations can result from shear, tension or high force compression with the resultant wound characteristics dependent on the mechanism of injury.

Penetrating: A penetrating wound can result from various mechanisms of injury and is described as a wound that enters the interior of an organ or cavity.

Puncture: A puncture wound is made by a sharp pointed object as it penetrates the skin and underlying tissues. Typically, there is relatively little tissue damage beyond the wound tract, however, the risks of contamination and infection can be significant.

Skin tear: A skin tear often results from trauma to fragile skin such as bumping into an object, adhesive removal, shear or friction forces. The severity of a skin tear can range from a flap-like tear, that may or may not remain viable, to full-thickness tissue loss.

Ulcers

Arterial Insufficiency Ulcers[1,2]

Wounds resulting from arterial insufficiency occur secondary to inadequate circulation of oxygenated blood (e.g., ischemia) often due to complicating factors such as atherosclerosis.

General Recommendations:

- Rest
- Limb protection
- Risk reduction education
- Inspect legs and feet daily
- Avoid unnecessary leg elevation
- Avoid using heating pads or soaking feet in hot water
- Wear appropriately sized shoes with clean, seamless socks

CONSIDER THIS
ASSESSING PROTECTIVE SENSATION[4]

The loss of protective sensation in individuals with peripheral neuropathy can significantly increase the risk of tissue damage. Monofilament testing is a reliable method of assessing and documenting changes in protective sensation. Monofilament testing kits contain a variety of filament thicknesses which are applied perpendicular to the skin and held in place for one second with enough force to bend the filament into a "C" shape (Fig. 7-2).

Failure to perceive the application of a 10 gm monofilament indicates a loss of protective sensation (e.g., inability to feel a small pebble in a shoe or a developing blister) and places a patient at increased risk for developing a neuropathic ulcer. Failure to perceive a 75 gm monofilament indicates that an area is insensate.[4]

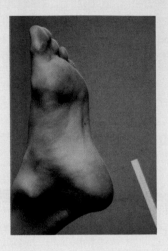

Fig. 7-2: A monofilament applied perpendicular to the target area.

Venous Insufficiency Ulcers[1,2]

Wounds resulting from venous insufficiency occur secondary to impaired functioning of the venous system resulting in inadequate circulation and eventual tissue damage and ulceration.

General Recommendations:

- Limb protection
- Risk reduction education
- Inspect legs and feet daily
- Compression to control edema
- Elevate legs above the heart when resting or sleeping
- Attempt active exercise including frequent range of motion
- Wear appropriately sized shoes with clean, seamless socks

Neuropathic Ulcers[1,2]

Neuropathic ulcers are a secondary complication usually associated with a combination of ischemia and neuropathy. Neuropathic ulcers are often associated with diabetes mellitus, however, any form of peripheral neuropathy poses an increased risk of wound development.

General Recommendations:

- Limb protection
- Risk reduction education
- Inspect legs and feet daily
- Inspect footwear for debris prior to donning
- Wear appropriately sized off-loading footwear with clean, cushioned, seamless socks

Pressure Ulcers[1,2]

Pressure ulcers, also referred to as decubitus ulcers, result from sustained or prolonged pressure on tissue at levels greater than that of capillary pressure. Skin covering bony prominences is particularly susceptible to localized ischemia and tissue necrosis due to pressure. Pressure injuries to deeper tissues may initially present as bruising or purple blisters under intact skin before opening to reveal full-thickness damage. Factors contributing to pressure ulcers include shearing forces, moisture, heat, friction, medications, muscle atrophy, malnutrition, and debilitating medical conditions. Valid and reliable pressure injury risk assessment tools are readily available (e.g., Braden Scale, Norton Scale) and typically include intervention recommendations based on the level of risk assessed.

General Recommendations:

- Repositioning every two hours in bed
- Management of excess moisture
- Off-loading with pressure relieving devices
- Inspect skin daily for signs of pressure damage
- Limit shear, traction, and friction forces over fragile skin

Characteristics of Lower Extremity Ulcers[1,2,4]

	Arterial Insufficiency Ulcers	Venous Insufficiency Ulcers	Neuropathic Ulcers
Location	Lower one-third of leg, toes, web spaces (distal toes, dorsal foot, lateral malleolus)	Proximal to the medial malleolus	Areas of the foot susceptible to pressure or shear forces during weight bearing
Appearance	Smooth edges, well defined; lack granulation tissue; tend to be deep	Irregular shape; shallow	Well-defined oval or circle; callused rim; cracked periwound tissue; little to no wound bed necrosis with good granulation
Exudate	Minimal	Moderate/heavy	Low/moderate
Pain	Severe	Mild to moderate	None, however dysesthesia may be reported
Pedal Pulses	Diminished or absent	Normal	Diminished or absent; unreliable ankle-brachial index with diabetes
Edema	Normal	Increased	Normal
Skin Temperature	Decreased	Normal	Decreased
Tissue Changes	Thin and shiny; hair loss; yellow nails	Flaking, dry skin; brownish discoloration	Dry, inelastic, shiny skin; decreased or absent sweat and oil production
Miscellaneous	Leg elevation increases pain	Leg elevation lessens pain	Loss of protective sensation

** Additional detail regarding pressure injury characteristics and the National Pressure Ulcer Advisory Panel (NPUAP) descriptions are found in the Wound Assessment section.

Wound Assessment

Wound Classification by Depth of Injury[4]

Wounds that are not categorized as pressure or neuropathic ulcers (e.g., skin tears, surgical wounds, venous stasis ulcers) are classified based on the depth of tissue loss.

Superficial wound

A superficial wound causes trauma to the skin with the epidermis remaining intact, such as with a non-blistering sunburn. A superficial wound will typically heal as part of the inflammatory process.

Partial-thickness wound

A partial-thickness wound extends through the epidermis and possibly into, but not through, the dermis. Examples include abrasions, blisters, and skin tears. A partial-thickness wound will typically heal by re-epithelialization or epidermal resurfacing depending on the depth of injury.

Full-thickness wound

A full-thickness wound extends through the dermis into deeper structures such as subcutaneous fat. Wounds deeper than 4 millimeters are typically considered full-thickness and heal by secondary intention.

Subcutaneous wound

Subcutaneous wounds extend through integumentary tissues and involve deeper structures such as subcutaneous fat, muscle, tendon or bone. Subcutaneous wounds typically require healing by secondary intention.

Wagner Ulcer Grade Classification Scale

Grade	Description
0	No open lesion, but may possess pre-ulcerative lesions; healed ulcers; presence of bony deformity
1	Superficial ulcer not involving subcutaneous tissue
2	Deep ulcer with penetration through the subcutaneous tissue; potentially exposing bone, tendon, ligament or joint capsule
3	Deep ulcer with osteitis, abscess or osteomyelitis
4	Gangrene of digit
5	Gangrene of foot requiring disarticulation

Wagner Ulcer Grade Classification System[1,2]

The Wagner Ulcer Grade Classification System categorizes dysvascular ulcers based on wound depth and the presence of infection. Most commonly associated with the assessment of diabetic foot ulcers, the scale can be appropriately used to categorize most ulcers arising from neuropathic, ischemic or arterial etiology.

Pressure Injury Staging

A pressure injury is localized damage to the skin and underlying soft tissue usually over a bony prominence or related to a medical or other device. The injury can present as intact skin or an open ulcer and may be painful. The injury occurs as a result of intense and/or prolonged pressure with or without shear. The tolerance of soft tissue for pressure and shear may also be affected by microclimate, nutrition, perfusion, and co-morbidities.

Stage 1 Pressure Injury: Non-blanchable erythema of intact skin

Intact skin with a localized area of non-blanchable erythema. Presence of blanchable erythema or changes in sensation, temperature, or firmness may precede visual changes. Color changes do not include purple or maroon discoloration; these may indicate deep tissue pressure injury.

Stage 2 Pressure Injury: Partial-thickness skin loss with exposed dermis

Partial-thickness loss of skin with exposed dermis. The wound bed is viable, pink or red, moist, and may also present as an intact or ruptured serum-filled blister. Adipose is not visible and deeper tissues are not visible. Granulation tissue, slough and eschar are not present. These injuries commonly result from adverse microclimate and shear over the pelvis and shear in the heel. This stage should not be used to describe moisture associated skin damage (MASD) including incontinence associated dermatitis (IAD), intertriginous dermatitis (ITD), medical adhesive related skin injury (MARSI), or traumatic wounds.

Stage 3 Pressure Injury: Full-thickness skin loss

Full-thickness loss of skin, in which adipose is visible in the ulcer and granulation tissue and epibole (rolled edges) are often present.

Slough and/or eschar may be visible. The depth of tissue damage varies by anatomical location; areas of significant adiposity can develop deep wounds. Undermining and tunneling may occur. Fascia, muscle, tendon, ligament, cartilage and/or bone are not exposed. If slough or eschar obscures the extent of tissue loss, this is an Unstageable Pressure Injury.

Stage 4 Pressure Injury: Full-thickness skin and tissue loss

Full-thickness skin and tissue loss with exposed or directly palpable fascia, muscle, tendon, ligament, cartilage or bone in the ulcer. Slough and/or eschar may be visible. Epibole (rolled edges), undermining and/or tunneling often occur. Depth varies by anatomical location. If slough or eschar obscures the extent of tissue loss this is an Unstageable Pressure Injury.

Unstageable Pressure Injury: Obscured full-thickness skin and tissue loss

Full-thickness skin and tissue loss in which the extent of tissue damage within the ulcer cannot be confirmed because it is obscured by slough or eschar. If slough or eschar is removed, a Stage 3 or Stage 4 pressure injury will be revealed. Stable eschar (i.e. dry, adherent, intact without erythema) on the heel or ischemic limb should not be softened or removed.

Deep Tissue Pressure Injury: Persistent non-blanchable deep red, maroon or purple discoloration

Intact or non-intact skin with localized area of persistent non-blanchable deep red, maroon, purple discoloration or epidermal separation revealing a dark wound bed or blood filled blister. Pain and temperature change often precede skin color changes. Discoloration may appear differently in darkly pigmented skin. This injury results from intense and/or prolonged pressure and shear forces at the bone-muscle interface. The wound may evolve rapidly to reveal the actual extent of tissue injury, or may resolve without tissue loss. If necrotic tissue, subcutaneous tissue, granulation tissue, fascia, muscle or other underlying structures are visible, this indicates a full-thickness pressure injury (Unstageable, Stage 3 or Stage 4). Do not use deep tissue pressure injury to describe vascular, traumatic, neuropathic, or dermatologic conditions.

Adapted from NPUAP's Pressure Ulcer Staging System, Revised 2016

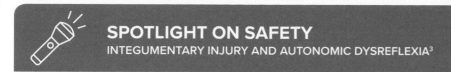

SPOTLIGHT ON SAFETY
INTEGUMENTARY INJURY AND AUTONOMIC DYSREFLEXIA[3]

Ingrown toenails, burns, pressure ulcers, blisters, and other integumentary trauma can trigger an episode of autonomic dysreflexia when occurring below the level of a patient's spinal cord injury.

Since this is a potentially life-threatening condition, it is important for therapists to recognize signs, symptoms, and causative factors of the condition as well as how to immediately and appropriately intervene. If symptoms do not begin to resolve after the patient has been assisted into a sitting position with catheter obstruction ruled out, the therapist should activate the emergency response system and begin to assess for other potential sources of noxious stimuli.

Bony Prominences Associated with Pressure Injuries[1]

Supine	Prone	Sidelying	Sitting (Chair)
Occiput	Forehead	Ears	Spine of the scapula
Spine of scapula	Anterior portion of acromion process	Lateral portion of acromion process	Vertebral spinous processes
Inferior angle of scapula	Anterior head of humerus	Lateral head of humerus	Ischial tuberosities
Vertebral spinous processes	Sternum	Lateral epicondyle of humerus	
Medial epicondyle of humerus	Anterior superior iliac spine	Greater trochanter	
Posterior iliac crest	Patella	Head of fibula	
Sacrum	Dorsum of foot	Lateral malleolus	
Coccyx		Medial malleolus	
Heel			

Exudate Classification[1]

Serous: Presents with a clear, light color and a thin, watery consistency. Serous exudate is considered to be normal in a healthy healing wound and is observed during the inflammatory and proliferative phases of healing.

Sanguineous: Presents with a red color and a thin, watery consistency. The red appearance of sanguineous exudate is due to the presence of blood which may become brown if allowed to dehydrate. Sanguineous exudate may be indicative of new blood vessel growth or the disruption of blood vessels.

Serosanguineous: Presents with a light red or pink color and a thin, watery consistency. Serosanguineous exudate is considered to be normal in a healthy healing wound and is typically observed during the inflammatory and proliferative phases of healing.

Seropurulent: Presents as cloudy or opaque, with a yellow or tan color and a thin, watery consistency. Seropurulent exudate may be an early warning sign of an impending infection and is always considered an abnormal finding.

Purulent: Presents with a yellow or green color and a thick, viscous consistency. Purulent exudate is generally an indicator of wound infection and is always considered an abnormal finding.

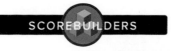

Necrotic Tissue Types[1,4]

Necrotic tissue is dead tissue resulting from the localized physiological and enzymatic changes associated with cell death. Necrotic tissue is often documented and named by the specific type observed, and may also be referred to as devitalized or nonviable tissue. The color, consistency, and adherence of necrotic tissue varies depending on other wound characteristics such as hydration and bacterial activity.

Eschar: Eschar is described as hard or leathery, black/brown, dehydrated tissue that tends to be firmly adhered to the wound bed.

Gangrene: Gangrene refers to the death and decay of tissue resulting from an interruption in blood flow to an area of the body. Some types of gangrene are also characterized by the presence of bacterial infection. Gangrene most commonly affects the extremities, but can also occur in muscles and internal organs.

Hyperkeratosis: Hyperkeratosis, also referred to as callus, is typically white/gray in color and can vary in texture from firm to soggy depending on the moisture level in surrounding tissue.

Slough: Slough is described as moist, stringy or mucinous, white/yellow tissue that tends to be loosely attached in clumps to the wound bed.

Wound Healing Interventions

Red-Yellow-Black System[2]		
Red-Yellow-Black System		
Color	**Wound Description**	**Goals**
Red	Pink granulation tissue	Protect wound; maintain moist environment
Yellow	Moist, yellow slough	Remove exudate and debris; absorb drainage
Black	Black, thick eschar firmly adhered	Debride necrotic tissue

Selective Debridement[2]

Selective debridement involves the removal of only nonviable tissues from a wound. The most common forms of selective debridement used by physical therapist assistants are enzymatic and autolytic.

Enzymatic Debridement

Enzymatic debridement refers to the topical application of an enzymatic preparation to necrotic tissue. Enzymatic debridement can be used on infected and non-infected wounds with necrotic tissue. This type of debridement may be used for wounds that have not responded to autolytic debridement or in conjunction with other debridement techniques. Enzymatic debridement can be slow to establish a clean wound bed and should be discontinued once devitalized tissue is removed to avoid damage to adjacent healthy tissue.

Autolytic Debridement

Autolytic debridement refers to the use of the body's own mechanisms to remove nonviable tissue. Common methods of autolytic debridement include the use of transparent films, hydrocolloids, hydrogels, and alginates. Autolytic debridement establishes a moist wound environment that rehydrates necrotic tissue and eschar, facilitating enzymatic digestion of the nonviable tissue. This type of debridement is non-invasive and pain free.

Autolytic debridement can be used with any amount of necrotic tissue, however, requires a longer healing period and should not be performed on infected wounds.

Non-selective Debridement[1,2,4]

Non-selective debridement involves the removal of both viable and nonviable tissues from a wound. Non-selective debridement is often termed "mechanical debridement" and is most commonly performed via wet-to-dry dressings, wound irrigation, and hydrotherapy (whirlpool).

Wet-to-dry Dressings

Wet-to-dry dressings refer to the application of a moistened gauze dressing over an area of necrotic tissue. The dressing is allowed to dry completely and is later removed, along with any necrotic tissue that has adhered to the gauze. Wet-to-dry dressings are most often used to debride wounds with moderate amounts of exudate and necrotic tissue. This type of debridement should be used sparingly on wounds containing both necrotic and viable tissue since granulation tissue will be traumatized in the process. Removal of dry dressings from granulation tissue may cause bleeding and be extremely painful.

Wound Irrigation

Wound irrigation removes necrotic tissue from the wound bed using pressurized fluid. Pulsatile lavage is an example of wound irrigation that uses a pressurized stream of irrigation solution. This type of debridement is most desirable for wounds that are infected or have loose debris. Many devices permit variable pressure settings and provide suction for the removal of exudate and debris.

Hydrotherapy

Hydrotherapy is most commonly employed using a whirlpool tank with agitation directed toward a wound requiring debridement. This process softens and loosens adherent necrotic tissue. Physical therapist assistants must be aware of potential hydrotherapy side effects such as maceration of viable tissue, edema from dependent lower extremity positioning, and systemic effects such as hypotension.

Modalities and Physical Agents[1,2,5]

Negative Pressure Wound Therapy (NPWT)

NPWT, also referred to as vacuum-assisted closure (V.A.C.), is a non-invasive wound care modality used to facilitate healing and manage drainage (Fig. 7-4). A sterile foam dressing is placed in the wound and sealed with an airtight secondary dressing which attaches via tubing to a vacuum pump with a reservoir container. Treatment protocols vary depending on wound characteristics.

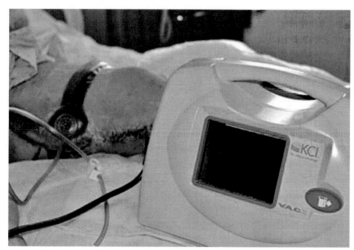

Fig. 7-4: Negative pressure wound therapy applied to the lower extremity.

Indications

Chronic or acute wounds which cannot be closed by primary intention such as dehisced surgical incisions, full-thickness wounds, partial-thickness burns, heavily draining granular wounds, flaps, grafts, and most ulcer types.

Contraindications

Malignancy within the wound, insufficient vascularity to sustain wound healing, large amounts of necrotic tissue with eschar present, untreated osteomyelitis, fistulas to organs or body cavities, exposed arteries or veins, and uncontrolled pain.

Advantages

- Provides management of wound drainage
- Maintains a moist wound environment

- Decreases interstitial edema
- Decreases bacterial colonization
- Increases capillary blood flow
- Increases granular tissue formation
- Enhances epithelial cell migration

Disadvantages

- Requires special supplies and training
- Treatment can be painful
- Not reimbursed in acute or long-term care settings

Hyperbaric Oxygen

Hyperbaric oxygen refers to the inhalation of 100% oxygen delivered at pressures greater than one atmosphere. Hyperbaric oxygen treatment is delivered in a closed chamber typically at pressures two to three times that of the atmosphere, effectively reducing edema and hyperoxygenating tissues.

Indications

Osteomyelitis, diabetic wounds, crush injuries, compartment syndromes, necrotizing soft tissue infection, thermal burns, radiation necrosis, and compromised flaps and grafts.

Contraindications

Terminal illness, untreated pneumothorax, active malignancy, pregnancy, seizure disorder, emphysema, and use of certain chemotherapy agents.

Advantages

- Antibiotic effects
- Stimulation of fibroblast production and collagen synthesis
- Stimulation of growth factor release and epithelialization

Disadvantages

- Specialized equipment is not widely available
- Cannot be used with active malignancy

Types of Dressings[1,2,4]

Dressings may be defined as either primary or secondary. A primary dressing is one that comes into direct contact with a wound. A number of primary dressings include a self-adhesive backing and do not require a secondary dressing. Secondary dressings are placed directly over the primary dressing to provide additional protection, absorption, occlusion, and/or to secure the primary dressing in place.

Alginates

Alginate dressings are derived from a seaweed extraction, specifically, the calcium salt component of alginic acid. Alginates are highly absorptive, but are also highly permeable and non-occlusive. As a result, they require a secondary dressing. Alginate dressings act as a hemostat and create a hydrophilic gel through the interaction of calcium ions in the dressing and sodium ions in the wound exudate.

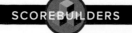

CONSIDER THIS
THERAPEUTIC MODALITIES WITH WOUND HEALING APPLICATIONS[1]

Therapeutic ultrasound applied at a low intensity with pulsed duty cycle has been shown to enhance all phases of wound healing. During the inflammatory and proliferative phases, fibroblast, endothelial, and white blood cell activity are stimulated by ultrasound. Ultrasound use during these early stages of repair has been shown to enhance the strength and elasticity of scar tissue. Recommended treatment protocols vary depending on the phase of healing and intended outcome (e.g., restarting the inflammatory phase of healing in a chronic ulcer vs. dispersing ecchymosis associated with skin tears or contusions to reduce pain and edema).

High-voltage pulsed current (HVPC) electrical stimulation has been shown to enhance healing in numerous types of wounds including chronic ulcers, burns, and donor and graft sites. The application of monophasic direct current stimulates angiogenesis and epithelial migration, decreases bacterial activity and wound pain, and increases oxygen perfusion and tensile strength. HVPC is typically applied using a sensory or sub-sensory intensity. Treatment protocols vary widely depending on the stage of healing or presence of infection.

Indications

Alginates are typically used on partial or full-thickness draining wounds such as pressure or venous insufficiency ulcers. Alginates are often used on infected wounds due to the likelihood of excessive drainage.

Advantages

- High absorptive capacity
- Enables autolytic debridement
- Offers protection from microbial contamination
- Can be used on infected or non-infected wounds
- Non-adhering to wound

Disadvantages

- May require frequent dressing changes based on level of exudate
- Requires a secondary dressing
- Cannot be used on wounds with an exposed tendon, joint capsule or bone

Foam Dressings

Foam dressings are comprised of a hydrophilic polyurethane base that contacts the wound surface and a hydrophobic outer layer. The dressings allow exudate to be absorbed into the foam through the hydrophilic layer. The dressings are most commonly available in sheets or pads with varying degrees of thickness. Semipermeable foam dressings are produced in adhesive and non-adhesive forms. Non-adhesive forms require a secondary dressing.

Indications

Foam dressings are used to provide protection and absorption over partial and full-thickness wounds with varying levels of exudate. They can also be used as secondary dressings over amorphous hydrogels.

Advantages

- Provides a moist environment for wound healing
- Available in adhesive and non-adhesive forms
- Provides prophylactic protection and cushioning
- Encourages autolytic debridement
- Provides moderate absorption

Disadvantages

- May tend to roll in areas of excessive friction
- Adhesive form may traumatize periwound area upon removal
- Lack of transparency makes inspection of wound difficult

Gauze

Gauze dressings are manufactured from yarn or thread and are the most readily available dressing used in inpatient environments. Gauze dressings come in many shapes and sizes (e.g., sheets, squares, rolls, packing strips). Impregnated gauze is a variation of woven gauze in which various materials such as petrolatum, zinc or antimicrobials have been added.

Indications

Gauze dressings are commonly used on infected or non-infected wounds of any size. The dressings can be used for wet-to-wet, wet-to-moist or wet-to-dry debridement.

Advantages

- Readily available and cost effective short-term dressings
- Can be used alone or in combination with other dressings and topical agents
- Can modify number of layers to accommodate for changing wound status
- Can be used on infected or non-infected wounds

Disadvantages

- Has a tendency to adhere to the wound bed traumatizing viable tissue on removal

- Highly permeable
- Requires frequent dressing changes
- Prolonged use decreases cost effectiveness
- Increased infection rate compared to occlusive dressings

Hydrocolloids

Hydrocolloid dressings consist of gel-forming polymers (e.g., carboxymethylcellulose, gelatin, pectin) backed by a strong film or foam adhesive. The dressing does not attach to the wound itself but instead anchors to the intact surrounding skin. The dressings absorb exudate by swelling into a gel-like mass and vary in permeability, thickness, and transparency.

Indications

Hydrocolloids are useful for partial and full-thickness wounds. The dressings can be used effectively with granular or necrotic wounds.

Advantages

- Provides a moist environment for wound healing
- Enables autolytic debridement
- Offers protection from microbial contamination
- Provides moderate absorption
- Does not require a secondary dressing
- Provides a waterproof surface

Disadvantages

- May traumatize surrounding intact skin upon removal
- May tend to roll in areas of excessive friction
- Cannot be used on infected wounds

Hydrogels

Hydrogels consist of varying amounts of water and gel-forming materials such as glycerin. The dressings are typically available in both sheet and amorphous forms.

Indications

Hydrogels are moisture retentive and commonly used on superficial and partial-thickness wounds (e.g., abrasions, blisters, pressure ulcers) that have minimal drainage.

Advantages

- Provides a moist environment for wound healing
- Enables autolytic debridement
- May reduce pressure and diminish pain
- Can be used as a coupling agent for ultrasound
- Minimally adheres to wound
- Some products have absorptive properties

Disadvantages

- Potential for dressings to dehydrate
- Cannot be used on wounds with significant drainage
- Typically requires a secondary dressing

Transparent Film

Transparent film dressings are thin membranes made from transparent polyurethane with water-resistant adhesives. The dressings are permeable to vapor and oxygen, but are largely impermeable to bacteria and water. They are highly elastic, conform to a variety of body contours, and allow easy visual inspection of the wound since they are transparent.

Indications

Film dressings are useful for superficial or partial-thickness wounds with minimal drainage (e.g., scalds, abrasions, lacerations).

Advantages

- Provides a moist environment for wound healing
- Enables autolytic debridement
- Allows visualization of the wound
- Resistant to shearing and frictional forces
- Cost effective over time

Disadvantages

- Excessive exudate accumulation can result in periwound maceration
- Adhesive may traumatize periwound area upon removal
- Cannot be used on infected wounds

CONSIDER THIS
COMBINATION DRESSINGS USING SILVER AND IODINE[1,2]

Silver and iodine are elemental broad-spectrum antimicrobial agents that have become valuable adjuncts to wound healing interventions. First used in topical applications (e.g., powder, ointment, cream), these elements control microorganism activity in wound beds without damaging viable tissue. Many silver and iodine-impregnated dressings also help to maintain a moist wound healing environment.

Absorbency and recommended frequency of dressing changes are product dependent with many requiring a secondary dressing.

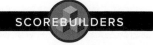

Moisture and Occlusion[2,4]

A dry wound bed slows normal metabolic functions, impeding the healing process. Dry peripheral tissues are at risk for developing cracks or fissures that can become open avenues for infection. Conversely, prolonged excessive moisture (e.g., from poorly managed exudate or incontinence) will cause maceration damage and erosion of intact peripheral tissues.

In an appropriately moist wound environment, macrophages appear earlier and in greater numbers helping to reduce the risk of infection. Collagen synthesis and epithelialization rate are enhanced, facilitating more rapid wound closure. In exuding wounds, moisture must be well managed to prevent damage to surrounding tissue. In dry wounds, moisture must be added in order to maintain hydration and sustain cellular activity. Maintaining an appropriately moist wound bed requires a delicate balance often necessitating specialized dressings to appropriately manage exudate and provide some level of occlusion.

Occlusion refers to the ability of a dressing to transmit moisture, vapor or gases between a wound bed and the atmosphere. A fully occlusive substance would be completely impermeable (e.g., latex gloves), while a non-occlusive substance would be completely permeable (e.g., gauze pads). Wound dressings are typically classified according to this occlusion continuum or by their moisture retention properties.

Dressings from Most Occlusive to Non-Occlusive	Dressings from Most to Least Moisture Retentive
Hydrocolloids	Alginates
Hydrogels	Semipermeable foams
Semipermeable foam	Hydrocolloids
Semipermeable film	Hydrogels
Impregnated gauze	Semipermeable films
Alginates	
Traditional gauze	

CONSIDER THIS
INCONTINENCE AND TISSUE INJURY[5]

Incontinence refers to the inability to control urination or defecation. A patient who is incontinent is at a significantly increased risk of tissue injury or in the presence of existing tissue injury, may experience additional complications including delayed healing.

- Urine and feces are typically acidic in composition and can contribute to tissue irritation and erosion.
- Skin shear and friction are increased in the presence of mild to moderate moisture.
- Macerated skin has decreased epidermal resilience to shear and friction forces.
- Harsh cleansers, hot water, and scrubbing will make delicate tissues more friable.
- Mild cleansers, warm water, and minimal friction should be used when cleansing to minimize irritation.
- Topical agents should be employed both to maintain the skin's natural moisture and act as a barrier to excessive moisture from incontinence.
- Emollient creams and ointments are typically better choices for skin moisturizers than watery lotions as they tend to have higher concentrations of solids and oils requiring less frequent reapplication and providing better barrier protection.

Skin Care Products[2,3]

Therapeutic moisturizers: (e.g., lotion, cream) Lotions are largely water-based and best used to replace skin moisture that has been lost either to the air or as a result of frequent hand washing. Creams are thicker water-based substances with higher concentrations of solids and oils than lotions, making the need for reapplication less frequent. Therapeutic moisturizers are intended to maintain the skin's natural moisture and prevent tissue cracking due to dryness, but do not typically protect the skin from excessive moisture.

Moisture barriers: (e.g., ointment) Moisture barriers are designed to adhere to the skin and repel excess moisture from protected areas. They are frequently used to protect surrounding skin from a heavily draining wound or perineal tissues from exposure to incontinence.

Liquid skin protectants: (e.g., skin sealant) Liquid skin protectant is applied to skin and when dry it creates a thin plastic film protecting the skin from adhesive-related tissue damage. This thin barrier also offers some degree of moisture protection. Skin protectant application varies slightly depending on packaging (e.g., swab, wipes, tube, bottle). Regardless, once applied to the skin it should be allowed to dry fully before an adhesive product is applied over it.

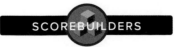

Skin cleansers: Skin cleansers are liquid agents typically intended for use on the skin of patients at risk for breakdown. Ingredients often have a pH balancing component that is especially beneficial for perineal cleansing in patients who are incontinent. Skin cleansers are designed to be less drying to the skin and more effective than usual soap or detergent skin products.

Wound cleansers: Wound cleansers vary from simple saline solutions to more complex compositions with cytotoxicity. Many wound cleansers have the potential to cause inflammation, however, this quality is product dependent. Wound cleansers are not typically designed to remove necrotic tissue, but rather associated wound substances such as foreign materials, exudate and dried blood.

Wound Terminology[1,2,4,5]

Contusion: An injury, usually caused by a blow, that does not disrupt skin integrity. The injury is characterized by pain, edema, and discoloration which appears as a result of blood seepage under the surface of the skin.

Dehiscence: The separation, rupture or splitting of a wound closed by primary intention. This disruption of previously approximated surfaces may be superficial or involve all layers of tissue.

Dermis: The vascular layer of skin located below the epidermis containing hair follicles, sebaceous glands, sweat glands, lymphatic and blood vessels, and nerve endings.

Ecchymosis: The discoloration occurring below intact skin resulting from trauma to underlying blood vessels and blood seeping into tissues. The discoloration is typically blue-black, changing in time to a greenish brown or yellow color. An area where ecchymosis is present is commonly referred to as a bruise.

Epidermis: The superficial, avascular epithelial layer of the skin that includes flat, scale-like squamous cells, round basal cells, and melanocytes which produce melanin and give skin its color.

Erythema: A diffuse redness of the skin often resulting from capillary dilation and congestion or inflammation.

Hematoma: A localized swelling or mass of clotted blood confined to a tissue, organ or space usually caused by a break in a blood vessel.

Hypergranulation: Increased thickness of the granular layer of the epidermis that exceeds the surface height of the skin.

Hyperpigmentation: An excess of pigment in a tissue that causes it to appear darker than surrounding tissues.

Hypertrophic scar: An abnormal scar resulting from excessive collagen formation during healing. A hypertrophic scar is typically raised, red, and firm with disorganized collagen fibers.

Keloid: An abnormal scar formation that is out of proportion to the scarring required for normal tissue repair and is comprised of irregularly distributed collagen bands. A keloid scar typically exceeds the boundaries of the original wound appearing red, thick, raised, and firm.

Maceration: The skin softening and degeneration that results from prolonged exposure to water or other fluids.

Normotrophic scar: A scar characterized by the organized formation of collagen fibers that align in a parallel fashion.

Turgor: The relative speed with which the skin resumes its normal appearance after being lightly pinched. Turgor is an indicator of skin elasticity and hydration and normally occurs more slowly in older adults.

Ulcer: An open sore or lesion of the skin accompanied by sloughing of inflamed necrotic tissue.

Burns

Types of Burns[6]

Thermal burn: Caused by conduction or convection. Examples include burns resulting from contact with a hot liquid, fire or steam.

Electrical burn: Caused by the passage of electrical current through the body. Typically there is an entrance and an exit wound. Complications can include cardiac arrhythmias, respiratory arrest, renal failure, neurological damage, and fractures. A burn caused by a lightning strike is an example of an electrical burn.

Chemical burn: Occurs when certain chemical compounds come in contact with the body. The reaction will continue until the chemical compound is diluted at the site of contact. Compounds that cause chemical burns include sulfuric acid, lye, hydrochloric acid, and gasoline.

Radiation burn: Occurs most commonly with exposure to external beam radiation therapy. DNA is altered in exposed tissues and ischemic injury may be irreversible. Complications may include severe blistering and desquamation, non-healing wounds, tissue fibrosis, permanent discoloration, and new malignancies.

Zones of Injury[3]

Zone of coagulation: The area of the burn that received the most severe injury with irreversible cell damage.

Zone of stasis: The area of less severe injury that possesses reversible damage and surrounds the zone of coagulation.

Zone of hyperemia: The area surrounding the zone of stasis that presents with inflammation, but will fully recover without any intervention or permanent damage.

Burn Classification[3,6]

The extent and severity of a burn is dependent on gender, age, duration of burn, type of burn, and affected area. Burns are most appropriately classified according to the depth of tissue destruction.

Superficial burn: A superficial burn involves only the outer epidermis. The involved area may be red with slight edema. Healing occurs without peeling or evidence of scarring in two to five days.

Superficial partial-thickness burn: A superficial partial-thickness burn involves the epidermis and the upper portion of the dermis. The involved area may be extremely painful and exhibit blisters. Healing occurs with minimal to no scarring in 5-21 days.

Deep partial-thickness burn: A deep partial-thickness burn involves complete destruction of the epidermis and the majority of the dermis. The involved area may appear to be discolored with broken blisters and edema. Damage to nerve endings may result in only moderate levels of pain. Hypertrophic or keloid scarring may occur. In the absence of infection, healing will occur in 21-35 days.

Full-thickness burn: A full-thickness burn involves complete destruction of the epidermis and dermis along with partial damage to the subcutaneous fat layer. The involved area typically presents with eschar formation and minimal pain. Patients with full-thickness burns require grafts and are susceptible to infection. Healing time varies significantly with smaller areas healing in a matter of weeks, with or without grafting, and larger areas requiring grafting and potentially months to heal.

Subdermal burn: A subdermal burn involves the complete destruction of the epidermis, dermis, and subcutaneous tissue. Subdermal burns may involve muscle and bone and as a result, often require multiple surgical interventions and extensive healing time.

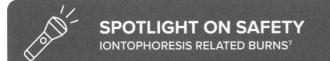

SPOTLIGHT ON SAFETY
IONTOPHORESIS RELATED BURNS[7]

Chemical burns from iontophoresis occur when skin pH increases or decreases beyond the range of normal tolerance. Chemically induced pH levels below 3 or greater than 5 can result in acidic or alkaline reactions, respectively.

Chemical burns are typically more severe under the negative electrode where pooling of the alkaline medium can occur. This can create a pH exceeding 9 which will quickly begin to erode the insulating epidermis. With skin resistance reduced, electrical current delivery increases, further accelerating skin erosion.

Factors contributing to chemical burns from iontophoresis include treatment delivered with excessive current, prolonged duration, and electrode placement over defective skin areas with lower resistance.

Poor iontophoresis electrode placement can contribute to a thermal burn in cases of excessive impedance or poor electrode contact.

Rule of Nines

Allows for a gross approximation of the percentage of the body affected by a burn. The rule of nines does not account for severity.

Adult Values

Head and neck	**9%**
Anterior trunk	**18%**
Posterior trunk	**18%**
Bilateral anterior arm, forearm, and hand	**9%**
Bilateral posterior arm, forearm, and hand	**9%**
Genital region	**1%**
Bilateral anterior leg and foot	**18%**
Bilateral posterior leg and foot	**18%**

Child Values

A child under one year has 9% taken from the lower extremities and added to the head and neck region. Each year of life, 1% is distributed back to the lower extremities until the age of nine when the head is considered to be the same proportion as an adult.

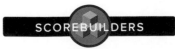

CONSIDER THIS
CALCULATING BURN SEVERITY[6]

Like the rule of nines, the Lund and Browder method also provides an estimated calculation of the extent of body surface area burned based on assigned percentages. This method, however, offers a more detailed calculation for children under the age of seven.

While both the rule of nines and the Lund and Browder method provide a gross surface area burned calculation method, neither offer indications of severity or prognosis. Prognostic burn indexes have been developed as more thorough evaluative tools used to predict medical attention needs, outcomes, and mortality by taking into account both the surface area burned and the severity of burns.

Anticipated Deformities Based on Burn Location

Area	Anticipated deformity	Splinting type
Anterior neck	Flexion with possible lateral flexion	Soft collar, molded collar, Philadelphia collar
Anterior chest and axilla	Shoulder adduction, extension, and medial rotation	Axillary or airplane splint, shoulder abduction brace
Elbow	Flexion and pronation	Gutter splint, conforming splint, three-point splint, air splint
Hand and wrist	Extension or hyperextension of the MCP joints; flexion of the IP joints; adduction and flexion of the thumb; flexion of the wrist	Wrist splint, thumb spica splint, palmar or dorsal extension splint
Hip	Flexion and adduction	Anterior hip spica, abduction splint
Knee	Flexion	Conforming splint, three-point splint, air splint
Ankle	Plantar flexion	Posterior foot drop splint, posterior ankle conforming splint, anterior ankle conforming splint

Scar Management[3,6]

Hypertrophic scarring is the result of an imbalance between collagen synthesis and lysis during healing, and can occur with any integumentary injury. The development of hypertrophic scarring is particularly common in relation to severe burn injuries. Complications of hypertrophic scarring may include contracture, adhesions, hypersensitivity, functional limitation, and poor cosmesis.

Scar assessment: Assessment devices, such as a tonometer, and rating scales aid in quantifying scar characteristics. A number of rating scales are available to objectively document observed characteristics. These tend to be more helpful in the assessment and re-assessment of an individual rather than for comparative assessment of a group. General characteristics that should be documented include location, sensation, texture, pigmentation, vascularity, pliability, and height.

Scar massage: Friction massage is advocated to loosen adhesions between cutaneous scar tissue and underlying structures. Reported benefits include decreased sensitivity and improved pliability. Caution should be taken not to begin scar massage too soon or too aggressively due to the risk of causing re-injury or re-initiating the inflammatory phase of healing. Massage techniques should be slow and firm using perpendicular, parallel, circular, and/or rolling strokes to mobilize tissue layers.

Compression garments: Compression therapy to reduce hypertrophic scarring is typically recommended for burns requiring greater than 14 days to heal. The use of sustained compression from 15-35 mm Hg is believed to create an environment that facilitates the balance of collagen synthesis and lysis, improving scar structure. Compression is applied by custom-made garments worn for 22-23 hours per day until the scar has matured. Silicone or foam inserts may be necessary to provide sufficient pressure over small areas or concave surfaces. For optimal effect, it is recommended that the use of compression garments begins between two weeks and two months after wound closure or grafting, continuing for up to two years.

CONSIDER THIS
DESENSITIZATION TECHNIQUES[8]

As with some patients status post amputation, patients who have sustained severe burns are susceptible to developing hypersensitivity that can become functionally limiting. Incorporating desensitization techniques into the plan of care and a patient's self-care routine can significantly improve a patient's tolerance to variable temperatures, touch, pressure, and vibration, thereby decreasing discomfort and improving functional abilities.

Desensitization interventions typically include variable texture, pressure, and vibratory sensations applied to the affected area by either rubbing, tapping or rolling motions. The use of particle contact (e.g., container of dry beans, popcorn kernels or fluidotherapy) can be beneficial in desensitizing distal extremities. Compression and TENS have also been shown to have clinical applications for desensitization goals.

It is recommended that desensitization interventions be performed for five to ten minutes, three to four times daily. Each session should begin with a sensation that is slightly irritating, but tolerable, and progress to more noxious stimuli. A textural progression may include: feather, cotton ball, chamois cloth, soft terry cloth, corduroy cloth, rough terry cloth, wool.

Skin Graft Terminology[6]

Allograft (homograft): A temporary skin graft taken from another human, usually a cadaver, in order to cover a large burned area.

Autograft: A permanent skin graft taken from a donor site on the patient's own body.

Donor site: A site where healthy skin is taken and used as a graft.

Escharotomy: A surgical procedure that opens or removes eschar from a burn site to reduce tension on a surrounding structure, relieve pressure from interstitial edema, and subsequently enhance circulation.

Full-thickness graft: A skin graft that contains the dermis and epidermis.

Heterograft (xenograft): A temporary skin graft taken from another species.

Mesh graft: A skin graft that is altered to create a mesh-like pattern in order to cover a larger surface area.

Recipient site: A site that has been burned and requires a graft.

Sheet graft: A skin graft that is transferred directly from the unburned donor site to the prepared recipient site.

Split-thickness graft: A skin graft that contains only a superficial layer of the dermis in addition to the epidermis.

Z-plasty: A surgical procedure to eliminate a scar contracture. An incision in the shape of a "z" allows the contracture to change configuration and lengthen the scar.

Integumentary Pathology[1,4,10]

Cellulitis

Cellulitis is a fast spreading inflammation that occurs as a result of a bacterial infection of the skin and connective tissues. It can develop anywhere under the skin, but will typically affect the extremities.

Etiology – Cellulitis is caused by particular bacterial infections including streptococci or staphylococci. Predisposing factors to cellulitis include an increased age, immunosuppression, trauma, the presence of wounds or venous insufficiency.

Signs and Symptoms – Symptoms may include localized redness that may spread quickly, skin that is warm or hot to touch, local abscess or ulceration, tenderness to palpation, chills, fever, and malaise.

Treatment – A patient with suspected cellulitis should be immediately referred to a physician for further assessment. Cellulitis requires pharmacological intervention using systemic antibiotics. Differential diagnosis should attempt to rule out deep vein thrombosis and contact dermatitis. Physical therapy may be warranted for wound care. Cellulitis can lead to sepsis or gangrene if not properly treated.

Contact Dermatitis

Contact dermatitis is a superficial irritation of the skin resulting from localized irritation (e.g., poison ivy, latex, soap, jewelry sensitivity). This condition can be acute or chronic based on exposure to the precipitating agent. Contact dermatitis is a very common skin disease that can occur at any age.

Etiology – Contact dermatitis occurs with exposure to mechanical, chemical, environmental or biological agents. Nickel, rubber, latex, and topical antibiotics are common precipitating agents.

Signs and Symptoms – Patients experience intense itching, burning, and red skin in areas corresponding to the location of the topical irritation. Edema may also occur in the area of sensitivity and symptoms can expand beyond the initial point of topical irritation.

Treatment – The focus of treatment should be on identifying and removing the source of irritation. Topical steroid application is commonly employed. Acute lesions should resolve with treatment once exposure to the external irritant has been removed.

Eczema

Eczema, also referred to as dermatitis, is used to describe a group of disorders that cause chronic skin inflammation typically due to an immune system abnormality, allergic reaction or external irritant.

Etiology – Eczema's etiology is based on the particular form of the disorder. Infants and children are at higher risk for eczema, however, many outgrow the condition with age. The geriatric population is also at an increased risk for many forms of eczema.

Signs and Symptoms – Red or brown-gray, itchy, lichenified skin plaques that may be exacerbated by some topical agents such as soaps and lotions. The younger population will also frequently experience oozing and crusting of the patchy areas of irritation.

Treatment – Pharmacological interventions are variable ranging from topical or oral corticosteroids to oral antibiotics and antihistamines. Cold compresses and other modalities may assist with reducing the itching. Stress management techniques and avoidance of extreme temperatures should be employed to avoid potential exacerbations of the condition.

Gangrene (Dry)

Gangrene is referred to as "dry" when there is a loss of vascular supply resulting in local tissue death. Fingers, toes, and limbs are most often affected. The hardened tissue is not painful, however, there may be significant pain at the line of demarcation. Dry gangrene typically develops slowly and in some cases results in auto-amputation.

Etiology – Dry gangrene occurs most commonly in blood vessel disease, such as diabetes mellitus or atherosclerosis. It develops when blood flow to an affected area is impaired, typically as a result of poor circulation. Infection is typically not present in dry gangrene, however, dry gangrene can progress to wet gangrene if infection occurs.

Signs and Symptoms – Dry gangrene presents as dark brown or black nonviable tissue that eventually becomes a hardened mass (mummified). The patient may complain of cold or numb skin and they may present with pain.

Treatment – Gangrene is a serious medical condition and requires immediate medical intervention. Depending on the severity, gangrene is treated by pharmacological intervention, surgery, and hyperbaric oxygen therapy.

Gangrene (Wet)

Gangrene is referred to as "wet" if there is an associated bacterial infection in the affected tissue. Gangrene may develop as a complication of an infected untreated wound. Swelling resulting from the bacterial infection causes a sudden stoppage of blood flow.

Etiology – Wet gangrene can develop after a severe burn, frostbite or injury and requires immediate treatment since it tends to spread very quickly and can be fatal. There is cessation of blood flow that starts a chain of events including invasion by bacteria at the affected site. As a result of the occluded blood supply, the white blood cells are unable to fight the infection.

Signs and Symptoms – swelling and pain at the site of infection, change in skin color from red to brown to black, blisters that produce pus, fever, and general malaise

Treatment – Wet gangrene is a serious medical condition and requires immediate medical intervention. Surgical debridement of the gangrene and intravenous antibiotic treatment are typical interventions for wet gangrene. Depending on the severity, gangrene is treated by pharmacological intervention, surgery, and hyperbaric oxygen therapy.

Psoriasis - Plaque

Plaque psoriasis is a chronic autoimmune disease of the skin and is the most common of the five types of psoriasis. T cells trigger inflammation within the skin and produce an accelerated rate of skin cell growth. The skin cells accumulate in raised red patches on the surface of the skin.

Etiology – Some patients have a genetic predisposition to plaque psoriasis. Other factors may trigger psoriasis, such as injury to the skin, insufficient or excess sunlight, stress, excessive alcohol, HIV infection, smoking, and certain medications.

Signs and Symptoms – The primary symptom is red raised blotches that typically present in a bilateral fashion for example over both knees or elbows. These plaques can appear anywhere on the body and will tend to itch and flake. Complications can include arthritis, pain, severe itching, secondary skin infections, and side effects secondary to pharmacological interventions.

Treatment – The primary goal for treatment of plaque psoriasis is to control the symptoms and prevent secondary infection. Treatment varies widely from topical applications to systemic medications and phototherapy. Plaque psoriasis is a life-long condition that can be effectively managed and controlled through the various stages and exacerbations.

Metabolic and Endocrine Systems

Metabolic System

Key Functions of the Metabolic System [11]

The metabolic system governs the chemical and physical changes that take place within the body enabling it to grow and function. Metabolism involves breakdown of the body's complex organic compounds in order to generate energy for all bodily processes. It also generates energy for the synthesis of complex substances that form tissues and organs. During metabolism, organic compounds are broken down by a process called catabolism, while anabolism is the process that combines simple molecules for tissue growth. Many metabolic processes are facilitated by enzymes. The overall speed at which an organism carries out its metabolic processes is termed its metabolic rate (or when the organism is at rest, its basal metabolic rate).

Metabolic System Pathology

Inherited Metabolic Disorders [10]

Metabolic disorders are classified by the particular building block that is affected. An enzyme deficiency leads to accumulation of the substrate and a subsequent deficiency in the intended enzyme's product. There are many different disorders that can occur genetically and these are grouped according to the substrate that has been affected (i.e., carbohydrates, amino acids). Inherited metabolic disorders can be diagnosed in utero via amniocentesis or chorionic villus sampling. Many inherited metabolic disorders will produce symptoms in a newborn including lethargy, apnea, poor feeding, tachypnea, vomiting, hypoglycemia, urine changes, and seizures. Symptoms that are immediately apparent indicate a more dangerous disorder.

Phenylketonuria (amino acid/organic acid metabolic disorder) [12]

Phenylketonuria (PKU) is a syndrome that consists of intellectual disability as well as behavioral and cognitive issues secondary to an elevation of serum phenylalanine. There is a deficiency in the enzyme phenylalanine hydroxylase. Normally, excessive phenylalanine is converted to tyrosine by phenylalanine hydroxylase. When this process does not occur and there is an excess of phenylalanine, the brain is the primary organ that becomes affected. Children in the United States are tested at birth for PKU and treated if necessary.

Etiology – This is an autosomal recessive inherited trait and is most common in Caucasian populations.

Signs and symptoms – Symptoms will typically present within a few months of birth as the phenylalanine accumulates. If left untreated, severe intellectual disability will occur. These children may also experience gait disturbances, hyperactivity, psychoses, abnormal body odor, and display features that are lighter in coloring when compared to other family members.

Treatment – Phenylketonuria is treated through dietary restriction of phenylalanine throughout the person's lifetime. Adequate prevention will avoid all manifestations of the disease.

Mitochondrial Disorders [10]

There are over one hundred different forms of mitochondrial disease and each produces a different spectrum of disability and clinical manifestations.

Etiology – Mitochondrial disorders result from genetically inherited or spontaneous mutations in the DNA that lead to impaired function of proteins found within the mitochondria.

Signs and symptoms – Symptoms vary depending on the type of mitochondrial disorder, however, can include loss of muscle coordination, muscle weakness, visual and hearing problems, learning disabilities, heart, liver, and kidney disease, respiratory, neurological, and gastrointestinal disorders, and dementia.

Treatment – These diagnoses are relatively new and treatment is as varied as the symptomatology and presentation of the disease. Treatment is aimed at alleviating the current symptoms and slowing the progression of the disease process.

Rehabilitation Considerations for Patients with Inherited Metabolic Disorders [10]

- Must have an awareness of dietary restrictions
- Patient and family training to prevent deleterious effects from the metabolic disease
- Adapt treatment to facilitate developmental milestones within patient tolerance

Acid-Base Metabolic Disorders [13]

The process of metabolism is regulated by the endocrine and nervous systems. The rate of metabolism can be influenced by body temperature, exercise, hormone activity, and digestion activity. If proper fluid or acid-base balance is compromised, it can alter metabolic function and cause many signs and symptoms of the dysfunction.

Metabolic Alkalosis [13]

Metabolic alkalosis is a condition that occurs when there is an increase in bicarbonate accumulation or an abnormal loss of acids. As a result, the pH rises above 7.45.

Etiology – Metabolic alkalosis commonly occurs when there has been continuous vomiting, ingestion of antacids or other alkaline substances or diuretic therapy. It may also be associated with hypokalemia or nasogastric suctioning.

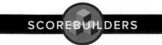

CONSIDER THIS
LOW BONE MASS[12]

Certain medical conditions may present with low bone mass as an associated clinical feature. A patient may report such conditions while detailing their medical history, but not be aware of the condition's potential influence on bone mass. Physical therapist assistants should be aware of such conditions, regardless of an accompanying osteopenia or osteoporosis diagnosis, in order to best incorporate preventative interventions and education into the plan of care.

Medical conditions which may cause low bone mass include: Cushing's syndrome, osteomalacia, hyperthyroidism, hyperparathyroidism, celiac disease, rheumatoid arthritis, renal failure, hypogonadism, and osteogenesis imperfecta.

Signs and symptoms – Symptoms include nausea, diarrhea, prolonged vomiting, confusion, muscle fasciculations, muscle cramping, neuromuscular hyperexcitability, convulsions, paresthesias, and hypoventilation. If left untreated the patient can become comatose, experience seizures, and respiratory paralysis.

Treatment – The most important interventions include managing the underlying cause, correcting coexisting electrolyte imbalances, and administering potassium chloride to the patient.

Rehabilitation Considerations for Patients with Acid-Base Disorders[10,13]

- Recognize higher risk populations for imbalances such as patients with renal, cardiovascular, pulmonary disease; burns, fever, and sepsis; patients on mechanical ventilation; diabetes mellitus; patients currently vomiting with diarrhea or enteric drainage

- Recognize signs of dehydration in a diabetic patient

- Injury prevention during involuntary muscular contractions secondary to metabolic alkalosis

- Recognize that patients using diuretic therapy may be at risk for potassium depletion

- Recognize that Trousseau's sign during blood pressure measurements may indicate calcium deficiency and the early stages of tetany

Metabolic Acidosis[13]

Metabolic acidosis is a condition that occurs when there is an accumulation of acids due to an acid gain or bicarbonate loss. As a result, the pH drops below 7.35.

Etiology – Metabolic acidosis commonly occurs with conditions such as renal failure, lactic acidosis, starvation, diabetic or alcoholic ketoacidosis, severe diarrhea or poisoning by certain toxins.

Signs and symptoms – Symptoms include compensatory hyperventilation, vomiting, diarrhea, headache, weakness and malaise, hyperkalemia, and cardiac arrhythmias. If left untreated the continued increase in acid can induce coma and eventual death.

Treatment – Treatment includes managing the underlying cause, correcting any coexisting electrolyte imbalances, and administering sodium bicarbonate.

Metabolic Bone Disease[10]

Metabolic bone disease is a classification for particular diagnoses where there has been a disruption in normal metabolism within the skeletal system. The skeletal system houses calcium and phosphorus. It also continuously balances the remodeling of the cortical and trabecular bone in order to optimize the structure of the skeleton. Disruption in the homeostasis of skeletal metabolic processes will result in deformity, bone loss, fracture, softening of the bone, arthritis, and pain.

Osteomalacia[10]

Osteomalacia is a metabolic condition where bones become soft secondary to a calcium or phosphorus deficiency. There is adequate bone matrix, however, there is insufficient calcification of the matrix due to the deficiency.

Etiology – Calcium is typically lost secondary to inadequate intestinal absorption and the phosphorus is lost secondary to an increase in renal excretion. A deficiency in vitamin D will also cause osteomalacia.

Signs and symptoms – Osteomalacia can include a vague presentation of aching, fatigue, and weight loss. Myopathy and sensory polyneuropathy may also occur along with periarticular tenderness and pain, thoracic kyphosis deformity, and bowing of the lower extremities. The patient may also struggle to perform transfers and assume a standing position.

Treatment – Specific intervention will focus on the underlying etiology. Increased nutrition is recommended and pharmacological intervention may include vitamin D or phosphate supplements.

Osteoporosis[10]

Osteoporosis is a metabolic condition that presents with a decrease in bone mass that subsequently increases the risk of fracture. Osteoporosis primarily affects trabecular and cortical bone where the rate of bone resorption accelerates while the rate of bone formation declines. Declining osteoblast function coupled with the loss of calcium and phosphate salts will cause the bones to become brittle.

Etiology – Primary osteoporosis can include idiopathic, post-menopausal or involutional (senile) osteoporosis. Secondary osteoporosis can occur as a result of another primary condition or with use of certain medications.

Signs and symptoms – Symptoms include compression and other bone fractures, low thoracic or lumbar pain, loss of lumbar lordosis, deformities such as kyphosis, decrease in height, dowager's hump, and postural changes.

Treatment – Management of primary osteoporosis includes vitamin and pharmacological intervention, proper nutrition, assistive and adaptive device prescription, and patient education. Surgical intervention may be required for fracture stabilization.

Paget's Disease[10]

Paget's disease is a metabolic condition characterized by heightened osteoclast activity. This process of excessive bone formation lacks true structural integrity. The bone appears enlarged, but lacks strength due to the high turnover of bone secondary to abnormal osteoclastic proliferation.

Etiology – This disease has a genetic component as well as geographical incidence, and most commonly affects patients over 50 years of age.

Signs and symptoms – Symptoms include musculoskeletal pain accompanied by bony deformities (kyphosis, coxa varus, bowing of the long bones, vertebral compression). The skull, clavicle, pelvis, femur, spine and tibia are common sites that will exhibit bony changes. Symptoms of advanced progression of the disease include continued pain, headache, vertigo, hearing loss, mental deterioration, fatigue, increased cardiac output, and heart failure (secondary to an increased cardiac output).

Treatment – Management relies heavily on pharmacological intervention using bisphosphonates in order to inhibit bone resorption and improve the quality of the involved bone. Exercise, weight control, and cardiac fitness are all key components in a program to maintain strength and motion.

CONSIDER THIS
OSTEOPOROSIS RISK FACTORS AND PREVENTION[12,14,15]

Bone mineral density (BMD) is used to diagnose osteoporosis and other low bone mass disorders. BMD is measured via dual-energy x-ray absorptiometry and expressed in terms of T-score and Z-score. T-score refers to how many standard deviations above or below average healthy young adult norms an individual's BMD is. Z-score refers to how many standard deviations above or below average age and gender adjusted norms an individual's BMD is. The World Health Organization reports that in women, a T-score lower than -1 standard deviation (SD) but greater than -2.5 SD is indicative of osteopenia. A score that is -2.5 SD or lower is indicative of osteoporosis, and a score at or below -2.5 SD with one or more related fractures is considered severe osteoporosis.

Physical therapists and physical therapist assistants are often the primary educators with patients who have either sustained or are at risk for osteoporotic fractures. Therapists should therefore have a sound understanding of non-modifiable and modifiable risk factors so that education topics and treatment planning may be adapted to address both.

Non-modifiable risk factors associated with the development of low bone mass include age, early menopause, history of previous fracture, slender build, family history of low bone mass, female gender, and being of either Asian or Caucasian descent. Certain conditions and medications, such as glucocorticoids, may also be considered non-modifiable if discontinuing such medications is medically ill-advised.

Modifiable risk factors associated with the development of low bone mass include insufficient dietary intake of vitamin D and calcium, estrogen deficiency, cigarette smoking, alcohol use in excess of two drinks per day, caffeine intake in excess of two servings per day, and sedentary lifestyle.

Treatment interventions and educational topics are similar for both osteopenia and osteoporosis. Prevention of osteoporosis associated fractures is a primary goal of therapeutic interventions for at-risk individuals of all ages. Specific interventions, however, may be emphasized or excluded depending on the patient's age and associated risk factors.

Interventions for Children and Adolescents

Osteoporosis prevention is important to begin during childhood by ensuring adequate nutrition, especially with regard to calcium intake, since malnutrition and undernutrition negatively impact bone development. Bone mass density typically peaks during an individual's mid-20's. Younger patients should be encouraged to participate regularly in physical activity to promote bone strength. The adverse effects of smoking and excessive alcohol consumption on bone development should also be addressed with younger patient populations. Adherence to recommendations may be the greatest challenge in addressing osteoporosis in younger populations.

Interventions for Adults

Once peak BMD has been reached, maintaining this during the processes of ongoing remodeling is paramount in minimizing the eventual imbalance between bone formation and remodeling. Maintaining good nutrition, including recommended calcium and vitamin D intake, is a key factor in managing the risk of osteoporotic fractures. Regular weight bearing exercise is strongly recommended in addition to avoiding smoking and heavy drinking. Postural education and fall prevention activities are also increasingly important during later years when fracture risk is heightened.

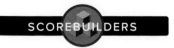

Rehabilitation Considerations for Patients with Metabolic Bone Disease[10]

- Must have awareness of signs of compression fracture and of patients at higher risk for all forms of fracture
- Focus on both resistance training and endurance training to build bone density and increase strength
- Avoid treatments that exacerbate the condition or place patients at risk for fracture

Metabolic System Terminology[10, 14-16]

Aerobic metabolism: The ATP producing metabolic processes that are dependent on oxygen transported via the circulatory system. Aerobic metabolic functions typically provide energy for low intensity and/or longer duration activities.

Anabolism: The metabolic process in which simple molecules (e.g., nucleic acids, polysaccharides, amino acids) are combined to create the complex molecules (e.g., proteins) needed for tissue and organ growth.

Anaerobic metabolism: Metabolic functions that do not require the presence of oxygen and produce energy for high intensity, shorter duration activities.

Adenosine triphosphate (ATP): The molecular unit within the body which transports the chemical compounds used for cellular metabolism.

Catabolism: The metabolic process in which complex materials (e.g., proteins, lipids) are broken down in the body for the purpose of creating and releasing heat and energy.

DNA (deoxyribonucleic acid): A double helix molecule that contains the genes that provide the blueprint for all of the structures and functions of a living being.

Gene: A fundamental unit of heredity.

Metabolism: The physical and chemical processes of cells burning fuel to produce and use energy. Examples include digestion, elimination of waste, breathing, thermoregulation, muscular contraction, brain function, and circulation.

Mitochondria: The part of the cell that is responsible for energy production. The mitochondria are also responsible for converting nutrients into energy and other specialized tasks.

Osteopenia: A condition presenting with low bone mass that is not severe enough to qualify as osteoporosis. Individuals with osteopenia may not have actual bone loss, but a naturally lower bone density than established norms.

Osteopetrosis: A group of conditions characterized by impaired osteoclast function which causes bone to become thickened but fragile. Osteopetrosis is an inherited condition that can vary widely in symptoms and severity.

pH: A measure of the hydrogen ion concentration in body fluid.

Endocrine System

Key Functions of the Endocrine System[12]

The endocrine system consists of endocrine glands (specialized ductless glands) that secrete hormones that travel through the bloodstream to signal specific target cells throughout the body. The hormones travel throughout the body to the target organs upon which they act. They will bind selectively to receptor sites on the surface of the receptor cells. The endocrine system and nervous system both function to achieve and maintain stability of the internal environment (homeostasis).

Glands of the Endocrine System[10,12]

Hypothalamus

The hypothalamus is located below the thalamus and cerebral hemisphere. It is responsible for regulation of the autonomic nervous system (body temperature, appetite, sweating, thirst, sexual behavior, rage, fear, blood pressure, sleep) and other endocrine glands through its impact on the pituitary gland.

Pituitary Gland

The pituitary gland is normally the size of a pea and is located at the base of the brain just beneath the hypothalamus. The pituitary gland is considered the most important part of the endocrine

system since it releases hormones that regulate several other endocrine glands. This "master gland" is influenced by factors such as seasonal changes or emotional stress. The pituitary gland secretes endorphins that act on the nervous system and reduce a person's sensitivity to pain. It also controls ovulation and works as a catalyst for the testes and ovaries to create sex hormones.

Thyroid Gland

The thyroid gland is located on the anterior and lateral surfaces of the trachea immediately below the larynx and is shaped like a "bow tie" or "butterfly" with two halves (lobes); a right lobe and a left lobe joined by an isthmus. The thyroid produces thyroxine and triiodothyronine that act to control the rate at which cells burn the fuel from food. An increase in thyroid hormones will increase the rate of the chemical reactions within the body.

Parathyroid Glands

There are four parathyroid glands found on the posterior surface of the thyroid's lateral lobes. These glands produce parathyroid hormone, which functions as an antagonist to calcitonin and is important for the maintenance of normal blood levels of calcium and phosphate. Normal clotting, neuromuscular excitability, and cell membrane permeability are dependent on normal calcium levels.

Adrenal Glands

The two adrenal glands are located on top of each kidney; the outer portion is called the adrenal cortex and the inner portion is called the adrenal medulla. The adrenal cortex produces corticosteroids that will regulate water and sodium balance, the body's response to stress, the immune system, sexual development and function, and metabolism. The adrenal medulla produces epinephrine that increases heart rate and blood pressure when there is an increase in stress.

Pancreas

The pancreas is located in the upper left quadrant of the abdominal cavity, extending from the duodenum to the spleen. The pancreas includes both endocrine and exocrine tissues. The islets of Langerhans are the hormone-producing cells of the pancreas. Alpha cells produce glucagon and beta cells produce insulin. These hormones work in combination to ensure a consistent level of glucose within the bloodstream and properly maintain stores of energy within the body.

Ovaries

The ovaries are located in the pelvic cavity on each side of the uterus. The ovaries provide estrogen and progesterone that contribute to regulation of the menstrual cycle and pregnancy. Estrogen is secreted by the ovarian follicles and is responsible for the development and maintenance of female sex characteristics such as breast development and the cycles of the female reproductive system. Progesterone is produced by the corpus luteum and functions to maintain the lining of the uterus at a level necessary for pregnancy.

Testes

The testes are located in the scrotum between the upper thighs. The testes secrete androgens (most importantly testosterone) that regulate body changes associated with sexual development and support the production of sperm.

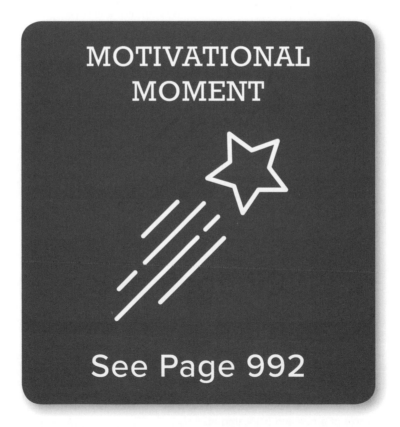

MOTIVATIONAL MOMENT

See Page 992

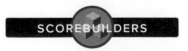

Endocrine System: Hormone, Function, and Regulation of Secretion[10,12]

Hormone	Function	Regulation of Secretion
Hypothalamus		
Growth hormone-releasing hormone Target: pituitary gland	Increases the release of growth hormone	Central nervous system feedback; circulating levels of hormones
Growth hormone-inhibiting hormone Target: pituitary gland	Decreases the release of growth hormone	Central nervous system feedback; circulating levels of hormones
Gonadotropin-releasing hormone Target: pituitary gland	Increases the release of luteinizing hormone and follicle-stimulating hormone	Central nervous system feedback; circulating levels of hormones
Thyrotropin-releasing hormone Target: pituitary gland	Increases the release of thyroid-stimulating hormone	Central nervous system feedback; circulating levels of hormones
Corticotropin-releasing hormone Target: pituitary gland	Increases the release of adrenocorticotropic hormone	Central nervous system feedback; circulating levels of hormones
Prolactin-releasing hormone Target: pituitary gland	Stimulates the release of prolactin	Central nervous system feedback; circulating levels of hormones
Prolactin-inhibitory factor; dopamine Target: pituitary gland	Decreases the release of prolactin	Central nervous system feedback; circulating levels of hormones
Pituitary		
Growth hormone Target: bone and muscle	Promotes growth and development; increases the rate of protein synthesis	Hypothalamus
Follicle-stimulating hormone Target: ovaries and testes	Promotes follicular development and the creation of estrogen in females; promotes spermatogenesis in males	Hypothalamus
Luteinizing hormone Target: ovaries and testes	Promotes ovulation along with estrogen/progesterone synthesis from the corpus luteum in females; promotes testosterone synthesis in males	Hypothalamus
Thyroid-stimulating hormone Target: thyroid gland	Increases the synthesis of thyroid hormones T3 and T4	Hypothalamus
Adrenocorticotropic hormone Target: adrenal cortex	Increases cortisol synthesis (adrenal steroids)	Hypothalamus
Prolactin Target: mammary glands	Allows for the process of lactation	Hypothalamus
Oxytocin Target: uterus and mammary glands	Increases contraction of uterine muscles; promotes release of milk from mammary glands	Nerve impulses from the hypothalamus; stretching of cervix; nipple stimulation
Antidiuretic hormone Target: kidneys	Increases water reabsorption; conserves water; increases blood pressure through stimulating contraction of muscles in small arteries	Decreased water content

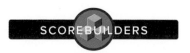

Hormone	Function	Regulation of Secretion
Adrenal Cortex		
Androgen Target: ovaries and testes	Increases masculinization; promotes growth of pubic hair in males and females	Influenced by the hypothalamic production and release of GnRH and luteinizing hormone (LH)
Aldosterone (mineralocorticoid) Target: kidneys	Increases reabsorption of sodium ions by the kidneys to the blood; increases excretion of potassium ions by the kidney into the urine	Low blood sodium level; high blood potassium level
Cortisol (glucocorticoid) Target: gastrointestinal system	Influences metabolism of food molecules; anti-inflammatory effect in large amounts	Adrenocorticotropic hormone
Adrenal Medulla		
Epinephrine Target: cardiovascular and metabolic systems	Increases heart rate and force of contraction; increases energy production; vasodilation in skeletal muscle	Sympathetic impulses from the hypothalamus in stress situations
Norepinephrine Target: cardiovascular and metabolic systems	Vasoconstriction in skin, viscera, and skeletal muscles	
Ovaries		
Estrogen, progesterone Target: uterus and mammary glands	Involved in regulation of the female reproductive system and female sexual characteristics	Cyclical rise and fall of hormone levels
Pancreas		
Glucagon Target: liver	Increases blood glucose by stimulating the conversion of glycogen to glucose	Hypoglycemia
Insulin Target: all body systems	Decreases blood glucose and increases the storage of fat, protein, and carbohydrates	Hyperglycemia
Parathyroids		
Parathormone Target: bone, kidney, intestinal mucosa	Increases blood calcium	Hypocalcemia
Testes		
Testosterone Target: pituitary gland	Involved in the process of spermatogenesis and male sexual characteristics	Influenced by pituitary release of LH
Thyroid		
Thyroxine (T4), Triiodothyronine (T3) Target: all tissues	Involved with normal development; increases cellular level metabolism	Thyroid-stimulating hormone
Calcitonin Target: plasma	Increases calcium storage in bone; decreases blood calcium levels	Hypercalcemia

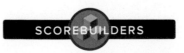

Endocrine System Pathology[10,12]

The endocrine system is multifaceted and can develop pathology in one or more areas due to hyperfunction or hypofunction of one or more glands. In many instances, it is the hypothalamus or the pituitary gland that affects the function of other endocrine glands when they experience direct or indirect dysfunction.

Hyperfunction of an endocrine gland: usually secondary to overstimulation of the pituitary gland. This can also occur due to hyperplasia or neoplasia of the gland itself.

Hypofunction of an endocrine gland: usually secondary to understimulation of the pituitary gland. This can also occur from congenital or acquired disorders.

Hypopituitarism: This condition occurs when there is a decreased or absent hormonal secretion from the anterior pituitary gland. This is a rare disorder and symptoms are dependent on the age of the affected person and deficit hormones. Typical disorders may include short stature (dwarfism), delayed growth and puberty, sexual and reproductive disorders, and diabetes insipidus. Treatment is also based on the deficit hormones and usually includes pharmacological replacement therapy.

Hyperpituitarism: This condition occurs when there is an excessive secretion of one or more hormones under the pituitary gland's control (frequently growth hormone that produces acromegaly in adults). Disorders and symptoms are dependent on the hormone(s) that are affected. Some disorders include gigantism or acromegaly, hirsutism, galactorrhea (abnormal lactation in males or females), amenorrhea, infertility, and impotence. Treatment is hormone and site dependent and can include tumor resection, surgery, radiation therapy, and hormone suppression or replacement (if gland becomes dysfunctional after treatment).

Rehabilitation Considerations for Patients with Pituitary Dysfunction[10]

- Ambulation/exercise encouraged within 24 hours of surgery (post tumor/gland removal)
- Must demonstrate increased awareness for signs of hypoglycemia
- Bilateral carpal tunnel syndrome, arthritis, osteophyte formation are common with hyperpituitarism
- Orthostatic hypotension may be present with hypopituitarism
- Bilateral hemianopsia that can occur with hypopituitarism requires special consideration during treatment

Adrenal Dysfunction

Addison's Disease[12]

Addison's disease is a form of adrenal dysfunction that presents with hypofunction of the adrenal cortex. Subsequently, there is decreased production of both cortisol (glucocorticoid) and aldosterone (mineralocorticoid).

Etiology – When the adrenal cortex produces insufficient cortisol and aldosterone hormones it is termed Addison's disease.

Signs and symptoms – Symptoms include a widespread metabolic dysfunction secondary to cortisol deficiency as well as fluid and electrolyte imbalances secondary to aldosterone dysfunction. The person may experience hypotension, weakness, anorexia, weight loss, altered pigmentation, and if left untreated this condition will result in shock and possible death.

Treatment – Treatment primarily consists of long-term pharmacological intervention using synthetic corticosteroids and mineralocorticoids.

Cushing's Syndrome[12]

Cushing's syndrome is a form of adrenal dysfunction that presents with hyperfunction of the adrenal gland, allowing for excessive amounts of cortisol (glucocorticoid) production.

Etiology – When the pituitary gland produces excessive adrenocorticotropic hormone (ACTH) with subsequent hypercortisolism, it is termed Cushing's syndrome.

Signs and symptoms – Symptoms evolve over years and can include persistent hyperglycemia, growth failure, truncal obesity, purple abdominal striae, "moon shaped face," "buffalo hump" posteriorly at the base of the neck, weakness, acne, hypertension, and male gynecomastia. Mental changes can include depression, poor concentration, and memory loss.

Treatment – Treatment may include pharmacological intervention to block the production of the hormones, radiation therapy, chemotherapy or surgery.

Rehabilitation Considerations for Patients with Adrenal Dysfunction[10]

- Recognize signs of stress or exhaustion and avoid treatments that exacerbate the condition
- Notify the physician with any signs of illness or increased intracranial pressure (e.g., papilledema); medications may need to be altered
- Orthostatic hypotension is common secondary to long-term cortisol therapy
- Report sleep disturbances to the physician
- Increased incidence of osteoporosis, bone fractures, degenerative myopathy, tendon ruptures, ataxic gait
- Delayed wound healing may be common

Thyroid Dysfunction[11]

Hypothyroidism: This condition occurs when there are decreased levels of thyroid hormones in the bloodstream, slowing metabolic processes within the body. Symptoms may include fatigue, weakness, decreased heart rate, weight gain, constipation, delayed puberty, and retarded growth and development. Common causes of hypothyroidism are Hashimoto's thyroiditis or an

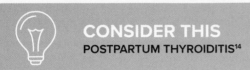

CONSIDER THIS
POSTPARTUM THYROIDITIS[14]

Postpartum thyroiditis refers to a painless inflammation of the thyroid occurring in some women after childbirth. The presentation of this condition is typically defined by two phases. Initially, a state of hyperthyroidism will present within the first one to four months following childbirth. This is followed by a shift to hypothyroidism four to eight months following delivery.

Signs of the hyperactive phase of postpartum thyroiditis may include tachycardia, unexplained weight loss, anxiety, irritability, fatigue, and heat sensitivity. Unfortunately, the initial signs of this hyperactive thyroid phase may be misinterpreted as typical postpartum symptoms, thereby delaying diagnosis. More frequently, postpartum thyroiditis is detected after the onset of the hypoactive phase. Symptoms in this phase are consistent with other hypothyroidism disorders including dry skin, hoarse voice, depression, cold sensitivity, and poor exercise tolerance. Risk factors for postpartum thyroiditis include a history of autoimmune disorders, thyroid dysfunction, prior postpartum thyroiditis or a family history of thyroid dysfunction. Blood tests are used to confirm a diagnosis in either phase.

Timely diagnosis and treatment of women with postpartum thyroiditis can impact both physical therapy outcomes and the patient's quality of life. Therapists should be cautious not to dismiss symptoms of fatigue and irritability as typical postpartum occurrences, especially if other signs of thyroid dysfunction can be identified. Therapists should also be mindful that pharmacological interventions (e.g., beta blockers, thyroid replacement hormones) may further influence a patient's exercise tolerance and anticipated outcomes.

underdeveloped thyroid gland. Treatment includes oral thyroid hormone replacement therapy.

Hyperthyroidism: This condition occurs when there are excessive levels of thyroid hormones in the bloodstream. Symptoms can include an increase in nervousness, excessive sweating, weight loss, increase in blood pressure, exophthalmos, myopathy, chronic periarthritis, and an enlarged thyroid gland. Treatment may include pharmacological intervention, radioactive iodine, and surgery.

Graves' Disease[10]

Graves' disease is the most specific cause of hyperthyroidism. Graves' disease is most common in women over age 20, however, it occurs in men as well and can affect any age group.

Etiology – Graves' disease is caused by an autoimmune disease in which certain antibodies produced by the immune system stimulate the thyroid gland causing it to become overactive.

Signs and symptoms – Symptoms are consistent with hyperthyroid presentation. The classic signs of Graves' disease include mild enlargement of the thyroid gland (goiter), heat intolerance, nervousness, weight loss, tremor, and palpitations.

Treatment – Management includes pharmacological intervention and/or removal of the thyroid gland using radiation or surgical intervention.

Hypothyroidism[17]	Hyperthyroidism[17]
Depression and/or anxiety, increased lethargy, fatigue, headache, slowed speech, slowed mental function, impaired short-term memory	Tremors, hyperkinesis, nervousness, increased DTRs, emotional lability, insomnia, weakness, atrophy
Proximal muscle weakness, carpal tunnel syndrome, trigger points, myalgia, increased bone density, cold intolerance, paresthesias	Chronic periarthritis, heat intolerance, flushed skin, hyperpigmentation, increased hair loss
Dyspnea, bradycardia, CHF, respiratory muscle weakness, decreased peripheral circulation, angina, increase in cholesterol	Tachycardia, palpitations, increased respiratory rate, increase in blood pressure, arrhythmias
Anorexia, constipation, weight gain, decreased absorption of food and glucose	Hypermetabolism, increased appetite, increased peristalsis, nausea, vomiting, diarrhea, dysphagia
Infertility, irregular menstrual cycle, increased menstrual bleeding	Polyuria, infertility, increased first trimester miscarriage, amenorrhea

Rehabilitation Considerations for Patients with Thyroid Dysfunction[10]

- Recognize reduced exercise capacity and fatigue are typical
- Avoid treatments that exacerbate the condition such as exercise in a hot aquatic or gym setting due to heat intolerance (Graves' disease)
- Avoid cardiovascular stress to eliminate secondary complications from hypotension, goiter, Graves' disease
- Provide close monitoring of vital signs
- Recognize the effects of radioiodine therapy
- Recognize the risk of rhabdomyolysis (hypothyroidism)

Parathyroid Dysfunction[10]

Hypoparathyroidism: This condition occurs due to hyposecretion or low-level production of parathyroid hormone by the parathyroid gland. Symptoms may include hypocalcemia, neurological symptoms such as seizures, cognitive defects, short stature, tetany, muscle pain, and cramps. Treatment of acute hypoparathyroidism requires rapid elevation in serum calcium levels through intravenous calcium. Long-term treatment includes pharmacological management and dietary modifications.

Hyperparathyroidism: This condition occurs due to excessive levels of hormone production by the parathyroid gland that leads to disruption of calcium, phosphate, and bone metabolism. Symptoms may include renal stones and kidney damage, depression, memory loss, muscle wasting, bone deformity, and myopathy. Acute treatment may include pharmacological intervention that produces an immediate lowering of serum calcium using diuretics or antiresorptive medications. Surgical intervention is usually required to remove the diseased parathyroid gland. Pharmacological intervention may be used prior to surgery or for long-term management.

Rehabilitation Considerations for Patients with Parathyroid Dysfunction[10]

- Must be familiar with all signs and symptoms of parathyroid dysfunction in order to refer patients to a physician if a change in their status occurs
- Recognize symptoms of excessive or inadequate pharmacological treatment and side effects of the agents
- Avoid treatments that exacerbate the condition
- Recognize effects of hypercalcemia (hyperparathyroidism) and hypocalcemia (hypoparathyroidism)
- Recognize the increased risk for fractures and effects from osteogenic synovitis (Achilles, triceps, and obturator tendons most affected)

Hypoparathyroidism[17]	Hyperparathyroidism[17]
Decreased bone resorption	Increased bone resorption
Hypocalcemia	Hypercalcemia
Elevated serum phosphate levels	Decreased serum phosphate levels
Shortened 4th and 5th metacarpals (pseudohypoparathyroidism)	Osteitis fibrosa, subperiosteal resorption, arthritis, bone deformity
Compromised breathing due to intercostal muscle and diaphragm spasms	Nephrocalcinosis, renal hypertension, and significant renal damage
Cardiac arrhythmias and potential heart failure	Gout
Increased neuromuscular activity that can result in tetany	Decreased neuromuscular irritability

Pancreas Dysfunction[12]

Type 1 Diabetes Mellitus (DM)

This form of DM occurs when the pancreas fails to produce enough or any insulin. This form of diabetes is normally diagnosed in childhood, but can occur at any age. It is also known as insulin-dependent diabetes or juvenile diabetes.

Etiology – The exact cause is unknown, but genetic predisposition in combination with exposure to a viral or environmental trigger is believed to cause an immune reaction that damages the pancreas with subsequent failure in secretion of endogenous insulin.

Signs and symptoms – Symptoms of DM include a rapid onset of symptoms, polyphagia, weight loss, ketoacidosis, polyuria, polydipsia, blurred vision, dehydration, and fatigue.

Treatment – Management includes exogenous insulin injections that are required to maintain proper glucose blood levels and avoid complications. Proper nutritional management is also required for blood glucose control. Insulin pumps may be indicated for continuous administration of insulin. Presently, there is no cure for type 1 DM and as a result, the goal is to control the regulation of blood glucose levels (Fig. 7-5).

Type 2 Diabetes Mellitus (DM)

This form of DM typically occurs in the population over the age of 45, however, there has been an increase in children diagnosed with type 2 DM secondary to a rise in childhood obesity. This form of DM typically retains the ability to produce some endogenous insulin.

Etiology – Type 2 DM occurs secondary to an array of dysfunctions resulting from the combination of resistance to insulin action and inadequate insulin secretion. This disorder is characterized by hyperglycemia when the body cannot properly respond to insulin. Obesity is found to contribute to this condition by increasing insulin resistance.

Signs and symptoms – Symptoms are relatively the same as with type 1, however, ketoacidosis does not occur since insulin is still typically produced.

Treatment – Treatment of type 2 diabetes includes blood glucose control through diet, exercise, oral medications or insulin injections when necessary.

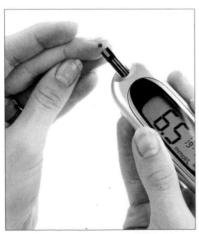

Fig. 7-5: Self-monitoring of blood glucose levels.

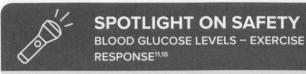

SPOTLIGHT ON SAFETY
BLOOD GLUCOSE LEVELS – EXERCISE RESPONSE[11,18]

For patients with diabetes mellitus (DM), an awareness of how to manage blood glucose levels is imperative to prevent the potentially life threatening effects of hyper or hypoglycemia. Both patients and therapists must be aware of the signs and symptoms of these emergent conditions, how to respond, and how therapy interventions may be either a causative or alleviating factor.

Hyperglycemia

Unaddressed hyperglycemia is a significant factor in the development of DM related complications. In addition to blood glucose measures, early signs of hyperglycemia that can occur when blood glucose is >180-200 mg/dl include increased thirst and frequent urination. Recognition of these early signs is crucial in preventing the dangerous onset of ketoacidosis, often referred to as a "diabetic coma." Most commonly occurring in patients with type 1 DM, ketoacidosis is a life-threatening condition requiring immediate medical attention. Symptoms include dyspnea, a fruity breath odor, dry mouth, nausea, vomiting, confusion, and an eventual loss of consciousness.

Hypoglycemia

It is equally important to recognize the initial signs of hypoglycemia so that early intervention may prevent more serious symptoms. Early signs of hypoglycemia that may occur when blood glucose is <70 mg/dl include hunger, sweating, shaking, dizziness, clumsiness, and headache. If unaddressed, patients who become hypoglycemic may lose consciousness, at which point immediate medical attention is necessary. Hypoglycemia is often counteracted simply by ingestion of a glucose or carbohydrate-rich substance (e.g., sugar, honey, juice, crackers). Patients with significant hypoglycemic issues may be advised by their physician to carry a glucose source or injectable glucagon with them at all times.

Exercise Response

A regular exercise program offers numerous benefits to patients with DM. The weight and stress management aspects of exercise are particularly beneficial with regard to controlling blood glucose levels. Physical and mental stressors have been shown to elevate blood glucose levels making long term management more challenging for patients with DM. Exercise provides positive dual influences of aiding stress management and increasing blood glucose uptake by the muscles without significantly impacting insulin levels. Therapists, however, must be alert to signs of exercise induced hypoglycemia which may occur with strenuous or prolonged exercise tasks. The risk of symptom onset can often be reduced by ingestion of a carbohydrate snack prior to exercise in order to compensate for increased glucose demands and/or increased insulin absorption.

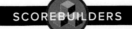

Type 1 Diabetes Mellitus[12] (insulin-dependent, juvenile diabetes)	Type 2 Diabetes Mellitus[12] (non-insulin dependent, adult onset diabetes)
Onset: usually less than 25 years of age	Onset: usually older than 45 years of age
Abrupt onset	Gradual onset
5-10% of all cases	90-95% of all cases
Etiology: destruction of islets of Langerhans cells secondary to possible autoimmune or viral causative factor	Etiology: resistance at insulin receptor sites usually secondary to obesity; ethnic prevalence
Insulin production: very little or none	Insulin production: variable
Ketoacidosis can occur	Ketoacidosis will rarely occur
Treatment includes insulin injection, exercise, and diet	Treatment includes weight loss, oral insulin, exercise, and diet

Rehabilitation Considerations for Patients with Diabetes Mellitus[10]

- Recognize the risk for peripheral neuropathies, small vessel angiopathy, tissue ischemia and ulceration, impaired wound healing, tissue necrosis, and amputation
- Recognize acute metabolic changes
- Recognize the signs of sudden hypoglycemia and necessary treatment
- Focus on consistent management of insulin intake, diet, and physical activity
- Provide education for proper skin care, shoe evaluation, and shoe wear

Gestational Diabetes

Gestational diabetes is a condition characterized by an increase in insulin resistance and therefore an increase in blood glucose levels that occurs during pregnancy. This condition generally develops in the last trimester. The etiology of the condition is not known, but it is thought that hormones that assist the fetus to grow and develop also lead to insulin resistance. Gestational diabetes occurs in about 4% of all pregnancies. The large majority of women with gestational diabetes return to normal glucose metabolism after the pregnancy. If glucose intolerance persists for more than six weeks after childbirth, the patient should be reclassified to another form of diabetes mellitus.

Babies born to women with gestational diabetes have increased glucose levels and are at an increased risk for macrosomia (i.e., larger than average size), which makes delivery more difficult and potentially more dangerous. The baby may also experience breathing difficulties, jaundice, and hypoglycemia following birth. In childhood and adolescence, these children are more likely to experience insulin resistance, obesity, behavior health issues such as hyperactivity disorders, and delays in gross and fine motor skills.

Diabetes Testing

There are several different methods of testing for diabetes mellitus (DM). Testing is generally performed on two different occasions to confirm a diagnosis of DM. Some of the various testing procedures include:

Fasting plasma glucose – Blood glucose testing that occurs at least eight hours after a patient's last intake of food or drink. Testing is positive for DM if the blood glucose level is >125 mg/dL (normal is <100 mg/dL).

Oral glucose tolerance test – Blood glucose testing that occurs two hours after ingestion of a sugary drink. Testing is positive for DM if the blood glucose level is 200 mg/dL or greater (normal is <140 mg/dL).

A1c testing – A blood test based on the attachment of glucose to hemoglobin that measures the patient's average blood glucose level over the past 2-3 months. Testing is positive for DM if the A1c level is 6.5% or greater (normal is <5.7%).

A diagnosis of DM may also be made if a patient has classic signs and symptoms of DM (e.g., polydipsia, polyuria) along with a casual (random) glucose test of 200 mg/dL or greater. Casual glucose testing can be performed at any time of day without regard to food or drink intake.

Testes and Ovaries Dysfunction[10]

Male hypogonadism: Primary hypogonadism is defined as a deficiency of testosterone secondary to failure of the testes to respond to FSH and LH (produced by the pituitary and hypothalamus). The most common cause of primary hypogonadism is Klinefelter's syndrome. Secondary hypogonadism occurs when there is a failure of the hypothalamus or pituitary to produce the hormones that will subsequently stimulate the production of testosterone. If a male experiences this prior to puberty, symptoms will include sparse body hair, underdevelopment of skeletal muscles, and long arms and legs secondary to a delay in the closure of the epiphyseal growth plates. Adult-onset testosterone deficiency will present with a decreased libido, erectile dysfunction, infertility, decreased cognitive skills, mood changes, and sleep disturbances. Treatment includes hormone replacement pharmacological intervention.

Female hypogonadism: Primary hypogonadism results if the gonad does not produce the amount of sex steroid sufficient to suppress secretion of LH and FSH at normal levels. The most common cause of primary hypogonadism is Turner syndrome. Secondary hypogonadism occurs when there is a failure of the hypothalamus or pituitary to produce the hormones that subsequently stimulate the production of estrogen. If a female experiences this prior to puberty symptoms will include gonadal dysgenesis, a short stature, failure to progress through puberty or primary amenorrhea, and premature gonadal failure. When hypogonadism occurs in postpubescent females, secondary amenorrhea is the primary symptom. Treatment includes hormone replacement pharmacological intervention.

Pharmacology - Endocrine Management[19]

Endocrine pharmacological intervention will either consist of replacement therapy that will provide the deficient hormones or hyperfunction therapy which inhibits the oversecretion of the target hormones. The following is an overview highlighting only the general process for treatment.

Bone Mineral Regulating Agents

Action: Bone mineral regulating agents attempt to enhance and maximize bone mass along with preventing bone loss or rate of bone reabsorption. Typical agents can include estrogens, calcium and vitamin D, bisphosphonates, calcitonin, and anabolic agents.

Indications: Paget's disease, osteoporosis, hyperparathyroidism, rickets, hypoparathyroidism, osteomalacia

Side effects: (agent dependent) gastrointestinal distress, dyspepsia, dysphagia, anorexia, bone pain, cardiac arrhythmias

Implications for PT: Patients with bone mineralization deficit are at risk for fracture and side effects from drug therapy. Therapists must be aware of potential side effects and should attempt to augment drug therapy through ambulation and other weight bearing activities that stimulate bone formation.

Examples: Fosamax, Boniva, Cibacalcin

Hormone Replacement Agents

Action: These agents restore normal endocrine function when endogenous production of a particular hormone is deficient or absent.

Indications: decrease in endogenous hormone secretion

Side effects: Vary by exogenous or synthetic hormone replacement used for treatment

Implications for PT: Therapists must be aware of signs and symptoms of hormone deficit and side effects of hormone therapy.

Examples: see specific hormone categories, pgs. 461-462

Hyperfunction Agents

Action: These agents manage hyperactive endocrine function to allow for inhibition of hormone function. This is accomplished through negative feedback loops or through hormone antagonists.

Indications: hyperactive or excessive endocrine function, excessive hormone levels

Side effects: Vary depending on the use of exogenous or synthetic hormone therapy

Implications for PT: Therapists must be aware of signs of hyperfunction of particular hormones and side effects from agents that attempt to regulate and normalize hormone functioning.

Examples: see specific hormone categories, pgs. 461-462

Gastrointestinal System

Gastrointestinal System

The gastrointestinal system is responsible for the process of digestion. It breaks down food into its components, absorbs nutrients, and discards the waste.

Gastrointestinal Anatomy and Function[10]

Upper GI	
Mouth	Initiation of mechanical and chemical digestion
Esophagus	Transports food from the mouth to the stomach
Stomach	Grinding of food, secretion of hydrochloric acid and other exocrine functions, secretion of hormones that release digestive enzymes from the liver, pancreas, and gallbladder to assist with digestion

Lower GI – Small Intestine	
Duodenum	Neutralizes acid in food from the stomach and mixes pancreatic and biliary secretions with food
Jejunum	Absorbs water, electrolytes, and nutrients
Ileum	Absorbs bile and intrinsic factors to be recycled

Lower GI – Large Intestine	
Ascending colon, Transverse colon, Descending colon, Sigmoid colon, Rectum, Anus	Continues to absorb water and electrolytes, stores and eliminates undigested food as feces

Gland Organs	
Gallbladder	Stores and releases bile into the duodenum to assist with digestion
Liver	Bile is produced and is necessary for absorption of lipid soluble substances, assists with red blood cell and vitamin K production, regulates serum level of carbohydrates, proteins, and fats
Pancreas	Exocrine - secretes bicarbonate and digestive enzymes into the duodenum; Endocrine - secretes insulin, glucagon, and other hormones into the blood to regulate serum glucose level

Gastrointestinal System Pathology

GI Components	Common Pathologies
Esophagus	Hiatal hernia, gastroesophageal reflux disease, esophageal cancer, dysphagia, esophageal varices, Barrett's esophagus
Stomach	Gastritis, peptic ulcer disease, gastric cancer, gastrointestinal hemorrhage, motility and emptying disorders
Intestines	Malabsorption syndrome, appendicitis, irritable bowel syndrome, Crohn's disease, ulcerative colitis, colon cancer, intestinal hernia, diverticular diseases
Rectum and anus	Rectal or anal cancer, hemorrhoids, anorectal fistula, rectal fissure
Gallbladder	Gallstones (cholelithiasis), cholecystitis, gallbladder cancer
Liver	Cirrhosis, jaundice, hepatitis (A, B, C, D, E, G), ascites, hepatic encephalopathy, liver cancer, hepatomegaly
Pancreas	Pancreatitis (acute and chronic), diabetes mellitus, pancreatic cancer

Rehabilitation Considerations for Patients with Gastrointestinal Disease[10]

- Recognize electrolyte imbalances from diarrhea, vomiting, and weight loss
- Recognize the potential for orthostatic hypotension secondary to electrolyte imbalances
- Increased risk for muscle cramping secondary to alteration in the sodium-potassium pumps
- Potential for difficulty swallowing secondary to disk protrusion or esophageal pathology
- Recognize that back pain and/or shoulder pain may be secondary to an acute ulcer or GI bleed
- Observation of Kehr's sign indicates free air or blood within the abdominal cavity

Esophagus

Gastroesophageal Reflux Disease (GERD)[10,17]

GERD is the result of an incompetent lower esophageal sphincter (LES) that allows reflux of gastric contents. This backwards movement of stomach acids and contents can cause esophageal tissue injury over time as well as other pathology. GERD is estimated to occur in 20-30% of adults and can be found in some newborns or infants.

Etiology – The etiologies of GERD include weakness of the LES, intermittent relaxation of the LES, direct damage of the LES through NSAIDs, alcohol, infectious agents, smoking, and certain prescription medications.

Signs and symptoms – Clinical symptoms include heartburn, regurgitation of gastric contents, belching, chest pain, hoarseness and coughing, esophagitis, and hematemesis. If GERD is left untreated, the patient may develop esophageal strictures, esophagitis, aspiration pneumonia, asthma, Barrett's esophagitis, and esophageal adenocarcinoma.

Treatment – Treatment is primarily through pharmacological intervention.

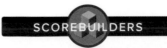

Rehabilitation Considerations for Patients with GERD[10,17]

- Avoid certain exercise secondary to an increase in symptoms with activity; recumbency will induce symptoms
- Recognize increased incidence of neck and head discomfort secondary to perception of a lump in the throat and subsequent compensation
- Left sidelying preferred since right sidelying may promote acid flowing into the esophagus
- Recognize conditions such as chronic bronchitis, asthma, and pulmonary fibrosis may all present with GERD
- Recognize that tight clothing, exercise, and constipation may all precipitate GERD
- Consider that certain positioning during postural drainage may encourage acid to move into the esophagus

Stomach

Gastritis[10,17]

Gastritis is the inflammation of the gastric mucosa or inner layer of the stomach. Symptoms are similar to GERD, however, they tend to have a higher intensity. Gastritis is classified as erosive or non-erosive based on the level and zone of injury.

Erosive Gastritis (acute gastritis)[10,17]

Etiology – Etiology includes bleeding from the gastric mucosa secondary to stress, NSAIDs, alcohol utilization, viral infection or direct trauma.

Signs and symptoms – Symptoms include dyspepsia, nausea, vomiting, and hematemesis. At times, the patient may be asymptomatic.

Treatment – Treatment is supportive with removal of the stimulus of the disease process and pharmacological intervention. Surgical procedures may be required if the bleeding continues.

Non-erosive Gastritis (chronic type B gastritis)[10,17]

Etiology – This condition is typically a result of a helicobacter pylori infection (H. pylori).

Signs and symptoms – The patient is usually asymptomatic but will show symptoms if the gastritis progresses.

Treatment – H. pylori is a carcinogen and must be treated aggressively. Pharmacological intervention is most common and typically includes a proton pump inhibitor and antibiotics.

Rehabilitation Considerations for Patients with Gastritis[10,17]

- Patients with gastritis secondary to chronic NSAID use may be asymptomatic
- Knowledge of blood in the stool should result in physician referral
- Educate each patient to take medications with food and avoid certain types of food and drink
- The patient should avoid all aspirin-containing compounds

Peptic Ulcer Disease[10,17]

Peptic ulcer disease is a condition where there is a disruption or erosion in the gastrointestinal mucosa. There is an imbalance between the protective mechanisms of the stomach and the secretion of acids within the stomach.

Etiology – Many ulcers are caused by the H. pylori infection and chronic NSAID use. Irritants that increase risk of ulcer include stress, alcohol, particular medications, foods, and smoking.

Signs and symptoms – Symptoms are dependent on the location and severity of ulceration (gastric or duodenal) and can include epigastric pain, burning or heartburn, nausea, vomiting, bleeding, bloody stools, and pain that comes in waves that is relieved by eating. Symptoms specific to the etiology of H. pylori can also include halitosis, rosacea, and flushing. Complications can include hemorrhage, perforation, obstruction (secondary to scarring), and malignancy.

Treatment – Treatment is primarily through pharmacological intervention, however, in more severe cases, surgical intervention may be required.

Rehabilitation Considerations for Patients with Peptic Ulcer Disease[10]

- Asymptomatic patients with history of ulcer should be monitored for signs of bleeding
- Fatigue level, pallor, and exercise tolerance must be monitored for signs of bleeding
- Recognize that heart rate increase or blood pressure decrease may be signs of bleeding
- Recognize that back pain is a sign of a perforated ulcer located on the posterior wall of the stomach and duodenum
- Recognize that pain that radiates from the midthoracic area to the right upper quadrant and shoulder may signify blood and acid within the peritoneal cavity secondary to a perforated and bleeding ulcer

Intestines

Irritable Bowel Syndrome (IBS)[10,17]

Irritable bowel syndrome consists of recurrent symptoms of the upper and lower gastrointestinal system that interfere with the normal functioning of the colon.

Etiology – The etiology is unknown, but one theory believes that the colon or large intestine may be sensitive to certain foods or stress. Other theories hypothesize that the immune system, serotonin, and bacterial infections may all be causative factors. IBS typically occurs in as many as 20% of adults, more commonly in females, and begins prior to the age of 30 in 50% of patients. Females have a slightly higher rate of incidence which may be triggered by food sensitivities, stress, anxiety, caffeine, smoking, alcohol or high fat intake.

Signs and symptoms – Symptoms can include abdominal pain, bloating or distention of the abdomen, nausea, vomiting, anorexia, changes in form and frequency of stool, and passing of mucus in the stool.

Treatment – IBS is normally a diagnosis of exclusion from other GI diagnoses and treatment is usually multifactorial. Change in lifestyle and nutrition, decrease in stress, pharmacological intervention, adequate sleep, exercise, and psychotherapy may all assist in alleviating symptoms. Patients with IBS should avoid large meals, milk, wheat, rye, barley, alcohol, and caffeine. Although the symptoms can be severe, it does not lead to serious disease. Symptoms can typically be controlled by diet, pharmacological intervention, and stress management.

Rehabilitation Considerations for Patients with Irritable Bowel Syndrome[10]

- Emphasize physical activity to assist with bowel function and relieve stress
- Emphasize breathing techniques to assist in stress reduction and with breath-holding patterns
- Recognize that biofeedback training may be beneficial

Diverticulitis[10,17]

Diverticulitis is the condition of having inflamed or infected diverticula. This occurs in approximately 20-25% of the population that has diverticulosis. Diverticulosis is the condition of having diverticula. These are pouch-like protrusions occurring in the colon. Approximately 10% of the population over 40 years of age develops diverticulosis. Approximately 80% of individuals with diverticulosis are asymptomatic, however, those with symptoms may experience bloating, mild cramping, and both diarrhea and constipation. Treatment includes an increased amount of dietary fiber (20-35 grams per day recommended) to avoid diverticulitis.

Etiology – The exact etiology of diverticulitis is unknown; however, a dominant theory is that the disease results from a low fiber diet.

Signs and symptoms – Abdominal pain is the primary symptom of diverticulitis. Tenderness over the left side of the lower abdomen, cramping, constipation or diarrhea, nausea, fever, chills, and vomiting can also occur.

Treatment – Treatment includes diet modification, controlling the underlying infection, and lowering internal colonic pressure through increased fiber intake. In more severe cases, a nasogastric tube may be required to give the intestines a rest. Surgical intervention is indicated for severe obstruction, perforation or necrosis. Complications can include bleeding infections, intestinal blockage, abscess, perforations or tears in the colon, fistulas or peritonitis.

Rehabilitation Considerations for Patients with Diverticular Disease[10]

- Physical activity assists the bowel function and is extremely important during periods of remission
- Breathing techniques will assist in stress reduction and with breath-holding patterns
- Avoid any increase in intra-abdominal pressure with exercise or activity
- Back pain and/or referred hip pain must be examined for possible medical diseases

---

Liver

Hepatitis[10,17]

Hepatitis is an inflammatory process within the liver. Viral hepatitis is most common and is classified as hepatitis A, B, C, D, E or G. Hepatitis A, B, and C are the most common and discussed briefly below.

Etiology – Many instances of hepatitis are viral in nature. Other etiologies include a chemical reaction, drug reaction or alcohol abuse. Other viruses that can cause hepatitis include Epstein-Barr virus, herpes virus I and II, varicella-zoster virus, and measles.

Signs and symptoms – Symptoms of hepatitis include fever, flu symptoms, abrupt onset of fatigue, anorexia, headache, jaundice, darkened urine, lighter stool, enlarged spleen and liver, and intermittent pruritus.

Treatment – Acute viral hepatitis usually resolves with medical treatment, but can become chronic in some cases. Chronic hepatitis may result in the need for liver transplant.

Hepatitis A (HAV)

Hepatitis A is a virus that affects the liver and its function. Transmission occurs by close personal contact with someone that has the infection or through the fecal-oral route (i.e., contaminated water and food sources). The flu-like symptoms represent an acute infection; this form does not progress to chronic disease or cirrhosis of the liver. Patients usually recover in six to ten weeks. Treatment is supportive and the virus is self-limiting.

Hepatitis B (HBV)

Hepatitis B is a virus that affects the liver and its function. Transmission of this virus occurs through the sharing of needles, intercourse with an infected person, exposure to an infected person's blood, semen or maternal-fetal exposure. Approximately 10% of cases progress to chronic hepatitis since the body cannot always rid itself of HBV. Treatment includes hepatitis B immunoglobulin (HBIG) for the unvaccinated patient within 24 hours of exposure. The patient should then receive the vaccination series at one and six months. If the patient is already vaccinated, they may require another dose of the HBV vaccine.

Hepatitis C (HCV)

Hepatitis C is a virus that affects the liver and its function. It is one of the primary etiologies for chronic liver disease and eventual liver failure. Transmission of this virus occurs through the sharing of needles, intercourse with an infected person, exposure to an infected person's blood, semen, body fluids or maternal-fetal exposure. The virus accounts for 90% of post transfusion hepatitis cases. Like hepatitis B, this virus is often asymptomatic and the acute infection can be mild. Patients with hepatitis C have an increased frequency of manifesting conditions such as Hashimoto's thyroiditis, diabetes mellitus, and corneal ulceration. Treatment may include the use of interferon alfa-2b to reduce the inflammation and liver damage but only a small percentage of patients with hepatitis C benefit from the medication. There is no vaccine to prevent this virus and no immunoglobulin fully effective in treating the infection. Chronic hepatitis occurs in 50% of cases and 20% of those cases progress to cirrhosis of the liver.

Pancreas
Diabetes Mellitus

Please refer to the endocrine section on page 466 and the clinical application templates on diabetes mellitus on pages 526 and 528.

Gallbladder
Cholecystitis and Cholelithiasis[10,17]

Cholecystitis refers to inflammation of the gallbladder that may be acute or chronic.

Etiology – The most common etiology is gallstones (cholelithiasis) that have become impacted within the cystic duct. Gallstones develop from hypomobility of the gallbladder, supersaturation of the bile with cholesterol or crystal formation from bilirubin salts.

Signs and symptoms – Many times gallstones are asymptomatic, however, the most common symptom is right upper quadrant pain. If the gallstone becomes lodged within the cystic duct, then the patient can experience many problems including severe right upper quadrant pain with muscle guarding, tenderness, and rebound pain. These symptoms can radiate to the interscapular region.

Treatment – Treatment is not recommended for the patient with asymptomatic gallstones, but a low-fat diet can decrease gallbladder stimulation if mild symptoms are present. If patients are symptomatic, a lithotripsy procedure can be used in an attempt to break up and dissolve the stones. Primary treatment is a laparoscopic cholecystectomy to remove the gallbladder and the lodged stones from the ducts.

Rehabilitation Considerations for Patients with Hepatitis[10]

- Health care workers that are at risk for contact with hepatitis should receive all immunizations for HBV, and if exposed to blood or body fluids of an infected person must receive immunoglobulin therapy immediately
- Standard precautions should be followed at all times for protection
- Enteric precautions are required for patients with hepatitis A and E
- Recognize that arthralgias may be noted, especially in older patients, and will not typically respond to traditional therapeutic intervention
- Energy conservation techniques and pacing skills should be incorporated into therapy
- Balance activities along with periods of rest, avoid prolonged bed rest, and provide patient education regarding signs of relapse or chronic hepatitis

---

Rehabilitation Considerations for Patients with Cholecystitis and Cholelithiasis[10]

- Must be familiar with all signs and symptoms of cholecystitis in order to refer patients to a physician if a change in their status occurs
- Post-surgical exercises and ambulation are appropriate post laparoscopic cholecystectomy such as breathing exercises, splinting while coughing, and mobility training

Pharmacology - Gastrointestinal Management[19]

Pharmacological intervention is normally related to gastrointestinal disorders that are caused by gastric acid secretion and abnormal food movement through the gastrointestinal tract.

Antacid Agents

Action: Antacid agents are used to chemically neutralize gastric acid and increase the intragastric pH. Primary antacids are classified as aluminum-containing, calcium carbonate-containing, magnesium-containing or sodium bicarbonate-containing.

Indications: episodic minor gastric indigestion or heartburn, peptic ulcer, gastroesophageal reflux disease (GERD)

Side effects: acid rebound phenomenon, constipation or diarrhea (depending on the antacid), may affect metabolism of other medication, electrolyte imbalances

Implications for PT: Since these agents are well tolerated, there are typically no side effects that interfere with physical therapy. Patients are more likely to participate in therapy with effective management of gastrointestinal issues using these agents.

Examples: Tums, Milk of Magnesia

Antibiotics

Action: Antibiotics are prescribed to treat H. pylori infection with the goal of facilitating more rapid healing of associated gastric ulcerations.

Indications: H. pylori bacteria

Side effects: hypersensitivity, diarrhea, nausea

Implications for PT: Physical therapist assistants should be aware of potential side effects in order to respond appropriately especially with regard to severe dermatologic and respiratory reactions which may be associated with hypersensitivity.

Examples: Tetracycline, Amoxicillin

Anticholinergics

Action: Anticholinergics block the effects of acetylcholine on parietal cells in the stomach and decrease the release of gastric acid.

Indications: gastric ulcers

Side effects: dry mouth, confusion, constipation, urinary retention

Implications for PT: Physical therapist assistants should be aware of potential side effects in order to respond appropriately to changes in cognition or complaints of dry mouth, constipation or urinary retention.

Examples: Gastrozepin

Antidiarrheal Agents

Action: Antidiarrheal agents are used to slow the serious debilitating effects of dehydration associated with prolonged diarrhea. There are multiple classes of antidiarrheal agents.

Indications: prolonged diarrhea

Side effects: constipation, abdominal discomfort

Implications for PT: Since these agents are well tolerated there are typically no side effects that interfere with physical therapy. Patients are more likely to participate in therapy with effective management of gastrointestinal issues using these agents.

Examples: Kapectolin, Pepto-Bismol

Antiemetic Agents

Action: Antiemetic agents are used to decrease symptoms of nausea and vomiting.

Indications: nausea associated with motion sickness, anesthesia, pain or oncology treatments

Side effects: side effects are agent dependent, but can include sedation, dysrhythmias, and pain.

Implications for PT: Antiemetic agents frequently cause sedative effects which can be limiting to physical therapy interventions. Many other antiemetic agents are typically well tolerated and should not significantly interfere with therapy interventions.

Examples: Scopolamine, Meclizine

Emetic Agents

Action: Emetic agents are used to induce vomiting.

Indications: to induce vomiting; usually after ingestion of a toxic substance

Side effects: dehydration, electrolyte imbalance, and upper GI erosion may occur with inappropriate or prolonged usage

Implications for PT: The medical concerns associated with administration of an emetic agent should be addressed prior to initiation or resumption of therapy interventions. Therapy should also be deferred if a patient is actively vomiting.

Examples: Apomorphine, Ipecac

H_2 Receptor Blockers

Action: H_2 receptor blockers bind specifically to histamine receptors to prevent the histamine-activated release of gastric acid normally stimulated during food intake.

Indications: dyspepsia, acute and long-term treatment of peptic ulcer, GERD

Side effects: headache, dizziness, mild gastrointestinal distress, tolerance, arthralgia, acid rebound with discontinuation of agent

Implications for PT: Since these agents are well tolerated there are typically no side effects that interfere with physical therapy. Patients are more likely to participate in therapy with effective management of gastrointestinal issues using these agents.

Examples: Tagamet, Pepcid

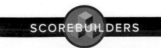

CONSIDER THIS
REFERRED VISCERAL PAIN MAY MIMIC MUSCULOSKELETAL CONDITIONS[17]

Visceral pain refers to pain caused by pathology in the visceral organs (e.g., organ cancer, small bowel obstruction, kidney stones). Pain originating from organs is often difficult to localize due to the tendency to perceive the pain in locations other than the organ source. Due to the overlap in sensory and visceral nerve pathways, symptoms will often refer to soft tissue within the dermatome that corresponds to the organ's spinal cord innervation. The left arm or jaw pain commonly associated with myocardial infarction is a well known example of referred visceral pain. With lesser known symptoms, however, referred pain patterns may result in a delayed diagnosis. Many referred visceral pain patterns mimic musculoskeletal symptoms. Therefore therapists must be diligent in assessing pain of an unknown origin. Since visceral pain is transmitted via the autonomic nervous system, this is especially true when pain is accompanied by autonomic responses such as nausea, vomiting, pallor or sweating.

Laxative Agents

Action: Laxative agents are used to facilitate bowel evacuation and should be used sparingly.

Indications: to promote defecation

Side effects: nausea, abdominal discomfort, cramping, electrolyte imbalance, dehydration, dependence with prolonged use

Implications for PT: If the laxative was recently ingested, physical discomfort may temporarily limit patient participation in therapy interventions. Patients may also express concern about treatment occurring in areas that do not have easy access to restroom facilities.

Examples: Citrucel, Colace

Proton Pump Inhibitors (PPI)

Action: Proton pump inhibitor agents inhibit the H+/K+ -ATPase enzyme, blocking secretions of acid from gastric cells into the stomach. These agents prevent erosive esophagitis and may also possess antibacterial effects against H. pylori.

Indications: dyspepsia, GERD

Side effects: acid rebound phenomenon when discontinued after prolonged use

Implications for PT: Since these agents are well tolerated, there are typically no side effects that interfere with physical therapy. Patients are more likely to participate in therapy with effective management of gastrointestinal issues using these agents.

Examples: Prevacid, Nexium

Abdominal Pain Quadrant and Potential Etiologies[17,20]

Left upper quadrant	Right upper quadrant	Left lower quadrant	Right lower quadrant
Gastric ulcer	Hepatomegaly	Perforated colon	Kidney stone
Perforated colon	Duodenal ulcer	Ileitis	Ureteral stone
Pneumonia	Cholecystitis	Sigmoid diverticulitis	Meckel diverticulum
Spleen injury	Pneumonia	Kidney stone	Appendicitis
Spleen rupture	Hepatitis	Ureteral stone	Cholecystitis
Aortic aneurysm	Biliary stones	Intestinal obstruction	Intestinal obstruction

Gastrointestinal System Terminology

Adhesion: Fibrous bands of tissue that bind together normally separate anatomic structures.

Ascites: Fluid in the peritoneal cavity, usually causing abdominal swelling.

Barium: A substance that, when swallowed or given rectally as an enema, makes the upper gastrointestinal tract visible on x-ray.

Biopsy: Removal of a sample of tissue taken from the body for study, usually under a microscope.

Colectomy: The surgical removal of part or all of the colon.

Colonoscopy: Visual inspection of the interior of the colon with a flexible, lighted instrument inserted through the rectum.

Colostomy: The surgical creation of an opening from the colon through the abdominal wall.

Constipation: Infrequent or difficult passage of stool, secondary to an increase in the hardness of the stool.

Diarrhea: Abnormal frequency or volume of stool that often appears as a symptom of certain gastrointestinal pathologies.

Endoscopy: A method of physical examination using a lighted, flexible instrument that allows a physician to examine the inside of the digestive tract.

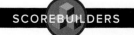

Enema: Injection of fluid into the rectum and colon to induce a bowel movement.

Esophagus: A muscular tube connecting the pharynx with the stomach.

Fecal diversion: Surgical creation of an opening of part of the colon or small intestine to the surface of the skin to allow for stool to exit the body.

Fecal incontinence: Inability to retain stool, resulting in leakage of stool from the rectum.

Fecal occult blood test: A lab test used to check a stool sample for blood.

Gas: A product of digestion that is made primarily of odorless vapors.

Gastrectomy: Surgical procedure in which all or part of the stomach is removed.

Gastric: Pertaining to the stomach.

Gastroscopy: Procedure to examine the upper gastrointestinal tract using an endoscope which is passed through the mouth and into the stomach.

Heartburn: A form of indigestion.

Helicobacter pylori: A type of bacterium that causes infection in the stomach. The bacterium is often the causative agent in peptic ulcers.

Ileocolectomy: Surgical removal of a section of the ileum and ascending colon.

Ileostomy: The surgical creation of an opening from the ileum through the abdominal wall.

Jaundice: A condition in which the skin and eyes turn yellow because of increased levels of bilirubin in the blood.

Laparoscopy: A surgical diagnostic procedure utilizing a fiber optic instrument inserted through the abdominal wall to view organs.

Large intestine: The portion of the digestive tract made up of the ascending colon, transverse colon, descending colon, sigmoid colon, and appendix. The large intestine receives the liquid contents from the small intestine and absorbs the water and electrolytes from this liquid to form feces or waste.

Laxative: Medications that increase the action of the intestines or stimulate the addition of water to the stool to facilitate bowel evacuation.

Peristalsis: Involuntary contraction and relaxation of the muscles of the intestines which propel food.

Polyps (colon): Small, non-cancerous growths on the inner lining of the colon.

Small intestine: The portion of the digestive tract that first receives food from the stomach. The small intestine is comprised of the duodenum, jejunum and ileum.

Stoma: An artificial opening of the intestine through the abdominal wall.

Thrombosis: The formation of a blood clot in a blood vessel.

Ulcers: A break in the lining of the stomach or in the duodenum.

Varices: Large, swollen veins that develop in the esophagus or stomach, often causing internal bleeding.

Vomiting: The forcible expulsion of the contents of the stomach through the mouth.

Genitourinary System

Genitourinary System

The genitourinary system consists of all the reproductive organs and the urinary organs. These are often considered together due to their common embryological origin.

Genitourinary Anatomy and Function

The genitourinary system is supported by the pelvic floor consisting of muscle, fascia, and ligament.

Muscles of the Pelvic Floor[20,21]	
Pelvic diaphragm	Levator ani: pubococcygeus, puborectalis, iliococcygeus, and coccygeus (ischiococcygeus)
Urogenital diaphragm	Deep transverse perineal, urethrae sphincter
Urogenital triangle	Female: bulbocavernosus, ischiocavernosus, superficial transverse perineal Male: bulbospongiosus, ischiocavernosus, superficial transverse perineal
Anal triangle	Internal anal sphincter, external anal sphincter

Genital System

The genital system consists of the male and female gonads and associated ducts, external genitalia, and associated hormones that all function for reproduction.

Female Genital System[20-22]	
External genitalia Mons pubis, labia majora, labia minora, clitoris, vestibule of vagina, bulbs of vestibule, greater vestibular (Bartholin's) glands, Skene's gland	• Provides protection and hydration of vaginal tissue and urethra
Vagina Musculomembranous tube connected to the cervix	• Receptacle for male sperm • Birth canal • Excretory duct for menstrual fluid
Uterus Hollow muscular organ	• Houses the fetus during development
Uterine tubes Extend laterally from the ovaries to the uterus	• Provides transport for the ovum from the ovary for fertilization and implantation within the uterus
Ovaries Almond-shaped glands suspended in the broad ligaments	• Produce hormones such as estrogen and progesterone • Storage of oocytes prior to ovulation

Male Genital System[20]	
Penis	• External genitalia that expels urine during voiding and semen during the act of copulation
Scrotum	• Cutaneous fibromuscular external sac for the testes, ductus deferens, epididymis, nerves, and blood vessels
Testes	• Produce sperm and hormones such as testosterone
Ductus/vas deferens	• Carries sperm from the testes to the seminal vesicle to form the ejaculatory duct
Epididymis	• Encased within the scrotum • Stores sperm
Seminal vesicles	• Internal tubes that secrete a thick fluid to combine with sperm within the ejaculatory duct
Prostate	• Internal organ lying inferior to the bladder • Produces and secretes fluid to combine with sperm, seminal vesicle fluid, and bulbourethral gland fluid to create semen

Renal System

The renal system consists of two kidneys, two ureters, the urinary bladder, and the urethra that function to form and eliminate urine.

Renal System[20,21]	
Kidneys	• Remove water, salt, and metabolic waste from the blood through excretion of urine • Contribute to homeostasis including: acid-base balance, regulation of electrolyte concentrations, control of blood volume, and regulation of blood pressure through the control of hormones secreted into the bloodstream
Ureters	• Muscular tubes connecting the kidneys to the urinary bladder to transport urine
Urinary bladder	• Temporary muscular reservoir for urine
Urethra	• Muscular tube for excretion of urine • Semen transport during ejaculation in males

CONSIDER THIS

GENITOURINARY SYSTEM SUPPORT STRUCTURE[20,21]

The pelvic floor muscles' primary functions include bladder/bowel control and sexual function. In addition, the pelvic floor muscles support the pelvic organs by holding the organs in position in conjunction with ligaments and surrounding fascia. The muscles are made up of two different fiber types, type I (slow twitch) and type II (fast twitch). When the pelvic floor muscles are weak or have poor endurance due to pregnancy, trauma, surgery, repetitive straining or genetics they are not able to support the pelvic organs leading to organ prolapse. Affected structures may include the bladder, uterus, cervix, intestines, and rectum. This may result in urgency, frequency, urinary or fecal incontinence due to the muscle imbalance during increased intra-abdominal pressure.

Genitourinary System Pathology

Genital Components	Common Pathologies[20,21]
Uterus	Cervical cancer*, endometriosis, uterine prolapse
Vagina	Dyspareunia, vulvodynia, vulvovaginal candidiasis (yeast infection)
Prostate	Prostatitis, prostate cancer*
Penis	Erectile dysfunction
Renal Components	**Common Pathologies[20,21]**
Kidneys	Glomerulonephritis, nephrolithiasis, renal failure
Bladder	Cystocele, dysuria, hematuria, interstitial cystitis, neurogenic bladder, nocturia, polyuria, urgency, frequency, urinary incontinence, urinary tract infections

*For more information on cervical and prostate cancer see pages 491-492.

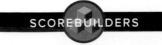

Kidneys
Renal Failure[10,24]

Renal failure is a condition where the kidneys experience a decrease in glomerular filtration rate and fail to adequately filter toxins and waste from the blood. There are two forms: acute renal failure and chronic renal failure.

Etiology – Renal pathology typically occurs secondary to diabetes mellitus or hypertension, but can also occur from poison, trauma, and genetics. The nephrons are usually damaged and they lose their ability to filter the blood. Renal failure can be classified as:

- Acute (damage occurs quickly)
- Chronic (damage occurs slowly)
- End-stage (nearly total or total renal failure, dialysis required)

Acute Renal Failure (ARF)

- Sudden decline in renal function
- Increase in BUN and creatinine
- Oliguria, hyperkalemia, sodium retention
- Prerenal etiology is secondary to a decrease in blood flow typically due to shock, hemorrhage, burn or pulmonary embolism
- Postrenal etiology is secondary to obstruction distal to the kidney due to neoplasm, kidney stone or prostate hypertrophy
- Intrarenal etiology is secondary to primary damage of renal tissue due to toxins, intrarenal ischemia or vascular disorders

Chronic Renal Failure (CRF)

- Progressive deterioration in renal function
- Diabetes mellitus
- Severe hypertension
- Glomerulopathies
- Obstructive uropathy
- Interstitial nephritis
- Polycystic kidney disease

Signs and symptoms – Symptoms of renal failure vary based on severity of the condition and can include nausea, vomiting, lethargy, weakness, hiccups, anorexia, ulceration within the GI tract, sleep disorders, headache, peripheral neuropathy, anemia, pruritus, osteomalacia, ecchymosis, pulmonary edema, seizures, and coma.

Treatment – Treatment of ARF includes management of primary etiology, pharmacological intervention, diuretics, nutritional support, hydration, hemodialysis and/or transfusions if applicable. Treatment of CRF includes conservative management and renal replacement therapy. Conservative management assists with slowing the process and assisting the body in its compensation. Nutritional support, hydration, avoidance of protein, and pharmacological intervention are usually the primary basis of intervention. Renal replacement therapy includes some form of hemodialysis and/or organ transplant. Peritoneal dialysis is a form of renal replacement therapy that uses the peritoneal cavity as a semi-permeable membrane between the dialysate fluid and blood vessels of the abdominal cavity.

Hemodialysis

Hemodialysis is a treatment process for patients with advanced and permanent kidney failure. Kidney failure creates excess toxic waste, increased blood pressure, retention of excess body fluids, and a decrease in red blood cell production. Hemodialysis removes the blood from the body along with waste, excess sodium, and fluids. The process cleanses the blood and returns it to the body. A patient requires this process on average three times per week and each visit requires three to five hours to complete the treatment. Side effects that may be associated with dialysis include anemia, renal osteodystrophy, pruritus (itching), sleep disorders ("restless legs"), and dialysis-related amyloidosis.

Rehabilitation Considerations for Patients with Renal Failure/Dialysis[10,24]

- Modify treatment plan based on fluid and electrolyte status
- Standard precautions should be followed at all times for protection
- Recognize patient's abilities post dialysis and potential for dehydration and hypotension
- Monitor vital signs closely, however, avoid placement of the blood pressure cuff over the fistula
- Avoid mobilization activities as they are contraindicated during dialysis
- Energy conservation techniques and pacing skills should be incorporated into therapy

Bladder
Neurogenic Bladder[10,24]

Neurogenic bladder is a dysfunction where there is damage to the cerebral control that allows for urinary dysfunction. If the urine cannot be properly released, there may be an increase in urinary tract infections and kidney damage.

Etiology – The etiology of neurogenic bladder can include diabetes, diminished bladder capacity, hyperactive detrusor muscle, CVA, other disease processes, infection, and nerve damage.

Signs and symptoms – Symptoms include frequent urinary tract infections, leakage of urine, inability to empty the bladder or loss of the urge to urinate when the bladder is full. Diagnosis should include an evaluation by a physician, X-rays, and urodynamics to assist with diagnosis.

Treatment – Management is dependent on the actual etiology with a goal of preventing bladder overdistention, UTIs, and renal damage. Patient education, bladder techniques, lower abdominal massage, temporary catheterization, pharmacological intervention, and a timed urination program may be indicated.

CONSIDER THIS
LIFESTYLE MODIFICATIONS TO ADDRESS BLADDER SYMPTOMS[24]

- Daily fluid intake should be 2,500 mL, or 10 cups, to regulate excessively high or low fluid intake.
- Reduce bladder irritants including carbonated, caffeinated, and alcoholic beverages, spicy foods, citrus, and artificial sweeteners. Caffeine reduction should be tapered slowly to avoid severe headaches.
- Schedule voiding for every 3-4 hours to reduce bladder distention. An average person voids 6-8 times in a 24-hour period. A bladder diary assists with baseline measurements and goal setting.
- Regulate bowel function to prevent constipation and straining during bowel movements by monitoring dietary fiber, fluid intake, and exercise.
- Avoid fluid intake 2-3 hours prior to bedtime to reduce nocturia.
- A smoking cessation program may decrease the occurrence of coughing and subsequent bladder leakage.
- A weight loss program, if moderately obese, may decrease pressure on the pelvic tissues and organs.

Urinary Incontinence[10,24]

Urinary incontinence is an involuntary loss of urine that is great enough to be problematic for the person and typically occurs when bladder pressure exceeds sphincter resistance. Below are four classifications of urinary incontinence. General treatment includes pelvic floor muscle training using biofeedback, lifestyle modifications, bladder retraining, prompted voiding programs, urge suppression strategies, myofascial release, visceral mobilization, body mechanics, abdominal strengthening, and stretching exercises of surrounding muscles. Pharmacological intervention to address urgency, injection therapy of a "bulking" agent, and surgical intervention for urethral and bladder positioning may also be indicated. These interventions may not apply to all types of urinary incontinence and should be determined on a per patient basis.

Stress Urinary Incontinence (SUI)

SUI is the loss of urine due to activities that increase intra-abdominal pressure, such as sneezing, coughing, laughing, running, and jumping. *Please refer to clinical application template on page 544 for more information.*

Urge Urinary Incontinence (UUI)

UUI is the loss of urine after a sudden, intense urge to void due to the detrusor muscle of the bladder involuntarily contracting during bladder filling. UUI is the most common incontinence in the geriatric population and among residents in long-term care facilities.

Etiology – The most common etiologies are detrusor muscle overactivity, overactive bladder also known as "urgency-frequency" syndrome, changes in the smooth muscle of the bladder, increased afferent activity, increased sensitivity of the detrusor to acetylcholine, and idiopathic. There is also association with the following neurological disorders: multiple sclerosis, spinal cord injury, cerebrovascular accident, and Parkinson's disease.

Signs and symptoms – For many people, UUI is triggered by certain events due to a conditioned reflex. Two of the most common triggers are "key-in-the-lock" when arriving home and running water.

Treatment – Behavior modification is the primary goal of treatment for this condition. Biofeedback, pelvic floor strengthening, and bladder retraining (scheduled voiding) are key components in resolving UUI. Pharmacological intervention may also be warranted.

SPOTLIGHT ON SAFETY
FUNCTIONAL INCONTINENCE AND AT-RISK POPULATIONS[2]

When working with patients within the acute care, long-term care or home care settings there are many factors contributing to functional incontinence that pose an added safety risk.

- Restricted mobility or dexterity: Patients may have difficulty or the inability to get to the bathroom in a timely fashion due to underlying physical disabilities or limitations such as a spinal cord injury, rheumatoid arthritis or acute illness.
- Environmental barriers: Patients may not be able to reach the restroom or toilet due to stairs, lack of handrails or narrow doorways that do not accommodate wheelchairs or walkers.
- Mental and psychosocial disability: Patients may not realize they have to urinate or may be confused over the location of the restroom.
- Pharmacological intervention: Patients may take medications that affect awareness, mobility, and dexterity.

Overflow Urinary Incontinence (OUI)

OUI is the loss of urine when the intra-bladder pressure exceeds the urethra's capacity to remain closed due to urinary retention.

Etiology – This condition is caused by outflow obstruction secondary to a narrowed or obstructed urethra that results from a prolapsed pelvic organ, a stricture, an enlarged prostate, chronic constipation or neurological disease.

Signs and Symptoms – Individuals who present with OUI may also experience difficulty initiating the urine stream. Once the stream is initiated, it is weak and presents with post void dribble.

Treatment – Treatment will likely include surgical intervention if there is an obstruction. If there is weakness of the detrusor muscles, double voiding is recommended for these patients as well as other strengthening measures. Failed intervention may result in intermittent catheterization.

Functional Urinary Incontinence (FUI)

FUI is the loss of urine due to the inability or unwillingness of a person to use the bathroom facilities prior to involuntary bladder release.

Etiology – A decreased level of mental awareness or a decrease in mobility are the two primary causative factors for FUI. FUI is rarely seen without another bladder issue or neurological involvement.

Signs and symptoms – These patients will typically present with impaired cognition and/or mobility and will experience incontinence secondary to the inability to successfully use a bathroom to void.

Treatment – Since there is typically no urologic pathology associated with functional incontinence, treatment should be directed to alleviate the underlying issue. Improving mobility, modifying clothing style, increasing independence with ambulation and with function will assist with decreasing functional incontinence. Patients may also require a behavioral toileting schedule or program to decrease incontinence.

Urinary Tract Infections (UTI)[10,24]

Urinary tract infections are very common and occur within the general population, however, there is a higher incidence in women and the geriatric population. UTIs can be classified as uncomplicated, complicated, recurrent or chronic.

Etiology – Urinary tract infections (UTI) occur when bacteria infiltrate the urethra (termed urethritis) or further into the bladder itself (cystitis). Untreated, this type of infection can spread and cause a kidney infection (pyelonephritis). Diagnosis is confirmed with urinalysis. Frequent UTIs may require ultrasound, intravenous pyelogram, and cystoscopy to further assess the function of the bladder.

Signs and symptoms – Symptoms of a UTI include increased frequency of urination, pain and/or burning with urination, cloudy urine, pressure above the pubic bone in women, shakiness, fever, back pain, and fatigue.

Treatment – Early treatment has the best results; delay in treatment may allow for serious infection to occur. Pharmacological treatment includes bacteria-specific antibiotics based on the bacteria found in the bladder. Patients are also encouraged to drink an excess of fluids to assist with treatment of the infection.

CONSIDER THIS
ADVANCED PHYSICAL THERAPY INTERVENTIONS[21,23,24]

Other treatment techniques that are not entry-level for pelvic floor dysfunction may include:

- Perineal massage both by the practitioner and patient

- Scar tissue massage both by the practitioner and patient

- Intravaginal soft tissue massage (also known as Thiele massage)

- Intravaginal trigger point release and myofascial release

- Intravaginal self-stretching techniques including the use of a dilator

- Prostate massage

These techniques may be used for, but are not limited to patients who have dyspareunia, vulvodynia, prostatitis, interstitial cystitis, urgency, urge incontinence, levator ani syndrome, coccydynia, and perineal pain from pregnancy.

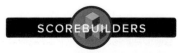

Obstetrics

Obstetric Pathology

Diastasis Recti[21,22,25]

Diastasis recti is a separation of the rectus abdominis muscle along the linea alba that can occur during pregnancy. Testing for diastasis recti should be performed on all pregnant women prior to prescribing exercises that require the use of the abdominals.

Etiology – The exact cause is unknown, however, theories indicate biomechanical and hormonal changes in women may cause the separation. The therapist must note how many fingers fit into the separation and modify treatment accordingly.

Signs and symptoms – A patient is considered to have diastasis recti if the therapist detects a separation greater than the width of two fingers when the woman lifts her head and shoulders off the plinth (Figs. 7-6, 7-7).

Treatment – Treatment will include stabilization and support with abdominal strengthening exercises, postural awareness exercises, and body mechanics training. A newborn can also have diastasis recti secondary to incomplete development, however, in infants this condition usually resolves itself without intervention.

Piriformis Syndrome[21]

Piriformis syndrome refers to a persistent, severe radiating low back and buttock pain spanning from the sacrum to the hip and posterior thigh. However, controversy exists over piriformis syndrome's efficacy as an accurate diagnosis.

Etiology – During pregnancy the piriformis may shorten or spasm due to postural changes and hip lateral rotation while walking.

Signs and symptoms – The primary symptom is sciatic paresthesia due to nerve entrapment as the sciatic nerve passes under or through the piriformis muscle.

Treatment – Manual techniques for correcting pelvic or sacral alignment such as muscle energy techniques, joint mobilization, self-correction techniques for alignment, heat application, deep tissue massage, myofascial release, strain-counterstrain, abdominal strengthening, stretching exercises for both the piriformis and surrounding muscles, body mechanics, and postural education.

Physiological and Postural Changes during Pregnancy[21,22,25]

- Weight gain between 25 and 35 pounds; anemia may occur
- Uterus ascends into the abdominal cavity becoming an abdominal organ
- Ribs expand to accommodate the uterine ascent; respiratory diaphragm elevates four centimeters
- Increased depth of respiration, tidal volume, and minute ventilation
- Increased oxygen consumption (15-20%), blood volume (40-50%), and cardiac output (30-60%)
- Hypotension in supine position during pregnancy from pressure on the inferior vena cava
- Abdominals become overstretched; ligaments become lax secondary to hormonal changes
- Joints may become hypermobile

Exercise & Pregnancy[21,22,25-27]

Pregnant women are encouraged to continue with exercise activity at a moderate rate during a low risk pregnancy. Guidelines permit women to remain at 50-60% of their maximal heart rate for approximately thirty minutes per session. Women must monitor their heart rate intermittently to ensure that they are maintaining their target heart rate. Non-weight bearing activities are preferred due to the continuous change in the center of gravity and balance. Loose clothing is advised to allow for adequate heat loss, and adequate fluids are required during exercise. Women should avoid becoming overtired and should not exercise in the supine position after the first trimester.

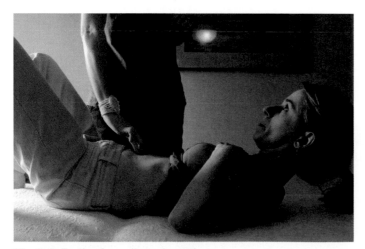

Fig. 7-6: Testing for a diastasis recti.

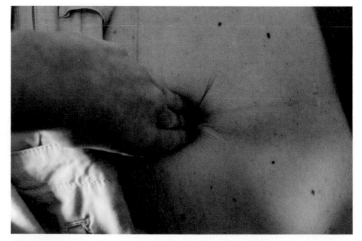

Fig. 7-7: A three finger separation at the linea alba.

CONSIDER THIS
BACK PAIN DURING PREGNANCY[21,22]

Back pain has been reported in 70% of pregnant women, ranging from minor strain to significant structural deformities. Back pain is often caused by physical changes associated with pregnancy including weight gain, altered muscle tone, increased lordosis, changes in center of gravity and laxity within pelvic ligaments. Typically excessive bending, lifting and walking can produce back pain especially if there is a history of prior back pain or obesity.

Minor back pain can be relieved through education related to body mechanics, postural awareness, and stretching and strengthening exercises to provide balance within musculature. More severe pain should not be dismissed as simply a side effect of pregnancy. Etiology of severe back pain may include pregnancy-induced osteoporosis, disk disease or herniated disk, vertebral osteoarthritis, and septic arthritis. Patients with both minor and severe back pain should be examined to determine if the source of the pain is mechanical, muscular, joint or discogenic.

SPOTLIGHT ON SAFETY
CONTRAINDICATIONS TO EXERCISE DURING PREGNANCY[27]

Participating in a wide range of recreational activities and exercise appears to be safe during and after pregnancy. Exercise programs are designed to minimize impairments and help maintain function during pregnancy. Certain circumstances exist where exercise is not safe during pregnancy. Below is a list of relative and absolute contraindications to exercise.

Relative
- Severe anemia
- Unevaluated maternal cardiac dysrhythmia
- Chronic bronchitis
- Poorly controlled type 1 diabetes
- Extreme morbid obesity
- Extreme underweight (BMI <12)
- History of extremely sedentary lifestyle
- Intrauterine growth restriction in current pregnancy
- Poorly controlled hypertension
- Orthopedic limitations
- Poorly controlled seizure disorder
- Poorly controlled hyperthyroidism
- Heavy smoker

Absolute
- Hemodynamically significant heart disease
- Restrictive lung disease
- Incompetent cervix/cerclage
- Multiple gestation at risk for premature labor
- Persistent second or third trimester bleeding
- Placenta previa after 26 weeks of gestation
- Premature labor during the current pregnancy
- Ruptured membranes
- Preeclampsia/pregnancy-induced hypertension

Pelvic Floor Muscle Exercises[21,25]

Once the pelvic floor muscles have been assessed for strength, an exercise routine can be created based on the findings. Some factors to consider are: position, endurance, and repetitions. Introduce new positions transitioning from gravity-assisted to standing as the strength and awareness of the pelvic floor muscles increase. The goal is for the patient to be able to perform the contractions with functional tasks.

Recommendations vary from 80-100 contractions per day combining quick, long hold, and functional contractions. Quick contractions are important to withstand increased intra-abdominal pressure. The patient typically begins with three sets of ten quick contractions daily, holding for two seconds and resting for four seconds. Long hold contractions are for endurance training and are important for maintaining proper posture and pelvic support. The patient typically begins with three sets of five long hold contractions daily, holding for five seconds and resting for ten seconds, gradually increasing the contraction time to ten seconds. Make sure the patient fully relaxes after each contraction. Variations of contractions will depend on each patient's diagnosis, awareness, and ability.

American College of Obstetricians and Gynecologists (ACOG) Recommendations for Exercise in Pregnancy and Postpartum[27]

1. During pregnancy, women can continue to exercise and derive health benefits even from mild to moderate exercise routines. Regular exercise (at least three times per week) is preferable to intermittent activity.

2. Women should avoid exercise in the supine position after the first trimester. Such a position is associated with decreased cardiac output in most pregnant women. Since the remaining cardiac output will be preferentially distributed away from splanchnic beds (including the uterus) during vigorous exercise, such regimens are best avoided during pregnancy. Prolonged periods of motionless standing should be avoided.

3. Women should be aware of the decreased oxygen available for aerobic exercise during pregnancy. They should be encouraged to modify the intensity of their exercise according to maternal symptoms. Pregnant women should stop exercising when fatigued and not exercise to exhaustion. Weight bearing exercises may, under some circumstances, be continued at intensities similar to those prior to pregnancy throughout pregnancy. Non-weight bearing exercises, such as cycling or swimming, will minimize the risk of injury and facilitate the continuation of exercise during pregnancy.

4. Morphologic changes in pregnancy should serve as a relative contraindication to types of exercise in which loss of balance could be detrimental to maternal or fetal well-being, especially in the third trimester. Further, any type of exercise involving the potential for even mild abdominal trauma should be avoided.

5. Pregnancy requires an additional 300 kcal/day in order to maintain metabolic homeostasis. Thus, women who exercise during pregnancy should be particularly careful to ensure an adequate diet.

6. Pregnant women who exercise in the first trimester should augment heat dissipation by ensuring adequate hydration, appropriate clothing, and optimal environmental surroundings during exercise.

7. Many of the physiological and morphological changes of pregnancy persist 4 to 6 weeks postpartum. Thus, pre-pregnancy exercise routines should be resumed gradually based upon a woman's physical capability.

From American College of Obstetricians and Gynecologists. Exercise During Pregnancy and the Postpartum Period. (Technical Bulletin No. 189). Washington, DC, copyrights ACOG, February 1994, with permission.

Pharmacology - Genitourinary Management[19]

Pharmacological intervention is used for treating bladder symptoms related to urgency, frequency, infection, and pain.

Diuretic Agents

See Cardiac pharmacology

Hormones

See Metabolic and Endocrine pharmacology

Overactive Bladder Agents

Action: Overactive bladder agents relieve the symptoms of an overactive bladder. This condition is noted by involuntary contractions of the bladder (detrusor muscle).

Indications: urinary urgency, urinary frequency, urge incontinence, nocturia

Side effects: widely vary based on drug classification; typically gastrointestinal distress, nausea, dizziness, photosensitivity, headache, constipation, pulmonary reactions

Implications for PT: Therapists should be aware of the adverse effects of these agents, however, these agents do not typically interfere with rehabilitation. A therapist should communicate any

SPOTLIGHT ON SAFETY
MANAGEMENT GUIDELINES AND PRECAUTIONS FOR HIGH-RISK PREGNANCIES[25]

A pregnancy is designated as high-risk based on complications from disease or pathology that place the mother and fetus at risk for illness or death. Medical intervention is focused on prevention of preterm delivery through the prescription of bed rest, activity restriction, and medications.

Physical therapy can enhance the well-being and quality of life of the pregnant woman with a high-risk pregnancy. The therapist should closely monitor the patient during all activities, reassess after each treatment, and develop an individualized exercise program addressing the patient's needs. The patient should also be instructed in self-monitoring techniques during activities to avoid adverse reactions.

The following guidelines can assist in working with high-risk patients:

- Left sidelying is the position of choice to reduce the pressure on the inferior vena cava, maximize cardiac output to enhance maternal and fetal circulation, and reduce the risk of incompetent cervix.
- Abdominal exercises may stimulate uterine contractions. The therapist should modify or discontinue the exercises.
- Keep exercises simple, slow, smooth, and with minimal exertion.
- Avoid the Valsalva maneuver by discontinuing activities that increase intra-abdominal pressure.
- Provide instruction on proper body mechanics and postural instruction to limit straining during abdominal contractions.
- Encourage maximum muscle efficiency during each movement.
- Educate the women about Cesarean delivery rehabilitation.
- Monitor and report any uterine contraction, bleeding or amniotic fluid loss.

signs of pulmonary impairment or distress to the physician.

Examples: Ditropan, Detrol

Urinary Anti-infective Agents

Action: Urinary anti-infective agents treat urinary tract infections, but are not traditional antibiotics or sulfonamide agents. These agents can be used independently or in combination to treat urinary infections.

Indications: cystitis, urinary urgency, burning with urination, urinary tract infection, nocturia

Side effects: widely vary based on drug classification; gastrointestinal distress, nausea, dizziness, photosensitivity, headache, constipation, rash

Implications for PT: Therapists should be aware of the adverse effects of these agents, however, these agents do not typically interfere with rehabilitation.

Examples: Cinobac, Furadantin

Genitourinary System Terminology[10,20,24]

Anuria: Inadequate urine output in a 24-hour period; less than 100 ml (e.g., severe dehydration, shock, end-stage renal disease).

Cystocele: Bulging of the bladder into the vagina.

Ectopic: Implantation of a fertilized ovum outside of the uterus. The fallopian tube is the most common site of an ectopic pregnancy.

Endometrium: The inner lining of the uterus that is shed monthly in response to hormonal influence.

Glomerular filtration rate: An estimate of the filtering capacity of the kidneys; volume of filtrate produced per minute by the kidneys.

Glomerulus: The specialized tuft of capillaries that are needed for the filtration of fluid as blood passes through the arterioles of the kidneys.

Hematuria: Presence of blood in the urine (e.g., cancer, faulty catheterization, serious disease).

Impotence: Impairment with ejaculation, orgasm, erection, and/or libido.

Nephrolithiasis: The condition of developing kidney stones. There are various types of crystal formations that create stones.

Nocturia: Urinary frequency at night (e.g., diabetes mellitus, congestive heart failure).

Oliguria: Inadequate urine output in a 24-hour period; less than 400 ml (e.g., acute renal failure, diabetes mellitus).

Polyuria: Large volume of urine excreted at one time (e.g., diabetes mellitus, chronic renal failure).

Radical mastectomy: A surgical procedure in which the entire breast, pectoral muscles, axillary lymph nodes, and some skin are removed usually secondary to breast cancer.

Rectocele: The bulging of the anterior wall of the rectum into the vagina secondary to weakening of the pelvic supporting structures.

Urea: Major nitrogen-containing end product of protein metabolism normally cleared from the blood by the kidney into the urine.

Urinary frequency: Voiding more than eight times in a 24-hour period. Etiology may include overactive bladder, reduced bladder capacity, painful bladder syndrome or increased urine output caused by uncontrolled diabetes mellitus.

Urinary urgency: The sudden desire to urinate that is stronger than usual and difficult to defer. Etiology may include detrusor overactivity, bladder infection, inflammation or the presence of a foreign body such as stones or tumors. Urgency may lead to urinary urge incontinence.

Lymphatic System

Anatomy and Physiology

The primary functions of the lymphatic system include collection and transportation of fluids and other materials that are not reabsorbed by the venous system, maintenance of fluid balance within the body, and immune system defense.

Lymph is the fluid transported by the lymphatic system. It originates as a component of the interstitial fluid and primarily consists of water, proteins, fatty acids, and cellular components. The lymphatic system consists of a network of both superficial and deep lymph vessels that transport lymph throughout the body.

The first lymph vessel within the lymphatic system is the smallest vessel and is known as the initial lymph vessel. These initial lymph vessels are located near blood capillaries and are responsible for collecting fluid from the interstitium that is not picked up by the venous system. The lymphatic system also transports the majority of extracellular proteins since they are often too large to be transported by the venous system. The lymphatic system is normally responsible for collecting 10-20% of the interstitial fluid, while the venous system collects the other 80-90%.

From the initial lymph vessels, lymph is transported towards larger lymph vessels known as lymph collectors. The lymph collectors then transport lymph to even larger lymph vessels known as lymphatic trunks. The two main lymphatic trunks are the right lymphatic duct, which drains lymph from the right arm and right side of the head, and the thoracic duct, which drains lymph from the remainder of the body. These vessels empty lymph directly into the venous system via the subclavian veins.

The lymphatic system is under the control of the autonomic nervous system, which produces contractions of smooth muscle within the lymph vessel walls to help move the lymph fluid along. Skeletal muscle contraction can also help to compress the lymph vessels and move lymph. One-way valves help maintain the unidirectional flow of lymph throughout the entire lymphatic system.

Lymph nodes are specialized structures contained throughout the lymphatic system, but found most commonly in the neck, axilla, chest, abdomen, and groin. The lymph nodes collect lymph from several adjacent areas and function primarily to filter waste products and foreign materials from the lymph (e.g., bacteria, viruses) and provide immune system defense with the use of T and B lymphocytes.

Lymphedema

Lymphedema is a chronic, incurable condition and is characterized by the accumulation of protein-rich fluid (i.e., lymph) in the body. The result is edema that typically presents in the extremities, but can occur anywhere in the body including the face, neck, abdomen, genitalia, and trunk. Fluid accumulation occurs secondary to damage to the lymph structures, which affects the normal flow of lymph. Lymphedema is categorized as either primary or secondary based on the etiology.

Primary lymphedema occurs due to an abnormal development of the lymphatic system. Though this may occur from birth, it may take several years before the patient becomes symptomatic. Abnormalities of the lymph system may include the absence of lymph vessels, a decrease in the number or size of lymph vessels, and/or an increased size of lymph vessels, which makes the valves incompetent.

Secondary lymphedema occurs as a result of some other disease or injury that causes damage to the lymphatic system. This may include trauma, surgery, radiation, tumor growth, multiparity, chronic venous insufficiency or infection. In the United States, breast cancer surgery and treatment is the most common cause for secondary lymphedema. When a patient has treatment for breast cancer, the risk for lymphedema increases significantly with axillary lymph node dissection and/or radiation therapy.

The primary sign of lymphedema is swelling in the extremities. Because the lymphatic system can no longer handle the volume of fluid that it normally would, excess fluid builds up in the interstitium and leads to enlargement of the affected limb. Patients will complain of achiness, fullness, and heaviness of the affected limb. As lymphedema progresses, the valves expand and become incompetent, which leads to further fluid accumulation. If the fluid stasis continues, the proteins begin to degrade which leads to the development of chronic inflammation and eventually fibrotic changes to the surrounding tissues. Fibrosis results in local hypoxia in the tissues, which causes further chronic inflammation and an increased risk for infection.

Physical Therapy Tests and Measures

Tests and measures used by therapists for lymphedema commonly include comparative measurements for limb size. Changes in limb size help determine the progression of the disease and the effectiveness of treatment. The most common method for measuring lymphedema is circumferential measurements.

Circumferences for Limb Edema[26]

Circumference measurements made at a number of points along the limb at specified distances from an anatomical landmark are an accepted technique to detect limb enlargement and to provide a quantitative assessment of changes in limb size due to edema, lymphedema, and joint effusion.

Procedure

- Measurements should be made on a measuring board.
- Measurements should be from a standard point of reference on the extremity that is replicable (e.g., every 5 or 10 centimeters along the extremity or a specified distance from a bony prominence).
- Seven circumferences are recommended for the upper and lower extremities to deduce that the fluid has been removed and not just redistributed.

Interpretation

The opposite limb, when available, is used for comparison. A difference of two or three centimeters between four comparative circumferences on bilateral upper extremities is evidence of lymphedema.

CONSIDER THIS
LYMPHEDEMA PREVENTION

Individuals at greater risk for lymphedema (e.g., lymph node removal, extensive chest surgeries, radiation therapy, obesity) can significantly limit their risk by following specific guidelines.

1. Avoid injury to the skin to help reduce the risk of infection. This may include treating cuts and abrasions properly, caution with use of razors or nail clippers, applying moisturizer to the skin, and avoiding skin punctures (e.g., blood draws) on the affected limb.
2. Avoid any constriction of the extremity. This may include wearing loose fitting clothing and avoiding having blood pressure measurements performed on the affected limb.
3. Diet and exercise to maintain a healthy weight. Being overweight significantly increases a patient's risk for developing lymphedema.
4. When exercising, carefully observe any changes in the size of the limb to ensure that increased activity is not causing negative side effects. It is also advisable to take frequent rest breaks during periods of intense activity.
5. Avoid extreme hot and cold temperatures as they can lead to fluctuations in limb edema.
6. Wear compression garments during periods of strenuous activity, when standing for prolonged periods of time or when traveling on an airplane.

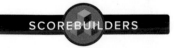

Staging of Lymphedema

Stage	Description
0	This stage is known as the latent (or preclinical) stage. There is no visible edema, though the transport capacity of the lymph system has been affected.
1	This stage is known as the reversible lymphedema stage. Pitting edema is present and increases with activity or heat, but will diminish with elevation and rest.
2	This stage is known as the spontaneously irreversible lymphedema stage. The edema is now non-pitting and does not change with elevation or rest. The skin begins to demonstrate fibrotic changes and the risk for infection increases. Stemmer's sign is positive at this stage.
3	This stage is known as the lymphostatic elephantiasis stage. It is characterized by extensive non-pitting edema, significant fibrotic changes to the skin, and the presence of papillomas, deep skinfolds, and hyperkeratosis. Infection is common at this stage. Stemmer's sign remains positive at this stage.

Classification for lymphedema[27]

Mild: < 3 centimeters difference between the affected and unaffected limbs

Moderate: 3 to 5 centimeters difference between the affected and unaffected limbs

Severe: > 5 centimeters difference between the affected and unaffected limbs

Other tests and measures that may be part of the examination include volumetric measurements, goniometry, manual muscle testing, pain assessment, sensory testing, skin inspection, bioelectrical impedance, and gait and balance assessments.

Treatment

Once a diagnosis has been made, formal intervention is recommended in order to assist patients in managing their symptoms at the lowest possible level. Early, appropriate intervention and ongoing self-care significantly decrease the risk of infection and other negative sequelae associated with poor symptom management. Complete decongestive therapy (CDT) is the standard of care for patients with lymphedema.

Complete Decongestive Therapy

CDT is a treatment model that occurs in two different phases. Phase I is the intensive acute treatment phase and is typically provided in an outpatient setting by a certified lymphedema therapist for 4-6 weeks. Phase II is the self-management phase and consists of long-term management of symptoms utilizing various components of CDT. CDT consists of manual lymphatic drainage, compression therapy, exercise, and skin care.

Manual lymphatic drainage: Manual lymphatic drainage (MLD) involves techniques designed to move lymph around blockages in the lymphatic system and into desired areas where it can be drained. Treatment should first be directed at uninvolved areas to prepare those areas for new lymph flow, then be directed towards the involved areas. It is important for therapists to know the location of lymph nodes since this will affect where they decide to perform manual strokes and in what direction.

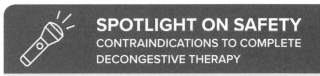

SPOTLIGHT ON SAFETY
CONTRAINDICATIONS TO COMPLETE DECONGESTIVE THERAPY

There are several precautions and relative contraindications to complete decongestive therapy. Failure to recognize the presence of these medical conditions has the potential to significantly compromise patient safety.

- Acute infection
- Cardiac edema
- Diabetes
- Hypertension
- Malignancy
- Renal insufficiency
- Deep vein thrombosis

Compression therapy: Compression therapy helps to maintain the reduction in edema that is achieved with MLD. Compression therapy helps reduce limb size by improving the reabsorption ability of the capillaries and reducing the filtration of fluids into the interstitium. It can also help soften fibrotic tissues that may have formed. In phase I treatment, compression bandages are typically used. Short-stretch bandages are used for treating lymphedema since they have a low resting pressure and therefore do not constrict lymph flow like long-stretch bandages would. In phase II treatment, a combination of compression garments (during the day) and compression bandages (during the night) are used. Compression garments should only be fitted once edema levels have plateaued.

Exercise: Exercise can help improve lymph flow by increasing lymph vessel contractions, increasing fluid uptake in the initial lymph vessels, improving the "muscle pump" to stimulate lymph flow, and increasing deep breathing which improves lymph flow in the thoracic duct. Because some patients can have a negative response to exercise, they must be monitored carefully when initiating an exercise program and their program should be gradually progressed. Low impact, aerobic activities are generally recommended at the onset since they are less likely to exacerbate the patient's lymphedema. Compression bandages/garments should be used when exercising.

Skin care: The skin is more prone to damage since the protein-rich fluid of lymphedema impairs immune system function allowing for bacterial and fungal growth. Infections can lead to worsening of a patient's lymphedema. Prevention is therefore of primary importance. The limb should be inspected and cleansed thoroughly each day and patients should frequently apply moisturizing lotion. Any soaps or moisturizers used should have a low or neutral pH to avoid damage to the skin.

Lymphatic Terminology

Hyperkeratosis: Thickening of the outermost layer of the skin, which is typically observed with stage 3 lymphedema.

Non-pitting edema: Fluid accumulation that is "harder" and not compressible when pressure is applied. This type of edema is observed in the later stages of lymphedema.

Papilloma: A benign wart-like skin growth that is typically observed with stage 3 lymphedema.

Pitting edema: Fluid accumulation that can be compressed and demonstrates an indentation with applied pressure. This type of edema may be observed in the early stages of lymphedema.

Spleen: An organ located in the upper left quadrant of the abdomen that is responsible for the filtration of red blood cells as well as the production of antibodies to help fight infection.

Stemmer's sign: A test used to aid in the diagnosis of lymphedema. Stemmer's sign is positive if the skin at the dorsal base of the second toe/finger can't be easily lifted away from the bone, which indicates thickening of the skin due to fibrotic changes.

Thymus: An organ located posterior to the sternum and anterior to the heart that produces T cells and T lymphocytes to help combat infection.

System Interactions

Oncology[28,29]

Cancer, malignancy, neoplasm, and tumor are all terms referring to abnormal uncontrolled cell growth within the body. There are more than one hundred different cancers of various types and tissue origins currently recognized, including lymphoma and hematologic cancers. Malignant cancer cells are characterized by their ability to grow uncontrollably, invade other tissues, remain undifferentiated, initiate growth at distant sites, and avoid detection and destruction by the body's immune system. The origins of malignant cells vary widely from environmental factors and lifestyle choices to genetic predisposition.

Carcinoma is a malignancy originating from the epithelial cells of organs. Carcinomas in specific organs may be named more specifically depending on the characteristics present. For example, large cell carcinoma, adenocarcinoma, and squamous cell carcinoma are all subsets of lung carcinoma. The American Cancer Society reports that at least 80% of all cancers in the United States are carcinomas.

Risk Factors[28]	
• Increasing age	• Poor diet
• Tobacco use	• Stress
• Alcohol use	• Occupational hazards
• Gender	• Ethnic background
• Virus exposure	• Genetic influence
• Environmental influence	• Sexual/reproductive behavior

General Signs and Symptoms of Cancer

C	–	Change in bowel/bladder routine
A	–	A sore that will not heal
U	–	Unusual bleeding/discharge
T	–	Thickening/lump develops
I	–	Indigestion or difficulty swallowing
O	–	Obvious change in wart/mole
N	–	Nagging cough/hoarseness

Unexplained weight loss, fatigue, anorexia, anemia, pain, and/or weakness are other general symptoms that may indicate cancer.[28]

Cancer Prevention[28]

Primary Prevention	• Elimination of modifiable risk factors • Use of natural agents (i.e., teas, vitamins) to prevent cancer • Cancer vaccine
Secondary Prevention	• Early detection • Selective preventative pharmacological agents (e.g., Tamoxifen) • Multifactorial risk reduction
Tertiary Prevention	• Prevent disability that can occur secondary to cancer and its treatment • Manage symptoms • Limit complications

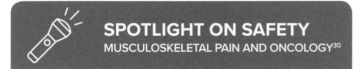

SPOTLIGHT ON SAFETY
MUSCULOSKELETAL PAIN AND ONCOLOGY[30]

Musculoskeletal pain complaints should not be taken lightly in oncology populations. Bony or soft tissue pain complaints can be heralding signs of disease progression or adverse treatment effects.

Bony pain complaints may relate to a primary site of malignancy, such as with osteosarcoma, or new metastasis to a bony area. New back pain complaints of unclear origin, for example, should be evaluated immediately as this pain may be indicative of spinal metastasis which may result in neurological deficits.

Soft tissue complaints may relate to medication side effects or physiological changes in the tissue itself as a result of oncological interventions. Women who have received radiation treatment for breast cancer and develop axillary web syndrome or radiation fibrosis, for example, may experience considerable discomfort along with palpable tissue changes and functional limitations in the affected upper quadrant.

Tissue and Tumor Classification[30]

Tissue Classification	Examples	Tumor Classification
Epithelium Protect, absorb, and excrete	– Skin – Lines internal cavities – Mucous membrane – Lining of bladder	Carcinoma Adenocarcinoma (glandular tissue)
Pigmented Cells	– Moles	Malignant melanoma
Connective Tissues Elastic, collagen, fibrous	– Striated muscle – Blood vessels – Bone – Cartilage – Fat – Smooth muscle	Sarcoma Fibrosarcoma Liposarcoma Chondrosarcoma Osteosarcoma Hemangiosarcoma Leiomyosarcoma Rhabdomyosarcoma
Nerve Tissues Neurons, nerve fibers, dendrites, glial cells	– Brain – Nerves – Spinal cord – Retina	Astrocytoma Glioma Neurilemma sarcoma Neuroblastoma Retinoblastoma
Lymphoid Tissues	– Wherever lymph tissue is present throughout the body – Lymph nodes – Spleen – Can appear in stomach, intestines, skin, CNS, bone, and tonsils	Lymphoma
Hematopoietic Tissues	– Bone marrow – Plasma cells	Leukemia Myelodysplasia Myeloproliferative syndromes Multiple myeloma

Diagnostic Tools[28]

• Family history	• Pap smear
• Physical examination	• Blood tests
• Radiography	• Biopsy
• CT scan	• Mammography
• Bone scan	• Endoscopy
• Stool guaiac	• Isotope scan

Staging[31,32]

The stage of a malignancy is determined by evaluating the extent of the disease, lymph node involvement, and existence of metastasis. Staging data is utilized in the selection of treatment interventions, to assist in goal setting, and in the prediction of outcomes and prognosis for both oncological and physical therapy interventions. Staging data and responses to treatment are also typically reported to a tumor registry. The aggregate data maintained by a tumor registry supplies medical providers with information regarding treatment outcomes that can be compared nationally. Numerous staging systems exist with some used for many cancer types and others being type specific such as for cancers of the blood or lymphatic system.

Oncology Pathology

Brain Cancer[10,32]

Brain cancer may occur as a primary tumor arising from astrocytes, meninges, nerve cells, or tissues within the brain. Metastatic brain cancer occurs when a brain tumor develops as a consequence of cancer in another primary area of the body.

Etiology – Most primary cancers outside of the brain metastasize to the brain during progression of the cancer.

Signs and symptoms – Symptoms are dependent on the location of the tumor and typically progress rapidly. Symptoms include headache, seizures, increased intracranial pressure, cognitive and emotional impairment, and decreased motor and sensory function.

Treatment – Surgical resection along with radiation or other combined therapies are typically indicated.

Breast Cancer[10,32]

Breast cancer is the most common female malignancy, but can also occur in men. The majority of cases are classified as adenocarcinoma and it is the second leading cause of female death from cancer. Common metastases are found in the lymph nodes, lungs, bones, skin, and brain. If the cancer recurs, it is usually within two years of the initial diagnosis.

Etiology – Risk factors include genetics, gender, age, menstrual history, and geography.

The TNM system is one of the most commonly used methods of determining tumor stage. The system describes a malignancy based on the size and extent of the primary tumor (T), lymph node involvement (N), and presence of metastasis (M). For most cancers, the TNM combination will correspond to a stage designation that further defines the severity of the disease. Lower numbered stages are considered to have a better overall prognosis.

National Cancer Institute Staging[31]

Stage	Definition
Stage 0	Early malignancy that is present only in the layer of cells in which it began. For most cancers, this is referred to as carcinoma in situ. Not all cancers have a stage 0.
Stage I	Malignancy limited to the tissue of origin with no lymph node involvement or metastasis.
Stage II	Malignancy spreading into adjacent tissues; lymph nodes may show signs of micrometastases.
Stage III	Malignancy that has spread to adjacent tissue showing signs of fixation to deeper structures. The likelihood of metastatic lymph node involvement is high.
Stage IV	Malignancy that has metastasized beyond the primary site, for example, to bone or another organ.

Adapted from National Cancer Institute, www.cancer.gov

Signs and symptoms – Breast cancer presents as a lump and is usually found by the woman. The mass is typically firm, irregular, and non-painful. The patient may also present with signs including nipple discharge, erythema or a change in breast shape.

Treatment – Treatment may include surgery, radiation, chemotherapy or hormonal manipulation. It is curable if diagnosed prior to metastases; survival rate decreases as the stage of the cancer increases. The current 5-year survival rate for localized tumors is 92%; this drops substantially if there is nodal involvement.

Bronchial Carcinoma[3]

Bronchial carcinoma refers to any epithelial carcinoma occurring in the bronchopulmonary tree. Cancers are broadly divided into two main groups: small cell lung carcinomas and non-small cell lung carcinomas, including squamous cell carcinoma, adenocarcinoma, and large cell carcinoma.

Etiology – Smoking is the primary cause of the majority of lung cancers, but it can occur in people who have never smoked or had prolonged exposure to secondhand smoke. In these cases, the exact etiology may be unknown.

Signs and symptoms – A new cough or changes in a chronic cough, coughing up blood, shortness of breath, wheezing, weight loss, and bone pain. Typically, signs and symptoms are not present until the disease is advanced.

CONSIDER THIS
EXERCISE GUIDELINES FOR PATIENTS UNDERGOING CANCER TREATMENT[30]

The combination of surgical, medical, and radiation oncology interventions can produce a variety of unpleasant symptoms which may significantly impact a patient's quality of life during treatment. Common side effects include pain, fatigue, depression, anxiety, altered body image, sleep disturbances, lymphedema, and gastrointestinal distress. With therapeutic exercise, therapists have the ability to positively impact both symptoms and quality of life. In planning exercise interventions, therapists should consider the following:

- Always check physician orders prior to treating a patient with bone metastases to verify weight bearing status and clearance to perform mobility
- Monitor a patient's blood values daily, especially platelet and hematocrit counts, to ensure that it is safe for the patient to participate in therapy activities
- Exercise should be conducted at a range of 40-65% of the peak heart rate, heart rate reserve, and VO_{2max} or below the anaerobic threshold
- During exercise, perceived exertion should not exceed a 12 using the Borg's Rating of Perceived Exertion Scale
- Treatment visits should be scheduled during the time of day when the patient's energy is at peak levels
- Treatment should be modified as needed to accommodate any side effects of medical treatment

Treatment – Surgery (wedge resection, segmental resection, lobectomy, pneumonectomy), chemotherapy, and radiation therapy.

Cervical Cancer[10,32]

Cervical cancer starts in the cells on the surface of the cervix, typically squamous cells. This precancerous condition is called dysplasia and is easily treatable. Annual cervical screening is recommended; diagnosis is made through a Pap test (smear). Prognosis is good with timely intervention. If dysplasia goes undetected, changes can develop into cervical cancer and metastasize to the bladder, intestines, lungs, and liver.

Etiology – The human papilloma virus (HPV) is the primary cause of cervical cancer; it is slow growing. Risk factors include smoking, maternal use of diethylstilbestrol (DES), African American ethnicity, oral contraceptive use, and certain sexually transmitted diseases.

Signs and symptoms – Asymptomatic during the early stages; however, symptoms can include abnormal bleeding, pelvic and low back pain, impairment with bladder and bowel function.

Treatment – Treatment is dependent on staging of the cancer and may include laser therapy, excision, cryotherapy or hysterectomy with adjunct chemotherapy or radiation.

Colorectal Cancer[10,32]

Colorectal cancer accounts for approximately 15% of cancer deaths annually. Adenocarcinoma and primary lymphoma account for the majority of intestinal cancers.

Etiology – Risk factors include increasing age, history of polyps, ulcerative colitis, Crohn's disease, family history, and a diet high in fat and low in fiber.

Signs and symptoms – Colon cancer does not provide early signs of disease and the most prominent symptom is a continuous change in bowel habits. Bright red blood from the rectum is another prominent sign of colon cancer. The patient may experience symptoms of fatigue, weight loss, anemia, and overt rectal bleeding.

Treatment – Treatment is based on the type and staging of the cancer and may include surgical resection of the tumor and potentially a portion of the bowel, with subsequent radiation therapy and/or chemotherapy; colostomy may be required. Prognosis is good for early diagnosis if the cancer is contained; prognosis is poor if it has metastasized.

Lung Cancer[10,32]

Lung cancer is cancer of the epithelium within the respiratory tract. It is the most frequent cause of death from all cancers. Rapid metastasis can occur through the pulmonary vascular system, adrenal gland, brain, bone, and liver.

Etiology – Risk factors include smoking, environment, geography, occupational hazards, age, and family history.

Signs and symptoms – Early symptoms include cough, sputum, and dyspnea. Progression may include symptoms of adventitious breath sounds, chest pain, and hemoptysis.

Treatment – There is a poor prognosis secondary to expedited metastasis (less than 14% for a five-year survival rate). Surgical intervention along with combination therapies may be required.

Lymphoma (Hodgkin, non-Hodgkin disease)[10,32]

Lymphoma is classified as cancer found in the lymphatic system and lymph tissues; lymphomas are categorized as Hodgkin disease or non-Hodgkin lymphoma.

Etiology – Risk factors for Hodgkin disease include association with Epstein-Barr virus, drug abuse, immunosuppressant use, obesity, chronic or autoimmune diseases. Risk factors for non-Hodgkin lymphoma include exposure to benzene (i.e., cigarette smoke), auto emissions, and pollution.

Signs and symptoms – A painless lump is typically the first sign and general symptoms include fever, chills, and fatigue. Hodgkin disease is distinguished by the presence of Reed-Sternberg cancer cells. Both forms can metastasize.

Treatment – Hodgkin disease is one of the most curable cancers depending on age, disease stage, overall health, and responsiveness to treatment. Treatment options are based on the patient's age and staging classification and include chemotherapy, radiation, stem cell transplant, and highly active antiretroviral therapy. Non-Hodgkin progression varies based on classification, co-morbidities, and treatment response.

Pancreatic Cancer[10,32]

Pancreatic cancer is a prominent type of cancer with an extremely high mortality rate. Cancer of the exocrine cells within the ducts is the most common form of pancreatic cancer. It will metastasize to the liver, lungs, pleura, colon, stomach, and spleen.

Etiology – Risk factors include tobacco use, gender, increasing age, and cholecystectomy.

Signs and symptoms – Symptoms are very vague during the initial stages of the disease which often results in delayed diagnosis. Common symptoms include weight loss, jaundice, and epigastric pain that can radiate to the thoracic region. Advanced cancer may present with severe pain that may indicate the cancer has metastasized.

Treatment – Treatment is usually directed to assist in the relief of symptoms. Pancreatic cancer has a very poor survival rate with a mortality rate of almost 100%. Surgical resection along with chemotherapy and radiation assist to relieve symptoms.

Prostate Cancer[10,32]

Adenocarcinoma is the most common type of prostate cancer. Prostate cancer typically affects men over 50 years old; it is the second highest cause of death from cancer in men. Diagnosis is found through prostate biopsy and prognosis is good with appropriate treatment. There is an approximate 10% fatality from this diagnosis.

Etiology – Risk factors include increased age, high fat diet, genetic predisposition, African American descent, and exposure to cadmium.

Signs and symptoms – Most times this is asymptomatic until the cancer reaches the advanced stages. Symptoms include urinary obstruction, pain, urgency, and decreased stream/flow of urine.

Treatment – Treatment varies and may include surgical incision of the prostate gland, radiation, or hormonal therapy; can metastasize to the bladder, musculoskeletal system, lungs, and lymph nodes.

Skin Cancer[10,32]

Basal Cell Carcinoma

Basal cell carcinoma is a slow growing form of skin cancer that rarely metastasizes. It originates from the epidermis and is the most common form of skin cancer.

Etiology – Sun exposure is a common cause, with risk factors including frequent sun exposure, light eyes, and fair skin.

Signs and symptoms – Open sores that can bleed or crust and remain for three or more weeks, reddish patches of skin, a shiny bump on the skin that is often pink, or a scar-like area that has poorly defined borders

Treatment – Prognosis is good; basal cell carcinoma can routinely be cured. Surgical excision may be required to remove the cancer cells.

Malignant Melanoma

Malignant melanoma originates from melanocytes and can be classified as: superficial spreading, nodular, lentigo maligna or acral lentiginous melanomas. Peak incidence is between 40-60 years of age. Early diagnosis is vital to prognosis, as it can spread and metastasize quickly. Areas of metastases include the brain, lungs, liver, bone, and skin.

Etiology – Risk factors for malignant melanoma include a history of blistering sunburns prior to 20 years of age, family history, immunosuppression, light eyes, fair skin, and a previous history of cancer.

Signs and symptoms – Lesions can be elevated on the surface of the skin and appear keratotic or scaly. Other symptoms when observing the skin or a mole may include asymmetry, irregular borders, varied color, and a diameter of greater than six millimeters.

Treatment – This form of cancer is 100% curable with early diagnosis. Excision may solely be required with early treatment. If melanoma has metastasized, surgical intervention along with combination therapies may be required.

Oncology Treatment Options[28,36,37]

Surgery

Surgery is often used to resect and excise a defined area of malignancy, but may be indicated for prophylactic, diagnostic, curative or palliative goals. Surgical interventions usually require a combination of other treatment modalities secondary to the potential for metastases. These adjunct therapies function to destroy any residual malignant cells. Common side effects include fatigue, pain, deformity, scar tissue formation, and infection.

Radiation

Radiation is administered as either ionizing radiation or particle radiation and can be delivered by teletherapy (external beam), brachytherapy (a sealed and/or implanted source) or system therapy (unsealed source). Radiation destroys the hydrogen bonds between the DNA strands of malignant cells. Radiation may be curative, adjuvant or palliative in its use. It may be used prior to surgical intervention, palliatively to shrink a malignant mass or post-surgically to ensure destruction of residual malignant cells. Radiation is most useful with localized malignancy. Common side effects include headache, bone marrow suppression, skin reactions, neuropathy, visual disturbances, nausea, vomiting, urinary frequency, diarrhea, delayed wound healing, and infection.

Chemotherapy

Chemotherapy consists of a group of drugs that are administered to destroy malignant cells. Chemotherapeutic agents include alkylating agents, antimetabolite agents, steroid hormones, plant

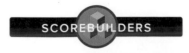

CONSIDER THIS
CHEMOTHERAPY RELATED ALTERED BLOOD COUNTS[38]

Many chemotherapeutic agents include side effects that alter a patient's normal blood count which may result in conditions such as anemia, thrombocytopenia, and neutropenia. These conditions are diagnosed based on the laboratory results from a complete blood count.

Anemia refers to hemoglobin and hematocrit levels below normal gender specific laboratory reference values. In severe cases, a blood transfusion may be necessary. Symptoms may include dyspnea, heart palpitations, and dizziness. Patients who are anemic are advised to change positions slowly, rest frequently during activity, and allow themselves full nights of sleep.

Thrombocytopenia refers to platelet levels below normal reference laboratory values. Patients with thrombocytopenia will bruise very easily. Other symptoms may include petechiae, epistaxis, bleeding gums, and black or bloody stool. Patients with thrombocytopenia are advised to consult a physician before using over the counter medications that may further affect platelets such as aspirin and ibuprofen. Other precautions include avoiding contact sports, working with or around sharp objects, and tight fitting clothing or accessories.

Neutropenia refers to a neutrophil count below normal laboratory reference values placing a patient at risk for developing a serious infection. The severity of neutropenia may be categorized as mild, moderate or severe. An individual's risk of infection is typically a factor of the severity and duration of neutropenia. Patients who are neutropenic do not typically present with observable signs or symptoms. In hospitals, patients with neutropenia are typically assigned a private room with precautions instituted to decrease a patient's risk of exposure to infection from visitors, staff or unhygienic conditions. Patients with neutropenia who are not in medical facilities are advised to maintain excellent hand and body hygiene, closely self monitor for signs and symptoms of infection, wear shoes even in the home, and avoid exposure to potentially infectious environmental factors (e.g., crowds or people with illnesses, litter boxes, bird cages, fish tanks, flowers and plants, stagnant water, manicures/pedicures, jacuzzis/hot tubs).

alkaloid agents, interferons, and antitumor antibiotics. Each class of chemotherapeutic agents has a different mechanism of action to destroy malignant cells. Chemotherapy is most useful with widespread and metastatic malignancies, but is also used to induce remission, cure and/or eradicate residual malignant cells. The drugs may be administered orally, subcutaneously, intramuscularly, intravenously or intracavitary. Common side effects include nausea, vomiting, electrolyte imbalance, sexual dysfunction, hair loss, pain, and a decrease in platelet, red, and white blood cell counts.

Biotherapy (Immunotherapy)

Biotherapy utilizes various agents and/or techniques to change the relationship between the malignancy and its host. Biologic response modifiers are commonly utilized for biotherapy and act to strengthen a patient's biological response to the malignant cells. Common agents or procedures used with this treatment include interferons, interleukin-2, bone marrow transplant, stem cell transplant, monoclonal antibodies, hormonal therapy, and colony-stimulating factors. Common side effects include fever, chills, nausea, vomiting, anorexia, central nervous system impairment, inflammatory reactions, leukopenia, and fatigue.

Antiangiogenic Therapy

Antiangiogenic therapy focuses on the use of thalidomide and its suppression of blood supply formation. It has had initial success in the treatment of multiple myeloma. There is research that supports blocking the process of growth, as opposed to destruction of an already formed mass, as a means of inhibiting growth of primary malignant masses.

SPOTLIGHT ON SAFETY
REHABILITATION CONSIDERATIONS FOR PATIENTS UNDERGOING CHEMOTHERAPY AND RADIATION[30]

- Strenuous activity should be initially avoided following implantation of radioactive seeds utilized for brachytherapy. Communication with the radiation oncologist and/or referring physician is imperative as further activity contraindications or precautions may be advised depending on the individual case.

- Skin tattoos are used to guide beam alignment with external beam radiation. Physical therapist assistants must be cautious and defer interventions which may alter the position of alignment tattoos (e.g., taping interventions, certain soft tissue or myofascial mobilizations).

- Irradiated skin requires special care to protect tissues prone to erythema, rash, and dry desquamation, as well as more painful wet desquamation and superficial burns.

- Massage and heat are contraindicated over irradiated areas for a minimum of 12 months.

- Certain chemotherapy agents may cause the patient to have a level of toxicity that requires staff and visitors to take additional precautions before making physical contact.

- Patient vomiting during therapy should be reported to the nurse/physician, especially if the patient is taking antiemetic medication to control nausea and vomiting.

Palliative Treatment[39,40]

Palliative treatment emphasizes symptom management as opposed to curative efforts. Palliative oncology interventions may include radiation, chemotherapy, physical therapy, chiropractic, acupuncture, alternative and homeopathic medicines, relaxation, biofeedback, pharmacological intervention, and hospice. Palliative treatment may be provided at any time in the disease process with goals of maintaining comfort and dignity through appropriate symptom management. Palliative services can be differentiated into patient support and caregiver support. Patient focused goals may include pain management, emotional and spiritual support, and management of symptoms such as confusion, fatigue, dyspnea, nausea, weakness, and bowel/bladder concerns. Caregiver support may include respite care, education, assistance with transportation, home management, and accessing social services.

Oncology Terminology[16,31,32]

Benign neoplasm: An abnormal cell growth that is usually slow growing and harmless, closely resembling the composition of adjacent tissues.

Cancer: A group of diseases characterized by uncontrolled cell proliferation with mutation and spreading of the abnormal cells. The etiology is based on the type and location of the cancer. The most common causes include cigarette smoking, diet and nutrition, chemical agents, physical agents, environmental causes, viral causes, and genetics.

Differentiated cells: Cells that have matured from a less specific to a more specific cell type.

Dysplasia: An abnormal development of cells or tissue that is often an early sign of neoplasia.

Hyperplasia: An increase in cell number that may be normal or abnormal depending on additional characteristics.

Malignant neoplasm: An abnormal uncontrolled cell growth that invades and destroys adjacent tissues and may metastasize to other sites and systems of the body.

Metaplasia: A change in a cell from one type to another that may be normal or abnormal.

SPOTLIGHT ON SAFETY
MODALITIES AND PALLIATIVE CARE[39]

Numerous electrotherapeutic, thermal, and mechanical modalities are considered to be contraindicated for use with the oncology population. Physical therapist assistants should be aware of the specifics of these contraindications in order to avoid limiting appropriate treatment options. For example, most heat and electrotherapeutic modalities are contraindicated for use over an active malignancy, but are not necessarily contraindicated for use elsewhere on the body. The therapist's ability to interpret information with respect to an individual's disease status, and when appropriate to seek physician guidance, is imperative when treating patients undergoing oncological interventions.

The use of heat and electrical modalities are typically contraindicated for direct use over malignancies due to the potential for facilitating growth of a malignant mass or hematogenous spread. With physician guidance, these contraindications often may be overlooked in lieu of palliative goals for terminally ill patients. This is especially true in hospice environments where curative efforts have been discontinued and end of life is imminent. However, therapists are advised to be mindful of and adhere to contraindications which may cause a terminally ill patient additional discomfort (e.g., the potential for neuromuscular electrical stimulation causing a pathological fracture in a patient with bone metastasis).

Tumor (neoplasm): An abnormal new growth of tissue that increases the overall tissue mass. Tumors are benign (non-cancerous) or malignant (cancerous) as well as primary or secondary. Primary tumors form from cells that belong to the area of the tumor. Secondary tumors grow from cells that have metastasized (spread) from another affected area within the body. Tumor classification is defined by cell type, tissue of origin, amount of differentiation, benign versus malignant, and anatomic site.

Undifferentiated cells: Cells which have not differentiated into a specific type (e.g., primitive, embryonic) or have no special structure or function.

CONSIDER THIS
"CHEMO BRAIN": COGNITIVE CHANGES ASSOCIATED WITH CANCER TREATMENT[42]

Many patients and medical professionals recognize that treatment related cognitive changes in the oncology population are common occurrences. Referred to as "chemo brain" or "chemo fog," these colloquial names are misleading as research has not definitively connected impaired cognition with chemotherapy interventions. A number of factors make defining "chemo brain" difficult. For example, many patients still perform well on formal cognitive assessments, and most do not undergo baseline cognitive testing prior to beginning cancer treatment. Likewise, it is difficult for researchers to truly delineate if cognitive changes are due to the disease process itself, the treatment interventions or side effects of treatment (e.g., depression, fatigue, hormonal changes, altered blood counts, stress). Common "chemo brain" complaints may include feelings of "foggy cognition," confusion, fatigue, limited attention span or short-term memory, and an unusual degree of difficulty with concentration, word finding, multi-tasking, and organization.[28]

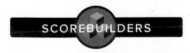

Psychological Disorders[10,32,43]

Affective Disorders

Affective disorders are classified by disturbances in mood or emotion. States of extreme happiness or sadness occur and mood can alternate without cause. These extreme emotions can become intense and unrealistic.

Bipolar

- Alternating periods of depression and mania
- Females are at greater risk; typically begins in a patient's twenties

Depression

- Slower mental and physical activity; poor self-esteem
- Immobilized from everyday activities; sadness, hopelessness, and helplessness
- Desire to withdraw; delusions in severe cases

Mania

- Constantly active
- Impulses immediately expressed
- Unrealistic activity
- Elation and self-confidence
- Disagreement with a patient may produce patient aggression
- Disorganized thoughts and speech
- Very few patients are diagnosed with only a manic disorder

Neuroses Disorders

Neuroses refer to a group of disorders that are characterized by individuals exhibiting fear and maladaptive strategies in dealing with stressful or everyday stimuli. Patients with neuroses are not dealing with psychosis, do not have delusions, and usually realize that they have a problem.

Anxiety Disorder

- Constant high tension; overreacts in certain instances
- Presents with apprehension and chronic worry
- Acute anxiety attacks
  - Lasts a few minutes in duration
  - Excitation of the sympathetic autonomic nervous system
  - Fear of impending doom or death
  - Shortness of breath, heart palpitations, dizziness, nausea
  - Initiated by unconscious and internal mechanisms

Obsessive-compulsive Disorder

- Obsessions – persistent thoughts that will not leave
- Compulsions – repetitive ritual behaviors the patient cannot stop performing
- Thoughts or ritual behaviors that interfere with daily living
- Unable to control irrational behavior
- Most commonly begins in young adulthood

Phobia Disorder

- Excessive fear of objects, occurrences or situations that is considerably out of proportion/irrational
- Fear creates difficulty in everyday life
- Subclassifications include agoraphobia, social phobia, and simple phobia; simple phobia is easiest to treat
- May develop from traumatic experiences, observation, classical conditioning

Personality Disorders

A personality disorder is classified by observing a patient's pattern of behavior, dysfunctional view of society, and level of sadness. Personality disorders are usually ongoing patterns of dysfunctional behavior.

Antisocial Behavior

- Results from particular causes (e.g., need for attention or involvement in a gang)
- Typically has some concern for others
- Blames other institutions (e.g., family, school) for their actions
- Symptoms are typically seen before 16 years of age
- Violates the rights of others; lacks responsibility and emotional stability

Borderline Behavior

- Instability in all aspects of life
- Can identify self from others
- Uses projection, denial, defensiveness; unpredictable mood or behavior
- Intense and uncontrolled anger; chronic feelings of emptiness

Narcissistic Behavior

- Incapable of loving others
- Self-absorbed; obsessed with success and power
- Unrealistic perception of self-importance

Psychopathic Personality

- Low morality, poor sense of responsibility, no respect for others
- Impulsive behavior for immediate gratification; high frustration
- Little guilt or remorse for all actions; inability to alter behavior, even with punishment
- Expert liar

Schizophrenia Disorders

Schizophrenia disorders are psychotic in nature and present with disorganization of thought, hallucinations, emotional dysfunction, anxiety, and perceptual impairments. Causative factors include traumatic events, genetic inheritance, biochemical imbalances, and environmental influence.

Catatonic Schizophrenia

- Motor disturbances with rigid posturing
- Episodes consist of uncontrolled movements, however, patients remain aware during episodes
- Medications are required to regulate episodes

Disorganized Schizophrenia

- Usually progressive and irreversible with inappropriate emotional responses; mumbled talking

Paranoid Schizophrenia

- Delusions of grandeur; delusions of persecution
- May believe they possess special powers

Somatoform Disorders

Somatoform disorders are classified based on the physical symptoms present in each disorder.

Conversion Disorder

- Physical complaints of neurological basis with no underlying cause
- Paralysis is the most common finding; other findings include deafness, blindness, paresthesia
- Freud believed this is mental anxiety transformed into physical symptoms
- Diagnosis can be made once testing is negative for physical ailments

Hypochondriasis Disorder

- Excessive fear of illness
- Believes that minor illnesses or medical problems indicate a serious or life threatening disease

Somatization Disorder

- Primarily in women, has familial association, and often chronic and long lasting
- Complaints of symptoms with no physiological basis
- Symptoms usually lead to medications and medical visits and alter the patient's life
- Resembles hypochondriasis disorder

Pharmacology - Psychiatric Management[19,43]

Antianxiety Agents

Action: Antianxiety agents collectively target the CNS through facilitating the effects of GABA or targeting dopamine and serotonin within the brain. Benzodiazepines, azapirones, and certain selective serotonin reuptake inhibitor (SSRI) antidepressants treat various anxiety disorders.

Indications: general anxiety disorder, social anxiety, panic disorder, obsessive-compulsive disorder, post-traumatic stress syndrome

Side effects: drowsiness, sedation, withdrawal symptoms including rebound anxiety

Implications for PT: Similar concerns as with sedative-hypnotic agents; therapists can also implement alternate methods to decrease stress and anxiety including exercise and physical activity, massage, relaxation techniques, and stress management education.

Examples: Xanax, Valium

Antidepressant Agents (Tricyclic, SSRI, MAOI, Other)

Action: Antidepressant agents are classified as tricyclic, monoamine oxidase inhibitors (MAOI), and selective serotonin reuptake inhibitors (SSRI), as well as miscellaneous agents that attempt to increase aminergic transmission and normalize neurotransmission activity.

Indications: depression, certain agents also treat anxiety disorders

Side effects: vary by class of drugs and by specific agent; sedation, blurred vision, tachycardia, dry mouth, insomnia, weight gain, sexual dysfunction

Implications for PT: Therapists should typically see improvement in a patient's affect with pharmacological treatment for depression. Therapists must be aware of side effects such as sedation, fatigue, hypertension or orthostatic hypotension. Therapists must also look for any signs of further depression or suicidal tendencies.

Examples: Elavil, Wellbutrin

Antipsychotic Agents (Neuroleptic Agents)

Action: Most antipsychotic agents block dopamine receptors and reduce the overactivity of dopamine typically transmitted in areas such as the limbic system. The agents will bind to the dopamine receptors, but will not allow for activation. There are traditional and newer "atypical" antipsychotic agents used for schizophrenia and other various psychosis disorders.

Indications: schizophrenia, various psychotic disorders, Alzheimer's disease (certain cases)

Side effects: traditional agents produce increased extrapyramidal (motor) side effects, tardive dyskinesia, pseudoparkinsonism, akathisia, sedation, constipation, dry mouth; atypical agents can produce substantial weight gain, diabetes mellitus, hyperlipidemia

Implications for PT: These agents assist patients to participate in physical therapy by decreasing their symptoms of psychoses and allowing for an increased attention span, diminished agitation and restlessness, improved sense of reality, and an overall normalization of their behavior and affect. The largest barrier is the influence of extrapyramidal effects on therapy. Early detection of these effects can allow for prompt medical and pharmacological management.

Examples: Haldol, Thorazine

Bipolar Disorder Agents

Action: Bipolar disorder agents focus on the prevention of manic episodes in order to avoid the extreme mood swings that follow. The primary agent used in this treatment is lithium. Certain antiseizure and antipsychotic medications may assist as mood stabilizers with bipolar disorder.

Indications: bipolar or manic-depressive disorders

Side effects: in general, gastrointestinal distress, tardive dyskinesia, fatigue, confusion, ataxia, nystagmus, lethargy, tremor, Parkinsonism, seizures, diabetes insipidus, toxicity, coma, risk of death

Implications for PT: Therapists should become familiar with the side effects of medications that treat bipolar disorder, especially symptoms of toxicity as it relates to lithium. Long-term use of lithium may result in osteoporosis which will impact the physical therapy plan of care.

Examples: Lithobid, Tegretol

Sedative-hypnotic Agents (Benzodiazepine and Non-benzodiazepine)

Action: Sedative agents produce a calming and relaxation while hypnotic agents induce sleep. Benzodiazepines have properties to promote sleep through increasing inhibitory effects at the CNS synapses where GABA (gamma-aminobutyric acid) is found. Non-benzodiazepines include barbiturates and other drugs that also provide CNS depression through the inhibitory effects of GABA.

Indications: anxiety, preoperative sedation, insomnia

Side effects: residual effects can produce drowsiness and decreased motor performance, anterograde amnesia, tolerance, dependency, rebound insomnia with withdrawal; barbiturates are highly addictive and can be fatal

Implications for PT: Therapists may find it beneficial to treat a patient when peak blood levels of the agent exist so that the patient is calm, relaxed, and can focus on the treatment regimen, however, this may become problematic if the patient experiences side effects of drowsiness and impairments in motor control. The risk of falling increases with use of these agents.

Examples: Halcion, Luminal

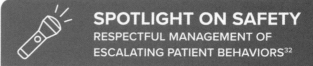

SPOTLIGHT ON SAFETY
RESPECTFUL MANAGEMENT OF ESCALATING PATIENT BEHAVIORS[32]

Patients with or without a psychiatric diagnosis may exhibit escalating behaviors from time to time. The financial, social, physical, and mental stress that accompanies injury or illness can be frustrating enough to cause even mild mannered patients to become agitated or combative. When dealing with patients in these challenging situations, therapists should be respectful in their de-escalation attempts, but also mindful of maintaining a safe environment for everyone involved.

Many health care facilities offer training in non-verbal de-escalation techniques which are helpful in defusing a potentially threatening situation. Guiding principles for safe use of these techniques include an understanding that attempting to reason with an escalating patient may make matters worse, and that calm reasoning in a threatening situation is counterintuitive to our own "fight or flight" response. Successful non-verbal de-escalation requires the provider to maintain self-control and a protective yet non-threatening physical presence while facilitating the de-escalation conversation.

Tips for interacting with an escalating patient:

- Be empathetic when setting boundaries
- Use a low, calm tone of voice when speaking
- Do not respond defensively to patient comments
- Offer choices, options or small concessions if appropriate
- Do not force constant eye contact, allow the patient to look away
- Be respectful and acknowledge the patient's complaints or frustration
- When speaking, wait for the patient to pause rather than raising your voice to be heard
- Be aware of your supportive resources, including the option to leave the area if necessary
- Avoid physical contact
- Do not turn your back to an agitated or escalating patient
- Do not allow an agitated or escalating patient to block your exit route
- Maintain more space than usual between yourself and the patient for safety
- Stand at an angle facing the patient so that it is easier to sidestep if necessary
- Always stay at the same eye level as the patient (e.g., both standing, both sitting)
- Keep hands out of your pockets both for self-protection and to avoid the appearance of concealment

Geriatrics

Gerontology is defined as the study of aging in older adults. By the year 2030 it is expected that 20% of the United States' population will be greater than 65 years of age. Adults 85 years of age or older are also expected to see a dramatic increase in their demographic representation due to improvements in health care and the aging of the baby-boomer generation. Knowing how to provide skilled care to an aging adult requires specific knowledge of the biological, psychological, and social influences affecting the patient.

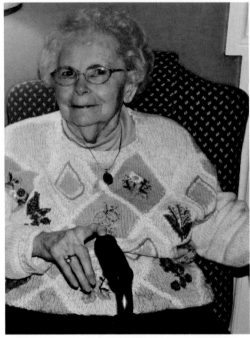

Fig. 7-8: An older adult at rest.

The Body Systems[10,53,54]

Individuals reach their greatest physical health in their 20s and early 30s. Afterwards, age-related changes begin to occur that result in a decrease in physical and cognitive functioning. Aging affects all physiologic processes within the body. The rate of age-related changes is relatively constant, though the patient is typically more symptomatic later in life. Many of the physiologic changes that occur with aging also occur with a decrease in activity, therefore exercise may help to attenuate some of these changes.

Musculoskeletal System

Age-related changes that occur within the musculoskeletal system lead to an overall decrease in a patient's physical functioning. Muscles atrophy and decrease in their ability to regenerate (i.e., sarcopenia), both of which result in a loss of strength. Additionally, the number of motor units decreases so that each motor neuron must innervate a larger number of muscle fibers, resulting in motor unit hypertrophy. An increase in fat mass occurs as an older adult's lean body mass decreases. This infiltration of fat is a predictor of mobility restriction.

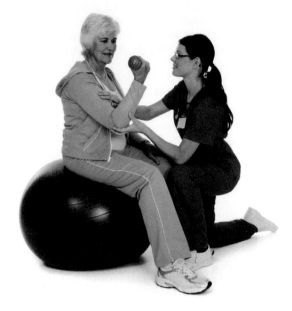

Fig. 7-9: An older adult exercising with assistance from a therapist.

Older adults also begin to experience a decrease in bone mass in their 40s or 50s, a change that occurs due to an increase in bone resorption without an equivalent increase in bone deposition. Due to the decrease in bone density, older adults are at a higher risk for fractures secondary to falls, especially when combined with sarcopenia. With increasing age, there are also changes noted in the patient's joints and connective tissues. Articular cartilage loses much of its water content and begins to degenerate leading to arthritis, especially in weight bearing joints. Connective tissues such as fascia, ligaments, and tendons lose their extensibility, which results in an overall decrease in the patient's range of motion and flexibility. Many of the changes that occur in the musculoskeletal system with aging can be mitigated with exercise.

Age-Related Changes Impacting the Musculoskeletal System

- Type IIb fibers are denervated and remaining motor units hypertrophy
- Decreased muscle mass (sarcopenia)
- Decreased velocity of muscular contraction
- Increased muscular fat infiltration
- Decreased skeletal bone mass after the fourth decade
- Women have lower bone mass compared to men
- Decreased articular cartilage thickness
- Increased collagen stiffness due to cross linkage between fibers

CONSIDER THIS
AGEISM[51]

Ageism is a form of discrimination based on stereotypes regarding age. While this can be directed at any specific age group, older adults often encounter prejudice because of myths and stereotypes perpetuated by cultural beliefs, personal beliefs, and media representations. Ageism can impact the ability of a caretaker or health professional to provide unbiased care, where treatment is instead based on preconceived notions. Examples include when a therapist refers to an older adult as "honey" or "sweetie," thereby infantilizing the older adult despite good intentions. Another example of ageism is when an older adult presents to physical therapy with a family member, and the therapist directs questions to the family member rather than the patient. This minimizes the patient's role in the rehabilitation program, potentially reducing their motivation. Finally, ageism can present itself as the routine delivery of care for all patients over a specific age, instead of applying sound principles of clinical decision making. Recognizing inherent beliefs and prejudices allow practitioners to provide objective, unbiased care, and meet the needs of the patient.

Neuromuscular and Nervous Systems

Changes with age occur in both the central and peripheral nervous systems. Changes in the central nervous system include an overall decrease in brain size due to atrophy of brain tissue and a decrease in nerve conduction velocity that results in an overall decrease in central processing. These changes can result in alterations with the patient's movement as well as their cognition. In the peripheral nervous system, there is also a decrease in processing time that affects nociceptors and other peripheral receptors. As a result, older adults have decreased ability to sense pain, decreased joint proprioception and coordination, decreased somatosensory input, impaired balance reactions and reflexes, and increased gait instability. Balance is also negatively affected by changes that occur within the vestibular system, primarily due to a loss of vestibular receptor cells. Combined with the musculoskeletal changes normally experienced with age, this leaves an older adult at greater risk for falls.

Age-Related Changes Impacting the Neuromuscular and Nervous Systems

- Decreased brain volume with an increased ventricular size
- Decreased peripheral nerve conduction velocity
- Decreased reaction speed

Cardiovascular and Pulmonary Systems

With increasing age, cardiac output decreases making older adults less tolerant to exercise secondary to decreased perfusion of the peripheral tissues. Several factors lead to this decrease in cardiac output, including decreased venous return, arteriosclerosis which increases afterload (especially in the aorta), fibrotic changes within the myocardium that make it less compliant, and a decreased response to cardiac hormones. However, if stroke volume can be maintained or increased as a result of exercise, overall cardiac output can be sustained despite the diminished maximum heart rate. Other changes in the cardiovascular system that occur with aging include increased blood pressure, an increased risk for postural hypotension, decreased resting heart rate, and an increased risk for cardiac

dysrhythmias. Due to these cardiovascular changes, older adults are at greater risk for stroke, coronary artery disease, and congestive heart failure. Greater than 50% of all older adults have some form of heart disease.

Age-Related Changes Impacting the Cardiovascular and Pulmonary Systems

- Increased cardiac afterload
- Increased calcification and fibrosis of heart valves
- Increased vascular tone leading to increased systolic blood pressure
- Decreased arterial elasticity and compliance
- Increased physiological "dead space"
- Decreased inspiratory muscle strength
- Decreased FEV_1
- Increased residual volume following maximal expiration

There are several changes within the pulmonary system that occur with aging that result in a decrease in overall gas exchange. The chest wall becomes stiffer and less compliant and the elasticity and recoil of the lungs also decreases. In combination with an increased thoracic kyphosis and weakened inspiratory muscles, these changes result in a diminished musculoskeletal pump. The result is a decrease in the vital capacity of the lungs. As vital capacity decreases, residual volume increases (since total lung capacity stays roughly the same). Other changes that occur in the pulmonary system include decreased number and size of alveoli, decreased expiratory flow rates, decreased ciliary function in the upper airways (which increases the risk for infections like pneumonia), and decreased strength and effectiveness of coughing.

Integumentary System

The integumentary system experiences several changes associated with aging. A decrease in thickness of the dermal layer as well as a loss of elastin fibers causes the skin to wrinkle and sag and makes it more prone to damage (e.g., bruising, cuts). Pressure ulcers are more common in this population, especially since vascular changes further delay wound healing. A reduction in blood vessels within the dermis makes the skin appear paler and also impairs thermoregulation. These changes make older adults more prone to hypothermia and hyperthermia. A decrease in the number and structure of sweat glands decreases perspiration and further impairs thermoregulation.

Age-Related Changes Impacting the Integumentary System

- Decreased autonomic regulation of thermoregulatory responses
- Decreased vascularity, thickness, and elasticity of the dermis
- Decreased sensory perception

Metabolic and Endocrine Systems

There are a variety of changes that occur within the metabolic and endocrine systems as a person ages. In general, basal metabolism decreases with age, which may be a result of the decrease in lean body mass. In the endocrine system, there is a general decrease in hormone production and function. Older adults tend to exhibit higher blood glucose levels secondary to a reduction in the number and function of beta cells within the pancreas as well as an increase in peripheral resistance to insulin. Loss of bone mass occurs secondary to an increase in bone resorption and has also been linked to hormonal changes, especially in older adult women.

Age-Related Changes Impacting the Metabolic and Endocrine Systems

- Decreased insulin sensitivity
- Decreased hepatic insulin release control
- Decreased sensitivity to beta-adrenergic stimulation

Gastrointestinal System

Physiologic changes with aging occur along the entire length of the gastrointestinal tract. Decreased taste and smell sensations may affect the patient's desire to eat. Decreased salivation leads to dry mouth, which may further affect a patient's appetite. This can result in malnutrition and dehydration, which will adversely affect all of the body's systems. Loss of motility (i.e., peristalsis) begins in the esophagus and continues throughout the digestive tract. In the esophagus, this can lead to dysphagia and gastroesophageal reflux disease. Intestinal motility issues are common (especially in the large intestine) and lead to an increased incidence of constipation and diverticulosis. Aging is also associated with a loss of control of the anal sphincters (i.e., internal, external), which increases the risk for fecal incontinence.

Age-Related Changes Impacting the Gastrointestinal System

- Decreased drug metabolism
- Increased risk of adverse side effects from medications
- Decreased gastric acid production
- Decreased bowel mobility

Genitourinary System

With increasing age, the kidneys become less effective at removing wastes from the blood. This occurs secondary to anatomic and physiologic changes such as decreased blood flow to the kidneys, fewer nephrons and glomeruli, and an overall decrease in the size of the kidney. Another change that occurs with aging is decreasing capacity of the bladder which increases the likelihood of urinary frequency and nocturia. Sensation associated with the need to urinate is often delayed or nonexistent in older adults, which results in an increased incidence of incontinence. Certain medical conditions such as Alzheimer's disease and Parkinson's disease result in detrusor muscle instability, which leads to an overactive bladder and urge incontinence. Conversely, some older adults require assistance to ambulate to the bathroom and may be unable to reach the bathroom before voiding (i.e., functional incontinence).

Age-Related Changes Impacting the Genitourinary System

- Increased incontinence
- Decreased kidney function and filtration rate
- Decreased bladder capacity

The Five Senses[53,54]

Hearing

The progressive loss of hearing experienced in older adults is called presbycusis. Older adults tend to have difficulty differentiating between sounds. For example, they often have trouble following a conversation when they are in a crowded room. When working with patients with hearing loss, the therapist should reduce background noise, speak loudly and slowly, and pronounce their words carefully. The therapist should attempt to communicate in a lower frequency range since older adults can distinguish lower frequencies better than higher frequencies.

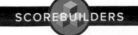

Vision

As an individual ages, the degree of visual impairment will increase. There are several specific changes that occur in the visual system with increased age. Visual acuity, the visual field, and peripheral vision all decrease. The pupils become smaller and are less responsive to changes in light, making it more difficult to see in the dark. Older adults have an increase in the amount of time it takes to accommodate to a brighter or darker environment. Common eye diseases that occur with aging include cataracts, glaucoma, macular degeneration, and diabetic retinopathy.

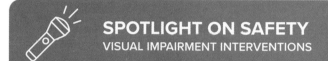

SPOTLIGHT ON SAFETY
VISUAL IMPAIRMENT INTERVENTIONS

Visual impairments can be mitigated through environmental and behavioral modifications that can reduce the risk of injury associated with visual decline.

- Use contrasting colors to highlight the edge of steps, thresholds, and transition areas.
- Remove throw rugs that are not secured at the edges to the floor.
- Use diffuse lighting instead of direct lighting throughout the home.
- Use night lights for maintaining low level illumination during the night.
- Allow for extra time when transitioning from a bright atmosphere to a dark atmosphere, and vice-versa, to accommodate to the change.
- Maintain clear hallways and rooms, including removing any wires across the walkway.
- Have handrails, preferably two, for stairwells both in and outside of the home.

Taste and Smell

The senses of taste and smell both interact to play a role in the enjoyment of food. With increasing age, the number and size of taste buds decrease resulting in a decreased sensitivity to all five tastes (e.g., sour, sweet). Additionally, less saliva is produced and causes a dry mouth, which can also decrease taste sensitivity. A decrease in the ability to detect odors also occurs with increased age. The combination of decreased taste and smell result in a diminished desire for older adults to eat, which can affect their nutritional health.

Touch

Older adults have decreased sensitivity to a variety of sensations including touch, pain, vibration, pressure, proprioception, and temperature. Changes in sensation make older adults more prone to injury (e.g., burns, pressure ulcers). A decrease in somatosensation contributes to balance impairments. These impairments can be exacerbated due to the influence of age-related visual impairments.

Cognition[51,53]

Memory

Memory loss is the most common cognitive impairment that is associated with aging. Memory is made up of numerous constructs, and only some of the facets of memory are affected by aging. Short-term memory is affected, and as a result older adults may have difficulty recalling information they have just learned. Working memory also declines in older age. This is the memory type where individuals use relevant information while in the middle of an activity (e.g., remembering items on a shopping list while shopping). Episodic memory (i.e., personally experienced events) tends to be affected to a greater degree than semantic memory (i.e., knowledge of facts) or procedural memory (i.e., performance of skills).

Attention

Older adults demonstrate significant loss of divided attention, which is the ability to process two or more sources of information at the same time. This is known as dual-tasking and a deficit in this ability can be associated with a greater risk for falls in older adults. They also show a decreased ability to switch their attention between two different tasks. However, other forms of attention do not show a decline with age, such as sustained attention (i.e., maintaining attention over a long period of time on a single task) and selective attention (i.e., the ability to disregard sources of information that are irrelevant to the task).

Intelligence

With increasing age, intelligence declines though this construct is difficult to study due to generational differences. General intelligence begins to decline sometime between the 50s and 70s. Crystalized intelligence, which is the accumulation of knowledge and skills, has the tendency to be maintained, or even improve, as an individual ages. However, fluid intelligence, which is the speed and ability to reason and problem solve, begins to decline.

Mild Cognitive Impairment

Mild cognitive impairment (MCI) is defined as having lower than expected cognitive performance when compared to others in the age group. It generally does not interfere with activities of daily living. Having MCI does not infer that an individual will progress towards developing dementia.

Dementia

Dementia is a process of cognitive decline that eventually influences the individual's ability to participate in daily activities. Difficulty comprehending language, impaired problem solving, behavioral disturbances, and memory deficits are all commonly associated with dementia. Alzheimer's disease, a progressive form of dementia, is found largely in older adults. The incidence of dementia is shown to increase with age.

Delirium

Delirium is different from dementia in that it is a transient state of fluctuating cognitive abilities. Memory, orientation, and arousal may all be affected. The condition is commonly experienced after a hospitalization, post-surgically, during the course of an untreated medical condition or as a side effect of certain medications. While the symptoms of delirium can mimic other conditions (e.g., dementia), it is important to consider that the patient's cognitive status may change from day to day. Risk factors for developing delirium include age greater than 70, having a diminished cognitive status, depression, and alcohol abuse.

Medication Safety[10,19,51]

Pharmacology Considerations in Geriatrics

Older adults process medication differently than younger adults, therefore an awareness of the pharmacokinetic and pharmacodynamic changes is necessary. This section discusses the differences experienced with aging and how they can impact patient care.

Pharmacokinetics

Pharmacokinetics is the study of what happens to the drug once it is in the human body. There are four major parameters that are influenced by pharmacokinetics: absorption, distribution, metabolism, and excretion. As an individual ages, the ability to process a drug changes and it can greatly influence the effect of the medication. Absorption refers to the movement of a drug into the bloodstream. Decreased acidity in the stomach, along with slower emptying times and decreased motility can alter the absorption of the drug.

Distribution of the medication refers to the transport of the drug to various tissues. Certain drugs are lipophilic or hydrophilic, and as such the distribution will be influenced based on the older adult's body composition. Considering older adults demonstrate a decrease in total body water, an increase in adipose tissue, and a decrease in muscle mass, certain drugs will be influenced greater by their distribution characteristics than others.

Metabolism is a component of drug clearance and it occurs primarily in the liver. Since metabolism of a drug is dependent on the mass of the liver, enzyme levels, and blood flow, any changes to the hepatic system can influence the body's ability to break down the drug.

The final component of pharmacokinetics is excretion. Excretion is primarily performed by the renal system. In the older adult, the kidneys have diminished ability to excrete drugs from the body due to decreases in kidney size, renal blood flow, and glomerular filtration rate. These changes result in medications acting for a longer period of time in the body (i.e., increased half-life), which can result in drug toxicity if dosages are not adjusted accordingly.

Pharmacodynamics

Pharmacodynamics refers to the study of how a drug exerts its therapeutic effects on the body at the cellular or organ level. Pharmacodynamics is influenced primarily by the age-related pharmacokinetic alterations to the body, but also by a decrease of neurotransmitters and receptors. When treating an older adult, a therapist must consider that the same dosage amount and time schedule will likely produce different effects based on variables such as age and body composition.

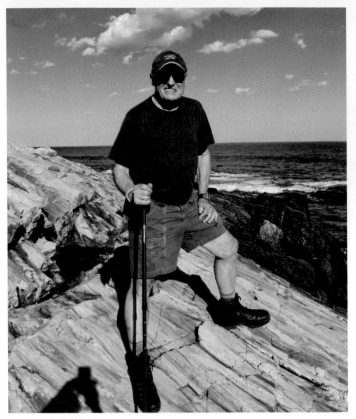

Fig. 7-10: An active older adult on a hike.

Polypharmacy

Polypharmacy can be defined as taking multiple medications. There are two primary forms of polypharmacy: rational and irrational. Rational polypharmacy is when an individual takes multiple medications to treat multiple medical issues, or to treat a single medical issue where each drug works together to control symptoms. Irrational polypharmacy occurs when excessive, duplicate or contraindicated medications are prescribed to treat a medical condition.

End-of-Life Care Terminology

Advance directives: Documents that are completed by a patient prior to the onset of an illness that dictate how the patient wants their end-of-life care to be carried out. Advance directives are important since illness may take away a patient's ability to communicate their wishes concerning their own health care as they get older. A durable power of attorney and a living will are two types of advance directives.

Do not resuscitate: A medical order written by a doctor that documents a patient's wishes to not be resuscitated with cardiopulmonary resuscitation (CPR) if they stop breathing or their heart stops beating. This order only applies to CPR; it does not apply to the administration of medication or other health care treatments.

Durable power of attorney: A legal document in which a patient authorizes another person to make their health care decisions when the patient can no longer make their own decisions.

Hospice: A form of palliative care for terminally ill patients who have a limited life expectancy that focuses on the management of their pain and other symptoms as well as the acceptance of their own death. The goal of hospice care is to allow the patient to remain in their home as they near death, though there are inpatient facilities that provide these services as well.

Living will: A legal document in which a patient dictates their preferences for health care treatment, which becomes especially important if the patient becomes terminally ill and can no longer express their wishes.

Palliative care: An approach to a patient's care (typically patients with serious illnesses) that aims to relieve their pain and suffering, as well as address any psychological, social, and spiritual problems, with the goal of improving the patient's quality of life.

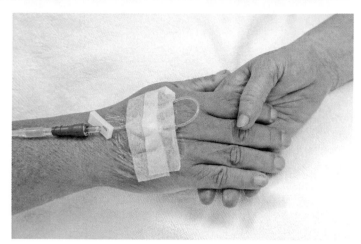

Fig. 7-11: A therapist holding the hand of an older adult.

Bariatrics[44-46]

Obesity refers to the state of excessive adipose tissue accumulation in the body contributing to a variety of chronic conditions that negatively impact multiple body systems and overall health. Obesity is most commonly the result of a prolonged imbalance between an individual's energy intake through diet and energy expenditure through activity and metabolic functions. The prevalence of obesity has reached pandemic proportions and has in recent years become viewed as a chronic progressive disease. Obesity is a modifiable morbidity and mortality risk factor second only to smoking.

Risk Factors for Developing Obesity[44-46]

• Sedentary lifestyle	• Medications that increase appetite or food cravings
• High glycemic diet	• Genetic or familial predisposition
• Environmental and lifestyle factors: smoking cessation, stress, history of abuse	• Underlying illness (e.g., hypothyroidism, polycystic ovary syndrome, Cushing's syndrome, Prader-Willi syndrome)

Anatomic and Physiologic Changes Commonly Associated with Obesity[45]

Cardiac	Cardiomyopathy (e.g., heart failure), abnormal ventricular remodeling (e.g., hypertrophy), atrial fibrillation, dysrhythmias
Pulmonary	Asthma, obstructive sleep apnea, hypoventilation syndrome
Kidneys	Decreased renal perfusion
Genitourinary	Urinary incontinence, infertility
Integumentary	Infection, hyperkeratosis, acanthosis nigricans
Vascular	Increased total blood volume, altered stroke volume and cardiac output, hypertension, venous insufficiency, varicosities
Musculoskeletal	Osteoarthritis, altered mobility patterns
Adipose tissue	Increased production of adipokines (e.g., leptin, interleukin-6, angiotensinogen)
Liver	Non-alcoholic fatty liver disease, non-alcoholic steatohepatitis
Pancreas	Insulin resistance, type 2 diabetes mellitus

CONSIDER THIS
CHILDHOOD OBESITY

The behaviors and systemic changes associated with childhood obesity can set children and adolescents on an unfortunate path toward lifelong health problems. The rise of childhood obesity has had a significant impact on the development of co-morbidities and risk factors previously associated only with adults (e.g., hypertension, type 2 diabetes mellitus, sleep disorders, metabolic syndrome). Adding to the physical health concerns of the condition, children and adolescents that are obese have also been shown to be at increased risk for a number of social and emotional issues including bullying, low self-esteem, depression, and behavioral problems.[47,48]

Because of the rapid developmental changes and variations in body type associated with this younger population, health care providers and caregivers must be cautious not to assume that all children who appear to be carrying extra weight are truly overweight or obese. At various points in normal development children and adolescents are expected to carry differing proportions of body fat. For parents, a conversation with their child's pediatrician is usually the best way to determine if the appearance of extra weight is truly a long term health concern. In general, a child is considered overweight if their age-appropriate BMI is between the 85th and 94th percentiles. Childhood obesity is characterized by an age-appropriate BMI greater than or equal to the 95th percentile.[49,50]

Behavioral risk factors for developing childhood obesity are similar to those in adult populations. Increased dietary intake, decreased activity levels, and psychological factors such as stress and boredom are most frequently attributed to childhood obesity. Some children may be more susceptible to weight gain due to genetic factors, however, genetic predisposition is often erroneously blamed for childhood obesity. Prader-Willi syndrome is an example of a condition where children are more likely to become obese. However, given the prevalence of childhood obesity, the greater influence of diet, activity, behavioral habits, and environmental factors must be both clearly acknowledged and addressed.[49,50]

Bariatric Interventions[45,46]

Medical Management: Due to the multi-system health risks associated with obesity, physician involvement is imperative for support on many levels. With physician monitoring, patients are more likely to have appropriate medical management of co-morbidities as well as access to education or program referrals which may assist in weight loss goals. For patients who do not elect to attempt weight loss, the physician role typically becomes more focused on the medical management of co-morbidities. Most bariatric surgical teams include a physician specialist, often an internist, responsible for the medical assessment and monitoring of patients throughout the weight loss process.

Behavioral Therapy: Typically there is some degree of psychological influence associated with the behaviors that lead to obesity. Identifying and addressing these influences can significantly improve long-term outcomes that could otherwise be limited by underlying issues of motivation and compliance. Behavioral therapy may be provided in individualized or support group formats with topics including stimulus control, goal setting and problem solving strategies, social support, and/or strategies to improve self-monitoring of dietary intake and physical activity. Patients hoping to undergo bariatric surgery are typically required to participate in some form of behavioral counseling prior to surgery.

Increased Activity: Increased activity levels are essential for long term weight loss and weight management. For obese individuals, increased activity in the first six months of weight loss efforts has not been shown to significantly impact weight reduction. Patient education and support should be offered so as to prevent frustration and diminished motivation in attempts to make long-term modifications in activity level. Patients should be advised to begin increasing activity levels with gentle modes of exercise, such as walking or swimming, performed at a tolerable pace. A general target of thirty minutes of increased activity daily is recommended and may be spread out into smaller intervals over the course of a day. Caution should be taken to prevent injury as intensity level and exercise duration increase. Research suggests that increased activity levels can positively influence the body's insulin sensitivity and fasting blood glucose to a measurable degree even in the absence of weight loss.

Dietary Modifications: In obese populations, a 500-1000 kcal/day reduction in dietary intake is usually sufficient to produce a 1-2 pounds per week weight loss. This rate can typically be maintained for six months before slowing or plateauing. Patients often have the misconception that reducing fat intake alone will produce the desired weight loss result. While this is a component of dietary modification, reduction of carbohydrate intake and overall calories are equally important. It is recommended that patients who are obese and wish to lose weight consult both a physician and dietician to ensure a medically safe and nutritionally sound approach to weight loss.

Pharmacology: The Food and Drug Administration (FDA) has approved a number of pharmacological weight loss agents for short-term adjunct use with diet, activity, and behavioral modifications. Classes of approved medications include appetite suppressants and lipase inhibitors. Appetite suppressants function to either reduce feelings of hunger or increase feelings of fullness. Lipase inhibitors decrease the body's ability to absorb dietary fats, thereby decreasing overall caloric intake. Though not specifically approved for weight loss by the FDA, some antidepressant, seizure, and diabetes medications are prescribed for short-term use to assist weight loss goals.

Community Resources: A variety of community-based weight loss programs are in existence, each with their own structured approach. Program commonalities include advocating increased activity and decreased caloric intake. Patients often cite geographical, philosophical or financial concerns as barriers to participating in a formal program. Well known community-based programs include Weight Watchers, Jenny Craig, Take Off Pounds Sensibly (TOPS), and Food Addicts Anonymous.

Bariatric Surgery: Bariatric surgery is a consideration for some patients who are morbidly obese and is often considered the intervention of last resort. Pre-operatively, patients must meet a number of requirements in order to be considered a surgical candidate. This typically includes a BMI greater than 40, or greater than 35 with additional co-morbidities, and evidence that other weight loss interventions have been largely unsuccessful. Most bariatric programs require a pre-operative commitment to support group attendance or individual counseling as well as some degree of substantive weight loss by more traditional methods. Pre- and post-operatively, a multidisciplinary team is responsible for providing support and assessing a number of pre-operative factors (e.g., co-morbidities, behavioral history, extent of adiposity). This bariatric specialty team commonly includes an internist, surgeon, psychologist, dietician, and program coordinator.

Nutrition[10,19,32]

Macronutrients

Macronutrients are the nutrients that have caloric value and provide the body with energy. These nutrients make up a greater proportion of our diet since they are needed in large amounts. The three macronutrients are carbohydrates, fats, and proteins.

Carbohydrates: Carbohydrates are the preferred fuel source for high-intensity exercise. Without adequate carbohydrate intake, the body will start to consume protein (i.e., muscle) as its fuel source. Carbohydrates can be broken down into simple and complex carbohydrates. Simple carbohydrates are made up of smaller molecules that increase blood glucose levels rapidly. Complex carbohydrates are made up of larger molecules that need to be broken down before they can be used, therefore they increase blood glucose levels much more slowly over a longer period of time. The glycemic index is a measure of how quickly a specific food will raise blood glucose levels.

Fats: Fats act as an energy reserve in the body and are the primary fuel source for low-intensity exercise. Fats also play a role in insulating the body, protecting organs, and assisting in the transport of fat-soluble vitamins. Fats are made up of fatty acids, which can be classified as saturated, monounsaturated or polyunsaturated. Saturated fats are commonly found in animal fats and tend to increase levels of bad cholesterol (i.e., low-density lipoprotein) within the body, while unsaturated fats are more commonly found in plant fats and tend to increase levels of good cholesterol (i.e., high-density lipoprotein).

Proteins: Proteins make up the structure of the body and are responsible for the growth and maintenance of the body's tissues. Proteins are abundant in collagen fibers which are present in structures such as skin, ligaments, and skeletal muscle. If the body is not receiving adequate carbohydrate or fat intake, protein may also be used as a fuel source. Proteins are made up of smaller subunits known as amino acids. There are 20 amino acids, 9 of which cannot be produced by the body and must be consumed in the diet (i.e., essential amino acids).

Vitamins

Vitamins are essential non-caloric nutrients that are required in small amounts for certain metabolic functions and cannot be manufactured by the body. Vitamins are most often classified as fat-soluble or water-soluble.

Fat-Soluble Vitamins

Fat-soluble vitamins include vitamins A, D, E, and K. Fat-soluble vitamins require protein carriers to move through body fluids and excesses are stored in the body. Since they are not water-soluble, it is possible that the vitamins may reach toxic levels.

Vitamin A

Vitamin A is essential to the eyes, epithelial tissue, normal growth and development, and reproduction.

- Common food sources containing vitamin A include green, orange, and yellow vegetables, liver, butter, egg yolks, and fortified margarine.
- Symptoms of deficiency include night blindness, rough and dry skin, and growth failure.
- Symptoms of toxicity include appetite loss, hair loss, and enlarged liver and spleen.

Vitamin D

Vitamin D increases the blood flow levels of minerals, notably calcium and phosphorus.

- Common food sources containing vitamin D include fortified milk, fish oils, and fortified margarine.
- Symptoms of deficiency include faulty bone growth, rickets, and osteomalacia.
- Symptoms of toxicity include calcification of soft tissues and hypercalcemia.

Vitamin E

Vitamin E functions as an antioxidant in cell membranes and is especially important for the integrity of cells that are constantly exposed to high levels of oxygen such as the lungs and red blood cells.

- Common food sources containing vitamin E include vegetable oils, wheat germ, nuts, and fish.
- Symptoms of deficiency include breakdown of red blood cells, however, this is relatively rare in adults.
- Symptoms of toxicity include decreased thyroid hormone levels and increased triglycerides.

Vitamin K

Vitamin K is necessary for the synthesis of at least two of the proteins involved in blood clotting.

- Common food sources containing vitamin K include dark green leafy vegetables, cheese, egg yolks, and liver.
- Symptoms of deficiency include hemorrhage and defective blood clotting.
- Toxicity has not been reported.

Water-Soluble Vitamins

Water-soluble vitamins are not stored in the body in any significant amount and therefore need to be included in the diet on a daily basis. Toxicity is less common than with fat-soluble vitamins.

Vitamin B2 (Riboflavin)

Vitamin B2 facilitates selected enzymes involved in carbohydrate, protein, and fat metabolism.

- Common food sources containing vitamin B2 include milk, green leafy vegetables, eggs, and peanuts.
- Symptoms of deficiency include inflammation of the tongue, sensitive eyes, and scaling of the skin.
- Toxicity has not been reported.

Vitamin B3 (Niacin)

Vitamin B3 facilitates several enzymes that regulate energy metabolism.

- Common food sources containing vitamin B3 include meats, whole grains, and white flour.
- Symptoms of deficiency include pellagra and gastrointestinal disturbances.
- Symptoms of toxicity include abnormal glucose metabolism, nausea, vomiting, and gastric ulceration.

Vitamin B6 (Pyridoxine)

Vitamin B6 is essential in the metabolism of proteins, amino acids, carbohydrates, and fat.

- Common food sources containing vitamin B6 include liver, red meats, whole grains, and potatoes.
- Symptoms of deficiency include peripheral neuropathy, convulsions, and depression.
- Symptoms of toxicity include sensory damage, numbness of the extremities, and ataxia.

Vitamin B12 (Cobalamin)

Vitamin B12 is essential for the functioning of all cells and aids in hemoglobin synthesis.

- Common food sources containing vitamin B12 include meats, whole eggs, and egg yolks.
- Symptoms of deficiency include pernicious anemia and various psychological disorders.
- Toxicity has not been reported.

Vitamin C

Vitamin C assists the body to combat infections and facilitates wound healing. The vitamin is necessary for the development and maintenance of bones, cartilage, connective tissue, and blood vessels.

- Common food sources containing vitamin C include citrus fruits, tomatoes, and cantaloupe.
- Symptoms of deficiency include anemia, swollen gums, loose teeth, and scurvy.
- Symptoms of toxicity include urinary stones, diarrhea, and hypoglycemia.

Biotin

Biotin is necessary for the action of many enzyme systems.

- Common food sources containing biotin include liver, meats, and milk.
- Symptoms of deficiency include anemia, depression, and muscle pain.
- Toxicity has not been reported.

Choline

Choline is a component of compounds necessary for nerve function and lipid metabolism.

- Choline is synthesized from methionine which is an amino acid.
- Symptoms of deficiency only occur when intake of methylamine is low.
- Toxicity has not been reported.

Folacin (Folic acid)

Folacin is involved in the formation of red blood cells and in the functioning of the gastrointestinal tract.

- Common food sources containing folacin include yeast, dark green leafy vegetables, and whole grains.
- Symptoms of deficiency include impaired cell division and alteration of protein synthesis.
- Toxicity has not been reported.

Pantothenic Acid

Pantothenic acid is an integral component of complex enzymes involved in the metabolism of fatty acids.

- Common food sources containing pantothenic acid include liver, eggs, and whole grains.
- Symptoms of deficiency include headache, fatigue, and poor muscle coordination.
- Symptoms of toxicity include diarrhea.

Minerals

Minerals are organic elements that fulfill essential roles in the metabolic process.

Major Minerals

Calcium (Ca)

Calcium facilitates muscle contraction and relaxation, builds strong bones and teeth, and aids in coagulation.

- Common food sources containing calcium include milk, green leafy vegetables, and soy products.
- Calcium deficiency may lead to poor bone growth, rickets, osteomalacia, and osteoporosis.
- Symptoms of toxicity include kidney stones.

Chloride (Cl)

Chloride facilitates the maintenance of fluid and acid-base balance.

- Common food sources containing chloride include table salt, fish, and vegetables.
- Chloride deficiency may lead to a disturbance of acid-base balance.
- Toxicity has not been reported.

Magnesium (Mg)

Magnesium builds strong bones and teeth, activates enzymes, and helps regulate heartbeat.

- Common food sources containing magnesium include raw dark vegetables, nuts, soybeans, milk, and cheese.
- Symptoms of deficiency include confusion, apathy, muscle weakness, and tremors.
- Symptoms of toxicity include increased calcium excretion.

Phosphorus (P)

Phosphorus strengthens bones, assists in the oxidation of fats and carbohydrates, and aids in maintaining acid-base balance.

- Common food sources containing phosphorus include milk, milk products, meats, whole grains, and soft drinks.
- Symptoms of deficiency include weakness, stiff joints, and fragile bones.
- Symptoms of toxicity include muscle spasms.

Potassium (K)

Potassium maintains fluid and acid-base balance.

- Common food sources containing potassium include apricots, bananas, oranges, grapefruit, and milk.
- Symptoms of deficiency include impaired growth and diminished heart rate.
- Symptoms of toxicity include hyperkalemia and cardiac disturbances.

Sodium (Na)

Sodium facilitates the maintenance of acid-base balance, transmits nerve impulses, and helps control muscle contractions.

- Common food sources containing sodium include salt and milk.
- Deficiency and toxicity have not been reported.

Sulfur (S)

Sulfur facilitates enzyme activity and energy metabolism.

- Common food sources containing sulfur include meat, eggs, milk, and cheese.
- Deficiency is extremely rare.
- Toxicity has not been reported.

Trace Minerals

Chromium (Cr)

Chromium controls glucose metabolism.

- Common food sources containing chromium include whole grains, meats, and cheese.
- Symptoms of deficiency include weight loss and central nervous system abnormalities.
- Symptoms of toxicity include liver damage.

Cobalt (Co)

Cobalt is an essential component of vitamin B12 and functions to activate enzymes.

- Common food sources containing cobalt include figs, cabbage, and spinach.
- Symptoms of deficiency include pernicious anemia.
- Symptoms of toxicity include polycythemia and increased blood volume.

Copper (Cu)

Copper facilitates hemoglobin synthesis and lipid metabolism.

- Common food sources containing copper include shellfish, liver, meat, and whole grains.
- Symptoms of deficiency include anemia, central nervous system abnormalities, and abnormal electrocardiograms.
- Symptoms of toxicity include Wilson's disease.

Fluorine (F)

Fluorine aids in the formation of bones and teeth and prevents osteoporosis.

- Common food sources containing fluorine include fish and water.
- Symptoms of deficiency include increased susceptibility of dental cavities.
- Symptoms of toxicity include fluorosis.

Iodine (I)

Iodine assists with the regulation of cell metabolism and basal metabolic rate.

- Common food sources containing iodine include iodized salt and seafood.
- Symptoms of deficiency may include goiters.
- Toxicity has not been reported.

Iron (Fe)

Iron assists in oxygen transport and cell oxidation.

- Common food sources containing iron include red meats and liver.
- Symptoms of deficiency include anemia.
- Symptoms of toxicity include hemochromatosis.

Manganese (Mn)

Manganese facilitates proper bone structure and functions as an enzyme component in general metabolism.

- Common food sources containing manganese include cereals and whole grains.
- There are no known symptoms of deficiency.
- Toxicity has not been reported.

Selenium (Se)

Selenium is a synergistic antioxidant with vitamin E.

- Common food sources containing selenium include meat, eggs, milk, seafood, and garlic.
- Symptoms of deficiency include Keshan's disease.
- Symptoms of toxicity include physical defects of fingernails and toenails, nausea, and abdominal pain.

Molybdenum (Mo)

Molybdenum is a component of three enzymes in particular, that are necessary for normal cell functioning.

- Common food sources containing molybdenum include meats, whole grains, and dark green vegetables.
- Symptoms of deficiency include vomiting and tachypnea.
- Toxicity has not been reported.

Zinc (Zn)

Zinc aids in immune function and cell division.

- Common food sources containing zinc include seafood, liver, milk, cheese, and whole grains.
- Symptoms of deficiency include depressed immune functions and impaired skeletal growth.
- Symptoms of toxicity include anemia, nausea, and vomiting.

Healthy Eating

MyPlate is a program created by the United States Department of Agriculture (USDA) that is designed to teach people how to create and maintain a healthy diet and healthy eating habits. General principles of MyPlate include making healthy choices from all of the food groups, eating the correct number of calories based on age, gender, size, and activity level, and limiting saturated fats, sodium, and added sugars. The MyPlate diet is broken down into six different food groups: fruits, vegetables, grains, protein foods, dairy, and oils.

Fruits: Any fruit or 100% fruit juice is considered to be in the "fruit" category. Whole fruits are a more ideal source of fruit when compared to fruit juices. Fruit intake should be 1.5-2 cups per day for an adult. A cup is equal to one cup of fruit or fruit juice or half a cup of dried fruit.

Vegetables: Any vegetable or 100% vegetable juice is considered to be in the "vegetable" category. Vegetables are categorized into five subgroups: dark green vegetables, starchy vegetables, red and orange vegetables, beans and peas, and other vegetables. A healthy diet should consist of a variety of these different vegetable subgroups. Vegetable intake should be 2.5-3 cups per day for an adult. A cup is equal to one cup of vegetables or vegetable juice or two cups of raw leafy green vegetables.

Grains: Any food made from wheat, barley, oats, cornmeal, rice or another cereal grain is considered to be in the "grain" category. Grains are divided into two subgroups: whole grains and refined grains. Whole grains contain the entire grain kernel; examples include whole wheat flour and oatmeal. Refined grains have been processed and only contain part of the grain kernel; examples include white flour and white rice. Grain intake should be 5-8 ounce equivalents per day for an adult. An ounce equivalent is equal to a slice of bread, one cup of cereal or half a cup of cooked pasta or rice. It is recommended that half of the grain intake come from whole grains.

Protein foods: Any food made from meat, poultry, seafood, eggs, soy products, beans and peas (also in the vegetable category), nuts, and seeds is considered to be in the "protein food" category. Protein intake should be 5-6.5 ounce equivalents per day for an adult. An ounce equivalent is equal to one ounce of meat, poultry or fish, an egg, half an ounce of nuts or seeds or a quarter cup of cooked beans. Protein intake should be varied among the different groups. Meat and poultry choices should be lean or low-fat. To limit sodium intake, nuts and seeds should be unsalted and processed meats should be limited.

Dairy: Fluid milk products and foods made from milk are considered to be in the "dairy" category. Dairy intake should be 3 cups per day for an adult. A cup is equal to one cup of milk or yogurt, 1.5 ounces of natural cheese or 2 ounces of processed cheese. It is recommended that most dairy choices be fat-free or low-fat.

Oils: Oils are fats that are liquid at room temperature. Oils are not a separate food group, though they do provide essential nutrients and are therefore important to consume. Oil intake should be 5-7 teaspoons per day for an adult. Commonly eaten oils include canola oil, olive oil, and safflower oil. Some foods are naturally high in oils, like fish, nuts, olives, and avocados. It is recommended that oils consumed in the diet should be high in unsaturated fats and low in saturated fats.

Pharmacology Basics[19,32]

Methods of Drug Administration

There are two basic methods for the administration of drugs:

- **Enteral Administration** – involves use of the gastrointestinal tract for administration of a drug.

- **Parenteral administration** – involves any form of drug administration that does not involve the gastrointestinal tract.

Enteral administration

Oral: Oral administration involves swallowing a medication so it passes through the esophagus and stomach and is eventually absorbed into the body by the intestines. It is the most common and easiest method for administering a drug. Absorption by the gastrointestinal tract allows for a gradual increase in drug levels within the body. A disadvantage to oral administration is that the compound must be lipid-soluble so that the intestinal tract can absorb it. Other disadvantages include gastric irritation from the drug, metabolism and degradation of a drug by the liver before reaching its target tissue, and factors that affect intestinal absorption and thus make bioavailability unpredictable.

Sublingual: Sublingual administration involves passage of a drug through the sublingual mucosa (under the tongue) or buccal mucosa (between the cheek and gums). After being absorbed, the drug travels from the venous circulation directly to the heart, where it enters the systemic circulation. Sublingual administration allows for faster introduction of a drug in cases of acute pain (e.g., angina) and allows drugs to bypass the liver so they are not overly metabolized before reaching their target tissue.

Rectal: Rectal administration involves the insertion of a suppository into the rectum and absorption of the drug within the rectal cavity. Rectal administration is advantageous for patients who cannot take drugs orally (e.g., unconscious, vomiting). As with sublingual medications, these drugs also bypass the liver. However, drugs are not absorbed as well through the rectal cavity when compared to sublingual and oral administrations.

Parenteral administration

Inhalation: Drugs can be inhaled for administration if they are in a gaseous or aerosol form. Inhalation is advantageous since the lungs have a large surface area for absorption and therefore the drug can enter the systemic circulation rapidly. A potential disadvantage of inhalation is that the respiratory tract can become irritated.

Topical: Topical administration involves application of a drug directly to the skin or mucous membranes. Because drugs are poorly absorbed through the skin into the systemic circulation, this method is reserved for treating localized skin, ear, eye or nose disorders. Mucous membranes have a larger capacity for drug absorption and thus drugs applied to mucous membranes (e.g., nasal mucosa) can be used to treat systemic conditions.

Transdermal: Transdermal administration involves application of a drug directly to the skin. Unlike topical administration, the intent is that the drug will absorb through the skin and enter the systemic circulation. Transdermal administration allows for a slow, controlled release of the drug into the circulation over a long period of time. This form of administration often occurs with the use of patches (e.g., fentanyl), though iontophoresis and phonophoresis also use the transdermal route.

Injection: There are a variety of administration methods that involve injection of a medication. Injection can be used to administer a drug either locally or systemically. A disadvantage is that injection is invasive and therefore can cause infection. The various forms of injection include:

- **Intravenous:** Intravenous (IV) administration involves injection of a medication into a peripheral vein so it can enter the bloodstream. An advantage of IV administration is that the drug can enter the circulation and reach the target tissue rapidly, though this can become dangerous if an inaccurate dosage is given. IV administration is a more accurate method of administering a drug since it is considered 100% bioavailable.

- **Intra-arterial:** Intra-arterial administration involves injection of a medication into an artery so that it can travel directly to the target tissue. This type of injection is difficult to perform, though may be necessary in instances where the drug is intended to act at a specific site without affecting other tissues (e.g., chemotherapy).

- **Subcutaneous:** Subcutaneous administration involves injection of a drug directly under the skin into the subcutaneous fat or connective tissue. This form of administration can be useful when a slow release of medication into the systemic circulation is required (e.g., insulin). Patients have the ability to self-administer these medications if they are trained. However, the rate of absorption of these drugs can be affected by a variety of factors. Some factors, such as immobility of the limb or the application of cold, may slow the absorption rate while other factors, such as massage or the application of heat, may speed absorption.

- **Intramuscular:** Intramuscular (IM) administration involves injection of a drug into skeletal muscle. IM injections are often used when treating localized muscular problems (e.g., botulinum toxin for spasticity). Absorption of a drug via IM injection is more rapid than subcutaneous injection, while still allowing for a steady release of the drug into the systemic circulation. A disadvantage of IM injections is that they tend to cause localized muscle soreness and pain at the site of injection.

CONSIDER THIS
FACTORS THAT AFFECT PHARMACOKINETICS

Age: As age increases, the incidence of adverse drug reactions tends to increase. There may be several reasons for this including a decrease in lean body mass, a decrease in serum proteins, a reduction in renal and liver function, and interactions with other drugs. Infants and young children also require alterations in dosing to avoid adverse reactions since their organs are not fully developed and are unable to metabolize drugs in the same manner.

Weight: Dosages are typically based on a 150-pound individual. Patients who fall far above or below this value may need their drug dosage altered to achieve the desired therapeutic effect.

Genetics: Because genes control the production of enzymes, genetic mutations may result in an abnormal response to the administration of a drug. Differences in drug effectiveness or the elimination of a drug may be seen among different ethnic groups.

Disease: Disease of the kidneys or liver can result in reduced ability to metabolize or eliminate a drug and may cause toxic effects. Viral infections may also affect a drug's half-life by exerting a negative effect on enzymatic activity.

Exercise: Exercise can affect many factors that have an influence on drug activity, including blood flow, pH, body temperature, gastrointestinal function, metabolism, and excretion. The effects of exercise on drug action can vary based on the type and intensity of exercise, the type of drug, the method of administration, and the dosing schedule. Because the interactions are so complex, there is not a clear consensus on the exact effects that exercise exerts on drug action.

Medications: The effectiveness of a drug may be altered when it is taken in combination with other drugs. These drug-drug interactions can be antagonistic or synergistic. For example, taking aspirin may reduce the effectiveness of a diuretic (i.e., antagonistic), or taking a sedative while also drinking alcohol may result in excessive central nervous system depression (i.e., synergistic).

Food: The presence of food in the stomach can slow the rate of absorption of a drug. Drugs may be taken on an empty stomach to speed their absorption into the bloodstream, while other drugs may be taken in combination with food to avoid gastric irritation. Specific food-drug interactions are generally insignificant, though there are several examples of foods that affect the bioavailability of a drug. Foods or beverages that are acidic (e.g., soda) may affect the absorption of some drugs within the gastrointestinal tract. Grapefruit juice is a commonly identified drink that affects enzymatic activity within the gastrointestinal tract and thus changes the metabolism of certain drugs.

Pharmacology Terminology

Bioavailability: Bioavailability refers to the percentage of a drug that makes it into the systemic circulation from the site of original administration. Bioavailability will vary depending on how much the drug becomes degraded before reaching the systemic circulation. A drug that is injected intravenously is 100% bioavailable.

Chemical name: The name for the drug's specific compound structure (e.g., N-acetyl-p-aminophenol).

Dose-response curve: The dose-response curve (Fig. 7-12) is a graphic representation of the relationship between the dosage of a drug and the body's response to that drug. As the dosage of a drug increases, more receptors for the drug become activated which increases the body's response to the drug. However, the body's response will plateau at a certain dosage. The dose-response curve can be used to compare the potency of two different drugs.

Generic name: The official name given to a drug that is derived from its chemical name (e.g., acetaminophen).

Half-life: The half-life of a drug refers to the rate of elimination of the drug. If a drug has a half-life of two hours and 4,000 units of the drug are administered initially, then only 2,000 units will remain after two hours, and only 1,000 units will remain after four hours.

Pharmacodynamics: The study of how a drug exerts its therapeutic effect on the body at the cellular or organ level.

DOSE-RESPONSE RELATIONSHIP

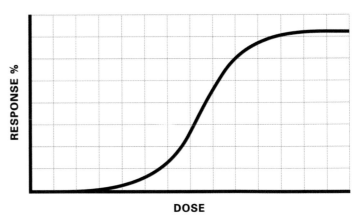

Fig. 7-12: A dose-response curve.

Pharmacotherapeutics: The division of pharmacology that deals with the use of drugs for preventing, treating, and diagnosing diseases.

Pharmacokinetics: The study of how drugs are absorbed, distributed, metabolized, and eliminated by the body.

Toxicology: The division of pharmacology that studies the adverse effects of drugs.

Trade name: The brand name of a drug that is assigned by the pharmaceutical company (e.g., Tylenol); there can be several trade names for a single drug if there are multiple companies manufacturing the same drug.

Pharmacology Effects on Specific Systems

Musculoskeletal System

General anesthesia: Therapists may encounter patients who are post-surgery and dealing with the side effects of general anesthesia. These effects can last for several days in some patients. Confusion and muscle weakness are two of the more common side effects associated with anesthesia. Since anesthesia can result in retained pulmonary secretions, the therapist may need to initiate breathing exercises or postural drainage with the patient.

Local anesthesia: Patients that receive a local or spinal nerve block during surgery may have diminished sensation and motor function following surgery. Exercise should be performed cautiously since the patient may not fully feel pain. Additionally, bracing may be needed during ambulation if the patient is lacking motor control.

Opioid analgesic agents: These drugs provide significant pain relief that may allow a patient to tolerate more aggressive physical therapy interventions. Therapy sessions should be scheduled to coincide with peak effectiveness of the drug. Side effects that may affect therapy interventions include sedation and respiratory depression.

Nonsteroidal anti-inflammatory agents: These drugs can provide analgesia while avoiding the side effects that are associated with opioid analgesics (e.g., sedation). However, these drugs will not provide the same level of pain relief as compared to opioid analgesics. The side effects associated with nonsteroidal anti-inflammatory drugs, primarily gastrointestinal discomfort, are unlikely to have a negative effect on physical therapy sessions.

Antiarthritic agents: Side effects of these drugs will vary depending on the specific drug that is administered. Glucocorticoid drugs have catabolic effects and can lead to the breakdown of tendon, bone or skin. Therapists should be cautious with aggressive stretching and strengthening exercises to eliminate the risk for fractures or soft tissue injuries. Care must also be taken when applying orthotic devices to prevent skin breakdown.

Neuromuscular and Nervous Systems

Antiepileptic agents: Cerebellar side effects (e.g., ataxia) are common with antiepileptic drugs and the loss of coordination may significantly affect therapeutic activities. Additionally, these drugs may cause specific skin conditions (e.g., dermatitis). Any modalities used in therapy that may exacerbate these conditions should be used cautiously.

Skeletal muscle relaxants: These drugs reduce muscle spasm and spasticity and therefore can improve a patient's ability to participate in and benefit from rehabilitation activities. However, these effects can be detrimental for patients who rely on spasticity to improve their function (e.g., using extensor tone to help with standing transfers). Physical therapy plays an important role in assisting these patients to adapt to a sudden decrease in spasticity by improving their strength and motor control.

Sedation and muscle weakness are common side effects of these drugs and should be taken into consideration when scheduling therapy sessions.

Anti-Parkinson's agents: Therapy sessions should be scheduled to coincide with maximum effectiveness of anti-Parkinson's drugs (roughly an hour after administration for levodopa). Therapists should closely monitor blood pressure for these patients since the drugs may produce orthostatic hypotension and increase the risk for falls.

Cardiovascular and Pulmonary Systems

Antihypertensive agents: Patients taking these drugs to lower blood pressure are at increased risk for orthostatic hypotension. Therapists should be alert for hypotensive symptoms, especially when patients are changing position. Interventions that cause widespread vasodilation, such as whirlpool therapy, should be avoided in patients who are taking vasodilating drugs. Patients taking beta blockers may have a diminished heart rate response to exercise, therefore other means of assessing exercise intensity (e.g., rating of perceived exertion) should be used.

Antianginal agents: Drugs taken to treat symptoms of angina pectoris can have a variety of effects on the cardiovascular system. Some patients will have an increase in exercise tolerance since they will not be limited by episodes of angina. Other patients, especially those taking beta blockers or calcium channel blockers, will have a diminished heart rate response to exercise and therefore may not be able to tolerate higher workloads. As stated with antihypertensive drugs, patients taking drugs to treat angina are also at an increased risk for orthostatic hypotension due to the vasodilating properties of the drug.

Antiarrhythmic agents: While these drugs are used to treat cardiac arrhythmias, they can sometimes lead to an increase in arrhythmias or a change in the type of arrhythmia the patient is experiencing. If beta blockers or calcium channel blockers are used to treat cardiac arrhythmias, therapists should be aware of the risk for orthostatic hypotension.

Congestive heart failure agents: Side effects of these drugs will depend on the specific drug used to treat congestive heart failure. Patients taking diuretics may experience fatigue and muscle weakness associated with diminished fluid and electrolyte levels, which may affect their ability to actively participate in therapy sessions. Vasodilating drugs will increase the risk for orthostatic hypotension and therefore exercise or modalities that produce widespread vasodilation should be avoided.

Anticoagulant agents: Patients taking anticoagulant drugs are at an increased risk for bleeding. Physical therapy interventions that increase the risk for tissue trauma, such as soft tissue massage or chest percussion, should be performed with caution. Likewise, wound care interventions (e.g., dressing changes) should be performed carefully to avoid excessive bleeding.

Respiratory agents: Patients who use bronchodilator drugs may experience cardiac arrhythmias, confusion, and tremors, all of which may be signs of toxicity and should be closely monitored by therapists. There are no significant side effects noted with the use of mucolytic and expectorant drugs, however, therapists should be aware of the patient's dosing schedule. Mucolytics and expectorants should be taken 30-60 minutes prior to chest physical therapy to maximize treatment effectiveness.

Other Systems

Sedative-hypnotic and antianxiety agents: These drugs initially create a calming effect that may make a patient more willing to participate in physical therapy. However, when the drugs reach their peak effectiveness, the patient may experience a level of drowsiness that makes it difficult to actively participate. Scheduling patients a few hours after taking these medications should be avoided since the therapy session will be less effective. It is also important to note that patients taking these medications have an increased risk for falls and subsequent injury.

Antidepressant agents: These drugs are associated with a variety of side effects that may negatively affect therapy sessions. Some antidepressant drugs, such as lithium and the tricyclics, produce sedation and muscle weakness, making it more difficult for a patient to actively participate in therapy sessions. Some antidepressants increase the risk for orthostatic hypotension, while others result in hypertension. Therapists should monitor patients' blood pressure regularly to avoid drastic increases or decreases during exercise.

Antipsychotic agents: The most common side effects associated with antipsychotic drugs are extrapyramidal symptoms, which are abnormal movement patterns such as dyskinesia or dystonia. Therapists should be alert for changes in the patient's posture, balance or movement pattern and notify personnel immediately.

Thyroid agents: Drugs used to treat hypothyroidism or hyperthyroidism often produce side effects associated with symptoms of the opposite condition. Therapists should avoid interventions that can exacerbate symptoms of thyroid dysfunction. For example, patients with hypothyroidism symptoms may have decreased cardiac function and may not tolerate heavy workloads.

Insulin replacement therapy: Patients taking insulin to control diabetes mellitus may experience symptoms of hypoglycemia, especially if they have not eaten or are participating in strenuous physical activity. Therapists should be aware of the signs of hypoglycemia (e.g., confusion, nausea) and monitor patients closely during and after therapy sessions.

Chemotherapy agents: These drugs can have a number of adverse side effects that will affect physical therapy treatment. The most significant side effect is severe fatigue that may make it impossible for a patient to participate in therapy sessions. It is important for the therapist to recognize that there will be days when the patient is unable to tolerate even a light therapy session. These drugs may also cause toxic effects on both the central and peripheral nervous systems. Therapists should be aware of any nervous system abnormalities that may affect treatment, such as peripheral neuropathy or ataxia.

GOLD Level Clinical Application Templates

Level Clinical Application Template Executive Summary

Arterial Insufficiency Ulcer

- Characterized by the narrowing of arterial vessels that impedes the delivery of oxygenated blood to tissues
- Peripheral artery disease is typically linked to the development of arterial insufficiency ulcers; risk factors include atherosclerosis, hypertension, obesity, diabetes mellitus, and smoking
- Typically heal by secondary intention with adequate blood supply and wound healing interventions

Breast Cancer

- May spread to the lymphatic system and commonly metastasizes to the brain, lungs, bones, adrenals, and liver
- Breast cancer makes up 30% of all female cancers and is the second leading cause of death for females in the United States
- Prognosis and ten-year survival rates for women are over 85% for stage I; 66% for stage II; 36% for stage III; and 7% for stage IV disease

Burn - Full Thickness

- Burn causes immediate cellular and tissue death and subsequent vascular destruction
- Eschar forms from necrotic cells and creates a dry and hard layer that requires debridement
- Absent sensation and pain due to destruction of free nerve endings, however, there may be pain from adjacent areas that experience partial-thickness burns

Burn - Partial Thickness

- Superficial partial-thickness burn involves the epidermis and upper portion of the dermis; deep partial-thickness burn involves the epidermis, majority of the dermis, and structures within the dermis
- Superficial partial-thickness burn is characterized by a red color that will blanch when touched; deep partial-thickness burn is characterized by red discoloration, however, it will not blanch
- Will typically heal without residual deficits in the absence of infection or other factors that may complicate or delay healing

Diabetes Mellitus - Type 1

- Insulin is functionally absent due to the destruction of the beta cells of the pancreas; where the insulin would normally be produced
- Starts in children ages four years or older, with the peak incidence of onset coinciding with early adolescence and puberty
- Common symptoms include polyuria, polydipsia, polyphagia, nausea, weight loss, fatigue, blurred vision, and dehydration

Level Clinical Application Template Executive Summary

Diabetes Mellitus - Type 2

- Characterized by an inappropriate cellular response to insulin, preventing adequate absorption of blood glucose; excess blood glucose results in a persistent hyperglycemic state
- May develop slowly prior to showing initial symptoms that can include polydipsia, polyuria, blurred vision, delayed healing, frequent infections, and acanthosis nigricans
- Medical management is typically focused on lifestyle changes and pharmaceutical intervention through various oral or injectable pharmacological agents

Fibromyalgia Syndrome

- Nonarticular rheumatic condition with pain caused by tender points within muscles, tendons, and ligaments
- Greater incidence in females (almost 75% of the cases) potentially affecting any age
- Widespread history of pain that exists in all four quadrants of the body (above and below the waist)

Lymphedema Post-Mastectomy

- Caused by an excess load of lymph fluid or inadequate transport capacity within the lymphatic system secondary to the loss of homeostasis
- Primary contributing factor in the development of lymphedema following a mastectomy is the damage and/or removal of the axillary lymph nodes and vessels
- Intervention should focus on manual lymph drainage, short stretch compression bandages, retrograde massage, exercise, compression therapy, and use of a mechanical pump

Neuropathic Ulcer

- Occurs most frequently in the diabetic population and are often referred to as diabetic ulcers
- At-risk areas include those that are routinely subjected to pressure during normal weight bearing, atypical stresses due to structural changes or improper fitting footwear
- Will typically heal by secondary intention with appropriate wound healing interventions and the absence of complications (e.g., infection, severe arterial insufficiency)

Osteoporosis

- Metabolic bone disorder where the rate of bone resorption accelerates while the rate of bone formation slows down
- Patients may complain of low thoracic or lumbar pain and experience compression fractures of the vertebrae
- Bone mineral density test accounts for 70% of bone strength and is the easiest way to determine osteoporosis

Level Clinical Application Template Executive Summary

Pressure Ulcer

- Unrelieved pressure deprives the tissues of oxygen which causes ischemia, subsequent cell death, and tissue necrosis
- High risk areas for pressure ulcers include the occiput, heels, greater trochanters, ischial tuberosities, sacrum, and epicondyles of the elbow
- Impaired cognition, poor nutrition, altered sensation, incontinence, decreased lean body mass, and infection contribute to the development of a pressure ulcer

Rheumatoid Arthritis

- Systemic autoimmune disorder of the connective tissue that is characterized by chronic inflammation within synovial membranes, tendon sheaths, and articular cartilage
- Incidence is three times greater in females than males and is diagnosed most frequently between 30-50 years of age
- Blood work assists with the diagnosis of rheumatoid arthritis through evaluation of the rheumatoid factor, white blood cell count, erythrocyte sedimentation rate, hemoglobin, and hematocrit values

Systemic Lupus Erythematosus

- Connective tissue disorder caused by an autoimmune reaction in the body
- Females are at greater risk than males with the most common age group ranging from 15-40 years of age
- Clinical presentation includes a red butterfly rash across the cheeks and nose, a red rash over light exposed areas, arthralgias, alopecia, pleurisy, kidney involvement, seizures, and depression

Urinary Stress Incontinence

- Occurs during activities where there is an increase in abdominal pressure through straining, sneezing, coughing or lifting
- Risk factors include pregnancy, vaginal delivery, episiotomy, prostate or pelvic surgery, aging, diabetes mellitus, central nervous system dysfunction, and recurrent urinary infection
- Accounts for 50-60% of all incontinence cases and is manifested solely by the involuntary loss of urine with any form of exertion or increased abdominal pressure

GOLD **Level Clinical Application Template Executive Summary**

Venous Insufficiency Ulcer

- Typically results from venous hypertension which may present idiopathically, secondary to valve incompetence or peripheral impedance
- Pain complaints are typically mild and relieved with elevation or use of compression garments
- Treatment of a venous insufficiency ulcer and the underlying pathology should allow for a normal course of recovery without residual deficits

DIAGNOSIS

What condition produces a patient's symptoms?

An arterial insufficiency ulcer is caused by inadequate perfusion of oxygenated blood in the affected tissue. Over time, diminished blood flow is no longer able to meet the metabolic demands of the tissue resulting in cell death and tissue necrosis. Arterial insufficiency ulcers typically occur due to underlying pathology such as progressive atherosclerosis or an arterial embolism.

An injury was most likely sustained to which structure?

An arterial insufficiency ulcer can affect different structures based on the depth of tissue injury. A superficial ulceration is associated with damage to the epidermis. Damage from a partial-thickness ulceration will extend through the epidermis and possibly into, but not through, the dermis. A full-thickness ulceration extends through the dermis and into deeper layers such as the subcutaneous fat layer.

INFERENCE

What is the most likely contributing factor in the development of this condition?

Peripheral artery disease (PAD) is typically linked to the development of arterial insufficiency ulcers. The condition is characterized by the narrowing of arterial vessels that impedes the delivery of oxygenated blood to tissues. Risk factors for the development of PAD include atherosclerosis, hypertension, obesity, diabetes mellitus, and smoking.

CONFIRMATION

What is the most likely clinical presentation?

A patient will typically develop an arterial insufficiency ulcer distally on the lower one-third of the lower extremity. Common sites include the dorsum of the foot, the lateral malleolus, and the toes. Wound edges may initially be slightly irregular, however, they soon progress to the more characteristic smooth and defined appearance. A clean wound bed is typically light pink in color though a grayish undertone may be observed. Minimal bleeding is noted with manipulation of the wound and debridement. Discoloration may be noted in the nails (e.g., yellow), nail beds (e.g., cyanotic), and surrounding skin (e.g., pale). Intact surrounding skin may be cool to the touch, thin, shiny, and hairless. Distal pulses are usually diminished or absent with palpation and often require assessment via Doppler ultrasound. In more advanced cases, muscle wasting may also be observed. Pain complaints are typically significant. Limb-related pain is most commonly positional, occurring when the limb is in a non-dependent position or with activity that results in intermittent claudication.

What laboratory or imaging studies would confirm the diagnosis?

Diagnosis of an arterial insufficiency ulcer is made based on the characteristics of the observed wound and diagnosis of the underlying condition. Duplex ultrasonography is the least invasive method of assessing arterial blood flow. It determines the speed and direction of blood flow and narrowing of the vessels. An angiogram (e.g., arteriogram, venogram) utilizes a contrast dye and x-ray imaging to identify narrowed, blocked, malformed or enlarged arterial vessels.

What additional information should be obtained to confirm the diagnosis?

The ankle-brachial index (ABI) assists in predicting the severity of arterial occlusion. An ABI of 0.79 or less is indicative of a moderate arterial blockage, increasing the likelihood of ulcer development and symptoms of intermittent claudication with activity.

EXAMINATION

What history should be documented?

Important areas to explore include past medical history, medications, family history, current symptoms, current health status, social history and habits, occupation, leisure activities, and social support system.

What tests/measures are most appropriate?

Anthropometric characteristics: circumferential measurements

Arousal, attention, and cognition: examine mental status, learning ability, memory, and motivation

Assistive and adaptive devices: analysis of components and safety of a device

Gait, locomotion, and balance: static and dynamic balance in sitting and standing, safety during gait with/without an assistive device

Integumentary integrity: skin assessment, assessment of sensation, assessment of wound characteristics, photographic documentation

Muscle performance: strength assessment, muscle tone assessment

Pain: pain perception assessment scale, visual analogue scale, claudication pain

Range of motion: active and passive range of motion

Reflex integrity: assessment of deep tendon reflexes

Self-care and home management: assessment of functional capacity

Ventilation, respiration, and circulation: assessment of pulse oximetry, palpation of pulses, capillary refill, ankle-brachial index

Arterial Insufficiency Ulcer   GOLD

What additional findings are likely with this patient?

Arterial insufficiency ulcers are likely to become chronic without adequate perfusion to the wound bed and surrounding tissue. Patients may develop multiple ulcers concurrently. Complications that may further impact healing include gangrene, osteomyelitis, sepsis, and pain.

MANAGEMENT

What is the most effective management of this patient?

Medical management typically includes monitoring the severity of the underlying disease process, counseling regarding modifiable risk factors, pharmaceutical intervention, and potential surgical intervention. Surgical debridement will typically convert a chronic ulceration to an acute wound thereby reactivating the normal healing process. In cases with more significant arterial occlusion, surgical revascularization (e.g., femoral-popliteal bypass) will typically allow the wound to heal. For larger wounds, grafting may be indicated once normal circulation has been restored. If vascular integrity cannot be restored, amputation is typically recommended. Physical therapy management emphasizes skin protection and wound healing interventions. The ulcer may require cleansing agents and/or debridement (e.g., enzymatic, mechanical, autolytic, sharp) and should be regularly monitored for signs of infection. Packing may be necessary to fill the wound space as part of the dressing application depending on the wound depth. Arterial insufficiency ulcers typically produce minimal exudate, therefore, it is important to select dressings which both protect the wound and assist in maintaining a moist wound healing environment. Photo documentation is recommended to supplement written documentation describing wound characteristics (e.g., area, depth, odor, exudate, color).

What home care regimen should be recommended?

The home care regimen is dependent on the size and characteristics of the arterial ulcer. Patients who do not require debridement may appropriately manage routine dressing changes at home. All patients should be diligent with hygiene and skin protection to limit the risk of infection.

OUTCOME

What is the likely outcome of a course of physical therapy?

An arterial insufficiency ulcer will typically heal by secondary intention with adequate blood supply and wound healing interventions. Patients typically will not experience residual deficits from the wound itself, but may have increased morbidity and mortality secondary to the underlying pathology.

What are the long-term effects of the patient's condition?

Treatment of an arterial insufficiency ulcer and the underlying pathology should allow for a normal course of recovery without residual deficits. Infection or other healing complications may require additional pharmacological, medical or surgical intervention. If infection is pervasive or vascular integrity cannot be adequately restored, additional ulcerations, gangrene or amputation may result.

COMPARISON

What are the distinguishing characteristics of a similar condition?

Venous insufficiency ulcers are typically the result of tissue changes associated with venous hypertension. These ulcers commonly develop in the distal lower extremities, as with arterial insufficiency ulcers, however, the underlying pathology and ulcer characteristics are markedly different. Venous insufficiency ulcers are typically shallow with irregular edges and moderate to heavy exudate. Pain complaints are usually mild to moderate, most notable with prolonged dependent positioning, and relieved with elevation. On examination, pedal pulses are typically intact, however, they may be difficult to assess if edema is significant. Skin is often dry and flaky with a brownish discoloration (e.g., hemosiderin staining). Specific wound care interventions emphasize skin and wound protection, establishing a clean wound bed, exudate management, and the selection of optimal primary and secondary dressings. Successful treatment typically will require some degree of graded compression to manage edema and support normal tissue healing. The regular use of compression is recommended to reduce the risk of future ulcer development.

CLINICAL SCENARIOS

Scenario One

A 91-year-old female is referred to physical therapy by her vascular surgeon for wound care. She has an ABI of 0.7 and small ulceration on her left great toe which is covered with firmly adhered eschar. The patient complains of significant pain during the examination. She resides with her daughter in a second floor apartment.

Scenario Two

A 67-year-old male is a two pack per day smoker with a history of hypertension and atherosclerosis. He has developed large ulcerations on the dorsum of his right foot and proximal to the lateral malleolus. The patient has an ABI of 0.45 and cyanotic nail beds. He is a general contractor and lives alone in a one story home.

DIAGNOSIS

What condition produces a patient's symptoms?

Breast cancer's primary symptom is a painless mass within the breast tissue. This mass is composed of malignant altered cells that proliferate and spread uncontrollably. A malignancy can occur anywhere within the breast tissue, however, the lump is usually found directly behind the areola in men and is usually located behind the areola or in the outer upper quadrant of the breast in women. There may or may not be generalized discomfort in the area of the mass.

An injury was most likely sustained to which structure?

Injury occurs initially at the cellular level within the breast tissue. Breast cancer either begins in the lobules, which are the milk producing glands, or in the ducts that bring the milk to the nipples. Breast cancer can spread into the lymphatic system and will commonly metastasize to the brain, lungs, bones, adrenals, and liver.

INFERENCE

What is the most likely contributing factor in the development of this condition?

The etiology of breast cancer is unknown, however, estrogen is believed to have some relationship to the disease process. Risk factors include gender, age, young menarche, late menopause, family history of breast cancer, high alcohol intake, high fat diet, radiation exposure, and past history of cancer. Breast cancer can occur in both males and females, however, males account for less than 1% of all breast cancer cases.

CONFIRMATION

What is the most likely clinical presentation?

Breast cancer makes up approximately 30% of all female cancers and is the second leading cause of death in female cancers within the United States. Approximately 70% of all breast cancer occurs in women over the age of 50. A patient with breast cancer will present with a lump in the breast that is noticed by a physician (10%) or by the patient through self-examination (90%). Breast cancer is initially otherwise asymptomatic. As the disease progresses the breast may become painful, change shape, bleed from the nipple, and dimple over the area of the mass. Symptoms associated with metastases may include bone pain, upper extremity edema, and weight loss.

What laboratory or imaging studies would confirm the diagnosis?

Mammography is used to detect the location and growth of a mass, however, definitive diagnosis of breast cancer is made only after microscopic examination of a suspected mass by needle or excision biopsy. Ultrasound can also be used to detect if a lump is filled with fluid or a solid mass. Sentinel lymph node mapping is used upon diagnosis to identify exact lymph node involvement.

What additional information should be obtained to confirm the diagnosis?

Additional information such as family history of cancer, past medical history, and history of self-examination is helpful in support of a definitive diagnosis. This information is usually obtained prior to mammography and biopsy.

EXAMINATION

What history should be documented?

Important areas to explore include past medical history, family history of cancer, medications, current health status, social history and habits, hand dominance, occupation, living environment, and social support system.

What tests/measures are most appropriate?

Aerobic capacity and endurance: assessment of vital signs at rest and with activity

Anthropometric characteristics: upper extremity circumferential measurements

Arousal, attention, and cognition: examine mental status, learning ability, memory, motivation

Community and work integration: analysis of community, work, and leisure activities

Gait, locomotion, and balance: assess static/dynamic balance in sitting and standing, safety during gait

Integumentary integrity: assessment for potential infection of surgical incision

Muscle performance: strength assessment

Pain: pain perception assessment scale, visual analogue scale

Range of motion: active and passive range of motion

Self-care and home management: assessment of self-care and home management skills, assessment of functional capacity, Barthel Index

Sensory integrity: assessment of superficial and combined sensations, proprioception, and kinesthesia

Breast Cancer   **GOLD**

What additional findings are likely with this patient?

Additional findings are dependent on the stage of the cancer (I, II, III, IV) and course of treatment. If a patient has undergone surgical resection or mastectomy the patient may experience pain, edema, fatigue, and psychological issues. Patients that are diagnosed with advanced breast cancer may experience pleural effusion, pathological fractures, and spinal compression.

MANAGEMENT

What is the most effective management of this patient?

The medical management of breast cancer is based on the size and the stage of the mass and corresponding involvement of the lymph nodes. Surgical management may range from excision of the mass (lumpectomy) to total radical mastectomy with axillary dissection. Chemotherapy, radiation therapy, and hormone therapies may be used in isolation or after a surgical procedure. Physical therapy may be indicated to assist with lymphedema management, post-surgical breathing exercises, positioning, pain management, strengthening and endurance activities, range of motion exercises, massage, intermittent compression, and patient education.

What home care regimen should be recommended?

A home care regimen should include education, positioning, and techniques to manage lymphedema. Range of motion exercises, energy conservation techniques, as well as general exercise and endurance activities should continue on a regular basis at home.

OUTCOME

What is the likely outcome of a course in physical therapy?

Physical therapy may be indicated for post-surgical management to assist with impairments and promote independence with self-care and functional skills.

What are the long-term effects of the patient's condition?

The long-term effects of breast cancer are varied. The risk of recurrence is always present and should be monitored closely. Post-surgical lymphedema may persist and require ongoing home management. Overall prognosis and ten-year survival rates for women are over 85% for stage I disease; 66% for stage II; 36% for stage III; and 7% for stage IV disease. The survival rate decreases as the tumor progresses and lymph nodes become involved. Overall mortality has decreased 1-2% annually within the United States secondary to changes in lifestyle, improved self-examination, earlier diagnosis, and better treatment.

COMPARISON

What are the distinguishing characteristics of a similar condition?

Fibrocystic breast disease (mammary dysplasia) usually occurs in both breasts and is characterized by nodular lumps within the breast tissue. The cysts are benign and become tender immediately prior to menstruation. Fibrocystic breast disease is the most common breast disorder in women. Other symptoms include aching and burning within the breast. Symptoms normally disappear after menstruation is over. Although benign, fibrocystic breast disease increases a patient's risk for breast cancer later in life.

CLINICAL SCENARIOS

Scenario One

A 65-year-old female is seen by a therapist 24 hours after total mastectomy. The patient was active prior to the surgery and walked for exercise two miles every day. The patient's past medical history is positive for fibrocystic breast disease, diabetes mellitus, and skin cancer. The patient reports pain with coughing. The patient resides alone in a retirement village and lost her husband to cancer last year. She has three supportive children that reside in the local area.

Scenario Two

A 45-year-old female is referred to outpatient physical therapy with lymphedema secondary to stage III breast cancer and radical mastectomy three months ago. The patient is fatigued and anxious about the increased size of her arm and limitation in range of motion. The patient runs a daycare center out of her home and is active in her church. Past medical history includes endometriosis and pharmacological treatment for depression.

Burn - Full-Thickness

DIAGNOSIS

What condition produces a patient's symptoms?

Full-thickness burns can be caused by thermal (fire, hot fluids, steam), chemical (acid, alkalis, vesicants) or electrical (lightning, high voltage, faulty wiring) agents. This severe burn causes immediate cellular and tissue death and subsequent vascular destruction. The patient will experience primary and secondary symptoms secondary to the extent and area of injury.

An injury was most likely sustained to which structure?

A full-thickness burn indicates complete destruction of the epidermis, dermis, hair follicle, and nerve endings within the dermis; and also affects the subcutaneous fat layer and underlying muscles, resulting in red blood cell destruction. There is irreversible damage sustained to all epithelial elements.

INFERENCE

What is the most likely contributing factor in the development of this condition?

The National Burn Information Exchange indicates that 75% of burns are a direct result of the patient's actions. There are approximately two million individuals burned annually with 70,000 hospitalized and 6,000-7,000 deaths. There is higher risk for burns in children between one and five years of age as well as individuals over 70 years of age. Burns are currently the third leading cause of accidental death in all age categories with males having a higher overall frequency of injury.

CONFIRMATION

What is the most likely clinical presentation?

A full-thickness burn is characterized by a variable appearance of deep red, black or white coloring. Eschar forms from necrotic cells and creates a dry and hard layer that requires debridement. Edema is present at the site of injury and in surrounding tissues. Hairs within the region of the burn are easily pulled from the follicle due to the destruction. An area of full-thickness burn does not have sensation or pain due to destruction of free nerve endings, however, there may be pain from adjacent areas that experience partial-thickness burns. During the initial stages the patient will experience thermoregulation impairment, shortness of breath, electrolyte disturbances, poor urine output, and variation in level of consciousness.

What laboratory or imaging studies would confirm the diagnosis?

Blood work should include a complete blood count, electrolytes, blood urea nitrogen, creatinine, bilirubin, and arterial blood gases. This will indicate baseline data, systemic changes, level of shock, and metabolic complications. Bronchoscopy and pulmonary function tests may be indicated to assess airway damage and pulmonary insufficiency.

What additional information should be obtained to confirm the diagnosis?

Diagnosis is primarily based on observation and assessment regarding the extent and depth of the burn. The rule of nines and the Lund-Browder charts grossly approximate the percentage of the body affected by a burn.

EXAMINATION

What history should be documented?

Important areas to explore include past medical history, mechanism of injury, medications, family history, type and percentage of burn, current symptoms and health status, social history and habits, occupation, leisure activities, and social support system.

What tests/measures are most appropriate?

Aerobic capacity and endurance: assessment of vital signs, perceived exertion scale, pulse oximetry

Anthropometric characteristics: circumferential measurements of affected areas

Arousal, attention, and cognition: examine mental status, learning ability, memory, motivation

Cranial nerve integrity: dermatome assessment

Gait, locomotion, and balance: static and dynamic balance in sitting and standing

Integumentary integrity: sensation assessment, assessment of burn, size, color, eschar, hair follicle integrity, wound mapping

Joint integrity and mobility: assessment of contracture, hypomobility of joints, soft tissue swelling

Muscle performance: strength and tone assessment

Pain: pain perception assessment scale, visual analogue scale to the area of the burn and surrounding tissues

Posture: analysis of resting and dynamic posture

Range of motion: active and passive range of motion

Reflex integrity: assessment of deep tendon and pathological reflexes (e.g., Babinski, ATNR)

Self-care and home management: functional capacity, Functional Independence Measure (FIM)

Ventilation, respiration, and circulation: cough and clearance of secretions, auscultation of the lungs, breathing patterns, respiratory muscle strength, accessory muscle utilization, vital capacity, pulse oximetry and palpation, pulmonary function testing

Burn - Full-Thickness

What additional findings are likely with this patient?

A patient with a full-thickness burn will present with multiple secondary effects based on the mechanism of the burn, size of the burn, and location of the burn. Infection, hypertrophic scarring, and contractures are the most common complications. Other secondary damage may include impairments of the cardiovascular system, renal system, gastrointestinal system, respiratory system and/or immune system. Damage to these vital areas can result in metabolic disorders, acidosis, sepsis, and dehydration.

MANAGEMENT

What is the most effective management of this patient?

The initial management includes medically stabilizing the patient followed by a full assessment of primary and secondary damage. This emergent phase lasts 48-72 hours and concludes with regaining capillary permeability and hemodynamic stability. An autograft procedure is usually required for full-thickness burns. The rehabilitation phase is a long-term commitment that includes all aspects of functional recovery. Physical therapy intervention begins immediately following skin grafting and includes wound care, pulmonary exercises, positioning, splinting, and immobilization for the first three to five days. A therapist will also provide education regarding skin care, positioning, and contracture prevention. Early ambulation and mobility activities should be incorporated as soon as possible in order to decrease complications such as atelectasis, pneumonia, and contracture. Continued physical therapy management will involve edema control, monitoring of any elastic garments, massage, stretching, hydrotherapy, ROM, debridement, relaxation techniques, progressive exercise, ambulation, and functional mobility training.

What home care regimen should be recommended?

A patient must continue with the established splinting and positioning schedule at home. Physical therapy may initially be warranted for continued pulmonary management, stretching, and functional mobility. A home program is vital to the patient's continued success and should include strengthening exercises, massage, scar management, positioning, and stretching. As the patient progresses, participation in wound management, activities of daily living, and functional activities should be incorporated into the daily routine.

OUTCOME

What is the likely outcome of a course in physical therapy?

Patient outcome is dependent on location, extent, and secondary complications of the burn. Physical therapy will provide the patient with education for an ongoing therapeutic program. Therapeutic exercise, stretching, compression garments, and other modalities will enhance the probability of a positive outcome.

What are the long-term effects of the patient's condition?

The mortality rate has decreased over the last two decades due to improvement in burn care, prevention of infection, and advances in grafting procedures. Mortality rates are highest for children under four and adults over 65 years of age. Overall prognosis is dependent on factors such as cardiac pathology, alcoholism, peripheral vascular disease, and obesity. Other factors that also require consideration are depression, social and emotional shock, and level of difficulty reintegrating into a daily routine (with employment, spouse, children, community). Long-term outcome is also based on the extent of secondary effects such as scarring and contractures. Garments may be worn up to two years after injury. Without significant complications a patient should achieve independence within a few months post injury.

COMPARISON

What are the distinguishing characteristics of a similar condition?

A superficial partial-thickness burn damages the epidermis and the papillary layer of the dermis (the dermis remains largely intact). This burn presents with blister formation, bright red coloring, intact blanching, moderate edema, and pain. The burn will heal without surgical intervention within 5-21 days with minimal to no scarring noted.

CLINICAL SCENARIOS

Scenario One

A 32-year-old female six weeks status post full-thickness burns to 50% of her right arm and 70% of her right leg is referred to physical therapy. She wears compression garments and has decreased range of motion. She resides alone in a two-story home and is employed as a cook.

Scenario Two

A three-year-old boy is referred to physical therapy 48 hours after an autograft for a full-thickness burn on the left side of his thorax. The chart review notes the mechanism of injury as pulling a cup of coffee off a table. Other medical history includes developmental delay, seizures, and hydrocephaly.

DIAGNOSIS

What condition produces a patient's symptoms?

Partial-thickness burns can be caused by thermal (e.g., fire, hot fluid, steam), chemical (e.g., acid, alkali, vesicant) or electrical (e.g., lightning, high voltage, faulty wiring) agents. They are differentiated as superficial partial-thickness and deep partial-thickness burns based on the depth of tissue destruction. The area and extent of the injury determine the primary and secondary symptoms experienced by the patient.

An injury was most likely sustained to which structure?

A superficial partial-thickness burn involves the epidermis and the upper portion of the dermis. Free nerve endings are exposed making this depth of burn extremely painful. A deep partial-thickness burn involves complete destruction of the epidermis, the majority of the dermis, and the structures within the dermis (e.g., hair follicles, sebaceous glands, sweat glands). As a result of damage to nerve endings, there is less pain than would be associated with a superficial partial-thickness burn. Irreversible epithelial damage is sustained with a deep partial-thickness burn which may result in hypertrophic or keloid scarring.

INFERENCE

What is the most likely contributing factor in the development of this condition?

The National Burn Information Exchange indicates that 75% of burns are a direct result of the patient's actions. There is a higher risk for burns in children between one and five years of age as well as individuals over 70 years of age. Burns are currently the third leading cause of accidental death in all age categories with males having a higher overall frequency of injury.

CONFIRMATION

What is the most likely clinical presentation?

A superficial partial-thickness burn is characterized by a red color that will blanch when touched and then return to red indicating that capillary refill is intact. Blisters and superficial moisture are typically present with hair follicles remaining intact. The preservation of deeper dermal tissues will allow for epithelial regeneration during healing. A deep partial-thickness burn is also characterized by red discoloration, however, when touched it will not blanch. This indicates the absence of capillary refill and damage to deeper blood vessels. Edema typically accumulates between the epidermal and dermal layers. Cellular necrosis is typical, especially in the upper dermal layer. Healing occurs either with scar tissue formation or grafting.

What laboratory or imaging studies would confirm the diagnosis?

Diagnosis of a partial thickness-burn is typically based on a physical examination. Depending on the total area burned and the depth of damage, the burn may still be considered quite severe. In this case, blood work (e.g., complete blood count, electrolytes, blood urea nitrogen, arterial blood gases) may be indicated to establish baseline data, systemic changes, level of shock, and metabolic complications. Bronchoscopy and pulmonary function tests may be indicated to assess airway damage and pulmonary insufficiency.

What additional information should be obtained to confirm the diagnosis?

Diagnosis is primarily based on observation and assessment regarding the extent and depth of the burn. The rule of nines and the Lund-Browder charts grossly approximate the percentage of the body affected by the burn. Prognostic burn indices provide a more thorough evaluative tool to assist caregivers in the prediction of medical attention needs, outcomes, and mortality by taking into account both the surface area burned and the severity of burns.

EXAMINATION

What history should be documented?

Important areas to explore include past medical history, medications, family history, current symptoms, current health status, social history and habits, occupation, leisure activities, and social support system.

What tests/measures are most appropriate?

Aerobic capacity and endurance: assessment of vital signs, perceived exertion scale, pulse oximetry

Anthropometric characteristics: circumferential measurements of affected areas

Arousal, attention, and cognition: examine mental status, learning ability, memory, and motivation

Cranial nerve integrity: dermatome assessment

Gait, locomotion, and balance: static and dynamic balance in sitting and standing

Integumentary integrity: sensation assessment, assessment of burn size, color, hair follicle integrity, surface characteristics (e.g., blisters), wound mapping

Joint integrity and mobility: assessment of contracture, joint hypomobility, soft tissue swelling

Muscle performance: strength and tone assessment

Pain: pain perception assessment scale, visual analogue scale for the burn and surrounding tissues

Posture: analysis of resting and dynamic posture

Range of motion: active and passive range of motion

Reflex integrity: assessment of deep tendon and pathological reflexes (e.g., Babinski, ATNR)

Self-care and home management: assessment of functional capacity, Functional Independence Measure (FIM), Barthel ADL Index

Ventilation, respiration, and circulation: assessment of cough and clearance of secretions, breathing patterns, respiratory muscle strength, accessory muscle utilization and vital capacity, pulse oximetry, palpation of pulses, pulmonary function testing, auscultation of the lungs

Burn - Partial-Thickness   GOLD

What additional findings are likely with this patient?

Partial-thickness burns may present with secondary effects based on the mechanism of the burn, the overall size, and the location of the burn. Infection, hypertrophic scarring, and contracture may occur with deep partial-thickness burns, but are not typically associated with superficial partial-thickness burns.

MANAGEMENT

What is the most effective management of this patient?

Medical management of a partial-thickness burn begins with a full assessment of primary and secondary damage. Since the dermis is not fully destroyed, the patient is typically able to maintain hemodynamic stability even with large areas affected. A superficial partial-thickness burn will typically re-epithelialize with little to no scarring within five to twenty-one days, though larger areas may require a longer period even with a normal healing progression. Management primarily involves protection of the damaged area and maintenance of an appropriate moisture balance with the use of specialized dressings and topical agents. Medical follow-up is not typically required unless the patient develops complications such as an infection. No additional consults, including physical therapy, are indicated. A deep partial-thickness burn will typically heal through the formation of scar tissue although in some cases may require grafting. Uncomplicated healing will typically occur within twenty-one to thirty-five days. Like superficial partial-thickness burns, tissue protection and maintenance of an appropriate moisture balance are emphasized and supported with the use of specialized dressings. A surgical consult may be indicated to determine if a skin graft is necessary. Physical therapy may be indicated to assist in preventing hypertrophic or keloid scarring and contractures if the burns include joint involvement. Physical therapy intervention may include edema management, splinting and positioning, scar mobilization techniques, massage, range of motion, stretching, dressing management, wound care, monitoring elastic garment use, and functional mobility training.

What home care regimen should be recommended?

A patient should continue with any established wound management, splinting, positioning, massage, exercise, and scar management techniques at home. This is especially important for patients with deep partial-thickness burns due to the increased likelihood of infection, scarring, and contractures. As the patient progresses, normal activities of daily living and functional activities should be resumed.

OUTCOME

What is the likely outcome of a course of physical therapy?

Physical therapy is not typically indicated for a patient with a superficial partial thickness wound. A patient with a deep partial-thickness wound may benefit from physical therapy to address wound and edema management and prevent the formation of hypertrophic or keloid scarring.

What are the long-term effects of the patient's condition?

Both types of partial-thickness burns will typically heal without residual deficits in the absence of infection or other factors that may complicate or delay healing (e.g., smoking, diabetes mellitus). A full functional return is expected.

COMPARISON

What are the distinguishing characteristics of a similar condition?

A subdermal burn is typically severe and life-threatening, involving the complete destruction of the epidermis, dermis, subcutaneous tissue, and larger blood vessels. The burned tissue has a charred appearance and is not painful due to the complete destruction of local nerve fibers. A subdermal burn may involve muscle and bone and as a result is highly susceptible to infection and other healing complications. Multiple surgical interventions (e.g., debridement, grafting) are typically required and associated with extensive healing times.

CLINICAL SCENARIOS

Scenario One

A 22-year-old female sunburns a large percentage of her body during a beach vacation. She reports significant skin discomfort and pain with even light palpation. Blisters have formed on her upper chest and forearms due to the extent of the sun damage. She is a college student who resides in student housing.

Scenario Two

A 43-year-old-male is referred to physical therapy for wound management. During a motorcycle accident he sustained a deep partial-thickness burn to his posterior-medial ankle from the tailpipe. His gait is antalgic and the physical therapist assistant observes both dorsiflexion and plantar flexion range of motion limitations at the ankle. The patient resides with his wife and two children and is employed as a lineman for a phone company.

Diabetes Mellitus - Type 1

DIAGNOSIS

What condition produces a patient's symptoms?

Type 1 diabetes mellitus (DM) is a multi-system disease with both biochemical and anatomical consequences. There is persistent hyperglycemia due to diminished or absent production of insulin. In type 1 DM, insulin is functionally absent due to the destruction of the beta cells of the pancreas where the insulin would normally be produced.

An injury was most likely sustained to which structure?

Type 1 DM is characterized as an autoimmune disease in which circulating insulin is very low or absent, plasma glucose is elevated, and the pancreatic beta cells fail to respond to all insulin producing stimuli. The pancreas shows lymphocytic infiltration and destruction of insulin-secreting cells of the islets of Langerhans, causing insulin deficiency. Patients need exogenous insulin to reverse this catabolic condition, prevent ketosis, decrease hyperglycemia, and normalize lipid and protein metabolism.

INFERENCE

What is the most likely contributing factor in the development of this condition?

The exact etiology of type 1 DM is unknown, however, there are several theories. It is an autoimmune process with a strong genetic component. It is also believed that the genetic predisposition in combination with an unknown factor, potentially environmental, triggers the ongoing cycle of destruction of the beta cells of the pancreas.

CONFIRMATION

What is the most likely clinical presentation?

Type 1 DM usually starts in children ages 4 years or older, with the peak incidence of onset at 11-13 years of age, coinciding with early adolescence and puberty. Also, a relatively high incidence exists in people in their late 30s and early 40s, when it tends to present in a less aggressive manner. The most common symptoms of type 1 DM are polyuria, polydipsia, and polyphagia, along with nausea, weight loss, fatigue, blurred vision, and dehydration. A fasting glucose reading of 126 mg/dl is also a sign of DM. The disease onset is usually sudden or within a short period of time. It is not unusual for type 1 DM to present with ketoacidosis.

What laboratory or imaging studies would confirm the diagnosis?

A test of blood glucose levels will be necessary. In asymptomatic patients, physicians use the American Diabetes Association (ADA) recommendation of two different fasting plasma glucose levels of greater than 125 mg/dl. In symptomatic patients, a random glucose of 200 mg/dl suggests DM. Other testing includes urinalysis for glucose, ketones, and protein and a white blood cell count as well as blood and urine cultures to rule out infection.

What additional information should be obtained to confirm the diagnosis?

A detailed history and exam should provide the physician with confirmation of the previously mentioned symptoms that present with type 1 DM. Diagnosis is based on one of the subsequent factors: fasting glucose levels, two-hour post-load glucose levels or symptoms of DM.

EXAMINATION

What history should be documented?

Important areas to explore include past medical history, medications, current health status, history of incontinence, recent polyuria, polydipsia, nocturia or weight loss, nutritional status, social history and habits, occupation, living environment, and social support system.

What tests/measures are most appropriate?

Arousal, attention, and cognition: examine mental status, learning ability, memory, motivation

Community and work integration: analysis of community, work, and leisure activities

Environmental, home, and work barriers: analysis of current and potential barriers or hazards

Gait, locomotion, and balance: static and dynamic balance in sitting and standing, safety during gait

Integumentary integrity: skin assessment, assessment of sensation

Motor function: equilibrium and righting reactions, coordination, posture and balance in sitting

Muscle performance: strength assessment, muscle tone assessment

Posture: analysis of resting and dynamic posture

Range of motion: active and passive range of motion

Self-care and home management: assessment of functional capacity, Functional Independence Measure

What additional findings are likely with this patient?

Complications of type 1 DM include hypoglycemia and hyperglycemia, diabetic ketoacidosis, increased risk of infections, cardiovascular and peripheral vascular disease, retinopathy, nephropathy, impotence, and acceleration of atherosclerosis. DM is the major cause of blindness in adults aged 20-74 years, as well as the leading cause of non-traumatic lower extremity amputation and end-stage renal disease.

MANAGEMENT

What is the most effective management of this patient?

Patients with type 1 DM require insulin therapy to control initial hyperglycemia and maintain serum electrolytes and hydration. At times, the first incidence of ketoacidosis is followed by a symptom-free period where patients do not need treatment. Pharmacological intervention includes the use of exogenous insulin per physician orders. Type 1 DM typically requires insulin delivery subcutaneously via continuous pump or self-administered injection. Supplemental insulin may also be delivered by oral or nasal route. Medical management should also include regular self-monitoring of blood glucose levels through finger stick samples and urine testing. Patient education and counseling is appropriate for nutritional components, weight loss if obese, the disease process, complications, medications, and long-term effects. Physical therapy may be indicated for a home exercise program and the patient may be seen intermittently for change and update of their program. Exercise is an important aspect in management of DM. Patients should be taught general exercise and strengthening, stretching, and self-monitoring of their cardiac status. The therapist should coordinate exercise sessions around the patient's meal schedule in order to avoid hypoglycemia and optimize exercise tolerance. Patients should exercise at 50-60% of their predicted maximum heart rate unless directed by a physician otherwise.

What home care regimen should be recommended?

A patient with type 1 DM requires a good nutritional program, regular self-monitoring of blood glucose levels, and adequate and consistent daily exercise.

OUTCOME

What is the likely outcome of a course in physical therapy?

Type 1 DM is the most common metabolic disease of childhood, with a yearly incidence of 15 cases per 100,000 people less than 18 years of age. Approximately one million Americans have type 1 DM, and physicians diagnose 10,000 new cases every year. Physical therapy may be indicated initially for a patient with goals of optimizing exercise endurance and implementing a home exercise program. Otherwise, patients are usually seen in physical therapy for co-morbidities or due to complications from DM. Physical therapy attempts to maximize patients' functional and health status, but cannot alter the disease process.

What are the long-term effects of the patient's condition?

Type 1 DM is associated with a high morbidity and premature mortality due to complications. As a result of these complications, people with diabetes have an increased risk of developing ischemic heart disease, cerebral vascular disease, peripheral vascular disease (that sometimes leads to amputation), chronic renal disease, reduced visual acuity and blindness, and autonomic and peripheral neuropathy.

COMPARISON

What are the distinguishing characteristics of a similar condition?

Type 2 DM is more common in the United States than type 1. Type 2 usually involves a defect in the insulin release sites within the pancreas or a resistance to the insulin due to impairment of the receptor sites in the peripheral tissues. In contrast to type 1, type 2 is usually diagnosed in a patient older than 40 years of age. This form of DM is significantly linked to a person's lifestyle, weight, and age. A patient with type 2 can present with the symptoms of type 1, but can also include paresthesias, visual changes, recurrent infections, inadequate wound healing, and cold extremities. In most cases, oral hypoglycemics are used instead of insulin injections.

CLINICAL SCENARIOS

Scenario One

A three-year-old girl is seen in physical therapy that has just been diagnosed with type 1 DM. She also has a greenstick fracture of the left tibia secondary to an auto accident, but otherwise is in good health. Her mother has stated that her blood sugar levels were not yet regulated and it has been difficult for the physician to find the correct amount and timing of insulin.

Scenario Two

A 35-year-old male was just diagnosed with type 1 DM after he visited his physician for a routine check-up. He did note polyuria, polydipsia, and visual changes over the last six months. He is referred to physical therapy for a home exercise program. The physician also recommended a nutritional consult as the patient is approximately 40 pounds overweight.

Diabetes Mellitus - Type 2

DIAGNOSIS

What condition produces a patient's symptoms?

Type 2 diabetes mellitus (DM) is a chronic disease with biochemical and anatomical consequences. Normally, insulin facilitates the absorption of glucose from the bloodstream into liver, fat, and muscle cells where it may be used immediately or stored for energy. Type 2 DM is characterized by an inappropriate cellular response to insulin, preventing adequate absorption of blood glucose. Excess blood glucose results in a persistent hyperglycemic state.

An injury was most likely sustained to which structure?

Type 2 DM is characterized by an alteration in the metabolism of glucose. This is typically due to either an inadequate supply or cellular resistance to insulin. Excess body fat interferes with the body's ability to metabolize insulin correctly and is often a key characteristic of type 2 DM. Decreased insulin production and the insulin resistance that may accompany it, may result from factors including stress, advanced age, sedentary lifestyle, comorbidities, and certain prescribed medications.

INFERENCE

What is the most likely contributing factor in the development of this condition?

Patients with a family history of type 2 DM, who are over 45 years of age or who are of African, Asian, Hispanic or American Indian descent are at increased risk for developing type 2 DM. Patients who are overweight, sedentary, pre-diabetic or had gestational diabetes are also at increased risk.

CONFIRMATION

What is the most likely clinical presentation?

Type 2 DM may develop slowly over time prior to manifestation of initial symptoms. Common symptoms include polydipsia, polyuria, blurred vision, delayed healing and frequent infections. Type 2 DM was formerly referred to as "adult onset diabetes mellitus," however, there has been a statistically significant rise in the incidence of type 2 DM in patients between 10 and 19 years of age over the last two decades. This is largely attributed to increasingly sedentary habits among adolescents and epidemic childhood obesity.

What laboratory or imaging studies would confirm the diagnosis?

A diagnosis of type 2 DM is based on blood glucose measures. The glycated hemoglobin (A1C) test measures the average blood glucose level over a two to three month period and is typically used to confirm the diagnosis. A random blood glucose measure of 200 mg/dL or higher is suggestive of DM. Fasting blood glucose measures greater than 125 mg/dL on two separate tests is considered to be indicative of DM. The rate of blood glucose metabolism may be more specifically assessed with an oral glucose tolerance test.

What additional information should be obtained to confirm the diagnosis?

A thorough history and examination should be performed to confirm relevant risk factors and rule out similar diagnoses.

EXAMINATION

What history should be documented?

Important areas to explore include past medical history, medications, current health status, history of incontinence, recent polyuria, polydipsia, nocturia, nutritional status, social history and habits, occupation, living environment, and social support system.

What tests/measures are most appropriate?

Arousal, attention, and cognition: examine mental status, learning ability, memory, motivation
Community and work integration: analysis of community, work, and leisure activities
Environmental, home, and work barriers: analysis of current and potential barriers or hazards
Gait, locomotion, and balance: static and dynamic balance in sitting and standing, safety during gait
Integumentary integrity: skin assessment, assessment of sensation
Motor function: equilibrium and righting reactions, coordination, posture and balance in sitting
Muscle performance: strength assessment, muscle tone assessment
Posture: analysis of resting and dynamic posture
Range of motion: active and passive range of motion
Self-care and home management: assessment of functional capacity, Functional Independence Measure

What additional findings are likely with this patient?

Complications of type 2 DM include hypoglycemia and hyperglycemia, increased risk of infections, cardiovascular and peripheral vascular disease, retinopathy, nephropathy, impotence, and acceleration of atherosclerosis. DM is the major cause of blindness in adults aged 20-74 years, as well as the leading cause of nontraumatic lower extremity amputation and end-stage renal disease.

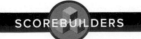

MANAGEMENT

What is the most effective management of this patient?

Medical management is typically focused on lifestyle changes and pharmaceutical intervention. Patient education and counseling are appropriate to address the disease process, nutrition, and long-term effects. Many patients are able to manage type 2 DM through lifestyle changes that impact modifiable risk factors. Increased physical activity increases insulin sensitivity, assisting cells to better absorb and utilize blood glucose as an appropriate source of energy. Stress management is also an important focus as prolonged stress can impact the body's ability to properly produce and metabolize insulin. Various oral or injectable pharmacological agents may be prescribed depending on individual factors. Patients should be instructed in general exercise, including strengthening and stretching activities. Education should address common signs and symptoms of hyperglycemia or hypoglycemia, foot care, susceptibility to infection, and the potential for delayed healing.

What home care regimen should be recommended?

A home care regimen should emphasize management of modifiable risk factors including nutrition, exercise, stress management, and self-monitoring for complications such as neuropathy, hyperglycemia, and hypoglycemia.

OUTCOME

What is the likely outcome of a course of physical therapy?

Physical therapy may be indicated initially to assist patients in optimizing outcomes relating to weight management, increasing activity levels, and stress management goals. Physical therapy should maximize function and support management of the condition. More commonly, patients are treated for comorbidities or complications that result from poor management of type 2 DM.

What are the long-term effects of the patient's condition?

In the United States, DM is the leading cause of kidney failure, new cases of blindness, and non-traumatic lower extremity amputation in adults. Type 2 DM accounts for greater than 90% of all DM cases diagnosed and is one of the conditions included in the diagnostic criteria for metabolic syndrome. Patients with type 2 DM are at an increased risk of developing numerous systemic comorbidities such as neuropathy, kidney damage, osteoporosis, and cardiac and vessel disease.

COMPARISON

What are the distinguishing characteristics of a similar condition?

Type 1 DM is less common in the United States than type 2. Type 1 is caused by a diminished or absent production of insulin due to destruction of the beta cells within the pancreas. In contrast to type 2, type 1 is typically diagnosed in adolescence, though some patients are diagnosed in adulthood (i.e., 30s to 40s). Though the exact etiology is unknown, it is thought to be an autoimmune condition that has both genetic and environmental influences. Signs and symptoms between the two conditions are similar, though a patient with type 1 DM is far more likely to experience diabetic ketoacidosis. Because patients with type 1 DM do not produce insulin, they require exogenous insulin, which is usually administered via self-injections.

CLINICAL SCENARIOS

Scenario One

A 65-year-old male with type 2 DM is being seen in physical therapy for balance training. Examination reveals that the patient has decreased protective sensation on the plantar surface of both feet and an inability to maintain static stance with his eyes closed. The patient's gait is slow and cautious and characterized by decreased step length.

Scenario Two

A 70-year-old female with type 2 DM is being seen in physical therapy for gait training with a new prosthesis. The patient had a transtibial amputation ten weeks ago and is just beginning to ambulate with a single point cane. The patient admits that they are not compliant with taking their medications or controlling their blood glucose levels.

DIAGNOSIS

What condition produces a patient's symptoms?

Fibromyalgia syndrome (FMS) is classified as a rheumatology syndrome or a nonarticular rheumatic condition. Pain is the primary symptom caused by tender points within muscles, tendons, and ligaments.

An injury was most likely sustained to which structure?

The exact etiology of FMS is unknown. Theories suggest potential biochemical, metabolic or immunologic pathology. Researchers believe it to be multifactorial in origin and suggest a link to a dysfunction within the stress system, autonomic nervous system, immune system and/or reproductive and hormone systems.

INFERENCE

What is the most likely contributing factor in the development of this condition?

Since the exact etiology of FMS is unknown there is speculation linking many factors to the development of this condition. Factors include diet, sleep disorders, viral infections, psychological distress, occupational and environmental factors, hypothyroidism, trauma, and potential hereditary links. Many individuals diagnosed with FMS note multiple causative factors, however, there are individuals diagnosed with FMS that possess none of the theorized causative factors.

CONFIRMATION

What is the most likely clinical presentation?

The American College of Rheumatology's data indicates that there are approximately six million individuals living with FMS, making it the most common musculoskeletal disorder in the United States. FMS has a greater incidence in females (almost 75% of the cases) and can affect any age, but most frequently is diagnosed between 14 and 68 years of age. FMS is diagnosed when a patient exhibits the criteria authored by the American College of Rheumatology. There is a widespread history of pain that exists in all four quadrants of the body (above and below the waist). The patient may also complain of fatigue, memory and visual impairment, sleep disturbances, irritable bowel syndrome, headaches, and anxiety/depression.

What laboratory or imaging studies would confirm the diagnosis?

FMS has been commonly misdiagnosed as myofascial pain, systemic lupus erythematosus, fibrositis, and chronic fatigue syndrome. There are no specific tests used to diagnose FMS. Radiographs are negative and blood work often appears normal except for a possible alteration in the levels of substance P. This substance is a chemical involved with pain transmission. Image studies and other lab testing are performed only for differential diagnosis.

What additional information should be obtained to confirm the diagnosis?

FMS is diagnosed according to the criteria from the American College of Rheumatology. A dolorimeter is used for reliability when testing the tender points by providing a consistent pressure (4 kg/cm^2). If the patient meets the criteria and has experienced symptoms for greater than three months, then a patient may be diagnosed with FMS. Diagnostic written tools that can assist with diagnosis include the Beck Depression Inventory and the Fibromyalgia Impact Questionnaire.

EXAMINATION

What history should be documented?

Important areas to explore include past medical history, medications, family history, current symptoms, current health status, social history and habits, occupation, leisure activities, and social support system.

What tests/measures are most appropriate?

Aerobic capacity and endurance: assessment of vital signs at rest and with activity, perceived exertion scale, pulse oximetry, auscultation of the lungs

Arousal, attention, and cognition: examine mental status, learning ability, memory, motivation

Community and work integration: analysis of community, work, and leisure activities

Environmental, home, and work barriers: analysis of current and potential barriers or hazards

Ergonomics and body mechanics: analysis of dexterity and coordination

Gait, locomotion, and balance: static and dynamic balance in sitting and standing, safety during gait

Integumentary integrity: skin assessment, assessment of sensation

Joint integrity and mobility: assessment of hypermobility and hypomobility of a joint, effusion, edema

Muscle performance: strength assessment, muscle tone assessment

Neuromotor development and sensory integration: analysis of reflex movement patterns, assessment of involuntary movements, sensory integration tests, gross and fine motor skills

Pain: pain perception assessment scale, visual analogue scale, assessment of muscle soreness and tender points

Posture: analysis of resting and dynamic posture

Range of motion: active and passive range of motion

Self-care and home management: assessment of functional capacity

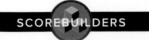

What additional findings are likely with this patient?

The aforementioned symptoms can progress over time. Certain symptoms intensify and cause the patient to lose functional independence secondary to increased pain, decreased range of motion, and severe fatigue.

MANAGEMENT

What is the most effective management of this patient?

FMS is best treated with a multidisciplinary approach including education, medical management, and exercise. Medical management will attempt to normalize various dysfunctions of the autonomic nervous system, hormonal imbalances, and metabolic abnormalities. Physicians must address sleep disorders (which can be common) and pharmacological intervention based on symptoms. Psychotherapy may be warranted for anxiety or depression and must incorporate stress management and coping strategies into the plan of care. Physical therapy intervention may include relaxation techniques, energy conservation, gentle stretching, moist heat, ultrasound, posture and body mechanics, biofeedback, and exercise to tolerance. Aquatic therapy is recommended to improve a patient's fitness level and an ergonomic evaluation should be performed at the patient's work place. This population should not work through pain. They require short exercise sessions initially (three to five minutes) due to a low tolerance for exertion.

What home care regimen should be recommended?

A home care regimen should include short duration exercise, aquatic therapy (if indicated), energy conservation strategies, the use of proper positioning, proper body mechanics, and gentle stretching. Patient education is the key to success. Exercises that strain muscles such as weight lifting should be avoided. A comprehensive plan should also include lifestyle management, nutritional support, and stress management.

OUTCOME

What is the likely outcome of a course in physical therapy?

A patient with FMS may benefit from multidisciplinary intervention. Patient compliance with a home program increases the overall success rate. In many cases, symptoms can remain unchanged even with intervention and patient compliance. Some patients will report improvement in areas of fatigue, sleep, and self-reported pain.

What are the long-term effects of the patient's condition?

FMS is presently not "curable." Many patients that have mild symptoms do not require multidisciplinary intervention and have a good long-term outcome. The majority of patients diagnosed with FMS exhibit moderate levels of symptoms and usually continue to experience these symptoms for years or even their entire lifetime.

COMPARISON

What are the distinguishing characteristics of a similar condition?

Myofascial pain syndrome (MPS) is often misdiagnosed for FMS. MPS is characterized by trigger points rather than tender points and lacks associated symptoms. MPS is a localized musculoskeletal condition that is specific to a muscle. FMS, on the other hand, is a systemic condition. MPS is usually caused by overuse, reduced muscle activity or repetitive motions.

CLINICAL SCENARIOS

Scenario One

A 32-year-old female recently diagnosed with FMS is seen in physical therapy. Her chief complaints are fatigue, pain throughout her body, and difficulty with sleeping which has affected her employment as a mail carrier. She has been on disability for the last six months and under a physician's care for depression.

Scenario Two

A 45-year-old construction worker is referred to physical therapy with diagnosis of FMS. His history reveals mild symptoms for the last year. He has seen specialists and was diagnosed last week by a rheumatologist. He exhibits tender points throughout his body and denies any sleep disturbances or other medical history. He is currently working and appears motivated for therapy.

Lymphedema Post-Mastectomy

DIAGNOSIS

What condition produces a patient's symptoms?

Lymphedema following a mastectomy is termed secondary lymphedema and is the result of damage to the lymphatic nodes and vessels during surgery. Excessive accumulation of lymph fluid within the soft tissues is caused by an excess load of lymph fluid or inadequate transport capacity within the lymphatic system secondary to the loss of homeostasis.

An injury was most likely sustained to which structure?

The lymphatic system is damaged as a result of the mastectomy, the surgical removal of the breast, whereby the lymph nodes and vessels are removed or damaged. The lymphatic system is unable to compensate, the lymph vessels dilate, and the valve flaps are not able to fully stop lymph flow. This allows for backflow of lymph into the tissues. This chain reaction causes further injury, chronic inflammation and progression including fibrosis, hypoxia within the tissues, and an increased risk of infection.

INFERENCE

What is the most likely contributing factor in the development of this condition?

The most likely contributing factor in the development of lymphedema following a mastectomy is the damage and/or removal of the axillary lymph nodes and vessels in an attempt to prevent the spread of breast cancer. If the lymphatic nodes have not been removed, but have received radiation they may stop functioning due to chronic inflammation, fibrosis, and scarring. Globally, the parasitic infection called filariasis is the most common cause of secondary lymphedema. The virus is carried by mosquitoes in regions such as Africa, India, and Malaysia. Other causes include severe infection, crush injuries, burns or repeated pregnancies. There are an estimated three million new cases of secondary lymphedema each year with approximately 30% of breast cancer survivors affected by this condition. Primary lymphedema statistics indicate 15% of the cases are present at birth and 75% of the cases are acquired from adolescence through midlife years. Females are affected more than males with a 4:1 ratio.

CONFIRMATION

What is the most likely clinical presentation?

The clinical presentation of lymphedema includes edema in an affected area/extremity that increases with dependent positioning. The patient usually does not experience pain, but rather a tight or heavy sensation. Lymphedema is classified into three stages that present differently based on the severity of the condition. Stage I is characterized by pitting edema that reduces with elevation overnight and does not exhibit any fibrotic changes. Stage II is identified by some fibrotic changes that begin to occur and an increase in non-pitting edema that does not reduce with elevation. Stage III is characterized by skin changes, frequent infections, and severe edema that is non-pitting and fibrotic.

What laboratory or imaging studies would confirm the diagnosis?

Diagnosis is confirmed through history, observation, and several diagnostic tools to rule out other potential disorders. A Doppler study of the affected area is able to rule out a deep vein thrombosis. A CT scan or MRI may be performed before treatment of lymphedema is initiated to rule out malignancy. A lymphoscintigram is a nuclear medicine procedure that tests the function of the lymphatic system.

What additional information should be obtained to confirm the diagnosis?

A medical evaluation should include a thorough history including all illnesses, hospitalizations, and surgeries. History should be noted regarding the current edema and its course. Date of onset, progression, and symptoms associated with the edema are important to attain and note in the patient's record.

EXAMINATION

What history should be documented?

Important areas to explore include past medical history and surgical history, medications, history of swelling, family history, current symptoms, current health status, living environment, social history and habits, occupation, and social support system.

What tests/measures are most appropriate?

Aerobic capacity and endurance: assessment of vital signs at rest and with activity, perceived exertion scale, pulse oximetry, auscultation of the lungs

Anthropometric characteristics: circumferential and volumetric measurements of involved areas, skinfold measurements

Arousal, attention, and cognition: examine mental status, learning ability, memory, motivation

Community and work integration: analysis of community, work, and leisure activities

Environmental, home, and work barriers: analysis of current and potential barriers or hazards

Gait, locomotion, and balance: static and dynamic balance in sitting and standing, safety during gait with/without an assistive device

Integumentary integrity: skin assessment, assessment of sensation, nailbed assessment

Joint integrity and mobility: soft tissue swelling and inflammation

Muscle performance: strength and tone assessment

Pain: pain perception assessment scale

Range of motion: active and passive range of motion

Lymphedema Post-Mastectomy   GOLD

Self-care and home management: assessment of functional capacity

Ventilation, respiration, and circulation: assessment of brachial and radial pulses, capillary refill assessment

What additional findings are likely with this patient?

Additional findings are based on the etiology, stage, and progression of the lymphedema. Complications can include ulcer formation, increased risk for fungal and bacterial infections, loss of range, fatigue, and fibrotic edema with atrophic skin changes. If left untreated a patient could progress to stage III "lymphostatic elephantiasis."

MANAGEMENT

What is the most effective management of this patient?

Effective medical management of secondary lymphedema may involve pharmacological intervention or natural substances that increase proteolysis and macrophage activity, however, there is no particular class of drugs that can "cure" lymphedema. Surgery is used in the treatment of severe lymphedema, but only achieves limited results since the cause remains unchanged. Physical therapy intervention usually follows a treatment approach termed complete decongestive therapy (CDT). The philosophy of lymphatic management includes patient education in skin care, hygiene, bandaging, self-massage, and exercise. Therapeutic intervention should focus on manual lymph drainage, short stretch compression bandages, retrograde massage, and exercise.

What home care regimen should be recommended?

A home care regimen is vital to the success of the CDT treatment of lymphedema. A patient must understand and comply with skin care, bandaging, self-massage, lymphatic drainage techniques, compression therapy, and an exercise program. Each patient must also understand the lifetime precautions that can increase lymphedema such as sunburn, air travel, excessive exercise, poor nutrition, and obesity.

OUTCOME

What is the likely outcome of a course in physical therapy?

Comprehensive lymphedema intervention such as CDT has shown significant reduction in lymphedema during treatment and continued reduction with an ongoing home program over time.

What are the long-term effects of the patient's condition?

Lymphedema is progressive if left untreated, but can be managed through intervention and education. Patients must comply with a home program and must remain aware of all activities that place the patient at an increased risk for lymphedema.

COMPARISON

What are the distinguishing characteristics of a similar condition?

Lipedema is a condition where there appears to be swelling throughout the bilateral lower extremities from the hips to the ankle joints. This swelling is actually subcutaneous adipose tissue. This condition is sometimes confused with lymphedema, but does not affect the lymphatic system. It most often occurs in women with hormonal disorders and is believed to have a family history in approximately 20% of the cases. Medical management treats the hormonal imbalance and assists with nutritional guidance to allow for effective weight management.

CLINICAL SCENARIOS

Scenario One

A 39-year-old female status post right mastectomy secondary to malignancy develops lymphedema in her right arm four months after surgery. She resides alone and is employed as a web design consultant. She complains of heaviness in the arm, but denies pain. She was referred by her oncologist for outpatient physical therapy.

Scenario Two

A 68-year-old male is seen in physical therapy with stage II lymphedema in his right lower extremity. He underwent total hip arthroplasty two months ago and experienced immediate swelling and discomfort. His history includes multiple abdominal surgeries with edema present after each surgery. He presents with non-pitting edema that does not reduce with elevation.

DIAGNOSIS

What condition produces a patient's symptoms?

A neuropathic ulcer typically develops due to a combination of peripheral neuropathy, atherosclerotic changes, and pressure. Neuropathic ulcers occur most frequently in the diabetic population and are often referred to as diabetic ulcers. This form of ulcer may also develop in association with other peripheral neuropathy etiologies.

An injury was most likely sustained to which structure?

A neuropathic ulcer can affect various tissue structures based on the depth of injury. A superficial ulceration is associated with damage to the epidermis only. Damage from a partial-thickness ulceration will extend through the epidermis and possibly into, but not through the dermis. A full-thickness ulceration extends through the dermis and into deeper layers such as the subcutaneous fat layer. Damage from a subcutaneous ulcer extends through all layers of integumentary tissue typically exposing deeper tissue layers such as tendon, muscle or bone.

INFERENCE

What is the most likely contributing factor in the development of this condition?

Neuropathic ulcers are most prevalent among patients with diabetes mellitus. Peripheral neuropathy impacts both motor and sensory function which contributes to the development of neuropathic ulcers. Motor neuropathy, for example, may cause weakness of the intrinsic foot muscles allowing the forefoot to splay during weight bearing and altering the fit of footwear. Decreased coordination within the muscles of the lower leg, ankle, and foot further contributes to increased stress over bony prominences during weight bearing. The loss of protective sensation impairs the patient's ability to detect discomfort from these altered physical pressures and is often the most significant contributing factor to ulcer development.

CONFIRMATION

What is the most likely clinical presentation?

A patient will typically develop a neuropathic ulcer in the distal lower extremity. At-risk areas include those that are routinely subjected to pressure during normal weight bearing, atypical stresses due to structural changes or improper fitting footwear. Common sites include the heel, tips of prominent toes, tips of hammer toes, plantar surface of the metatarsal heads, dorsal aspect of hammer toes, and bunions. The wound typically presents with a well-defined oval or round shape surrounded by a rim of hypertrophic callus. The wound bed typically shows evidence of granular tissue with little evidence of necrosis. Exudate production is typically minimal. Pain complaints are minimal, however, dysesthesia may be reported. Surrounding intact skin tends to be shiny, dry, and inelastic. Distal pulses may be diminished or absent. Ankle-brachial index measures may be unreliable especially for patients with diabetes mellitus who are likely to develop vessel rigidity. The loss of protective sensation is a significant characteristic and should be well documented.

What laboratory or imaging studies would confirm the diagnosis?

A neuropathic ulcer is diagnosed primarily based on the physical characteristics of the ulcer and the diagnosis of underlying conditions. Laboratory blood analysis may be warranted to assist in identifying the etiology of the ulcer, ruling out infection, and identifying additional conditions which may impede wound healing. Imaging is typically utilized to determine vascular integrity, to rule out infection or to identify bony changes such as demineralization or deformity which may contribute to ulcer formation.

What additional information should be obtained to confirm the diagnosis?

A complete medical history should be obtained to assist in identifying conditions which may contribute to the development of an ulcer or impede ulcer healing. Both the ulcer and general condition of the extremities should be thoroughly examined. Testing to determine the extent of the peripheral neuropathy and potential vascular insufficiency should also be performed.

EXAMINATION

What history should be documented?

Important areas to explore include past medical history, medications, family history, current symptoms, current health status, social history and habits, occupation, leisure activities, and social support system.

What tests/measures are most appropriate?

Anthropometric characteristics: circumferential measurements

Arousal, attention, and cognition: mental status, learning ability, memory, motivation, and level of consciousness

Assistive and adaptive devices: analysis of components and safety of a device

Gait, locomotion, and balance: static and dynamic balance in sitting and standing, safety during gait with/without an assistive device

Integumentary integrity: skin assessment, assessment of sensation, Wagner Ulcer Grade Classification Scale, assessment of wound characteristics, exudate, surrounding skin, photo documentation

Joint integrity and mobility: assessment of hypermobility and hypomobility of a joint, swelling and inflammation

Muscle performance: strength assessment, muscle tone assessment, signs of muscle atrophy

Orthotic, prosthetic, and supportive devices: analysis of components of a device, analysis of movement while wearing a device

Pain: pain perception assessment scale, visual analogue scale

Range of motion: active and passive range of motion
Reflex integrity: assessment of deep tendon and pathological reflexes (e.g., Babinski, ATNR)
Self-care and home management: assessment of functional capacity
Sensory integrity: assessment of proprioception and kinesthesia, Semmes-Weinstein monofilament testing
Ventilation, respiration, and circulation: pulse oximetry, palpation of pulses, ankle-brachial index, capillary refill

What additional findings are likely with this patient?

Neuropathic ulcer staging is based on the extent of soft tissue and osseous involvement. Neuropathic ulcers which extend to bony surfaces are associated with a high risk of osteomyelitis. Physical examination is likely to reveal numerous abnormalities associated with peripheral neuropathy and arterial changes. Neuropathic ulcers are often slow to heal due to the systemic impact of the associated underlying conditions.

MANAGEMENT
What is the most effective management of this patient?

Medical management typically emphasizes management of contributing factors (e.g., blood glucose, hypertension, hyperlipidemia, obesity, atherosclerosis, renal insufficiency) through lifestyle modifications (e.g., dietary changes, stress management) and pharmaceutical intervention. Pharmaceutical interventions specifically directed toward wound management may include the use of platelet-derived growth factors (PDGF) or, in the presence of infection, antimicrobial or antibiotic agents. Activity restrictions, total contact casting or specialized footwear may be indicated to protect the extremity as the wound heals. Surgical management may include debridement for wounds with heavy necrosis, grafting for non-healing wounds, stabilization or revision of bony structures to reduce pressure points, and restoration of vascular integrity. Physical therapy management emphasizes skin protection through footwear assessment, moisturizers, skin inspection, and wound healing interventions. The ulcer may require cleansing agents and/or debridement (enzymatic, autolytic, mechanical non-selective or sharp) and should be closely monitored for signs of infection. Deep wounds or those with significant tunneling or tracts may specifically benefit from debridement by means of pulsatile lavage and packing may be indicated as a part of the dressing application. Neuropathic ulcers do not typically produce significant volumes of exudate, therefore, if a neuropathic ulcer begins to produce significant volumes of exudate, infection should be ruled out. If an infection is confirmed, the use of dressings impregnated with antimicrobial or antibiotic agents (e.g., silver or iodine) may be indicated. Dressings should be selected to appropriately manage the increased exudate and prevent maceration of adjacent tissue. For more severe wounds, healing interventions may also include vacuum-assisted closure or hyperbaric oxygen treatment. Photo documentation is recommended to supplement written documentation describing wound characteristics.

What home care regimen should be recommended?

The home care regimen is dependent on the size and characteristics of the neuropathic ulcer. Many patients who do not require debridement may appropriately manage routine dressing changes at home. All patients should be diligent with skin hygiene, protection, and inspection to limit the risk of infection and the formation of additional wounds.

OUTCOME
What is the likely outcome of a course of physical therapy?

A neuropathic ulcer will typically heal by secondary intention with appropriate wound healing interventions and the absence of complications (e.g., infection, severe arterial insufficiency). Patients will not typically experience residual deficits from the wound itself, but may have increased morbidity and mortality risks associated with the underlying pathology.

What are the long-term effects of the patient's condition?

Treatment of a neuropathic ulcer and the underlying pathology should allow for a normal course of recovery without residual deficits. Complicated wounds may require additional orthotic, pharmacological, medical or surgical intervention.

COMPARISON
What are the distinguishing characteristics of a similar condition?

A pressure ulcer results from ischemia that is caused by unrelieved tissue pressure. Pressure ulcers typically occur over bony prominences that are likely to be subjected to sustained pressure such as the sacrum or heels. Pressure ulcers are staged based on the depth of tissue damage and may vary widely in their general characteristics.

CLINICAL SCENARIOS

Scenario One

A 44-year-old male with peripheral neuropathy develops a neuropathic ulcer on the plantar surface of the third metatarsal head. The patient is a postal carrier and resides alone. He attempted to manage the wound, however, examination reveals visible bone at the base of the wound bed and moderate production of purulent exudate.

Scenario Two

A 63-year-old patient was diagnosed with type 1 diabetes mellitus as an adolescent. The patient has an extensive history of non-compliance resulting in visual deficits, Charcot foot deformity, and a neuropathic ulcer on the plantar surface of the midfoot. The patient resides alone in an apartment building with an elevator.

DIAGNOSIS

What condition produces a patient's symptoms?

Osteoporosis is a metabolic bone disorder where the rate of bone resorption accelerates while the rate of bone formation slows down; osteoclast activity exceeds osteoblast activity. This reduction of bone mass decreases the overall bone density and strength. Primary osteoporosis includes classifications such as idiopathic osteoporosis, involutional (senile) osteoporosis, and postmenopausal osteoporosis. Secondary osteoporosis occurs due to a primary disease process or as a result of taking certain medications.

An injury was most likely sustained to which structure?

Osteoporosis primarily affects trabecular bone in a postmenopausal patient, however, is primarily seen in both trabecular and cortical bone in the geriatric population. Impaired bone formation due to declining osteoblast function in addition to the loss of calcium and phosphate salts within the bone structure cause brittle and porous bones that easily fracture. All bones can be affected with fractures of the vertebrae, distal radius/ulna, and femoral neck being the most common.

INFERENCE

What is the most likely contributing factor in the development of this condition?

The exact cause of primary osteoporosis is unknown, however, risk factors include inadequate dietary calcium, smoking, excessive caffeine, high intake of alcohol or salt, small stature, Caucasian race, inactive lifestyle, family history or history of chronic disease. Secondary osteoporosis may be caused by prolonged drug therapies of heparin or corticosteroid use, endocrine disorders, malnutrition, and other disease processes. Postmenopausal osteoporosis targets women approximately 50-60 years of age. Involutional (senile) osteoporosis usually targets men and women >70 years of age. Idiopathic osteoporosis can occur in both genders at all ages.

CONFIRMATION

What is the most likely clinical presentation?

Osteoporosis is the most frequently seen metabolic bone disease that affects approximately 10 million individuals within the United States. The prevalence is expected to increase with the increase in the aging population. A patient diagnosed with osteoporosis may complain of low thoracic or lumbar pain, experience compression fractures of the vertebrae, and complain of back pain. Vertebral and other crush fractures may occur with little to no trauma. Pain is acute and increases with weight bearing and palpation. A patient may also present with deformities such as kyphosis, Dowager's hump, a decrease in height, and other postural changes.

What laboratory or imaging studies would confirm the diagnosis?

There is not an accurate measure of overall bone strength or standards for routine screening that have been established, however, X-rays are taken to investigate the amount of degeneration and the decrease in density of a particular area. A bone mineral density test accounts for 70% of bone strength and is the easiest way to determine osteoporosis. Photon absorptiometry is used to measure bone mass particularly of the vertebrae, hips, and extremities. Quantitative CT scans may be used to aid diagnosis by examining the bone density of the spine.

What additional information should be obtained to confirm the diagnosis?

Differential diagnosis including lab testing and urinalysis must exclude other disease processes through examination and testing. A patient's past medical history, current symptoms, and location of pain all play a role in diagnosing osteoporosis.

EXAMINATION

What history should be documented?

Important areas to explore include past medical history, medications, family history, current symptoms, current health status, social history and habits, occupation, leisure activities, and social support system.

What tests/measures are most appropriate?

Aerobic capacity and endurance: assessment of vital signs at rest and with activity, perceived exertion scale

Arousal, attention, and cognition: examine mental status, learning ability, memory, motivation

Assistive and adaptive devices: analysis of components and safety of a device

Environmental, home, and work barriers: analysis of current and potential barriers or hazards

Ergonomics and body mechanics: analysis of dexterity and coordination

Gait, locomotion, and balance: static and dynamic balance in sitting and standing, safety during gait with/without an assistive device, Berg Balance Scale, functional capacity evaluation

Integumentary integrity: skin and sensation assessment

Motor function: coordination, posture/balance in sitting

Muscle performance: strength of active range of motion only

Pain: pain perception scale, visual analogue scale

Posture: analysis of resting and dynamic posture

Range of motion: active range of motion

Self-care and home management: assessment of functional capacity

What additional findings are likely with this patient?

Once osteoporosis progresses in severity it can affect areas other than weight bearing bones such as the skull, long bones, and ribs. Spontaneous fractures and skeletal deformities may increase due to the continuing bone loss. A single fracture significantly increases the risk for subsequent fractures and skeletal deformities such as kyphosis.

MANAGEMENT

What is the most effective management of this patient?

Effective management of osteoporosis includes vitamin and pharmaceutical supplements, proper nutrition, education and physical therapy intervention. Hormone replacement therapy is recommended for postmenopausal patients. Calcium supplements, vitamin D, Raloxifene, and Fosamax (prevents bone resorption) may be recommended in the treatment of osteoporosis. Physical therapy intervention should include patient education regarding exercise, positioning, pain management, nutrition, and fall prevention. Physical therapy should include an exercise program that emphasizes weight bearing activities as tolerated. A patient may require a corset or lumbar support if at risk for vertebral fractures and many patients will require training with an assistive device. Aquatic therapy will assist with conditioning, however, should not replace weight bearing activities. Surgical intervention may be indicated for a patient requiring fracture stabilization.

What home care regimen should be recommended?

The home care regimen for osteoporosis includes a consistent home exercise program that combines exercise, walking, and other activities within a patient's tolerance. Exercise is crucial to slow the bone resorption process and increase bone development. Patients should be educated to avoid heavy resistive exercise, excessive flexion during exercise or household activities, and the use of ballistic movements. Light resistance such as small dumbbells or Theraband can be used with caution after consulting with the physician.

OUTCOME

What is the likely outcome of a course in physical therapy?

Physical therapy should prescribe an exercise program that the patient can follow independently. Patient education should allow for independent decision making regarding proper nutrition and activities that incorporate precautions and fall prevention techniques. This level of patient competency should assist in decreasing the risk of fractures and other complications. Physical therapy cannot cease the process, but can empower the patient to effectively manage this bone disorder.

What are the long-term effects of the patient's condition?

Osteoporosis will create thin and porous bones that will fracture easily and result in direct and indirect complications. Deformity and pain can become long-term effects of osteoporosis. Early detection and management of osteoporosis is important to limit the long-term effects of the disease.

COMPARISON

What are the distinguishing characteristics of a similar condition?

Paget's disease (osteitis deformans) is a chronic bone disease of unknown etiology where there is thickened, spongy, and abnormal bone formation. Large multinucleated osteoblasts, fibrous tissue, and thickened lamellae and trabeculae form and create weak and brittle bones. Bone pain, headache, hearing loss, fatigue, and stiffness are some early characteristics of Paget's disease. Progression of the disease includes bowing of long bones, an increase in skull size, bone deformities, and fractures (especially of the vertebrae).

CLINICAL SCENARIOS

Scenario One

A 63-year-old female is seen in outpatient physical therapy for a home exercise program. She is postmenopausal and does not take hormone replacement therapy. She has been recently diagnosed with osteoporosis and x-rays revealed three old vertebral fractures. The patient's major complaints are pain and stiffness.

Scenario Two

A 92-year-old male was admitted to the hospital for internal fixation of a femoral neck fracture. The patient's history reveals osteoporosis, diabetes, and anxiety. He wants to be discharged home to care for his cat. The physician orders are for physical therapy two times per week with the goal of returning home alone.

Pressure Ulcer

DIAGNOSIS

What condition produces a patient's symptoms?

A pressure ulcer is a type of ulcer or wound caused by unrelieved pressure to a specific area that results in damage to the underlying tissues. The unrelieved pressure deprives the tissues of oxygen, which causes ischemia to the site, subsequent cell death, and tissue necrosis. A definition of unrelieved pressure is >32 mm Hg of pressure to an area for more than two hours.

An injury was most likely sustained to which structure?

A pressure ulcer can affect different structures based on the degree or staging of the ulcer. Damage can be contained to only the epidermis in stage I ulcers, while stage IV ulcers will include damage to the epidermis, dermis, the fascia and deeper, potentially damaging muscles, ligaments, tendons and/or bones. The most high risk areas for pressure ulcers include the occiput, heels, greater trochanters, ischial tuberosities, sacrum, and epicondyles of the elbow.

INFERENCE

What is the most likely contributing factor in the development of this condition?

A pressure ulcer can occur at any time secondary to unrelieved pressure, but there are certain populations and risk factors that are associated with its development. Immobility is a leading factor and is seen with populations such as spinal cord injury, other paralysis, and hemiplegia. Impaired cognition, poor nutrition, altered sensation, incontinence, decreased lean body mass, and infection are other contributing factors in the development of a pressure ulcer. At the cellular level, the interface pressure, shear and/or friction are the contributing factors in the development of a pressure ulcer.

CONFIRMATION

What is the most likely clinical presentation?

A patient will usually develop a pressure ulcer over a bony prominence with common sites including the greater trochanter, ischium, sacrum, and heel. A stage I pressure ulcer is classified as an area of nonblanchable erythema of intact skin. There may also be an increase in warmth to the site or altered coloration. Stage II is classified as a partial thickness wound involving the epidermis, dermis or both. This ulcer does not extend through the entire dermis. Stage III is classified as an ulcer that has extended into subcutaneous tissue, but not through fascia. Stage IV is classified as an ulcer that extends through the fascia and deeper. It is a full thickness wound that may damage muscles, bones, ligaments and/or tendons. Pressure ulcers will vary in color, odor, drainage, and volume.

What laboratory or imaging studies would confirm the diagnosis?

A diagnosis is made from visual inspection, however, blood studies such as a CBC, electrolyte, and protein levels, as well as tests for bacteremia or sepsis may be indicated. Urinalysis and stool samples may be indicated to determine contributing factors in the development of the ulcer. Coagulation studies and tissue sampling may also be indicated.

What additional information should be obtained to confirm the diagnosis?

Extensive examination and photography of the site are necessary for accurate baseline data. A patient's history and current status are also important factors in designing the plan of care. Diagnosis of staging of the ulcer requires the use of the Braden Scale, Gosnell Scale or Norton Scale along with baseline measurements of size and depth of the ulcer.

EXAMINATION

What history should be documented?

Important areas to explore include past medical history, medications, current health status, history of incontinence, nutritional status, social history, living environment, occupation, and social support system.

What tests/measures are most appropriate?

Aerobic capacity and endurance: assessment of vital signs at rest and with activity

Arousal, attention, and cognition: examine mental status, learning ability, memory and motivation

Environmental, home, and work barriers: analysis of current and potential barriers or hazards

Gait, locomotion, and balance: static and dynamic balance in sitting and standing, safety during gait with/without an assistive device

Integumentary integrity: skin assessment, assessment of sensation, Braden Scale, Norton Scale, photography of ulcer, eschar, granulation formation, Gosnell Scale

Joint integrity and mobility: assessment of hypermobility and hypomobility of a joint, soft tissue swelling and inflammation

Muscle performance: strength assessment

Pain: pain perception assessment scale, visual analogue scale

Posture: analysis of resting and dynamic posture

Range of motion: active and passive range of motion

Sensory integrity: proprioception and kinesthesia

Pressure Ulcer

What additional findings are likely with this patient?

Complications that may prevent healing of the ulcer include infection, osteomyelitis, sepsis, pain, spasticity, malnutrition, incontinence, and depression. Patients at high risk may also develop multiple ulcers at once.

MANAGEMENT

What is the most effective management of this patient?

Patient and caregiver education for the prevention of subsequent pressure ulcers is very important and should include skin inspection, positioning, and pressure relief techniques. The use of pressure reducing devices such as seat cushions, multipodus boots or specialized mattresses is also an important aspect to the overall care of ulcers. Pharmacological intervention may include antimicrobials and antibiotics to fight infection and allow for proper healing. Dressings for the ulcer may include nonocclusive or occlusive types of dressings. Nonocclusive dressings include dry to dry, wet to wet, wet to dry or composite dressings. Occlusive dressings include semipermeable films, hydrocolloids, hydrogels, semipermeable foams, and alginates. The ulcer may require cleansing agents, and/or debridement (enzymatic, mechanical non-selective or sharp). Mobility training and proper positioning for the patient will also be vital in order to decrease forces of shear and friction upon the site of the ulcer. A general exercise program should be initiated as well as mobility training to tolerance. Skin inspection should be provided daily and photography should be documented regularly to track the progress of healing. Patients should avoid the use of hot water and the use of massage surrounding the site. The therapist should promote proper positioning techniques (such as positioning of the bed at less than a 45 degree angle) in order to decrease friction and shear forces.

What home care regimen should be recommended?

The home care regimen is dependent on the size and staging of the pressure sore. The patient should continue with the appropriate schedule for dressings and follow physician orders. The patient should maintain an appropriate activity level, use correct positioning, and receive adequate protein and calorie intake to assist with the healing process. The patient should use a mild cleansing agent, dry and wrinkle free sheets for their bed, and appropriate moisturizers.

OUTCOME

What is the likely outcome of a course in physical therapy?

The care of ulcers is estimated to cost $6 billion dollars annually which makes this diagnosis the most costly preventable injury. Approximately 60,000 patients die annually due to secondary complications from ulcers. However, many people that develop a pressure ulcer completely recover with no residual impairments.

What are the long-term effects of the patient's condition?

Treatment of a pressure ulcer should provide a normal path of recovery without any residual deficits. If there is infection or complications to healing, the patient may have to undergo additional treatment such as further pharmacological intervention or surgical procedures. If the patient is in a high risk group for skin breakdown the patient may require the ongoing use of a pressure relief seating system or air mattress for the bed.

COMPARISON

What are the distinguishing characteristics of a similar condition?

A neuropathic ulcer is an ulcer that develops due to the lack of neural function, which occurs commonly in patients with diabetes mellitus. Other high risk groups include spinal cord injury, stroke, spina bifida, sensory neuropathies, and tumors. The feet are the prime region for neuropathic ulcers in the diabetic patient. These ulcers occur in areas of weight bearing where there are mechanical shear forces such as under the metatarsal heads. These ulcers are usually round in shape and are not painful. It is believed that these ulcers occur not only due to motor neuropathy, but also impairment of the sensory and autonomic systems. Approximately 15% of patients with diabetes mellitus will develop a foot ulcer. Treatment is usually the same as with a pressure ulcer, but care must be taken to continually assess progress since there is usually motor and sensory damage surrounding the ulcer site.

CLINICAL SCENARIOS

Scenario One

A 31-year-old male has been in the hospital for four weeks secondary to a motor vehicle accident. He was in a coma for ten days and was required to stay in bed due to multiple fractures for three of the four weeks. He developed a stage two pressure ulcer on his right heel and has orders for whirlpool treatment. He is being discharged home alone in two weeks to his two-story home and is currently NWB on the right lower extremity and WBAT on the left lower extremity.

Scenario Two

An 85-year-old female is admitted to the hospital due to a stage four pressure ulcer on her sacrum. She had been cared for at home by her husband since her stroke four months ago. The husband states that the wife remained in bed most of the time, has lost over 30 pounds, and presents with some mild cognitive deficits.

Rheumatoid Arthritis

DIAGNOSIS

What condition produces a patient's symptoms?

Rheumatoid arthritis (RA) is a systemic autoimmune disorder of the connective tissue that is characterized by chronic inflammation within synovial membranes, tendon sheaths, and articular cartilage. The acute and chronic inflammatory changes produce the symptoms of this condition.

An injury was most likely sustained to which structure?

Smaller peripheral joints are usually the first to be affected by RA, however, all connective tissue may become involved. Inflammation is present within the synovial membrane and granulation tissue forms as a result of the synovitis. The granulation tissue and protein degrading enzymes erode articular cartilage resulting in destruction, adhesions, and fibrosis within the joint.

INFERENCE

What is the most likely contributing factor in the development of this condition?

The etiology of RA is unknown, however, there appears to be evidence of genetic predisposition with viral or bacterial triggers. Approximately 80% of individuals diagnosed with RA possess a positive rheumatoid factor (RF). RF represents the presence of autoantibodies that conflict with immunoglobulin antibodies found in the blood. The incidence of RA in women is three times greater than the incidence in men.

CONFIRMATION

What is the most likely clinical presentation?

RA affects approximately 1-2% of the population within the United States or two million individuals (1.5 million women, 600,000 men). This condition is characterized by periods of exacerbations and is diagnosed most frequently between 30 and 50 years of age. RA will vary in onset and progression from patient to patient. Onset of RA may be sudden or develop over a period of weeks. Early characteristics include fatigue, bilateral involvement, tenderness of smaller joints, and low-grade fever. Patients often experience pain with motion, stiffness including prolonged morning stiffness, and progression of symptoms to larger synovial joints. In late stages of the disease the heart can become affected and deformities, subluxations, and contractures can occur.

What laboratory or imaging studies would confirm the diagnosis?

Blood work assists with the diagnosis of RA through evaluation of the rheumatoid factor (RF), white blood cell count, erythrocyte sedimentation rate, hemoglobin, and hematocrit values. A synovial fluid analysis evaluates the content of synovial fluid within a joint. X-rays can be used to evaluate the joint space and the extent of decalcification.

What additional information should be obtained to confirm the diagnosis?

Physical examination and patient history of symptoms are required to confirm the diagnosis. The American Rheumatoid Association has designed diagnostic criteria for RA that can be used as a guide to determine a definite, possible, probable or classic diagnosis.

EXAMINATION

What history should be documented?

Important areas to explore include past medical history, family history, medications, current symptoms and health status, living environment, social history and habits, occupation, and social support system.

What tests/measures are most appropriate?

Aerobic capacity and endurance: assessment of vital signs at rest and with activity, timed walk, VO_{2max}

Anthropometric characteristics: circumferential measurements of all affected joints

Arousal, attention, and cognition: examine mental status, learning ability, memory, motivation

Community and work integration: analysis of community, work, and leisure activities

Ergonomics and body mechanics: analysis of dexterity and coordination

Environmental, home, and work barriers: analysis of current and potential barriers or hazards

Gait, locomotion, and balance: safety during gait with/ without an assistive device, Functional Ambulation Profile, gait over level/unlevel surfaces, visual inspection of gait with and without shoes

Integumentary integrity: skin and sensation assessment

Joint integrity and mobility: assessment of joint hypomobility, soft tissue inflammation, presence of deformity, active joint count, articular tenderness

Motor function: equilibrium and righting reactions, motor assessment scales, coordination, posture and balance in sitting, physical performance scales

Muscle performance: break testing of isometric contractions, manometer method of strength testing

Orthotic, protective, and supportive devices: potential utilization of bracing, analysis of movement while wearing a device

Pain: pain perception assessment scale

Range of motion: active and passive range of motion

Self-care and home management: assessment of functional capacity

Sensory integrity: assessment of sensation, kinesthesia, and proprioception

What additional findings are likely with this patient?

Extraarticular manifestations with RA can include pericarditis, anemia, tearing of tendons and musculature, osteoporosis, swan neck and/or boutonniere deformities, compression neuropathies, peripheral neuropathies, depression, pleurisy, skin changes, and anorexia.

MANAGEMENT

What is the most effective management of this patient?

Early medical management of a patient with RA is critical to improve the long-term outcomes of the disease. Medical treatment will focus on pain relief, reduction of edema, and preservation of joint integrity. Pharmacological intervention is required to decrease inflammation and retard the progression of the disease. NSAIDs, corticosteroids, and disease-modifying medications such as methotrexate are indicated. Physical therapy management during the acute stage or exacerbation includes patient education regarding regular rest, pain relief, relaxation, positioning, joint protection techniques, splinting, energy conservation, and body mechanics. Treatment may include gentle massage, hydrotherapy, hot pack, paraffin or cold modalities, gentle isometrics, and instruction in the use of assistive devices. Treatment during the acute stage should avoid resistive exercise, deep heating modalities, and any form of active stretching since these activities will further exacerbate the arthritis. Physical therapy management during the chronic stage or remission focuses on improving overall functional capacity, endurance, and strength. Treatment consists of low-impact conditioning through swimming or the stationary bicycle. Gentle stretching may be indicated to maintain available range of motion, however, aggressive stretching is contraindicated.

What home care regimen should be recommended?

A home care regimen for a patient with RA must maintain a delicate balance between activity and rest. The patient should perform low-level exercise, utilize relaxation and energy conservation techniques, and use splints as needed. The patient should recognize when total rest is indicated due to an acute exacerbation.

OUTCOME

What is the likely outcome of a course in physical therapy?

Physical therapy cannot halt the progression of RA, however, it can improve a patient's ability to function. Physical therapy may be indicated intermittently throughout the disease process with goals that focus on pain relief, relaxation, improving motion, and preventing deformity.

What are the long-term effects of the patient's condition?

RA is a chronic disease process that currently does not have a known cure, progresses at a varied rate, creates irreversible damage and deformity, and results in disability. As the disease progresses there is bilateral and symmetrical involvement of joints. Systemic effects include insomnia, fatigue, and organ involvement including the heart and lungs.

COMPARISON

What are the distinguishing characteristics of a similar condition?

Osteoarthritis is a chronic degenerative condition that usually develops secondary to repetitive trauma, disease or obesity. The hyaline cartilage in the joint softens and breaks apart allowing bone-to-bone contact that results in joint deformity, crepitus, impaired range of motion, and pain. Pain typically increases with prolonged activity. Joints become swollen and tender and joint deformity develops. Women have a slightly greater risk for OA than men. Surgical procedures including osteotomy and joint replacement may be indicated if conservative treatment is unsuccessful.

CLINICAL SCENARIOS

Scenario One

A 38-year-old female diagnosed with RA is seen in an outpatient clinic. The patient history reveals fatigue and malaise for two to three weeks and pain in the fingers and wrists. The patient has difficulty caring for herself at home and is on medical leave from her job. The patient does not have any other significant past medical history and resides alone.

Scenario Two

A 74-year-old male diagnosed with RA is treated by a therapist. The patient presents with multi-joint involvement, deformities of the hands and feet, poor endurance, stiffness, and pain. The patient is ambulatory, however, is currently in a wheelchair secondary to pain from an exacerbation. The patient is oriented and has a history of COPD.

Systemic Lupus Erythematosus

DIAGNOSIS

What condition produces a patient's symptoms?

Systemic lupus erythematosus (SLE) is a connective tissue disorder caused by an autoimmune reaction in the body. The primary manifestation of the condition is the production of destructive antibodies that are directed at the individual's own body. The chronic inflammatory disorder produces a variety of symptoms depending on the severity and extent of involvement.

An injury was most likely sustained to which structure?

SLE is an autoimmune disorder that creates high levels of autoantibodies (antinuclear antibodies) that attack various cells and tissues within the body. The autoantibodies form immune complexes that produce an inflammatory response and cause further tissue destruction. Proliferation of immune complexes precipitates inflammation responses that in turn destroy cells, tissues, and organs. Specific injury is organ or system dependent depending on which areas of the body are affected by SLE.

INFERENCE

What is the most likely contributing factor in the development of this condition?

The exact etiology of SLE is unknown, however, it is described as an immunoregulatory disturbance from genetic, environmental, viral, and hormonal contributing factors. Environmental factors associated with SLE include ultraviolet light exposure, infection, antibiotics (specifically penicillin and sulfa drugs), extreme stress, immunization, and pregnancy. SLE can occur at any age, but the most common age group is 15 to 40 years of age. The disorder is 10-15 times more common in women.

CONFIRMATION

What is the most likely clinical presentation?

There are an estimated 1.4 million individuals diagnosed with SLE in the United States. A patient with SLE will have diverse symptoms based on the involvement of the connective tissue throughout the body. Symptoms will appear with exacerbations and disappear with remissions throughout the course of the disease. Symptoms such as arthralgias, malaise, and fatigue may persist even during a remission period. A patient may initially see a physician for symptoms that include fever, malaise, rash, arthralgias, headache, and weight loss. Common clinical presentation throughout the course of SLE includes a red butterfly rash across the cheeks and nose, a red rash over light exposed areas, arthralgias, alopecia, pleurisy, kidney involvement, seizures, depression, fibromyalgia, and cardiac involvement. SLE can affect the skin, joints, kidneys, lungs, heart, and other organs and tissues within the body. Patients can also have CNS involvement that can lead to neuropsychiatric manifestations that present with depression, irritability, emotional instability, and seizures.

What laboratory or imaging studies would confirm the diagnosis?

Microscopic fluorescent techniques are indicated to detect the presence of the antinuclear antibody (ANA) within the blood. A positive ANA test warrants an additional test for antideoxyribonucleic acid antibodies. These two tests in combination with the physical presentation support the presence of SLE. Other testing including erythrocyte sedimentation rate, complete blood count, and urinalysis.

What additional information should be obtained to confirm the diagnosis?

The American Rheumatism Association has designated criteria to confirm the diagnosis of SLE. A patient requires at least four of fourteen characteristics that occur during the same period of time. A patient evaluation including a thorough history and current symptoms assists with confirming a diagnosis of SLE.

EXAMINATION

What history should be documented?

Important areas to explore include past medical and family history, medications, current symptoms and health status, living environment, social history and habits, occupation, and social support system.

What tests/measures are most appropriate?

Aerobic capacity and endurance: assessment of vital signs at rest/activity, auscultation of the lungs/heart

Arousal, attention, and cognition: examine mental status, learning ability, memory, motivation

Assistive and adaptive devices: analysis of components and safety of a device

Community and work integration: analysis of community, work, and leisure activities

Environmental, home, and work barriers: analysis of current and potential barriers or hazards

Ergonomics and body mechanics: analysis of dexterity and coordination

Gait, locomotion, and balance: static/dynamic balance in sitting and standing, safety during gait, Tinetti Performance Oriented Mobility Assessment, Berg Balance Scale, Functional Ambulation Profile

Integumentary integrity: skin assessment, assessment of sensation, presence and assessment of rash

Joint integrity and mobility: soft tissue swelling and inflammation, presence of deformity

Motor function: posture and balance

Muscle performance: strength assessment

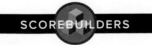

Systemic Lupus Erythematosus   GOLD

Neuromotor development and sensory integration: analysis of reflex movement patterns, sensory integration tests, gross and fine motor skills
Orthotic, protective, and supportive devices: potential utilization of bracing
Pain: pain perception assessment scale
Range of motion: active and passive range of motion
Self-care and home management: assessment of functional capacity

What additional findings are likely with this patient?

SLE can produce skeletal deformities such as ulnar deviation and subluxed interphalangeal joints. Kidney involvement and cardiovascular impairments such as endocarditis, myocarditis, and pericarditis can occur during an exacerbation. Patients that experience nephritis, myocarditis or neurological implications have a poor prognosis. Modifiable risk factors for exacerbation include high stress, limited emotional and social support, and psychological distress.

MANAGEMENT

What is the most effective management of this patient?

Medical management of SLE focuses on reversing the autoimmune response in order to avoid complications and exacerbations of symptoms. Pharmacological intervention for a patient with mild SLE will include salicylates, Indomethacin or NSAIDs. Antimalarial medications, corticosteroids, and immunosuppressive therapy may be used. General management of SLE includes good nutrition, ongoing medical supervision, and avoidance of ultraviolet exposure. Physical therapy intervention is usually indicated after a period of exacerbation and includes a slow resumption of physical activity, energy conservation techniques, gradual endurance activities and significant patient education regarding skin care, pacing, exercise, and strengthening to tolerance.

What home care regimen should be recommended?

A home care regimen during an acute exacerbation of SLE should include relaxation and energy conservation techniques, stress reduction strategies, therapeutic exercise as tolerated, and pain management.

OUTCOME

What is the likely outcome of a course in physical therapy?

Physical therapy cannot cease or alter the clinical course of SLE, however, it may assist in controlling the debilitating effects during an acute phase/exacerbation of the disease. Goals include focus on pain relief, relaxation, strengthening, and preventing deformity.

What are the long-term effects of the patient's condition?

The clinical course of SLE is highly unpredictable. A patient may only exhibit symptoms for skin and joint involvement or may exhibit multi-system involvement. Periods of remission may last years and the prognosis depends on the severity and the extent of the disease process. The overall prognosis for SLE is good, although in rare cases the disease process can remain acute and become fatal within a short period of time. There is a high ten-year survival rate with SLE. Death is usually attributed to kidney failure or secondary infections.

COMPARISON

What are the distinguishing characteristics of a similar condition?

Systemic sclerosis, also termed scleroderma, is a chronic disease that primarily affects the skin, but can involve articular structures and internal organs. There is long-term hardening and shrinking of the affected connective tissues. The two subtypes of this disease are systemic scleroderma and localized scleroderma. Etiology is unknown and the disease varies in course (months, years or a lifetime) and progression.

CLINICAL SCENARIOS

Scenario One

A 25-year-old female is referred to physical therapy for a therapeutic exercise program. The patient was diagnosed last year with SLE and has not exercised since that time. The patient is currently taking corticosteroids and antimalarial medications to manage a recent exacerbation.

Scenario Two

A 43-year-old female was seen in outpatient physical therapy to assist with pain management. The patient was diagnosed five years ago with SLE and has recently experienced increased difficulty using her hands secondary to deformity and pain. The patient's goal is to reduce the pain in her hands.

Urinary Stress Incontinence

DIAGNOSIS

What condition produces a patient's symptoms?

Urinary incontinence is the involuntary loss of urine. There are five classifications that include functional incontinence, stress incontinence, urge incontinence, mixed incontinence, and overflow incontinence. Urinary stress incontinence may occur during activities when there is an increase in abdominal pressure through straining, sneezing, coughing or lifting.

An injury was most likely sustained to which structure?

Urinary stress incontinence usually occurs from loss of strength and/or integrity of the contractile and noncontractile tissues that maintain bladder control. Urinary stress incontinence is caused by weakness of the pelvic floor musculature (urogenital diaphragm, levator ani muscle group), damage of the pudendal nerve, malposition of the urethra, and/or urethral sphincter incompetence.

INFERENCE

What is the most likely contributing factor in the development of this condition?

Risk factors for the development of urinary stress incontinence include pregnancy, vaginal delivery, episiotomy, prostate or pelvic surgery, aging, diabetes mellitus, central nervous system and peripheral nervous system dysfunction, and recurrent urinary tract infections. A prolapsed bladder, uterus or bowel may contribute to leakage and is seen in women that have had multiple vaginal deliveries. Medications that treat other illnesses can sometimes contribute to incontinence especially with the older population. Obesity is another risk factor that is believed to increase the risk of stress incontinence due to increased intra-abdominal pressure and the effect of obesity on the neuromuscular function of the genitourinary tract.

CONFIRMATION

What is the most likely clinical presentation?

It is estimated that approximately 10 million adults experience some form of urinary incontinence. Urinary stress incontinence accounts for 50-60% of all incontinence cases and is manifested solely by the involuntary loss of urine with any form of exertion or increased abdominal pressure. The amount of urine that leaks is typically less than 50 milliliters with coughing, sneezing or straining. Physical activity or exercise can also produce leakage due to exertion with these activities. Other manifestations may include dribbling of urine, urgency, frequency, nocturia, and a weak stream while voiding.

What laboratory or imaging studies would confirm the diagnosis?

Cystometry is used to evaluate bladder capacity, control, contractility, and sensation. During this procedure, provocative stress testing will be performed when stress incontinence is suspected. Urodynamic testing observes the stability of the bladder and electromyography observes bladder contractions. Urinalysis is used for differential diagnosis to rule out infection, diabetes, and other conditions.

What additional information should be obtained to confirm the diagnosis?

Urinary stress incontinence can be determined through history, pelvic examination, and noted loss of urine with straining activities. The Marshall-Marchetti test utilizes finger elevation of the paraurethral vaginal tissues at the neck of the bladder in order to stop the leakage of urine during coughing, sneezing or straining. Baseline exam should include the amount of time that a patient can hold urine, repetitions performed of a holding contraction, and the amount of pelvic floor contractions a patient can perform.

EXAMINATION

What history should be documented?

Important areas to explore include past medical history, childbirth history, medications, current health status, fluid intake, social history, occupation, living environment, and social support system.

What tests/measures are most appropriate?

Aerobic capacity and endurance: assessment of vital signs at rest and with activity, perceived exertion scale

Arousal, attention, and cognition: examine mental status, learning ability, memory, motivation, Urge Impact scale

Community and work integration: analysis of community, work, and leisure activities

Environmental, home, and work barriers: analysis of current and potential barriers or hazards

Ergonomics and body mechanics: analysis of dexterity and coordination, assessment of lifting techniques (intra-abdominal pressure)

Integumentary integrity: skin assessment, examination of the pelvic floor

Muscle performance: strength assessment of the pelvic floor and abdominal muscles, muscle tone assessment

Pain: pain perception assessment scale

Posture: analysis of resting and dynamic posture

Range of motion: active and passive range of motion

Self-care and home management: assessment of functional capacity, bladder diary, fluid intake

Urinary Stress Incontinence   GOLD

What additional findings are likely with this patient?

A patient with urinary stress incontinence may be at increased risk for a urinary tract infection with subsequent skin breakdown. Pelvic floor weakness, uterine prolapse, and kidney infection may all relate to urinary stress incontinence. A patient that has poor diet and nutrition, constipation, inadequate hydration, and urinary frequency will further promote incontinence.

MANAGEMENT

What is the most effective management of this patient?

Medical management of urinary incontinence usually consists of conservative measures (physical therapy) as a first line of defense followed by pharmacological and surgical interventions depending on the underlying cause and response to conservative treatment. Physical therapy intervention for pelvic floor muscle weakness that is tested as 0/5 – 2/5 includes biofeedback, electrical stimulation, bladder retraining, and therapeutic exercise. Pelvic floor muscle strengthening at this level includes facilitation and tapping of the pelvic floor muscles, overflow exercises using the buttocks, adductors, and lower abdominals, and implementation of Kegel exercises. Physical therapy intervention for pelvic floor muscle weakness that is tested as 3/5 – 5/5 includes continued biofeedback and bladder retraining, weighted vaginal cones for resistance training, and implementation of pelvic floor muscle exercise during activities.

What home care regimen should be recommended?

A home care regimen for a patient with urinary stress incontinence should emphasize an active exercise program that includes pelvic floor strengthening in order to regain control of the flow of urine. Patients are encouraged to perform the recommended exercises throughout the day and integrate the pelvic exercises during activities that may trigger an increase in abdominal pressure within their daily routine. In addition to exercise, patients are advised to make behavioral and dietary modifications based on their personal bladder diary.

OUTCOME

What is the likely outcome of a course in physical therapy?

Outpatient physical therapy for urinary stress incontinence should alleviate pelvic floor weakness and involuntary leakage of urine within eight to twelve weeks. If a patient requires surgical intervention or presents with multiple impairments then physical therapy may be warranted for a longer period of time to assist with gaining bladder control.

What are the long-term effects of the patient's condition?

The long-term effects of urinary stress incontinence depend on the exact cause for the incontinence and the responsiveness to therapeutic intervention. Some patients do not have any long-term effects upon successful completion of physical therapy while other patients do not benefit from physical therapy intervention and require surgical intervention for the underlying cause. Compliance with the home exercise program is required when the underlying cause is weakness of the pelvic floor musculature. Research indicates that in an older population approximately 50% of all admissions to skilled nursing facilities have a direct relationship to unresolved urinary incontinence and impairments.

COMPARISON

What are the distinguishing characteristics of a similar condition?

Bowel incontinence can occur from birth defects, trauma to the rectum, spinal cord injuries, fecal impaction, and tumor. Conservative treatment is preferred and includes diet, pharmacological agents, and strengthening of the sphincter muscles through exercise, electrical stimulation, and biofeedback. Surgical intervention may be warranted.

CLINICAL SCENARIOS

Scenario One

A 32-year-old female is referred to physical therapy with a diagnosis of incontinence. The patient gave birth to her fourth child six weeks ago. The patient reports involuntary leakage of urine with exertion. The patient has no significant past medical history, however, reports that she is very anxious about participating in physical therapy.

Scenario Two

A 68-year-old female complains to her doctor during her annual examination that she has difficulty controlling her bladder since a kidney infection six months ago. The patient states that she is unable to hold her urine if she sneezes or coughs and cannot perform any activity of exertion without wearing feminine pads due to leakage. The physician referred the patient to physical therapy for Kegel exercises.

DIAGNOSIS

What condition produces a patient's symptoms?

A venous insufficiency ulcer typically results from venous hypertension which may present idiopathically, secondary to valve incompetence (e.g., damaged from a deep vein thrombosis) or peripheral impedance (e.g., obesity). The resultant distension of the capillary beds impedes the exchange of oxygen and nutrients at the capillary level. This results in relative stasis of the interstitial fluid and significant edema. Over time, increased protein and fibrinogen content in the interstitium facilitates fibrotic changes further impeding capillary exchange. The formation of an ulcer results from a combination of increased tissue pressure that decreases skin resilience and endothelial damage that allows enzyme and free radical leakage into the tissue.

An injury was most likely sustained to which structure?

A superficial ulceration is associated with damage to the epidermis only. Damage from a partial-thickness ulceration will extend through the epidermis and possibly into, but not through, the dermis. A full-thickness ulceration extends through the dermis and into deeper layers such as the subcutaneous fat layer. Damage from a subcutaneous ulcer extends through all layers of integumentary tissue typically exposing tendon, muscle or bone.

INFERENCE

What is the most likely contributing factor in the development of this condition?

A venous insufficiency ulcer forms as a result of an underlying condition which impedes normal venous blood flow and capillary exchange. Diagnoses of venous hypertension and chronic venous insufficiency are commonly associated with venous insufficiency ulcers. Patients who are obese are more likely to develop a venous insufficiency ulcer.

CONFIRMATION

What is the most likely clinical presentation?

A patient will typically develop a venous insufficiency ulcer on the medial surface of the lower leg in the area between the mid-calf and malleolus. Venous insufficiency ulcers are typically larger in area and more shallow in depth than arterial or neuropathic ulcers. Wound borders are typically irregular. The wound bed is typically moist with evidence of red granulation tissue. The wound bed may initially be obscured by a moist layer of yellow-white slough requiring debridement. Both the wound borders and bed will typically bleed easily with disruption (e.g., palpation, debridement, dressing changes) due to distended and fragile superficial capillaries. Serous or serosanguineous exudate is typically moderate to heavy. Signs of stasis dermatitis may be observed in the surrounding skin including a dry, flaky appearance and a ruddy, brownish skin discoloration termed hemosiderin staining. Distal lower extremity pulses are typically intact and pain complaints are typically mild and associated with the increased tissue tension caused by edema. Pain complaints are typically relieved with elevation or use of compression garments.

What laboratory or imaging studies would confirm the diagnosis?

A diagnosis of venous insufficiency ulcer is made based on the characteristics of the observed wound and diagnosis of the underlying condition. Duplex ultrasonography produces two-dimensional color images and is the least invasive method of assessing venous blood flow.

What additional information should be obtained to confirm the diagnosis?

An ankle-brachial index (ABI) should be obtained since compression is typically desirable when treating a venous insufficiency ulcer. The use of compression may be limited or contraindicated depending on the severity of occlusion.

EXAMINATION

What history should be documented?

Important areas to explore include past medical history, medications, family history, current symptoms, current health status, social history and habits, occupation, leisure activities, and social support system.

What tests/measures are most appropriate?

Anthropometric characteristics: circumferential measurements

Arousal, attention, and cognition: examine mental status, learning ability, memory, and motivation

Assistive and adaptive devices: analysis of components and safety of a device

Gait, locomotion, and balance: static and dynamic balance in sitting and standing, safety during gait with/without an assistive device

Integumentary integrity: skin assessment, assessment of sensation, assessment of wound characteristics, photo documentation, assessment of edema

Pain: pain perception assessment scale, visual analogue scale

Range of motion: active and passive range of motion

Reflex integrity: assessment of deep tendon reflexes

Self-care and home management: assessment of functional capacity

Ventilation, respiration, and circulation: assessment of pulse oximetry, palpation of pulses, capillary refill, ankle-brachial index

Venous Insufficiency Ulcer   GOLD

What additional findings are likely with this patient?

With chronic venous insufficiency, the same conditions that impede capillary exchange are also likely to locally overwhelm the lymphatic system. With impaired lymphatic function, the patient is at increased risk for developing a significant infection (e.g., cellulitis, wound infection, osteomyelitis). Impaired lymphatic function is also associated with fibrotic tissue changes. Over time, this may further limit normal exchange functions of both the capillaries and lymphatic vessels.

MANAGEMENT

What is the most effective management of this patient?

Medical management typically includes monitoring the severity of the underlying disease process and counseling regarding modifiable risk factors (e.g., weight, edema management). Other medical interventions may include procedures that either chemically (e.g., sclerotherapy) or thermally (e.g., ablation) close abnormal veins thereby redirecting venous blood return to better functioning vessels. Pharmacological intervention may include diuretics, antibiotics or antimicrobial agents. Surgical intervention typically targets the underlying pathology and may include vein stripping, bypass, valve repair, angioplasty or stent placement. Grafting may be indicated when the wound bed is unable to support normal healing and conservative measures have failed. Physical therapy management emphasizes edema management, skin protection, and wound healing interventions. Successful healing of venous insufficiency ulcers typically will include graded compression (e.g., garments, bandaging, Unna boot). The surrounding skin should be kept well moisturized and appropriate exudate management is essential to prevent breakdown of surrounding tissue. The ulcer may require cleansing agents and/or debridement (enzymatic, mechanical non-selective, sharp or autolytic). A venous insufficiency ulcer typically produces moderate to heavy volumes of exudate, therefore, it is important to select dressing components which protect the wound and maintain an appropriate moisture balance. Photo documentation is recommended to supplement written documentation describing wound characteristics (e.g., area, depth, odor, exudate, color).

What home care regimen should be recommended?

The home care regimen is dependent on the size and characteristics of the venous insufficiency ulcer. Patients who do not require debridement may appropriately manage routine dressing changes at home. All patients should be diligent with edema management, hygiene, and skin protection to limit the risk of infection.

OUTCOME

What is the likely outcome of a course of physical therapy?

A venous insufficiency ulcer will typically heal by secondary intention with appropriate management and an uncomplicated course of healing. Patients will not typically experience residual deficits from the wound itself, but may have increased morbidity and mortality risks associated with the wound's underlying pathology.

What are the long-term effects of the patient's condition?

Treatment of a venous insufficiency ulcer and the underlying pathology, in addition to edema management, should allow for a normal course of recovery without residual deficits. Infection or other complications to healing may require additional pharmacological, medical or surgical intervention. If infection is pervasive, osteomyelitis or sepsis may result.

COMPARISON

What are the distinguishing characteristics of a similar condition?

An arterial insufficiency ulcer is typically the result of inadequate perfusion of oxygenated blood causing cell death and tissue necrosis. Ulcers typically form on the distal lower extremities with smooth borders giving the wound a punched out appearance. Exudate is typically minimal, however, pain may be severe especially when the limb is not in a dependent position. On examination, pedal pulses are typically diminished. Skin is cool with a shiny, hairless appearance. Specific wound care interventions emphasize skin and wound protection as well as maintenance of a moist wound environment to facilitate healing. Medical or surgical intervention is typically required to address decreased blood supply to the area before healing can be supported.

CLINICAL SCENARIOS

Scenario One

A 53-year-old morbidly obese male presents with multiple small venous insufficiency ulcers on both lower legs. The wound beds are clean and granulating, however, exudate regularly saturates the gauze dressings. The patient reports that the ulcers have not healed in six months. The patient must walk distances with his job and does not have proper footwear.

Scenario Two

A 68-year-old active female is diagnosed with venous hypertension due to valve incompetence. She is referred to physical therapy for wound management after developing a shallow lower extremity ulceration. The wound bed is loosely covered in moist yellow-white slough and exudate is primarily serous.

SILVER Level Clinical Application Templates

SILVER   Level Clinical Application Template Executive Summary

Ankylosing Spondylitis

- Systemic condition characterized by inflammation of the spine and the larger peripheral joints
- Males are at two to three times greater risk than females with peak onset observed between 20-40 years of age
- Clinical presentation initially includes recurrent and insidious onset of back pain, morning stiffness, and impaired spinal extension

Cellulitis

- Refers to a noncontagious bacterial skin infection occurring in the dermal and subcutaneous layers
- Typically presents with visible signs of inflammation including localized redness, warmth, tenderness, and edema that progressively worsens
- Early detection and treatment are vital in reducing complications and systemic infection; untreated cellulitis can spread, causing potentially fatal septicemia

Complex Regional Pain Syndrome

- Increase in sympathetic activity causes a release of norepinephrine in the periphery and subsequent vasoconstriction of blood vessels resulting in pain and an increase in sensitivity to peripheral stimulation
- Affects all age groups, but is most likely found in individuals 35-60 years of age with females being three times more likely to be affected than males
- Patients experience intense burning and chronic pain in the affected extremity that eventually spreads in a proximal direction

Human Immunodeficiency Virus

- Primary risk factors for contracting HIV include unprotected sexual intercourse (anal or vaginal), intravenous drug use, or mother to fetus transmission
- Without treatment, HIV advances in three stages: 1) acute HIV infection, 2) clinical latency, and 3) AIDS (acquired immunodeficiency syndrome)
- Leading cause of death for patients with the virus are, in order of prevalence, AIDS-related (i.e., opportunistic infections), non-AIDS-defining cancers, liver disease, and cardiovascular disease

Juvenile Rheumatoid Arthritis

- Autoimmune disorder found in children less than 16 years of age that occurs when the immune cells mistakenly begin to attack the joints and organs causing local and systemic effects throughout the body
- Girls have a higher incidence of JRA and are most commonly diagnosed as toddlers or in early adolescence
- Clinical symptoms include persistent joint swelling, pain, and stiffness

Ankylosing Spondylitis

DIAGNOSIS

What condition produces a patient's symptoms?

Ankylosing spondylitis (AS), also known as Marie-Strumpell disease, is a systemic condition that is characterized by inflammation of the spine and larger peripheral joints. The chronic inflammation causes destruction of the ligamentous-osseous junction with subsequent fibrosis and ossification of the area.

An injury was most likely sustained to which structure?

AS primarily affects the sacroiliac joint, intervertebral disks, spine, costovertebral and apophyseal joints, connective tissue, and larger peripheral joints (hips, knees, and shoulders). Ossification can occur within all affected joints resulting in pain and deformity.

INFERENCE

What is the most likely contributing factor in the development of this condition?

AS is a progressive systemic disorder with uncertain etiology. Research supports the possibility of genetic inheritance combined with environmental influence. Gender, race, age, and family history are all factors to consider regarding risk for developing AS. A person born with a histocompatibility antigen HLA-B27 has a high risk for the disease. Approximately 80-90% of patients with AS are HLA-B27 positive, but only 2% of individuals that are HLA-B27 positive develop AS. HLA-B27 is found in 8.5% of Caucasians and only 2.5% of African Americans. Men are at a two to three times greater risk than women and onset is typically seen between twenty and forty years of age.

CONFIRMATION

What is the most likely clinical presentation?

A patient with early AS will present with recurrent and insidious episodes of low back pain, morning stiffness, impaired spinal extension, and limited range of motion in the affected joints for over a three-month period of time. As the disease progresses pain will become severe, consistent, and extending to the midback, and sometimes towards the neck. The natural lumbar curve will eventually flatten due to muscle spasms. Other manifestations include fixed flexion at the hips, spinal kyphosis, fatigue, weight loss, and peripheral joint involvement. If the costovertebral joints are affected a patient will present with impaired chest mobility, compromised breathing, and decreased vital capacity.

What laboratory or imaging studies would confirm the diagnosis?

X-ray of the spine may be negative in the initial stage of AS but with progression will reveal areas of erosion, demineralization, calcification, and syndesmophyte formation (ossification of the outside of the intervertebral disks). In the later stages of the disease x-ray will reveal fusion of the sacroiliac joint, calcification of apophyseal joints and spinal ligaments, and a bamboo appearance of the spine. Blood work can be used to rule out other diseases and assists with the diagnosis since the majority of patients with AS possess the HLA-B27 antigen and approximately 40% have an elevated erythrocyte sedimentation rate.

What additional information should be obtained to confirm the diagnosis?

Physical examination may reveal joint tenderness, pain, and/or limitation of the sacroiliac joint and the spine. Family inheritance and a thorough history of a patient's symptoms assist with the diagnosis of AS.

MANAGEMENT

What is the most effective management of this patient?

The goals of medical management are to reduce inflammation, maintain functional mobility, and relieve pain. Pharmacological intervention may include NSAIDs, disease-modifying drugs such as methotrexate, analgesics, and specifically Indomethacin to relieve pain. Physical therapy intervention should include postural exercises emphasizing extension, general range of motion, pain management, and energy conservation techniques. Low-impact and aerobic exercise with emphasis on extension and rotation are appropriate for a patient with AS. High-impact and flexion exercises are contraindicated. Patient education should include posture retraining, positioning for sleeping, and lifting techniques. Excessive exercise should be avoided as it can increase the inflammatory response and injury. Swimming is a highly recommended activity. Surgical intervention is rarely indicated to correct or stabilize a musculoskeletal deformity.

What home care regimen should be recommended?

A home care regimen for a patient with AS should include a daily low-impact therapeutic exercise program. Range of motion should focus on spinal movement in all directions. The patient requires a firm sleeping surface and competence with proper positioning and use of pillows to maintain optimal alignment. Ongoing breathing exercises and posture retraining will assist with overall level of function.

OUTCOME

What is the likely outcome of a course in physical therapy?

Physical therapy cannot modify the progression of AS, however, it may assist to alleviate pain and improve a patient's functional capacity. A patient may require physical therapy on an intermittent basis for secondary complications throughout the disease process.

What are the long-term effects of the patient's condition?

AS progresses slowly over a fifteen to twenty-five year period and may remain isolated to the spine and sacroiliac joint or spread to larger peripheral joints. Stiffness and joint limitation are common long-term effects of AS that can negatively impact a patient's functional mobility. The extent of disability varies greatly with only 1% of patients experiencing complete remission. Normal course includes periods of exacerbations and remissions. Hip disease with AS is a marker for a severe form of AS and is more likely to occur in a patient that is diagnosed at a young age.

Cellulitis   **SILVER**

DIAGNOSIS

What condition produces a patient's symptoms?

Cellulitis refers to a noncontagious bacterial skin infection occurring in the dermal and subcutaneous layers. Streptococcus and Staphylococcus microbes are most commonly associated with cellulitis. Other microbes including pneumococcus, pseudomonas, and clostridium may also cause cellulitis.

An injury was most likely sustained to which structure?

The integumentary system functions to protect underlying tissues from external debris and infectious microbes. When there is compromise of this protective barrier (e.g., insect bite, surgical wound, abrasion), vulnerable tissues are more easily exposed to bacteria resulting in infection. Without timely treatment the infection can spread to adjacent tissues and systemically through the bloodstream and lymphatic system. Repeated cellulitis infections and the associated edema can cause permanent damage to the lymphatic system.

INFERENCE

What is the most likely contributing factor in the development of this condition?

The body's immune response prevents external microbes from causing infection in exposed tissues. Patients with a weakened immune system secondary to medication (e.g., corticosteroids, chemotherapy agents) or other medical conditions (e.g., HIV, leukemia) are more susceptible to cellulitis. High-risk patients also include those with conditions that impede immune responses due to impaired blood or lymphatic flow (e.g., chronic venous insufficiency, lymphedema, obesity). Although a break in the skin's protective barrier is typically associated with cellulitis, some patients, such as those with diabetes, may develop cellulitis without an identifiable cause.

CONFIRMATION

What is the most likely clinical presentation?

Cellulitis typically presents with visible signs of inflammation including localized redness, warmth, tenderness, and edema that progressively worsens. Red streaks leading away from the primary site of infection, weeping, and serous drainage may also be observed. As the condition worsens, other systemic signs and symptoms of infection may develop including fever, aches, chills, and swollen or tender lymph nodes.

What laboratory or imaging studies would confirm the diagnosis?

Blood sample analysis may be used to evaluate the patient's white blood cell count. When elevated, it is suggestive of infection, but alone is not conclusive. A wound culture can assist in identifying the specific infectious microbe present so that treatment can be specifically targeted.

What additional information should be obtained to confirm the diagnosis?

A thorough medical history should be obtained, including a detailed history of current symptoms and the identification of known cellulitis risk factors. Physical examination should include an examination of the integumentary system.

MANAGEMENT

What is the most effective management of this patient?

Early detection is important to prevent the infection from spreading systemically. Pharmacological intervention with antibiotic therapy is the primary mode of medical management. The antibiotic selected will vary depending on the type of bacteria involved. Typically, antibiotics are administered orally, allowing the patient to self-medicate and care for themselves. In more severe cases (e.g., patients who are immunocompromised or have a high fever), inpatient treatment and intravenous antibiotics may be required. Physical therapy interventions may be indicated if an integumentary injury requires ongoing wound care. Patients who demonstrate functional limitations due to pain from severe inflammation are likely to benefit from adaptive equipment instruction to assist with mobility or self-care activities until symptoms resolve. Education regarding risk reduction, skin protection, and appropriate skin hygiene practices may also be components of a physical therapy plan of care.

What home care regimen should be recommended?

With antibiotic intervention, symptoms should begin to resolve within a few days. Until this time, rest and elevation of the affected area may assist in reducing edema and discomfort caused by inflammation. Skin protection and skin hygiene are important both while recovering and after symptoms have resolved to prevent recurrence in at-risk patients. Patients should be educated regarding risk factors, appropriate care following future skin compromise, and early recognition of signs or symptoms suggesting recurrence.

OUTCOME

What is the likely outcome of a course of physical therapy?

Physical therapy interventions for cellulitis are primarily palliative to assist in improving comfort and function during recovery. Appropriate antibiotic intervention will typically resolve symptom complaints and any associated limitations.

What are the long-term effects of the patient's condition?

Recurrences of cellulitis are common among patients with comorbidities that increase the risk of infection. Early detection and treatment are vital in reducing complications and systemic infection. Untreated cellulitis can spread, causing potentially fatal septicemia.

Complex Regional Pain Syndrome

DIAGNOSIS

What condition produces a patient's symptoms?

Complex regional pain syndrome is usually found in an extremity that has experienced some form of trauma. Symptoms result from a disturbance in the functioning of the sympathetic nervous system. The increase in sympathetic activity causes a release of norepinephrine in the periphery and subsequent vasoconstriction of blood vessels. This results in pain and an increase in sensitivity to peripheral stimulation.

An injury was most likely sustained to which structure?

Complex regional pain syndrome results from injured sensory nerve fibers at one somatic level that initiates sympathetic efferent activity that affects many segmental levels. The extremity of origin sustains injury as well as areas adjacent to the extremity.

INFERENCE

What is the most likely contributing factor in the development of this condition?

The exact etiology of complex regional pain syndrome is unknown, however, predisposing factors include trauma, surgery, CVA, TBI, repetitive motion disorders, and lower motor neuron and peripheral nerve injuries. Complex regional pain syndrome is reported to occur following 5% of all injuries. While many cases of complex regional pain syndrome resolve, others progress and become a disabling disorder. Complex regional pain syndrome can affect all age groups but is most likely found in the age group of 35-60 years with females three times more likely to be affected by complex regional pain syndrome than males.

CONFIRMATION

What is the most likely clinical presentation?

A patient with complex regional pain syndrome will experience intense, burning, and chronic pain in the affected extremity that will eventually spread proximally. Early in the syndrome, the degree of pain is greater than expected based on the amount of trauma that the tissue sustained. Edema, thermal changes, discoloration, stiffness, and dryness are seen during stage I (acute stage) of complex regional pain syndrome. Progression to stage II (dystrophic stage) is characterized by worsening and constant pain, continued edema, and trophic skin changes. X-rays may reveal bone loss, osteoporosis, and subchondral bone erosion in the affected extremity. Stage III (atrophic stage) is characterized by pain that continues to spread, hardened edema, decreased limb temperature, and atrophic changes to fingertips or toes. X-rays at this stage may reveal demineralization and ankylosis. Motor disorders such as tremor, spasms, and atrophy may also be present throughout each stage of complex regional pain syndrome.

What laboratory or imaging studies would confirm the diagnosis?

Imaging studies that can assist with the diagnosis of complex regional pain syndrome include x-rays, thermographic studies, a three-phase bone scan, and laser Doppler flowmetry.

What additional information should be obtained to confirm the diagnosis?

Complex regional pain syndrome is diagnosed primarily through a complete physical examination and a patient's complete medical history including a history and course of illness.

MANAGEMENT

What is the most effective management of this patient?

Complex regional pain syndrome requires prolonged medical management. Treatment is based on identifying the underlying cause and stage of complex regional pain syndrome at the time of diagnosis. Pharmacological intervention may include NSAIDs and corticosteroids for pain relief in early stages. Amitriptyline may be used for sleep and calcium channel blockers used for increasing peripheral circulation. Baclofen has been used as a long-term intervention to assist motor function. Bisphosphonate administration is warranted in later stages to combat bone loss. Surgical interventions such as sympathetic blocks or a sympathectomy are used to alleviate pain. Physical therapy intervention is a key component in the management of complex regional pain syndrome. Pain control, patient education, skin care, joint mobilization, desensitization, and functional activity training are vital to the program. Modalities, pool therapy, relaxation training, and a home program all assist a patient with management of this syndrome.

What home care regimen should be recommended?

A home program is vital to the management of complex regional pain syndrome. Stretching and ROM, light weight bearing activities, ice and/or heat, TENS, and light exercise for conditioning are all key components of a home program. The patient must be educated and encouraged to use the involved extremity as tolerated. Edema management using a pump or compression garments may be indicated. Functional activities must also be encouraged.

OUTCOME

What is the likely outcome of a course in physical therapy?

Overall prognosis is better for a patient that begins treatment early in the cycle of the disease process. Physical therapy attempts to break the pain cycle and allows for a patient to continue with functional activities. Outcome is also dependent on a patient's motivation to maintain all aspects of a home program.

What are the long-term effects of the patient's condition?

Complex regional pain syndrome can spontaneously resolve, continue with ongoing symptoms that can last for years or follow a pattern of remissions and recurring symptoms that develop from subsequent injuries. A patient's long-term outcome is dependent on how early the complex regional pain syndrome was detected and treated. Research indicates a better prognosis if treatment is initiated within the first six months of the disease process.

DIAGNOSIS

What condition produces a patient's symptoms?

The human immunodeficiency virus (HIV) is a retrovirus that initially invades and destroys cells within the immune system, specifically CD4+ T-lymphocytes (T-cells). This virus also affects monocytes, macrophages, and B-cells. Once the T-cells decrease beyond a specific level a patient will begin to demonstrate symptoms of the HIV infection.

An injury was most likely sustained to which structure?

HIV infects T-cells within the immune system. Other cells that eventually house HIV include monocytes, macrophages, microglia, cervical cells, and epithelial cells of the GI tract. HIV uses and destroys the cells that possess the antigen CD4 on their surface in order to replicate HIV, and as a result the immune system becomes weaker and unable to function.

INFERENCE

What is the most likely contributing factor in the development of this condition?

HIV is transmitted through contact with blood, semen, vaginal secretions, and breast milk. Contact can be sexual, perinatal or through contact with blood or body fluids that carry infected cells. Risk factors for contracting HIV include unprotected sexual relations, intravenous drug use or mother to fetus transmission. The largest risk factors for HIV transmission are unprotected sex among men having sex with men (MSM), unprotected sex between men and women, and intravenous drug use with a shared needle.

CONFIRMATION

What is the most likely clinical presentation?

The incidence of newly diagnosed cases of HIV is approximately 50,000 per year within the United States. Without treatment, HIV advances in three stages: Acute HIV infection, Clinical Latency/Asymptomatic HIV, and AIDS. Stage 1: Acute HIV infection: This stage occurs 2-4 weeks after initial transmission. Patients can range from being asymptomatic to experiencing severe flu-like symptoms including fever, rash, myalgia, arthralgia, and headaches. During this stage, large amounts of the virus are being produced, CD4 cells fall rapidly, and the patient is at the highest risk of transmitting the virus to others. Stage 2: Clinical latency/Asymptomatic HIV/Chronic HIV infection: Patients on antiretroviral therapy (ART) can live with clinical latency for several decades as the treatment keeps the virus in check. Clinical latency for people not taking ART typically lasts 10 years before progressing to AIDS. Stage 3: AIDS: When the number of CD4 cells falls below 200 cells/mm^3 and the person has other AIDS-defining illnesses, a person is considered to have progressed to AIDS. Without treatment, people typically survive with AIDS about 3 years. Once a person has an opportunistic illness, life expectancy without treatment falls to about 1 year. Manifestations of HIV may lead to other infections, malignancies, neurological dysfunction, cognitive decline, and cardiopulmonary pathologies.

What laboratory or imaging studies would confirm the diagnosis?

HIV is diagnosed through various blood tests such as the enzyme-linked immunosorbent test or Western blot test. Once diagnosed the lab results can also assist with classifying the stage of HIV infection.

What additional information should be obtained to confirm the diagnosis?

Definitive diagnosis is made through blood tests, however, the physician should ascertain accurate medical and social history. Accurate drug use and sexual partner history will allow for appropriate patient education in order to cease the spread of the virus. A positive diagnosis will allow the patient to notify others at risk.

MANAGEMENT

What is the most effective management of this patient?

Early detection is important so that pharmacological intervention can be initiated and slow the progression of the virus. There is no cure for HIV, however, proper medical intervention can allow the virus to remain a manageable chronic condition. With proper medical management, people living with HIV have equal life expectancies as their HIV-negative counterparts. Current guidelines recommend antiretroviral therapy for all HIV-infected individuals, regardless of CD4 count, to reduce HIV-related morbidity and mortality. The goal of drug therapy is to significantly decrease the virus' ability to replicate, and therefore decrease the progression of the disease. Physical therapy intervention may be indicated during the course of HIV/AIDS due to secondary impairments. Physical therapy goals and intervention include the promotion of optimal fitness, flexibility, energy conservation, stress management, ADL equipment, relaxation, aquatic therapy, modalities, positioning, pain management, breathing exercises, and neurological rehabilitation.

What home care regimen should be recommended?

A patient with HIV must follow a home regimen including medication, proper nutrition and sleep, and fitness in order to remain as healthy as possible. A physical therapy home program can also minimize the negative effects on functional ability and improve the overall independence and quality of life.

OUTCOME

What is the likely outcome of a course in physical therapy?

Physical therapy may be warranted for periods of time throughout the progression of HIV/AIDS. Physical therapy cannot alter the progression of the virus, but can foster improvement in functional mobility, conditioning, and overall independence.

What are the long-term effects of the patient's condition?

The World Health Organization estimates 36.9 million people living with HIV/AIDS worldwide. Studies indicate that psychosocial factors influence progression of the virus as well as survival. Presently, the leading causes of death, in order of prevalence, AIDS-related (i.e., opportunistic infections), non-AIDS-defining cancers, liver disease, and cardiovascular disease.

Juvenile Rheumatoid Arthritis

DIAGNOSIS

What condition produces a patient's symptoms?

Juvenile rheumatoid arthritis (JRA) is a form of arthritis found in children less than 16 years of age. JRA causes inflammation and stiffness to multiple joints for a period of greater than six weeks. The inflammatory process affects the tissues surrounding the affected synovial joints causing symptoms of JRA.

An injury was most likely sustained to which structure?

JRA, like adult rheumatoid arthritis, is an autoimmune disorder that occurs when the immune cells mistakenly begin to attack the joints and organs causing local and systemic effects throughout the body. The severity of ongoing injury is based on the specific classification and subtype of the disease.

INFERENCE

What is the most likely contributing factor in the development of this condition?

The etiology for JRA is currently unknown. Research postulates that JRA develops in children with a genetic predisposition for the disease. The predisposition may be triggered by environmental factors or a viral or bacterial infection. Girls have a higher incidence of JRA and it is found to begin most commonly in the toddler or adolescent.

CONFIRMATION

What is the most likely clinical presentation?

JRA is an umbrella term for three specific classifications and subtypes of childhood arthritis. Classification is based on the number of joints involved, symptoms, presence of the rheumatoid factor (RF) or antinuclear antibody (ANA), and systemic involvement. General symptoms include persistent joint swelling, pain, and stiffness. Pauciarticular JRA involves four or less joints, is asymmetric, and is usually a mild form of JRA. This is the most common form of JRA and accounts for 50% of the cases, with girls under eight most likely to develop this subtype. ANA can also be found in 20-30% of patients and correlates with eye disease. Polyarticular JRA involves more than four joints, is usually symmetrical, involves the joints of the hands and feet as well as larger joints, and has potential for severe destruction. This subtype accounts for 30-40% of the cases and children may have the IgM rheumatoid factor (RF) similar to adult RA. Systemic JRA accounts for 10-20% of the cases and is otherwise known as Still's disease. Onset includes a high fever, chills, and a rash that may last for weeks, followed by severe myalgia and polyarthritis. This form presents with severe extraarticular manifestations including anemia, hepatosplenomegaly, lymphadenopathy, pericarditis, and myocarditis. Most children in this subtype are negative for RF or ANA antibodies. About 25% experience severe and unremitting arthritis.

What laboratory or imaging studies would confirm the diagnosis?

There is not a single test to identify the presence of JRA. Blood tests may include serum evaluation to measure inflammation and detect RF, ANA or HLA-B27 (human leukocyte antigen). Only a small percentage of patients with JRA possess RF or ANA. An erythrocyte sedimentation rate (ESR or "sed rate") may also indicate rheumatic disease. Other tests or procedures may be used to rule out other conditions such as Lyme disease, lupus, infection, and cancers.

What additional information should be obtained to confirm the diagnosis?

Diagnosis is made largely through physical examination, a patient's past and present medical status, and meeting the criteria set forth by the American Rheumatoid Association regarding the diagnosis and classification of JRA.

MANAGEMENT

What is the most effective management of this patient?

A pediatric rheumatologist is ideal to direct a multidisciplinary team in the complex care of JRA. Primary goals of treatment are to maintain a high level of physical functioning and quality of life. Pharmacological intervention may include NSAIDS, immunosuppressive medications, disease-modifying antirheumatic drugs, and corticosteroids. Physical therapy intervention is a key component and should include range of motion, exercise, and pain control. Functional mobility, strengthening, endurance, and aerobic training will assist a patient in overall function. Range of motion exercises, modalities, splints and orthotics, patient/family education, and the integration of recreational activities should optimize the quality of life. Surgical intervention is sometimes warranted for severe contractures or irreversible joint destruction. Soft tissue release, supracondylar osteotomy, and arthroplasty are the most common surgical procedures.

What home care regimen should be recommended?

A home care regimen should provide an individualized exercise program. The program should be simple and take no more than 20 minutes to complete in order to optimize compliance. Swimming is also a beneficial activity for a child with JRA.

OUTCOME

What is the likely outcome of a course in physical therapy?

Physical therapy may be indicated periodically throughout a patient's childhood based on symptoms and complications. Ongoing education and revision of a home program is vital to promote patient compliance. Physical therapy outcome is variable depending on the severity of the patient's symptoms.

What are the long-term effects of the patient's condition?

Long-term effects of JRA are dependent on subtype, symptoms, and any complications encountered. Some patients "outgrow" JRA and are not affected as adults while others experience pain and other manifestations of the disease on a consistent and long-term basis.

| BRONZE | Level Clinical Application Templates

BRONZE Level Clinical Application Template Executive Summary

Addison's Disease

- Adrenal insufficiency that occurs due to dysfunction of the adrenal cortex resulting in decreased production of glucocorticoid and mineralocorticoid hormones
- Glucocorticoid hormones assist in regulation of cardiovascular function, metabolism, and stress; mineralocorticoid hormones assist in regulation of fluid and electrolyte balances
- Laboratory results of the rapid adrenocorticotropic hormone (ACTH) test are considered to be definitive in the diagnosis of Addison's disease

Appendicitis

- An inflammation of the inner lining of the appendix which may spread to other areas
- Abdominal pain is most commonly reported with symptoms beginning as either umbilical or gastric pain that migrates to the right lower quadrant
- Examination findings typically include abdominal rebound tenderness, pain with percussion, guarding, and rigidity

Chronic Fatigue Syndrome

- Complex condition with an unknown etiology; potential etiologies include a viral origin, an immune response to inflammation with the nervous system, or a combination of lifestyle factors
- Best managed using a multidisciplinary approach including education, medical management, cognitive behavioral therapy, and exercise
- There is no cure; symptom presentation, progression, and resolution can be highly variable making outcomes difficult to predict

Crohn's Disease

- A specific form of inflammatory bowel disease in which the lining of the gastrointestinal (GI) tract becomes abnormally inflamed
- Typical signs and symptoms range from mild to significantly debilitating to life-threatening
- Symptoms may develop gradually or rapidly and typically include abdominal pain, cramping, diarrhea, blood in the stool, GI tract ulcers, diminished appetite, and weight loss

Cushing's Syndrome

- Results from abnormally high levels of cortisol which may occur due to endogenous overproduction of cortisol or excessive exogenous use of corticosteroids
- Typically present with hallmark physical signs including weight gain, purple striae, and a ruddy complexion
- May be diagnosed by laboratory analysis of cortisol levels in urine, saliva or blood

Diastasis Recti

- Refers to a separation of the right and left sides of the rectus abdominis
- The condition is not exclusively seen in women who are pregnant, however, there is a significant prevalence among this population
- Most patients improve with conservative treatment focused on corrective exercise and do not suffer long-term functional deficits associated with the condition

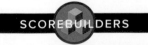

Level Clinical Application Template Executive Summary

Diverticular Disease

- Benign condition characterized by the presence of outpocketings of the colon wall (i.e., diverticula)
- Risk factors include constipation, a diet low in fiber, obesity, a lack of exercise, connective tissue disorders, and advanced age
- Patients are often asymptomatic, though may experience abdominal pain and tenderness, fever, nausea, vomiting, constipation or diarrhea

Gastroesophageal Reflux Disease

- Gastroesophageal reflux refers to the abnormal movement of partially digested solids, liquids, and gastric acid from the stomach into the esophagus
- Most common complaints include heartburn, acid reflux, nausea after eating, and feeling as though food remains trapped in the esophagus
- Typically diagnosed by reported symptoms and physical examination with additional testing for patients who do not respond to initial treatment

Gout

- Considered a complex form of arthritis resulting from an abnormally high uric acid level (hyperuricemia) in the body
- Greater prevalence among males with the great toe, knee, and ankle being the most commonly affected joints; may present as a chronic condition or a series of acute attacks
- Identification of uric acid crystals in synovial fluid, collected via synovial biopsy, may be used to confirm the diagnosis

Graves' Disease

- Most common form of hyperactive thyroid disorder and is the result of an autoimmune attack on the thyroid gland causing overproduction of the hormone thyroxine (T4)
- General complaints may include heat intolerance, increased appetite, increased sweating, frequent bowel movements, physical fatigue, weakness, tremor, weight loss, and insomnia
- Typically responds well to pharmacological intervention that regulates T4 hormone production

Irritable Bowel Syndrome

- Characterized by gastrointestinal distress and alterations in bowel habits, such as constipation and diarrhea, which may be triggered by foods, stress or illness
- There are three main types of the condition: diarrhea-predominant, constipation-predominant, and alternating diarrhea and constipation symptoms
- Diagnosis is based on symptoms and the exclusion of other similar conditions

Lung Cancer

- Smoking, or exposure to smoke, is the leading cause of lung cancer
- Signs and symptoms that may suggest lung cancer include wheezing, coughing, hemoptysis, shortness of breath, chest pain, weight loss, fever, clubbing of the fingernails, and fatigue
- X-ray imaging is often used to detect an abnormal mass or nodule within the lungs, though computed tomography may be used to detect smaller lesions that cannot be seen on x-ray

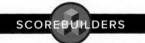

BRONZE Level Clinical Application Template Executive Summary

Malignant Melanoma

- A form of skin cancer considered to be especially serious due to the high likelihood of metastasis that develops in the melanin-producing cells responsible for giving skin its color
- The first sign is a suspicious change in the appearance of a freckle or mole through asymmetry, irregular borders, uneven coloration or increased diameter
- Diagnosis of malignant melanoma is typically confirmed by an analysis of biopsied tissue

Metabolic Acidosis

- A state in which the pH of body fluids is abnormally low, which may result from overproduction or inadequate excretion of hydrogen ions or excessive excretion of bicarbonate ions
- Common signs and symptoms include tachypnea, confusion, and lethargy, though other signs and symptoms may present depending on the underlying pathology
- Laboratory analysis of arterial blood gases, serum electrolytes, and urine pH are used to identify abnormal acidity and differentiate between respiratory and metabolic acidosis

Metabolic Alkalosis

- A state in which the pH of body fluids is abnormally elevated, which may result from inadequate excretion of bicarbonate ions, ingestion of large amounts of bicarbonate or excessive excretion of hydrogen ions
- Common signs and symptoms include bradypnea and symptoms of hypokalemia (e.g., weakness, myalgia, polyuria), though other signs and symptoms may present depending on the underlying pathology
- Laboratory analysis of arterial blood gases, serum electrolytes, and urine pH are used to identify abnormal alkalinity and differentiate between respiratory and metabolic alkalosis

Peptic Ulcer Disease

- Peptic ulcers form when the balance of protective and erosive factors is disrupted to such an extent that epithelial injury occurs and subsequent erosion extends to the muscularis mucosa
- Primary symptom of a burning epigastric pain that occurs after eating; other symptoms include dyspepsia, chest discomfort, heartburn, fatty food intolerance, and hematemesis
- Upper GI endoscopy is typically the diagnostic tool of choice allowing for visualization and tissue biopsy

Prostate Cancer

- Prostate cancer is generally a slow-growing cancer, though it can metastasize to other parts of the body, especially the lymph nodes and bones
- Symptoms are more likely to be present in the advanced stages of the disease and may include difficulty urinating, nocturia, erectile dysfunction, blood in the urine or semen, pelvic or low back pain, and bone pain, if metastasized
- The prostate-specific antigen (PSA) test is a blood test used to determine the presence of elevated levels of PSA, which can be indicative of prostate cancer

Level Clinical Application Template Executive Summary

Ulcerative Colitis

- An inflammatory bowel disease that results in chronic inflammation and the formation of ulcers in the large intestine
- Symptoms may include abdominal pain and cramping, diarrhea, blood in the stools, urgency to defecate, weight loss, fatigue, and fever
- The best test for diagnosing ulcerative colitis is endoscopy, which allows for direct visualization of the colon

Urinary Tract Infection

- The urinary tract is normally a sterile environment, but under certain conditions infectious organisms from internal or external sources can proliferate and cause infection
- Characterized by a strong and persistent urge to urinate, as well as a burning sensation with urination
- Urinalysis and urine culture are most commonly used to diagnose a urinary tract infection, however, patients who suffer recurrent urinary tract infections may require more invasive diagnostic testing

Uterine Cancer

- The most common type of uterine cancer affects the endometrium, which is thought to occur when an imbalance of hormones causes the endometrium to grow thicker
- Unexpected vaginal bleeding is the most common symptom associated with uterine cancer, especially when it occurs after menopause
- The only method to confirm the diagnosis of uterine cancer is through a tissue biopsy, which is obtained during a procedure known as dilation and curettage

Addison's Disease

DIAGNOSIS

What condition produces a patient's symptoms?

Addison's disease refers to a specific form of adrenal insufficiency that occurs due to dysfunction of the adrenal cortex resulting in decreased production of glucocorticoid (e.g., cortisol) and mineralocorticoid (e.g., aldosterone) hormones. Glucocorticoid hormones assist with regulation of cardiovascular function, metabolism, and the body's response to stress. Mineralocorticoid hormones assist in the regulation of fluids and electrolytes.

An injury was most likely sustained to which structure?

The most common etiology of Addison's disease is idiopathic autoimmune adrenocortical insufficiency. The chronic condition is the result of an abnormal autoimmune response which causes atrophy, fibrosis, and infiltration of lymphocytes within the adrenal cortex. Etiologies of acute Addison's disease include stress due to infection, trauma, emotional distress, adrenal hemorrhage, and adrenal artery embolism or thrombosis.

CONFIRMATION

What is the most likely clinical presentation?

Characteristics of Addison's disease typically mimic signs and symptoms of glucocorticoid and mineralocorticoid deficiency. Hyperpigmentation of the skin and mucous membranes is typically the first symptom to present, with changes most notable over areas frequently exposed to the sun. Vitiligo, gastrointestinal symptoms, syncope, weakness, fatigue, and myalgias are also common. Idiopathic autoimmune Addison's disease is most prevalent among females, typically between 30 and 50 years of age. Patients may experience an adrenal crisis presenting with significant nausea and vomiting while appearing confused and cyanotic. Abdominal symptoms may be acute including abdominal distention, pain, and tenderness.

What laboratory or imaging studies would confirm the diagnosis?

Laboratory results of the rapid adrenocorticotropic hormone (ACTH) test are considered to be definitive in the diagnosis of Addison's disease. Other laboratory studies may include a complete metabolic panel, complete blood count, antibody testing, and thyroid-stimulating hormone (TSH) test.

What additional information should be obtained to confirm the diagnosis?

A complete medical history should be obtained. Information regarding a familial history of adrenal insufficiency and commonly occurring comorbidities such as Graves' disease, type 1 diabetes mellitus or celiac disease should also be reviewed.

Appendicitis

DIAGNOSIS

What condition produces a patient's symptoms?

Appendicitis refers to an inflammation of the inner lining of the appendix which may spread to other areas. The inflammation may occur for a number of reasons, however, infection and obstruction of the appendiceal lumen are among the most commonly reported causes. Both etiologies result in increased pressure as bacteria multiply and fluids stagnate within the appendix. Eventually, the walls of the appendix become ischemic compromising their integrity and allowing for bacterial invasion which can lead to perforation, gangrene, peritonitis or abscess.

An injury was most likely sustained to which structure?

The appendix extends from the cecum as a worm-like projection. Though its position is not fixed, it is most commonly located in a dorsomedial position in the right lower quadrant. The actual position of an individual's appendix can considerably alter the clinical presentation of appendicitis.

CONFIRMATION

What is the most likely clinical presentation?

Presentation may vary depending on the age of the patient, position of the appendix, and degree of inflammation. Abdominal pain is most commonly reported with symptoms beginning as either umbilical or gastric pain that migrates to the right lower quadrant. Patients will often try to remain still, lying down with the hips flexed in an attempt to avoid exacerbating movements. Nausea, vomiting, and anorexia are also often reported. The duration of symptoms is typically less than 48 hours in adults, but may be longer in elderly patients or in instances when the appendix has perforated. Examination findings typically include abdominal rebound tenderness, pain with percussion, guarding, and rigidity.

What laboratory or imaging studies would confirm the diagnosis?

Laboratory tests are utilized to confirm the presence of infection or inflammation. Tests typically include a complete blood count, C-reactive protein test, urinalysis, and in some cases liver and pancreatic function tests. Imaging studies such as ultrasonography, CT scan, and MRI may be used.

What additional information should be obtained to confirm the diagnosis?

A thorough medical and symptom history should be obtained to assist in ruling out similar diagnoses. Specific questions regarding recent gastroenterologic and genitourinary conditions should be included as well as a gynecologic history for female patients.

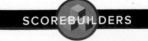

Chronic Fatigue Syndrome   BRONZE

DIAGNOSIS

What condition produces a patient's symptoms?

Chronic fatigue syndrome (CFS) is a complex condition with unknown etiology. Potential etiologies include a viral origin, an immune response to inflammation within the nervous system or a combination of lifestyle factors (e.g., stress, environment), non-modifiable factors (e.g., age, genetics), and comorbidities.

An injury was most likely sustained to which structure?

Since the exact etiology of CFS is unknown, the condition cannot be linked specifically to one structure or system.

CONFIRMATION

What is the most likely clinical presentation?

Patients must meet several specific criteria in order to meet the diagnostic criteria set forth by the Centers for Disease Control and Prevention. These criteria include a history of at least six months of unexplained, prolonged, and severe fatigue that is not relieved by rest. This must be accompanied by at least four of eight additional symptoms, including self-reported memory or concentration deficits severe enough to interfere with daily activities, persistent or recurrent sore throat, painful or enlarged axillary or cervical lymph nodes, unexplained muscle pain, migrating joint pain without visible signs of inflammation, complaints of malaise lasting more than 24 hours after physical or mental exertion, and headache that exhibits changes in pattern or severity.

What laboratory or imaging studies would confirm the diagnosis?

The etiology of CFS is unknown, therefore no specific diagnostic tests exist to confirm the diagnosis. Since CFS is considered a diagnosis of exclusion, laboratory and imaging studies are frequently used to rule out other conditions known to produce severe and prolonged fatigue (e.g., hypothyroidism, multiple sclerosis, cancer, mononucleosis).

What additional information should be obtained to confirm the diagnosis?

A thorough medical history should be obtained to assist in ruling out other conditions that may mimic the symptoms of CFS, including psychological disorders, sleep apnea, eating disorders, substance abuse, and morbid obesity. Additional diagnostic testing may be warranted if a specific alternative pathology is suspected.

Crohn's Disease   BRONZE

DIAGNOSIS

What condition produces a patient's symptoms?

Crohn's disease is a specific form of inflammatory bowel disease in which the lining of the gastrointestinal (GI) tract becomes abnormally inflamed. Symptoms can involve any aspect of the GI tract, however, typically present in lower structures (e.g., small bowel, colon). Symptom complaints are typically associated with an exacerbation of the inflammatory process or complications such as fibrosis or obstruction.

An injury was most likely sustained to which structure?

The etiology of Crohn's disease is idiopathic, but likely the result of an imbalance between anti-inflammatory and pro-inflammatory mediators within the GI tract. Structural injury typically begins with ulceration, hyperemia, and edema of the GI tract's superficial mucosal lining. The inflammatory process may cause adhesions, fibrosis, thickening, and may also spread to deeper mucosal layers forming granulomas or abscesses.

CONFIRMATION

What is the most likely clinical presentation?

The typical signs and symptoms range from mild to significantly debilitating to life-threatening. Symptoms may develop gradually or rapidly and typically include abdominal pain, cramping, and diarrhea. Other symptoms may include blood in the stool, GI tract ulcers, diminished appetite, and weight loss. Over time, some patients may develop complications including anal fissures, intestinal fistula, malnutrition, and bowel obstruction. The chronic inflammatory process may also precipitate symptoms such as gallstones, kidney stones, arthritis, and osteoporosis. Children with Crohn's disease typically experience delays in normal growth and development.

What laboratory or imaging studies would confirm the diagnosis?

Blood tests may be utilized to determine the presence of infection, anemia or abnormal antibodies and also typically include a fecal occult blood test. Invasive imaging procedures such as colonoscopy and sigmoidoscopy allow for lower GI visualization and the collection of tissue samples. X-ray, MRI, and CT scan may be visually enhanced using barium to assist in the identification of affected intestinal segments.

What additional information should be obtained to confirm the diagnosis?

A medical history should be completed to rule out similar diagnoses such as colon cancer, irritable bowel syndrome, and diverticulitis. Patients with a family history of Crohn's disease, who smoke, or who maintain a diet high in fat are at greater risk for developing the condition.

BRONZE   Cushing's Syndrome

DIAGNOSIS

What condition produces a patient's symptoms?

Cortisol is a glucocorticoid hormone produced by the adrenal cortex which assists in the regulation of cardiovascular function, metabolism, and the body's response to stress. Cushing's syndrome is a condition resulting from abnormally high levels of cortisol due to endogenous overproduction of cortisol or excessive exogenous use of corticosteroids.

An injury was most likely sustained to which structure?

The most common endogenous etiology of hypercortisolism is a pituitary or adrenal gland tumor. Pituitary tumors are typically benign and linked to increased production of the adrenocorticotropic hormone (ACTH) which stimulates cortisol overproduction. This condition is termed Cushing's syndrome. A benign adrenal cortex tumor may also cause cortisol overproduction independent of ACTH influence. Less common endogenous etiologies include genetics and malignancy. Exogenous etiologies are linked to high doses of corticosteroids typically used for inflammatory conditions.

CONFIRMATION

What is the most likely clinical presentation?

Patients with Cushing's syndrome typically present with hallmark physical signs including weight gain, purple striae, and a ruddy complexion. Weight gain is accompanied by increased adipose tissue distribution in the face (e.g., "moon face"), upper back (e.g., "buffalo hump"), torso (e.g., central obesity), and supraclavicular region. Other symptoms include fatigue, depression, emotional lability, excessive hair growth, bruising, and proximal muscle weakness. Systemically, Cushing's syndrome may contribute to conditions such as hypertension, diabetes mellitus, peptic ulcer disease, osteopenia, and immune system impairment. There is a significantly greater prevalence among women with the onset of symptoms between 25 and 40 years of age.

What laboratory or imaging studies would confirm the diagnosis?

Cushing's syndrome may be diagnosed by laboratory analysis of cortisol levels in urine, saliva or blood. Laboratory studies detailing the body's response to a low dose of dexamethasone, alone or in combination with ACTH stimulation, are also considered to be diagnostically valid.

What additional information should be obtained to confirm the diagnosis?

A thorough medical history and physical examination should be completed to rule out similar diagnoses and identify characteristics commonly associated with the condition.

BRONZE   Diastasis Recti

DIAGNOSIS

What condition produces a patient's symptoms?

Diastasis recti refers to a separation of the right and left sides of the rectus abdominis. This is typically the result of anteriorly directed sustained internal pressure which weakens and eventually splits the connective tissue between the two sides of the muscle. The result is an alteration in the alignment and mechanics of the rectus abdominis which may lead to trunk instability and, in severe cases, abdominal hernia.

An injury was most likely sustained to which structure?

The medial aspects of the right and left rectus abdominis are connected by a fibrous band extending from the xiphoid process to the pubic symphysis. This seam of connective tissue is referred to as the linea alba. Sustained pressure within the abdomen that is directed anteriorly weakens the fibers of the linea alba causing it to stretch and in some cases split. This may occur in a segment of the fibrous line or along the full length depending on the duration and force of the pressure.

CONFIRMATION

What is the most likely clinical presentation?

The degree of muscle separation is highly variable. A visible separation can be observed in one or more positions (e.g., sitting, standing, supine), though this varies widely based on the patient's body morphology. Abdominal weakness, decreased lumbar stability, and low back pain complaints are often noted due to the altered mechanics associated with the rectus separation. Abdominal pain may be present if excessive stretching has caused microtearing within the muscle tissue.

What laboratory or imaging studies would confirm the diagnosis?

There are no specific laboratory or imaging tests used to diagnose diastasis recti.

What additional information should be obtained to confirm the diagnosis?

A thorough medical history and physical examination should be completed. Diastasis recti is typically diagnosed on the basis of the physical examination. The patient should be positioned in hooklying and asked to lift their head and shoulders from the supporting surface. While in this position, a palpable separation of greater than two finger widths is considered to signify the presence of diastasis recti.

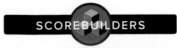

Diverticular Disease   BRONZE

DIAGNOSIS

What condition produces a patient's symptoms?

Diverticulosis is a benign condition characterized by the presence of outpocketings of the colon wall (i.e., diverticula). The condition develops secondary to increased pressure within the colon. Diverticulitis is the condition characterized by the inflammation or infection of the diverticula. Risk factors for this condition include constipation, a diet low in fiber, obesity, a lack of exercise, connective tissue disorders (e.g., Marfan syndrome, Ehlers-Danlos syndrome), and advanced age.

An injury was most likely sustained to what structure?

The condition is characterized by outpocketings of the colon wall, most often in the sigmoid colon. When the colon experiences an increase in pressure, pockets develop in areas where the wall of the colon is weak (i.e., herniations). If these pockets become further damaged or rupture, they may become infected (i.e., diverticulitis).

CONFIRMATION

What is the most likely clinical presentation?

Patients with diverticulosis will likely be asymptomatic. They may experience abdominal pain and tenderness (often in the left lower quadrant), fever, nausea, vomiting, constipation or diarrhea. More serious complications of the condition include rectal bleeding, colonic obstruction, and infection of the abdominal cavity.

What laboratory or imaging studies would confirm the diagnosis?

Computed tomography is the most commonly used tool to identify the presence of diverticulitis. A colonoscopy can be performed to directly visualize the diverticula and surrounding structures, though it should not be conducted during or shortly after an acute episode of diverticulitis.

What additional information should be obtained to confirm the diagnosis?

A thorough medical history and physical examination should be performed to rule out other pathologies that may cause abdominal pain. The physical examination would include palpation of the abdomen to check for areas of tenderness.

Gastroesophageal Reflux Disease   BRONZE

DIAGNOSIS

What condition produces a patient's symptoms?

Gastroesophageal reflux occurs in the upper gastrointestinal tract and refers to the abnormal movement of partially digested solids, liquids, and gastric acid from the stomach into the esophagus. This back flow of highly acidic stomach contents irritates the lining of the esophagus causing acid indigestion. Occasional reflux is common, however, chronic recurrences are typically indicative of gastroesophageal reflux disease (GERD).

An injury was most likely sustained to which structure?

The esophagus has both an upper esophageal sphincter (UES) and a lower esophageal sphincter (LES) which function to prevent regurgitation. A weak or abnormally functioning LES that fails to close completely will allow stomach contents to reflux into the esophagus. Persistent reflux, as is characteristic of GERD, can cause significant irritation of the esophageal lining and eventual esophagitis leading to more severe damage and additional symptoms such as esophageal erosion and bleeding.

CONFIRMATION

What is the most likely clinical presentation?

Patients with GERD can present with a variety of symptoms that typically occur more than twice weekly and interfere to some degree with daily life. The most common complaints include heartburn, acid reflux, nausea after eating, and feeling as though food remains trapped in the esophagus. Other symptoms may include a sour taste in the mouth, dysphagia, chest pain, dry cough, hoarseness, and the sensation of a lump in the throat. GERD symptoms are often increased with bending, stooping or supine positioning and tend to worsen at night.

What laboratory or imaging studies would confirm the diagnosis?

A barium swallow with x-ray imaging of the upper GI tract may be used to identify structural or anatomical problems within the esophagus. An upper GI endoscopy may be used to visualize and identify esophageal irritation or damage. GERD is typically diagnosed by reported symptoms and physical examination with additional testing pursued in patients who do not respond to initial treatment.

What additional information should be obtained to confirm the diagnosis?

A thorough medical history should be obtained with a detailed symptom history. Patients at increased risk for developing GERD include those who are obese, pregnant, use cigarettes, abuse alcohol or present with a hiatal hernia or scleroderma.

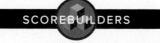

BRONZE   Gout

DIAGNOSIS

What condition produces a patient's symptoms?

Gout is a complex form of arthritis resulting from an abnormally high uric acid level in the body. This most commonly occurs secondary to the underexcretion of uric acid, but can also result from overproduction of uric acid or a combination of both. As uric acid levels increase around joints, needle-like crystals form and accumulate causing inflammation and joint swelling.

An injury was most likely sustained to which structure?

Uric acid is formed as the body breaks down foods that are high in purine. The etiology of hyperuricemia is often idiopathic, however, a number of medical conditions (e.g., ketoacidosis, hypothyroidism) and side effects of certain medications are also associated with hyperuricemia. Some individuals with hyperuricemia fail to develop symptoms of gout while others may be asymptomatic for years prior to the first acute gout attack. Structural damage is more commonly associated with chronic gout.

CONFIRMATION

What is the most likely clinical presentation?

Gout has a significantly greater prevalence among males with the great toe, knee, and ankle being the most commonly affected joints. Gout may present as a chronic condition or a series of acute attacks. An acute attack typically involves a single joint and presents with signs of inflammation including pain, redness, and warmth. Pain tends to be severe and is described as throbbing, crushing or excruciating. The onset of acute symptoms typically begins with a rapid progression of discomfort, often occurring at night time, which then gradually eases over time. In chronic gout, multiple joints tend to be affected with less intense symptoms. Chronic gout may go unrecognized initially with symptoms attributed to arthritis. Firm, lumpy deposits of uric acid that form under the skin, referred to as tophi, are typically associated with chronic gout.

What laboratory or imaging studies would confirm the diagnosis?

The identification of uric acid crystals in synovial fluid, collected via synovial biopsy, may be used to confirm the diagnosis. Abnormal systemic levels of uric acid may be assessed through laboratory analysis of blood and urine samples.

What additional information should be obtained to confirm the diagnosis?

A thorough medical history and physical examination should be completed. Conditions such as obesity, kidney disease, diabetes mellitus or insipidus, leukemia, and sickle cell anemia are associated with an increased incidence of gout.

BRONZE   Graves' Disease

DIAGNOSIS

What condition produces a patient's symptoms?

Graves' disease is the most common form of hyperactive thyroid disorder and is the result of an autoimmune attack on the thyroid gland causing overproduction of the hormone thyroxine (T4). Abnormally high levels of T4 increase the body's metabolic rate producing subsequent symptoms. The etiology of Graves' disease is currently unknown.

An injury was most likely sustained to which structure?

The thyroid gland is a part of the endocrine system, located anteriorly in the neck just below the larynx. It is butterfly-shaped and responsible for the release of the T4 and triiodothyronine (T3) hormones which control metabolism and influence factors such as weight, mood, and general energy levels. Patients with Graves' disease have an abnormal presence of the thyroid-stimulating hormone receptor antibody (TRAb). TRAb mimics the effect of the thyroid-stimulating hormone (TSH) released by the pituitary gland that results in an increased production of T4.

CONFIRMATION

What is the most likely clinical presentation?

Patients with Graves' disease typically present with a variety of multi-systemic symptoms. General complaints may include heat intolerance, increased appetite, increased sweating, frequent bowel movements, physical fatigue, weakness, tremor, weight loss, and insomnia. Visual complaints typically stem from exophthalmos, which may cause excessive tear production, double vision, light sensitivity, and eye irritation. Cardiopulmonary complaints may include dyspnea with exertion, palpitations, tachycardia, and arrhythmias. Cognitive changes may include increased anxiety, mental fatigue, and difficulty with concentration.

What laboratory or imaging studies would confirm the diagnosis?

Graves' disease is typically diagnosed through blood analysis of T3 and T4 hormone levels as well as TSH released by the pituitary gland. An elevated T4 level in combination with low TSH is considered indicative of Graves' disease. Thyroid function may be further evaluated via a radioactive iodine uptake test. A high uptake of radioactive iodine is indicative of excess T4 production, as occurs with Graves' disease.

What additional information should be obtained to confirm the diagnosis?

A thorough medical history should be obtained and physical examination completed, including a detailed assessment of reported symptoms.

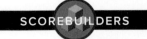

Irritable Bowel Syndrome

DIAGNOSIS

What condition produces a patient's symptoms?

Irritable bowel syndrome (IBS) is a condition characterized by gastrointestinal distress and alterations in bowel habits, such as constipation and diarrhea. The exact etiology of IBS is not known. Theories include an overgrowth of bacteria in the small intestine and altered signaling between the brain and gastrointestinal tract. Triggers for the condition include foods, stress, and illness.

An injury was most likely sustained to what structure?

IBS is a condition that affects the gastrointestinal tract, specifically the large intestine. The walls of the intestines are lined with muscular layers which contract and relax to pass food along the tract. When the contractions are longer or stronger than normal, symptoms of gastrointestinal distress (e.g., bloating, flatulence) may result. When the contractions are too weak, stools may become hard and dry and lead to constipation. Unlike other gastrointestinal disorders (e.g., Crohn's disease, ulcerative colitis), IBS does not result in structural changes to the intestinal tissue.

CONFIRMATION

What is the most likely clinical presentation?

IBS is characterized by abdominal pain and discomfort, bloating, flatulence, and constipation and/or diarrhea. There are three main types of the condition: diarrhea-predominant (IBS-D), constipation-predominant (IBS-C) or alternating diarrhea and constipation symptoms (IBS-A). Typically, IBS is a chronic condition that will require lifetime management of symptoms.

What laboratory or imaging studies would confirm the diagnosis?

There are no laboratory or imaging studies that diagnose IBS. Colonoscopy or computed tomography may be performed to rule out other conditions that produce abdominal pain and gastrointestinal distress. Blood tests and stool tests may also be performed for this reason.

What additional information should be obtained to confirm the diagnosis?

A thorough medical history and physical examination should be performed since this condition is diagnosed based on symptoms and the exclusion of other similar conditions. Abdominal pain that improves with defecation and changes in stool consistency are two symptoms that often suggest the presence of IBS.

Lung Cancer

DIAGNOSIS

What condition produces a patient's symptoms?

Lung cancer is a malignant tumor within the lungs that is characterized by uncontrolled cell growth. Smoking or exposure to smoke is the leading cause of lung cancer. Approximately 10-15% of lung cancer occurs in individuals that have never smoked. Other causes of lung cancer may include genetic factors and exposure to radon gas, asbestos or air pollution.

An injury was most likely sustained to what structure?

Lung cancer arises when carcinogens damage the epithelial cells of the lungs. Initially, the body is able to repair the cell damage, though cumulative damage causes genetic mutation to the DNA of the cells and leads to development of a tumor. As the cells divide and proliferate, they may metastasize to other areas of the body. Lung cancer metastasizes early, making it a very difficult cancer to treat. Common locations of metastasis include the adrenal glands, liver, brain, and bones.

CONFIRMATION

What is the most likely clinical presentation?

Signs and symptoms that may suggest lung cancer include wheezing, coughing, hemoptysis, shortness of breath, chest pain, weight loss, fever, clubbing of the fingernails, and fatigue. Signs and symptoms often only present in the more advanced stages of the disease, which results in a poor prognosis.

What laboratory or imaging studies would confirm the diagnosis?

X-ray imaging is often used to detect an abnormal mass or nodule within the lungs, though computed tomography may be used to detect smaller lesions that cannot be seen on x-ray. If cancer is suspected, a tissue biopsy may be performed to determine the presence of malignant cells. If the patient presents with a cough that produces sputum, the sputum can also be tested to identify the presence of malignant cells. A bone scan may be performed to determine the level of metastasis.

What additional information should be obtained to confirm the diagnosis?

A thorough medical history and physical examination is helpful in identifying signs and symptoms that may be suspicious for lung cancer. Once lung cancer has been diagnosed, the physician will "stage" the cancer (i.e., the extent of metastasis) to determine what treatment is most appropriate.

BRONZE   Malignant Melanoma

DIAGNOSIS

What condition produces a patient's symptoms?

Malignant melanoma is a form of skin cancer considered to be especially serious due to the high risk of metastasis. The cancer develops in the melanin-producing cells responsible for giving skin its color. The disease is most commonly diagnosed among patients with light complexions. Visible changes in skin markings may be more difficult to detect in darker skin tones leading to a delay in diagnosis and a less favorable prognosis.

An injury was most likely sustained to which structure?

Injury occurs at the cellular level with an alteration in melanocyte DNA causing cell overproduction and the formation of a malignant mass. The exact etiology of this abnormality is unclear, however, exposure to ultraviolet radiation is regarded to be the most significant risk factor.

CONFIRMATION

What is the most likely clinical presentation?

Most melanomas develop in areas of skin that have been extensively exposed to ultraviolet radiation such as the face, chest, back, arms, and legs. Typically, the first sign of melanoma is a suspicious change in the appearance of a freckle or mole. Asymmetry, irregular borders, uneven coloration or increased diameter of a skin marking may all be signs of malignancy. Many melanomas do not exclusively occur in areas exposed to ultraviolet radiation. Occurrences in these areas are often difficult to detect due to limited visibility or overlooked due to their uncommon location. Consequently, detection is often delayed increasing the likelihood of metastasis occurring before a diagnosis is made.

What laboratory or imaging studies would confirm the diagnosis?

A diagnosis of malignant melanoma is typically confirmed by an analysis of biopsied tissue. The type of biopsy utilized depends on the location, type of skin involved, and specific presentation. If melanoma is confirmed, a sentinel node biopsy is typically recommended to determine if the cancerous cells have metastasized to nearby lymph nodes.

What additional information should be obtained to confirm the diagnosis?

A thorough medical history and physical examination should be completed. Factors that increase the risk of developing melanoma include living at high altitudes close to the equator, history of sunburns or ultraviolet radiation exposure, excessive number of moles, fair skin, weakened immune system, and a family history of melanoma. Regular skin examinations are recommended for early identification of suspicious skin marks.

BRONZE   Metabolic Acidosis

DIAGNOSIS

What condition produces a patient's symptoms?

Metabolic acidosis refers to a state in which the pH of body fluids is abnormally low indicating acidemia. This may result from overproduction or inadequate excretion of hydrogen ions (H+) or excessive excretion of bicarbonate ions (HCO_3-). Conditions such as ketoacidosis and lactic acidosis are common forms of metabolic acidosis related to H+ overproduction. Impaired kidney function is most often associated with metabolic acidosis due to inadequate H+ excretion. The kidneys may also play a role in excessive HCO_3- excretion, however, severe diarrhea is more often the etiology of excessive HCO_3- excretion.

An injury was most likely sustained to which structure?

Metabolic acidosis is not an independent disease process, but rather a symptom of some other underlying condition or disease. Injuries sustained vary with the etiology of the acidosis.

CONFIRMATION

What is the most likely clinical presentation?

Tachypnea is often observed as the body tries to regulate its acid-base balance by inducing respiratory alkalosis through hyperventilation. Confusion or lethargy is likely to occur as acid levels increase. Other signs and symptoms are typically related more to the underlying pathology than the resultant acid-base imbalance. Depending on the etiology, metabolic acidosis can cause a variety of nonspecific symptoms including tinnitus, cardiac arrhythmia, chest pain, headache, visual changes, vomiting, abdominal pain, generalized weakness, and hyperventilation. Metabolic acidosis may present as either an acute or chronic condition and can be fatal if left untreated.

What laboratory or imaging studies would confirm the diagnosis?

Laboratory analysis of arterial blood gases, serum electrolytes, and urine pH are used to identify abnormal acidity and differentiate between respiratory and metabolic acidosis.

What additional information should be obtained to confirm the diagnosis?

A thorough medical history should be obtained in order to identify conditions which may contribute to systemic H+ increases (e.g., uncontrolled diabetes, alcoholism, salicylate poisoning), inadequate H+ excretion (e.g., renal failure) or excessive HCO_3- loss (e.g., severe diarrhea, intestinal fistula).

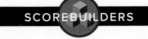

Metabolic Alkalosis   BRONZE

DIAGNOSIS

What condition produces a patient's symptoms?

Metabolic alkalosis refers to a state in which the pH of body fluids is abnormally elevated indicating alkalemia. This typically results from inadequate excretion of bicarbonate ions (HCO_3^-), ingestion of large amounts of bicarbonate (e.g., antacids) or excessive excretion of hydrogen ions (H^+). Renal dysfunction is typically the etiology of metabolic alkalosis due to inadequate HCO_3^- excretion. Metabolic alkalosis due to excessive H^+ excretion is most frequently attributed to the use of diuretics or activities that decrease the body's volume of acidic substances (e.g., gastric acid) such as vomiting and nasogastric suctioning.

An injury was most likely sustained to which structure?

Metabolic alkalosis is not an independent disease process, but rather a symptom of some other underlying condition or disease. Injuries sustained vary with the etiology of the alkalosis.

CONFIRMATION

What is the most likely clinical presentation?

Bradypnea is typically observed as the body tries to regulate its acid-base balance by inducing respiratory acidosis through hypoventilation. In patients with other pulmonary impairments, this may also cause hypoxemia. In severe cases, metabolic alkalosis can cause seizure, tetany, altered mental status or arrhythmia. Patients with metabolic alkalosis typically present with symptoms of hypokalemia (e.g., weakness, myalgia, polyuria). Other signs and symptoms tend to be nonspecific and related more to the underlying pathology of the acid-base imbalance. Metabolic alkalosis may present as either an acute or chronic condition and can be fatal if untreated.

What laboratory or imaging studies would confirm the diagnosis?

Laboratory analysis of arterial blood gases, serum electrolytes, and urine pH are used to identify abnormal alkalinity and differentiate between respiratory and metabolic alkalosis.

What additional information should be obtained to confirm the diagnosis?

A thorough medical history should be obtained in order to identify conditions which may contribute to systemic increases in HCO_3^- (e.g., blood transfusion, significant alkali ingestion) or decreases in H^+ (e.g., bulimia, hypertension).

Peptic Ulcer Disease   BRONZE

DIAGNOSIS

What condition produces a patient's symptoms?

Peptic ulcer disease affects the gastrointestinal (GI) tract and encompasses both gastric and duodenal ulcers. H. pylori infection and use of high-dose NSAIDs are the two most prevalent etiologies linked to peptic ulcer disease. Other etiologies include psychological stress, advanced age, genetics, and certain comorbidities (e.g., COPD, celiac disease, Crohn's disease).

An injury was most likely sustained to which structure?

The protective lining of the stomach and duodenum is comprised of various cells which normally prevent the erosion of the underlying tissue. Peptic ulcers form when the balance of these protective and erosive factors is disrupted to such an extent that epithelial injury occurs and subsequent erosion extends to the muscularis mucosa.

CONFIRMATION

What is the most likely clinical presentation?

Patients with peptic ulcer disease typically present with the gnawing or burning epigastric pain that occurs after eating. Other general symptoms include dyspepsia, chest discomfort, heartburn, and hematemesis. Patients with a bleeding ulcer may also present with symptoms of anemia. A patient with a gastric ulcer will typically report pain shortly after eating, while a patient with a duodenal ulcer will typically report pain two to three hours after a meal often waking at night with pain. Patients who present with sudden or more severe symptoms may have developed a perforated ulcer and should be promptly evaluated by a physician. Symptoms of perforation include abdominal guarding, rigidity or rebound tenderness with palpation, and a more generalized but sharp abdominal pain that worsens with movement. The condition should be considered emergent if perforation is suspected and the patient displays any signs of septic shock such as anuria, hypotension or tachycardia.

What laboratory or imaging studies would confirm the diagnosis?

Upper GI endoscopy is typically the diagnostic tool used for visualization and tissue biopsy. This tool may also be used to rule out gastric cancer or H. pylori infection.

What additional information should be obtained to confirm the diagnosis?

A thorough medical history should be completed to assist in ruling out similar diagnoses and identifying factors which may contribute to the development or exacerbation of peptic ulcer disease.

DIAGNOSIS

What condition produces a patient's symptoms?

Prostate cancer is the growth of malignant cancer cells within the prostate gland. There is no known etiology for prostate cancer, but factors increasing the risk for acquiring prostate cancer include advanced age, African American descent, family history of prostate or breast cancer, and obesity.

An injury was most likely sustained to what structure?

The prostate is a gland found in the male reproductive system that is responsible for the production of seminal fluid. Prostate cancer is generally a slow-growing cancer, though it can metastasize to other parts of the body, especially the lymph nodes and bones.

CONFIRMATION

What is the most likely clinical presentation?

In its early stages, prostate cancer is generally asymptomatic. Symptoms are more likely present during the advanced stages of the disease. Because of the prostate's position surrounding the urethra, prostate cancer may result in difficulty urinating, nocturia, erectile dysfunction, blood in the urine or semen, pelvic or low back pain, and bone pain, if metastasized.

What laboratory or imaging studies would confirm the diagnosis?

The prostate-specific antigen (PSA) test is a blood test used to determine the presence of elevated levels of PSA, which may be indicative of prostate cancer. If prostate cancer is suspected, a physician may decide to perform a tissue biopsy of the prostate to further assist with diagnosis. Imaging studies that may be used include transrectal ultrasound or magnetic resonance imaging.

What additional information should be obtained to confirm the diagnosis?

A thorough medical history and physical examination should be performed to rule out other similar conditions (e.g., benign prostatic hypertrophy) and assist with diagnosis. The physical examination involves a prostate examination to determine abnormalities in the texture, shape or size of the prostate gland.

DIAGNOSIS

What condition produces a patient's symptoms?

Ulcerative colitis is an inflammatory bowel disease that results in chronic inflammation and the formation of ulcers in the gastrointestinal tract. There is no known etiology for this condition, though it is thought to be an autoimmune condition that results from an exaggerated response to a bacterium or virus. There is also a presumed genetic component to the condition.

An injury was most likely sustained to what structure?

Ulcerative colitis affects the innermost lining of the large intestine (most often the sigmoid colon) and rectum, as opposed to Crohn's disease which may affect any portion of the gastrointestinal tract. The severity of the patient's symptoms is directly related to the extent of the colon that is affected.

CONFIRMATION

What is the most likely clinical presentation?

The clinical presentation will be determined by the location and severity of inflammation. Signs and symptoms may include abdominal pain and cramping, diarrhea, blood in the stools, urgency to defecate, weight loss, fatigue, and fever. Symptoms are often intermittent, alternating between periods of exacerbation and remission. Because the condition is considered an autoimmune disorder, other systemic symptoms can also occur (e.g., arthritic joints, skin disorders, visual issues).

What laboratory or imaging studies would confirm the diagnosis?

The primary test for diagnosing ulcerative colitis is endoscopy, which allows for direct visualization of the colon. Biopsies of the mucosa may also be performed to definitively diagnose the condition. Other testing may include stool samples and blood tests.

What additional information should be obtained to confirm the diagnosis?

A thorough medical history and physical examination should be performed to rule out the presence of other similar conditions (e.g., Crohn's disease, irritable bowel syndrome, diverticulitis).

Urinary Tract Infection   BRONZE

DIAGNOSIS

What condition produces a patient's symptoms?

The urinary tract is normally a sterile environment. Under certain conditions, however, infectious organisms from internal or external sources can proliferate causing a urinary tract infection (UTI). The Escherichia coli (E. coli) bacteria and the sexually transmitted microorganisms chlamydia and mycoplasma are most commonly associated with UTI.

An injury was most likely sustained to which structure?

The urinary system is comprised of the kidneys and ureters in the upper urinary tract and the bladder and urethra in the lower urinary tract. An infection can occur anywhere within the system although the lower urinary tract is more commonly involved. A UTI may be more specifically named based on the location of the infection.

CONFIRMATION

What is the most likely clinical presentation?

A UTI is typically characterized by a strong and persistent urge to urinate, as well as a burning sensation with urination. Frequent voiding tends to produce only small volumes of cloudy, strong smelling urine. Other general symptoms that may be associated with UTI include fever and body aches. Cognitive changes are commonly observed in elderly and cognitively impaired patients.

UTIs are more prevalent among women, especially those who are pregnant or menopausal due to the associated hormonal and body chemistry changes.

What laboratory or imaging studies would confirm the diagnosis?

Urinalysis and urine culture are most commonly used to diagnose a UTI. Urinalysis details the urine's physical (e.g., color, clarity, odor), microscopic (e.g., white blood cell, red blood cell, and bacterial counts), and chemical (e.g., acidity, concentration, glucose level) characteristics with comparison to established norms. A urine culture is used to identify the specific organism causing the infection so that treatment interventions may be targeted accordingly. Patients who suffer recurrent UTIs may require more invasive diagnostic testing.

What additional information should be obtained to confirm the diagnosis?

A thorough medical history should be obtained. Patients with urinary catheters are at an increased risk of developing a UTI as are those with conditions which impede the normal flow of urine (e.g., benign prostate hypertrophy, kidney stones) or impact kidney function (e.g., diabetes mellitus).

Uterine Cancer   BRONZE

DIAGNOSIS

What condition produces a patient's symptoms?

Uterine cancer (i.e., endometrial cancer) is the malignant growth of any cells that comprise the tissue of the uterus. The exact etiology of uterine cancer is unknown, though risk factors for the disease involve elevated levels of estrogen without similar levels of progesterone. Common risk factors include advanced age, obesity, diabetes, family history of uterine cancer, radiation therapy to the pelvis, medications (e.g., estrogen, tamoxifen), early onset of menstruation or late onset of menopause, and nulliparity.

An injury was most likely sustained to what structure?

The most common type of uterine cancer affects the endometrium, which is the inner lining of the uterus. When there is an imbalance of hormones (i.e., estrogen and progesterone), the endometrium becomes thicker over time. As the condition progresses, cancerous cells may start to develop. If metastasized, these cancerous cells can invade the lymph nodes, lungs, liver, bones or brain.

CONFIRMATION

What is the most likely clinical presentation?

Unexpected vaginal bleeding is the most common symptom associated with uterine cancer, especially when it occurs after menopause. Other signs and symptoms may include abnormal

menstrual cycles (in premenopausal women), vaginal discharge (in postmenopausal women), pelvic or lower abdominal pain, painful urination, and painful intercourse.

What laboratory or imaging studies would confirm the diagnosis?

The only method to confirm the diagnosis of uterine cancer is through a tissue biopsy, which is obtained during a procedure known as dilation and curettage. The physician may perform a transvaginal ultrasound or hysteroscopy for imaging. Diagnostic imaging can also be used (e.g., MRI, CT scan) to determine if the cancer has metastasized.

What additional information should be obtained to confirm the diagnosis?

A thorough medical history and physical examination should be performed to rule out the presence of other similar conditions (e.g., endometriosis). The physical examination will typically involve a pelvic examination, in which the physician palpates for changes in the size, shape or consistency of the uterus.

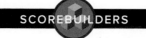

Other Systems Essentials

Integumentary System

1. The integumentary system or "skin" is the largest organ of the body and consists of dermal and epidermal layers, hair follicles, nails, sebaceous glands, and sweat glands.

2. The normal phases of healing are overlapping and progressive beginning with an inflammatory response and ending with scar maturity.

3. Healing can occur through primary, secondary or tertiary intention. Most wounds requiring formal wound care interventions will heal by secondary intention.

4. Maintaining the balance of moisture in and around healing wounds is paramount. A wound that is too dry will have delayed healing; a wound with excessive moisture is at risk for additional tissue deterioration.

5. Infection is the most common cause of wound chronicity.

6. Certain types of wound exudate typically occur during the various stages of wound healing while others may be signs of impending infection or other complications.

7. Ulcers have primary classification as arterial, venous, neuropathic or pressure. Causative factors are ulcer specific and treatment is dependent on classification and severity of the ulcer.

8. Wounds that are not classified as pressure or neuropathic can be classified by depth of tissue loss.

9. Wound color, depth, exudate, and infection status must be considered in order to select the most appropriate wound dressing for a patient.

10. Wagner Ulcer Grade Classification System categorizes dysvascular ulcers based on wound depth and the presence of infection.

11. Pressure injury staging typically includes stage 1,2,3,4, Suspected Deep Tissue Injury, and Unstageable.

12. Exudate is typically classified as serous, sanguineous, serosanguineous, seropurulent, and purulent.

13. Physical therapist assistants provide selective debridement through sharp, enzymatic or autolytic debridement interventions. Non-selective debridement typically includes wet-to-dry dressings, hydrotherapy, and wound irrigation interventions.

14. Modalities and physical agents such as negative pressure wound therapy, hyperbaric oxygen, and growth factors promote and facilitate healing, improve oxygenation and blood flow, increase collagen synthesis, minimize edema, and decrease drainage from the wound.

15. Therapeutic modalities such as ultrasound and high-voltage pulsed current have clinical applications and parameters which can assist through all stages of healing.

16. A fully occlusive substance would be completely impermeable while a non-occlusive dressing permits bacteria and fluid contamination of the wound bed increasing the risk for infection and delaying the healing process.

17. Classification of dressings includes hydrocolloids, hydrogels, foam dressings, transparent film, gauze, and alginates. Each dressing classification has advantages and disadvantages and is used based on the wound characteristics and goals for the dressing.

18. The major classifications of burn injury include thermal, electrical, chemical, and radiation burns. The extent of burn-related tissue damage in each zone of injury will significantly impact the overall healing prognosis.

19. The level of pain secondary to a burn varies based on the depth of the burn with superficial partial-thickness burns typically exhibiting the highest level of pain.

20. The rule of nines is well recognized for its use in estimating the amount of total surface area damaged by a burn injury. However, this calculation does not reflect wound severity and therefore cannot predict prognosis or outcomes.

21. Numerous scar assessment scales are available to assess characteristics such as scar height, thickness, pliability, banding/adherence, color, vascularity, texture, and size.

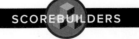

Other Systems Essentials

22. Burns sustained in proximity to joints are at particular risk for developing limiting contractures as patients will tend to assume a position of comfort. Splints should be used to support limbs in a neutral or slight stretch position to prevent deformity.

23. Principles of burn scar management, such as scar massage and desensitization techniques, are valuable tools for managing non-burn related scars that may be painful or otherwise restrictive.

Metabolic and Endocrine

24. The metabolic system is responsible for generating the energy required to fuel all bodily functions.

25. Catabolism refers to metabolic processes which provide heat and energy to the body while anabolism refers to processes involved with tissue growth and repair.

26. Inherited metabolic disorders, though present at birth, may not immediately show symptoms.

27. Metabolic acidosis occurs when the body's pH drops below 7.35 as a result of an acid and bicarbonate imbalance which allows acid to accumulate.

28. Metabolic alkalosis occurs when the body's pH rises above 7.45 as a result of a bicarbonate and acid imbalance which allows bicarbonate to accumulate.

29. Osteoporosis or osteopenia may be an underlying clinical feature of various other metabolic or systemic disorders.

30. A diagnosis of osteopenia may not be due to bone loss, but rather a naturally occurring bone density that is lower than established norms.

31. General classes of hormones controlled by the endocrine system include prostaglandins, catecholamines, and insulin.

32. Endocrine pathology most commonly relates to either hyper or hypofunction of endocrine glands and the effect of their targeted hormone secretions.

33. Patients with hyperthyroidism may present with exercise limitations associated with heat intolerance caused by hypermetabolism.

34. Patients with hypothyroidism often present with limited exercise tolerance due to a hypofunctioning metabolism and subsequent energy deficits.

35. Untreated, both hyperglycemia and hypoglycemia are life threatening conditions.

36. Type 1 diabetes mellitus occurs when the pancreas fails to produce insulin to regulate blood glucose levels in the body.

37. Type 2 diabetes mellitus occurs when the body becomes insulin resistant and is unable to effectively utilize the insulin that is present to control blood glucose levels.

38. Patients with diabetes mellitus must be cautious to avoid becoming hypoglycemic with exercise as a result of increased glucose uptake with increased muscle activity.

39. Patients with type 1 diabetes mellitus are at the greatest risk for becoming hyperglycemic and developing life threatening ketoacidosis.

Gastrointestinal

40. The gastrointestinal system is responsible for the process of digestion. It breaks down food into its components, absorbs nutrients, and discards the waste.

41. Diverticula, or pouch-like protrusions that occur in the colon, can become infected causing diverticulitis. A high fiber diet will help to avoid this condition.

42. The hepatitis B vaccine is administered in three doses and may be used prophylactically or as treatment for an unvaccinated patient who has been exposed.

43. Health care workers that are at risk for contact with hepatitis should receive all immunizations for HBV, and if exposed to blood or body fluids of an infected person must receive immunoglobulin therapy immediately.

44. Therapists must be diligent in assessing pain of an unknown origin. This is especially true when pain is accompanied by autonomic responses such as nausea, vomiting, pallor or sweating.

45. For numerous gastrointestinal disorders, lifestyle changes are the primary intervention recommended for symptom management.

Other Systems Essentials

Genitourinary

46. The pelvic floor complex attaches to the pelvis and serves the genitourinary system through three primary functions: support, sphincteric function, and sexual function.

47. The genitourinary system consists of female and male genital organs and the urinary organs.

48. Physical therapy intervention for all bladder pathologies includes behavioral modification to address healthy bladder habits.

49. A woman's body transitions through multiple physiological and postural changes during pregnancy that may lead to impairments and functional limitations.

50. Relative and absolute contraindications need to be considered when developing an exercise program for a pregnant woman.

51. The goal of pelvic floor muscle strengthening exercises is to be able to perform a contraction during functional tasks.

Lymphatic

52. The lymphatic system is responsible for collecting and transporting fluids that are not collected by the venous system, as well as immune system defense for the body.

53. Lymphedema is a chronic, incurable condition and is characterized by the accumulation of protein-rich fluid (i.e., lymph) in the body, especially in the extremities.

54. Primary lymphedema occurs due to abnormal development of the lymphatic system, while secondary lymphedema occurs as a result of some other disease or injury that causes damage to the lymphatic system (e.g., mastectomy, radiation therapy).

55. Signs and symptoms of lymphedema can range from mild pitting edema that reverses with elevation and rest to severe non-pitting edema that results in fibrotic changes to the skin and an increased risk for infections.

56. Complete decongestive therapy is the standard of care for patients with lymphedema, which consists of manual lymphatic drainage, compression therapy, exercise, and education in proper skin care.

57. Circumferential measurements are commonly used by therapists to determine the progression of lymphedema and the effectiveness of treatment.

58. Lymphedema is not curable, however, symptoms can be managed if patients are treated early and maintain ongoing self-care using the principles of complete decongestive therapy.

Oncology

59. Cancers are typically named based on the cell type involved and the tissue of origin.

60. A significant percentage of cancer related risk factors are modifiable.

61. The American Cancer Society names cancer as the leading cause of death in the United States.

62. Musculoskeletal pain in patients with cancer may be indicative of metastasis and should be promptly evaluated.

63. Physical therapist assistants should be aware of the general signs and symptoms of cancer and refer patients back to the referring physician when signs and symptoms are observed in patients without a cancer diagnosis.

64. Staging of a malignancy is most commonly based on factors relating to the size of the primary tumor, lymph node involvement, and the presence of metastasis.

65. Staging assists multidisciplinary care providers to establish an optimal plan of care with appropriate goals and interventions.

66. Patients being treated for a cancer diagnosis with chemotherapy, radiation, and/or surgical interventions are at an increased risk for developing lymphedema.

67. Palliative treatment emphasizes symptom relief and may be provided in any care setting at any time during the course of a disease process.

68. Hospice care includes palliative interventions and goals, but is specifically reserved for patients at the end of life when curative efforts are no longer being pursued.

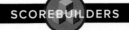

Other Systems Essentials

69. The usual modality contraindications relating to a cancer diagnosis may be occasionally disregarded in lieu of palliative goals for some patients at the end of life.

70. Cognitive changes related to oncological interventions are widely recognized and acknowledged despite limited definitive research on the subject.

71. The prevention of infection in patients who are neutropenic is imperative to prevent potentially life threatening complications.

Psychological Disorders

72. Affective disorders relate to changes in mood or emotion and include depression, mania, and bipolar disorder.

73. Neuroses disorders are characterized by irrational fears or maladaptive responses to everyday stimuli and include phobias, psychogenic amnesia, multiple personality, obsessive-compulsive, anxiety, and dissociative disorders.

74. Somatoform disorders are classified by the presenting physical characteristics and include somatization, conversion, and hypochondriasis disorders.

75. Schizophrenic disorders are psychotic in nature and vary widely in presentation. Classifications of schizophrenia include catatonic, paranoid, disorganized, and undifferentiated.

76. Personality disorders are classified based on behavior patterns and include psychopathic, antisocial, narcissistic, and borderline personalities.

77. The side effects of numerous medications can have a significant impact on a patient's willingness and ability to effectively participate in physical therapy treatment.

Geriatrics

78. Ageism can impact the ability of a caretaker or health professional to provide unbiased care, instead basing their treatment on preconceived notions.

79. Older adults experience specific age-related changes that impact the five senses (hearing, vision, taste and smell, touch, cognition).

80. Older adults are at an increased risk of experiencing medication-related problems such as non-adherence and adverse drug reactions.

81. Older adults process medication differently than younger adults, therefore it is critical to be aware of pharmacokinetic and pharmacodynamic changes.

Bariatrics

82. The morphological distribution of a patient's adipose tissue often correlates to their overall health risk factors.

83. Therapists may be the first health care providers to initiate a conversation about weight loss with a patient and should therefore be well informed of both appropriate community and medical resources so that a referral may be made as needed.

84. Failure to address psychological influences associated with obesity, or eating disorders of any kind, will limit the potential for positive long-term success.

85. Significant weight loss cannot be achieved or maintained in a healthful way through a single mode of intervention.

86. With regard to weight loss, an individual's readiness and commitment to altering behavior is a significant factor in predicting long-term outcomes and success.

87. Options for bariatric surgical interventions vary from minimally invasive, reversible procedures to highly invasive procedures which significantly impact the body's anatomy and gastrointestinal function.

88. When initiating an exercise program for a morbidly obese patient special care should be taken to prevent injury and ensure safe, appropriate systemic responses.

Nutrition

89. Macronutrients are the nutrients that provide the body with energy and consist of carbohydrates, fats, and proteins.

90. Carbohydrates are the energy source for high-intensity exercise, fats are the energy source for low-intensity exercise, and proteins are responsible for the growth and maintenance of the body's tissues.

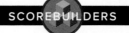

Other Systems Essentials

91. Vitamins are commonly classified as either fat-soluble or water-soluble.

92. Fat-soluble vitamins are more likely to reach toxic levels in the body.

93. Water-soluble vitamins are not stored in significant amounts within the body.

94. Some complementary and alternative medicine supplements can interfere with the action of pharmaceutical agents and reach toxic levels within the body.

95. Minerals and vitamins are necessary to support the body's metabolic functions.

96. MyPlate is a program that is designed to teach people how to create and maintain a healthy diet and includes recommendations for intake of the six major food groups: fruits, vegetables, grains, protein foods, dairy, and oils.

97. The nutrition label on food and drink products should be used to determine the health content of the product and will include information such as the number of calories, macronutrients, and micronutrients that the product contains.

Pharmacology Basics

98. Drugs can be administered via enteral routes (i.e., within the gastrointestinal tract) or parenteral routes (i.e., outside the gastrointestinal tract).

99. Oral administration is the most common type of enteral administration since it is easy for the patient to perform this method on their own and it allows for a slow, controlled release of the drug into the patient's system.

100. Intravenous injection is a common form of drug administration that allows for rapid administration of a drug to the target tissue and is one of the only methods that ensures 100% bioavailability of the drug.

101. There are several factors that can affect how a drug acts within the body, including a patient's age, weight, and ethnicity, the presence of disease or infection, drug-drug interactions, and food-drug interactions.

Other Systems Proficiencies

1. Integumentary Anatomy

Select the appropriate term for each of the specified locations. Answers must be selected from the Word Bank and can be used only once.

Word Bank: adipose tissue, arrector pili muscle, blood supply, dermis, epidermis, hair follicle, nerve, nerve ending, sebaceous gland, subcutaneous fatty tissue, sweat duct, sweat gland

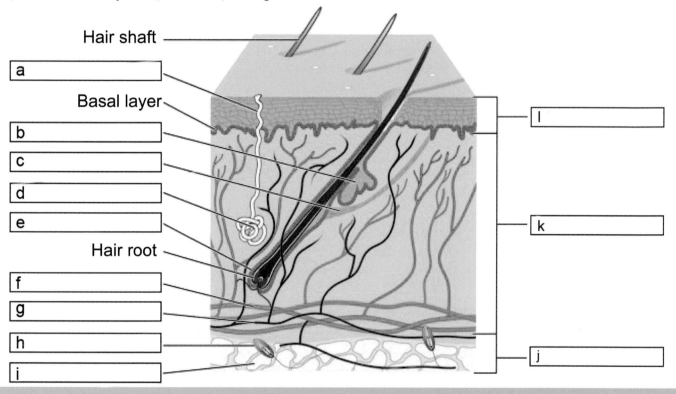

Hair shaft

a

Basal layer

b

c

d

e

Hair root

f

g

h

i

l

k

j

2. Ulcer Characteristics

Identify the type of ulcer that is most associated with the supplied description. Answers must be selected from the Word Bank and can be used more than once.

Word Bank: arterial, neuropathic, venous

Type of Ulcer	Clinical Finding
a	ulcer located proximal to the medial malleolus
b	normal pedal pulse
c	leg elevation diminishes pain
d	absence of pain
e	evidence of increased edema
f	evidence of hair loss in tissue

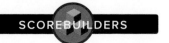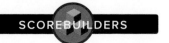

Other Systems Proficiencies

3. Pressure Injury Staging

Identify the pressure injury stage that is most associated with the supplied description. Answers must be selected from the Word Bank and can be used more than once.

Word Bank: 1, 2, 3, 4

Stage	Clinical Finding
a	slough is present, but does not obscure depth of tissue loss
b	subcutaneous fat is visible, but bone, tendon or muscles are not exposed
c	extends into the joint capsule
d	intact skin with non-blanchable redness
e	tunneling with muscle visible
f	intact serum filled blister
g	shallow ulcer with a red wound bed

4. Pressure Injuries

Identify the position or positions, most likely to cause a pressure injury over the identified bony prominence. The number of desired responses for each bony prominence is identified in parentheses. Answers must be selected from the Word Bank and can be used more than once.

Word Bank: sidelying, sitting, supine, prone

Bony Structure	Position(s)	
patella	a	(1)
dorsum of foot	b	(1)
ear	c	(1)
ischial tuberosity	d	(1)
vertebral spinous process	e	(2)
sternum	f	(1)
head of fibula	g	(1)
anterior superior iliac spine	h	(1)

Other Systems Proficiencies

5. Debridement

Classify each of the debridement techniques as selective or non-selective debridement.

Type of Debridement	Classification
autolytic	a
enzymatic	b
hydrotherapy	c
wet-to-dry	d
wound irrigation	e

6. Wound Terminology

Identify the wound terminology most closely associated with the supplied description. Answers must be selected from the Word Bank and can be used only once.

Word Bank: contusion, dehiscence, ecchymosis, erythema, hematoma, keloid, maceration, turgor

Terminology	Description
a	The separation, rupture or splitting of a wound closed by primary intention.
b	A diffuse redness of the skin often resulting from either capillary dilation and congestion or inflammation.
c	Skin softening and degeneration that results from prolonged exposure to water or other fluids.
d	A localized swelling or mass of clotted blood confined to a tissue, organ or space usually caused by a break in a blood vessel.
e	The discoloration occurring below intact skin resulting from trauma to underlying blood vessels and blood seeping into tissue.
f	An abnormal scar formation that is out of proportion to the scarring required for normal tissue repair.
g	The relative speed with which the skin resumes its normal appearance after being lightly pinched.
h	An injury, usually caused by a blow, that does not disrupt the skin integrity.

Other Systems Proficiencies

7. Rule of Nines

Identify the percentage of the total body surface affected based on the description of the area involved. Answers must be selected from the Word Bank and can be used more than once. Not all answers will be used.

Word Bank: 10%, 18%, 19%, 22.5%, 23.5%, 28%, 36%, 54%, 55%, 63%, 64%

	% of Body	Areas Affected
a		anterior right arm, forearm, and hand; anterior trunk
b		bilateral legs and feet
c		anterior trunk, genital region, bilateral legs and feet
d		posterior head and neck; posterior trunk
e		bilateral arms, forearms, and hands; entire trunk
f		genital region, anterior left leg and foot

8. Integumentary System Basics

Mark each statement as True or False. If the statement is False, correct the statement in the space provided.

	True/False	Statement
a		A patient with a deep partial-thickness burn would typically experience more pain than a patient with a superficial partial-thickness burn.
	Correction:	
b		Patients with venous insufficiency ulcers should avoid unnecessary leg elevation.
	Correction:	
c		Enzymatic debridement refers to the use of the body's own mechanisms to remove nonviable tissue.
	Correction:	

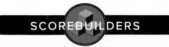

Other Systems Proficiencies

True/False	Statement
d	The epidermis thickens as part of the aging process, making it more resilient and therefore less susceptible to injury from friction and shear.
Correction:	
e	Healing by primary intention permits wounds to close on their own without superficial closure.
Correction:	
f	Patients with arterial insufficiency ulcers should avoid heating pads or soaking their feet in hot water.
Correction:	
g	A full-thickness burn involves complete destruction of the epidermis and dermis, along with partial damage to the subcutaneous fat layer.
Correction:	
h	The goal of treatment with a wound classified as "Red" using the Red-Yellow-Black System is to remove exudate and debris.
Correction:	
i	A superficial partial-thickness burn involves the epidermis and the upper portion of the dermis.
Correction:	
j	A grade of 3 on the Wagner Ulcer Grade Classification scale is indicative of a superficial ulcer not involving subcutaneous tissue.
Correction:	

Other Systems Proficiencies

9. Pathology of the Metabolic and Endocrine Systems

Identify the appropriate medical condition based on the supplied descriptions. Answers must be selected from the Word Bank and can only be used once.

Word Bank: Cushing's syndrome, Graves' disease, Klinefelter's syndrome, osteoporosis, Paget's disease, phenylketonuria, diabetes mellitus - type 1

	Pathology	Description
a		Adrenal dysfunction that produces excessive cortisol as well as a "moon-shaped face" and "buffalo hump."
b		Metabolic bone disease that affects trabecular and cortical bone resulting in decreased bone mass and increased risk for fracture.
c		Hypofunction of the pancreas where there is failure to produce adequate endogenous insulin.
d		Primary hypogonadism that presents with a deficiency of testosterone secondary to a failure of the testes to respond to follicle stimulating and luteinizing hormones.
e		Autosomal recessive inherited trait in which an enzyme deficiency permits excessive phenylalanine accumulation within the brain.
f		Autoimmune disease that produces thyroid hypersecretion resulting in heat intolerance, tremor, weight loss, and nervousness.
g		Metabolic bone disease characterized by heightened osteoclast activity resulting in excessive bone formation that lacks true structural integrity.

10. Metabolic Acidosis versus Metabolic Alkalosis

Identify characteristics of each condition. Answers must be selected from the Word Bank and can be used only once.

Word Bank: <7.35, >7.45, compensatory hyperventilation, continuous vomiting, potassium chloride, renal failure, slowed breathing, sodium bicarbonate

Metabolic Acidosis		Metabolic Alkalosis
a	Possible etiologies	e
b	pH	f
c	Symptoms	g
d	Treatment	h

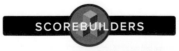

Other Systems Proficiencies

11. Glands of the Endocrine System and Hormones Secreted

Identify the endocrine gland or associated hormones. Answers must be selected from the Word Bank and can be used only once.

Word Bank: adrenal gland, estrogen and progesterone, glucagon and insulin, parathyroid gland, testes, thyroxine and triiodothyronine

Endocrine Gland		Associated Hormones
a		testosterone and other androgens
	ovaries	b
	thyroid	c
	pancreas	d
e		parathyroid hormone
f		corticosteroids and epinephrine

12. Diabetes: Type 1 or Type 2

Identify the characteristic as Type 1 or Type 2 diabetes mellitus. Answers must be selected from the Word Bank and can be used more than once.

Word Bank: Type 1, Type 2

Type	Characteristic
a	treatment includes insulin injections or insulin pump
b	etiology unclear, but a genetic predisposition with a viral or environmental trigger is believed to facilitate onset
c	typically controlled through diet, exercise, and oral medications
d	obesity contributes to the condition by increasing insulin resistance
e	increased incidence in children due to rise in childhood obesity
f	typically there is some ongoing production of endogenous insulin
g	exogenous insulin injections are typically required
h	ketoacidosis rarely occurs
i	5-10% of all cases of diabetes mellitus
j	gradual onset
k	destruction of the islet of Langerhans cells

Other Systems Proficiencies

13. Other Systems Basics

Mark each statement as True or False. If the statement is False, correct the statement in the space provided.

True/False	Statement
a	Catabolism is the process that combines simple molecules for tissue growth.
Correction	
b	Hormones secreted by endocrine glands travel through the bloodstream and signal specific target organs in order to maintain homeostasis of the internal environment.
Correction	
c	Norepinephrine is the catecholamine that creates the "fight or flight" response.
Correction	
d	Gastroesophageal reflux disease occurs as the result of an incompetent lower esophageal sphincter and allows for backwards movement of stomach acids into the esophagus.
Correction	
e	Diverticulitis is a condition with inflamed diverticula (pouch-like protrusions within the colon).
Correction	
f	The ovaries provide storage of oocytes prior to ovulation and secrete both estrogen and progesterone.
Correction	
g	Diastasis recti is the separation of the rectus abdominis along the linea alba.
Correction	

Other Systems Proficiencies

True/False	Statement
h	Hypertension in supine during late pregnancy is secondary to compression of the inferior vena cava.
Correction	
i	Incompetent cervix, placenta previa, restrictive lung disease, and preeclampsia are absolute contraindications for exercise during pregnancy.
Correction	
j	A melanoma is a malignancy originating from connective tissues such as fat, cartilage, bone or muscle.
Correction	
k	Affective disorders include diagnoses such as obsessive-compulsive, anxiety, and phobia disorders.
Correction	
l	A body mass index of greater than 30 is indicative of obesity.
Correction	

Other Systems Proficiencies

14. Other Systems Terminology

Identify the term most closely associated with the supplied description. Answers must be selected from the Word Bank and can be used only once.

Word Bank: anorexia nervosa, gastritis, gene, hypoglycemia, insulin, lymphoma, mitochondria, neoplasm, osteopenia, pH

	Terminology	Description
a		self-imposed starvation that results in impairment or "shut down" of systemic processes
b		the measure of the hydrogen ion concentration in body fluid
c		a fundamental unit of heredity
d		a group of oncology diagnoses referring to cancers that involve uncontrolled lymphocyte proliferation in the lymph nodes
e		a part of the cell that is responsible for energy production
f		an abnormal new growth of tissue that can be classified as benign or malignant
g		a condition that presents with decreased bone mass, but not severe enough to be classified as osteoporosis
h		a condition where blood sugar levels decrease below 70 mg/dL
i		inflammation of the gastric mucosa of the inner layer of the stomach
j		hormone secreted by the islets of Langerhans within the pancreas

Other Systems Proficiencies

15. Staging of Cancer

Identify the appropriate sequence of staging based on the supplied description. Answers must be selected from the Word Bank and can be used only once.

Word Bank: 0, I, II, III, IV

Stage	Description
a	Malignancy that has spread to adjacent tissue showing signs of fixation to deeper structures. The likelihood of metastatic lymph node involvement is high.
b	Malignancy that has metastasized beyond the primary site, for example, to bone or another organ.
c	Malignancy spreading into adjacent tissues; lymph nodes may show signs of micrometastases.
d	Early malignancy that is present only in the layer of cells in which it began. For most cancers, this is referred to as carcinoma in situ.
e	Malignancy limited to the tissue of origin with no lymph node involvement or metastasis.

16. Pharmacology for Other Systems

Identify the appropriate medication based on the supplied descriptions. Answers must be selected from the Word Bank and can be used only once.

Word Bank: antacid agents, bipolar disorder agents, bone mineral regulating agents, chemotherapy, emetic agents, endocrine hyperfunction agents, insulin, laxative agents, proton pump inhibitors

Drug	Action
a	prevents histamine-activated release of gastric acid
b	administered to destroy malignant cells
c	administered as mood stabilizers preventing manic episodes and extreme swings in mood
d	facilitate bowel evacuation
e	administered via injection to maintain blood glucose levels
f	used to induce vomiting
g	promote inhibition of hormone function
h	chemically neutralize gastric acid and increase the intragastric pH
i	enhance and maximize bone mass while preventing bone loss or rate of bone reabsorption

Other Systems Proficiencies

17. Vitamins and Potential Food Sources

Identify the appropriate vitamin based on the supplied potential food sources. Answers must be selected from the Word Bank. Each answer can be used only once.

Word Bank: A, B12, C, D, E, K

Vitamin	Potential Food Sources
a	fortified milk, fish oils, salmon
b	green, orange, yellow vegetables, liver
c	citrus fruits, tomatoes, cantaloupe
d	vegetable oils, nuts, fish
e	meats, whole eggs
f	dark green leafy vegetables, cheese, egg yolks

18. Minerals and their Function

Identify the appropriate mineral based on the supplied function. Answers must be selected from the Word Bank. Each answer can be used only once.

Word Bank: calcium, chromium, copper, iodine, iron, sodium, sulfur, zinc

Mineral	Function
a	assists with glucose metabolism
b	facilitates the maintenance of acid-base balance, transmits nerve impulses, and assists to control muscle contractions
c	facilitates muscle contraction and relaxation, builds strong bones, aids in coagulation
d	facilitates enzyme activity and energy metabolism
e	assists with regulation of cell metabolism and basal metabolic rate
f	facilitates hemoglobin synthesis and lipid metabolism
g	assists in oxygen transport and cell oxidation
h	aids in immune function and cell division

Other Systems Answer Key

1. Integumentary Anatomy

a.   sweat duct

b.   sebaceous gland

c.   arrector pili muscle

d.   sweat gland

e.   hair follicle

f.   blood supply

g.   nerve

h.   nerve ending

i.   adipose tissue

j.   subcutaneous fatty layer

k.   dermis

l.   epidermis

2. Ulcer Characteristics

a.   venous

b.   venous

c.   venous

d.   neuropathic

e.   venous

f.   arterial

3. Pressure Injury Staging

a.   3

b.   3

c.   4

d.   1

e.   4

f.   2

g.   2

4. Pressure Injuries

a.   prone

b.   prone

c.   sidelying

d.   sitting

e.   supine, sitting

f.   prone

g.   sidelying

h.   prone

5. Debridement

a.   selective

b.   selective

c.   non-selective

d.   non-selective

e.   non-selective

6. Wound Terminology

a.   dehiscence

b.   erythema

c.   maceration

d.   hematoma

e.   ecchymosis

f.   keloid

g.   turgor

h.   contusion

7. Rule of Nines

a.   22.5%

b.   36%

c.   55%

d.   22.5%

e.   54%

f.   10%

8. Integumentary System Basics*

a.   FALSE: Correction - A patient with a deep partial-thickness burn would typically experience less pain than a patient with a superficial partial-thickness burn.

b.   FALSE: Correction - Patients with venous insufficiency ulcers should elevate the legs when possible.

c.   FALSE: Correction - Autolytic debridement refers to the use of the body's own mechanisms to remove nonviable tissue.

d.   FALSE: Correction - The epidermis thins as part of the aging process, making it less resilient and therefore more susceptible to injury from friction and shear.

e.   FALSE: Correction - Healing by secondary intention permits wounds to close on their own without superficial closure.

f.   TRUE

g.   TRUE

h.   FALSE: Correction - The goal of treatment with a wound classified as "Red" using the Red-Yellow-Black System is to protect the wound and maintain a moist wound environment.

i.   TRUE

j.   FALSE: Correction - A grade of 3 on the Wagner Ulcer Grade Classification scale is indicative of a deep ulcer with osteitis, abscess or osteomyelitis.

*The correction presented for each false statement is an example of several possible corrections.

Other Systems Answer Key

9. Pathology of the Metabolic and Endocrine Systems

a. Cushing's syndrome
b. osteoporosis
c. diabetes mellitus - type 1
d. Klinefelter's syndrome
e. phenylketonuria
f. Graves' disease
g. Paget's disease

10. Metabolic Acidosis versus Metabolic Alkalosis

a. renal failure
b. <7.35
c. compensatory hyperventilation
d. sodium bicarbonate
e. continuous vomiting
f. >7.45
g. slowed breathing
h. potassium chloride

11. Glands of the Endocrine System and Hormones Secreted

a. testes
b. estrogen and progesterone
c. thyroxine and triiodothyronine
d. glucagon and insulin
e. parathyroid gland
f. adrenal gland

12. Diabetes: Type 1 or Type 2

a. Type 1
b. Type 1
c. Type 2
d. Type 2
e. Type 2
f. Type 2
g. Type 1
h. Type 2
i. Type 1
j. Type 2
k. Type 1

13. Other Systems Basics

a. FALSE: Correction - Catabolism is the process of breaking down organic compounds during metabolism.
b. TRUE
c. FALSE: Correction - Epinephrine is the catecholamine that creates the "fight or flight" response.
d. TRUE
e. TRUE
f. TRUE
g. TRUE
h. FALSE: Correction - Hypotension in supine during late pregnancy is secondary to compression of the inferior vena cava.
i. TRUE
j. FALSE: Correction - A sarcoma is a malignancy originating from connective tissues such as fat, cartilage, bone or muscle.
k. FALSE: Correction - Neuroses disorders would include diagnoses such as obsessive-compulsive, anxiety, and phobia disorders. Affective disorders include depression, mania, and bipolar disorders.
l. TRUE

*The correction presented for each false statement is an example of several possible corrections.

14. Other Systems Terminology

a. anorexia nervosa
b. pH
c. gene
d. lymphoma
e. mitochondria
f. neoplasm
g. osteopenia
h. hypoglycemia
i. gastritis
j. insulin

Other Systems Answer Key

15. Staging of Cancer

a. III

b. IV

c. II

d. 0

e. I

16. Pharmacology for Other Systems

a. proton pump inhibitors

b. chemotherapy

c. bipolar disorder agents

d. laxative agents

e. insulin

f. emetic agents

g. endocrine hyperfunction agents

h. antacid agents

i. bone mineral regulating agents

17. Vitamins and Potential Food Sources

a. D

b. A

c. C

d. E

e. B12

f. K

18. Minerals and their Function

a. chromium

b. sodium

c. calcium

d. sulfur

e. iodine

f. copper

g. iron

h. zinc

Other Systems References

1. Sussman C, Bates-Jensen B. *Wound Care: A Collaborative Practice Manual for Health Professionals*. Fourth Edition. Wolters Kluwer Health/Lippincott Williams & Wilkins. 2012.

2. Irion G. *Comprehensive Wound Management*. Second Edition. SLACK Inc. 2010.

3. O'Sullivan S, Schmitz T, Fulk G. *Physical Rehabilitation: Assessment and Treatment* Fifth Edition. F.A. Davis Company. 2014.

4. Baranoski S, Ayello EA. *Wound Care Essentials: Practice Principles.* Second Edition. Lippincott Williams & Wilkins. 2008.

5. Milne CT, Corbett LQ, Dubuc DL. *Wound, Ostomy, and Continence Nursing Secrets*. Hanley & Belfus. 2003.

6. Herdon DN. *Total Burn Care*. Third Edition. Saunders Elsevier. 2007.

7. Prentice W. *Therapeutic Modalities in Rehabilitation*. Fifth Edition. McGraw-Hill Inc. 2018.

8. Stanley BG, Tribuzi SM. *Concepts in Hand Rehabilitation*. F.A. Davis Company. 1992.

9. Trofino RB. *Nursing Care of the Burn-Injured Patient*. F.A. Davis Company. 1991.

10. Goodman C, Fuller KS. *Pathology: Implications for the Physical Therapist*. Fourth Edition. W.B. Saunders Company. 2015.

11. Gould BE, Dyer RM. *Pathophysiology for the Health Professions*. Fourth Edition. Saunders Elsevier. 2011.

12. McDermott MT. *Endocrine Secrets*. Fifth Edition. Mosby Elsevier. 2009.

13. *Fluids & Electrolytes: An Incredibly Easy Pocket Guide*. Lippincott Williams & Wilkins. 2006.

14. About Osteoporosis. National Osteoporosis Foundation Website. http://www.nof.org/aboutosteoporosis. Updated 2010. Accessed September 15, 2010.

15. About Osteoporosis. International Osteoporosis Foundation Website. http://www.iofbonehealth.org/health-professionals/about-osteoporosis.html. Updated 2010. Accessed September 15, 2010.

16. *Stedman's Medical Dictionary*. 27th Edition. Lippincott Williams & Wilkins. 2000.

17. Goodman C, Heick J, Lazaro R. *Differential Diagnosis for Physical Therapists – Screening for Referral*. Sixth Edition. Elsevier. 2018.

18. Blood Glucose Control. American Diabetes Association Website. http://www.diabetes.org/living-with-diabetes/treatment-and-care/blood-glucose-control/?utm_source=WWW&utm_medium=DropDownLWD&utm_content=BGC&utm_campaign=CON. Accessed October 4, 2010.

19. Ciccone C. *Pharmacology in Rehabilitation*. Fifth Edition. F.A. Davis Company. 2016.

20. Moore K, Dalley A. *Clinically Oriented Anatomy*. Seventh Edition. Lippincott Williams & Wilkins. 2013.

21. Stephenson R, O'Connor L. *Obstetric and Gynecologic Care in Physical Therapy*. Second Edition. Slack Inc. 2000.

22. Cunningham FG, Leveno KJ, Bloom SL, Hauth JC, Rouse DJ, Spong CY. *Williams Obstetrics*. 23rd Edition. McGraw Hill Medical. 2010.

23. Gibbs RS, Karlan BY, Kaney AF, Nygaard I. *Danforth's Obstetrics and Gynecology*. Tenth Edition. Lippincott Williams & Wilkins. 2008.

24. Newman DK, Wein AJ. *Managing and Treating Urinary Incontinence*. Second Edition. Health Professions Press. 2009.

25. Kisner C, Colby L, Borstad J. *Therapeutic Exercise Foundations and Techniques*. Seventh Edition. F.A. Davis Company. 2018.

26. American College of Sports Medicine. *ACSM's Resource Manual for Guidelines for Exercise Testing and Prescription*. Seventh Edition. Lippincott Williams & Wilkins. 2014.

27. American College of Obstetricians and Gynecologists: Exercise During Pregnancy and the Postpartum Period, ACOG Committee Opinion No. 267. Obstet Gynecol 2002; 99: 171-173.

28. Gates RA, Fink RM. *Oncology Nursing Secrets*. Third Edition. Mosby Elsevier. 2008.

29. Disease Information. Leukemia and Lymphoma Society Website. http://www.leukemia-lymphoma.org/all_toplevel.adp?item_id=4187. Accessed September 24, 2010.

30. Schneider CM, Dennehy CA, Carter SD. *Exercise and Cancer Recovery*. Human Kinetics Publishing. 2003.

31. Staging: Questions and Answers. National Cancer Institute Website. http://www.cancer.gov/cancertopics/factsheet/Detection/staging. Reviewed September 22, 2010. Accessed September 29, 2010.

32. *The Merck Manual*. 18th Edition. Merck Research Laboratories. 2006.

33. Foldi M, Foldi E. *Foldi's Textbook of Lymphology for Physicians and Lymphedema Therapists*. Second Edition. Mosby Elsevier. 2006.

34. Tecklin J. *Pediatric Physical Therapy*. Fifth Edition. Lippincott Williams & Wilkins. 2015.

35. Palisano R, Orlin M, Shreiber J. *Campbell's Physical Therapy for Children*. Fifth Edition. Elsevier. 2017.

36. Paz J, West MP. *Acute Care Handbook for Physical Therapists*. Fourth Edition. W. B. Saunders Company. 2014.

Other Systems References

37. Cancer Facts and Figures 2010. American Cancer Society Website. http://www.cancer.org/acs/groups/content/@epidemiologysurveilance/documents/document/acspc-026238.pdf. Reviewed 2010. Accessed September 24, 2010.

38. Understanding Your Complete Blood Count. Clinical Center National Institute of Health Website. http://www.cc.nih.gov/ccc/patient_education/pepubs/cbc97.pdf. Updated November 2008. Accessed September 26, 2010.

39. Cooper J. *Occupational Therapy in Oncology and Palliative Care*. Second Edition. John Wiley & Sons. 2007.

40. JAMA Patient Page: Palliative Care. Journal of the American Medical Association Website. http://jama.ama-assn.org/cgi/reprint/296/11/1428.pdf. Updated September 20, 2006. Accessed September 26, 2010.

41. Chemotherapy Principles: An Indepth Discussion. American Cancer Society Website. http://www.cancer.org/Treatment/TreatmentsandSideEffects/TreatmentTypes/Chemotherapy/ChemotherapyPrinciplesAnIn-depthDiscussionoftheTechniquesanditsRoleinTreatment/index. Updated September 28, 2010. Accessed October 1, 2010.

42. Chemo Brain. Mayo Clinic Website. http://www.mayoclinic.com/health/chemo-brain/DS01109. Updated October 10, 2010. Accessed October 15, 2010.

43. Bickley L. *Bates' Guide to Physical Examination and History Taking*. Twelfth Edition. Wolters Kluwer. 2017.

44. American College of Sports Medicine. *ACSM's Resource Manual for Guidelines for Exercise Testing and Prescription*. Seventh Edition. Lippincott Williams & Wilkins. 2014.

45. Alvarez A, Brodsky JB, Lemmens HJM, Morton JM. *Morbid Obesity: Peri-operative Management*. Second Edition. Cambridge University Press. 2010.

46. Clinical Guidelines on the Identification, Evaluation, and Treatment of Overweight and Obesity in Adults: The Evidence Report. National Heart, Lung, and Blood Institute Website. http://www.nhlbi.nih.gov/guidelines/obesity/ob_gdlns.pdf. 1998.

47. Childhood Obesity: Risk Factors. Mayo Clinic Website. http://www.mayoclinic.com/health/childhood-obesity/DS00698/DSECTION=risk%2Dfactors. Reviewed October 9, 2010. Accessed October 14, 2010.

48. Childhood Overweight and Obesity. Centers for Disease Control Website. http://www.cdc.gov/obesity/childhood/index.html. Reviewed March 31, 2010. Accessed October 9, 2010.

49. Childhood Obesity. Mayo Clinic Website. http://www.mayoclinic.com/health/childhood-obesity/DS00698. Updated October 9, 2010. Accessed October 11, 2010.

50. Childhood Overweight and Obesity. Centers for Disease Control and Prevention Website. http://www.cdc.gov/obesity/childhood/index.html. Updated March 31, 2010. Accessed September 24, 2010.

51. Robnett R, Chop W. *Gerontology for the Healthcare Practitioner*. Third Edition. Jones & Bartlett Publishing. 2015.

52. Lewis C, Bottomley J. *Geriatric Rehabilitation: A Clinical Approach.* Third Edition. Prentice Hall. 2007

53. Guccione A, Wong R, Avers D. *Geriatric Physical Therapy*. Third Edition. Mosby. 2011.

54. Kauffman T, Scott R, Barr J. *A Comprehensive Guide to Geriatric Rehabilitation*. Third Edition. Elsevier. 2014.

8

Equipment, Devices, and Technologies; Therapeutic Modalities

Scott Giles

Equipment, Devices, and Technologies represents approximately 7 - 9 questions (4.7% - 6%) on the NPTE-PTA.

Scott Giles

Therapeutic Modalities represents approximately 9 - 11 questions (6% - 7.33%) on the NPTE-PTA.

CHAPTER 8
Equipment, Devices, and Technologies; Therapeutic Modalities

Mobility

Preparation for Treatment

In order to create an effective and successful treatment environment, the patient must be informed regarding all expectations of the upcoming treatment as well as have all questions answered prior to initiating the actual hands-on intervention. The therapist must obtain informed consent from the patient and document consent in the patient's chart. The therapist must also determine if there are any potential limitations to treatment due to a patient's religious or cultural beliefs. The patient must be notified as to appropriate clothing for therapy, and subject areas such as draping must also be discussed prior to the initiation of therapy in order to ensure a patient's comfort during treatment.

Draping

Draping is a technique utilized by health care providers to ensure the patient's privacy and modesty when treating particular areas of the body. Draping assists to keep the patient warm during treatment, adequately expose the area of treatment, and protect open areas, wounds, scars, and the patient's personal belongings from being soiled or injured during treatment. Draping materials may include gowns, towels, and sheets that must be secured in a manner that will properly expose the area of the body that requires treatment, while maintaining a patient's modesty and overall level of comfort during treatment.

Bed Mobility Guidelines[1,2]

- A patient that is dependent must be repositioned in bed at least every two hours
- Skin should be inspected for redness or breakdown with each position change
- A dependent patient must be lifted when changing positions in order to avoid shearing of the skin across the bed
- Use pillows, towels or blankets when positioning a patient in order to support and maintain a particular position
- A patient should always be encouraged to participate in all mobility and positioning
- Practice moving segmentally from one side of the bed to the other
- Utilize the "bridging" position of hip flexion and knee flexion with feet flat on the surface to assist with movement and rolling
- Move from a supine to sitting position by rolling into sidelying and placing the feet over the edge; with assist as needed
- All components of bed mobility are complete only when the patient ends in a comfortable and safe position

Transfers

Communication During Transfers

The patient should be informed about the transfer itself and their responsibility during the transfer. The explanation should be understood by the patient and should occur prior to performing the transfer.

Commands and counts are used to synchronize the actions of the participants involved in the transfer. The therapist at the head of the patient should give the commands during transfers when more than one person is involved (Fig. 8-1).

Levels of Physical Assistance[1,3]

Independent: The patient does not require any assistance to complete the task.

Supervision: The patient requires a therapist to observe throughout completion of the task.

Contact Guard: The patient requires the therapist to maintain contact with the patient to complete the task. Contact guard is usually needed to assist if there is a loss of balance.

Minimal Assist: The patient requires 25% assist from the therapist to complete the task.

Moderate Assist: The patient requires 50% assist from the therapist to complete the task.

Maximal Assist: The patient requires 75% assist from the therapist to complete the task.

Dependent: The patient is unable to participate and the therapist must provide all of the effort to perform the task.

Transfer Guidelines

- Evaluate the patient's level of cognition and mobility
- When in doubt, utilize a second person to maintain patient/therapist safety
- Obtain all appropriate equipment prior to initiating the transfer
- Utilize a safety belt
- Educate the patient regarding the expectations and transfer sequence through verbal explanation and demonstration
- Instruct the patient in smaller segments of the transfer, if necessary, prior to performing the entire transfer all at once
- Position yourself correctly around the patient and maintain a large base of support; use proper body mechanics throughout the transfer

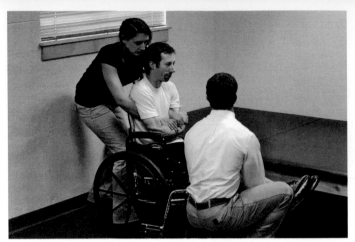

Fig. 8-1: The therapist at the head verbally initiates the transfer.

- Vary the amount of assistance as needed
- Utilize manual contacts with the patient to direct their participation during the transfer
- Complete the transfer with the patient positioned comfortably and safely

Types of Transfers[1,3]

Dependent Transfers
Three-person carry/lift

The three-person carry or lift is used to transfer a patient from a stretcher to a bed or treatment plinth. Three therapists carry the patient in a supine position; one therapist supports the head and upper trunk, the second therapist supports the trunk, and the third supports the lower extremities. The therapist at the head is the one to initiate commands. The therapists flex their elbows that are positioned under the patient and roll the patient on their side towards them. The therapists then lift on command and move in a line to the destination surface, lower, and position the patient properly.

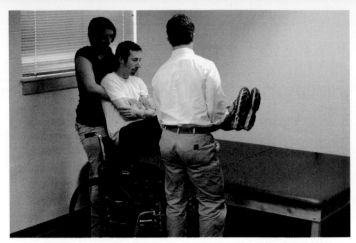

Fig. 8-2: The therapists lift the patient from the wheelchair in a coordinated fashion.

Two-person lift

The two-person lift is used to transfer a patient between two surfaces of different heights or when transferring a patient to the floor. Standing behind the patient, the first therapist should place their arms underneath the patient's axilla. The therapist should grasp the patient's left forearm with their right hand and grasp the patient's right forearm with their left hand. The second therapist places one arm under the mid to distal thighs and the other arm is used to support the lower legs. The therapist at the head usually initiates the command to lift and transfer the patient out of the chair to the destination surface (Figs. 8-1, 8-2, 8-3, 8-4).

Dependent squat pivot transfer

The dependent squat pivot transfer is used to transfer a patient who cannot stand independently, but can bear some weight through the trunk and lower extremities. The therapist should position the patient at a 45-degree angle to the destination surface. The patient places their upper extremities on the therapist's shoulders, but should not be allowed to pull on the therapist's neck. The

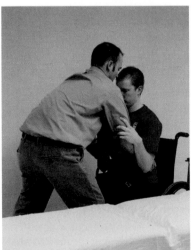

Fig. 8-5: A therapist prepares to initiate a dependent squat pivot transfer.

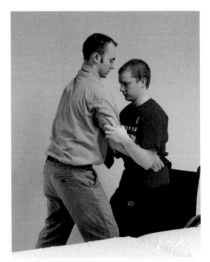

Fig. 8-6: The therapist moves the patient from the chair to a supported squatting position. The patient can bear some weight through the lower extremities.

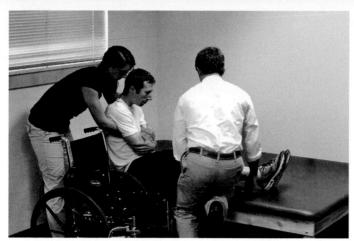

Fig. 8-3: The patient is slowly lowered to the mat table.

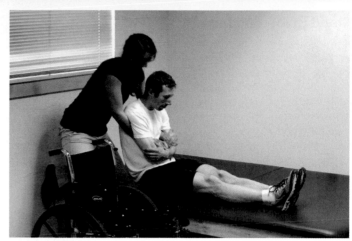

Fig. 8-4: The patient must be in a comfortable and safe position before the therapist concludes the transfer.

therapist should position the patient at the edge of the surface, hold the patient around the hips and under the buttocks, and block the patient's knees in order to avoid buckling while standing. The therapist should utilize momentum, straighten their legs, and raise the patient or allow the patient to remain in a squatting position. The therapist should then pivot and slowly lower the patient to the destination surface (Figs. 8-5, 8-6, 8-7, 8-8).

Hydraulic lift

The hydraulic lift is a device used for dependent transfers when a patient is obese, there is only one therapist available to assist with the transfer or the patient is totally dependent. The hydraulic lift needs to be locked in position before the transfer. The therapist positions a webbed sling under the patient and attaches the S-ring to the bars on the lift. Once all attachments are checked, the therapist should pump the handle on the device in order to elevate the patient. When the patient is elevated, the therapist can navigate the lift with the patient to the destination surface. The chains should be removed once the patient has been transferred, however, the webbed sling should remain in place in preparation for the return transfer.

Assisted Transfers
Sliding board transfer

The sliding board transfer is used for a patient who has some sitting balance, some upper extremity strength, and can adequately follow directions. The patient should be positioned at the edge of the wheelchair or bed and should lean to one side while placing one end of the sliding board sufficiently under the proximal thigh. The other end of the sliding board should be positioned on the destination surface. The patient should not hold onto the end of the sliding board in order to avoid pinching the fingers. The patient should place the lead hand four to six inches away from the sliding board and use both arms to initiate a push-up and scoot across the board. The therapist should guard in front of the patient and assist as needed as the patient performs a series of push-ups across the board. The therapist should be careful to avoid direct contact between the patient's skin and the sliding board to avoid shearing force and potential skin breakdown.

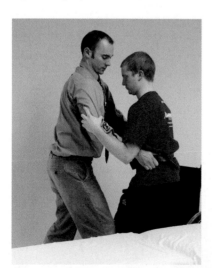

Fig. 8-7: The therapist blocks the patient's knees in order to provide additional stability during the transfer.

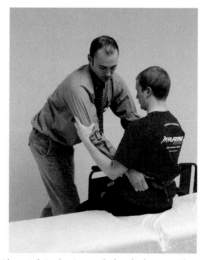

Fig. 8-8: The therapist pivots and slowly lowers the patient to the plinth.

Stand pivot transfer

The stand pivot transfer is used when a patient is able to stand and bear weight through one or both of the lower extremities. The patient must possess functional balance and the ability to pivot. Patients with unilateral weight bearing restrictions or hemiplegia may utilize this transfer and lead with the uninvolved side. The transfer may also be used therapeutically, leading with the involved side for a patient post CVA. A patient should be positioned at the edge of the wheelchair or bed to initiate the transfer. The therapist can assist the patient to keep their feet flat on the floor while bringing the head and trunk forward. The therapist should assist the patient as needed with their feet. The therapist must guard or assist the patient through the transfer and instruct the patient to reach back for the surface before they begin to sit down. Once the stand pivot is performed, the therapist should assist as needed to ensure control with lowering the patient to the destination surface.

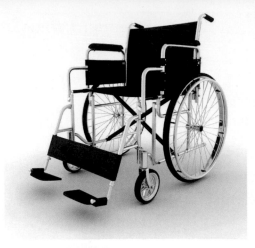

Fig. 8-9: A manual wheelchair.

Stand step transfer

The stand step transfer is used with a patient who has the necessary strength and balance to weight shift and step during the transfer. The patient requires guarding or supervision from the therapist and performs the transfer as a stand pivot transfer except the patient actually takes a step to maneuver and reposition their feet instead of a pivot.

Wheelchairs

Wheelchairs can be manually propelled or externally powered. Manual wheelchairs require patients to possess sufficient strength to propel the wheelchair independently (Fig. 8-9). Powered wheelchairs are propelled by an external energy source, usually a battery, that provides stored energy to one or more belts that propel the wheelchair (Fig. 8-10). Considerations when selecting an appropriate wheelchair include the patient's physical needs, physical abilities, cognition, coordination, and endurance.

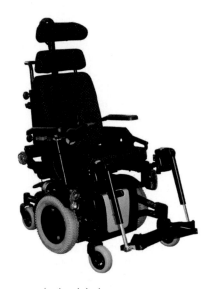

Fig. 8-10: A powered wheelchair.

Wheelchair Measurements

A = total height

B = seat depth

C = armrest height

D = seat height from floor

E = seat and back width

F = back height

Fig. 8-11: Common wheelchair measurements.[4]

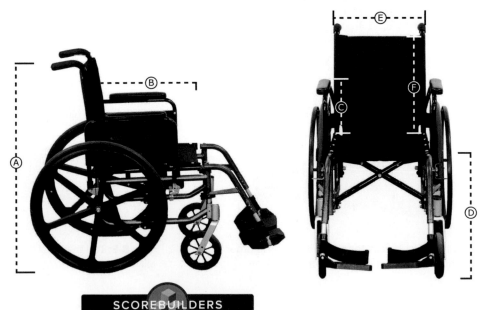

Standard Wheelchair Measurements for Proper Fit[1]

Measurement	Instructions	Average Adult Size
Seat Height	Measure from the user's heel to the popliteal fold and add 2 inches to allow clearance of the footrest.	19.5 to 20.5 inches
Seat Depth	Measure from the user's posterior buttock, along the lateral thigh to the popliteal fold; then subtract approximately 2 inches to avoid pressure from the front edge of the seat against the popliteal space. **Fig. 8-12:** A therapist assesses the depth of a wheelchair.	16 inches
Seat Width	Measure the widest aspect of the user's buttocks, hips or thighs and add approximately 2 inches. This will provide space for bulky clothing, orthoses or clearance of the trochanters from the armrest side panel. **Fig. 8-13:** A therapist assesses the width of a wheelchair.	18 inches
Back Height	Measure from the seat of the chair to the floor of the axilla with the user's shoulder flexed to 90 degrees and then subtract approximately 4 inches. This will allow the final back height to be below the inferior angles of the scapulae. (Note: This measurement will be affected if a seat cushion is to be used. The person should be measured while seated on the cushion or the thickness of the cushion must be considered by adding that value to the actual measurement.)	16 to 16.5 inches
Armrest Height	Measure from the seat of the chair to the olecranon process with the user's elbow flexed to 90 degrees and then add approximately 1 inch. (Note: This measurement will be affected if a seat cushion is to be used. The person should be measured while seated on the cushion or the thickness of the cushion must be considered by adding that value to the actual measurement.)	9 inches above the chair seat

From Pierson, FM: Principles and Techniques of Patient Care. W.B. Saunders Company, Philadelphia 2002, p.168, with permission.

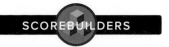

Common Components of Wheelchair Prescription[5-8]

Wheelchair Component	Clinical Indication
Wheelchair Frame	
Ultralight frame	Patient is highly active with no need for postural supports; used for sports
Standard or lightweight frame	Patient is able to self propel using both upper extremities; adequate lower extremity ROM and sitting ability for comfortable seating
Hemi frame	Patient is able to self propel using lower extremities
One-hand drive frame	Patient is able to self propel using one upper extremity
Amputee frame	Patient is able to self propel, but center of gravity is shifted posteriorly due to amputation
Power wheelchair	Patient is not able to self propel, but is able to safely operate a power mobility device; patient may have transfer, sitting and/or upper extremity functional limitations
Geri chair	Patient is not able to self propel or safely operate a power mobility device; requires assistance for seated mobility
Reclining frame	Patient is unable to perform weight shifting tasks and/or is unable to sit upright for extended periods; moderate to severe trunk involvement
Backward tilt-in-space frame	Patient is unable to sit upright or perform weight shifts, but also has issues with sliding or extensor tone
Back Inserts	
Sling back	Patient requires no postural support and has no neuromuscular deficits; not typically intended for long term use
Planar back insert	Patient requires mild to moderate trunk support due to tone, strength or deformity related postural concerns
Curved back insert	Patient requires moderate trunk support due to tone, strength or deformity related postural concerns
Custom molded insert	Patient requires significant trunk support due to severe postural concerns
Seat Inserts	
Sling seat	Patient requires no postural support and has no neuromuscular deficits; not typically intended for long term use
Planar seat	Patient has no seated deformity

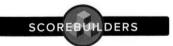

Common Components of Wheelchair Prescription[5-8]

Wheelchair Component	Clinical Indication
Curved seat	Patient requires mild to aggressive supportive curvature to provide increased contact between the lower body and seat
Custom molded seat	Patient requires customized seat support to correct for pelvic obliquity or a fixed asymmetrical deformity
Armrests	
Removable	Patient transfers via slide board or two person maximal assist; patient requires access to wheels for propulsion
No armrests	Patient does not require any upper extremity or trunk support
Full length arms	Patient performs sit to stand transfers; patient requires additional postural support; patient utilizes a lap board
Fixed/non-removable	Patient requires durable upper extremity support
Wheel locks/brakes	
Toggle/lever brakes (push or pull)	Patient has coordinated motor ability to operate brakes
Brake extension	Patient requires additional leverage to operate a toggle/lever brake; patient has limited ability to reach brake mechanism
Attendant operated brakes	Patient does not possess the ability to safely or independently operate brakes
Handrims	
Small diameter	Patient has adequate strength to efficiently propel chair without adaptation; typically suggested for patients requiring speed for tasks
Large diameter	Patient has some degree of weakness in the upper extremities; typically suggested for patients requiring the ability to propel with more power
Rim projections	Patient has grip deficits or hand deformity which limits the ability to functionally grip rims
Covered rims	Patient requires assist for adequate grasp or friction when hands are in contact with wheel rims

Common Components of Wheelchair Prescription[5-8]

Wheelchair Component	Clinical Indication
Footrests	
Standard	Patient has full ROM available through feet and ankles
Adjustable angle	Patient has some degree of deformity in feet and/or ankles
One-piece footboard	Patient requires a supportive surface to maximize strength and/or stability; patient requires additional lateral foot support
Power Mobility Controls	
Joystick control	Joysticks options vary widely and can be adapted for operation by numerous body parts (e.g., hand, chin, foot)
Proportional control	Allows user to modulate speed of device based on the displacement of the joystick; 360 degree directionality
Non-proportional control	Device moves at a pre-set speed regardless of joystick displacement; user must release joystick in order to change directions
Sip-and-puff control	A switch based system often used for patients with high level spinal cord injuries; patient controls direction based on the force of inhalation/exhalation into a small tube positioned near the patient's mouth
Head control	Head controls may be proportional or non-proportional and operate via an electronic switch system; configurations vary
Other Considerations	
Bariatric wheelchair	Bariatric wheelchairs are available in a variety of weight ratings and dimensions to accommodate patient needs. Weight limits for bariatric wheelchairs typically range between 300 and 1,000 pounds.
Solid cushions (viscoelastic, polyurethane or honeycomb foam)	Solid cushions vary greatly in density and stiffness depending on the product selected. Solid cushions are typically lightweight, however, can produce high shear forces. Examples include Sunmate, Stimulite, and T-foam cushions.
Liquid cushions (gel or water filled)	Liquid cushions vary greatly in the density and stiffness depending on the product selected. Liquid cushions are typically heavier than other alternatives, but serve to limit shear forces. Examples include Jay, Flo-fit, Avanti, and Action cushions.
Air filled cushions	Air filled cushions vary in average shear forces depending on the product selected. Common characteristics include being lightweight with pressure influenced by altitude. Air filled cushions require diligent monitoring of inflation levels. Examples include the Roho and Bye Bye Decubiti cushions.

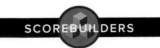

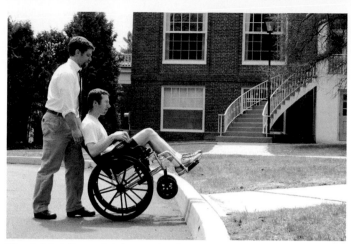

Fig. 8-14: A therapist tips a wheelchair backwards.

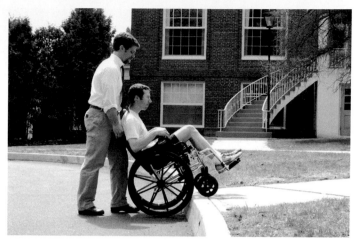

Fig. 8-15: The wheelchair is moved forward until the rear wheels come in contact with the curb.

Wheelchair Mobility[1,3]

Ascending a curb with a forward approach

1. Elevate the front casters of the wheelchair by tipping the wheelchair backwards (Fig. 8-14).

2. Move the wheelchair forward until the rear wheels are in contact with the curb and the casters are above the curb (Fig. 8-15).

3. Lower the casters on the elevated surface and ascend the curb with the real wheels until the rear wheels and the casters are in contact with the elevated surface (Figs. 8-16, 8-17).

Ascending a curb with a backward approach

1. Position the patient facing away from the curb.

2. Standing on the upper surface, lift and roll the rear wheels backward up the curb.

3. Continue to roll the wheelchair backwards until the casters are in contact with the upper surface.

Descending a curb with a forward approach

1. Position the casters close to the elevated edge of the curb.

2. Tip the wheelchair backwards and slowly roll the wheelchair forward until the rear wheels are in contact with the lower surface.

3. Gently lower the casters to the lower surface.

Descending a curb with a backward approach

1. Position the patient facing away from the curb.

2. Move the wheelchair backwards and slowly lower the rear wheels to the lower surface maintaining contact with the curb.

3. Continue to roll the wheelchair backwards and gently lower the casters to the lower surface.

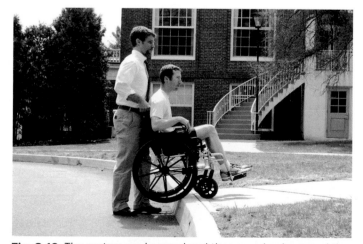

Fig. 8-16: The casters are lowered and the rear wheels ascend the curb.

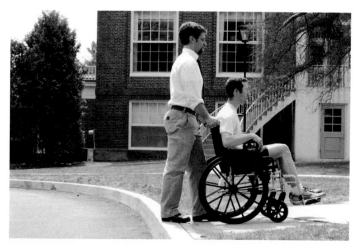

Fig. 8-17: The rear wheels and casters are positioned on the elevated surface.

CONSIDER THIS
EQUIPMENT FOR ACTIVITIES OF DAILY LIVING[9]

Physical therapist assistants should be aware of equipment available to assist patients to perform activities of daily living as effectively and efficiently as possible. The most appropriate equipment for each patient will depend on the patient's medical status and their current living condition.

A listing of some of the more commonly used equipment for activities of daily living is presented.

Bed safety rails - Externally applied rails assist patients with bed mobility.

Button hook - A device that allows individuals with limited dexterity to button clothing using a handheld device. Individuals unable to utilize the device effectively can use Velcro instead of buttons.

Commode chair - A chair with a cut out seat for personal hygiene and a removable pan for commode use. The device is elevated above the level of a standard commode and the armrests increase safety during transfers.

Door knob extenders - A device that increases leverage when opening and closing doors making it easier for individuals with diminished strength and dexterity to function independently.

Grab bars - Stable, mounted bars designed to provide individuals with a handgrip for added stability during functional tasks.

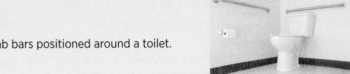

Fig. 8-18: Grab bars positioned around a toilet.

Handwriting aids - Writing devices can be enlarged using a triangular grip or cylindrical foam. This adaptation makes it easier for patients with limited dexterity and pinch strength to write.

Long straw - A long plastic straw enables individuals to drink from a glass without lifting the glass from the surface.

Reacher - The device consists of a long, lightweight aluminum surface with a trigger which activates a grip closure enabling an individual to reach upward or downward without excessive bending.

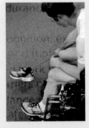
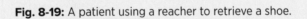

Fig. 8-19: A patient using a reacher to retrieve a shoe.

Rocker knife - This type of knife has a curved blade with an enlarged handle which allows an individual to cut food using a rocking motion.

Sock aids/shoe aids - Devices designed to assist individuals to independently apply socks and shoes using some type of a plastic or wire frame. The devices work by maintaining the sock in an open position or providing a funnel for the patient to use when placing the foot into a shoe.

Tub bench - A bench that allows an individual to sit on a firm, stable surface when bathing.

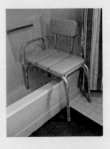

Fig. 8-20: A tub bench positioned in a bath tub.

Zipper pull - A device that allows individuals with inadequate strength in the arms and fingers to pull a zipper using a loop.

Ambulation

Assistive Devices

Primary indications for using an assistive device during ambulation include:

- Decreased weight bearing on the lower extremities
- Muscle weakness of the trunk or lower extremities
- Decreased balance or impaired kinesthetic awareness
- Pain

Assistive Device Selection[1,3,10]

Parallel Bars

Parallel bars provide maximum stability and security for a patient during the beginning stages of ambulation or standing. Proper fit includes bar height that allows for 20-25 degrees of elbow flexion while grasping on the bars approximately four to six inches in front of the body. A patient must progress out of the parallel bars as quickly as possible to increase overall mobility and decrease dependence using the parallel bars.

Walker

A walker can be used with all levels of weight bearing. The walker has a significant base of support and offers good stability (Fig. 8-21). The walker should allow for 20-25 degrees of elbow flexion to ensure proper fit. The standard walker has many variations including rolling, hemi, reciprocal, folding, or adjustable walker with brakes, upper extremity attachments and/or a seat platform. The walker is used with a three-point gait pattern.

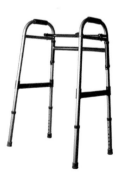

Fig. 8-21: A standard walker.

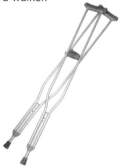

Fig. 8-22: Axillary crutches.

Axillary Crutches

Axillary crutches can be used with all levels of weight bearing, however, require higher coordination for proper use (Fig. 8-22). Proper fit includes positioning with the crutches six inches in front and two inches lateral to the patient. The crutch height should be adjusted no greater than three finger widths from the axilla (Fig. 8-23). The handgrip height should be adjusted to the ulnar styloid process and allow for 20-25 degrees of elbow flexion while grasping the handgrip (Fig. 8-24). A platform attachment can be utilized with this device. Axillary crutches can be used with two-point, three-point, four-point, swing-to, and swing-through gait patterns.

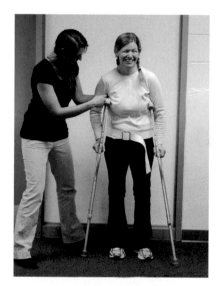

Fig. 8-23: A therapist assesses crutch height by determining the distance from the top of the crutch to the base of the axilla.

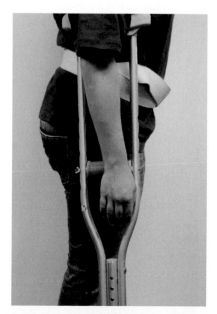

Fig. 8-24: The handgrip of an axillary crutch should be at the approximate level of the ulnar styloid process.

Lofstrand (forearm) Crutches

Lofstrand crutches can be used with all levels of weight bearing, however, require the highest level of coordination for proper use (Fig. 8-25). Proper fit includes 20–25 degrees of elbow flexion while holding the handgrip with the crutches positioned six inches in front and two inches lateral to the patient's foot. The arm cuff should be positioned one to one and one half inches below the olecranon process so it does not interfere with elbow flexion. A platform attachment can be utilized with this device if necessary. The Lofstrand crutches can be used with two-point, three-point, four-point, swing-to, and swing-through gait patterns.

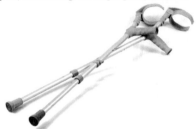

Fig. 8-25: Lofstrand crutches.

Cane

A cane provides minimal stability and support for patients during ambulation activities. The straight cane provides the least support and is used primarily for assisting with balance. A straight cane should not be utilized for patients that are partial weight bearing. The small base and large base quad canes provide a larger base of support and can better assist with limiting weight bearing on an involved lower extremity and improving balance on unlevel surfaces, curbs, and stairs. The cane is typically used on the opposite side of an involved lower extremity. Proper fit includes standing the cane at the patient's side and adjusting the handle to the level of the wrist crease at the ulnar styloid (Fig. 8-26). The patient should have 20–25 degrees of elbow flexion while grasping the handgrip. The straight cane can be used with the two-point, four-point, modified two-point, and modified four-point gait patterns.

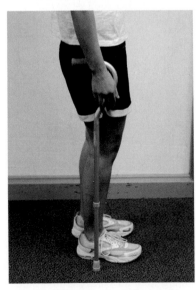

Fig. 8-26: The handle of a cane should be at the approximate level of the ulnar styloid process.

Levels of Weight Bearing[3]

Non-weight bearing (NWB): A patient is unable to place any weight through the involved extremity and is not permitted to touch the ground or any surface. An assistive device is required.

Toe touch weight bearing (TTWB): A patient is unable to place any weight through the involved extremity, however, may place the toes on the ground to assist with balance. An assistive device is required.

Partial weight bearing (PWB): A patient is allowed to put a particular amount of weight through the involved extremity. The amount of weight bearing is expressed as allowable pounds of pressure or as a percentage of total weight. A therapist must monitor the amount of actual weight transferred through the involved foot during partial weight bearing (Fig. 8-27). An assistive device is required.

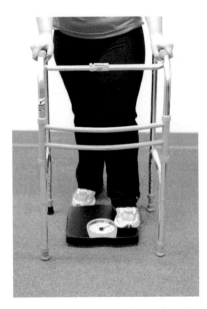

Fig. 8-27: A patient using a scale to determine the approximate amount of weight bearing.

Weight bearing as tolerated (WBAT): A patient determines the proper amount of weight bearing based on comfort. The amount of weight bearing can range from minimal to full. An assistive device may or may not be required.

Full weight bearing (FWB): A patient is able to place full weight on the involved extremity. An assistive device is not required at this level, but may be used to assist with balance.

Guarding

Guarding During Ambulation

A therapist must consider the patient's size, weight, and level of impairment prior to initiating ambulation activities. The following are general guarding recommendations:

- Stand to the side (usually the affected side) and slightly behind the patient.

- Grasp the safety belt with one hand; place the other hand on the patient's shoulder.

- Avoid grasping the arm since it can interfere with the patient's ability to use the extremity.

- Move the lead foot forward when the patient moves; the back leg should advance as the patient ambulates.

- Attempt to anticipate potential hazards during ambulation and take appropriate precautions when possible.

- Utilize a second therapist when needed.

Gait Patterns[1,3]

An appropriate gait pattern is determined by the amount of weight bearing permitted and the severity of the patient's overall condition. Commonly used gait patterns include two-point, three-point, four-point, swing-to, and swing-through.

Two-point gait

This is a pattern in which a patient uses two crutches or canes. The patient ambulates moving the left crutch forward while simultaneously advancing the right lower extremity and vice versa. Each step is one point and a complete cycle is two points.

Three-point gait

This pattern can be seen with a walker or crutches. It involves one injured lower extremity that may have decreased weight bearing. The assistive device is advanced followed by the injured lower extremity and then the uninjured lower extremity. The assistive device and each lower extremity are considered separate points.

Four-point gait

This pattern is very similar to the two-point pattern. The primary difference is that the patient does not move the lower extremities simultaneously with the device, but rather waits and advances the opposite leg once the crutch/cane has been advanced. This gait pattern may be prescribed when a patient exhibits impaired coordination, balance or significant strength deficits. Each advancement of the crutch or cane as well as the bilateral lower extremities indicates a single point, thus allowing for a four-point gait pattern.

Swing-to gait

A gait pattern where a patient with trunk and/or bilateral lower extremity weakness, paresis or paralysis uses crutches or a walker and advances the lower extremities simultaneously only to the point of the assistive device.

Swing-through gait

A gait pattern where the patient performs the same sequence as a swing-to gait pattern, however, advances the lower extremities beyond the point of the assistive device.

Guarding During Curbs and Stairs[1,11]

Ascending

- When using a handrail, stand to the opposite side and behind the patient.

- When a handrail is not available, stand behind the patient slightly toward the affected side (Fig. 8-28).

- Grasp the safety belt with one hand and have the opposite hand available to support the trunk as needed.

- The therapist should position one foot on the step the patient is starting from and the other on the step below. The therapist should maintain a wide base of support.

- Remain static when the patient is moving, then advance keeping the feet in stride position.

Descending

- When using a handrail, stand to the opposite side and in front of the patient.

- When a handrail is not available, stand in front of the patient slightly toward the affected side.

- Grasp the safety belt with one hand and have the opposite hand available to support the trunk as needed.

- The therapist should position one foot on the step the patient will step to and the other on the step below. The therapist should maintain a wide base of support.

- Remain static when the patient is moving, then advance keeping the feet in stride position.

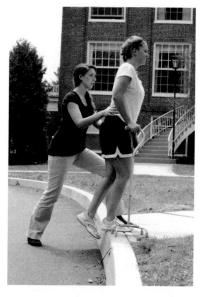

Fig. 8-28: A patient ascending a curb with a quad cane.

CONSIDER THIS
ASCENDING AND DESCENDING STAIRS WITH AN ASSISTIVE DEVICE[1,11]

Patients can ascend and descend stairs with a number of different assistive devices. Regardless of the specific assistive device utilized, when ascending stairs the patient should place the uninvolved lower extremity on the higher stair since it will generate the force needed to propel the body. The involved lower extremity and the assistive device then move to the same stair. When descending stairs, the uninvolved lower extremity generates the force needed to lower the involved extremity with the assistive device to the next step.

Additional factors for therapists to consider when using various assistive devices on stairs are listed.

Walker

Ascending - The patient should place the walker on the opposite side of the handrail and turn the walker sideways. The patient should then grasp the handrail with one hand and the top of the walker's handpiece with the other hand. Using the handrail and walker for stability, the patient takes a step up with the uninvolved extremity. The involved extremity is then advanced to the same step and the walker follows.

Descending - The walker is positioned in a similar manner as described previously. The patient uses the handrail and top of the walker for stability while lowering the involved lower extremity. The uninvolved lower extremity is then lowered and the walker follows.

Axillary Crutches

Ascending - The patient should use the handrail and turn the crutch sideways. This will result in the patient grasping the handrail and the crutch with the same hand. The patient should use the handrail and advance the uninvolved lower extremity to the next step. The patient will then advance the involved lower extremity followed by the other crutch.

Descending - The patient uses the handrail and turns the crutch sideways as described previously. The patient lowers the involved lower extremity and the crutch to the next step followed by the uninvolved extremity.

The patient may alternately elect to ascend and descend stairs holding the handrail with one hand and the two crutches in the other hand.

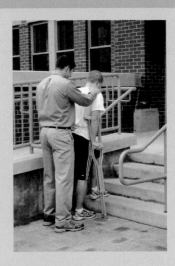

Fig. 8-29: A patient ascending stairs with axillary crutches using the alternate method.

Cane

Ascending - The patient should use the handrail and turn the cane sideways. This will result in the patient grasping the handrail and the cane with the same hand. The patient should use the handrail and advance the uninvolved lower extremity to the next step. The patient will then advance the involved lower extremity.

Descending - The patient uses the handrail and turns the cane sideways as described previously. The patient lowers the involved lower extremity to the next step followed by the uninvolved extremity.

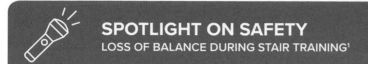

SPOTLIGHT ON SAFETY
LOSS OF BALANCE DURING STAIR TRAINING[1]

Therapists take many precautions to avoid unnecessary safety risks when instructing patients in a variety of functional activities. Despite these precautions, on occasion adverse events still occur. In these instances, therapists must be prepared to take immediate action to avoid or minimize the potential impact of an adverse event.

The most appropriate therapist action when a patient experiences a loss of balance during stair training is described. The descriptions are based on the therapist being positioned behind the patient when ascending the stairs and in front of the patient when descending the stairs.

Forward loss of balance

Ascending: Pull backwards on the safety belt and attempt to move the trunk backwards with the opposing hand. If the patient cannot regain balance, transition the patient toward the handrail or lower the patient slowly toward the stairs.

Descending: Use one hand to apply a posterior directed force to the patient's trunk. The therapist may elect to use both hands to stabilize the patient or may use one hand to grasp the handrail while stabilizing the trunk with the opposing hand. If the patient cannot regain balance, the therapist should attempt to move them to a sitting position.

Backward loss of balance

Ascending: Attempt to stabilize the patient's trunk by applying an anterior directed force while maintaining a wide base of support. If the patient cannot regain balance, transition the patient toward the handrail or lower the patient slowly toward the stairs.

Descending: Pull forwards on the safety belt using one hand to grasp the handrail. If the patient cannot regain balance, transition the patient toward the handrail or attempt to move them to a sitting position.

Sideways loss of balance toward the therapist

Ascending: Use one hand or your trunk to stabilize the patient and use the other hand to grasp the handrail. If the patient cannot regain balance, transition the patient toward the handrail or lower the patient slowly toward the stairs.

Descending: Use one hand or your trunk to stabilize the patient and use the other hand to grasp the safety belt or handrail. If the patient cannot regain balance, transition the patient toward the handrail or attempt to move them to a sitting position.

Sideways loss of balance away from the therapist

Ascending: Use one hand to pull the safety belt toward you and use the other to stabilize the trunk or grasp the handrail. If the patient cannot regain balance, transition the patient toward the handrail or lower the patient slowly toward the stairs.

Descending: Use one hand to pull the safety belt toward you and use the other to stabilize the trunk or grasp the handrail. If the patient cannot regain balance, transition the patient toward the handrail or attempt to move them to a sitting position.

Medical Equipment

Feeding Devices[1,12]

Nasogastric tube (NG tube)

A nasogastric tube is a plastic tube inserted through a nostril that extends into the stomach. The device is commonly used for short-term liquid feeding, medication administration or to remove gas from the stomach. The position of the tube in the nostril and back of the throat can inhibit a cough and be irritating for the patient.

Gastric tube (G tube)

A gastric tube is a tube inserted through a small incision in the abdomen into the stomach. The tube can be used for long-term feeding in the presence of difficulty with swallowing due to an anatomic or neurologic disorder or to avoid the risk of aspiration.

Jejunostomy tube (J tube)

A jejunostomy tube is a tube inserted through endoscopy into the jejunum via the abdominal wall. The tube can be used for long-term feeding for patients that are unable to receive food by mouth.

Intravenous system (IV)

An intravenous system consists of a sterile fluid source, a pump, a clamp, and a catheter to insert into a vein (Fig. 8-30). An intravenous system can be used to infuse fluids, electrolytes, nutrients, and medication. Intravenous lines are most commonly inserted into superficial veins such as the basilic, cephalic or antecubital. Intravenous infusion lines permit nutrients to be introduced when the gastrointestinal tract is not able to digest and absorb food.

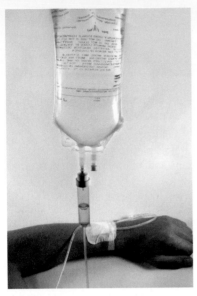

Fig. 8-30: An intravenous system.

Monitoring Devices[1,12,13]

Arterial line

An arterial line is a monitoring device consisting of a catheter that is inserted into an artery and attached to an electronic monitoring system. An arterial line is used to measure blood pressure or to obtain blood samples. The device is considered to be more accurate than traditional measures of blood pressure and does not require repeated needle punctures. If an arterial line is displaced, a therapist should apply direct pressure to limit blood loss and call for assistance.

Central venous pressure catheter

A central venous pressure catheter is used for measuring pressures in the right atrium or the superior vena cava by means of an indwelling venous catheter and a pressure manometer. It is used to evaluate the right ventricular function, right atrial filling pressure, and circulating blood volume. The use of the catheter significantly reduces the need for repeated venipuncture.

Indwelling right atrial catheter (Hickman)

An indwelling right atrial catheter is inserted through the cephalic or internal jugular vein and threaded into the superior vena cava and right atrium. The catheter is used for long-term administration of substances into the venous system such as chemotherapeutic agents, total parenteral nutrition, and antibiotics.

Intracranial pressure monitor

An intracranial pressure monitor measures the pressure exerted against the skull using pressure sensing devices placed inside the skull. Excessive pressure can be produced by a closed head injury, cerebral hemorrhage, overproduction of cerebrospinal fluid or brain tumor. Types of intracranial pressure monitors include epidural sensor, subarachnoid bolt, and intraventricular catheter.

Oximeter

An oximeter is a photoelectric device used to determine the oxygen saturation of blood. The device is most commonly applied to the finger or the ear. Oximetry is often used by therapists to assess activity tolerance. Therapists should monitor changes in oxygen saturation during exercise and position changes.

Pulmonary artery catheter (Swan-Ganz catheter)

A pulmonary artery catheter is a soft, flexible catheter that is inserted through a vein into the pulmonary artery. The device is used to provide continuous measurements of pulmonary artery pressure. The patient should avoid excessive movement of the head, neck, and extremities to avoid disrupting the line at the insertion site.

Oxygen Therapy[1,12]

Nasal cannula

A nasal cannula consists of tubing extending approximately one centimeter into each of the patient's nostrils. The tubing is connected to a common tube that is attached to an oxygen source. This method of oxygen therapy is capable of delivering up to six liters of oxygen per minute.

Oronasal mask

An oronasal mask consists of a facepiece designed to cover the nose and mouth with small vent holes to expel exhaled air along with a breathing tube and connector. The device is used most often for oxygen therapy, however, can be used to administer medications, mucolytic detergents, or humidity, by the use of an accessory nebulizer.

Tent

An oxygen tent refers to a canopy placed over the head and shoulders or the entire body for the purpose of delivering oxygen at a higher level than normal.

Tracheostomy mask

A tracheostomy mask is placed over a stoma or tracheostomy for the purpose of administering supplemental oxygen. The mask is held in place by an elastic strap placed around the patient's neck.

Skeletal Traction[12]

Balanced suspension

Balanced suspension traction requires pins, screws, and wires to be surgically inserted into bone for the purpose of applying a traction force using an externally applied weight. This type of traction is most often utilized with comminuted femur fractures. Balanced suspension traction requires prolonged immobilization and therefore increases the incidence of secondary complications such as contractures or skin breakdown.

External fixation

External fixation refers to a surgical procedure where holes are drilled into uninjured areas of bone surrounding the fracture. The fracture is then set in the desired anatomical configuration using specialized wires, pins, bolts, and screws. An external frame is used to maintain the bony fragments in the desired alignment (Fig. 8-31). External fixation enhances stability and allows for earlier mobility while maintaining the desired alignment.

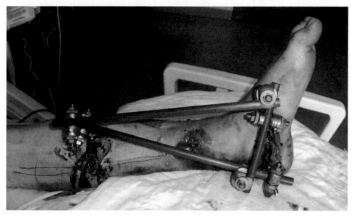

Fig. 8-31: An external fixation device applied to a tibial fracture sustained in a motor vehicle accident.

Internal fixation

Internal fixation refers to a surgical procedure that attempts to promote the healing process of bone without appliances being applied external to the skin. Common types of internal fixation include metal plates, rods, wires, screws, and nails. Internal fixation is often employed with comminuted or displaced fractures. The procedure provides needed stability to healing joints which allows earlier mobility and less postoperative complications.

Urinary Catheters[1,12]

External catheter

An external catheter is applied over the shaft of the penis and is held in place by a padded strap or adhesive tape.

Foley catheter

A Foley catheter is an indwelling urinary tract catheter that has a balloon attachment at the indwelling end. The balloon which is filled with air or sterile water must be deflated before the catheter can be removed.

Suprapubic catheter

A suprapubic catheter is an indwelling urinary catheter that is surgically inserted directly into the patient's bladder. Insertion of a suprapubic catheter is performed under general anesthesia.

Miscellaneous[1,12]

Chest tube

A chest tube is a flexible plastic tube that is inserted through an incision into the side of the chest. The tube uses a suction system to remove air, fluid or pus from the intrathoracic space. A chest tube can cause significant discomfort and result in inhibition of a cough, deep breathing, and mobility.

Mechanical ventilator

A mechanical ventilator produces a controlled flow of gas into a patient's airways. The flow of gas provides positive pressure that produces lung inflation. Patients with acute illness, trauma, and severe chronic illness may require mechanical ventilation. The most common type of ventilators include volume cycled and pressure cycled. Volume cycled ventilators deliver a predetermined amount of gas based on the patient's needs during the inspiratory phase. This type of ventilation is most commonly used for patients that require long-term support. Pressure cycled ventilators deliver a predetermined maximum pressure of gas during respiration. When the established pressure is reached, the inspiratory phase ends. The expiratory phase is passive with both volume cycled and pressure cycled ventilators.

Ostomy device

An ostomy device provides a method for collection of waste from a surgically produced opening in the abdomen. The removal of the waste occurs through a stoma extending into the small intestine. The waste is collected in a plastic bag or pouch covering the stoma. Ostomy systems are typically air and water-tight and allow the user to lead an active normal lifestyle.

Diagnostic Imaging[12,14,30]

Arteriography

Arteriography (i.e., angiography) is an invasive procedure that uses x-ray imaging and an injected contrast dye to visualize blood vessels (Fig. 8-32). This technique can visualize the major systemic arteries as well as the arterial systems that perfuse the major organs (e.g., brain, heart). A catheter is inserted into an artery, either at the groin or in the arm, and is guided up to the heart. The test can be used to identify arteriosclerosis, aneurysm, vascular malformations, tumors or blockages.

Advantages:

- useful in the diagnosis of vascular abnormalities

Disadvantages:

- invasive procedure
- contrast dye may cause an allergic reaction

Arthrography

Arthrography is an invasive procedure that uses x-ray imaging and an injected contrast dye to visualize joint structures. A long needle is used to inject the dye directly into the joint (i.e., direct arthrography). Alternatively, the dye can be injected into a blood vessel and then absorbed into the joint space (i.e., indirect arthrography). X-rays are then taken with the joint in different positions. Arthrography is useful in identifying pathology of joint structures (e.g., ligament damage, capsular tears). Soft tissue disruption can be identified by leakage of fluid from the joint cavity. The test is commonly used at peripheral joints such as the hip, knee, ankle, shoulder, elbow, and wrist. Arthrography is commonly used with x-ray imaging, though it can also be used with fluoroscopy, MRI, and CT imaging.

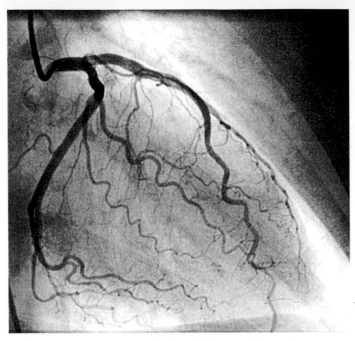

Fig. 8-32: Blood vessels as depicted using arteriography.

Advantages:

- provides a more detailed image of a joint compared to a standard x-ray

Disadvantages:

- invasive procedure
- contrast dye may cause an allergic reaction (especially with indirect arthrography)
- patient may experience joint swelling after the procedure
- not recommended for patients with active arthritis or joint infection

Bone scan

A bone scan (i.e., skeletal scintigraphy) is an invasive procedure used specifically to provide detailed information on bony structures, such as stress fractures, infection, and bone cancer or metastasis (Fig. 8-33). A bone scan involves the injection of a radionuclide into the body. The body is then scanned with a gamma camera to see which bones have taken up the radioactive material. The image produced during the scan shows areas that have high levels of bone remodeling since the radionuclide is taken up by the osteoblast cells within the bone. Bone scans can identify bone disease or stress fractures with as little as 4-7% bone loss.

Advantages:

- provides information on bone pathology that is not identified on x-ray
- low dose of radiation used
- less expensive than PET scans

Disadvantages:

- invasive procedure
- requires a 2-3 hour waiting period between injection and imaging
- patient must lie still for long periods of time
- radionuclide may cause an allergic reaction
- not recommended for patients who are pregnant

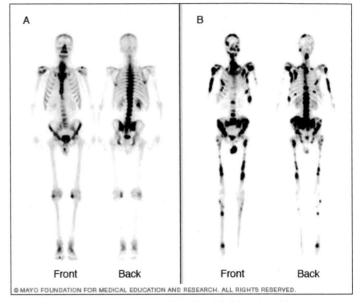

Fig. 8-33: Bone scan images depicting high levels of bone remodeling.

Computed tomography

Computed tomography (CT) is a non-invasive imaging procedure in which x-ray images are taken from multiple angles using a large circular scanner (Fig. 8-34). The images are then combined using computer analysis to produce cross-sectional images. Some types of CT scans use a contrast medium, which can be swallowed or injected, to improve the image quality. CT scans produce images of any structure within the body and therefore have a wide range of uses. CT scans are most commonly used to diagnose spinal lesions and in diagnostic studies of the brain.

Advantages:

- offers quick results and is useful in emergent situations
- generates images of multiple structures at the same time
- produces more detailed images than x-ray

Disadvantages:

- uses a higher dosage of radiation than other imaging techniques
- not recommended for patients who are pregnant
- contrast dye may cause an allergic reaction
- patient is in a small space and may become claustrophobic

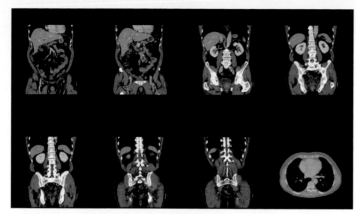

Fig. 8-34: Computed tomography image series.

Electrocardiography

Electrocardiography (ECG) is a procedure used to record the electrical activity of the heart. This form of diagnostic imaging is covered in detail in Chapter 6: Cardiovascular and Pulmonary Systems.

Electroencephalography

Electroencephalography (EEG) is a non-invasive procedure used to record the electrical activity of the brain. Several electrodes are placed on the scalp and are used to record the electrical impulses that result from brain activity. The electrical activity is recorded and displayed as characteristic waveforms on a monitor. Brain disorders, such as epilepsy or narcolepsy, can be diagnosed based on abnormalities in these waveforms. Evoked potential studies are a form of EEG in which brain activity is measured in response to various stimuli (e.g., light, sound).

Advantages:

- useful in diagnosing brain disorders by measuring electrical activity directly as opposed to measuring blood flow or metabolic activity
- noninvasive procedure
- detects changes over the course of milliseconds, as opposed to seconds or minutes with other imaging techniques (e.g., MRI)
- costs less than other imaging techniques

Disadvantages:

- less effective at providing information on exact location of the pathology compared to other imaging techniques (e.g., MRI)
- several factors can affect the accuracy of the results (e.g., medications, caffeine, hypoglycemia, hair products, small movements)
- in some patients with epilepsy, use of an evoked potential study may cause a seizure

Electromyography

Electromyography (EMG) is the recording of the electrical activity of a selected muscle or muscle groups at rest and during voluntary contraction. This form of diagnostic imaging is covered in detail in Chapter 8: Equipment, Devices, and Technologies; Therapeutic Modalities.

Fluoroscopy

Fluoroscopy is designed to show motion within the body with the use of x-ray imaging and injection of a contrast dye. The technique permits objects placed between a fluorescent screen and a roentgen tube to become visible. Instead of a single x-ray image being taken, the x-ray beam is passed through the body continuously to allow for the visualization of movement. Fluoroscopy can show motion within joints or movement of the dye within the digestive tract. A barium swallow exam is a specific type of fluoroscopy procedure used to assess the gastrointestinal tract. The procedure can also be used during the insertion of medical devices (e.g., pacemakers).

Advantages:

- can visualize movement within the body

Disadvantages:

- invasive procedure
- higher dose of radiation than x-rays
- not recommended for patients who are pregnant
- contrast dye may cause an allergic reaction

Lumbar puncture

Lumbar puncture is an invasive procedure that is used to diagnose problems with the spine or brain. The procedure is performed by inserting a needle into the subarachnoid space in the lumber spine and drawing cerebrospinal fluid (CSF) out to be tested. Lumbar puncture can be used to diagnose conditions such as encephalitis, meningitis, and Guillain-Barre syndrome. Lumbar puncture can also be used to measure the pressure of the CSF.

Advantages:

- useful in diagnosing a variety of brain and spinal cord pathologies

Disadvantages:

- invasive procedure
- should not be performed in the presence of increased intracranial pressure
- leakage of CSF can cause a headache
- small risk of bleeding occurring in epidural and subarachnoid spaces
- patient must remain inactive after the procedure

Magnetic resonance imaging

Magnetic resonance imaging (MRI) is a noninvasive procedure that utilizes magnetic fields and radio waves to produce cross-sectional images of the body (Figs. 8-35, 8-36). The MRI scanner is a large cylindrical device with a hollow tunnel in the center where the patient lies. MRI can be used to visualize almost any structure within the body, but is most often used for imaging soft tissue structures, such as muscles, menisci, ligaments, tumors, and internal organs. MRI provides excellent contrast detail, therefore contrast dyes rarely need to be used, though they may still be used in certain types of imaging to improve the image quality.

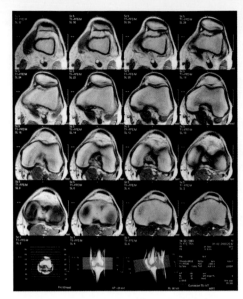

Fig. 8-35: Magnetic resonance imaging of the knee.

Advantages:

- useful in imaging a wide variety of structures, especially soft tissue structures
- noninvasive procedure
- does not use radiation
- safe for use on patients who are pregnant
- contrast dye used is unlikely to cause an allergic reaction

Disadvantages:

- cannot be used if there is metal in the body
- interferes with functioning of internal devices (e.g., pacemaker, cochlear implant)
- patient must lie still for long periods of time
- patient is in a small space and may become claustrophobic
- high cost compared to other tests

Myelography

Myelography is an invasive procedure that combines x-ray/fluoroscopy or computed tomography with use of a contrast dye to evaluate spinal structures, specifically the spinal cord, nerve roots, and meninges. The contrast dye is injected directly into the epidural space by lumbar puncture. Myelography is used to identify bone displacement, spinal stenosis, disk herniation, spinal cord compression, infection/inflammation of the meninges or tumors.

Advantages:

- provides better detail of spinal structures than x-ray
- provides imaging of spinal structures for those patients who cannot have MRI
- low dose of radiation

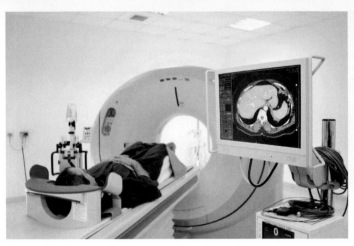

Fig. 8-36: A magnetic resonance imaging unit.

Disadvantages:

- invasive procedure
- contrast dye may cause an allergic reaction
- may cause headache if cerebrospinal fluid leaks out
- small risk of seizure since dye is injected into cerebrospinal fluid

Nerve conduction velocity test

A nerve conduction velocity (NCV) test is a procedure used to determine the extent of nerve damage by measuring the speed of an electrical impulse through the nerve. Two surface electrodes are attached on the skin over the course of the nerve. The first electrode stimulates the nerve while the second electrode measures the speed of the electrical impulse. NCV is often used in conjunction with electromyography testing. Performing both tests allows the health care practitioner to determine if the condition is related to nerve pathology or muscle pathology. NCV is helpful in the diagnosis of conditions such as Guillain-Barre syndrome, carpal tunnel syndrome, and peripheral neuropathy.

Advantages:

- effective at diagnosing nerve-related pathology
- noninvasive procedure
- offers quick results

Disadvantages:

- precautions need to be taken for patients with a pacemaker

Positron emission tomography

Positron emission tomography (PET) is an invasive procedure that uses radiography and an injected radionuclide to determine the metabolic activity of an organ or tissue. The radionuclide is attached to a substance that would be used by the organ of interest (e.g., attached to glucose when studying the brain). A scanner is used to determine the amount of radionuclide taken up by the organ, thereby determining how metabolically active the organ is. PET is commonly used in oncology to identify malignant tumors, though it is also used in the neurology (e.g., identifying brain diseases) and cardiology (e.g., identifying impaired blood flow) fields. PET has more recently been used in conjunction with CT scan to provide greater detail on tumors and other lesions.

Advantages:

- images the function of an organ as opposed to just its anatomy
- detects pathological changes at the cellular level
- identifies the onset of disease processes before other imaging techniques
- low dose of radiation

Disadvantages:

- invasive procedure
- radionuclide may cause an allergic reaction
- not recommended for patients who are pregnant
- results may be affected by high blood glucose levels, medications, caffeine, alcohol or tobacco
- patient must lie still for long periods of time
- patient is in a small space and may become claustrophobic

Ultrasound

Ultrasound is a noninvasive procedure that uses sound waves to produce images of structures within the body, especially the internal organs (e.g., liver, kidneys). A transducer is placed on the skin and sends sound waves into the body, where they reflect off the internal structures and are then received and processed by the transducer. This information is converted into an image based on the different speeds at which the sound waves travel. Ultrasound shows not only an image of a structure, but also the movement of that structure since it is performed in real time. Doppler ultrasound is a specific form of ultrasound that evaluates blood flow in the major veins, arteries, and cerebrovascular system. In comparison to a standard ultrasound, Doppler ultrasound can provide auditory output in addition to the visual projection.

Advantages:

- shows movement of internal structures in real time
- noninvasive procedure
- does not use radiation
- can be used on patients who are pregnant
- safer and less expensive than other procedures (e.g., arteriography)

Disadvantages:

- quality of images highly dependent on the skill of the operator
- cannot image structures filled with air (e.g., stomach, intestines) or structures behind bone (e.g., brain)
- not as effective for patients who are obese due to subcutaneous fat

Venography

Venography is an invasive procedure that uses x-ray imaging and an injected contrast dye to visualize the venous system. A catheter is inserted into a vein in the foot so that the contrast dye can be injected. This test is most often used for visualizing the veins in the leg, though it can also be used for the upper extremities or the inferior vena cava. Venography is helpful for diagnosing deep vein thrombosis, tumors, valve dysfunction or other pathology of the venous system.

Advantages:

- effective in visualizing the venous system
- low dose of radiation

Disadvantages:

- invasive procedure
- contrast dye may cause an allergic reaction

X-ray

X-ray is a radiographic image commonly used to assist with the diagnosis of issues related to the bones, such as fractures, dislocations, arthritis, and bone infections (Fig. 8-37). Chest x-rays may be performed to help diagnose lung conditions, such as pneumonia or chronic obstructive pulmonary disease. An x-ray uses radiation to penetrate the body and create a two-dimensional picture. Structures with low density (e.g., soft tissue structures) do not absorb x-rays as well and therefore do not show up on a radiograph. X-ray produces only two-dimensional images and as a result often requires images to be taken in multiple planes in order to visualize a lesion's location and size.

Advantages:

- useful in diagnosing bone and joint pathology
- noninvasive procedure
- low dose of radiation
- low cost and rapid results

Disadvantages:

- cannot image soft tissue structures
- not recommended for patients who are pregnant

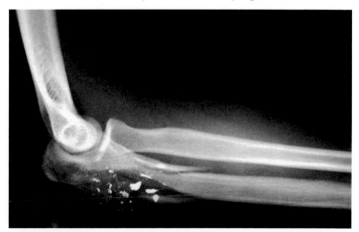

Fig. 8-37: An x-ray image depicting a comminuted fracture.

Therapeutic Modalities

Therapeutic modalities is a broad term describing a variety of agents used in the rehabilitation of patients. Therapeutic modalities include thermal agents (e.g., hot pack, ultrasound), mechanical agents (e.g., traction, compression), and electromagnetic agents (e.g., electrical stimulation, diathermy). In a rehabilitation program, therapeutic modalities are primarily used as adjuncts to other interventions, such as therapeutic exercise.

Indications for Therapeutic Modalities[16,17,18]

Inflammation and repair: Modalities can alter circulation, chemical reactions, flow of body fluids, and cell function throughout all phases of healing. Modalities can enhance and accelerate the healing process and reduce the risk of adverse effects associated with inflammation.

Pain: Modalities can assist with controlling pain by altering the origin of the pain or altering the process of pain perception.

Restriction in motion: Modalities are used to enhance extensibility of collagen to allow for greater range of motion and tolerance to stretch.

Abnormal tone: Modalities can influence tonal abnormalities that are due to pain, musculoskeletal pathology or neurological pathology. Alterations in nerve conduction, pain, and biomechanical properties of muscle can normalize tone and enhance functional outcomes.

Principles of Heat Transfer[16,18]

Therapeutic modalities result in the transfer of heat to or from a patient's body. Heating agents transfer heat to the body, while cooling agents transfer heat away from the body. Methods of heat transfer include conduction, convection, conversion, evaporation, and radiation.

Conduction

Conduction refers to the gain or loss of heat resulting from direct contact between two materials at different temperatures. Heat is conducted from a material of higher temperature to a material of lower temperature. Heat transfer continues until the temperature and speed of molecular movement of both materials become equal. The rate of heat transfer will accelerate when there is a large temperature difference between a heating or cooling agent and the body part being treated. Materials with high thermal conductivity transfer heat faster than those with low thermal conductivity. For example, water transfers heat faster than air since it possesses higher thermal conductivity. Metal has extremely high thermal conductivity, which is the rationale for removing all metal jewelry prior to initiating treatment with a conductive thermal agent.

Examples of modalities that utilize conduction include hot pack, cold pack, paraffin, ice massage, and Cryo Cuff.

Convection

Convection refers to the gain or loss of heat resulting from air or water moving in a constant motion across the body. Since the thermal agent is in motion and new parts of the agent are constantly coming into contact with the target area, heating by convection is capable of transferring large amounts of heat. For example, blood circulating in the body maintains body temperature by convection. As a result, when circulation is compromised, the relative risk of thermal injury significantly increases.

Examples of modalities that utilize convection include fluidotherapy, hot whirlpool, and cold whirlpool.

Conversion

Conversion refers to heating that occurs when nonthermal energy (e.g., mechanical, electrical) is absorbed into tissue and transformed into heat. The rate of heat transfer with conversion is determined by the power of the energy source. For example, the power of ultrasound would be determined by the selected intensity. Heating by conversion is not affected by the temperature of the thermal agent as it is with conduction and convection. Heat transfer does not require direct contact between the thermal agent and the target area, however, it does require a medium that allows transmission of the particular type of energy. In the case of ultrasound, the medium may be gel, lotion or water.

Examples of modalities that utilize conversion include diathermy and ultrasound.

Evaporation

Evaporation refers to the transfer of heat that occurs as a liquid absorbs energy and changes form into a vapor. In the case of a vapocoolant spray, the liquid spray is applied to a patient's body. The vapocoolant spray is then heated by the warmer skin of the body, causing the liquid to change into a vapor. The evaporation of sweat is another example of this cooling phenomenon.

An example of a modality that utilizes evaporation is vapocoolant spray.

Radiation

Radiation refers to the direct transfer of heat from a radiation energy source of higher temperature to one of cooler temperature. In order for heating by radiation to occur, there must be a difference in temperature between the energy source and the target area. This difference must exist without the energy source being in direct contact with the target area. The rate of heat transfer will be influenced by a number of factors including the intensity and size of the energy source, the target area, the angle of the radiation in relation to the target area, and the distance between the energy source and the target area.

Examples of modalities that utilize radiation include infrared lamp, laser, and ultraviolet light.

Examples of Heat Transfer by Category

Conduction	Convection	Conversion	Evaporation	Radiation
Cold pack	Cold whirlpool	Diathermy	Vapocoolant spray	Infrared lamp
Cryo Cuff	Fluidotherapy	Ultrasound		Laser
Ice massage	Hot whirlpool			Ultraviolet light
Hot pack				
Paraffin				

Cryotherapy

Cryotherapy refers to the local or general use of low temperatures in rehabilitation. Cryotherapy generates therapeutic effects by influencing hemodynamic (e.g., blood flow), metabolic (e.g., metabolic rate), and neuromuscular processes (e.g., nerve conduction velocity). Common examples of modalities used for cryotherapy include ice massage, cold pack, cold bath, controlled cold compression unit, Cryo Cuff, and vapocoolant spray. The type of cryotherapeutic agent selected is influenced by numerous variables including the size of the target area, anatomical location, desired magnitude of cooling, and the patient's medical history.

Therapeutic Effects[16,18]

- Decreased blood flow to the treatment area
- Decreased edema
- Decreased local temperature
- Decreased metabolic rate
- Decreased nerve conduction velocity
- Decreased tone
- Increased pain threshold

Indications[16,18]

- Abnormal tone
- Acute or chronic pain
- Acute or subacute inflammation
- Bursitis
- Muscle spasm
- Musculoskeletal trauma
- Myofascial trigger points
- Tendonitis
- Tenosynovitis

Contraindications[16,18]

- Cold intolerance
- Cold urticaria
- Cryoglobulinemia
- Infection
- Over an area of compromised circulation
- Over regenerating peripheral nerves
- Paroxysmal cold hemoglobinuria
- Peripheral vascular disease
- Raynaud's phenomenon
- Skin anesthesia

Ice Massage

Ice massage is typically performed by freezing water in a paper cup and then applying the ice directly to the treatment area. A wooden tongue depressor can be frozen in water to form an ice popsicle. Ice massage is ideal for small or contoured areas and is easily integrated into a home exercise program. In addition to the anti-inflammatory effects, ice massage can be used as a stimulus to facilitate a desired motor response in patients with impaired motor control. In this scenario, ice is applied with direct pressure over a muscle belly for 3-5 seconds or quickly stroked over the targeted muscle belly to enhance contraction.[16]

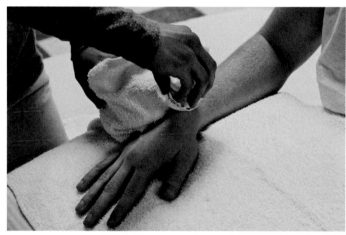

Fig. 8-38: Using a towel to absorb excess water during ice massage.

Ice massage should be applied with the patient in a relaxed and comfortable position. Clothing and jewelry should be removed from the treatment area. The top third of the paper cup should be removed leaving the base of the cup covered for the therapist or patient to grip. A towel should be used to absorb dripping water as melting occurs. Ideally, the body part to be treated should also be elevated (Fig. 8-38).

The ice should be applied using small, overlapping circles or strokes. An area 10 cm by 15 cm can be covered in 5-10 minutes (Fig. 8-39).[17] Patients will typically progress through a series of unique sensations during ice massage including Intense cold, burning, aching, and analgesia.[17] These sensations are thought to be caused by increased stimulation of thermal receptors and pain receptors, followed by blocking of sensory nerve conduction as the tissue temperature decreases.

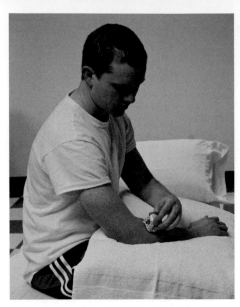

Fig. 8-39: Ice massage being self administered.

Ice massage should continue until the patient reports analgesia. The exact amount of time for analgesia to occur will depend largely on the size of the treatment area, however, 5-10 minutes is typically adequate.[17] Maintaining skin temperature above 59 degrees Fahrenheit will minimize the risk of damaging tissue or producing frostbite.[16]

Ice massage typically cools tissues more rapidly than other types of cryotherapy, including an ice pack or ice bag. The therapist should inspect the skin during treatment and after the completion of treatment. Normally, the skin should appear to be red or dark pink. An abnormal response is most often noted by the presence of wheals or a rash.[16]

Cold Pack

A cold pack typically contains silica gel and is available in a variety of shapes and sizes. The gel remains in a semisolid form even at relatively low temperatures, which allows the cold pack to conform to the contour of the body. Cold packs are typically stored in a

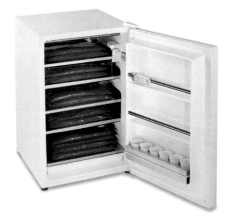

Fig. 8-40: A specialized cooling unit containing cold packs and cups for ice massage. Courtesy Chattanooga, a DJO Global Company.

specialized cooling unit at approximately 25 degrees Fahrenheit (Fig. 8-40).[17] Cold packs should be cooled for at least 30 minutes between uses and for two or more hours prior to the initial use.[17]

The therapist should thoroughly inspect the targeted area prior to initiating treatment. Clothing and jewelry should be removed from the treatment area. If edema is present, the involved extremity can be elevated. The cold pack should be applied over a moist, cold towel to increase the initial magnitude of cooling (Fig. 8-41). The moist towel increases the conduction by minimizing the influence of air, which is a poor conductor.[17] Warm water can be used to moisten the towel when using a cold pack on a patient who is sensitive to cold, since it allows for a more gradual onset of cold. The cold pack can be applied using an elastic wrap to increase the surface contact between the cold pack and the target area. The patient should be given a bell or another type of call device in the event they need assistance during treatment.

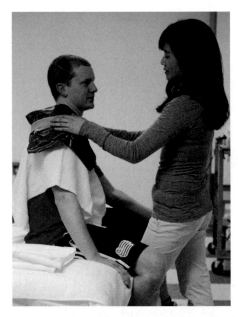

Fig. 8-41: Application of a cold pack to a patient's shoulder.

A cold pack should be applied for approximately 20 minutes.[18] Applying a cold pack for this duration reduces the temperature of the skin and subcutaneous tissues up to two centimeters in depth. Additional treatment time may be necessary when applying the cold pack over bandages or other types of wraps to allow the cold to adequately penetrate through the additional layers. The therapist should inspect the skin during and after the completion of treatment. Normally, the skin should appear red or dark pink. An abnormal response is most often noted by the presence of wheals or a rash.[16]

Cold packs can be applied every one to two hours for the reduction of inflammation and pain control. Patients can use a variety of substitute cryotherapeutic agents at home, such as a bag of frozen vegetables or a plastic bag filled with crushed ice.

Application may extend to 30 minutes if the treatment goal is spasticity reduction.[17] In this scenario, the skin would require inspection every ten minutes. Treatment beyond 20 minutes may require replacing the original cold pack.

Cold Bath

A cold bath is commonly used for the immersion of the distal extremities. Unlike many other forms of cryotherapy, a cold bath allows for circumferential contact with the cooling agent. In the presence of edema, therapists should be mindful of the influence of a gravity-dependent position on the involved extremity during treatment.

A cold bath requires water temperature ranging from 55-64 degrees Fahrenheit.[19] A whirlpool or container of water with crushed ice can be used (Fig. 8-42). The body part should be immersed for 15-20 minutes to attain the desired therapeutic effects.[19] The lower the temperature selected, the shorter the duration of treatment. The intervention is often used as a component of a home exercise program.

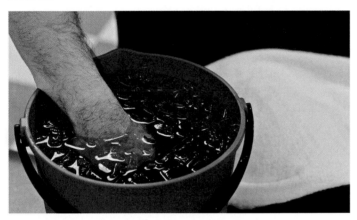

Fig. 8-42: Immersion of a hand in a cold bath.

Controlled Cold Compression Unit

A controlled cold compression unit circulates cooled water through a sleeve that is applied to an extremity. The water can be maintained at temperatures ranging from 50-77 degrees Fahrenheit.[19] Compression is applied intermittently by inflating the sleeve with air with the goal of controlling inflammation and reducing edema in the extremity. In post-operative situations, the sleeve may be placed on the patient's involved extremity immediately after surgery. The combined use of cold and compression is more effective than cold or compression alone in controlling inflammation.[18]

Cryo Cuff

A Cryo Cuff is a cold water circulating unit that combines the benefits of cold with compression. The Cryo Cuff consists of a nylon sleeve that is connected to a specialized gallon container via a plastic tube. Water from the container flows via gravity into the sleeve when the gallon container is elevated approximately 15-18 inches above the level of the sleeve (Fig. 8-43). This action provides cooling from the cold water and compression from the increased pressure in the sleeve. The water is drained from the sleeve via gravity by placing the container below the level of the sleeve (Fig. 8-44). The water in the container must be recooled periodically in order to maintain the desired therapeutic temperature.

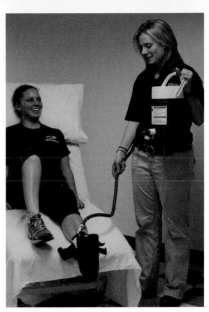

Fig. 8-43: Filling an ankle Cryo Cuff.

The device can provide hours of mild cooling at levels far below the intensity of other cryotherapeutic agents, such as ice massage or cold packs.[20] The Cryo Cuff is most commonly used on the knee, however, it is available for a number of other areas of the body including the shoulder and the ankle. The device is commonly employed post-operatively with the goal of decreasing pain and the need for analgesic medications.

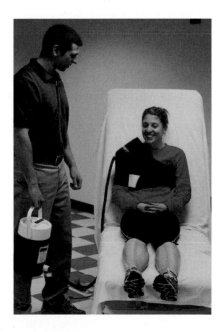

Fig. 8-44: Draining water from a shoulder Cryo Cuff.

CONSIDER THIS
CRYOTHERAPY AGENTS - ADVANTAGES AND DISADVANTAGES[16,17,18]

There are a variety of cryotherapy agents that provide similar therapeutic effects. Therapists should consider the nuances associated with the patient's current condition, as well as the advantages and disadvantages of each cryotherapy agent, when selecting an appropriate mode of intervention.

The following table illustrates several advantages and disadvantages of commonly used cryotherapy agents.

Cryotherapy Agent	Advantages	Disadvantages
Ice massage	Effective for small or irregular areas Target area can be observed during treatment Short duration of treatment Available for home use	Intensity of cooling may not be tolerated by the patient Time consuming for large areas Requires active participation from the therapist or patient
Cold pack	Covers moderate to large areas Can be applied in conjunction with elevation Available for home use	May not maintain good contact on small or severely contoured areas Patient may not tolerate the weight of the pack Difficult to observe target area directly during treatment
Cold bath	Effective for cooling the distal extremities Allows for circumferential contact with water Available for home use	Requires the extremity to remain in a gravity-dependent position
Controlled cold compression unit	Allows simultaneous application of cold and compression Temperature and compression force can be accurately controlled Can be combined with other interventions, such as electrotherapy	Difficult to observe target area directly during treatment Limited to extremity use
Cryo Cuff	Allows simultaneous application of cold and compression Provides hours of mild cooling Available for home use	Difficult to precisely control temperature and compression force
Vapocoolant spray	Localized area of application Brief duration of cooling Effectively treats trigger points Increases range of motion	Difficult to apply spray uniformly Risk of frostbite if skin is not rewarmed between repeated treatments Limited in scope of use

Vapocoolant Spray[16,18,20]

A vapocoolant spray produces rapid cooling through evaporation, with temperature changes occurring superficially in the epidermis. This therapeutic modality is most commonly used in the treatment of trigger points, which are described as deep and hypersensitive, localized spots in a muscle that cause a referred pain pattern. Vapocoolant sprays produce a counter-irritant stimulus to the cutaneous thermal afferent nerves that overlay the muscles. This causes a reduction in motor neuron activity and a decrease in the resistance to stretch. This may break the pain cycle and allow the muscle to be stretched to its normal length.

The use of vapocoolant spray to treat trigger points is often termed "spray and stretch" based on the work of Janet Travell. When using spray and stretch, therapists should identify the trigger point and make three to four sweeps with the spray in the direction of the muscle fibers. The spray must be applied in one direction only and not in a back and forth motion. Special care must be taken to cover the patient's eyes, nose, and mouth if spraying near the face. The spray should be applied at a 30 degree angle at a distance of 12-18 inches from the skin.

Stretching should begin while applying the spray and continue after the spray has been applied (Fig. 8-45).[18] Repeated applications during the same treatment are safe if the skin is rewarmed between applications.

When using vapocoolant sprays to increase range of motion without the presence of trigger points, the spray is applied along the muscle from the proximal to the distal attachment. Clinical conditions that may respond to treatment with vapocoolant sprays include torticollis, neck or low back pain caused by muscle spasm, acute bursitis, and hamstrings tightness.

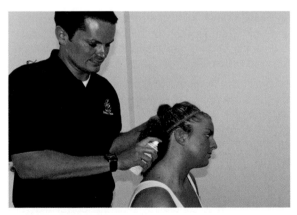

Fig. 8-45: Vapocoolant spray applied to the right upper quadrant.

Superficial Thermotherapy

Superficial thermotherapy refers to the local or general use of high temperatures in rehabilitation with the goal of increasing skin temperature and superficial subcutaneous tissue to depths of up to two centimeters. Superficial thermotherapy generates therapeutic effects by influencing hemodynamic (e.g., blood flow), metabolic (e.g., metabolic rate), and neuromuscular processes (e.g., nerve conduction velocity). Common examples of modalities used for superficial thermotherapy include hot packs, warm water baths, fluidotherapy, infrared lamp, and paraffin. Relative changes in skin temperature and superficial subcutaneous tissue will be influenced by the intensity of the heating agent, duration of the exposure, and thermal conductivity of the tissues.

Therapeutic Effects[16,18]	
• Decreased muscle spasm • Decreased tone • Increased blood flow to the treatment area • Increased capillary permeability • Increased collagen extensibility	• Increased local temperature • Increased metabolic rate • Increased muscle elasticity • Increased nerve conduction velocity • Increased pain threshold
Indications[16,18]	
• Abnormal tone • Decreased range of motion • Muscle guarding • Muscle spasm	• Myofascial trigger points • Subacute or chronic pain • Subacute or chronic inflammatory conditions
Contraindications[16,18]	
• Acute musculoskeletal trauma • Arterial disease • Bleeding or hemorrhage • Over an area of compromised circulation	• Over an area of malignancy • Peripheral vascular disease • Thrombophlebitis

Hot Packs

A hot pack consists of a canvas or nylon-covered pack filled with bentonite, a hydrophilic silicate gel that provides a moist heat. The size and shape of the hot pack varies depending on the size and contour of the treatment area. A standard size hot pack measures 12 inches by 12 inches and is used for the majority of body segments. A double size hot pack measures 24 inches by 24 inches and is generally used for the low back or buttocks. A cervical hot pack measures 6 inches by 18 inches.

Hot packs transmit heat to the body through conduction, since hot packs have a much higher temperature than the surface of the skin. The primary therapeutic effects include decreased pain, increased tissue extensibility, and reduced muscle spasm. A hot pack is easy to use, inexpensive, and can cover large areas. Limitations of hot packs include the need for close monitoring of the skin, the inability to maintain total contact in contoured areas, and the patient's inability to move during treatment.

Hot packs are stored in water between 158 and 167 degrees Fahrenheit.[16] The water is housed in a thermostatically controlled container that maintains the water at a relatively constant

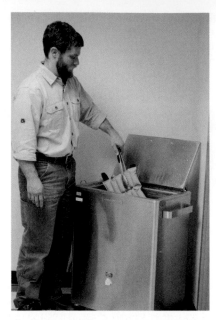

Fig. 8-46: Hot pack removal from a hydrocollator unit using tongs.

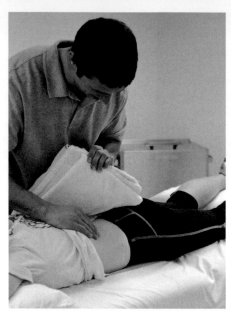

Fig. 8-47: Skin checks should be performed frequently when using hot packs.

temperature. The hot pack should be removed from the container with tongs due to the high water temperature (Fig. 8-46). The therapist should thoroughly inspect the target area prior to initiating treatment. Clothing and jewelry should be removed from the target area. Application requires six to eight layers of towels between the hot pack and skin.[16] If commercial hot pack covers are used, they typically are equivalent to two to three layers of towels.

The hot pack should be applied on top of the treatment area. The therapist should not permit the patient to lie on top of the hot pack since this action tends to remove some of the water from the hot pack, which can result in an accelerated rate of heating and an increased risk for burns. In addition, lying directly on the hot pack can reduce local circulation through compression of vessels resulting in reduced circulatory convective cooling.[17] If a patient cannot tolerate the weight of the hot pack directly on the target area (e.g., the low back while positioned in prone), the hot pack can be applied in sidelying with a strap or tied sheet.

The patient should feel a mild to moderate heating sensation from the hot pack.[17] Skin checks for excessive redness, blistering or other signs of a burn are required after five minutes (Fig. 8-47). The treatment area of fair-skinned individuals may turn bright pink or red, while darker-skinned individuals may exhibit areas of lighter or darker color. The maximum surface temperature is reached within 6-8 minutes, making it critical to perform frequent skin checks during the first 10 minutes of treatment.[17] The patient should be given a bell or another type of call device in the event that they need assistance during treatment.

Hot packs require approximately 15-20 minutes to achieve the desired effects.[18] If a patient reports that the heat is too intense, the therapist may elect to add towel layers. If the patient reports insufficient warming, the therapist may elect to remove towels prior to administering a hot pack at the next treatment session. Towels should not be removed during the current session since

the increased skin temperature may diminish the patient's thermal sensitivity and the ability to accurately assess the intensity of the heat. A hot pack can take up to two hours to initially heat in the hydrocollator unit and 30 minutes to reheat after use.

Fluidotherapy

Fluidotherapy consists of a container that circulates warm air and small cellulose particles (Fig. 8-48). The superficial heating modality generates dry heat through forced convection. The dry cellulose medium does not irritate the skin and allows for higher treatment temperatures than hydrotherapy. Fluidotherapy units come in a variety of sizes and shapes and are most often used to treat the distal extremities.

The therapist must thoroughly inspect the area to be treated and have the patient remove all clothing and jewelry. The extremity is placed into the container and a protective shield is applied to prevent the escape of the cellulose particles. Direct contact between the skin and the cellulose particles is desired since this will maximize heat transfer. Open wounds should be covered with a plastic barrier to prevent the cellulose particles from becoming embedded in the wound bed.

The fluidotherapy unit contains a separate portal that provides the therapist with access to the extremity during treatment. The temperature should be set between 100-118 degrees Fahrenheit.[16] The maximum temperature rise during treatment occurs after approximately 15 minutes. Treatment time is usually 15-20 minutes.[18] The level of agitation (i.e., air speed) can be controlled for patient comfort or for use as part of a desensitization program. Some units provide other treatment options including the ability to preheat or select a pulse mode. The therapeutic effects of fluidotherapy include the promotion of tissue healing, skin desensitization, and edema management.

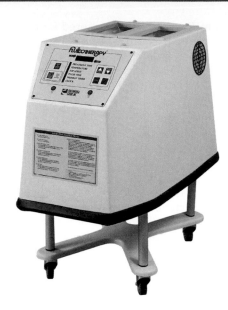

Fig. 8-48: A fluidotherapy unit. Courtesy Chattanooga, a DJO Global Company.

Heated air is circulated in the unit causing cellulose particles to become suspended and move rapidly within the unit. The result is a fluidized bed of cellulose particles that take on the properties of a liquid. Patients often report that the body part feels like it is suspended in a moving liquid. Patients can perform active exercise of the distal extremity during treatment, however, therapists should avoid placing the extremity in a gravity-dependent position whenever possible.[19]

Infrared Lamp

An infrared lamp produces superficial heating of tissue through radiant heat. Infrared radiation has a wavelength that lies between visible light and microwaves on the electromagnetic spectrum. Infrared lamps used in the clinical setting have a wavelength ranging from 780 to 1500 nanometers.[16] The majority of infrared radiation is absorbed within the first few millimeters of human tissue. Human skin allows maximum penetration of infrared radiation with a wavelength of 1200 nm.[16]

Infrared allows for constant observation of the skin since it does not require contact with the treatment area. The main therapeutic effect is the enhancement of soft tissue healing. The amount of tissue temperature increase is directly proportional to the amount of radiation that penetrates the tissue. The amount of radiation is influenced by the power and wavelength of the radiation, the distance of the radiation source from the target area, the angle of incidence, and the absorption coefficient of the target area.[16]

The therapist must thoroughly inspect the area to be treated and have the patient remove all clothing and jewelry. Opaque goggles should be worn by the therapist and the patient to avoid potential irradiation of the eyes. The patient should be positioned approximately 20 inches from the source to produce a comfortable level of warmth.[18] Protective toweling should be applied to tissues outside of the target area. Optimal absorption occurs when the infrared radiation strikes perpendicular to the target area. Darker tissue absorbs more radiation than lighter tissue.

The therapist should record the distance from the infrared lamp to the target area. The patient should be periodically monitored during the session and instructed to avoid moving closer or further away from the lamp since this will alter the amount of radiation reaching the target area. Treatment duration is generally 15-30 minutes and is influenced by the distance from the infrared lamp to the target area.[16] Infrared radiation tends to dry the skin more than other superficial heating agents and results in uneven heating when the target area is nonuniform.

Paraffin

Paraffin wax is a commonly used heating source for the distal extremities. There are several internal characteristics of paraffin that make it an effective superficial heating agent. Paraffin has a low melting point that can be lowered further by adding mineral oil. As a result, paraffin can provide a more even distribution of heat to areas, such as the fingers and toes. Secondly, paraffin has a low specific heat, that enhances a patient's ability to tolerate heat from paraffin compared to heat from water at the same temperature.

Therapists must have patients remove jewelry and thoroughly wash the body part being treated to minimize the chance of paraffin bath contamination. Paraffin cannot be applied to areas with open wounds or infected skin lesions. The temperature of the paraffin mixture should be maintained between 113 and 122 degrees Fahrenheit.[16]

There are three methods of paraffin application: dip-wrap, dip-reimmersion, and paint application.

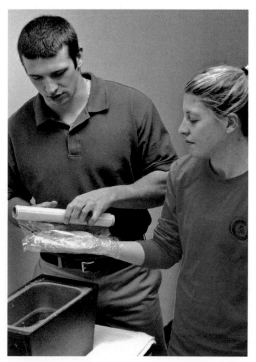

Fig. 8-49: Application of a plastic wrap to the hand following paraffin application.

Dip-wrap: The patient is required to maintain a static position as the distal extremity dips into the paraffin bath and is removed. After waiting briefly for the paraffin to harden, the extremity should be redipped 6-10 times and then immediately placed into a plastic bag (Fig. 8-49).[16] A towel should be wrapped around the bag to slow the paraffin cooling. The paraffin should be left in place for 10-15 minutes.[16]

Dip-reimmersion: After the initial 6-10 dips, the distal extremity should remain in the paraffin bath for the duration of treatment. The paraffin unit should be turned off during the treatment session to prevent the sides and the bottom of the unit from becoming too hot. It may also be necessary to use a temperature closer to the lower limit (i.e., 113 degrees Fahrenheit) since the affected extremity will remain in the bath for up to 20 minutes.[16]

Paint application: The paint method is used for body parts that cannot be immersed into the paraffin bath. A layer of paraffin is painted on the body with a brush. After a few seconds, 6-10 additional layers are applied. The area is then covered by a plastic bag or plastic wrap with a towel wrapped around it as described in the dip-wrap method. The paraffin should be left in place for approximately 20 minutes.[16]

Removal of the paraffin is the same for all forms of application. Paraffin should be peeled off after treatment and either placed back into the container to melt or discarded.[18] A paraffin bath can be reused unless it becomes contaminated. Some paraffin units have the ability to elevate the temperature to 212 degrees Fahrenheit, which will destroy bacteria that can grow in the paraffin.[18] In the absence of contamination, the contents of the paraffin bath must be changed at least every six months.

CONSIDER THIS
DOCUMENTATION OF THERAPEUTIC MODALITIES

The primary purpose of physical therapy patient care documentation is to communicate relevant information to other health care providers who are concurrently treating the same patient. The failure to document relevant patient care information in a clear, objective, and timely manner can result in professional negligence.

Documentation of therapeutic modalities must provide other health care providers with a clear understanding of the intervention performed and the associated parameters used. Appropriate documentation will allow another therapist treating the same patient to perform the identical intervention.

Relevant information when documenting therapeutic modalities includes:

- Body part to be treated (e.g., knee, anterior thigh, low back)
- Modality used (e.g., ultrasound, TENS)
- Treatment duration (e.g., 10 minutes, 20 minutes)
- Parameters (e.g., intensity, duty cycle, pulse rate)
- Patient response to treatment (e.g., skin color, pain level, sensitivity)
- Outcome measure (e.g., goniometry, circumferential measurements, visual analogue pain scale)

The following is an example of a documented ultrasound treatment in S.O.A.P. note format. Abbreviations were not used in the S.O.A.P. note below to increase clarity.

S: Patient reports the absence of knee pain during a recent exercise session.

O: Ultrasound to the anterior midline of the knee over the peri-patellar tendon region at 0.5 W/cm2, pulsed 20% duty cycle, 7 minutes.

A: Patient tolerated treatment without adverse effects.

P: Continue ultrasound treatment as described for three additional sessions. Continue to increase the intensity of exercise activities.

Deep Thermotherapy

Deep thermotherapy refers to the local or general use of energy (i.e., sound, electromagnetic) in rehabilitation with the goal of increasing tissue temperature.[16,18] Deep heating agents are capable of heating to depths of three to five centimeters.[21] Deep thermotherapy generates therapeutic effects by influencing mechanical (e.g., microstreaming), muscular (e.g., muscle heating), connective tissue (e.g., tendon, ligament), hemodynamic (e.g., blood flow), metabolic (e.g., metabolic rate), and neuromuscular processes (e.g., nerve conduction velocity).[16,18] Common examples of modalities used for deep thermotherapy include ultrasound and diathermy.

Relative changes in tissue temperature will be influenced by the intensity of the heating agent, the duration of the exposure, and the thermal conductivity of the tissues.

Ultrasound

Ultrasound is a common deep heating agent that transfers heat through conversion and elevates tissue temperature to depths up to five centimeters (Fig. 8-50). The modality uses high frequency acoustic mechanical vibrations to produce thermal and nonthermal effects. Ultrasound has a frequency above 20,000 hertz (Hz).[16] Therapeutic ultrasound typically has a frequency between 0.75 and 3 megahertz (MHz).[18]

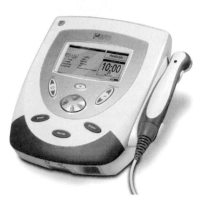

Fig. 8-50: An ultrasound machine. Courtesy Chattanooga, a DJO Global Company.

An ultrasound machine uses an alternating electrical current, generated at the same frequency as the crystal resonance, to create a mechanical vibration of the piezoelectric crystal located in the transducer. This action converts electrical energy to acoustic energy and generates ultrasound at the desired frequency.

Thermal effects[16,18]

Thermal effects of ultrasound include acceleration of metabolic rate, modulation of pain, reduction of muscle spasm, decreased joint stiffness, alteration of nerve conduction velocity, increased circulation, and increased soft tissue extensibility. The extent of the thermal effects is dependent on the intensity, duration, and frequency selected.

Nonthermal effects[16,18]

Nonthermal effects of ultrasound include increased cell and skin membrane permeability, increased intracellular calcium levels, facilitation of tissue repair, and promotion of normal cell function. The nonthermal effects occur as a result of cavitation and acoustic microstreaming.

Indications[16,18]

• Acute and post-acute conditions (ultrasound with nonthermal effects)	• Dermal ulcers
	• Joint contracture
• Calcium deposits	• Muscle spasm
• Chronic inflammation	• Myofascial trigger points
• Delayed soft tissue healing	• Pain
	• Plantar warts
	• Scar tissue
	• Tissue regeneration

Contraindications[16,18]

• Acute and post-acute conditions (ultrasound with thermal effects)	• Over epiphyseal areas in young children
• Areas of active bleeding	• Over eyes, heart, and genitalia
• Areas of decreased temperature sensation	• Over methyl methacrylate cement or plastic
• Areas of decreased circulation	• Over pelvic, lumbar or abdominal areas in pregnant women
• Deep vein thrombosis	• Over a pacemaker
• Infection	• Thrombophlebitis
• Malignancy	• Vascular insufficiency
• Over breast implants	
• Over carotid sinus or cervical ganglia	

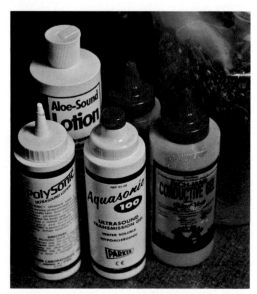

Fig. 8-51: Coupling agents used with ultrasound.

Cavitation refers to the formation of gas-filled bubbles that expand and compress secondary to pressure changes caused by ultrasound.[18] Cavitation can be classified as stable or unstable. During stable cavitation, the bubbles oscillate in size in response to pressure changes, but do not burst. During unstable cavitation, the bubbles change in size over several cycles and then suddenly burst. Unstable cavitation is possible with high intensity, low frequency ultrasound, however, it does not typically occur with therapeutic ultrasound. Acoustic microstreaming refers to the unidirectional movement of fluids along the boundaries of cell membranes caused by ultrasound.[18]

Ultrasound Parameters

Technique

A transducer housing a piezoelectric crystal is used to administer ultrasound. Transducers vary in size, but most often range from 5-10 cm². Ultrasound waves do not travel through air and, as a result, a coupling agent is required. Coupling agents are designed to decrease acoustical impedance by eliminating as much air as possible between the transducer and the target area. Coupling agents can be direct or indirect and include gels, gel pads, mineral oil, water, and lotions (Fig. 8-51).

Direct coupling agents (e.g., gel, lotion) should be applied to the treatment area and the transducer before the power is turned on. The face of the transducer must be parallel with the surface of the skin so that ultrasound waves will be introduced at a 90 degree angle.[18] Failure to maintain the integrity of the transducer-skin interface will result in a large percentage of the ultrasound energy being reflected and may damage the ultrasound's piezoelectric crystal.

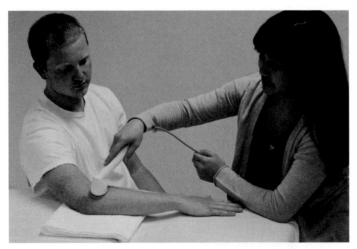

Fig. 8-52: Ultrasound applied to the dorsal surface of the forearm.

Indirect coupling agents are often employed when the treatment area is excessively small, irregularly shaped or unable to tolerate direct pressure from the transducer. Water immersion is an indirect coupling method requiring the treatment area to be immersed in a basin of water (Fig. 8-54). The basin should be made of rubber or plastic to minimize the amount of reflection present with metals. The transducer should be moved parallel to the treatment surface at a distance of 0.5 - 3.0 centimeters away from the skin.[21] Air bubbles occurring on the transducer and the patient's skin should be wiped away by the therapist since they will interfere with

ultrasound transmission.[17] Increased intensity, as much as 50%, may be necessary when using the underwater technique due to dispersion and ultrasound energy absorption by the water. Other methods of indirect coupling include gel or water-filled bladders and gel pads. This type of indirect coupling is often referred to as "cushion contact."

Administration of ultrasound can occur with a stationary or moving (i.e., dynamic) technique (Fig. 8-52). The stationary technique is used sparingly in clinical practice due to the potential for uneven heating and other undesirable effects, such as subjective reports of pain or tissue damage. Justification for use of the stationary technique may include a very small treatment area or when pulsed ultrasound is used with low intensity. When using a moving technique the transducer should be moved slowly in a small, rhythmical pattern. Longitudinal stroking or overlapping circular motions are the most common application method (Fig. 8-53). The transducer should be moved at an approximate rate of 4 centimeters per second.[16]

Intensity

Intensity measures the quantity of energy delivered per unit area. The power generated from ultrasound is not uniform and therefore, some portions of the ultrasound beam are more intense than others as it leaves the transducer. Effective radiating area (ERA) refers to the area of the transducer that transmits ultrasound energy.[16] The ERA is always smaller than the total size of the transducer head. Spatial-averaged intensity refers to the intensity of the ultrasound beam averaged over the area of the transducer.[18] It is computed by dividing the power output in watts by the total effective radiating area of the soundhead in cm². Spatial-averaged intensity is labeled as intensity on an ultrasound unit and is expressed in watts per square centimeter (W/cm²). Spatial-peak intensity refers to the intensity of the ultrasound beam at its highest point.[18]

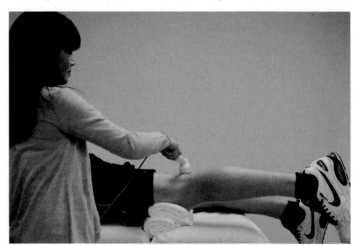

Fig. 8-53: Ultrasound applied to the posterior knee region combined with gravity assisted passive stretching.

Beam nonuniformity ratio (BNR) is the ratio between the spatial-peak intensity and spatial-averaged intensity. The BNR is derived from the intrinsic factors and quality of the piezoelectric crystal. The higher the quality of the crystal, the lower the BNR. A lower BNR is more favorable since patients will be less likely to experience hot spots and discomfort during treatment.[20] The BNR of an ultrasound unit is required to be listed on the device for consumer education and awareness. BNR values should range between 2:1 and 8:1, however, most devices often fall in the 5:1 or 6:1 range.[21] The higher the beam nonuniformity ratio, the more critical it is to move the transducer more rapidly to avoid undesirable effects, such as pain, caused by periosteal irritation.[16]

Frequency

Frequency is the primary determinant in the depth of ultrasound penetration. Attenuation is a term that describes the inevitable decrease in energy intensity as the ultrasound travels through various tissues. Tissues that are high in water content, such as blood plasma, have a low rate of absorption while more dense tissues high in protein, such as bone, have a high rate of absorption.[18]

Ultrasound delivered at a higher frequency is absorbed more rapidly than ultrasound delivered at a lower frequency. As a result, ultrasound at higher frequencies affects more superficial tissues and ultrasound at lower frequencies affects deeper tissues. A frequency setting of 1 MHz is used for deeper tissues (up to five centimeters) while a setting of 3 MHz is used for more superficial tissues (one to two centimeters).[18]

Duty Cycle

Ultrasound can be administered using a continuous or pulsed mode. In continuous mode, ultrasound intensity remains constant throughout the treatment. In pulsed mode, the ultrasound intensity is periodically interrupted. The portion of treatment time that ultrasound is generated during the entire treatment is referred to as the duty cycle.

$$\text{Duty cycle} \ = \ \frac{\text{on time}}{\text{on time} + \text{off time}} \quad (*100)$$

Duty cycle is calculated by dividing the time sound is delivered (on time) by the total time (on time + off time).[17] For example, if the on time was 1 msec and the off time was 4 msec, the duty cycle would be 20%.

Continuous ultrasound (i.e., 100% duty cycle) generates constant ultrasound waves producing thermal effects at higher intensities and nonthermal effects at lower intensities. Continuous ultrasound is more effective in elevating tissue temperature, while pulsed ultrasound minimizes the thermal effects.

Pulsed ultrasound with a duty cycle of 20% generates ultrasound 20% of the total treatment time (on time + off time). Pulsed ultrasound results in a reduced average heating of the tissues and is therefore used primarily for nonthermal effects. When using pulsed ultrasound for nonthermal effects, most resources recommend a 20% or lower duty cycle.

The duty cycle impacts the total quantity of energy generated. Ultrasound using a pulsed mode requires an intensity measure that takes the duty cycle into consideration. Spatial-temporal averaged intensity refers to the ultrasound beam averaged over the on time and off time of the pulse.[16] This measure allows therapists to compare energy outputs between continuous and pulsed ultrasound, however, it is not frequently used in clinical practice. Instead, therapists often describe the intensity based on the spatial-averaged intensity and then specify a duty cycle.

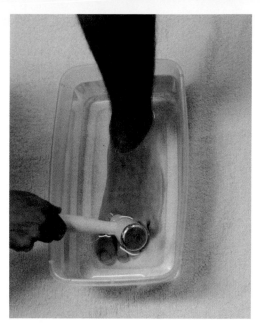

Fig. 8-54: Ultrasound applied to the dorsal surface of the foot using water immersion.

Duration

Duration of ultrasound is determined based on a number of variables including the size of the treatment area, the depth of penetration, and the desired therapeutic effects. An area two to three times the size of the transducer typically requires a duration of five minutes.[17,18] Longer duration may be necessary when using lower intensities or lower frequencies or when the therapeutic objective is higher tissue temperatures. Ultrasound should not be used to treat areas larger than four times the effective radiating area (ERA) of the transducer. Areas larger than this would require excessively long treatment times making the application of ultrasound impractical.

Number of Treatments

The number of ultrasound treatments is primarily dependent on the established therapeutic objectives, the level of acuity, and the patient response. Ultrasound using thermal effects is usually applied later in the healing process and is most commonly administered two to three times a week. Ultrasound using nonthermal effects is usually applied earlier in the healing process, as frequently as once a day. A positive response to ultrasound should be evident within three sessions. Failure to observe a desired response within this time frame provides justification to change the ultrasound parameters or select an alternate intervention. Research has indicated that more than 14 ultrasound treatments within a single episode of care can reduce red and white blood cell counts.[18]

Patient Safety and Effectiveness

Safe and effective ultrasound treatment is dependent on the therapist's ability to identify relevant contraindications to ultrasound and select appropriate treatment parameters. The therapist must comfortably position the patient and seek feedback from the patient throughout the course of treatment. The therapist should periodically inspect the patient's skin during treatment and attempt to determine the relative effect of the intervention. The effectiveness of ultrasound can be assessed through a variety of subjective and objective measures. Examples of positive findings include decreased pain, diminished tenderness to palpation, increased range of motion, and enhanced functional levels.

Ultrasound units must be inspected by qualified personnel at the manufacturer's recommended interval or minimally on an annual basis. Many of the parameters, including intensity output, must conform to established performance standards.

Phonophoresis

Phonophoresis describes the use of ultrasound for the transdermal delivery of medication. Ultrasound enhances the distribution of medication through the skin, provides a high concentration of the drug directly to the treatment site, and avoids risks that may be associated with the injection of medication.[18] Medications regularly used in phonophoresis include anti-inflammatory agents and analgesics. Phonophoresis can be used with both continuous and pulsed techniques. Phonophoresis is not likely to produce burns or damage skin since the technique transports whole molecules instead of ions into the body's tissue (i.e., iontophoresis). Therapists using phonophoresis must carefully select coupling agents that are effective conductors of acoustic energy and are compatible with the medication selected. There is a limited amount of evidence in the literature that supports the efficacy of phonophoresis.

Diathermy

Diathermy is a deep heating agent that converts high frequency electromagnetic energy into therapeutic heat (Fig. 8-55). Electrical energy produces a molecular vibration within tissue that generates heat and elevates tissue temperature.

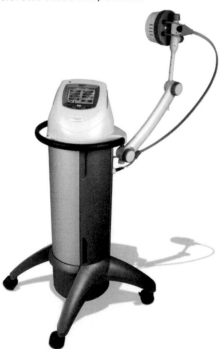

Fig. 8-55: A diathermy unit. Courtesy Chattanooga, a DJO Global Company.

Therapeutic Effects[16,18]

• Altered cell membrane function	• Increased muscle elasticity
• Increased collagen extensibility	• Increased nerve conduction velocity
• Increased edema	• Increased pain threshold
• Increased metabolic rate	• Increased temperature
	• Vasodilation

Indications[16,18]

• Bursitis	• Joint stiffness
• Chronic inflammation	• Muscle guarding
• Chronic inflammatory pelvic disease	• Myofascial trigger points
• Decreased collagen extensibility	• Pain
• Degenerative joint disease	• Peripheral nerve regeneration
• Increased metabolism	• Tissue healing

Contraindications[16,18]

• Acute infection	• Malignant area
• Acute inflammation	• Moist wound dressing
• Cardiac pacemaker	• Over a hemorrhagic region
• Hemophilia	• Over the eyes
• Internal and external metal objects	• Over the testes
• Intrauterine device	• Pain and temperature sensory deficits
• Ischemic tissue	
• Low back, abdomen or pelvis of a pregnant woman	

Shortwave diathermy can be delivered in a continuous or pulsed mode. A pulsed mode is typically utilized to attain nonthermal effects while a continuous mode is used for thermal effects. Pulsed diathermy is produced by discontinuing the output of continuous shortwave diathermy at regular intervals. The output during the on time is adequate to produce tissue heating, however, the length of the off time allows the heat to dissipate.

The most common frequency used for shortwave diathermy is 27.12 MHz.[17] Shortwave diathermy can utilize a capacitance technique or inductance technique. Capacitive plate applicators produce a high frequency electrical current that alternates between the plates. The patient becomes part of the electrical circuit and the oscillation of ions increases tissue temperature.

Inductive coil applicators utilize a coil that generates alternating electric current, creates a magnetic field perpendicular to the coil, and produces eddy currents within the tissues. Eddy currents cause the oscillation of ions that increase tissue temperature. Inductive coil applicators are bundled as cables that wrap around an extremity or as a drum applicator.

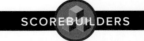

CONSIDER THIS
HEATING AGENTS - ADVANTAGES AND DISADVANTAGES[16,17,18]

Therapists should consider the nuances associated with the patient's current condition and the advantages and disadvantages of each heating agent when selecting an appropriate intervention.

The following table illustrates several advantages and disadvantages of commonly used heating agents.

Heating Agent	Advantages	Disadvantages
Fluidotherapy	Temperature and agitation of the dry particles can be controlled Patient can perform active exercise during treatment Minimal pressure applied to the treatment area Can be used for desensitization of distal extremities	Constant heat source can result in overheating Some patients are intolerant of the dry particles and the enclosed container Some units require the extremity to be in a dependent position
Hot pack	Moist, comfortable heat Variety of shapes and sizes Available for home use	May not maintain good contact on small or contoured areas Patient may not tolerate the weight of the pack Difficult to observe target area directly during treatment
Infrared lamp	Target area can be observed during treatment Does not require direct contact with the treatment area	Difficult to ensure uniform heating in all treatment areas Difficult to localize to a specific treatment area Tends to dry the skin more than other superficial heating agents
Paraffin	Low specific heat allows for application at higher temperatures than water Low thermal conductivity allows for slower heating of tissues which reduces the risk of overheating Maintains good contact with contoured areas Oils used in the wax add moisture to the skin	Effective only in distal extremities Risk of cross-contamination if the paraffin is reused Cannot be used over an open skin lesion
Diathermy	Capable of reaching deeper tissues Can produce thermal and nonthermal effects Covers large areas Heat is applied in a more uniform fashion since the application is performed statically Rate of tissue cooling is slower than other deep heating agents	Difficult to target small treatment areas effectively Requires patient to subjectively classify their heat sensation response Relatively large number of contraindications
Ultrasound	Capable of reaching deeper tissues Can produce thermal and nonthermal effects Amount of energy delivered per unit area can be quantified Covers small areas effectively Short duration of treatment	May not maintain good contact on small or contoured areas causing uneven heating Patient may not tolerate direct contact with the ultrasound transducer Rate of tissue cooling is faster than other deep heating agents

Capacitive Plate Method[16]

- Metal encased in a plastic housing produces an electric field from one plate to the other
- Field radiation consists of a strong electrical field and a weak magnetic field
- Heating pattern is superficial with the majority of energy absorbed within the skin
- Application is generally over areas of low fat content

Inductive Coil Method[16]

- Rigid metal encased coil produces a magnetic field perpendicular to the coil
- Field radiation consists of a strong magnetic field and a weak electrical field
- Heating pattern is deeper with the majority of energy absorbed within the deeper structures (i.e., tissues with the highest electrical conductivity, such as muscle and synovial fluid)
- Application is generally over areas of high water content

A therapist should first select the most appropriate diathermy technique and device based on patient examination. The patient must remove all metal and jewelry in the area surrounding the treatment site. The therapist should position the patient and clean and dry the patient's skin thoroughly. Nonmetal clothing does not need to be removed before treatment since the magnetic fields will penetrate through clothing, however, when using continuous mode, clothes should be removed so that sweat can be absorbed with towels.

When using an inductive applicator, the therapist must wrap the coils around the extremity that has been covered by a towel. When using a drum, the therapist should place the drum directly over the treatment area. When using a capacitive applicator, place the two plates over both sides of the treatment area ensuring equal distance from the plates to the skin (2-10 centimeters).[16] The patient must remain in the same position throughout treatment for complete and consistent heating.

The amount of energy delivered and corresponding temperature increase can be variable with continuous diathermy. As a result, therapists need to rely on the patient's subjective heat sensation response. The following dosage guidelines are commonly used in clinical practice.

Dose I – No sensation of heat

Dose II – Mild heating sensation

Dose III – Moderate heating sensation

Dose IV – Vigorous heating that is tolerable below the pain threshold

The patient should have a call bell and should be checked within the first few minutes of treatment. Treatment time with diathermy is approximately 20 minutes for thermal effects and may last as long as 30-60 minutes for nonthermal effects.[16]

Diathermy is not used as commonly as other therapeutic modalities, however, there are several scenarios where the use of diathermy may be particularly beneficial. These include when an increase in temperature is required at tissue depths greater than those achieved with superficial heating agents and when the target area will not tolerate direct contact from a thermal agent.

Diathermy also offers several potential advantages compared to ultrasound. Diathermy can effectively heat surfaces of up to 25 times the size of a typical ultrasound transducer.[18] Heat is applied to the target area in a more uniform fashion with diathermy since the application is performed statically. In addition, the rate of tissue cooling following heating with diathermy is significantly slower than the rate of tissue cooling with ultrasound. As a result, the therapist has additional time to perform interventions that are enhanced by the increased tissue temperature (e.g., stretching).

Additional Physical Agents

Ultraviolet Light

Ultraviolet light is a form of energy that is used therapeutically and is divided into UV-A, UV-B, and UV-C according to wavelength and location on the electromagnetic spectrum.[17] Ultraviolet light is absorbed one to two millimeters into the skin and is most commonly used to treat skin disorders.

Therapeutic Effects[16,18]

• Bacteriocidal effects	• Increased pigmentation
• Exfoliation	• Thickening of the epidermis
• Facilitate healing	• Vitamin D production

Indications[16,18]

• Acne	• Psoriasis
• Chronic ulcer/wound	• Sinusitis
• Osteomalacia	• Vitamin D deficiency

Contraindications[16,18]

• Areas receiving radiation	• Photosensitive medications
• Diabetes mellitus	• Skin cancer
• Herpes simplex	• Systemic lupus erythematosus
• Pellagra	• Tuberculosis

Ultraviolet Dosage

The ultraviolet dosage is classified according to the patient's response. Dosage categories include:[16]

Dose	Description
Suberythemal dose	The absence of erythema 24 hours after ultraviolet exposure.
Minimal erythemal dose	The smallest dose that produces erythema that appears in 1-8 hours and fades without trace within 24 hours.
First-degree erythemal dose	A dose that results in erythema that lasts 1-3 days with clear redness and mild desquamation. The dose is approximately 2.5 times the minimal erythemal dose and should be used only if the target area is less than 20% of the total body surface.
Second-degree erythemal dose	A dose that results in intense erythema, edema, peeling, pigmentation, and itching. The dose is approximately five times the minimal erythemal dose.
Third-degree erythemal dose	A dose that results in erythema with severe blistering, peeling, and exudation. The dose is approximately 10 times the minimal erythemal dose and should be used on areas less than 10 square inches.

Treatment parameters are based on diagnosis, desired effects, and minimal erythemal dose. Sensitivity to radiation varies greatly from person to person and is primarily influenced by age, pigmentation, prior exposure to ultraviolet radiation, and the use of photosensitive medications.

The therapist must thoroughly inspect the area to be treated and have the patient remove all jewelry. Polarized goggles should be worn by the therapist and the patient. A therapist should initially determine the patient's minimal erythemal dose (MED). The MED is tested by placing a piece of paper with five one-inch cut outs over a patient's anterior forearm. The patient should have all other non-treatment areas covered. Once the lamp is warmed up it should be positioned at a 90-degree angle to the area of treatment (for maximum absorption) and at a distance between 24 and 40 inches from the forearm.[18] The squares should be exposed sequentially in 15 second increments for 15, 30, 45, 60, and 75 seconds.[18] Visual inspection after an 8-hour period will determine the MED. The MED for patients being treated with psoralen-based topical and systemic drugs should be determined after the patient has taken psoralen orally or bathed in psoralen.

Parameters including distance from the lamp, position of the lamp at a 90-degree angle to the treatment site, and the MED must remain consistent over the course of treatment. The treatment time should increase each consecutive treatment day. Patients will build up tolerance to ultraviolet radiation with repeated exposure due to darkening of the skin with tanning and thickening of the skin caused by epidermal hyperplasia. Instead of increasing the treatment time, the therapist may elect to move the lamp closer to the target area. The intensity of the radiation reaching the target area increases as the lamp moves closer according to the inverse square law. For example, the intensity of the radiation increases by a multiple of four if the distance from the lamp to the target area is halved.

The therapist should utilize a stopwatch and continue with ongoing visual inspection during all treatment sessions. The response to ultraviolet radiation must be reassessed if an alternate lamp is used in a subsequent session since even a slight difference in the frequency of the radiation can significantly change the patient response.

Hydrotherapy

Hydrotherapy transfers heat through conduction or convection and is administered in tanks of varying size, ranging from extremity whirlpools to Olympic size pools. The main therapeutic effects of hydrotherapy include wound care, unloading of weight, and reduction of edema. The specific equipment and parameters used depend on the treatment objectives and site of the pathology.

Therapeutic Effects[16,18]	
• Decreased abnormal tone	• Pain relief
• Increased blood flow	• Relaxation
• Increased core temperature	• Vasodilation
	• Wound debridement

Indications[16,18]	
• Arthritis	• Joint stiffness
• Burn care	• Muscle spasm/spasticity
• Edema	• Muscle strain
• Decreased range of motion	• Pain
• Desensitization of residual limb	• Sprain
	• Wound care

Contraindications[16,18]	
• Advanced cardiovascular or pulmonary disease	• Incontinence
	• Maceration
• Active bleeding	• Peripheral vascular disease
• Diminished sensation	• Renal infection
• Gangrene	• Severe infection
• Impaired circulation	• Severe mental disorders

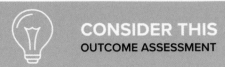

CONSIDER THIS
OUTCOME ASSESSMENT

Therapists must continually assess the effectiveness of selected interventions, including therapeutic modalities. There are a variety of subjective and objective measures that can assist the therapist to determine the relative value of each intervention.

Consider the following scenarios:

Scenario 1

A physical therapist assistant administers continuous ultrasound at 1.4 W/cm^2 for seven minutes to the right shoulder of a patient diagnosed with adhesive capsulitis.

1. Administer a visual analogue pain scale prior to and at the conclusion of treatment.
2. Perform periodic shoulder goniometric measurements to quantify the relative change in range of motion.

Scenario 2

A physical therapist assistant administers an ice pack to the knee of a patient positioned in supine with the lower extremity elevated. The patient is two weeks status post anterior cruciate ligament reconstruction.

1. Perform circumferential measurements at predetermined knee landmarks at regular intervals.
2. Administer a visual analogue pain scale prior to and at the conclusion of treatment.

It is often difficult to discern the effectiveness of a given intervention in isolation since, in most cases, patients are treated with several interventions addressing the same therapeutic objective. Despite this fact, it remains important for therapists to attempt to assess the relative effectiveness of selected interventions.

Properties of Water[22]

Buoyancy

Archimedes' principle of buoyancy states that there is an upward force on the body when immersed in water equal to the amount of water that has been displaced by the body.

Resistance

Water molecules tend to attract to each other and provide resistance to movement of the body in water. The resistance of water increases in proportion to the speed of motion.

Specific Gravity

The specific gravity of water is equal to 1.0. The human body varies based on size and somatotype, but typically it has a specific gravity of less than 1.0 (average .974). Therefore, a person will generally float when fully submerged in water.

Specific Heat

The specific heat is the measure of the ability of a fluid to store heat. This is calculated as the amount of thermal energy required to increase the fluid's temperature by one unit. Water has a specific heat of 1.0 calorie/gram while air has a specific heat of .001 calorie/gram. Water, therefore, retains heat 1,000 times more than an equivalent volume of air.

Total Drag Force

The total drag force is comprised of profile drag, wave drag, and surface drag forces. This is a hydromechanic force exerted on a person submerged in water that normally opposes the direction of the body's motion.

Viscosity

Viscosity refers to the magnitude of the cohesive forces between the molecules specific to the fluid. The greater the viscosity of the fluid, the greater the force required to create movement in the fluid.

Water Motion

The primary determinants of water motion include speed, viscosity, and turbulence. The movement of water includes laminar flow and turbulent flow. Laminar flow occurs when each particle of a fluid follows a smooth path without crossing paths. Typically, laminar flow rates are slow since when water moves quickly even minor oscillations create uneven flow. Turbulent flow occurs when fluids flow in erratic, small whirlpool-like circles called eddy currents or eddies. Movement in water at rest will encounter minimal turbulence. Movement against turbulent water will encounter greater resistance.

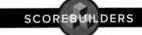

Types of Hydrotherapy Equipment

Extremity tank[17]

An extremity tank is used for a distal upper or lower extremity. Approximate dimensions for an extremity tank are a depth of 18-24 inches, a length of 28-32 inches, and a width of 15 inches (10-45 gallons).

Lowboy tank[17]

A lowboy tank is used for larger parts of the extremities and permits long sitting with water up to the midthoracic level. Approximate dimensions for a lowboy tank are a depth of 18 inches, a length of 52-65 inches, and a width of 24 inches (90-105 gallons).

Highboy tank[17]

A highboy tank is used for larger parts of the extremities and the trunk. This tank permits sitting in chest-high water with the hips and knees flexed (Fig. 8-56). Approximate dimensions for the highboy tank are a depth of 28 inches, a length of 36-48 inches, and a width of 20-24 inches (60-105 gallons).

Hubbard tank[16]

The Hubbard tank is used for full-body immersion. Approximate dimensions for the Hubbard tank are a depth of four feet, a length of eight feet, and a width of six feet. Contraindications specific to full-body immersion include unstable blood pressure and incontinence. The temperature should not exceed 100 degrees Fahrenheit (425 gallons).

Therapeutic pool[16]

A therapeutic pool is used for exercising in a water medium. The temperature should range from 79-97 degrees Fahrenheit depending on patient age, health status, and goals.

Treatment Temperature Guidelines	
Degrees F	**Purpose**
32 - 79 °F	Acute inflammation of distal extremities
79 - 92 °F	Exercise
92 - 96 °F	Wound care, spasticity
96 - 98 °F	Cardiopulmonary compromise, treatment of burns
99 - 104 °F	Pain management
104 - 110 °F	Chronic rheumatoid or osteoarthritis, increased range of motion

Adapted from Cameron M: *Physical Agents in Rehabilitation: From Research to Practice*, Third Edition, WB Saunders Company, 2008.

Whirlpool

A whirlpool consists of a tank that holds water with an attached motor, called a turbine, that provides agitation and aeration to create the "whirlpool effect." The turbine assembly typically allows the height and the lateral position of the turbine to be adjusted. This feature allows the therapist to direct the flow of water directly toward or away from the body part being treated. Whirlpools come in a variety of sizes and can accommodate an isolated body part or the entire body.

Prior to treatment the therapist should explain the sensations the patient will experience during treatment. Water temperature should be selected based on the patient diagnosis and goals. The therapist should assist the patient into a comfortable position and turn on the turbine. The patient's vital signs and reported level of comfort should be periodically assessed. Treatment time ranges between 10 and 30 minutes.[17] Exercise can be performed during whirlpool treatment as indicated. After treatment, dry and inspect the treated area. The tank must be thoroughly cleaned after each use with a disinfectant and antibacterial agent.

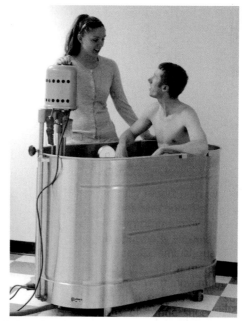

Fig. 8-56: A patient immersed in a whirlpool tank.

Pool Therapy

Advantages of pool therapy include decreased weight bearing due to buoyancy, improved therapist handling, enhanced control over the amount of resistance during exercise, and diminished risk of falling with activity. The therapist should assist the patient as needed into the pool and throughout treatment. The therapist must remain with the patient and monitor vital signs and tolerance to activity. Recommended populations for pool therapy include patients with arthritis, musculoskeletal injuries, neurological deficits, spinal cord injury, CVA, multiple sclerosis, and selected cardiopulmonary diagnoses.

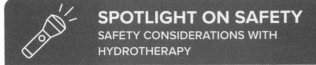

SPOTLIGHT ON SAFETY
SAFETY CONSIDERATIONS WITH HYDROTHERAPY

All physical therapy interventions, including hydrotherapy, have inherent safety risks. It is essential for therapists to be aware of potential risks in order to ensure patient safety and limit any potential liability. This section identifies specific risks associated with hydrotherapy and offers proactive strategies to assist therapists to minimize their level of risk.

Drowning

Personnel in charge of therapeutic pools should be trained in personal water safety techniques, as well as current cardiopulmonary resuscitation and first aid. The pool area should be equipped with emergency equipment including a spine board, blanket, life ring, and resuscitation devices. The entire staff should be aware of the facility's emergency action plan and be aware of the supervisory needs of each patient.

Electrical safety

All electrical equipment should be inspected by qualified personnel according to the manufacturer's recommendations. Ground fault circuit interrupters (GFCI) are required for all hydrotherapy units. GFCIs are designed to cut off electrical supply to equipment when any form of leakage or ground-fault is identified. Whirlpool tanks should be properly grounded and should use a hospital grade plug for the turbine.

Burns

Therapists must carefully screen patients to identify any potential contraindications to hydrotherapy. Therapists treating patients with a warm or hot whirlpool must correctly determine an appropriate temperature range to achieve the established therapeutic objectives. Prior to immersing the body part in water, the therapist must measure the temperature of the water. Therapists must be aware of medical and environmental conditions that may compromise a patient's ability to adequately dissipate heat.

Fainting

Patients are at an increased risk for fainting due to hypotension when large body areas are immersed in warm or hot water. This risk can be exaggerated in an aquatic environment due to the relative increase in ambient temperature. Patients taking antihypertensive medications such as beta blockers are also at an increased risk for becoming hypotensive. To minimize this risk, therapists should closely monitor patients during hydrotherapy and only immerse body parts in water that require treatment.

Falls

The presence of water on floors can result in a slippery surface that places patients at an increased risk of falling. Therapists should be diligent to dry any wet surfaces once they are identified.

Contrast Bath

A contrast bath utilizes alternating heat and cold in order to decrease edema in a distal extremity (Fig. 8-57). The alternating vasodilation and vasoconstriction is theorized to allow the benefits of heat, such as decreased pain and increased flexibility, while avoiding the risk of increased edema. The technique provides good contact over irregularly shaped areas, allows for movement during treatment, and assists with pain management. Limitations of contrast baths include potential intolerance to cold, dependent positioning, and a lack of credible research supporting the efficacy of contrast baths.

The therapist should position the patient so that both baths are easily accessible for the patient. The treatment should begin with the patient's distal extremity immersed in the hot bath with a temperature between 104-106 degrees Fahrenheit for 3-4 minutes.[17] The patient should then place the distal extremity into the cold bath with a temperature between 50 and 60 degrees Fahrenheit for one minute.[17] The patient should repeat this hot/cold sequence for 25-30 minutes.[16] The degree of temperature increase desired often determines whether the treatment ends in the hot or cold water.

Contrast baths are utilized primarily with arthritis of the smaller joints, musculoskeletal sprains and strains, complex regional pain syndrome, and residual limb desensitization.

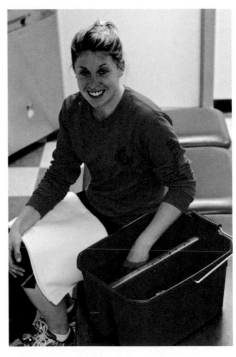

Fig. 8-57: A patient immersing their hand in hot water as part of a contrast bath.

Mechanical Agents

Traction

Traction is a modality that applies forces to the body to separate joint surfaces and decrease pressure. The force can be applied manually by the therapist, passively by the patient or mechanically by a machine. Types of traction include manual traction, mechanical traction, positional traction, gravity-assisted traction, and inversion traction. Traction is indicated for many diagnoses and allows for variation and adjustment of the established protocol based on individual patient needs. Traction affects many of the body's systems and requires ongoing monitoring and reassessment of treatment parameters.

Therapeutic Effects[16,18]

• Decreased disk protrusion • Decreased pain • Increased joint mobility • Increased muscle relaxation	• Increased soft tissue elasticity • Promote arterial, venous, and lymphatic flow

Indications[16,18]

• Disk herniation • Joint hypomobility • Muscle guarding • Muscle spasm • Narrowing of the intervertebral foramen • Nerve root impingement	• Osteophyte formation • Spinal ligament and other connective tissue contractures • Subacute joint inflammation • Subacute pain

Contraindications[16,18]

• Acute inflammation • Acute sprains or strains • Aortic aneurysm • Bone diseases • Cardiac or pulmonary problems • Conditions where movement significantly increases symptoms • Conditions where movement is contraindicated • Dislocation • Fracture • Hiatal hernia • Increased pain or radicular symptoms with traction • Infections in bones or joints	• Meningitis • Osteoporosis • Peripheralization of symptoms • Positive alar ligament test* • Positive vertebral artery test* • Pregnancy** • Rheumatoid arthritis–advanced* • Subluxation • Temporomandibular joint pain or dysfunction (use of halter)* • Trauma–if diagnostic tests have not ruled out other medical conditions • Tumors • Vascular conditions • Vertebral joint instability

* Cervical traction only   **Lumbar traction only

Mechanical Lumbar and Cervical Traction Procedures

Lumbar Traction

Procedure for mechanical lumbar traction

1. Determine the patient position

Mechanical lumbar traction is performed with the patient in a supine or prone position. The position chosen is often based on the medical diagnosis and patient tolerance. A flexed position of the spine (i.e., traction in supine) results in greater separation of the posterior structures including the facet joints and intervertebral foramen.[18] An extended position of the spine (i.e., traction in prone) results in greater separation of the anterior structures including the disk spaces.[18]

Traction is most often performed in the supine position, however, the prone position offers the therapist the opportunity to apply other modalities simultaneously and assess the amount of spinous process separation.

Certain medical diagnoses are characteristically treated in a specific position. For example, spinal stenosis is most often treated with a flexed spine since this position increases the intervertebral foramen opening.[17] Disk protrusions are most often treated with the patient positioned in prone since the spine can extend and the forces on the disk are directed anteriorly.[17] This is beneficial since the majority of disk herniations occur in a posterolateral direction.

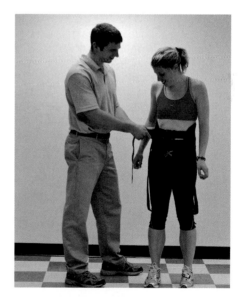

Fig. 8-58: Application of a traction harness.

2. Apply the traction harness

Mechanical lumbar traction requires the use of a traction harness. The harness is necessary to stabilize the trunk while the lumbar spine is placed under traction. The non-slip belt surface should be applied directly on the patient's skin in a standing position (Fig. 8-58).[18] This will allow the harness to better adhere to the skin and allow the therapist to adequately secure the harness with minimal active patient participation. The traction harness can also be applied by placing it on the traction table and having the patient lie on top of it. Once secured, the traction harness should be connected to the traction unit (Fig. 8-59).

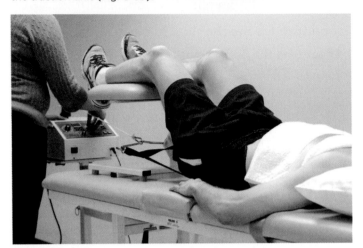

Fig. 8-59: A therapist setting the parameters for mechanical lumbar traction.

3. Select the traction parameters

Static versus intermittent traction

Traction can be applied in a static or intermittent form. Static refers to consistent force being applied throughout the treatment. Static traction may be desirable if the patient's symptoms are slightly exaggerated by movement.[17] Intermittent refers to varying force applied throughout the treatment. Intermittent traction may be desirable for joint mobilization or for patients who cannot tolerate static traction.[17] Intermittent traction requires the therapist to select the amount of force used during the hold and relax periods. The maximum force is applied during the hold period and the minimum force is applied during the relax period. The force during the relax period usually approximates 50% of the force used during the hold period.[16] There is little evidence to guide the timing of the hold and relax periods. The relax period should be relatively short, but must provide a sufficient interval to allow the patient to feel relaxed prior to the next traction cycle.

Force

The force of lumbar traction is dependent on the goals of treatment and is influenced by a number of variables including friction. Friction refers to the force that arises to oppose motion. The amount of friction when performing lumbar traction can be approximated by using the coefficient of friction, which refers to the constant frictional forces when applying traction between surfaces. The coefficient of friction of the human body on a mattress is 0.5.[17] The amount of friction can be estimated by multiplying the percentage of the body weight below L3 (i.e., 50%) and the coefficient of friction (0.5). The result is 25%, meaning that a force of approximately 25% of the patient's body weight is necessary to overcome the force of friction.[17]

The use of a split traction table can eliminate the majority of friction between the patient's body and the treatment table. When the two sections of the split traction table are unlocked and

traction is applied, the lower portion of the table slides away from the upper portion. If intermittent traction is used, the table should be split during the second or third hold period when the traction approaches its maximum force.[16]

The literature varies in the exact amount of force necessary when performing mechanical lumbar traction. The majority of sources indicate that a maximum of 30 pounds should be used for the initial traction session.[18] A force of 25% of total body weight may be adequate to stretch soft tissue and treat muscle spasm or disk protrusion.[16] A force of approximately 50% of the body weight is required for actual separation of the vertebrae.[18]

Many traction units provide therapists with the option to progressively increase or decrease the traction force in a series of predetermined steps. The gradual increase or decrease in pressure may be more comfortable for a patient since it allows the patient to gradually accommodate to the traction force and therefore, stay more relaxed throughout the duration of treatment.

Duration

The research does not offer specific guidance on the duration of lumbar traction. In general, treatment times vary from 5-30 minutes.[16] When treating disk-related symptoms, treatment time is generally 10 minutes or less and may extend up to 30 minutes with other spinal conditions.[18] Patient tolerance and changes in symptoms are the primary determining factors when selecting the duration of traction.

Cervical Traction

Procedure for mechanical cervical traction

1. Determine the patient position

Mechanical cervical traction is performed with the patient in a supine or sitting position. The position chosen is often based on the medical diagnosis and patient tolerance. A supine position is used more often since the traction force does not have to overcome the force exerted by gravity and the position allows the patient to attain a more relaxed state, minimizing the opposition to force. A flexed position of the spine results in greater separation of the posterior structures including the facet joints and intervertebral foramen.[16] An extended position of the spine results in greater separation of the anterior structures including the disk spaces.[16]

In a supine position, the therapist can adjust cervical flexion, rotation, and sidebending to focus on a specific target area and to promote comfort. In sitting, the amount of cervical flexion and extension can be controlled to a limited extent by the direction the patient is positioned in relation to the traction force. A patient positioned toward the traction force will exhibit more flexion than a patient positioned away from the traction force.

The relative amount of flexion in the cervical spine allows therapists to target specific spinal levels: upper cervical spine = 0-5 degrees of flexion; midcervical spine = 10-20 degrees of flexion; lower cervical spine = 25-35 degrees of flexion.[17]

2. Apply the head halter

Mechanical cervical traction requires the use of a head halter or padded board attached to a frictionless trolley that moves up and down a bar attached to the traction unit. The head halter is necessary to stabilize the head while the cervical spine is placed under traction (Fig. 8-60). The head halter should be applied so that the majority of traction pull is placed on the occiput and not the chin.[16] Therapists must be extremely careful when using the head halter since the device can place considerable force on the temporomandibular joints.

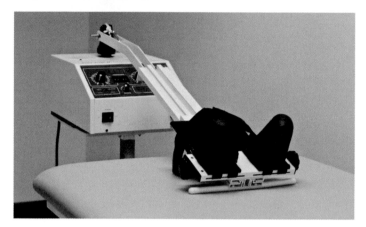

Fig. 8-60: A mechanical cervical traction unit.

3. Select the traction parameters

Static versus intermittent traction

The therapist should select static or intermittent traction. Intermittent traction may be more effective for reducing pain and increasing cervical range of motion.

Force

The force of cervical traction is dependent on the goals of treatment and is influenced by a number of variables including patient position. The literature varies as to the exact amount of force necessary when performing mechanical cervical traction. The majority of sources indicate that a force of up to 10 pounds should be used for the initial traction session.[16] A force of 7-10% of a patient's body weight (11-15 pounds) may be adequate to stretch soft tissue or treat muscle spasm and disk protrusion.[16] A force of 13-20% of a patient's body weight (20-30 pounds) may be necessary for joint distraction.[16] A traction force applied to the cervical spine should typically not exceed 30 pounds.

Duration

The research does not offer specific guidance on the duration of mechanical cervical traction. In general, treatment time varies from 5-30 minutes.[16] When treating disk-related symptoms, treatment time is generally 10 minutes or less, but may extend up to 30 minutes with other spinal conditions.[18] Patient tolerance and changes in symptoms are the primary determining factors when deciding the duration of traction.

Patient safety for mechanical lumbar and cervical traction

The therapist should assess the patient's initial response to traction within the initial five minutes of treatment. If the patient's symptoms worsen or peripheralize, the traction should be temporarily discontinued. The therapist may attempt to modify the traction

parameters, however, if undesirable symptoms persist, traction is not likely a viable treatment option. The patient should be supplied with a call bell or safety switch to turn off the traction in the event that traction increases symptoms or becomes uncomfortable.

Compression

Compression refers to the application of a mechanical force to increase pressure on the treated body part. Compression works to keep venous and lymphatic flow from pooling in the venous system and interstitial space.

Therapeutic Effects[16,18]	
• Control of peripheral edema • Management of scar formation • Prevention of deep vein thrombosis	• Promote lymphatic and venous return • Shaping of the residual limb
Indications[16,18]	
• Edema • Hypertrophic scarring • Lymphedema	• New residual limb • Risk for deep vein thrombosis • Stasis ulcers
Contraindications[16,18]	
• Circulatory obstruction • Deep vein thrombosis • Heart failure • Infection of treated area	• Malignancy of treated area • Unstable or acute fracture • Pulmonary edema

Static Compression

Static compression can be used to shape residual limbs, control edema, prevent abnormal scar formation, and reduce the risk of deep vein thrombosis. Examples of static compression devices include compression bandages and compression garments.

Compression bandages

Compression bandages increase external pressure on a body part by exerting resting pressure and working pressure. Resting pressure is produced when an elastic bandage is placed on stretch.[16] Pressure can be exerted when the patient is active or at rest. Working pressure is produced by an active muscle contracting against an inelastic bandage.[16] Pressure is only exerted when the patient is active.

Compression bandages are designed to offer greater pressure distally than proximally and must be applied using a figure-eight pattern. The bandages should not be applied in a circular pattern since this can result in uneven pressure and may actually inhibit edema management. In some instances, a liner may be applied under the bandages to minimize the probability of the bandages slipping on the skin.

There are a variety of different types of compression bandages including:

Long-stretch bandages provide the greatest resting pressure and are capable of applying 60-70 mm Hg of pressure.[16] The elasticity of the bandage allows them to extend up to 200% of their pre-stretch length.[16] This type of bandage provides very little working pressure since the bandages stretch when the muscles expand. Long-stretch bandages are most often used to apply compression in patients who are immobile.

Short-stretch bandages produce low pressure at rest and high working pressure when the muscles expand. These bandages can be moderately effective while a patient is active or at rest since they produce both resting and working pressure. Short-stretch bandages are most often used during exercise.[16] Patients must have a functional calf muscle and a functional gait pattern to maximally benefit from short-stretch bandages in the lower extremities.[16] The bandages are not effective in a flaccid or inactive limb.

Multi-layered bandages produce moderate to high resting pressure through the use of several bandages containing elastic and inelastic layers. The multiple layers of bandages provide protection, absorption, and compression. Multi-layered bandages are most commonly used to treat venous stasis ulcers.[16]

Semirigid bandages most often consist of treated gauze applied to a distal extremity. The treated gauze is initially wet and later dries into a hardened form. The bandages are often used in the treatment of venous stasis ulcers. An Unna boot is an example of a semirigid bandage made of zinc oxide impregnated gauze. The boot is capable of providing a sustained compression force of 35-40 mm Hg.[16]

Compression garments

Compression garments provide varying degrees of resting pressure and working pressure through elasticity. Compression garments are most often used to control edema, limit scar formation after burns, and improve venous circulation in active patients.[16,23] The garments consist of off-the-shelf and custom fit offerings for all parts of the body. Off-the-shelf garments (e.g., antiembolism stockings) provide a compression force of 16-18 mm Hg and are used to prevent deep vein thrombosis in patients on bed rest.[16] The stockings should be worn at all times unless bathing. Compression garments offering 20-30 mm Hg pressure are used for scar tissue control while 30-40 mm Hg pressure is typically required for edema control.[23]

Compression garments should be fit when the level of edema is minimal. An appropriately fit compression garment will fit tightly to the affected body part and can be challenging for some patients to don and doff without assistance. The average life expectancy of a compression garment is six months, although changes may be required sooner if there is a significant change in the size of the limb.[16]

Intermittent Compression

Intermittent compression refers to the use of compression at specified cyclical intervals to control edema. Intermittent compression is most often delivered using an intermittent pneumatic compression pump.

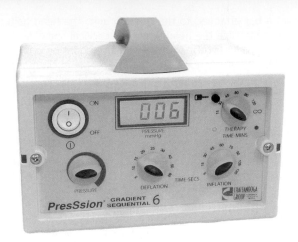

Fig. 8-61: An intermittent compression unit. Courtesy Chattanooga, a DJO Global Company.

Intermittent pneumatic compression pump

Intermittent compression with a pneumatic device is primarily used to reduce chronic or post-traumatic edema. The therapist has the ability to adjust treatment parameters including inflation pressure, on/off ratio, and total treatment time (Fig. 8-61).

The therapist must ask the patient to remove all jewelry and ensure appropriate fit of the compression sleeve prior to treatment. The patient should be placed in a comfortable position with the extremity elevated. Blood pressure and girth measurements should be recorded. The therapist should then apply a stockinette over the extremity and adjust the compression sleeve. The literature provides little definitive guidance on parameters such as on/off time, inflation time, and deflation time. As a result, patient comfort and the desired therapeutic effects are often the most important variables to consider.

Inflation pressure generally ranges from 30-80 mm Hg and typically should not exceed the patient's diastolic blood pressure.[16] Arterial capillary pressure is approximately 30 mm Hg, and therefore, inflation pressure below this value will not typically have any significant therapeutic value. Inflation pressure greater than the patient's systolic blood pressure may restrict arterial blood flow and create a medical emergency.

Treatment of the upper extremities generally requires 30-60 mm Hg of inflation pressure while treatment of the lower extremities generally requires 40-80 mm Hg of inflation pressure.[16] Treatment time varies from 30 minutes to four hours based on diagnosis. Intermittent compression is utilized from three times per week up to four times per day.[16] The patient should have a call bell and be monitored throughout treatment. When treatment is complete, the therapist should reassess the extremity and measure blood pressure. Girth measurements should be recorded and compared to the values obtained before treatment.

Compression may be coupled with therapeutic cold and electrical stimulation.[18] When using electrical stimulation in combination with compression, the current intensity should be adjusted only after the sleeve is fully inflated since this can significantly impact electrode contact with the skin.

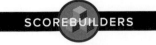

Continuous Passive Motion Machine

The continuous passive motion machine (CPM) is a mechanical device designed to provide continuous motion for a particular joint using a predetermined range and speed (Fig. 8-62). Robert Salter first developed this device based on research that continuous passive motion had beneficial healing effects for injured joints and surrounding soft tissues. Subsequent studies examining the efficacy of using a CPM versus not using a CPM vary in conclusion.[23] Some studies show no significant difference in short-term outcomes for CPM use versus alternate forms of early motion. Others show benefits from using CPM including earlier motion of joints resulting in shorter hospitalizations. The primary indication for CPM is to improve range of motion that may have been impaired secondary to a surgical procedure. Any joint may be indicated for CPM, however, the knee is the most commonly treated.

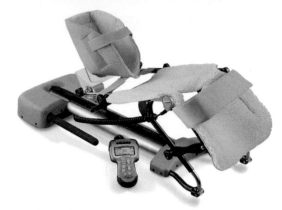

Fig. 8-62: A continuous passive motion machine. Courtesy Chattanooga, a DJO Global Company.

Therapeutic Effects	
• Decrease post-operative pain • Improve the rate of recovery • Increase range of motion	• Lessen the debilitating effects from immobilization • Reduce edema by assisting venous and lymphatic return • Stimulate tissue healing

Indications	
• Pain • Limited range of motion • Edema	• Susceptibility to contractures or adhesions • Muscle or joint stiffness

Contraindications	
• Increase in pain after use • Particular anticoagulants may increase the risk for intracompartment hematoma	• Unwanted translation of opposing bones

A continuous passive motion machine is often utilized immediately after surgery. The patient's joint must be aligned with the fulcrum of the CPM in order to receive effective and safe treatment. Proximal and distal stabilization straps stabilize the patient's upper and lower leg in the device and assist to maintain the desired alignment. The patient must be instructed in the use of the CPM and all associated safety information.

Specific protocols apply for each individual joint regarding time of use and degrees of motion. Initially, a small arc of motion is utilized and patients gradually increase the range of motion as tolerated or as allowed based on their current medical status. A rate of two cycles per minute typically allows patients to tolerate the CPM without difficulty. CPMs may be utilized at home after discharge from the hospital. A patient or caregiver must be independent with the CPM protocol for home use.

Electrotherapy

Electrotherapy is a commonly used therapeutic modality capable of producing a wide variety of therapeutic effects including muscle strengthening, pain management, muscle re-education, and stimulation of denervated muscle. Therapists must possess a thorough understanding of the mechanism by which electrical stimulation affects tissue as well as the advantages and disadvantages of the various electrotherapeutic agents available.

Therapeutic Effects[16,17,18,21]	
• Decreased edema • Decreased pain • Eliminate disuse atrophy • Facilitate bone repair • Facilitate wound healing	• Improved range of motion • Increased local circulation • Muscle re-education • Muscle strengthening • Relaxation of muscle spasm

Indications[16,17,18,21]	
• Bell's palsy • Decreased range of motion • Facial neuropathy • Fracture • Idiopathic scoliosis • Joint effusion • Labor and delivery	• Muscle atrophy • Muscle spasm • Muscle weakness • Open wound/ulcer • Pain • Stress incontinence • Shoulder subluxation

Contraindications[16,17,18,21]	
• Cardiac arrhythmia • Cardiac pacemaker • Malignancy • Osteomyelitis • Over a pregnant uterus	• Over carotid sinus • Patient with a bladder stimulator • Phlebitis • Seizure disorders

Muscle and Nerve Cell Excitation

Physical therapist assistants must possess a thorough understanding of muscle and nerve cell membranes and their response to electrical stimulation. Muscles and nerve cells are excitable because of the ability to produce action potentials. Action potentials refer to the recorded change in the electrical potential between the inside and outside of a nerve cell.[18] The muscle and nerve cell membranes regulate the exchange of substances between the inside of the cell and the environment outside of the cell. The potential difference in the concentration and permeability of sodium and potassium ions is termed the resting potential. Creating an impulse in a muscle or nerve cell requires the resting potential to be reduced below a threshold level causing changes in the membrane's permeability. The described change creates an action potential that results in depolarization. For an action potential to be evoked using electrical stimulation, the amplitude of the stimulus and pulse duration must be sufficient to overcome the established threshold.

Principles of Electricity

Current (i.e., electrical) refers to the directed flow of charge from one place to another. In order to produce electrical current, there must be a source of electrons, a material that allows passage of the electrons (i.e., conductor), and a driving force of electrons (i.e., electromotive force).[17,18] Current is measured in amperes. One ampere is equal to 6.25×10^{18} electrons per second. A milliampere is one thousandth of an ampere, while a microampere is one millionth of an ampere.[18]

Voltage is a measure of electromotive force or the electrical potential difference.[17,18] Electrons will only flow between two points when there is a difference in the quantity of electrons between the two points. The magnitude of the difference between the positive and negative poles is the voltage. Voltage is measured in volts.

Resistance describes the ability of a material to oppose the flow of ions through it. Resistance is measured in ohms.[17,18] The resistance of a material can be calculated using Ohm's law.

$$\text{Resistance} = \frac{\text{Voltage}}{\text{Current}}$$

Ohm's law states that the current in a conductor varies in proportion to the voltage and inversely with the resistance.[17] An electromotive force of one volt is required to drive one ampere of current across a resistance of one ohm.

Therapeutic Currents

Direct current[17,18]

Direct current is characterized by a constant flow of electrons from the anode (i.e., positive electrode) to the cathode (i.e., negative electrode) for a period of greater than one second without interruption (Fig. 8-63). Polarity remains constant and is determined by the therapist based on treatment goals. Direct current can be modulated for therapeutic use by interrupting the current flow after one second, reversing the polarity or gradually increasing or decreasing the amplitude. Clinically, direct current is most often used with iontophoresis.

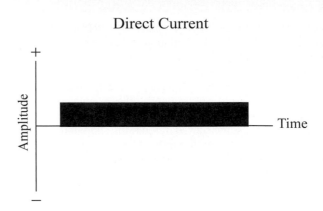

Direct Current

Fig. 8-63: Direct current is characterized by a constant flow of electrons from the anode to the cathode.

Alternating current[17,18]

Alternating current is characterized by polarity that continuously changes from positive to negative with the change in direction of current flow (Fig. 8-64). Alternating current is biphasic, symmetrical or asymmetrical, and is characterized by a waveform that is sinusoidal in shape. The frequency of cycles of alternating current is measured in cycles per second or hertz. Alternating current is used most frequently in a modulated form as burst or time-modulated.

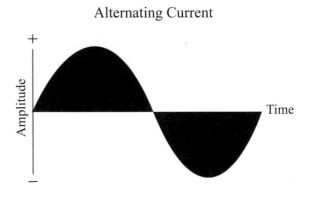

Alternating Current

Fig. 8-64: Alternating current is characterized by a continuous bidirectional flow of current.

Pulsatile current[17,18]

Pulsatile current is characterized by the non-continuous flow of direct or alternating current. A pulse is defined as a discrete electrical event separated from other pulses by a period of time in which no electrical activity exists. Most pulse waveforms are either monophasic or biphasic. Monophasic pulsed current has one phase for each pulse and therefore, the waveform is either positive or negative (Fig. 8-65). Monophasic pulsed current produces a polarity effect since the current flows through the tissues in only one polarity (i.e., positive or negative) for a given period of time.

Biphasic pulsed current has two phases, one which is positive and one which is negative (Fig. 8-66). Biphasic waveforms can be described as symmetric or asymmetric and balanced or unbalanced (Fig. 8-67).

Monophasic Pulsatile Current

Fig. 8-65: Monophasic pulsatile current has one phase for each pulse.

Biphasic Pulsatile Current

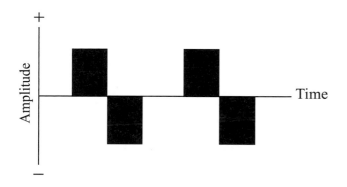

Fig. 8-66: Biphasic pulsatile current has two phases for each pulse.

Balanced and Unbalanced Current

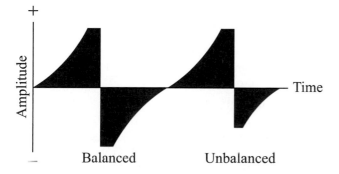

Fig. 8-67: Balanced and unbalanced biphasic pulsatile current.

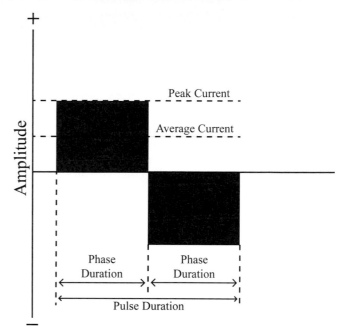

Fig. 8-68: Characteristics of pulsatile current.

Waveforms of Therapeutic Currents[18]

An oscilloscope can be used to create a graphical representation of the shape, direction, amplitude, duration, and pulse frequency of the electrical current being produced by an electrotherapeutic device. On an oscilloscope, an individual waveform is referred to as a pulse. Waveforms of monophasic, biphasic, and pulsatile currents include sine, square, rectangular or spiked (Fig. 8-69).

Waveforms

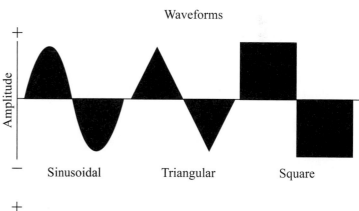

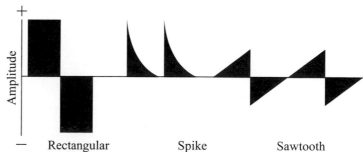

Fig. 8-69: Common types of electrical waveforms.

Electrodes

Administering electrical current to a body requires the use of at least two electrodes of opposing charges. When direct current or a monophasic pulsed waveform is used, one electrode will remain the cathode (negative) and the other the anode (positive) throughout the treatment. In an alternating current, the cathode and anode are constantly changing.

Proper cleaning of the skin and electrode application will facilitate conductance and limit impedance. Prior to applying the electrodes, the patient's skin must be thoroughly cleansed with soap and water or a suitable cleansing wipe. Ideally, hair should be removed from the identified treatment area, however, this is not required.

Electrodes are typically flexible with a self-adhesive gel coating and are intended for one time use. Reusable electrodes are typically made of carbon-silicon rubber. This type of electrode requires application of a gel or coupling spray to ensure appropriate contact. Since they are not self-adhesive, reusable electrodes must be secured on the patient with tape or elastic straps. Therapists should closely monitor the patient's skin since it is fairly common to develop irritation under the electrodes. Some patients may also exhibit an allergic reaction to the material or selected polymers from an electrode.[16] In these instances, the therapist may elect to utilize a different type of electrode, modify the location of the electrode placement or discontinue treatment.

Small electrodes are used for electrotherapy treatments for small areas of the body or small muscles that require relatively low levels of stimulation. Large electrodes are used for larger areas of the body or larger muscles of the body that require high levels of stimulation.[17] Current density is influenced by the size of the electrodes and the distance they are apart. When the same size electrodes are used, the current density under each electrode is the same. When unequal size electrodes are used, the current will be more concentrated in the smaller electrode. Current density can also refer to the concentration of current within the tissues.[20] If the electrodes are in close proximity, the current is more dense in the superficial tissues. If the electrodes are relatively farther apart, the current is more dense in the deeper tissues.[20]

Characteristics of Electrical Current Based on Electrode Size

Small Electrodes	Large Electrodes
Increased current density	Decreased current density
Increased impedance	Decreased impedance
Decreased current flow	Increased current flow

Electrode Placement

The two primary methods of electrode placement are monopolar and bipolar.

Monopolar technique: The stimulating or active electrode is placed over the target area. A second dispersive electrode is placed at another site away from the target area. Typically, the active electrode is smaller than the dispersive electrode. This technique is used with wounds, iontophoresis, and in the treatment of edema.[24]

Bipolar technique: Two active electrodes are placed over the target area. Typically, the electrodes are equal in size. This technique is used for muscle weakness, neuromuscular facilitation, spasms, and range of motion.[24]

Parameters of Electrical Stimulation

The law of Dubois Reymond specifies that the effectiveness of a current to target specific excitable tissue is dependent on three major factors:[20]

1. Adequate intensity to reach the threshold (i.e., amplitude)
2. Current onset fast enough to reduce accommodation (i.e., rise time)
3. Duration long enough to exceed the capacitance of the tissue (i.e., phase duration)

The specific parameters selected for electrotherapy determine the anticipated therapeutic effects. Common parameters available on most electrotherapy devices include:

Amplitude[16,18]

Amplitude refers to the magnitude of current. Average amplitude refers to the average amount of current supplied over a period of time, while peak amplitude refers to the maximum positive or negative point from zero where the pulse is maintained.[20] The peak amplitude must be large enough to exceed the threshold for the nerve or muscle cell. Amplitude controls are often labeled intensity or voltage and can be expressed in volts, microvolts or millivolts. The higher the amplitude, the greater the peak amplitude.

Rise time[16,18]

Rise time is the time it takes for the current to move from zero to the peak intensity within each phase (Fig. 8-71). Fast rise times are necessary with low capacitance tissues, such as large motor nerves. Rise times are typically very short, ranging from nanoseconds to milliseconds. By observing the graphical representation of a given pulse generated from an oscilloscope, therapists can gain a general sense of the rise time. For example, a sine wave would exhibit a more gradual increase in amplitude compared to a rectangular wave which has an almost instantaneous increase in amplitude. Decay time is the time it takes for the current to move from the peak intensity to zero.

Phase duration[16,18]

Phase duration is the amount of time it takes for one phase of a pulse. The phase begins when the current departs from the zero line and ends as the current returns to the zero line. Pulse duration is the amount of time it takes for two phases of a pulse with biphasic current (Fig. 8-68). In monophasic current, the phase duration and the pulse duration are the same. If the current is biphasic, there are two phase durations for each pulse. The length of the phase duration must be sufficient to exceed the capacitance of the targeted nerve in order to cause an action potential. Phase duration is typically measured in microseconds. The interpulse interval is the time between two successive phases of a pulse.

Frequency[16,18]

Frequency determines the number of pulses delivered through each channel per second. Frequency controls are often labeled as rate and are expressed in pulses per second or hertz. The frequency affects the number of action potentials elicited during the stimulation. Although the same number of fibers are recruited, a higher frequency causes them to fire at a more rapid rate.

Current modulation[18,24]

Current modulation refers to any alteration in the amplitude, duration or frequency of the current during a series of pulses or cycle.

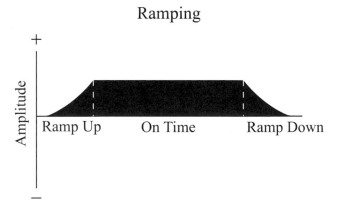

Ramping

Fig. 8-70: Current modulation using a ramp.

Common categories of modulation include bursts, interrupted pulses, and ramps (Fig. 8-70). Bursts occur when pulsed current flows for several milliseconds and then ceases to flow for several milliseconds in a repeated cycle. The minimal length of the interruptions is too short to allow for a true interruption of muscle contraction. Interrupted pulses allow for a true

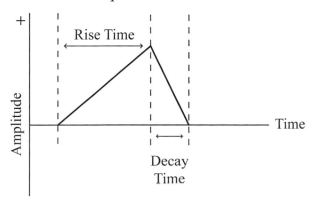

Time Dependent Characteristics

Fig. 8-71: Determining rise time and decay time.

interruption by using an on time and off time. This type of modulation is commonly used with muscle strengthening due to the necessity for a rest period. Ramps allow current amplitude to gradually increase to a preset maximum and then gradually decrease. Ramping is commonly used to make the onset of stimulation more comfortable and is frequently utilized with muscle strengthening.[24]

Neuromuscular Electrical Stimulation

Neuromuscular electrical stimulation (NMES) is a technique used to facilitate skeletal muscle activity (Fig. 8-72). Stimulation of an innervated muscle occurs when an electrical stimulus of appropriate intensity and duration is administered to the corresponding peripheral nerve. Electrical stimulation of a denervated muscle has been used in an attempt to maintain the muscle, however, there is little documented evidence that supports this treatment option. Functional electrical stimulation (FES) uses electrical stimulation to create or enhance the performance of a functional activity.[17] An example of FES is the stimulation of the anterior tibialis to produce dorsiflexion during the swing phase of gait.

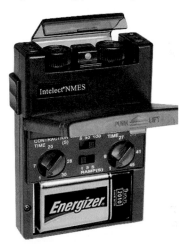

Fig. 8-72: A neuromuscular electrical stimulation unit. Courtesy Chattanooga, a DJO Global Company.

NMES is a commonly used therapeutic technique to facilitate the return of controlled functional muscular activity or to maintain postural alignment until recovery occurs. When performing NMES the patient should be positioned comfortably (Fig. 8-73). The therapist should place the electrodes over the muscle to be stimulated so that the electrodes are aligned in parallel. This alignment will allow the current to travel parallel to the direction of the muscle fibers. Ideally, one of the electrodes should be placed over the muscle's motor point since this will produce the strongest contraction with the least amount of current. The electrodes should be separated by a minimum of two inches.[17]

Parameters for applying NMES for muscle strengthening

Current amplitude: The amount of current amplitude is dependent on the desired strength of the contraction (Fig. 8-74). For example, a therapist would want a much more forceful muscle contraction for a patient participating in general muscle strengthening than for a patient recovering from a recent surgery.

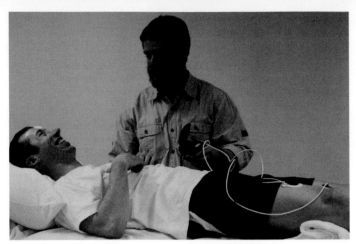

Fig. 8-73: A therapist discussing the use of a neuromuscular electrical stimulation unit with a patient.

Pulse duration: The pulse duration should be high enough to overcome the relatively low capacitance of motor nerve fibers. Despite the low capacitance, the relative depth of the muscle fibers requires a high pulse duration.[20] Patients often find shorter pulse durations more comfortable when targeting smaller muscles and longer pulse durations more comfortable when treating larger muscles.[17] Therapists should recognize that as the pulse duration is shortened, a greater current amplitude will be required to produce the same strength of contraction.

Frequency: The frequency should be sufficient to produce a tetanic contraction. A smooth tetanic contraction is usually produced at a frequency of 35-50 pulses per second.[20] Higher frequencies will not produce a stronger contraction, but instead will promote more rapid fatigue.

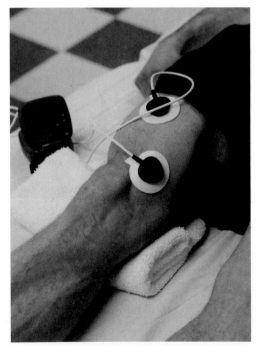

Fig. 8-74: A forceful quadriceps femoris contraction using a neuromuscular electrical stimulation unit.

Duty cycle: A duty cycle must be used when applying NMES to provide the muscle with relaxation time and limit the influence of fatigue. On time should range from 6-10 seconds while off time should be approximately five times longer.[20] The therapist may elect to decrease the length of the off time in subsequent sessions based on patient progress.

Ramp time: A ramp allows current amplitude to gradually increase to a preset maximum and then gradually decrease. Ramping is commonly used to make the onset of stimulation more comfortable when performing muscle strengthening. Based on an on time of 6-10 seconds, a ramp up time of 1-4 seconds would be recommended.

Treatment time: Patients should complete a minimum of 10 contractions and a maximum of 20 contractions. Based on typical on and off times, performing 10 contractions would take approximately 10 minutes while 20 contractions would take 20 minutes. Treatment should ideally take place a minimum of three times per week.[18]

Transcutaneous Electrical Nerve Stimulation (TENS)

Transcutaneous electrical nerve stimulation is widely used for acute and chronic pain management. Areas of use include obstetrics, temporomandibular joint pain, and post-operative pain. The main therapeutic effects of TENS include pain relief through the gate control theory of pain or the endogenous opiate pain control theory. TENS units are portable and indicated for home use (Fig. 8-75). The most commonly used modes of TENS include conventional, acupuncture-like, brief intense, and noxious.[16,25]

Conventional TENS[17,21,24]

Conventional TENS is characterized by delivery of electrical pulses having short duration and high frequency with low current amplitude. The current amplitude should be sufficient to generate a sensory response, but should be below the motor threshold. Electrodes should be placed over the painful area. The majority of patients report a mild tingling sensation under and between the electrodes. Pain relief is usually brief and only occurs when the current is being generated. Conventional TENS is most often used to relieve pain during activities of daily living. Treatment time is highly variable depending on the duration of the activity.

Acupuncture-like TENS[17,21,22]

Acupuncture-like TENS is characterized by the delivery of electrical pulses that have long duration and low frequency with moderate current amplitude. The current amplitude should be sufficient to generate muscle twitching. Electrodes should be placed over the area of pain or a related area, such as an acupuncture point. The majority of patients report the stimulus as uncomfortable or burning. Pain relief can last for several hours after stimulation. Acupuncture-like TENS is most often used for patients requiring longer lasting pain relief. It is not often used during activities of daily living since the muscle twitching can interfere with functional tasks. Treatment time is usually 20-45 minutes.

Common TENS Techniques and Recommended Parameters[17]

Technique	Amplitude	Pulse Frequency	Pulse Duration	Treatment Time
Conventional	Sufficient for a sensory response	High (30-150 pps)	Short (50-100 µsec)	Variable based on the duration of the activity
Acupuncture-like	Sufficient to produce muscle twitching	Low (2-4 pps)	Long (100-300 µsec)	20-45 minutes
Brief Intense	Sufficient for strong paresthesia or a motor response	High (60-200 pps)	Long (150-500 µsec)	15 minutes
Noxious	Highest tolerated stimulus	High or Low	Long (250 µsec up to 1 second)	30-60 seconds for each point

Adapted from Michlovitz S: *Thermal Agents in Rehabilitation,* Fourth Edition, FA Davis Company, 2005

**This table demonstrates a typical range for each type of TENS, however, there are discrepancies that exist from author to author regarding the appropriate settings for TENS. Given this fact, it is more important to have a basic understanding of TENS parameters (e.g., short, long, low, high) than it is to memorize an exact pulse frequency or pulse duration.

Brief intense TENS[17,21,24]

Brief intense TENS is characterized by delivery of electrical pulses having long duration and high frequency with moderate current amplitude. This mode of TENS is referred to as brief intense TENS since the application is shorter and the current amplitude is higher than some of the other presented modes. The current amplitude should be sufficient for strong paresthesia or a motor response. Brief intense TENS is often used to minimize pain during therapeutic activities that may be painful. Treatment time is usually 15 minutes.

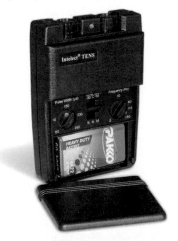

Fig. 8-75: A transcutaneous electrical nerve stimulation unit. Courtesy Chattanooga, a DJO Global Company.

Noxious TENS[17,24]

Noxious TENS is characterized by high density current that is described by patients as uncomfortable or painful. This mode of TENS is administered with a small probe type applicator or electrode. Stimulation is delivered in 30-60 second intervals to motor, acupuncture or trigger points. Noxious level stimulation should be applied to patients only after the therapist has thoroughly explained the expected sensation.[17]

The waveforms used are monophasic pulsatile current or biphasic pulsatile current with a spiked, square, rectangular or sine waveform. Electrode placement may be based on sites of nerve roots, trigger points, acupuncture sites or key points of pain and sensitivity.[24] Net polarity is normally equal to zero. If the waveform is unbalanced there will be an accumulation of charges that will lead to skin irritation under the electrodes.

Interferential Current

Interferential current combines two medium frequency alternating waveforms that are biphasic. The two waveforms are delivered through two sets of electrodes from separate channels of the same stimulator. When the currents intersect, they produce a higher amplitude when both currents are in the same phase and a lower current when they are in opposite phases. This continuous sequence produces envelopes of pulses known as beats.[16] Interferential current is often comfortable for patients since a low amplitude current is delivered through the skin and a higher amplitude current is delivered to deeper tissues. Interferential current is most often used for pain relief, increased circulation, and muscle stimulation.[20]

Methods of Interferential Current Delivery

Bipolar delivery[20]

Bipolar delivery utilizes two electrodes connected to a single channel with two medium sinusoidal currents. The interference between the two currents creates an amplitude modulated interferential current with a beat frequency (beats per second). The beat frequency is the net difference between the two currents. The bipolar method allows for the interferential current to be modulated prior to delivery of the current to the electrodes. Bipolar delivery creates an oval-shaped field of interferential current.

Quadripolar delivery[20]

Quadripolar delivery utilizes four electrodes with each pair connected to a single channel. The interference between the currents using this method occurs at the level of the treatment area within the targeted tissues. When the currents intersect at a 90 degree angle, the maximum resultant amplitude occurs halfway between the two lines of current. The current treatment area creates a four-leaf clover shaped treatment field within the area between all four electrodes (Fig. 8-76).

Quadripolar with automatic vector scan[21]

The quadripolar method with automatic vector scan is used when there is a need to increase the size of the field of current that is created by the quadripolar method. One of the circuits is allowed to vary in amplitude and this allows the field pattern to automatically rotate between the two lines of current. The field is circular in shape, as opposed to the cloverleaf, and allows for an overall larger field of current.

Some interferential units include suction electrodes that attach to the skin surface through mild suctioning. This feature can be desirable since the electrodes stay in place throughout treatment without having to be strapped to the body surface. Interferential current can be used in combination with other modalities, such as ice or heat. Treatment time is variable and is primarily influenced by the established goals (e.g., pain relief, increased circulation, muscle stimulation).

Interferential Current

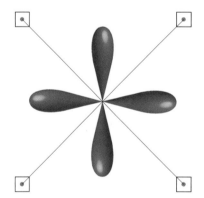

Fig. 8-76: Interaction of two medium frequency alternating wave-forms using interferential current with a quadripolar technique.

Iontophoresis

Iontophoresis is the process by which ions are introduced into the body through the skin by means of continuous direct current electrical stimulation (Fig. 8-77). Iontophoresis is based on the theory that like charges repel and, as a result, ions in a solution of similar charge will move away from the electrical source and into the body. Positively charged ions are carried into the body's tissue from the positive pole (anode) and negatively charged ions are carried into the body's tissue from the negative pole (cathode). The rate of ion delivery is determined by the concentration of the ion, the pH of the solution, the current density, and the duration of the treatment.[18] The specific therapeutic effects of iontophoresis are determined based on the ion selected.

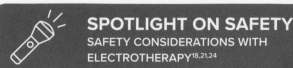

SPOTLIGHT ON SAFETY
SAFETY CONSIDERATIONS WITH ELECTROTHERAPY[18,21,24]

Electrical equipment used in health care can pose a significant potential risk to both the patient and therapist. Therapists should be aware of these potential risks in order to ensure safety and limit any potential liability. This section identifies several safe practices that minimize risk when using electrotherapy.

- All electrotherapy equipment should be inspected by qualified personnel at or before the manufacturer's suggested service dates.
- Any electrotherapy equipment that may have been damaged (e.g., dropped on the floor) or is functioning improperly should be inspected by qualified personnel before subsequent use.
- Ensure all line-powered equipment has a testing seal (maximum leakage of a current < 1 milliampere).
- A sticker should be placed on equipment noting the last inspection/maintenance date.
- Maintain an updated log for all equipment used in the physical therapy department.
- Maintain electrotherapy equipment operation manuals in an accessible location for staff members to use as a resource.
- Electrotherapy equipment should only be used by qualified personnel who have read the operating manual and are familiar with how to properly operate the equipment.
- All electrotherapy devices should have a hospital grade three-pronged plug that has a safety ground attached to an earth ground.
- Electrical outlets should be equipped with ground fault circuit interrupters (GFCIs). GFCIs are designed to cut off electrical supply to equipment when any form of leakage or ground-fault is identified.
- Extension cords or multiple adapters should not be used.
- Plugs should be removed from the wall by gripping and pulling the plug and not by pulling the cable.
- Unplug all powered-line devices at the end of each day.
- Always turn the intensity dial to zero before unplugging electrotherapy equipment.
- Instruct patients to avoid all contact with the controls of an electrotherapy device unless otherwise instructed.
- Thoroughly instruct patients on the type of sensations typically experienced with a specific electrotherapy device.
- Avoid placing containers of liquid (e.g., coffee, soda) on top of the casing of electrical equipment.
- Keep electrotherapy equipment 3-5 meters from each other when in use to minimize the possibility of electrical interference.

Indications[16,17,18]	
• Pain	• Keloids
• Calcium deposits	• Muscle spasm
• Fungal infection	• Myositis ossificans
• Hyperhidrosis	• Plantar warts
• Inflammation	• Scar tissue
• Ischemia	• Wounds
Contraindications[16,17,18]	
• Drug allergies	• Skin sensitivity reactions to specific ions

The amount of electricity used when performing iontophoresis is measured in milliamp minutes (mA-min). This value is often termed "dosage" and is determined by multiplying current amplitude and time. Dosage ranges from 40-80 mA-min with iontophoresis.[16,17]

A dosage of 40 mA-min could be delivered in 10 minutes with a current amplitude of 4.0 mA. The same dosage could be delivered using a lower current amplitude with a longer duration. A lower current amplitude and a longer duration will be less likely to cause skin irritation or burns.[17]

The current amplitude should be adjusted to be comfortable for the patient. Current amplitudes typically range from 1.0-4.0 mA.[16,17] Once the current amplitude is determined, the therapist can select an appropriate amount of time to ensure the appropriate mA-min dosage level. Many iontophoresis units will automatically calculate the duration of the treatment session based on the preset dosage and the current amplitude.

Iontophoresis procedures

The therapist must identify any known patient allergies or the potential for adverse reactions based on the ion used. The skin should be thoroughly cleaned with soap or isopropyl alcohol. The patient should be positioned comfortably, but should not lie on top of the electrodes. The unit should be set to continuous direct current. Polarity should be set to the same polarity as the ion solution.[16] The ion solution is placed into a small chamber located on a self-adhesive electrode placed at the treatment site.

The electrode containing the ion solution is referred to as the active electrode.[18] A second electrode, referred to as the dispersive electrode, is placed away from the active electrode. The recommended spacing between the active and dispersive electrodes should be minimally equivalent to the diameter of the active electrode.[18] As the spacing between the electrodes increases, the current density in the superficial tissues decreases, resulting in a diminished risk for burns. Smaller electrodes have higher current density and are often used to treat a specific lesion, while larger electrodes are used when the treatment area is less well defined.[18]

The therapist should make sure the electrodes are appropriately secured and slowly increase the intensity towards a maximum of four milliamperes. Treatment should last 10-20 minutes.[18] Additional time may be required for treatment at an intensity of less than

four milliamperes. The therapist must monitor the patient every 3-5 minutes during treatment to ensure that the patient is not exhibiting signs of skin irritation or burns under the electrode.[18]

Acidic reaction: A patient may have an acidic reaction from the iontophoresis treatment as a result of hydrochloric acid forming under the positive electrode (anode).[18]

Alkaline reaction: A patient may have an alkaline reaction from the iontophoresis treatment as a result of sodium hydroxide forming under the negative electrode (cathode).

Acidic and alkaline reactions often cause significant discomfort, skin irritation or chemical burns.[18]

The likelihood of a burn can be decreased by increasing the size of the cathode relative to the anode, decreasing the current density, and increasing the space between the electrodes.[18]

Upon completion of treatment, the therapist must slowly decrease the intensity and remove the electrodes. It is common for patients to have redness of the skin under the active electrode. In some cases, the active electrode can be left in place for 12-24 hours after treatment to facilitate further diffusion of ions through the skin.

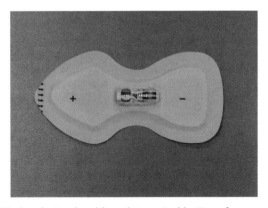

Fig. 8-77: An electrode with an integrated battery for iontophoresis drug delivery.

The frequency of treatment depends on the ion selected, the underlying condition, patient tolerance, and the relative effectiveness of the treatment.[17] Iontophoresis should be applied no more frequently than every other day due to the potential side effects from using direct current.[17] A therapist should be able to make a relative determination of the effectiveness of iontophoresis within three to five treatment sessions.

Ions Used with Iontophoresis[16,17,18]

Medication	Indications	Polarity
Acetic acid	Calcific deposits, myositis ossificans	Negative
Calcium chloride	Scar tissue, keloids, muscle spasms	Negative
Copper sulfate	Fungal infection	Positive
Dexamethasone	Inflammation	Negative
Iodine	Scars, adhesive capsulitis	Negative
Lidocaine	Analgesia, inflammation	Positive
Magnesium sulfate	Muscle spasms, ischemia	Positive
Salicylates	Muscle and joint pain, plantar warts	Negative
Zinc oxide	Healing, dermal ulcers, wounds	Positive

Biofeedback

Biofeedback refers to the use of instrumentation to bring specific events to conscious awareness (Fig. 8-78). Biofeedback can be utilized to receive information related to motor performance, kinesthetic performance or physiological response.[16] Electromyographic biofeedback is the most commonly used biofeedback modality in the clinical setting. Biofeedback allows patients to make small changes in performance and receive immediate feedback. By successfully rewarding small changes incrementally, larger changes can potentially be achieved.

Biofeedback does not measure muscle contraction, but rather the electrical activity associated with muscle contraction. There is not a standard measurement scale when reporting electrical activity using a biofeedback unit. The electrical activity is most commonly presented as visual and/or auditory feedback. Visual feedback is often presented as a series of colored lights that go on and off in a linear fashion based on the strength of the incoming signal. Auditory feedback is often presented as a buzzing, clicking or beeping sound that changes in intensity as the strength of the incoming signal increases or decreases.

Prior to treatment the therapist should ensure that the patient's skin is clean and dry. Biofeedback requires the use of surface electrodes which provide less specific information than indwelling electrodes, however, surface electrodes are more effective in quantifying muscle activity in several muscles or a group of muscles. The electrodes can be disposable or non-disposable.

Disposable electrodes typically are designed with the appropriate amount of gel and an adhesive that allows the electrode to firmly adhere to the skin. Non-disposable electrodes require gel and need to be adequately secured to the skin by the therapist.

Therapeutic Effects[18,20]

• Decreased accessory muscle use • Decreased muscle spasm • Decreased pain	• Improved muscle strength • Muscle relaxation • Neuromuscular control

Indications[18,20]

• Bowel incontinence • Cerebral palsy • Hemiplegia • Impaired motor control • Muscle spasm	• Muscle weakness • Pain • Spinal cord injury • Urinary incontinence

Contraindications[18,20]

• Conditions where muscle contraction is detrimental	• Skin irritation at the electrode site

The two active electrodes should be placed parallel to the muscle fibers and close to each other.[18] The reference or ground electrode can be placed anywhere on the body, but is often secured between the two active electrodes. The signals are transmitted to a differential amplifier and information is conveyed through visual and auditory feedback. The described setup can minimize "noise," which refers to the extraneous electrical activity not produced by the contraction of the muscle.

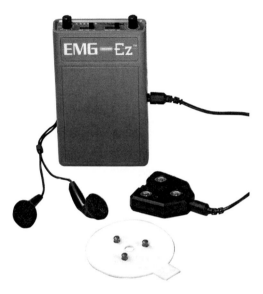

Fig. 8-78: A biofeedback unit. Courtesy Chattanooga, a DJO Global Company.

The therapist can control the relative signal sensitivity during treatment. A high sensitivity will detect extremely small amounts of electrical activity while a low sensitivity setting will detect only large amounts of electrical activity. As a result, high sensitivity settings are used when the treatment objective is relaxation and low sensitivity settings are used when the treatment objective is muscle re-education.[18]

Muscle relaxation

The treatment for muscle relaxation requires a high sensitivity setting with active electrodes initially positioned close to each other. As the patient improves with relaxation, the electrodes should be placed further apart and the sensitivity setting should be increased. A decrease in audio or visual feedback would be considered a positive sign. The patient may also benefit from adjunct relaxation techniques, such as imagery. Treatment duration of 10-15 minutes is usually adequate to attain relaxation.

Muscle re-education

The treatment for muscle re-education should begin with the patient performing a maximal muscle contraction. The sensitivity of the biofeedback unit should be set at a low sensitivity setting and adjusted so that the patient can perform the repetitions at a ratio of two-thirds of the maximal muscle contraction. Isometric contractions should continue for 6-10 seconds with relaxation in between each contraction. An increase in audio or visual feedback

would be considered a positive sign. Treatment duration for a single muscle group is 5-10 minutes.[18] As the patient is able to demonstrate greater recruitment of the target muscle, more complex activities are added to the program.

Massage

Massage is a manual therapeutic modality that produces physiologic effects through different types of stroking, rubbing, and pressure (Fig. 8-79). Massage is capable of producing mechanical and reflexive effects.

Therapeutic Effects[27,28,29]	
• Altered pain transmission • Decreased anxiety and tension • Decreased muscle atrophy • Decreased muscle spasm • Facilitate healing • Improved circulation	• Increased lymphatic circulation • Loosen adhesions • Reduction of edema • Relaxation • Removal of metabolic waste • Stimulate reflexive effects
Indications[27,28,29]	
• Adhesion • Bursitis • Decreased range of motion • Edema • Intermittent claudication • Lactic acid excess • Migraine or headache	• Muscle spasm and cramping • Pain • Raynaud's phenomenon • Scar tissue • Tendonitis • Trigger point
Contraindications[27,28,29]	
• Acute injury • Arteriosclerosis • Cancer • Cellulitis	• Embolus • Infection • Thrombus

Massage Parameters[28]

There are a variety of different massage techniques described in the literature. Each technique varies in relation to a number of important variables.

Direction – The general movement pattern of the massage stroke. Direction can be described as centrifugal or centripetal. Centrifugal is moving from the center of the body out. Centripetal is moving in from the extremities toward the center of the body.

Duration – The length of time a massage technique is performed. Duration is highly variable depending on the characteristics of the massage technique, established therapeutic objectives, and patient tolerance.

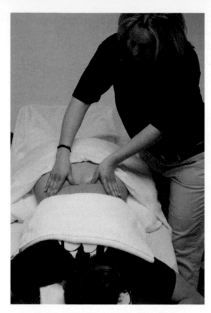

Fig. 8-79: Application of massage to the low back of a properly draped patient.

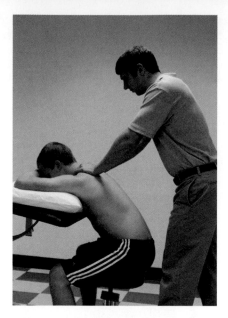

Fig. 8-80: Massage applied to the upper back of a patient in supported sitting.

Frequency – The rate at which the massage technique repeats itself in a given time frame. The variety of massage techniques are repeated several times prior to transitioning to a different technique.

Pressure – The relative amount of compressive stress applied to the body. Pressure is usually described by terms such as light, moderate, deep or variable (Fig. 8-80).

Rhythm – The relative regularity of the massage technique. A massage technique applied at regular consistent intervals would be considered rhythmic. If the technique was applied at inconsistent intervals, it would be considered non-rhythmic.

Speed – The general rate the therapist's hands move. Speed is usually described as slow, moderate, fast or variable.

Massage Techniques[27,28,29]

Effleurage

Effleurage is a massage technique that is characterized by a light stroke that produces a reflexive response. The technique is performed at the beginning and end of a massage to allow the patient to relax. Strokes should be directed towards the heart. Effleurage can also be applied as a deep stroke to produce both a mechanical and a reflexive response.

Friction

Friction is a massage technique that incorporates small circular motions over a trigger point or muscle spasm. This is a deep massage technique that penetrates into the depth of a muscle and attempts to reduce edema, loosen adhesions, and relieve muscle spasm. Friction massage is used frequently with chronic inflammation or with overuse injuries (Fig. 8-81).

Petrissage

Petrissage is a massage technique described as kneading, where the muscle is squeezed and rolled under the therapist's hands. The goal of petrissage is to loosen adhesions, improve lymphatic return, and facilitate removal of metabolic waste from the treatment area. Petrissage should be performed in a distal to proximal sequence. Petrissage can be performed with two hands over larger muscle groups or with as few as two fingers over smaller muscles.

Tapotement

Tapotement is a massage technique that provides stimulation through rapid alternating movements such as tapping, hacking, cupping, and slapping. The primary purpose of tapotement is to enhance circulation and stimulate peripheral nerve endings.

Vibration

Vibration is a massage technique that places the therapist's hands or fingers firmly over an area and utilizes a rapid, shaking motion that causes vibration to the treatment area. The therapist initiates this motion from the forearm while maintaining firm contact on the treatment area. Vibration is used primarily for relaxation.

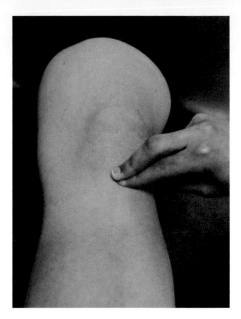

Fig. 8-81: Transverse friction massage applied to the patellar tendon.

The therapist's hands must be clean, dry, and warm. A therapist will typically use a lubricant to reduce friction on the skin during massage. The primary exception to using lubricant would be when performing friction massage. The lubricant should be applied to the therapist's hands and gently warmed by rubbing the hands together prior to patient application.

The therapist must be positioned in an efficient posture during treatment to maintain the required pressure and rhythm based on the goals of treatment. The massage should start with the effleurage technique. The amount of time required for each treatment is dependent on the body part and therapeutic goal. Generally, the back requires 15 minutes as opposed to a smaller area or joint that requires 8-10 minutes. The intensity should progressively increase and then decrease, using effleurage again to end the treatment session.

Massage Procedure

Prior to initiating massage, a therapist must obtain patient consent. Components of consent when performing massage would minimally include:

1. A description of the proposed massage.

2. The relative risks and benefits.

3. The expectations of the patient during the massage.

4. The opportunity to consent to or refuse the proposed intervention.

Massage should occur in a room with air temperature of 72-75 degrees Fahrenheit.[28] This temperature range will allow the patient to relax and minimize undesired muscular tension. The patient should be comfortably positioned and properly draped prior to the initiation of treatment. Standard bed linens are most often used for draping. The therapist should attempt to leave only the area of the body being massaged exposed, while the remainder of the body should be draped. Pillows, towels, bolsters, foam, and blankets can be used to ensure patient comfort.

MOTIVATIONAL MOMENT

See Page 994

Equipment, Devices, and Technologies; Therapeutic Modalities Essentials

Equipment, Devices, and Technologies

1. Communication between the therapist and patient is essential in performing safe and effective mobility tasks.

2. A patient who is dependent should be repositioned at least every two hours to prevent skin breakdown.

3. Shear and friction forces should be minimized during mobility and transfer tasks to prevent integumentary injury.

4. The level of physical assistance required during a mobility or transfer task is a function of the amount of assistance the therapist must provide in order for the patient to safely complete the task.

5. Levels of physical assistance for transfers include independent, supervision, contact guard, minimal assist, moderate assist, maximal assist, and dependent.

6. Dependent transfers may be performed either with physical assistance from staff or a mechanical lift device.

7. Dependent transfers include three-person carry/lift, two-person lift, dependent squat pivot transfer, and hydraulic lift.

8. Assisted transfers include sliding board transfer, stand pivot transfer, and stand step transfer.

9. The adult standard wheelchair seat specifications are 18 inches wide, 16 inches deep, and 20 inches high.

10. A patient's physical and mental abilities and limitations must be considered when making recommendations for wheelchair prescription.

11. Parallel bars provide the most stable environment for patients who are beginning to initiate standing and ambulation activities.

12. Levels of weight bearing include non-weight bearing, toe touch weight bearing, partial weight bearing, weight bearing as tolerated, and full weight bearing.

13. An appropriately fit walker, crutches or cane requires 20-25 degrees of elbow flexion.

14. A straight cane is not appropriate for patients who are partial weight bearing.

15. When using an assistive device, the gait pattern utilized should be dependent on the patient's weight bearing status and overall condition.

16. Gait patterns include two-point, three-point, four-point, swing-to, and swing-through.

17. Guidelines for guarding a patient during ambulation activities may require modification or the assist of a second therapist depending on the patient's size, impairments, and abilities.

18. During stair training, the physical therapist assistant should be positioned behind the patient while ascending and in front of the patient when descending.

19. An arterial line is a monitoring device consisting of a catheter that is inserted into an artery. The device is used to measure blood pressure or to obtain blood samples.

20. A nasal cannula is a commonly used device for oxygen therapy, capable of delivering up to six liters of oxygen per minute.

21. A suprapubic catheter is an indwelling urinary catheter that is surgically inserted directly into the patient's bladder.

22. Doppler ultrasonography is a non-invasive test that evaluates blood flow in the major veins, arteries, and cerebrovascular system.

23. Magnetic resonance imaging is a non-invasive technique that utilizes magnetic fields to produce an image of bone and soft tissue.

Therapeutic Modalities

24. Methods of heat transfer include conduction, convection, conversion, evaporation, and radiation.

25. Ice massage should be applied using small, overlapping circles or strokes. An area 10 centimeters by 15 centimeters can be covered in 5 to 10 minutes.

26. Patients typically progress through a series of different sensations during ice massage including intense cold, burning, aching, and analgesia.

27. Ice massage typically cools tissues more rapidly than other types of cryotherapy such as an ice pack or ice bag. The cold pack should be applied over a moist cold towel to increase the initial magnitude of cooling.

28. Cold baths allow for circumferential contact with the cooling agent, however, they require the lower extremity to be in a gravity-dependent position.

Equipment, Devices, and Technologies; Therapeutic Modalities Essentials

29. Controlled cold compression units combine cryotherapy and compression. The units allow therapists to precisely control the temperature of the cold and the amount of compression.

30. A Cryo Cuff is a commercially available device used to provide mild cooling and compression. The device consists of a nylon sleeve connected to a container using a plastic tube.

31. Vapocoolant sprays produce very rapid cooling through evaporation with temperature changes occurring only in the epidermis. The primary use of vapocoolant sprays is to treat trigger points.

32. Relative changes in surface tissue temperature will be influenced by the intensity of the heating agent, time of the exposure, and thermal conductivity of the tissues.

33. Superficial heating agents produce the largest temperature elevation within 0.5 centimeters from the skin surface.

34. Application of a hot pack requires six to eight towel layers. If commercial hot pack covers are used, they typically are equivalent to two or three layers of towels.

35. A patient should not lie on top of a hot pack since this tends to remove water from the hot pack. This can result in an accelerated rate of heating and an increased risk of burns.

36. Fluidotherapy is a superficial heating agent that generates dry heat through forced convection by circulating warm air and small cellulose particles.

37. An infrared lamp produces superficial heating of tissue through radiant heat. Optimal absorption occurs when the infrared radiation strikes the target area perpendicularly.

38. Paraffin has a low specific heat which enhances a patient's ability to tolerate heat compared to heat from water at the same temperature.

39. Paraffin can be applied using the dip-wrap method, dip-reimmersion method or paint application method.

40. Thermal effects of ultrasound include acceleration of metabolic rate, modulation of pain, reduction of muscle spasm, decreased joint stiffness, alteration of nerve conduction velocity, increased circulation, and increased soft tissue extensibility.

41. Nonthermal effects of ultrasound include increased cell and skin membrane permeability, increased intracellular calcium levels, facilitation of tissue repair, and promotion of normal cell function.

42. A frequency setting of 1 MHz when using ultrasound is used for deeper tissues (up to five centimeters) while a setting of 3 MHz is used for more superficial tissues (one to two centimeters).

43. An area two to three times the size of the ultrasound transducer typically requires a duration of five minutes.

44. The duty cycle of ultrasound is calculated by dividing the time during which sound is delivered (on time) by the total time (on time + off time) and multiplying the result by 100.

45. Phonophoresis is not likely to produce burns or damage skin since the technique transports whole molecules instead of ions into the body's tissue.

46. Shortwave diathermy can be delivered in a continuous or pulsed mode. A pulsed mode is typically utilized to attain nonthermal effects while a continuous mode is used for thermal effects.

47. The patient's subjective heat sensation response is used to estimate the amount of energy delivered and corresponding temperature increase with continuous diathermy.

48. The minimal erythemal dose refers to the smallest dose of ultraviolet light needed to produce an area of mild redness within eight hours of ultraviolet exposure that disappears within 24 hours after exposure.

49. The properties of water essential for physical therapist assistants to understand include buoyancy, resistance, specific gravity, specific heat, total drag force, and viscosity.

50. Hydrotherapy can be administered using a variety of equipment including an extremity tank, lowboy tank, highboy tank, Hubbard tank, and therapeutic pool.

51. A flexed position of the spine results in greater separation of the posterior structures including the facet joints and intervertebral foramen when using mechanical lumbar traction. An extended position of the spine results in greater separation of the anterior structures including the disk spaces.

52. Static traction may be desirable for more acute conditions or if the patient's symptoms are slightly exaggerated by movement.

Equipment, Devices, and Technologies; Therapeutic Modalities Essentials

53. Intermittent traction may be desirable for joint mobilization or for patients who cannot tolerate static traction.

54. A force of 25% of a patient's body weight may be adequate to treat muscle spasm, disk protrusion, and stretch soft tissue when using mechanical lumbar traction. A force of up to 50% of the body weight is required for actual separation of the vertebrae.

55. A supine position is used more often for cervical traction since the traction force does not have to overcome the force exerted by gravity.

56. A force of 7-10% of a patient's body weight (11-15 pounds) may be adequate to treat muscle spasm, stretch soft tissue, and reduce disk protrusion using cervical traction.

57. A force of 13-20% of a patient's body weight (20-30 pounds) may be necessary for joint distraction using cervical traction.

58. Compression garments are most often used to control edema, limit scar formation after burns, and improve venous circulation in active patients.

59. An intermittent pneumatic compression pump is primarily used to reduce chronic or post-traumatic edema and requires adjusting the parameters of inflation pressure, on/off ratio, and total treatment time.

60. A patient's joint must be aligned correctly with the axis of the CPM to receive safe and effective treatment. A rate of two cycles per minute allows most patients to tolerate the CPM without difficulty.

61. For an action potential to be evoked using electrical stimulation, the amplitude of the stimulus and pulse duration must be sufficient to overcome the established threshold.

62. Direct current is characterized by a constant flow of electrons from the anode to the cathode (for a period of greater than one second) without interruption.

63. Alternating current is characterized by polarity that continuously changes from positive to negative with a change in direction of current flow.

64. Pulsatile current is characterized by the non-continuous flow of direct or alternating current.

65. Small electrodes exhibit increased current density, increased impedance, and decreased current flow. Large electrodes exhibit decreased current density, decreased impedance, and increased current flow.

66. The effectiveness of a current to target specific excitable tissue is dependent on adequate intensity to reach the threshold, current onset fast enough to reduce accommodation (i.e., rise time), and duration long enough to exceed the capacitance of the tissue (i.e., phase duration).

67. Neuromuscular electrical stimulation (NMES) is a technique used to facilitate skeletal muscle activity. Functional electrical stimulation (FES) uses electrical stimulation to create or enhance the performance of a functional activity.

68. The most commonly used modes for TENS include conventional, acupuncture-like, brief intense, and noxious.

69. Interferential current combines two medium frequency alternating waveforms that are biphasic. Interferential current is most often used for pain relief, increased circulation, and muscle stimulation.

70. Iontophoresis is based on the theory that like charges repel and as a result, ions in a solution of similar charge will move away from the electrical source and into the body. The rate of ion delivery is determined by the concentration of the ion, the pH of the solution, the current density, and the duration of the treatment.

71. The likelihood of a burn using iontophoresis can be decreased by increasing the size of the cathode relative to the anode, decreasing the current density, and increasing the space between the electrodes.

72. Biofeedback can be utilized to receive information related to motor performance, kinesthetic performance or physiological response. A high sensitivity setting will detect extremely small amounts of electrical activity while a low sensitivity setting will detect only large amounts of electrical activity.

73. Descriptive characteristics of massage techniques include direction, duration, frequency, pressure, rhythm, and speed.

74. Commonly used massage techniques include effleurage, friction, petrissage, tapotement, and vibration.

Equipment, Devices, and Technologies; Therapeutic Modalities Proficiencies

Equipment, Devices, and Technologies Proficiencies

1. Levels of Physical Assistance

Identify the level of physical assistance associated with each of the descriptions. Answers must be selected from the Word Bank and can be used only once.

Word Bank: dependent, independent, maximal assist, minimal assist, moderate assist, supervision

Level	Description
a	The patient requires a therapist to observe throughout the completion of the task.
b	The therapist exerts all of the effort to perform the task.
c	The patient requires 50% assist from the therapist to complete the task.
d	The patient does not require any assistance to complete the task.
e	The patient requires 25% assist from the therapist to complete the task.
f	The patient requires 75% assist from the therapist to complete the task.

2. Wheelchair Measurements

Identify the most appropriate wheelchair component associated with each of the obtained measurements. Answers must be selected from the Word Bank and can be used only once. Secondly, identify the final value in inches for each component based on the obtained measurement.

Word Bank: armrest height, back height, seat depth, seat height, seat width

Component	Obtained Measurement	Final Value
a	7 inches from the seat of the chair to the olecranon process with the elbow flexed to 90 degrees.	b
c	18 inches from the user's heel to the popliteal fold.	d
e	18 inches from the posterior buttock, along the lateral thigh to the popliteal fold.	f
g	20 inches from the seat of the chair to the floor of the axilla with the user's shoulder flexed to 90 degrees.	h
i	17 inches represents the widest aspect of the user's buttocks, hips or thighs.	j

Equipment, Devices, and Technologies; Therapeutic Modalities Proficiencies

Equipment, Devices, and Technologies Proficiencies

3. Levels of Weight Bearing

Identify the level of weight bearing associated with each of the descriptions. Answers must be selected from the Word Bank and can be used only once.

Word Bank: full weight bearing, non-weight bearing, partial weight bearing, toe touch weight bearing, weight bearing as tolerated

Level	Description
a	A patient using axillary crutches is able to transmit approximately 25% of their weight through the involved lower extremity.
b	A patient uses a single cane during ambulation.
c	A patient is permitted to vary the amount of weight bearing based on their relative comfort level and the amount of pain present.
d	A patient is unable to transmit weight through the involved lower extremity, but may place a portion of the involved foot on the ground to assist with balance.
e	A patient is unable to transmit weight through the involved extremity or have the foot come in contact with the floor.

4. Assistive Device Selection

Identify the most appropriate assistive device for each patient based on the supplied description. Answers must be selected from the Word Bank and can be used only once.

Word Bank: axillary crutches, cane, Lofstrand crutches, parallel bars, walker

Level	Description
a	A 34-year-old male in an acute care hospital prepares to ambulate for the first time following a compound tibia fracture treated with internal fixation.
b	An 83-year-old female that often experiences transient periods of dizziness while walking in the home.
c	A 21-year-old female that is toe touch weight bearing following a grade II knee sprain.
d	A 74-year-old female that experiences subtle balance changes when walking on uneven ground.
e	A 28-year-old male that is partial weight bearing on the right ankle following an ankle sprain. The patient is unable to tolerate pressure in the axillary region due to recent removal of a benign cyst.

Equipment, Devices, and Technologies; Therapeutic Modalities Proficiencies

Equipment, Devices, and Technologies Proficiencies

5. Wheelchair Frame

Identify the most appropriate wheelchair frame for each patient based on the supplied description. Answers must be selected from the Word Bank and can be used only once.

Word Bank: amputee frame, hemi frame, one-hand drive frame, power wheelchair frame, reclining frame, ultralight frame

Frame	Description
a	Patient is able to independently propel the wheelchair, however, the center of gravity is shifted posteriorly.
b	Patient is able to independently propel the wheelchair using one or both of the lower extremities.
c	Patient is involved in sports activities without the need for postural supports.
d	Patient is able to independently propel the wheelchair using one upper extremity.
e	Patient is unable to independently propel the wheelchair.
f	Patient is unable to sit upright for extended periods of time.

Equipment, Devices, and Technologies;
Therapeutic Modalities Proficiencies

Equipment, Devices, and Technologies Proficiencies

6. Equipment and Devices Basics

Mark each statement as True or False. If the statement is False, correct the statement in the space provided.

	True/False	Statement
a		A dependent squat pivot transfer is used to transfer a patient who cannot stand independently and is unable to bear any weight through the lower extremities.
	Correction:	
b		The standard adult wheelchair has 16 inches of seat width, 18 inches of seat depth, and 20 inches of seat height.
	Correction:	
c		Wheelchair seat depth is determined by measuring from the posterior buttock, along the lateral thigh to the popliteal fold and adding two inches.
	Correction:	
d		An appropriately fit axillary crutch should result in the patient having 20-25 degrees of elbow flexion when grasping the hand grip.
	Correction:	
e		A custom molded wheelchair seat is warranted for patients with pelvic obliquity or fixed asymmetrical deformity.
	Correction:	

Equipment, Devices, and Technologies; Therapeutic Modalities Proficiencies

Equipment, Devices, and Technologies Proficiencies

True/False	Statement
f	A cane can be used to improve balance in patients that are partial weight bearing.
Correction:	
g	Lofstrand crutches can be used with a variety of gait patterns including four-point, swing-to, and swing-through.
Correction:	
h	A gastric tube is a plastic tube inserted through a nostril that extends into the stomach.
Correction:	
i	A suprapubic catheter is applied over the shaft of the penis and is held in place by a padded strap or adhesive tape.
Correction:	
j	Myelography utilizes a contrast medium that is injected into the epidural space by spinal puncture.
Correction:	

Equipment, Devices, and Technologies; Therapeutic Modalities Proficiencies

Therapeutic Modalities Proficiencies

7. Heat Transfer

Identify the type of heat transfer utilized by each therapeutic modality. Answers should be selected from the Word Bank. Answers can be used more than once.

Word Bank: conduction, convection, conversion, evaporation, radiation

Modality	Heat Transfer
fluidotherapy	a
paraffin	b
vapocoolant spray	c
hot pack	d
whirlpool	e
ultrasound	f
diathermy	g
ice massage	h
ultraviolet light	i

8. Therapeutic Effects of Cryotherapy

Potential therapeutic effects of cryotherapy are listed. Mark each statement as True or False.

True/False	Effects
a	increased metabolic rate
b	decreased nerve conduction velocity
c	decreased tone
d	decreased pain threshold
e	decreased blood flow to the treatment area

Equipment, Devices, and Technologies; Therapeutic Modalities Proficiencies

Therapeutic Modalities Proficiencies

9. Indications/Contraindications of Cryotherapy

Mark each condition as an indication or contraindication of cryotherapy.

	Indication/Contraindication	Condition
a		bursitis
b		infection
c		cold urticaria
d		tendonitis
e		tenosynovitis
f		skin anesthesia
g		Raynaud's phenomenon
h		muscle spasm

10. Cooling Agents Matching

Assign each of the descriptions to the most appropriate cooling agent. More than one of the descriptions may apply to each cooling agent. The number of desired responses for each cooling agent is identified in parentheses.

1. Effective for small and irregular contoured areas
2. Allows simultaneous application of cold and compression
3. Short duration time (i.e., 10 minutes or less)
4. Unable to observe target area during treatment
5. Difficult to apply spray uniformly
6. Requires the extremity to be in a gravity dependent position

Cooling Agent		Description	
cold bath	a		(1)
controlled cold compression unit	b		(2)
Cryo Cuff	c		(2)
ice massage	d		(2)
vapocoolant spray	e		(1)

Equipment, Devices, and Technologies; Therapeutic Modalities Proficiencies

Therapeutic Modalities Proficiencies

11. Therapeutic Effects of Superficial Thermotherapy

Potential therapeutic effects of superficial thermotherapy are listed. Mark each statement as True or False.

	True/False	Effects
a		increased tone
b		decreased collagen extensibility
c		increased pain threshold
d		decreased nerve conduction velocity
e		increased metabolic rate

12. Indications/Contraindications of Superficial Thermotherapy

Mark each condition as an indication or contraindication of superficial thermotherapy.

	Indication/Contraindication	Condition
a		decreased range of motion
b		over an area of malignancy
c		subacute or chronic pain
d		muscle spasm
e		arterial disease
f		subacute or chronic inflammatory conditions
g		peripheral vascular disease
h		thrombophlebitis

Equipment, Devices, and Technologies; Therapeutic Modalities Proficiencies

Therapeutic Modalities Proficiencies

13. Heating Agents Matching

Assign each of the descriptions to the most appropriate heating agent. More than one of the descriptions may apply to each heating agent. The number of desired responses for each heating agent is identified in parentheses.

1. Can produce thermal and nonthermal effects
2. Provides a moist, comfortable heat
3. Tends to dry skin
4. Useful for desensitization of the distal extremities
5. Does not require direct contact with the treatment area
6. May serve to moisturize the skin
7. Capable of reaching deeper tissues

Heating Agent	Description	
diathermy	a	(2)
fluidotherapy	b	(1)
hot pack	c	(1)
infrared lamp	d	(2)
paraffin	e	(1)
ultrasound	f	(2)

Equipment, Devices, and Technologies; Therapeutic Modalities Proficiencies

Therapeutic Modalities Proficiencies

14. Parameters and Procedures

Mark each statement as True or False. If the statement is False, correct the statement in the space provided.

	True/False	Statement
a		The Cryo Cuff should be held approximately 6-8 inches above the level of the sleeve during filling.
	Correction:	
b		A vapocoolant spray should be applied perpendicular to the direction of the muscle fibers.
	Correction:	
c		6-8 layers of towels are necessary for hot pack application.
	Correction:	
d		Ultrasound frequency of 3 MHz heats deep tissue (up to 5 cm), while 1 MHz heats superficial tissue (1-2 cm).
	Correction:	
e		The temperature of a paraffin bath should be maintained between 107 and 112 degrees Fahrenheit.
	Correction:	
f		A 20% duty cycle with an on time of 1 second would have an off time of 5 seconds.
	Correction:	
g		An area two to three times the size of the ultrasound transducer typically requires a treatment duration of five minutes.
	Correction:	

Equipment, Devices, and Technologies; Therapeutic Modalities Proficiencies

Therapeutic Modalities Proficiencies

True/False	Statement
h	A patient's subjective heat sensation response is an important factor when determining the amount of energy delivered with diathermy.
Correction:	
i	The minimal erythemal dose is characterized by a dose that results in erythema that lasts 1-3 days with clear redness and mild desquamation.
Correction:	
j	Buoyancy refers to the magnitude of the cohesive forces between the molecules specific to the fluid.
Correction:	
k	Hot packs are required to be in place for 5-10 minutes to achieve the desired therapeutic effects.
Correction:	
l	An infrared lamp's primary therapeutic effect is the enhancement of deep tissue healing.
Correction:	
m	During application of fluidotherapy, patients can perform active exercises of the distal extremity.
Correction:	
n	The rate of tissue cooling following heating with diathermy is significantly slower than the rate of tissue cooling with ultrasound.
Correction:	
o	Ultraviolet light is absorbed 1-2 centimeters into the skin.
Correction:	

Equipment, Devices, and Technologies; Therapeutic Modalities Proficiencies

Therapeutic Modalities Proficiencies

15. Electrotherapy Terminology

Identify the electrotherapy term most closely associated with the supplied description. Answers must be selected from the Word Bank and can be used only once.

Word Bank: alternating current, current, direct current, frequency, phase duration, pulsatile current, pulse duration, resistance, rise time, voltage

Terminology	Description
a	The time it takes for the current to move from zero to the peak intensity within each phase.
b	Characterized by a constant flow of electrons from the anode (i.e., positive electrode) to the cathode (i.e., negative electrode) for a period of greater than one second without interruption.
c	The number of pulses delivered through each channel per second.
d	The ability of a material to oppose the flow of ions through it.
e	Characterized by polarity that continuously changes from positive to negative with the change in the direction of current flow.
f	The amount of time it takes for two phases of a pulse with biphasic current.
g	A measure of the electromotive force or the electrical potential difference.
h	Characterized by the non-continuous flow of direct or alternating current.
i	The directed flow of charge from one place to another.
j	The amount of time it takes for one phase of a pulse.

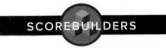

SCOREBUILDERS

Equipment, Devices, and Technologies; Therapeutic Modalities Proficiencies

Therapeutic Modalities Proficiencies

16. Electrical Current and Electrode Size

Identify the relevant influence of small electrodes versus large electrodes on selected elements of electrical current. Place the word "increased" or "decreased" in each of the blank cells.

	Small Electrodes	Large Electrodes
current density	a	b
impedance	c	d
current flow	e	f

17. TENS Parameters

Identify the specific TENS technique most closely associated with the supplied description. The specific technique should be selected from the Word Bank. A specific technique can be used more than once or not at all.

Word Bank: acupuncture-like, brief intense, conventional, noxious

Technique	Description
a	characterized by high pulse frequency and short pulse duration
b	often administered with a small probe applicator
c	the duration is 30-60 seconds for each point
d	the amplitude is sufficient for strong paresthesia
e	characterized by high density current that is described as uncomfortable or painful
f	the amplitude is sufficient for a sensory response
g	characterized by high pulse frequency and long pulse duration with moderate current amplitude

Equipment, Devices, and Technologies; Therapeutic Modalities Proficiencies

Therapeutic Modalities Proficiencies

18. Massage Techniques

Identify the specific massage technique most closely associated with the supplied description. Answers must be selected from the Word Bank and can be used only once.

Word Bank: effleurage, friction, petrissage, tapotement, vibration

Technique	Description
a	A technique described as kneading, where the muscle is squeezed and rolled under the therapist's hands.
b	A technique that provides stimulation through rapid alternating movements such as tapping, hacking, cupping, and slapping.
c	A technique characterized by a light stroke that produces a reflexive response.
d	A technique that incorporates small circular motions over a trigger point or muscle spasm.
e	A technique that places the therapist's hands or fingers firmly over an area and utilizes a rapid, shaking motion.

Equipment, Devices, and Technologies; Therapeutic Modalities Answer Key

Equipment, Devices, and Technologies

1. Levels of Physical Assistance
a. supervision
b. dependent
c. moderate assist
d. independent
e. minimal assist
f. maximal assist

2. Wheelchair Measurements
a. armrest height
b. 8 inches
c. seat height
d. 20 inches
e. seat depth
f. 16 inches
g. back height
h. 16 inches
i. seat width
j. 19 inches

3. Levels of Weight Bearing
a. partial weight bearing
b. full weight bearing
c. weight bearing as tolerated
d. toe touch weight bearing
e. non-weight bearing

4. Assistive Device Selection
a. parallel bars
b. walker
c. axillary crutches
d. cane
e. Lofstrand crutches

5. Wheelchair Frame
a. amputee frame
b. hemi frame
c. ultralight frame
d. one-hand drive frame
e. power wheelchair frame
f. reclining frame

6. Equipment and Devices Basics*
a. FALSE: Correction: A dependent squat pivot transfer is used to transfer a patient who cannot stand independently, but is able to bear some weight through the trunk and lower extremities.
b. FALSE: Correction: The standard adult wheelchair has 18 inches of width, 16 inches of depth, and 20 inches of height.
c. FALSE: Correction: Wheelchair seat depth is determined by measuring from the posterior buttock, along the lateral thigh to the popliteal fold and subtracting two inches.
d. TRUE
e. TRUE
f. FALSE: Correction: A cane can be used to improve balance, however, does not permit partial weight bearing.
g. TRUE
h. FALSE: Correction: A gastric tube is a tube inserted through a small incision in the abdomen into the stomach.
i. FALSE: Correction: A suprapubic catheter is an indwelling urinary catheter that is surgically inserted directly into a patient's bladder.
j. TRUE

*The correction presented for each false statement is an example of several possible corrections.

Therapeutic Modalities

7. Heat Transfer
a. convection
b. conduction
c. evaporation
d. conduction
e. convection
f. conversion
g. conversion
h. conduction
i. radiation

8. Therapeutic Effects of Cryotherapy
a. FALSE
b. TRUE
c. TRUE
d. FALSE
e. TRUE

Equipment, Devices, and Technologies; Therapeutic Modalities Answer Key

9. Indications/Contraindications of Cryotherapy

a. indication
b. contraindication
c. contraindication
d. indication
e. indication
f. contraindication
g. contraindication
h. indication

10. Cooling Agents Matching

a. 6
b. 2,4
c. 2,4
d. 1,3
e. 5

11. Therapeutic Effects of Superficial Thermotherapy

a. FALSE
b. FALSE
c. TRUE
d. FALSE
e. TRUE

12. Indications/Contraindications of Superficial Thermotherapy

a. indication
b. contraindication
c. indication
d. indication
e. contraindication
f. indication
g. contraindication
h. contraindication

13. Heating Agents Matching

a. 1,7
b. 4
c. 2
d. 3,5
e. 6
f. 1,7

14. Parameters and Procedures*

a. FALSE - Correction: The Cryo Cuff should be held 15-18 inches above the level of the sleeve during filling.

b. FALSE - Correction: A vapocoolant spray should be applied parallel to the direction of the muscle fibers.

c. TRUE

d. FALSE - Correction: Ultrasound frequency of 3 MHz heats superficial tissue (1-2 cm), while 1 MHz heats deep tissue (up to 5 cm).

e. FALSE - Correction: The temperature of a paraffin bath should be maintained between 113 and 122 degrees Fahrenheit.

f. FALSE - Correction: A 20% duty cycle with an on time of 1 second would have an off time of 4 seconds (duty cycle = on time / on + off time x 100).

g. TRUE

h. TRUE

i. FALSE - Correction: First-degree erythemal dose is characterized by a dose that results in erythema that lasts 1-3 days with clear redness and mild desquamation.

j. FALSE - Correction: The supplied definition describes viscosity. The principle of buoyancy states that there is an upward force on the body when immersed in water equal to the amount of water that has been displaced by the body.

k. FALSE - Correction: Hot packs are required to be in place for 15-20 minutes to achieve desired therapeutic effects.

l. FALSE - Correction: An infrared lamp's main therapeutic effect is the enhancement of superficial tissue healing.

m. TRUE

n. TRUE

o. FALSE - Correction: Ultraviolet light is absorbed 1-2 millimeters into the skin.

*The correction presented for each false statement is an example of several possible corrections.

Equipment, Devices, and Technologies; Therapeutic Modalities Answer Key

15. Electrotherapy Terminology
a.   rise time
b.   direct current
c.   frequency
d.   resistance
e.   alternating current
f.   pulse duration
g.   voltage
h.   pulsatile current
i.   current
j.   phase duration

16. Electrical Current and Electrode Size
a.   increased
b.   decreased
c.   increased
d.   decreased
e.   decreased
f.   increased

17. TENS Parameters
a.   conventional
b.   noxious
c.   noxious
d.   brief intense
e.   noxious
f.   conventional
g.   brief intense

18. Massage Techniques
a.   petrissage
b.   tapotement
c.   effleurage
d.   friction
e.   vibration

Equipment, Devices, and Technologies; Therapeutic Modalities References

Equipment, Devices, and Technologies References

1. Fairchild S, O'Shea R, Washington R. *Pierson and Fairchild's Principles and Techniques of Patient Care*. Sixth Edition. Elsevier. 2018.

2. *Nurse's 3-Minute Clinical Reference*. Second Edition. Lippincott Williams & Wilkins. 2007.

3. Minor M, Minor S. *Patient Care Skills*. Seventh Edition. Prentice Hall. 2014.

4. Roy S, Wolf S, Scalzitti, D. *The Rehabilitation Specialist's Handbook*. Fourth Edition. F.A. Davis Company. 2013.

5. Batavia M. *The Wheelchair Evaluation: A Clinician's Guide*. Second Edition. Jones and Bartlett Publishers. 2010.

6. Cook AM, Hussey SM, Polgar JM. *Cook & Hussey's Assistive Technologies: Principles and Practice.* Mosby Elsevier. 2008.

7. Olson DA, DeRuyter F. *A Clinician's Guide to Assistive Technology*. Mosby Elsevier. 2002.

8. Tan J. *Practical Manual of Physical Medicine and Rehabilitation*. Second Edition. Mosby Inc. 2006.

9. Pendleton H, Schultz-Krohn W. *Occupational Therapy Practice Skills for Physical Dysfunction*. Sixth Edition. Mosby. 2006.

10. Cameron M, Monroe L. *Physical Rehabilitation: Evidence-Based Examination, Evaluation, and Intervention*. W.B. Saunders Company. 2007.

11. Prentice W, Voight M. *Techniques in Musculoskeletal Rehabilitation*. McGraw-Hill Inc. 2008.

12. Paz J, West MP. *Acute Care Handbook for Physical Therapists*. Fourth Edition. W.B. Saunders Company. 2014.

13. Hillegass E, Sadowsky S. *Essentials of Cardiopulmonary Physical Therapy*. Fourth Edition. W.B. Saunders Company. 2017.

14. Magee D. *Orthopedic Physical Assessment*. Sixth Edition. W.B. Saunders Company. 2014.

15. Dutton M. *Orthopaedic Examination, Evaluation, and Intervention*. Fourth Edition. McGraw-Hill Inc. 2017.

Equipment, Devices, and Technologies; Therapeutic Modalities References

Therapeutic Modalities References

16. Cameron M. *Physical Agents in Rehabilitation: An Evidence-Based Approach to Practice.* Fifth Edition. Elsevier. 2018.

17. Bellew J, Michlovitz S, Nolan T. *Modalities for Therapeutic Intervention.* Sixth Edition. F.A. Davis Company. 2016.

18. Prentice W. *Therapeutic Modalities in Rehabilitation.* Fifth Edition. McGraw-Hill Inc. 2018.

19. Bracciano A. *Physical Agent Modalities. Theories and Application for the Occupational Therapist.* Second Edition. Slack Inc. 2008.

20. Denegar C. *Therapeutic Modalities for Musculoskeletal Injuries.* Second Edition. Human Kinetics. 2005.

21. Belanger AY. *Evidence-Based Guide to Therapeutic Physical Agents.* Lippincott Williams & Wilkins. 2003.

22. Ruoti RG, Morris DM. *Aquatic Rehabilitation.* Lippincott Williams & Wilkins. 1997.

23. Cameron M, Monroe L. *Physical Rehabilitation: Evidence Based Examination, Evaluation, and Intervention.* W.B. Saunders Company. 2007.

24. Nelson R, Hayes K, Currier D. *Clinical Electrotherapy.* Third Edition. Appleton & Lange. 1999.

25. Kitchen S. *Electrotherapy. Evidence-Based Practice.* Churchill Livingstone. 2002.

26. Robinson A, Snyder-Mackler L. *Clinical Electrophysiology.* Third Edition. Williams & Wilkins. 2007.

27. De Domenico G, Wood E. *Beard's Massage.* Fifth Edition. W.B. Saunders Company. 2007.

28. Fritz S. *Mosby's Fundamentals of Therapeutic Massage.* Second Edition. Mosby, Inc. 2000.

29. Houglum P. *Therapeutic Exercise for Athletic Injuries.* Human Kinetics. 2001.

30. McKinnis L. *Fundamentals of Musculoskeletal Imaging.* Fourth Edition. F.A. Davis. 2014.

9

SAFETY AND PROTECTION; PROFESSIONAL RESPONSIBILITIES; RESEARCH

Scott Giles
Michael Fillyaw

Safety and Protection represent approximately 4 - 6 questions (2.7% - 4%) on the NPTE-PTA.

Professional Responsibilities represent approximately 3 - 4 questions (2% - 2.7%) on the NPTE-PTA.

Research and Evidence-based Practice represent approximately 2 - 3 questions (1.3% - 2%) on the NPTE-PTA.

Contributors

Shawn Paquette

CHAPTER 9
Safety and Protection; Professional Responsibilities; Research

Safety and Protection

Infection Control

Infectious Disease

Infectious disease is defined as a condition where an organism invades a host and develops a parasitic relationship with the host. The invasion and multiplication of the microorganisms produces an immune response with subsequent signs and symptoms.

Potential Symptoms of Infectious Disease

• Fever, chill, malaise	• Headache
• Rash, skin lesion	• Stiff neck
• Bleeding from gums	• Myalgia
• Joint effusion	• Convulsions
• Diarrhea	• Confusion
• Frequency, urgency	• Tachycardia
• Cough, sore throat	• Hypotension
• Nausea, vomiting	

Chain of Transmission for Infection

1. Causative agent, bacteria, pathogen, virus
2. Reservoir of humans, animals, inanimate objects
3. Portal of exit through blood, intestinal tract, respiratory tract, skin/mucous membrane, open lesion, excretions, tears or semen
4. Transmission through airborne, contact, vector, vehicle or droplet modes
5. Portal of entry through non-intact skin, blood, mucous membrane, inhalation, ingestion or percutaneous injection
6. Susceptible host regarding age, health status, nutrition, and environmental status

Standard Precautions[3,4]

Standard Precautions are revised guidelines that update Universal Precautions and are designed for the care of all patients in hospitals regardless of infection or diagnosis.

These precautions combine Universal and body substance isolation precautions and apply to all blood/body fluids, secretions, and excretions.

Hand Washing

✓ Use plain soap for routine hand washing; use an antimicrobial agent for specific incidences based on the established infection control policy (Fig. 9-1).

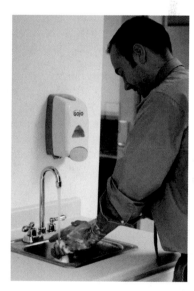

Fig. 9-1: A therapist washing his hands prior to initiating treatment.

Gloves

✓ Wear gloves when touching all body fluids, blood secretions, excretions, and contaminated items.

✓ Change gloves between tasks with a patient after coming in contact with infectious material. Remove gloves immediately, avoid touching non-contaminated items, and wash hands at that time.

Mask

✓ Wear a mask/eye protection/face shield for protection during activities that are at risk for splashing of any body fluids.

Gown

✓ Wear a gown for protection during activities that are at risk for splashing of any body fluids. Remove gown immediately and wash hands.

Patient Care Equipment

✓ Handle all patient equipment in a manner that prevents transfer of microorganisms.

✓ Ensure that all reusable equipment is properly sanitized prior to reuse.

Occupational Health and Bloodborne Pathogens

✓ Vigilance is required when handling/disposing of sharp instruments. Never recap needles or remove syringes by hand. All sharps disposals should use puncture-resistant containers.

✓ Mouthpieces, resuscitation bags, and ventilation devices should be used as an alternative to mouth-to-mouth resuscitation.

Transmission-based Precautions[3,4]

Transmission-based precautions are updated guidelines for the particular care of specified patients infected with epidemiologically important pathogens transmitted by airborne, droplet or contact modes. These are additional precautions that should be implemented in addition to Standard Precautions.

Airborne Precautions

Airborne precautions reduce the risk of airborne transmission of infectious agents through evaporated droplets in air or dust particles containing infectious agents.

• Private room with monitored negative air pressure

• Six to twelve air changes within the room per hour

• Room door should remain closed with patient remaining within the room

• Respiratory protection worn when entering the room

• Limit patient's transport outside of the room for only essential purposes; patient should wear a mask during transport

Examples
Measles, varicella, tuberculosis

Droplet Precautions

Droplet precautions reduce the risk of droplet transmission of infectious agents through contact of the mucous membranes of the mouth and nose, contact with the conjunctivae, and through coughing, sneezing, talking or suctioning. This transmission requires close contact, as the infectious agents do not suspend in the air and travel only three feet or less.

• Private room

• May share a room with a patient that has an active infection of the same microorganism

• Maintain at least three feet between the patient and any contact (patient, staff, visitor)

• Room door may remain open

• Wear a mask when working within three feet of the patient

• Limit the patient's transport outside of the room for only essential purposes; patient should wear a mask during transport

Examples
Bacterial include: Haemophilus influenzae (including meningitis, pneumonia, sepsis), Neisseria meningitidis (including meningitis, pneumonia, sepsis), diphtheria, mycoplasma pneumonia, pertussis, streptococcal (group A)
Viral include: Adenovirus, influenza, mumps, parvovirus B19, rubella

Contact Precautions

Contact precautions reduce the risk of transmission of infectious agents through direct or indirect contact. Direct contact involves skin-to-skin transmission; indirect contact involves a contaminated intermediate object, usually within the patient's environment.

• Private room

• May share a room with a patient that has an active infection of the same microorganism

• Use of gloves when entering the room

• Change of gloves after direct contact with infectious material

• Take gloves off prior to leaving the room and perform proper hand washing technique

• Wear a gown if you will have substantial close contact with the patient and remove the gown prior to leaving the room

• Limit patient's transport outside of the room for essential purposes only

• Dedicate non-critical patient care equipment to one patient, do not share between patients or disinfect properly prior to using the equipment again

Examples
Gastrointestinal, respiratory, skin or wound infections, multi-drug resistant bacteria, Clostridium difficile, enterohemorrhagic Escherichia coli, Shigella, hepatitis A (for incontinence/diapered), parainfluenza virus or enteroviral infection (infants/young children), diphtheria, herpes simplex virus, impetigo, pediculosis, scabies, zoster, viral hemorrhagic infections (Ebola)

Nosocomial Infections[4]

A term used to describe an infection that is acquired during a hospitalization. The primary factor in the prevention of nosocomial infections is proper hand washing. Staff must also follow standard precautions and all infection control procedures at all times.

The CDC Guidelines for Isolation Precautions in Hospitals is a document that outlines the guidelines from collaboration between the Centers for Disease Control and Prevention (CDC) and the Hospital Infection Control Practices Advisory Committee (HICPAC). This document describes infection control within the hospital setting and provides strategies for surveillance, prevention, and control of nosocomial infections within the hospital setting.

Application of Sterile Protective Garments[3]

Gowns

- ✓ Hold gown firmly away from the sterile field
- ✓ Shake gown open so it unfolds and keep hands above waist level
- ✓ Touch only the inside of the gown as you place both arms into the sleeves
- ✓ Stop when hands reach the sleeve cuff
- ✓ The gown is tied in back

Sterile Gloves

- ✓ Use the gown's sleeve cuffs as mittens and open the glove pack
- ✓ The sterile glove has a fold at the wrist where the inside (exposed) of the glove is not sterile
- ✓ Grasp the right glove with the left hand (still using the sleeve cuff as a mitten) and pull it on over the open end of the gown sleeve
- ✓ The first three fingers of the right hand should reach under the fold (touching the sterile portion of the left glove) and hold the glove while the left hand positions inside the glove
- ✓ Once both gloves are donned, the left glove can unfold the right glove's cuff

Cap and Mask

- ✓ Wash hands
- ✓ Avoid contact with the hair while applying the cap
- ✓ All hair must be contained within the cap
- ✓ Apply a mask, if necessary, by first positioning the mask over the bridge of the nose
- ✓ The mask should fit securely over the nose and mouth
- ✓ Secure the upper ties behind the head and the lower ties behind the neck

Sterile Field Guidelines[3]

- ✓ All items on a sterile field must be (and remain) sterile
- ✓ The edges of all packaging of sterile items become non-sterile once the package is opened
- ✓ Sterile gowns are only considered sterile in the front from the waist level upwards, including the sleeves
- ✓ Only the top surface of the table or sterile drape is considered sterile, with the outer one-inch of the field considered non-sterile
- ✓ Avoid all unnecessary activity around the sterile field
- ✓ Do not talk, sneeze or cough, as it will contaminate the sterile field
- ✓ Do not turn your back to a sterile field as the back of the gown is not sterile; constant observation of the sterile field is required
- ✓ If an object on the sterile field becomes contaminated, the field is considered non-sterile and should be discarded
- ✓ Sterile fields should never be left unattended and should be prepared as close to the treatment time as possible in order to further avoid contamination
- ✓ Any item that positions or falls below waist level is considered contaminated

Infection Control Terminology

Asepsis: The elimination of the microorganisms that cause infection and the creation of a sterile field.

Contamination: A term used to describe an area, surface or item coming in contact with something that is not sterile. Contamination assumes an environment that contains microorganisms.

Hand washing: Hand washing is an important technique for asepsis. Hands should be washed with warm water and soap after jewelry has been removed. Washing should occur for a minimum of 30 seconds. Rinse thoroughly and use a paper towel to turn off water.

Medical asepsis: A technique that attempts to contain pathogens to a specific area, object or person. A primary goal is to reduce the spread of pathogens. Example: A patient with tuberculosis is hospitalized and kept in isolation.

Personal protective equipment (PPE): Items that are worn and used as barriers to protect someone who is assisting a patient with a potentially infectious disease. Personal protective equipment includes gowns, lab coats, masks, gloves, goggles, spill kits, and mouthpieces.

Sterile field: A sterile field is used to maintain surgical asepsis. A sterile field is a designated area that is considered void of all contaminants and microorganisms. There are standard and required protocols that must be followed in order to develop and maintain a sterile field.

Surgical asepsis: A state in which an area or object is without any microorganisms. Example: A sterile field.

Emergent Conditions

Allergic Reaction

Recognition: A mild to moderate allergic reaction is typically not life-threatening and may include itchy skin, skin redness, rash, hives, areas of swelling, itchy and watery eyes, runny nose, sneezing, and headache. A severe allergic reaction may include swelling of the face or mouth, difficulty swallowing or speaking, wheezing and difficulty breathing, chest tightness and pressure, tachycardia, abdominal pain, nausea and vomiting, altered mental status, and dizziness or syncope. Common allergens include pollen, dust, eggs, shellfish, milk, wheat, soy, nuts, insect stings, chemicals, latex, and medications.

Response: A severe allergic reaction can be life-threatening and requires prompt medical attention. The therapist should first try to remove the source of the allergic reaction if possible. The therapist should check the patient's airway to assess if it is compromised and begin cardiopulmonary resuscitation if necessary. If the patient uses an emergency allergy medication (e.g., EpiPen), the therapist should assist the patient to ingest or inject the medication. If the patient is having trouble breathing, the patient should not take medications orally. Emergency medical services should be called if the patient is having difficulty breathing or swallowing.

Autonomic Dysreflexia

Recognition: This condition is commonly seen in patients with a complete spinal cord injury above the level of T6 in response to some noxious stimulus (e.g., bladder distention, tight clothing). Signs and symptoms include severe hypertension, bradycardia, profuse sweating above the level of the lesion, headache, nausea, piloerection, and red and blotchy skin.

Response: The patient should first be placed in an upright position (e.g., sitting, semirecumbent) and the therapist should attempt to identify and remove the noxious stimulus. For example, a kink in the catheter may prevent urine from draining from the bladder and cause a systemic response. The therapist should then monitor the patient's vital signs and call for medical assistance.

Burns

Recognition: There are several causative factors that can result in burns including heat, chemicals, and electricity. The therapist should identify the source of the burn, the location, and extent of the burn. Burns can be classified according to depth and according to the surface area affected (e.g., rule of nines).

Response: The therapist should initially attempt to remove the source of the burn if still present. If the burn has been caused by a chemical, water should be used to dilute the substance. However, be cautious not to wash the chemical onto an unaffected portion of skin. Also, if the chemical is a dry powder, it should be brushed off the skin. If it is a thermal burn, run the affected part under a cool tap for several minutes. However, if the burn covers a large surface area, cold water should not be used as this can increase the risk for hypothermia. If it is an electrical burn, assess the patient's heart rate and respiration and monitor for signs of cardiac arrest.

For all burns, the therapist should remove any clothing or jewelry near the burn, however, should not attempt to remove clothing if it has become part of the wound. A clean towel or dressing should be placed over the wound to prevent infection. If the burn is extensive, involves the face, hands, perineum or feet or involves the respiratory system, emergency medical services should be called.

Concussion

Recognition: A concussion is a mild traumatic brain injury that occurs secondary to a blow to the head. Signs and symptoms include loss of memory, confusion, drowsiness, behavior or personality changes, light or noise sensitivity, headache, impaired vision, nausea or vomiting, lack of coordination, dizziness, and loss of consciousness. Symptoms typically occur immediately after the injury, however, they can also occur hours or days later.

Response: If a patient demonstrates signs and symptoms of a concussion, they should not be allowed to return to physical activity until cleared by a medical professional. Emergency medical services should be contacted immediately if the patient demonstrates any of the following symptoms: extreme drowsiness or loss of consciousness, a headache that will not improve, one pupil that is larger than the other, slurred speech, weakness, numbness, loss of coordination, repeated vomiting or nausea, convulsions or seizures, and increasing confusion, restlessness or agitation.

Fractures

Recognition: Observe the site of the injury and the position of the extremity. A visible deformity and the presence of bruising and/or swelling may indicate that a fracture has occurred. Other signs and symptoms include pain, tenderness, and limited movement.

Response: Peripheral pulses and sensation should be assessed distal to the injury to determine the extent of injury to nerves and blood vessels. The therapist should apply support to the site with a firm object (e.g., flat piece of wood) to stabilize the position of the extremity. The splint should immobilize the affected area as well as the adjacent joints. The patient should avoid movement of the extremity and the therapist should not try to realign the fracture. If the fracture site is open, cover it with a sterile towel or dressing. If a spinal fracture is suspected, do not move the patient.

Heat Illness

Recognition: The two primary types of heat illness are heat exhaustion and heat stroke. Heat exhaustion is a less serious condition, but can progress to heat stroke, which is a medical emergency if not treated properly. The signs and symptoms of heat exhaustion include profuse sweating, moist and pale skin, nausea, headache, dizziness, muscle cramps, weakness, rapid and shallow breathing, and a weak and rapid pulse. The signs and symptoms of heat stroke include dry skin, a flushed color, nausea, headache, labored breathing, a strong and rapid pulse, elevated temperature, contraction and dilation of the pupils, convulsions, altered mental status, and possible loss of consciousness.

Response: For any form of heat illness, the patient should be placed in a shaded or covered area and the therapist should monitor vital signs. Remove or loosen any outer clothing layers and use an ice bag or cold compress on the patient's forehead, neck, and/or groin. Water or a solution with electrolytes can be given if the person is still conscious. Do not give the patient salt tablets as this can negatively affect the electrolyte balance. Emergency medical services should be called if the patient is experiencing heat stroke or if their condition is worsening.

Heart Attack/Cardiac Arrest

Recognition: The onset of a heart attack may be sudden or gradual. Signs and symptoms typically include chest discomfort that may feel like pressure, squeezing, fullness or pain. This discomfort may spread to the arms, back, neck, jaw or stomach. Other signs and symptoms include shortness of breath, abnormal heart rate and blood pressure, sweating, nausea, lightheadedness, and anxious behavior. If a heart attack progresses to cardiac arrest, there will be a sudden loss of responsiveness and/or consciousness.

Response: If a patient is experiencing a heart attack or cardiac arrest, the therapist should first determine if the patient is responsive. If unresponsive, the therapist should call emergency medical services and have a second person locate an automated external defibrillator (AED). Cardiopulmonary resuscitation (CPR) should be initiated until an AED or emergency medical personnel arrive. An AED should be used once five cycles of CPR have been completed. To use the AED, the therapist should expose the patient's chest so the pads can be applied. Once ready the AED will analyze the patient's heart rhythm. The therapist should follow the prompts from the AED. If the AED plans to "shock" the patient, the therapist should move away from the patient and clear the immediate area.

Hypothermia/Frostbite

Recognition: Hypothermia occurs when a person has been exposed to cold temperatures for a prolonged period of time. Signs and symptoms of hypothermia include shivering, exhaustion, decreased motor function, slurred speech, drowsiness, confusion, memory loss, and decreased vital signs. Infants will present with low energy and their skin will be cold and bright red. When exposed to freezing temperatures, frostbite may occur. Symptoms of frostbite include white or grayish-yellow skin that is numb and feels firm or waxy.

Response: The therapist should assess the patient's body temperature via palpation, as well as assess the patient's verbal and motor responses. To treat hypothermia, the patient should be moved into a warm room and remove any wet clothing. The therapist should attempt to warm the patient, starting with the core of the body, with dry towels or blankets or with skin-to-skin contact. If the patient loses consciousness or if their body temperature is below 95 degrees Fahrenheit, emergency medical services should be contacted immediately. For cases of frostbite, the affected area should be immersed in warm (not hot) water or be warmed using body heat. Massage should not be used over the affected areas since the additional pressure can increase the amount of tissue damage.

Insulin-related Illness

Recognition: Hypoglycemia is caused by low blood glucose and has a rapid onset. Signs and symptoms include pale and moist skin, rapid heart rate, shallow breathing, dizziness, headache, altered vision, hunger, excited and agitated behavior, confusion, seizure, and loss of consciousness. Hyperglycemia is caused by elevated blood glucose and has a slower onset. When hyperglycemia is left untreated for long periods of time, it can lead to ketoacidosis and diabetic coma, which are life-threatening conditions. Signs and symptoms of hyperglycemia include thirst, frequent urination, and glucose in the urine. Symptoms of ketoacidosis include fruity smelling breath, deep, labored breathing, nausea and vomiting, and a dry tongue.

Response: In cases of hypoglycemia, the patient should ingest some form of sugar (e.g., orange juice). If the patient is not conscious, an intravenous glucose injection should be administered by a medical professional. The patient should rest as much as possible until blood glucose levels have returned to normal. In cases of ketoacidosis, emergency medical services should be called as the patient will likely need to be injected with insulin. The therapist should avoid giving the patient any form of sugar.

Laceration (External Bleeding)

Recognition: Lacerations can vary in severity depending on the size, depth, and location of the laceration. Arterial bleeding is characterized by spurting blood that is bright red in appearance, while venous bleeding is characterized by flowing blood that is more purple in appearance.

Response: A therapist should apply gloves if available before applying pressure to the wound with a sterile towel. Direct pressure should be maintained over the laceration until bleeding ceases. If arterial bleeding occurs, then intermittent pressure may need to be applied to the artery just proximal to the site of the injury. If blood flow is excessive, the extremity should be elevated above the level of the heart. Prolonged pressure with use of a tourniquet should be avoided. Emergency medical services should be called if a cut is bleeding severely, blood is spurting out or the bleeding does not stop after ten minutes of steady pressure.

Obstructed Airway

Recognition: Ask the patient if they are choking. If they can speak, cough or breathe, do not attempt to intervene, but stay close by. If they cannot speak, cough or breathe, the therapist should provide assistance.

Response: The therapist should first check the patient's mouth and attempt to remove any foreign objects. The therapist should then position themselves behind the patient with their hands clasped (i.e., one hand in a closed fist with the other hand covering it) over the patient's abdomen (i.e., above the umbilicus and below the diaphragm). The therapist then gives forceful, abrupt thrusts inward and upward. This is done until the object becomes dislodged. If the patient becomes unconscious, the patient should be placed in supine and the therapist should perform rescue breathing and abdominal thrusts. When treating a child under the age of one, the child should be placed in a recumbent prone position over the therapist's forearm with the head supported while the therapist provides four forceful blows to the interscapular region with the heel of the hand. The therapist then turns the child over and provides four thrusts to the lower sternum with two fingers. This cycle is repeated until the object is expelled.

Orthostatic Hypotension

Recognition: Orthostatic hypotension occurs when a patient attempts to stand from a sitting or supine position. As a result of reduced venous return, perfusion of the brain decreases and results in symptoms of dizziness or syncope. Other symptoms may include weakness, altered vision, nausea, and confusion.

Response: Treatment for this condition is similar to that of shock, in that the patient should be positioned in a supine position with the legs elevated so that the blood supply can better perfuse the brain.

Pulmonary Embolism

Recognition: The common signs and symptoms of a pulmonary embolism include shortness of breath, a cough (sometimes with bloody sputum), and chest pain that worsens with deep breathing. Other signs and symptoms may include lightheadedness or dizziness, tachypnea, a rapid and irregular heart rate, fever, diaphoresis, anxious behavior, cyanosis, clammy skin, and leg pain and swelling.

Response: Emergency medical services should be called immediately, especially if the onset of symptoms is sudden. The therapist should continue to monitor vital signs until emergency medical personnel arrive.

Seizures

Recognition: There are several different types of seizures including myoclonic, tonic, clonic, tonic-clonic, atonic, and absence. Each form of seizure will present differently. Symptoms may include convulsions, muscle rigidity, loss of consciousness, jerking movements or loss of muscle tone.

Response: The therapist should place the patient in a safe location and position without trying to constrain the patient's movements. The patient's respiratory rate and quality should be monitored. The therapist should ensure that the airway stays patent, though an object should not be placed in the patient's mouth. When the convulsions subside, the patient's head should be turned to one side in case vomiting occurs.

Shock

Recognition: Shock is caused by the loss of perfusion to the body's organs, often from excessive bleeding, excessive heat or movement from a supine to a vertical position. Signs and symptoms of shock include pale, moist, cool skin, diaphoresis, shallow and irregular breathing, a weak and rapid pulse, hypotension, low body temperature, weakness, dizziness, nausea and vomiting, dilated pupils, anxiety, altered mental status, and syncope.

Response: The therapist should initially attempt to remove the source of the shock, as well as monitor the patient's blood pressure, heart rate, and respiration. Cardiopulmonary resuscitation should be performed if necessary. The patient should be placed in supine with the feet elevated above the level of the head, assuming they do not have injuries to the head, spine, trunk or legs. For comfort, a cold compress may be applied to the forehead or a blanket may be used to prevent loss of body heat. The patient should avoid exertion until symptoms have been relieved.

Stroke

Recognition: Signs and symptoms typically include drooping or numbness on one side of the face, numbness or weakness of one arm, slurred speech, altered vision, headache, dizziness, lack of coordination, confusion, and loss of consciousness.

Response: If the therapist recognizes that a stroke is occurring, emergency medical services should be called immediately. The therapist should note the time that the initial symptoms appeared since treatment is dependent on the amount of time that has elapsed. If the patient's symptoms go away after a few minutes, they should still seek treatment since they have likely experienced a transient ischemic attack, which is also a serious condition.

SPOTLIGHT ON SAFETY
SUMMARY OF KEY BASIC LIFE SUPPORT COMPONENTS FOR ADULTS, CHILDREN, AND INFANTS

Component	Adults	Children	Infants
Recognition	Unresponsive (all ages)		
	No breathing or no normal breathing (i.e., only gasping)	No breathing or only gasping	
	No pulse palpated within 10 seconds for all ages (HCP only)		
CPR sequence	Compression – Airway – Breathing		
Compression rate	100 - 120/min		
Compression depth	At least 2 inches (5 cm)	At least 1/3 AP depth About 2 inches (5 cm)	At least 1/3 AP depth About 1.5 inches (4 cm)
Chest wall recoil	Allow complete recoil between compressions HCPs rotate compressors every 2 minutes		
Compression interruptions	Minimize interruptions in chest compressions Attempt to limit interruptions to <10 seconds		
Airway	Head tilt–chin lift (HCP suspected trauma: jaw thrust)		
Compression-to-ventilation ratio (until advanced airway placed)	30:2 1 or 2 rescuers	30:2 Single rescuer 15:2 2 HCP rescuers	
Ventilations: when rescuer is untrained or trained and not proficient	Compressions only		
Ventilations with advanced airway (HCP)	1 breath every 6-8 seconds (8-10 breaths/minute) Asynchronous with chest compressions About 1 second per breath Visible chest rise		
Defibrillation	Attach and use an AED as soon as available. Minimize interruptions in chest compressions before and after shock. Resume CPR beginning with compressions immediately after each shock.		

AED = automated external defibrillator; AP = anterior-posterior; CPR = cardiopulmonary resuscitation; HCP = healthcare provider

From: American Heart Association Guidelines for CPR and ECC. American Heart Association Web site, www.heart.org.

Ergonomics

Ergonomic Guidelines[1]

Workstation Recommendations

- ✓ 18-20 inch monitor
- ✓ Easily adjustable monitor to angle or tilt
- ✓ Split keyboard preferred
- ✓ Adjustable feet for the keyboard
- ✓ Monitor display should be directed ten degrees below the horizontal
- ✓ Monitor should be placed at least twenty inches away from the eyes
- ✓ Chair should swivel 360 degrees for easy access
- ✓ Wrist rests should match the front edge of the keyboard in order to maximize comfort
- ✓ Hands-free telephone set preferred
- ✓ Use a mouse that contours to the hand
- ✓ 30 second exercise break every hour while at a desk
- ✓ Space under the desk should be at least 30 inches wide, 19 inches deep, and 27 inches in height; there should be 2-3 inches between the top of the thighs and the desk

Workstation Posture

Head: level, facing forward, in line with trunk

Shoulders: relaxed, arms at side

Elbows: remain close to trunk, bent 90-120 degrees

Forearms, wrists, hands: parallel to the floor, straight

Trunk: maintain normal curves of the spine with appropriate lumbar support, shoulders and pelvis are level

Hips, thighs: well supported with contoured seat, parallel to the floor

Knees: maintain a level position with a 90 degree angle of flexion, knees generally at the same height as the hips

Feet: place feet flat on the floor or supported in a slight incline

Body Mechanics[2,3]

A therapist must consistently use proper body mechanics when treating patients and avoid unnecessary stress and strain by maintaining proper alignment within the musculoskeletal system.

Principles of Proper Body Mechanics

- Use the shortest lever arm possible
- Stay close to the patient when possible
- Use larger muscles to perform heavy work
- Maintain a wide base of support
- Avoid any rotary movement when lifting
- Attempt to maintain your center of gravity and the patient's center of gravity within the base of support

Lifting Guidelines[2,3]

- ✓ Always attempt to increase your base of support
- ✓ Maintain a proper lumbar curve as you lift
- ✓ Pivot your feet when lifting; do not twist your back to turn
- ✓ Maintain a slow and consistent speed while lifting
- ✓ Only lift an object as a last resort

Deep Squat Lift (Figs. 9-2, 9-3, 9-4)

1. Begin with the hips below the level of the knees
2. Assume a wide base of support
3. Straddle the object
4. Grasp the object from each side or from beneath
5. The trunk should remain vertical
6. Maintain a lumbar lordosis and anterior pelvic tilt

Half-Kneeling Lift (Figs. 9-5, 9-6, 9-7, 9-8)

1. Begin in a half-kneel position
2. The bottom leg should be positioned behind and to the side of the object
3. Maintain a normal lumbar lordosis
4. Lift the object onto the knee and draw it closer to the trunk
5. Continue the lift by holding the object close as you assume a standing position

One Leg Stance Lift

1. Used for lifting light objects that can be lifted with one extremity
2. Face the object in a lunge position
3. Shift weight onto the forward extremity
4. Flex the forward extremity and lower to reach the object
5. The hind leg rises off the ground to counterbalance the shift in weight
6. Maintain a neutral spine throughout the lift

Power Lift

1. Begin with the hips above the level of the knees
2. Assume a wide base of support behind the object with the feet parallel to each other
3. Grasp the object from each side or from underneath
4. The trunk should remain in a vertical position
5. Maintain a lumbar lordosis and anterior tilt

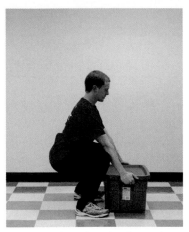

Fig. 9-2: A patient begins a deep squat lift with the hips below the knees.

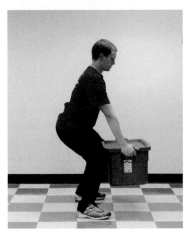

Fig. 9-3: The patient lifts the container while maintaining the trunk in a vertical position.

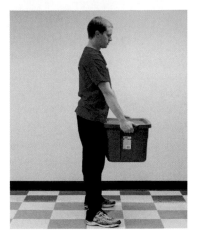

Fig. 9-4: The patient completes the lift by achieving a fully erect position.

Traditional Lift

1. Begin with the lower extremities in a full squat facing the object

2. The feet are positioned in an anterior-posterior manner on each side of the object

3. Grasp the object and flex the upper extremities to initiate the lift

4. Use bilateral lower extremities to provide the work of the lift

5. Keep the object close to the trunk during the lift

6. Maintain normal lumbar lordosis

7. Do not lift with the back

Pushing or Pulling an Object

✓ Use a semi-squat position to push or pull

✓ Apply the force parallel to the surface that the object should be moved upon

✓ Exert an initial force that is adequate to overcome the counterforce of inertia and friction

✓ Attempt to push, pull, slide or roll the object prior to lifting or carrying an object

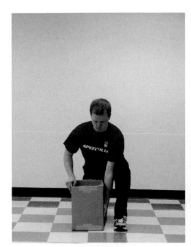

Fig. 9-5: The patient begins a half-kneeling lift while grasping the box in a half-kneeling position.

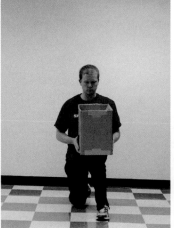

Fig. 9-6: The patient lifts the box onto the knee while maintaining normal lordosis.

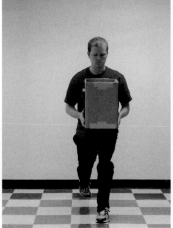

Fig. 9-7: The patient gradually assumes a standing position.

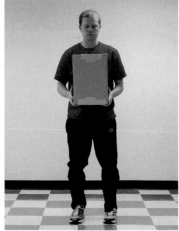

Fig. 9-8: The patient completes the lift by achieving a fully erect position.

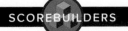

Professional Responsibilities

Accessibility

Americans with Disabilities Act[1,2]

The Americans with Disabilities Act is designed to provide a clear and comprehensive national mandate for the elimination of discrimination. The Americans with Disabilities Act is federal legislation that was signed into law on July 26, 1990.

The Americans with Disabilities Act is divided into five titles:

Title I	Employment
Title II	Public Services
Title III	Public Accommodations
Title IV	Telecommunications
Title V	Miscellaneous

The Americans with Disabilities Act applies primarily, but not exclusively, to "disabled" individuals. An individual is "disabled" if they meet at least one of the following criteria:

- They have a physical or mental impairment that substantially limits one or more of their major life activities.
- They have a record of such an impairment.
- They are regarded as having such an impairment.

The Employment provisions (Title I) apply to employers of fifteen employees or more. The Public Accommodations provisions (Title III) apply to all businesses, regardless of the number of employees.

Employers are required to make reasonable accommodations for qualified individuals with a disability, who are defined by the Americans with Disabilities Act as individuals who satisfy the job-related requirements of a position held or desired, and who can perform the "essential functions" of such position with or without reasonable accommodation. The Americans with Disabilities Act does not require employers to make accommodations that pose an "undue hardship." "Undue hardship" is defined as significantly difficult or expensive accommodations.

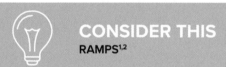

CONSIDER THIS
RAMPS[1,2]

Individuals unable to utilize stairs often rely on ramps. A ramp should possess twelve inches of horizontal run for each inch of vertical rise which is equivalent to an 8.3% grade (Fig. 9-9).

Ramp Specifications

Landing

Rise

Landing

Horizontal Run

Fig. 9-9: A diagram of a ramp depicting the relative relationship of rise to run.

Percent grade reflects the angle of inclination. A percent grade of 100% would be completely vertical and a percent grade of 0% would be completely horizontal. The percent grade is determined by taking the rise, dividing the value by the run, and then multiplying the number by 100 to convert the value to a percentage.

A ramp should be a minimum of 36 inches wide and should be equipped with handrails if the ramp has a rise of greater than 6 inches or a horizontal run of greater than 72 inches. The ramp should have a level landing at the top and bottom. If a ramp changes direction, the landing area must be a minimum of five feet by five feet (i.e., 60 inches x 60 inches).

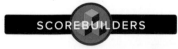

Accessibility Requirements[1,2,5]

Doorway (Fig. 9-10)	Minimum 32 inch width Maximum 24 inch depth
Threshold	Less than ¾ inch for sliding doors Less than ½ inch for other doors
Carpet	Requires ½ inch pile or less
Hallway clearance (Fig. 9-10)	36 inch width
Wheelchair turning radius (U-turn) (Fig. 9-11)	60 inch width 78 inch length
Forward reach in wheelchair (Fig. 9-12)	Low reach 15 inches High reach 48 inches
Side reach in wheelchair	Reach over obstruction to 24 inches
Bathroom sink	Not less than 29 inch height Not greater than 40 inches from floor to bottom of mirror or paper dispenser 17 inch minimum depth under sink to back wall
Bathroom toilet	17-19 inches from floor to top of toilet Not less than 36 inch grab bar length Grab bars should be 1¼ - 1½ inches in diameter 1½ inch spacing between grab bars and wall Grab bar placement 33-36 inches up from floor level
Hotel	Approximately 2% total rooms must be accessible
Parking space	96 inch width 240 inch length Approximately 2% of the total spaces must be accessible

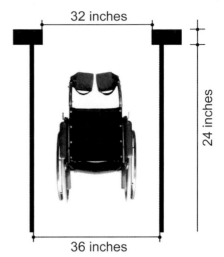

Fig. 9-10: An overhead image of the minimum required doorway width and hallway width.

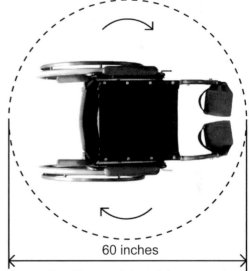

Fig. 9-11: An overhead image of the minimum required width for turning a wheelchair.

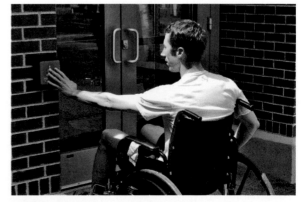

Fig. 9-12: A patient in a wheelchair activating an automatic door opener.

Documentation[6,7]

Purpose of Documentation

- Communicate with other treating professionals
- Assistance with discharge planning
- Reimbursement
- Assistance with utilization review
- A legal document regarding the course of therapy

Types of Documentation

Record

- An increase in specialization of care and multidisciplinary treatment increases the need for medical records to serve as a means of communication among clinicians.
- Progress notes and referrals related directly to patient care are examples of clinical records.
- Departmental statistics and records are examples of administrative records.

Referral

- Acceptable forms of referral range from a signed prescription form to a highly structured checklist. The referral must include the name of the patient and be signed and dated by the referring physician.
- Referrals commonly include some indication as to the number and frequency of treatments desired and any special precautions or instructions.

Progress Note

- Improvement of patient care is the most important function of progress notes.
- Progress notes allow members of all health services to know what the patient is accomplishing in each given area.
- Progress notes should contain patient identification, the date, and the signature of the therapist.
- Progress notes should be written when the patient's condition changes during the course of treatment.
- Specific frequency of progress notes is usually dictated by department policy.
- Appropriate forms of documentation include diagrams, videotapes, and flow sheets as well as many other less frequently used media.

S.O.A.P. Note

A commonly used record to write daily notes is the S.O.A.P. note. S.O.A.P. stands for:

- **S:** Subjective
- **O:** Objective
- **A:** Assessment
- **P:** Plan

Subjective: Refers to information the patient communicates to the therapist. This could include social or medical history not previously recorded. It could also include the patient's statements or complaints.

Objective: Refers to information the therapist observes. Common examples include range of motion measurements, muscle strength, and functional abilities. It also includes manual techniques and equipment used during treatment.

Assessment: Allows the therapist to express their professional opinion. Changes in the treatment program are often expressed in this section.

Plan: Includes ideas for future physical therapy sessions. Frequency and expected duration of physical therapy services can also be incorporated into this section.

Discharge Summary

A discharge summary should provide a capsule view of the patient's progress during therapy. The discharge summary is usually conducted on the day of the patient's last therapy session.

CONSIDER THIS
DOCUMENTATION RECOMMENDATIONS[9]

Physical therapists and physical therapist assistants are responsible for completing daily documentation on patients throughout the episode of care. Documentation should be completed in a timely manner and accurately describe the patient's status, physical therapy management, and outcome of care.

The American Physical Therapy Association provides therapists with insight on how to improve physical therapy documentation and promote reimbursement from third party payers.

Top 10 Tips for Defensible Documentation	Top 10 Payer Complaints Regarding Documentation
1. Limit use of abbreviations	1. Poor legibility
2. Date and sign all entries	2. Incomplete documentation
3. Document legibly	3. No documentation for date of service
4. Report progress towards goals regularly	4. Abbreviations, too many, cannot understand
5. Document at the time of the visit when possible	5. Does not demonstrate skilled care
6. Clearly identify note types (e.g., progress reports, daily notes)	6. Documentation does not support the billing code
7. Include all related communications	7. Does not support medical necessity
8. Include missed or cancelled visits	8. Does not demonstrate progress
9. Demonstrate skilled care and medical necessity	9. Repetitious daily notes showing no change in patient status
10. Demonstrate discharge planning through the episode of care	10. Interventions with no clarification of time, frequency, duration

Symbols Commonly Used in Clinical Practice

Symbol	Meaning	Symbol	Meaning
=	Equal	±	Very slight trace or reaction, indefinite
≠	Unequal	+	Slight trace or reaction, positive, plus excess, acidic reaction
>	Greater than	++	Trace or notable reaction
<	Less than	+++	Moderate amount of reaction
↑	Increase	++++	Large amount or pronounced reaction
↗	Increasing	#	Number, pound, has been given or done
↓	Decrease	→	Yields, leads to
↘	Decreasing	←	Resulting from or secondary to
−	Negative, minus, deficiency, alkaline reaction	1°, 2°	Primary, secondary

From Miller-Keane: Encyclopedia and Dictionary of Medicine, Nursing, and Allied Health. W.B. Saunders Company, Philadelphia 1997, p.1802, with permission.

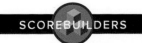

Military Time

The 24-hour clock (military time) is used to standardize time in the medical record.

Standard Time	Military Time
Noon	1200 hours
1:00 PM	1300 hours
2:00 PM	1400 hours
3:00 PM	1500 hours
4:00 PM	1600 hours
5:00 PM	1700 hours
6:00 PM	1800 hours
7:00 PM	1900 hours
8:00 PM	2000 hours
9:00 PM	2100 hours
10:00 PM	2200 hours
11:00 PM	2300 hours
Midnight	2400 hours

Measurement

Length	
1 cm	= 0.3937 inch
1 m	= 39.37 inches = 3.28 ft = 1.09 yds
1 km	= 0.62 mile
1 inch	= 2.54 centimeters (cm) = 25.4 millimeters (mm) = 0.0254 meters (m)
1 foot	= 30.48 cm = 304.8 mm = 0.304 m
1 mile	= 5280 ft = 1760 yds = 1609.35 m = 1.61 kilometers (km)

Temperature	
0°C	= 32°F = 273°K
100°C	= 212°F
°C	= (°F - 32) x 5/9
°F	= (°C x 9/5) + 32

Weight	
1 ounce (oz)	= 0.0625 pounds (lb) = 28.35 grams (g) = 0.028 kilograms (kg)
1 pound (lb)	= 16 oz = 454 g = 0.454 kg
1 g	= 0.035 oz = 0.0022 lb = 0.001 kg
1 kg	= 35.27 oz = 2.2 lb = 1000 g

Energy and Work	
1 kcal	= 3086 foot-pounds (ft/lbs) = 426.4 kilogram-meter (kg-m) = 4.184 kilojoules (kJ)
1 kJ	= 1000 joules (J) = 0.239 kcal
1 liter O_2 consumed	= 5.05 kcal = 15.575 ft/lbs = 2153 kg-m = 21.237 kJ
1 MET	= 3.5 mL O_2/kg-min = 0.0175 kcal/kg = 0.0732 kJ/kg
1 ft-lb	= 0.1383 kg-m
1 kg-m	= 7.23 ft/lbs

Metric versus United States Units of Measure			
1 inch =	2.54 centimeters	1 kilogram =	2.2 pounds
1 foot =	30.5 centimeters	1 pound =	4.45 Newtons
1 mile =	1.61 kilometers	1 liter =	.2642 gallons
1 meter =	3.28 feet	1 milliliter =	.0338 ounce
1 gram =	.0353 ounce	1 gallon =	3.785 liters
1 ounce =	28.35 grams	1 calorie =	4.18 Joules
1 pound =	454 grams		
°C =	(°F - 32) X 5/9	Boiling =	212 °F/100°C
°F =	(°C x 9/5) + 32	Freezing =	32 °F/0 °C

Management

Quality Management Process[12,13]

- Review selected patient medical records
- Prioritize adverse event outcomes
- Conduct a thorough review of care
- Identify problematic areas of care
- Develop a plan to change identified aspects of care
- Implement the plan
- Monitor the plan
- Determine if the implemented change results in a measurable difference

Quality Improvement[12,13]

Quality improvement is a form of objective self-examination designed to improve the quality of services. Quality measures should assess the structure, process, and outcome of physical therapy care. According to the American Physical Therapy Association structure, process, and outcome are defined as follows:

Structure

A review of structure is an assessment of organization, staffing and staff qualifications, rules and policies governing physical work, records, equipment, and physical facilities. The assessment may include a judgment of the adequacy as well as the presence of the element of structure being examined.

Process

Process assessment is based on the degree or extent to which the therapist conforms to accepted professional practices in providing services. The various approaches to care and their application, efficacy, adequacy, and timeliness are considered. A process review requires that considerable attention be given to developing and specifying the standards to be used in the assessment.

Outcome

Outcome assessment is based on the condition of the patient at the conclusion of care in relation to the goals of treatment. Assessment of outcome provides a means of reviewing the practitioner, the services, and events that led to the results of care. The results of outcome assessment ultimately may lead to the evaluation of the basic treatment procedures and modalities of physical therapy and validation of the approaches to patient care. Outcomes are the ultimate manifestations of effectiveness and quality of care.

Models of Disability

The Nagi Model[14]

This model was originally designed in 1965 by a social worker named Saad Nagi as an alternative to the medical model of disease. It describes health status as a product of the relationship between health and function and is defined by four primary concepts:

Pathology: An interruption or interference in the body's normal processes and the simultaneous efforts of the systems to regain homeostasis. Pathology occurs at the cellular level.

Impairment: The loss or abnormality at the tissue, organ or body system level. This can be of an anatomic, physiologic, mental or emotional nature. Each pathology will present with an impairment, however, impairments can exist without pathology (e.g., congenital defects). Impairments occur at the organ level.

Functional Limitation: The inability to perform an action or skill in a normal manner due to an impairment. Functional limitations are at the level of the whole person.

Disability: Any restriction or inability to perform a socially defined role within a social or physical environment due to an impairment. Environmental barriers impose disability.

Example: A patient with progressive weakness presents with paralysis of the trunk and lower extremities. The patient is diagnosed with a T12 spinal cord tumor. The patient utilizes a wheelchair for mobility and requires assistance with self-care. Prior to hospitalization, the patient worked as a delivery man.

Pathology: Spinal cord tumor at T12

Impairment: Loss of motor function below T12

Functional Limitation: Unable to ambulate

Disability: Cannot continue to work as a delivery person

International Classification of Functioning, Disability and Health (ICF) Model[15]

The International Classification of Functioning, Disability and Health (ICF) is a classification of health and health-related domains. These domains are classified from body, individual, and societal perspectives by means of two lists: one list of body functions and structure and one list of domains of activity and participation. Since an individual's functioning and disability occurs in a context, the ICF also includes a list of environmental factors.

The ICF is the World Health Organization's (WHO) latest framework, endorsed in 2001, for measuring health and disability at both individual and population levels. The WHO's previous model, known as the ICIDH, was defined by the primary concepts of disease, impairment, disability, and handicap. The WHO is also responsible for the creation and implementation of the International Classification of Diseases (ICD-10).

The ICF's constructs acknowledge that every human being can experience some degree of disability. It shifts focus from cause to impact and takes into account the social aspects of disability and acknowledges environmental factors that can impact a person's functioning.

ICF Primary Concepts:

Body Functions: physiological functions of body systems including psychological functions

Body Structures: anatomical parts of the body such as organs, limbs and their components

Impairments: problems in body function or structure such as a significant deviation or loss

Activity: the execution of a task or action by an individual

Participation: involvement in a life situation

Activity Limitations: difficulties an individual may have in executing activities

Participation Restrictions: problems an individual may experience in involvement in life situations

Environmental Factors: physical, social, and attitudinal environment in which people live

Categories that fall under each domain include:

Body Function

- Mental functions
- Sensory functions and pain
- Voice and speech functions
- Functions of the cardiovascular, hematological, immunological, and respiratory systems
- Functions of the digestive, metabolic, and endocrine systems
- Genitourinary and reproductive functions
- Neuromuscular and movement-related functions
- Functions of the skin and related structures

Body Structure

- Structures of the nervous system
- The eye, ear, and related structures
- Structures involved in voice and speech
- Structures of the cardiovascular, immunological, and respiratory systems
- Structures related to the digestive, metabolic, and endocrine systems
- Structures related to the genitourinary and reproductive systems
- Structures related to movement
- Skin and related structures

Activities and Participation

- Learning and applying knowledge
- General tasks and demands
- Communication
- Mobility
- Self-care
- Domestic life
- Interpersonal interactions and relationships
- Major life areas
- Community, social, and civic life

Environmental Factors

- Products and technology
- Natural environment and human-made changes to environment
- Support and relationships
- Attitudes
- Services, systems, and policies

Example: A patient status post motor vehicle accident diagnosed with C6 complete tetraplegia is wheelchair dependent for mobility and resides in a town without public transportation. He was very active in his church choir and taught Sunday school prior to his motor vehicle accident.

Health Condition: Complete spinal cord injury - tetraplegia

Impairment: Paralysis

Activity Limitation: Incapable of using public transportation

Participation Restriction: Lack of accommodations in public transportation leads to no participation in religious activities

Ethics

"Morality cannot be legislated, but behavior can be regulated. Judicial decrees may not change the heart, but they can restrain the heartless."   —*Martin Luther King Jr.*

Ethics is a branch of philosophy that emphasizes morality, justice, honesty, right versus wrong, and free will. Ethics is defined as a principle of good conduct or a body of right principles and specific moral choices. We respond to each instance that we face as health care providers based on specific moral choices. These are specific to each person and are based on cultural, religious, environmental, and personal values.

Ethical Principles and Terminology[10,11]

Autonomy: Requires that the wishes of competent individuals must be honored. Autonomy is often referred to as self-determination.

Beneficence: A moral obligation of health care providers to act for the benefit of others.

Confidentiality: The holding of professional secrets or discussions. Keeping client information within appropriate limits.

Duty: The obligations that individuals have to others in society.

Fidelity: Related to confidentiality and is defined as the moral duty to keep commitments that have been promised.

Justice: The quality of being just and fair; righteousness.

Nonmaleficence: The obligation of health care providers to above all else, do no harm.

Paternalism: A term used when someone fails to recognize another individual's rights and autonomy.

Rights: The ability to take advantage of a moral entitlement to do something or not to do something.

Veracity: Obligation of health care providers to tell the truth.

Ethical Issues

Professional Behaviors

✓ Organization	**L-** Listen
✓ Professional presentation	**E-** Explain
✓ Dependability	**A-** Acknowledge
✓ Initiative	**R-** Recommend
✓ Empathy	**N-** Negotiate
✓ Cooperation	
✓ Clinical reasoning	
✓ Written communication	
✓ Verbal communication	

Malpractice[11]

Claims of malpractice usually stem from the theory of negligence. Negligence describes a substandard level of care for the particular profession. Negligence deals with a particular conduct, not state of mind.

In order to prove malpractice through negligence, there are four elements:

1. A duty to act in a particular manner
2. Conduct that breaches that particular duty
3. Damage that occurs from that conduct
4. Conduct that is substandard, causing injury

Legal

Health Insurance Portability and Accountability Act

The Health Insurance Portability and Accountability Act (HIPAA) is a law that was passed in 1996 with the purpose of setting guidelines for the protection of patients' health information. This law applies to all covered entities, including health plans, health care providers, and billing services. Within Title II of HIPAA, there are several separate "rules" that dictate how protected health information (PHI) can be used.

PHI is considered to be any individually identifiable health information that is used by a covered entity. Individually identifiable health information is any health information that relates to the patient's health condition, the provision of their care or the payment for services, and that can be linked to the patient via a patient identifier (e.g., name, address, social security number, birthdate).

The Privacy Rule sets guidelines for the disclosure of PHI as needed for efficient and effective patient care. For example, health care providers can share PHI with other health care providers to facilitate treatment without the consent of the patient. At the same time, the Privacy Rule ensures that the patient's PHI is properly protected and the patient has rights concerning their own PHI. For example, when disclosing PHI, a covered entity must disclose only the minimum information that is necessary to facilitate treatment. Additionally, covered entities must maintain patient confidentiality at all times by de-identifying PHI, unless patient identification is necessary.

The Security Rule deals specifically with how electronic PHI should be protected and is divided into administrative, physical, and technical safeguards. Administrative safeguards address how the covered entity will protect electronic PHI, including creating policies and procedures and training staff members. Physical safeguards focus on controlling physical access to electronic PHI, including limiting access to the health care facility as well as limiting access to employee workstations. Technical safeguards include protecting access to electronic devices (e.g., use of passwords) and protecting information that is transmitted electronically.

OSHA

The Occupational Safety and Health Act is a law that was passed in 1970 to help protect employees from being physically harmed in the workplace. The law created the Occupational Safety and Health Administration (OSHA), an agency that sets and enforces workplace safety and health standards. These standards may include:

- Limiting exposure to hazardous chemicals
- Creating a materials safety data sheet
- Use of personal protective equipment
- Creating emergency action plans
- Providing protection against falls
- Keeping record of workplace injuries and illnesses

In addition to having a safe workplace, employees also have other rights. Employers must provide training for their employees concerning any and all workplace hazards. Additionally, employees have the right to file a complaint with OSHA without workplace retaliation.

Sexual Harassment

Sexual harassment is a form of discrimination that is based on a person's sex/gender. This type of harassment was made illegal in Title VII of the Civil Rights Act of 1964. Sexual harassment may include unwelcome sexual advances, requests for sexual favors or other verbal and physical conduct of a sexual nature. To be considered sexual harassment, the conduct must interfere with an individual's employment or work performance or must create a hostile or intimidating work environment.

There are many scenarios in which sexual harassment may occur. The perpetrator may be a boss or supervisor, though is not always in a position of power over the victim. Additionally, victims may include the person being harassed and other individuals who find the conduct offensive. The perpetrator can be a man or a woman, and the victim does not necessarily have to be a person of the opposite gender.

In cases of sexual harassment, the victim should attempt to inform the perpetrator that the behavior is unwelcome and that it needs to stop. The victim should file an official complaint with their employer if the behavior continues. Retaliation against employees that file a complaint is illegal. Prevention is the best tool in stopping sexual harassment. Employers should provide training on sexual harassment and establish an effective grievance process.

Elements of a Risk Management Program

- Management involvement
- Risk management organization
- Incident reporting and investigation
- Inspections
- Communications

Recommendations to Avoid Litigation[11]

- Conduct a thorough examination
- Seek consultation when in doubt
- Check the condition of your equipment
- Instruct patients thoroughly
- Keep the referring physician informed
- Obtain proper consent for treatment
- Do not delegate to unqualified individuals
- Keep accurate and timely written records

Legal Terminology[11]

Abandonment: Unacceptable one-sided termination of services by a health care professional without patient consent or agreement.

Administrative law: Administrative agencies at the federal and state level develop rules and regulations to supplement statutes and executive orders.

Common law: Refers to court decisions in the absence of statutory law. Common law often creates legal precedent in areas where statutes have not been enacted.

Constitutional law: Involves law that is derived from the federal Constitution. The United States Supreme Court is responsible for ultimately interpreting and enforcing the Constitution.

Informed consent: The patient is required to sign a document and give permission to the health care professional to render treatment. This should be obtained from the patient in accordance with the standards of practice prior to initiation of treatment. The patient has the right to full disclosure of treatment procedures, risks, expected outcomes, and goals.

Malpractice: The failure to exercise the skills that would normally be exercised by other members of the profession with similar skills and training. This can include areas of professional negligence, breach of contract issues, and intentional conduct by a health care professional.

Negligence: The failure to do what a reasonable and prudent person would ordinarily have done under the same or similar circumstances for a given situation. In order to prove negligence, the plaintiff must prove all of the following:

- There was a duty owed to the plaintiff by the defendant.
- There was a breach of that duty under conditions that constituted negligence and the negligence was the proximate cause of the breach.
- There was damage to the plaintiff's person or property.

Risk management: The identification, analysis, and evaluation of risks and the selection of the most advantageous method for treating them.

Statutory law: Congress and state legislatures are responsible for enacting statutes. Examples of federal statutes affecting health care include the Americans with Disabilities Act and the Family and Medical Leave Act.

Tort: A private or civil wrong or injury, involving omission and/or commission.

Delegation and Supervision[16]

Direction and Supervision of the Physical Therapist Assistant

Physical therapists have a responsibility to deliver services in ways that protect the public safety and maximize the availability of their services. They do this through direct delivery of services in conjunction with responsible utilization of physical therapist assistants who assist with selected components of intervention. The physical therapist assistant is the only individual permitted to assist a physical therapist in selected interventions under the direction and supervision of a physical therapist.

Direction and supervision are essential in the provision of quality physical therapy services. The degree of direction and supervision necessary for assuring quality physical therapy services is dependent upon many factors, including the education, experiences, and responsibilities of the parties involved, as well as the organizational structure in which the physical therapy services are provided.

Regardless of the setting in which the physical therapy service is provided, the following responsibilities must be borne solely by the physical therapist:

1. Interpretation of referrals when available.
2. Initial examination, evaluation, diagnosis, and prognosis.
3. Development or modification of a plan of care which is based on the initial examination or reexamination and which includes the physical therapy goals and outcomes.
4. Determination of when the expertise and decision-making capability of the physical therapist requires the physical therapist to personally render physical therapy interventions and when it may be appropriate to utilize the physical therapist assistant. A physical therapist shall determine the most appropriate utilization of the physical therapist assistant that provides for the delivery of service that is safe, effective, and efficient.
5. Reexamination of the patient/client in light of their goals, and revision of the plan of care when indicated.
6. Establishment of the discharge plan and documentation of discharge summary/status.
7. Oversight of all documentation for services rendered to each patient/client.

The physical therapist remains responsible for the physical therapy services provided when the physical therapist's plan of care involves the physical therapist assistant to assist with selected interventions. Regardless of the setting in which the service is provided, the determination to utilize physical therapist assistants for selected interventions requires the education, expertise, and professional judgment of a physical therapist as described by the *Standards of Practice, Guide to Professional Conduct,* and *Code of Ethics.*

In determining the appropriate extent of assistance from the physical therapist assistant (PTA), the physical therapist considers:

- The PTA's education, training, experience, and skill level.
- Patient/client criticality, acuity, stability, and complexity.
- The predictability of the consequences.
- The setting in which the care is being delivered.
- Federal and state statutes.
- Liability and risk management concerns.
- The mission of physical therapy services for the setting.
- The needed frequency of reexamination.

Physical Therapist Assistant

Definition: The physical therapist assistant is a technically educated health care provider who assists the physical therapist in the provision of physical therapy. The physical therapist assistant is a graduate of a physical therapist assistant associate degree program accredited by the Commission on Accreditation in Physical Therapy Education (CAPTE).

Utilization: The physical therapist is directly responsible for the actions of the physical therapist assistant related to patient/client management. The physical therapist assistant may perform selected physical therapy interventions under the direction and at least general supervision of the physical therapist. In general supervision, the physical therapist is not required to be on-site for direction and supervision, but must be available at least by telecommunications. The ability of the physical therapist assistant to perform the selected interventions as directed shall be assessed on an ongoing basis by the supervising physical therapist. The physical therapist assistant makes modifications to selected interventions either to progress the patient/client as directed by the physical therapist or to ensure patient/client safety and comfort.

The physical therapist assistant must work under the direction and at least general supervision of the physical therapist. In all practice settings, the performance of selected interventions by the physical therapist assistant must be consistent with safe and legal physical therapist practice, and shall be predicated on the following factors: complexity and acuity of the patient's/client's needs; proximity and accessibility to the physical therapist; supervision available in the event of emergencies or critical events; and type of setting in which the service is provided.

When supervising the physical therapist assistant in any off-site setting, the following requirements must be observed:

1. A physical therapist must be accessible by telecommunications to the physical therapist assistant at all times while the physical therapist assistant is treating patients/clients.

2. There must be regularly scheduled and documented conferences with the physical therapist assistant regarding patients/clients, the frequency of which is determined by the needs of the patient/client and the needs of the physical therapist assistant.

3. In those situations in which a physical therapist assistant is involved in the care of a patient/client, a supervisory visit by the physical therapist will be made:

    a. Upon the physical therapist assistant's request for a reexamination, when a change in the plan of care is needed, prior to any planned discharge, and in response to a change in the patient's/client's medical status.

    b. At least once a month, or at a higher frequency when established by the physical therapist, in accordance with the needs of the patient/client.

    c. A supervisory visit should include:

        i. An on-site reexamination of the patient/client.

        ii. On-site review of the plan of care with appropriate revision or termination.

        iii. Evaluation of need and recommendation for utilization of outside resources.

HOD P06-05-18-26 Updated: 08/07/12 American Physical Therapy Association, web site 2017.

Health Care Professionals[17]

Audiologists

Audiologists assess patients with suspected hearing disorders. The audiologist can educate patients on how to make the best use of their available hearing and assist them in selecting and fitting appropriate aids. Audiologists are required to possess a master's degree or equivalent. The vast majority of states require audiologists to obtain a license to practice.

Chiropractors

Chiropractors diagnose and treat patients whose health problems are associated with the body's muscular, nervous, and skeletal systems. Patient care activities include manually adjusting the spine, ordering and interpreting X-rays, performing postural analysis, and administering various physical agents. Chiropractors are required to complete a four-year chiropractic curriculum leading to the Doctor of Chiropractic degree. All states require chiropractors to obtain a license to practice.

Home Health Aides

Home health aides provide health-related services to the elderly, disabled, and ill in their homes. Patient care activities include performing housekeeping duties, assisting with ambulation or transfers, and promoting personal hygiene. A registered nurse, physical therapist, or social worker is often the health care professional that assigns specific duties and supervises the home health aide. The federal government has established guidelines for home health aides whose employers receive reimbursement from Medicare. The National Association for Home Care offers voluntary national certification for home health aides.

Licensed Practical Nurses

Licensed practical nurses care for the sick, injured, convalescent, and disabled under the direction of physicians and registered nurses. Patient care activities include taking vital signs, performing transfers, applying dressings, administering injections, and instructing patients and families. In some states, licensed practical nurses can administer prescribed medications or start intravenous fluids. Experienced licensed practical nurses may supervise nursing assistants and aides. Educational programs for licensed practical nurses are approximately one year in length and include classroom study and supervised clinical practice. All states require a license to practice.

Medical Assistants

Medical assistants perform routine administrative and clinical tasks in a medical office. Administrative duties include answering telephones, updating patient files, completing insurance forms, and scheduling appointments. Clinical duties include taking medical histories, measuring vital signs, and assisting the physician during treatment. Educational programs for medical assistants are typically one to two years in length.

Occupational Therapists

Occupational therapists help people improve their ability to perform activities of daily living, work, and leisure skills. The educational preparation of occupational therapists emphasizes the social, emotional, and physiological effects of illness and injury. Occupational therapists most commonly work with individuals who have conditions that are mentally, physically, developmentally or emotionally disabling. Occupational therapists can enter the field with bachelors, masters, or doctoral degrees. All states require occupational therapists to obtain a license to practice.

Occupational Therapy Aides

Occupational therapy aides work under the direction of occupational therapists to provide rehabilitation services to persons with mental, physical, developmental or emotional impairments. Occupational therapy aides often prepare materials and assemble equipment used during treatment and may be responsible for a variety of clerical tasks. The majority of training for occupational therapy aides occurs on the job.

Occupational Therapy Assistants

Occupational therapy assistants work under the direction of occupational therapists to provide rehabilitation services to persons with mental, physical, developmental or emotional impairments. Occupational therapy assistants perform a variety of rehabilitative activities and exercises as outlined in an established treatment plan. To practice as an occupational therapy assistant, individuals must complete an associate's degree or certificate program from an accredited academic institution. Occupational therapy assistants are regulated in the majority of states.

Physical Therapists

Physical therapists provide services to help restore function, improve mobility, relieve pain, and prevent or limit permanent physical disabilities of patients suffering from injuries or disease. Physical therapists engage in examination, evaluation, diagnosis, prognosis, and intervention in an effort to maximize patient outcomes. Physical therapists currently enter the field with a doctorate degree.

Physical Therapy Aides

Physical therapy aides are considered support personnel who may be involved in support services directed by physical therapists. Physical therapy aides receive on the job training under the direction and supervision of a physical therapist and are permitted to function only with continuous on-site supervision by a physical therapist or in some cases, a physical therapist assistant. Support services are limited to methods and techniques that do not require clinical decision making by the physical therapist or clinical problem solving by the physical therapist assistant.

Physical Therapist Assistants

Physical therapist assistants perform components of physical therapy procedures and related tasks selected and delegated by a supervising physical therapist. Physical therapist assistants may modify an intervention only in accordance with changes in patient status and within the established plan of care developed by the physical therapist. Physical therapist assistants are the only paraprofessionals that perform physical therapy interventions. Typically, physical therapist assistants have an associate's degree from an accredited physical therapist assistant program. The vast majority of states require physical therapist assistants to obtain a license to practice.

Physicians

Physicians diagnose illnesses and prescribe and administer treatment for people suffering from injury or disease. The term physician encompasses both the Doctor of Medicine (MD) and the Doctor of Osteopathic Medicine (DO). The role of the MD and DO are very similar, however, the DO tends to place special emphasis on the body's musculoskeletal system, preventive medicine, and holistic patient care. All states require physicians to obtain a license to practice.

Physician Assistants

Physician assistants provide health care services with supervision by physicians. The supervising physician and established state law determine the specific duties of the physician assistant. In the vast majority of states physician assistants may prescribe medication. Physician assistants work with the supervision of a physician. All states require physician assistants to obtain a license to practice.

Psychologists

Psychologists use various techniques including interviewing and testing to advise people how to deal with problems of everyday life. In the health care setting, psychologists may be involved in counseling programs designed to help people achieve goals such as weight loss or smoking cessation. A doctoral degree is usually required for employment as a licensed clinical or counseling psychologist. All states require psychologists to obtain a license to practice.

Recreational Therapists

Recreational therapists provide treatment services and recreation activities to individuals with disabilities or illness. In acute care hospitals and rehabilitation hospitals, recreational therapists work closely with other health care professionals to treat and rehabilitate individuals with specific medical conditions. In long-term care settings, recreational therapists function primarily by offering structured group sessions emphasizing leisure activities. Recreational therapists are required to have a bachelor's degree in order to be eligible for certification as certified therapeutic recreation specialists.

Registered Nurses

Registered nurses work to promote health, prevent disease, and help patients cope with illness. Patient care activities are extremely diverse including tasks such as assisting physicians during treatments and examinations, administering medications, recording symptoms and reactions, and instructing patients and families. Registered nurse programs include associates, bachelors, and diploma programs. All states require registered nurses to obtain a license to practice.

Respiratory Therapists

Respiratory therapists evaluate, treat, and care for patients with breathing disorders. The vast majority of respiratory therapists are employed in hospitals. Patient care activities include performing postural drainage techniques, measuring lung capacities, administering oxygen and aerosols, and analyzing oxygen and carbon dioxide concentrations. Educational programs for respiratory therapists are offered by hospitals, colleges, universities, vocational-technical institutes, and the military. The vast majority of states require respiratory therapists to obtain a license to practice.

Social Workers

Social workers help patients and their families to cope with chronic, acute or terminal illnesses and attempt to resolve problems that stand in the way of recovery or rehabilitation. A bachelor's degree is often the minimum requirement to qualify for employment as a social worker, however, in the health field, the master's degree is often required. All states have licensing, certification or registration requirements for social workers.

Speech-Language Pathologists

Speech-language pathologists evaluate speech, language, cognitive-communication, and swallowing skills of children and adults. The majority of practitioners provide direct clinical services to individuals with communication disorders. Speech-language pathologists are required to possess a master's degree or equivalent. The vast majority of states require speech-language pathologists to obtain a license to practice.

Regulatory Groups

American Physical Therapy Association (APTA): The APTA is the professional organization that represents physical therapists, physical therapist assistants, and physical therapy students. The goal of the APTA is to advance physical therapist practice, education, and research and increase the awareness of how physical therapy can play a role in health care. The APTA is responsible for creating and promoting ethical principles and standards of conduct for physical therapy practitioners and for influencing public policy that will affect the practice of physical therapy. Each state has its own APTA chapter, and there are also several special-interest sections (e.g., orthopedics, women's health) that exist within the APTA.

Federation of State Boards of Physical Therapy (FSBPT): The FSBPT is an organization that aims to protect the public by ensuring that physical therapists and physical therapist assistants provide safe and competent physical therapy services. They create the National Physical Therapy Examinations and determine necessary scoring requirements for PTs and PTAs to obtain licensure.

State licensing boards: State licensing boards are responsible for providing professional licenses to physical therapists and physical therapist assistants. Eligibility to acquire a license can vary widely from state to state, but it is generally based on a criminal background check, completion of an accredited physical therapy or physical therapist assistant educational program, and the ability to pass the National Physical Therapy Examinations provided by the FSBPT. State licensing boards also create and maintain the rules surrounding licensure renewal.

Commission on Accreditation of Rehabilitation Facilities (CARF): CARF is a nonprofit organization that provides accreditation services for institutions that provide health and human services, which may include behavioral health services, aging services, medical rehabilitation facilities, and opioid treatment programs. Institutions that are accredited by CARF commit to providing high quality health care services to ensure the satisfaction of consumers.

The Joint Commission: The Joint Commission, formerly the Joint Commission on Accreditation of Healthcare Organizations (JCAHO), is a nonprofit organization that provides accreditation and certification services to a variety of health care organizations, which may include hospitals, doctor's offices, nursing homes, home care companies, and behavioral health facilities. Organizations that are accredited by the Joint Commission agree to meet certain performance standards in their provision of health care services to ensure that members of the public are receiving the highest quality health care.

Health Care Settings

Acute care: This type of care is typically provided in a hospital for patients who have a serious injury or medical condition or who are recovering from a surgery. The inpatient stay is as short as possible; patients are typically discharged as soon as they are medically stable and able to transfer to a rehabilitation hospital, a skilled nursing facility, or home.

Long-term acute care: This type of care is provided for patients who need an extended hospital stay due to a chronic illness or injury. These patients require constant medical supervision (e.g., patient needing mechanical ventilation) and thus are not ready to be discharged to another facility. These types of facilities may be stand-alone hospitals or may exist as a unit within an acute care hospital.

Acute rehabilitation: This type of care occurs in a specific type of hospital that requires patients to participate in therapies (e.g., physical, occupational, speech) for at least three hours a day. Patients recovering from an injury or surgery are often discharged to a rehabilitation hospital from an acute care hospital once they are medically stable. The goal of this setting is to improve the patient's function so they can be discharged back to their home, though some patients may need long-term care in a nursing facility.

Sub-acute rehabilitation: This type of care provides similar services as an acute rehabilitation hospital, though the intensity of rehabilitation services is less. This setting is appropriate for patients of a lower functional level who need therapy services, but cannot tolerate three hours of therapy each day (i.e., receive one to two hours per day).

Nursing home: This type of care occurs in an inpatient setting that provides care for patients who are at a lower functional level and require assistance with their activities of daily living. These patients no longer need to be in a hospital, but they still require medical care and supervision that cannot be provided at home. Care may be provided on a long-term basis or for short periods of time (e.g., post-operative). A skilled nursing facility is a specific type of nursing home that provides skilled nursing and rehabilitation services.

Hospice care: This type of care is provided to patients who have an incurable disease and are nearing the end of their life. Health care in this setting is focused on managing a patient's pain and maximizing their function. Hospice care is often provided in a patient's home, though there are inpatient facilities that also provide these services.

Home health: In this setting, rehabilitation and nursing services are provided in the patient's home as opposed to an inpatient or outpatient setting. This setting is appropriate for patients who no longer need the constant medical care and supervision of an inpatient setting, but who are still limited in their physical ability to access outpatient services (e.g., unable to drive, inability to walk community distances).

Ambulatory care: This type of outpatient care is designed for patients that are typically at a higher functional level. The patients are well enough that they can travel to the clinic to attend their treatment session and return home the same day. Outpatient physical therapy is usually provided in a private practice clinic or in a hospital's outpatient department.

Physical Therapy Practice

The Physical Therapist Patient/Client Management Model[14]

Examination: The process of obtaining a history, performing a systems review, and selecting and administering tests and measures to gather data about the patient/client. The initial examination is a comprehensive screening and specific testing process that leads to a diagnostic classification. The examination process also may identify possible problems that require consultation with, or referral to, another provider.

Evaluation: A dynamic process in which the physical therapist makes clinical judgments based on data gathered during the examination. This process also may identify possible problems that require consultation with, or referral to, another provider.

Diagnosis: Both the process and the end result of evaluating examination data, which the physical therapist organizes into defined clusters, syndromes or categories to help determine the prognosis (including the plan of care) and the most appropriate intervention strategies.

Prognosis (including plan of care): Determination of the level of optimal improvement that may be attained through intervention and the amount of time required to reach that level. The plan of care specifies the interventions to be used and their timing and frequency.

Intervention: Purposeful and skilled interaction of the physical therapist with the patient/client and, if appropriate, with other individuals involved in the care of the patient/client, using various physical therapy methods and techniques to produce changes in the condition that are consistent with the diagnosis and prognosis. The physical therapist conducts a re-examination to determine changes in patient/client status and to modify or redirect intervention. The decision to re-examine may be based on new clinical findings or on lack of patient/client progress. The process of re-examination also may identify the need for consultation with, or referral to, another provider.

Outcomes: Results of patient/client management, which include the impact of physical therapy interventions in the following domains: pathology/pathophysiology (disease, disorder or condition); impairments, functional limitations and disabilities, risk reduction/prevention, health, wellness, and fitness; societal resources; and patient/client satisfaction.

From Guide to Physical Therapist Practice 3.0. American Physical Therapy Association, 2014.

Preamble

The Standards of Ethical Conduct for the Physical Therapist Assistant (Standards of Ethical Conduct) delineate the ethical obligations of all physical therapist assistants as determined by the House of Delegates of the American Physical Therapy Association (APTA). The Standards of Ethical Conduct provide a foundation for conduct to which all physical therapist assistants shall adhere. Fundamental to the Standards of Ethical Conduct is the special obligation of physical therapist assistants to enable patients/clients to achieve greater independence, health and wellness, and enhanced quality of life.

No document that delineates ethical standards can address every situation. Physical therapist assistants are encouraged to seek additional advice or consultation in instances where the guidance of the Standards of Ethical Conduct may not be definitive.

Standards of Ethical Conduct for the Physical Therapist Assistant

Standards

Standard #1: Physical therapist assistants shall respect the inherent dignity, and rights, of all individuals.

1A. Physical therapist assistants shall act in a respectful manner toward each person regardless of age, gender, race, nationality, religion, ethnicity, social or economic status, sexual orientation, health condition, or disability.

1B. Physical therapist assistants shall recognize their personal biases and shall not discriminate against others in the provision of physical therapy services.

Standard #2: Physical therapist assistants shall be trustworthy and compassionate in addressing the rights and needs of patients/clients.

2A. Physical therapist assistants shall act in the best interests of patients/clients over the interests of the physical therapist assistant.

2B. Physical therapist assistants shall provide physical therapy interventions with compassionate and caring behaviors that incorporate the individual and cultural differences of patients/clients.

2C. Physical therapist assistants shall provide patients/clients with information regarding the interventions they provide.

2D. Physical therapist assistants shall protect confidential patient/client information and, in collaboration with the physical therapist, may disclose confidential information to appropriate authorities only when allowed or as required by law.

Standard #3: Physical therapist assistants shall make sound decisions in collaboration with the physical therapist and within the boundaries established by laws and regulations.

3A.   Physical therapist assistants shall make objective decisions in the patient's/client's best interest in all practice settings.

3B.   Physical therapist assistants shall be guided by information about best practice regarding physical therapy interventions.

3C.   Physical therapist assistants shall make decisions based upon their level of competence and consistent with patient/client values.

3D.   Physical therapist assistants shall not engage in conflicts of interest that interfere with making sound decisions.

3E.   Physical therapist assistants shall provide physical therapy services under the direction and supervision of a physical therapist and shall communicate with the physical therapist when patient/client status requires modifications to the established plan of care.

Standard #4: Physical therapist assistants shall demonstrate integrity in their relationships with patients/clients, families, colleagues, students, other health care providers, employers, payers, and the public.

4A.   Physical therapist assistants shall provide truthful, accurate, and relevant information and shall not make misleading representations.

4B.   Physical therapist assistants shall not exploit persons over whom they have supervisory, evaluative or other authority (e.g., patients/clients, students, supervisees, research participants, or employees).

4C.   Physical therapist assistants shall discourage misconduct by health care professionals and report illegal or unethical acts to the relevant authority, when appropriate.

4D.   Physical therapist assistants shall report suspected cases of abuse involving children or vulnerable adults to the supervising physical therapist and the appropriate authority, subject to law.

4E.   Physical therapist assistants shall not engage in any sexual relationship with any of their patients/clients, supervisees, or students.

4F.   Physical therapist assistants shall not harass anyone verbally, physically, emotionally, or sexually.

Standard #5: Physical therapist assistants shall fulfill their legal and ethical obligations.

5A.   Physical therapist assistants shall comply with applicable local, state, and federal laws and regulations.

5B.   Physical therapist assistants shall support the supervisory role of the physical therapist to ensure quality care and promote patient/client safety.

5C.   Physical therapist assistants involved in research shall abide by accepted standards governing protection of research participants.

5D.   Physical therapist assistants shall encourage colleagues with physical, psychological, or substance-related impairments that may adversely impact their professional responsibilities to seek assistance or counsel.

5E.   Physical therapist assistants who have knowledge that a colleague is unable to perform their professional responsibilities with reasonable skill and safety shall report this information to the appropriate authority.

Standard #6: Physical therapist assistants shall enhance their competence through the lifelong acquisition and refinement of knowledge, skills, and abilities.

6A.   Physical therapist assistants shall achieve and maintain clinical competence.

6B.   Physical therapist assistants shall engage in lifelong learning consistent with changes in their roles and responsibilities and advances in the practice of physical therapy.

6C.   Physical therapist assistants shall support practice environments that support career development and lifelong learning.

Standard #7: Physical therapist assistants shall support organizational behaviors and business practices that benefit patients/clients and society.

7A.   Physical therapist assistants shall promote work environments that support ethical and accountable decision-making.

7B.   Physical therapist assistants shall not accept gifts or other considerations that influence or give an appearance of influencing their decisions.

7C.   Physical therapist assistants shall fully disclose any financial interest they have in products or services that they recommend to patients/clients.

7D.   Physical therapist assistants shall ensure that documentation for their interventions accurately reflects the nature and extent of the services provided.

7E.   Physical therapist assistants shall refrain from employment arrangements, or other arrangements, that prevent physical therapist assistants from fulfilling ethical obligations to patients/clients.

Standard #8: Physical therapist assistants shall participate in efforts to meet the health needs of people locally, nationally, or globally.

8A.   Physical therapist assistants shall support organizations that meet the health needs of people who are economically disadvantaged, uninsured, and underinsured.

8B.   Physical therapist assistants shall advocate for people with impairments, activity limitations, participation restrictions, and disabilities in order to promote their participation in community and society.

8C.   Physical therapist assistants shall be responsible stewards of health care resources by collaborating with physical therapists in order to avoid overutilization or underutilization of physical therapy services.

8D.   Physical therapist assistants shall educate members of the public about the benefits of physical therapy.

Health Insurance

There are three major classifications of health insurance companies. They include private health insurance companies, independent health plans, and government health insurance.

Private Health Insurance Companies

Private health insurance companies include stock companies, mutual companies, and non-profit insurance plans. Reimbursement for physical therapy services is usually on a fee for service basis.

Stock companies: Operated nationally and are owned by independent stockholders.

Mutual companies: Operated nationally and are owned by the individual policyholders.

Non-profit insurance plans: Operate in a specific geographic region and are subject to specific state regulations. They are classified as tax exempt due to their non-profit status.

Independent Health Plans[20,21]

Independent health plans are organized into various groups. Health maintenance organizations and self-insurance plans are examples of independent health plans. Reimbursement is typically based on fee for service or a predetermined fixed fee.

Managed care: A concept of health care delivery where subscribers utilize health care providers that are contracted by the insurance company at a lower cost. Health maintenance organizations (HMO) and preferred provider organizations (PPO) are two examples of a managed care system. This concept attempts to attain the highest quality of care at the lowest cost.

Health maintenance organization: Subscribers to these insurance plans agree to receive all of their health care services through the predetermined providers of the HMO. The primary physician of the subscriber controls health care access through a referral system. Cost containment is a high priority and subscribers cannot receive care from providers outside of the plan except in an emergency.

Preferred provider organization: Subscribers can choose their health care services from a list of providers that contract with the insurance plan. These contracts provide extreme discounts for health care. Subscribers can use a health care provider that is not associated with the PPO, however, they will absorb a greater portion of the cost.

Consolidated Omnibus Budget Reconciliation Act (COBRA): A law passed that requires an employer to allow an employee to remain under an employer's group plan for a period of time after the loss of a job, death of a spouse, a decrease in hours or a divorce. The employee may be required to pay the employer's portion of the premiums for their insurance coverage as well as their own portion.

Fee for Service versus Managed Care[20,21]

Fee for Service:	Managed Care:
Payers assume primary financial risk	Providers share in financial risk
Provides enrollees with freedom of choice	Services provided by a specific pool of providers
Unlimited access to specialty providers	Primary care provider serves as a gatekeeper
Co-payments often in the form of 80% / 20%	Provides services for a fixed, prepaid monthly fee
Limited internal/external cost controls	Formal quality assurance and utilization review
Minimal emphasis on health promotion and education	Health education and preventive medicine emphasized

Government Health Insurance[12,20,21]

Government health insurance programs such as Medicare and Medicaid are administered by the federal government. The government uses private contractors to manage the payment process of each health plan.

Medicare

Medicare provides health insurance for individuals over 65 years of age and the disabled. Medicare is a nationwide program operated by the Centers for Medicare and Medicaid Services.

Established in 1966, Medicare was the second mandated health insurance program in the United States (Workers' Compensation was the first). In 1972 Medicare coverage was expanded to include certain categories of the disabled, renal dialysis, and transplant patients.

Medicare Part A:

Provides benefits for care provided in hospitals, outpatient diagnostic services, extended care facilities, hospice, and short-term care at home required by an illness for which the patient is hospitalized.

Enrollment in Medicare Part A is automatic and funding is through payroll taxes.

Medicare Part B:

Provides benefits for outpatient care, physician services, and services ordered by physicians such as diagnostic tests, medical equipment, and supplies.

Enrollment in Medicare Part B is voluntary and funding is through premiums paid by beneficiaries and general federal tax revenues.

The Medicare program requires beneficiaries to share in the costs of health care through deductibles and coinsurance.

- Deductibles require beneficiaries to reach a predetermined amount of personal expenditure each 12 month period before Medicare payment is activated.

- Coinsurance requires that 20% of the costs for hospitalization is covered by the patient.

Medicare sets limits on the total days of hospital care that will be paid based on a lifetime pool of days limit. Medicare payments for post hospital stays in extended care facilities are limited to 100 days.

Providers are reimbursed for Medicare services through intermediaries such as Blue Cross.

Medicaid

Medicaid provides basic medical services to the economically indigent population who qualify by reason of low income or who qualify for welfare or public assistance benefits in the state of their residence. Medicaid is a jointly funded program through the federal and state governments.

Established in 1965, Medicaid is funded through personal income, corporate, and excise taxes. Federal and state support is shared based on the state's per capita income.

Rate setting formulas, procedures, and policies vary widely among states. All state Medicaid operations must be approved by the Centers for Medicare and Medicaid Services. The Medicaid program reimburses providers directly.

The Medicaid program covers inpatient and outpatient hospital services, physician services, diagnostic services, nursing care for older adults, home health care, preventative health screening services, and family planning services.

Workers' Compensation

First designed in 1911 to provide protection for employees that were injured on the job. This legislation provides continued income as well as paid medical expenses for employees injured while working. Workers' compensation is a joint federal and state program that is regulated at the state level. Recently, case managers have assisted this process by monitoring the rehabilitation process and controlling potential abuse.

Employers with 10 or more employees or high-risk employers must pay a percentage of each employee salary to the workers' compensation board of the state. The exact payment is based on the risk rating of the job or institution.

Reimbursement Coding

Current Procedural Terminology Codes

Current Procedural Terminology (CPT) codes are procedure codes used by physical therapists and other health care professionals to describe the interventions that were provided to a given patient. The majority of codes used by physical therapists are in the CPT 97000 series. Examples of commonly used CPT codes by physical therapists include: 97530 – Therapeutic Activities; 97035 – Ultrasound; 97012 – Traction, mechanical. CPT is a registered trademark of the American Medical Association.

In January 2017, three new CPT codes were created for billing evaluations (as opposed to one previously). The new codes were created to account for evaluating patients of different complexities, and they are as follows: 97161 (low complexity), 97162 (moderate complexity), and 97163 (high complexity). There is also a new code that is replacing the old code for re-evaluations (97164).

There are two types of CPT codes: timed and untimed. Timed codes are billed based on the amount of time spent performing that intervention, generally one unit per 15-minute interval. If a patient performs therapeutic exercise for 45 minutes, they would be billed for three units of that code (i.e., 97110). Untimed codes are billed for one unit regardless of the time spent performing the intervention. For example, whether a patient has unattended electrical stimulation (i.e., CPT code 97014) for 15 minutes or 30 minutes, they will still only be billed one unit for that code.

When using timed codes, Medicare (and other insurance companies that follow Medicare guidelines) state that at least eight minutes of an intervention must be performed to bill a unit of that code. To calculate the total number of units, take the total time spent performing the intervention and divide by 15. If there is a remainder of eight or greater, an extra unit can be billed for that code. For example, if a therapist performs manual therapy for 40 minutes, they should bill for three units of that code (40/15 = 2 units and 10 extra minutes), since the remaining extra time is greater than eight minutes.

Reimbursement rates for CPT codes vary widely according to the insurance company that is being billed. Each insurance company creates a contract with the medical facility to dictate what they will be willing to pay for each code. Though a therapist may bill the exact same treatment codes to two different insurance companies, the reimbursement rates from those two companies may be drastically different.

International Classification of Diseases

The International Classification of Diseases (ICD) codes are designed to describe a patient's infirmity through specific categories based on etiology and affected anatomical systems. ICD-10 was the 10th revision of this ICD coding system and it officially replaced ICD-9 in 2015. The change to ICD-10 included an overall expansion in the number of possible codes, a switch from numeric to alphanumeric coding (e.g., 755.12 vs. M25.712), and a switch from 5-character codes to 6-character codes (or 7-character, in some cases). The increase in the number of codes occurred due to the addition of symptom-based codes (e.g., M25.651 for "stiffness of the right hip"), the addition of codes defining the external cause of the injury (e.g., W10.1 for "fall from a sidewalk curb") and social circumstance it occurred in (e.g., Y93.66 for "soccer"), and a new option for defining laterality (i.e., coding right vs. left). Physicians are required to make the medical diagnosis, however, in some cases a physical therapist may need to utilize the ICD manual to determine an appropriate ICD code. This action is within a physical therapist's scope of practice and would not be considered equivalent to making a medical diagnosis.

Functional Limitation Reporting

Starting on July 1, 2013, the Centers for Medicare and Medicaid Services (CMS) began to collect data on the functional level of patients being treated in any setting that provides outpatient therapy services. Physical therapists dictate the patient's functional level using G-codes, as well as modifiers that explain the severity of the patient's functional impairment (e.g., 25% impaired). These codes must be reported at the onset of treatment, at certain specified intervals during treatment (e.g., every tenth visit), and at discharge. With each reporting, the provider must indicate the patient's current functional status as well as the desired goal status. Therapists must provide documentation that supports the codes that were selected. Use of standardized functional assessment tools as well as objective data gained from the physical examination may assist the therapist in determining the patient's severity of impairment.

Teaching & Learning

Maslow's Hierarchy of Needs[22]

Maslow's hierarchy of needs hypothesizes that there is a hierarchy of biogenic and psychogenic needs that individuals must progress through. In order to move to a higher level of needs, an individual must attain the objectives associated with the previous level. In essence, an individual must achieve basic or fundamental needs before moving to upper level needs.

Self-actualization needs: The need to realize one's full potential as a human being.

Esteem needs: The need to feel good about oneself and one's capabilities, to be respected by others, and to receive recognition and appreciation.

Affiliative needs: The need for security, stability, and a safe environment.

Physiological needs: The need for basic things necessary in order to survive such as food, water, and shelter.

Classical Conditioning (Pavlov)[22]

Classical conditioning is a process where learning occurs when an unconditioned stimulus (food) is repeatedly preceded by a neutral stimulus (bell). The neutral stimulus serves as a conditioned stimulus and the learned reaction that results is termed the conditioned response. In order to maintain a conditioned response, the conditioned and unconditioned stimuli must occasionally be paired.

Operant Conditioning (B.F. Skinner)[22]

Operant conditioning is a process where learning occurs when an individual engages in specific behaviors in order to receive certain consequences.

Positive reinforcement: Administering desirable consequences to individuals who perform a specific behavior.

Negative reinforcement: Removing undesirable consequences from individuals who perform a specific behavior.

Extinction: Removing selected variables that reinforce a specific behavior.

Punishment: Administering negative consequences to individuals who perform undesirable behaviors.

Reinforcement Frequency and Schedules

Continuous reinforcement: A behavior is reinforced every time it occurs.

Partial reinforcement: A behavior is reinforced intermittently.

Fixed-interval schedule: The period of time between the occurrences of each instance of reinforcement is fixed or set.

Variable-interval schedule: The amount of time between reinforcements varies around a constant average.

Levels of Prevention

Health care prevention is defined as the actions taken to reduce the potential risks to one's health. Prevention activities fall into one of three categories: primary, secondary or tertiary.

Primary prevention: Interventions that occur before the onset of a disease or condition with the goal of preventing the disease/condition. This may be accomplished by preventing exposure to substances that may cause a disease or by modifying behavior to prevent risk factors associated with a disease.

  Examples: receiving immunizations, educating patients on exercise and healthy eating, legislation aimed at banning the use of hazardous materials

Secondary prevention: Interventions that aim to diagnose a condition early in its onset and prevent complications from occurring. Though this form of prevention cannot stop the onset of disease, it can stop or slow the progression of the disease by treating it early.

  Examples: screening adolescents for scoliosis, performing self-testicular examinations, blood glucose testing for diabetes

Tertiary prevention: Interventions that occur after a disease has already been diagnosed with the goal of minimizing the long-term effects of the disease. This form of prevention typically occurs once a patient has already become symptomatic. The goal is to help the patient manage their condition and maximize their quality of life.

  Examples: rehabilitation after a spinal cord injury, palliative care for end-of-life patients, support groups for patients with HIV

CONSIDER THIS
CULTURAL INFLUENCES

Culture is characterized by the set of shared beliefs, values, attitudes, and customs that exist within a specific ethnic, religious or social group. As the cultural makeup of the United States becomes more diverse, it is important that health care professionals have an understanding of how a patient's unique culture may impact their health care experience. The following factors should be considered when working with patients of different cultural backgrounds.

Communication: Many Americans speak English as a second language or may not speak English at all. It is important for these patients to have adequate access to interpreter services so that they can effectively communicate with their health care provider. Therapists should realize that even with the use of an interpreter, some information can still be lost in translation, which could influence the patient's treatment. In addition to language barriers, other aspects of communication may vary from one culture to another, such as nonverbal communication, the use of silence during conversations, and the appropriateness of eye contact. In some cultures, patients choose to avoid any form of conflict with authority figures. A patient may disagree with their treatment plan but never verbalize it, which likely will lead to poor patient compliance.

Social roles: A patient's social role within their family or relationship may affect how they approach health care decisions. In some cultures, a patient may rely heavily on their family in the decision-making process. In other cultures, the patriarchal figure may be the sole party responsible for making health care decisions. It is important for therapists to include family members in appropriate aspects of a patient's care.

Modesty: Cultural influences may affect a patient's comfort level when it comes to being touched by their health care provider or being physically close to the provider. In some cultures, being touched by someone of the opposite gender is unacceptable. Before working with someone, it is important for the therapist to determine the patient's level of modesty to allow for maximum patient comfort during treatment.

Health care beliefs: A patient's culture may affect how they view their diagnosis and how they approach treatment for their diagnosis. Patients with strong religious beliefs may assume that their condition is controlled by a higher power and thus they may deny formal treatment. Other cultures may choose to seek treatment, though they may do so through "alternative" forms of medicine (e.g., herbal remedies, acupuncture). This may be done in isolation, or in conjunction with conventional treatments. In some cultures, reporting pain is considered a sign of weakness. These patients may appear to have a higher pain tolerance or neglect to report some of their symptoms, which could negatively impact their recovery.

End-of-life care: The approach towards a patient's end-of-life care may vary depending on the patient's cultural background. Some religions encourage prolonging a patient's life through whatever medical interventions are available, while other religions oppose this practice and believe the patient should die "naturally" (e.g., taking a comatose patient off life support). Cultural traditions may also dictate where a terminally ill patient chooses to spend their remaining days (e.g., hospital, home).

Patient Education

Adult Learning

- Therapists must strive to make patient education sessions practical and useful for the patient.

- Failure to identify the relevance of the presented information will promote disinterest and decrease compliance.

Guidelines to Promote Adult Learning

- Design learning activities that will incorporate the patient's past experiences.

- Encourage the learner to play an active role in their educational program.

- Attempt to demonstrate the relevance of selected learning activities.

- Provide ample opportunities for practice and feedback.

- Recognize skill acquisition or objective improvement in patient performance.

Domains of Learning

Domains of learning are educational terms that describe various aspects of human behavior. The three most commonly recognized domains of learning are the cognitive, psychomotor, and affective domains. Recognizing the various levels of each of the domains can assist therapists to plan appropriate patient learning activities.

Affective domain: The affective domain is primarily concerned with attitudes, values, and emotions.

The domain consists of five specific levels: receiving, responding, valuing, organization, and characterization.

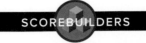

Cognitive domain: The cognitive domain is primarily concerned with knowledge and understanding.

The domain consists of six specific levels: knowledge, comprehension, application, analysis, synthesis, and evaluation.

Psychomotor domain: The psychomotor domain is primarily concerned with physical action or motor skill.

The domain consists of seven specific levels: perception, set, guided response, mechanism, complex overt response, adaptation, and origination.

Learning Style

Therapists can often obtain information related to a patient's preferred learning style by asking a few basic questions.

- Do you prefer to learn new information by observing, reading, listening or experiencing?
- Are you more comfortable learning in an active or passive manner?
- What increases your motivation to learn?

Teaching Methods

Individual

- Therapists most commonly instruct patients on an individual basis.
- The individual approach allows the therapist to focus on the needs of the learner and is the model of choice when the objectives of the session are unique to an individual patient.
- The individual approach allows the therapist to strengthen the patient/therapist bond and provides additional opportunities for specific feedback.

Group

- Therapists often instruct patients in a group.
- Group teaching may occur with patients, family members, staff, and support persons.
- Group teaching can be difficult if patients are not supportive of each other or if the learning needs of the group are diverse.
- Some patients may be intimidated by selected group members and tend to withdraw, while others may attempt to take control of the group.
- Since individuals typically receive less individual attention in a group, it is critical for the therapist to regularly assess individual patient progress.
- Group teaching allows participants to support each other in the educational process and permits therapists to effectively use scarce resources such as time or money.
- Patients participating in group activities often feel a sense of camaraderie interacting with others who have similar personal experiences.

Patient Communication[24,25]

- Verbal commands should focus the patient's attention on specifically desired actions.
- Instruction should remain as simplistic as possible and should not incorporate confusing medical terminology.
- The therapist should describe to the patient the general sequence of events that will occur prior to initiating treatment.
- The therapist should ask the patient questions during treatment in order to establish a rapport with the patient and to provide feedback as to the status of the current treatment.
- The therapist should speak clearly and vary their tone of voice as required by the situation.

Guidelines for Effective Patient Education[10,25]

- Attempt to establish a positive rapport with the patient.
- Assess the patient's readiness and motivation to learn.
- Attempt to identify the patient's preferred learning style and available resources.
- Identify potential barriers to patient progress.
- Design an individualized education program for the patient based on their medical condition and personal goals.
- Coordinate education with the other members of the health care team.
- Focus the majority of available time on the most important concepts.
- Provide clear and succinct communication to the patient.
- Use repetition to improve patient learning.
- Provide frequent feedback to the patient.
- Utilize appropriate teaching resources to facilitate patient learning.
- Assess the effectiveness of patient education.
- Modify the patient education program based on the assessment results.

Principles of Motivation[25,26]

- Readiness to learn significantly influences motivation.
- Individuals respond differently to selected motivational strategies.
- Success is more motivating than failure.
- Internal motivation has a greater potential to contribute to meaningful and lasting change than external motivation.
- A positive patient/therapist relationship enhances motivation.
- Limited anxiety may serve to motivate, while excessive anxiety may debilitate.
- Affiliation and approval can be motivating.

Culture[26]

- Understanding cultural differences in patients can assist therapists to function as more effective educators.
- Patient culture is influenced and shaped by society, community, family, personal values, and attitudes.
- Language barriers, nonverbal communication, and limited personal experience can serve as obstacles when educating patients with significant cultural differences.
- Therapists should embrace cultural diversity and avoid efforts to make patients conform to any particular norm or standard.
- Therapists must be cautious when interpreting specific language or behavior and avoid labeling patients as unmotivated or disinterested.
- Therapists should use available resources such as experienced staff members, interpreters or consultants as necessary to achieve desired outcomes.

Designing Effective Patient Education Materials

- Design the materials to convey only the necessary information.
- Emphasize essential information.
- Utilize active instructions such as "you" and avoid passive terms such as "patient."
- Larger print may be more desirable than smaller print.
- Avoid long sentences or complex medical terminology.
- Pictures or graphics should be used where appropriate to complement written information.
- Incorporate answers to frequently asked questions.
- Written materials should flow in a logical sequence.
- Written materials should utilize a reading level appropriate for the target audience.

Teaching Guidelines for Specific Patient Categories[25,26,27]

Therapists often vary their approach when educating patients of various ages and abilities. It is difficult to develop recommendations that apply to all patients in a given category, however, the following represent general guidelines for therapists to consider when treating selected patient categories.

Infants/Children

- Therapists should try to make therapy sessions with infants/children interactive.
- Sessions should include structured play and should be of relatively short duration.
- Frequent breaks and positive reinforcement will serve to increase the patient's level of participation.

Adolescents

- Therapists should try to assume the role of an advocate when working with adolescents.
- It is important for therapists to establish patients' trust and incorporate patient goals into the plan of care.
- Adolescents prefer to be treated like adults and may resent the presence of parents during therapy sessions.
- Therapists should provide patients with clear and concise instructions and offer frequent positive reinforcement.

Adults

- Therapists should involve adults in determining education outcomes.
- The education program should be compatible with the patient's daily routine and goals.
- Emphasizing the relevance of educational activities will serve to increase patient compliance.
- Therapists should be aware of the available patient support system and identify any barriers to progress.

Elderly

- Therapists may find it necessary to introduce new information gradually when working with the elderly.
- Special attention should be paid to identify signs of hearing loss or visual impairments.
- The elderly population often benefits from the social benefits of group activities.
- Education sessions for the elderly should not be longer in duration, however, the achievement of selected outcomes may require additional sessions.

Terminally Ill

- Therapists should incorporate patient goals as an integral component of any educational session for patients with terminal illness.
- Family members and other support personnel should be encouraged to participate in the educational session, however, it is important to provide the patient with the opportunity to make independent decisions whenever possible.
- Goals for the terminally ill patient often include maximizing function, safety, and comfort.
- Therapists may alter their teaching methods based on the current mental and physical well-being of the patient.

Cognitively Impaired

- The therapist should focus on the education of the caregiver and incorporate the patient whenever possible.
- When incorporating the patient in the session, instructions should be clear and concise and should be summarized through demonstration and pictures.
- Therapists should encourage the patient to compensate for any memory deficit.

Illiteracy

- Therapists should attempt to determine the literacy level of their patients.
- If a patient is determined to be illiterate, the therapist may elect to modify language to use basic wording and short sentences.
- Demonstration, repetition, and pictures should be incorporated into educational sessions.
- Therapists may include more detailed written information in educational sessions if the patient has adequate support at home.

Stages of Dying[10,24]

Elizabeth Kubler-Ross identified five stages in coming to terms with death after interviewing a large number of terminally ill patients. The stages Kubler-Ross identified were denial, anger, bargaining, depression, and acceptance.

Denial

The denial stage is characterized by a failure of the individual to believe that their condition is terminal. Therapists should attempt to establish trust with a patient in this stage and avoid trying to make the patient accept their condition.

Anger

The anger stage is characterized by frustration and negative emotional feelings often directed at anyone the individual comes in contact with. Individuals often ask "Why me?" Therapists should avoid taking the anger personally and recognize that expressing anger is often a useful step for the individual to move beyond this stage.

Bargaining

The bargaining stage is characterized by the individual trying to negotiate with fate. The individual may try to make a deal with a higher being based on good behavior, compliance with an exercise program or dedication of their life to a specific cause. Therapists should facilitate discussion with the patient and serve as a good listener.

Depression

The depression stage is characterized by the individual expressing the depths of their anguish. The individual is often deeply depressed and may show little interest in any form of medical intervention. Therapists should listen to the individual and exhibit a great deal of patience during this stage.

Acceptance

The acceptance stage is characterized by the individual coming to terms with their fate. The individual may attempt to resolve any unfinished business and may experience a sense of inner peace. Therapists should encourage the individual and family to ask questions and attempt to spend meaningful time with the individual.

Education Concepts

Team Models[28]

Unidisciplinary: A single discipline provides patient care services.

Multidisciplinary: Several different disciplines are involved in providing patient care, however, the disciplines tend to function independently and communication occurs primarily through the medical record.

Interdisciplinary: Several different disciplines are involved in providing patient care. The disciplines function independently, however, they routinely report to each other and may coordinate patient care.

Transdisciplinary: Numerous disciplines function as a collective unit to provide patient care services. Team goals are established rather than individual discipline goals and as a result, discipline specific boundaries tend to erode.

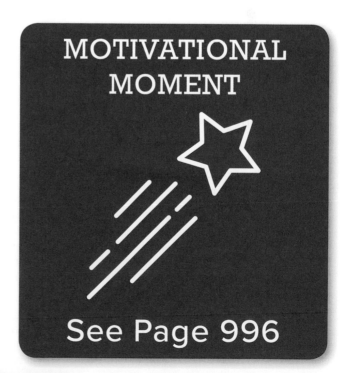

MOTIVATIONAL MOMENT

See Page 996

Research

Evidence-Based Practice (EBP)

Evidence-based medicine has been defined as the integration of the best clinically relevant research with clinical expertise and patient values.[29] In recognition of the movement's adoption by other health care practitioners, the concept has evolved into evidence-based practice (EBP). The term "practice" recognizes the expansion of the framework to physical therapy, nursing, and other aspects of health care beyond medicine.

Best research evidence refers to clinically relevant, patient-centered clinical research about the accuracy of diagnostic tests, prognostic factors, and the efficacy of interventions. Clinical expertise refers to the clinician's use of past experiences to make clinical judgments. Patient values refer to the preferences and expectations of the patient that are considered in clinical decisions about health care.[29] In physical therapy, the goal of evidence-based practice is to help therapists make sense of knowledge derived from research and use the information as a basis for making decisions about their patients.

Steps to Practicing Evidence-Based Physical Therapy[29]

1. Identify a problem or area of uncertainty about prevention, diagnosis, prognosis or therapy.
2. Formulate a focused clinical question for a specific patient problem.
3. Search the literature for relevant clinical articles to answer that question.
4. Critically appraise each article to determine its validity (closeness to the truth), impact (size of the effect), and applicability (usefulness in clinical practice).
5. Integrate the relevant findings in clinical practice along with clinical expertise and patient values.
6. Assess the outcomes of the selected action.

Levels of Evidence for Articles about Therapy/Intervention

The hierarchy of "levels of evidence" refers to how different categories of studies are ranked and should be considered when decisions need to be made about interventions. To evaluate the strength of the different types of clinical evidence, studies or clinical trials are ranked according to the strength of the design (Fig. 9-13).[35] In many cases, it is not possible to find the best level of evidence to answer a particular research question. In these instances, a clinician will need to consider moving down the pyramid to other types of studies, however, clinicians must be aware of the limitations incurred as the strength of the evidence diminishes.

Systematic Review

A comprehensive review of the medical literature that uses explicit methods to systematically search, identify, appraise, and summarize all literature on a specific issue. For example, a Cochrane Systematic Review is a type of review aimed at providing evidence specifically in health care and health policy.[29]

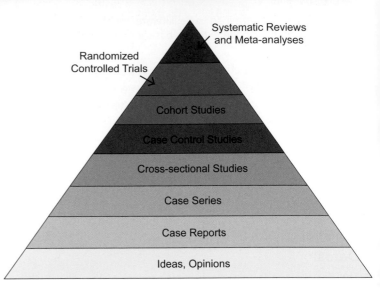

Fig. 9-13: Levels of evidence pyramid for studies about interventions.

Meta-analysis

A systematic review that uses a statistical technique to derive an estimate of effect size by combining the results of several randomized controlled trials to determine the overall effectiveness of a treatment. This strategy can minimize the problem of small sample size from individual studies since the pooling of trials increases the overall sample size.[36]

Randomized Controlled Trial (RCT)

A form of experimental research used to assess the relative effect of a specific intervention compared to a control condition. Patients are randomized into a control group and at least one experimental group. The control group receives either no treatment or a standard default treatment. Ideally, the groups will be identical except for the intervention they have been randomized to receive. Random assignment reduces the risk of bias and increases the probability that differences between the groups can be attributed to the intervention.[33]

Cohort Study

A type of longitudinal, observational study in which individuals with a risk factor or exposure are followed over time to compare the occurrence of a disease in the exposed group to that of the group of unexposed individuals. The measure of association between exposure and disease in cohort studies is the relative risk (i.e., the ratio of the incidence rate of exposed individuals to that of the controls). Cohort studies can be performed prospectively or retrospectively from historical records. Limitations of cohort studies include the excessive length of time a study can take and the influence of other lifestyle variables that invariably result in the two groups being uniquely different.[36]

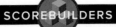

Case Control Study

A type of retrospective, observational study in which individuals who already have a particular disease are matched with a comparison group of individuals without the disease. The history of exposure or other characteristics prior to the onset of the disease is recorded through interview and other sources and compared between the two groups. The control group provides an estimate of the frequency and amount of exposure in subjects in the population without the disease being studied. The measure of association between exposure and occurrence of disease in case control studies is the odds ratio (i.e., the ratio of odds of exposure in diseased subjects to the odds of exposure in non-diseased subjects).[36]

Cross-Sectional Study

A type of observational study where the data or observations are made at only one point in time and all subjects are tested at relatively the same time.[5] A cross-sectional study aims to describe relationships between a disease or condition and factors of interest that exist in a specified population at a given time. These studies can describe the prevalence of disease or conditions and demonstrate associations, but they cannot distinguish between newly occurring and long-established conditions, nor can they identify causal relationships about what may have precipitated the disease or condition.

Case Report or Case Series

A case report is an in-depth description of an individual's condition or response to treatment. A case series consists of a collection of observations of similar cases. Case reports may be used to generate theories and hypotheses for future research. They cannot test hypotheses or establish cause-and-effect relationships.[36]

Types of Research

A number of methods are used to classify research. One way is to view research along a continuum reflecting the type of question the research is intended to answer. On this continuum, research is classified as descriptive, experimental or exploratory.[36]

Descriptive research: Recording, analyzing, and interpreting conditions that exist for the purpose of classification and understanding a clinical phenomenon.

Experimental research: Comparing two or more conditions for the purpose of determining cause-and-effect relationships between independent and dependent variables.

Exploratory research: Examines the dimensions of a phenomenon of interest and its relationships to other factors.

Ethics of Human Subjects Research

Belmont Report: In 1974, the National Research Act established the National Commission for the Protection of Human Subjects of Biomedical and Behavioral Research. This Commission, in turn, published The Belmont Report which articulated the three ethical principles that guide human subjects' research:[37]

- **Respect for persons:** Refers to the individual's right of self-determination and the right to make decisions about their medical care as an autonomous person. Respect for persons requires that people with diminished autonomy be provided special protection.

- **Beneficence:** Refers to the obligation of the researcher to provide for the well-being of their subjects and to maximize the possible benefits and minimize the possible harm in research.

- **Justice:** Refers to the fair treatment of subjects including the equitable distribution of burdens and benefits in research.

Confidentiality: An ethical principle that requires the researcher to not disclose any information revealed by the subject or discovered by the researcher to ensure that data is accessible only to authorized individuals.

Human subject: A living individual about whom an investigator conducting research obtains data through intervention or interaction with the individual or identifiable private information.[37]

Informed consent: The process by which a person is given important facts about the possible risks, benefits, and limits of the procedure, treatment, trial or testing before deciding whether or not to participate.[37]

Institutional Review Board (IRB): A group of scientists and non-scientists charged with protecting the rights and welfare of persons participating in research and authorized to review and approve research involving human subjects.[37]

Types of Data and Measurement

Data

Data are the numeric and non-numeric information that represent the quantitative or qualitative attributes of an object, event or person.[38] Types of data include:

Qualitative data: Also known as categorical data, these data represent different categories distinguished by a non-numeric characteristic.[38] Examples include eye color, blood type, and hand dominance.

Quantitative data: Data consisting of numbers that represent counts or measurements.[38] A measurement is the numeral assigned to an object, event or person, or the category to which an object, event or person is assigned according to rules.[11]

Scales of Measurement

Nominal: Also known as the classification scale because the values of the variable are mutually exclusive and exhaustive categories, so that each object or person can be assigned to only one category. Nominal scales are qualitative rather than quantitative. Examples of nominal scale measurements in physical therapy include blood type, type of breath sound, and type of arthritis.[39]

Ordinal: This scale of measurement is also known as a ranking scale. The data are ranked on the basis of a property of the variable, but the intervals between the ranks may not be equal or known. Examples of ordinal scale measurements in physical therapy include manual muscle test grades, levels of assistance, pain, and joint laxity grades.[39]

CONSIDER THIS
INFORMED CONSENT

In keeping with the principle of Respect for Persons, researchers must obtain the informed consent of the subject or the subject's legally authorized representative under circumstances that provide the opportunity to consider whether or not to participate without undue influence or coercion. Informed consent should contain all of the following:[37]

1. A statement that the study involves research.
2. An explanation of the purpose(s) of the research.
3. A description of the procedures to be followed, including the duration of participation, and identification of any experimental procedures.
4. A description of any reasonably foreseeable risks or discomforts to the subject.
5. A description of any benefits to the subject or to others that may reasonably be expected.
6. A disclosure of any appropriate alternative procedures or treatments that might be advantageous.
7. A description of who will have access to records that identify the subjects, and how confidentiality of those records will be maintained.
8. For research involving greater than minimal risk, an explanation of any compensation and an explanation of any medical treatments that are available if injury occurs, and what they consist of, or where further information may be obtained.
9. Identification of whom to contact for answers to questions about the research and subjects' rights, and whom to contact in the event of a research-related injury to the subject, along with contact information.
10. A statement that participation is voluntary and that the subject may refuse to participate or discontinue participation at any time without penalty.

Interval: A measurement scale where the intervals between adjacent values are equal, but there is no true zero point. Examples of interval scale measurements in physical therapy include temperature (e.g., body, skin, whirlpool) on the Fahrenheit or Celsius scale and some developmental and functional status tests.[39]

Ratio: A measurement scale where the intervals between adjacent values are equal and there is a true zero point. Examples of ratio scale measurements in physical therapy include range of motion (degrees), distance walked (m), time to complete an activity (s), and nerve conduction velocity (m/sec).[39]

Measurement Reliability

Reliability is the reproducibility or repeatability of measurements.[39] Examples of different forms of reliability include:

Alternate forms reliability: Also known as parallel forms reliability, it assesses the consistency or agreement of measurements obtained with different forms of a test. Alternate forms reliability is essential if the different forms of the test are to be used interchangeably.[39] For example, different forms of standardized tests like the SAT, GRE, and NPTE can be administered each year as long as the different versions of the tests are considered equivalent measures.

Internal consistency: The extent to which items or elements that contribute to a measurement reflect one basic phenomenon or dimension.[39] For example, in physical therapy, a functional assessment scale should only include items that relate to patients' physical function.[36]

Intrarater reliability: The consistency or equivalence of repeated measurements made by the same person over time.[39]

Interrater reliability: The consistency or equivalence of measurements made by more than one person. Interrater reliability indicates the agreement of measurements taken by different examiners.[39]

Test-retest reliability: The consistency or equivalence of repeated measurements made on the same individual on separate occasions.[39] Test-retest reliability can be affected by the interval between tests, effects of fatigue or learning, and changes in the characteristic being measured.[36]

Measurement Validity

Validity is the degree to which a useful or meaningful interpretation can be inferred from a measurement.[39] Examples of different types of measurement validity include:

Face validity: The degree to which a measurement appears to test what it is supposed to.[36] Although face validity is insufficient documentation of validity, it is an important form of validity because patients may not be compliant with repeated testing if they don't see how the measurements derived from the tests relate to their specific problem.

Content validity: The degree to which a measurement reflects the meaningful elements of a construct and the items in a test adequately reflect the content domain of interest and not extraneous elements.[39] For example, the McGill Pain Questionnaire may have greater content validity than a visual analogue pain scale because, in addition to pain intensity, it assesses the location, quality, and duration of pain.[36]

Construct validity: The degree to which a theoretical construct is measured by a test or measurement. Evidence of construct validity is through logical argument based on theoretical and research

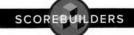

evidence.[39] For example, manual muscle test (MMT) scores would have construct validity as indicators of innervation status of muscle if there was a relationship between MMT scores and the results of electromyographic testing.

Criterion-related validity: The validity of the measurement is established by comparing it to either a different measurement often considered to be a "gold standard" or data obtained by different forms of testing.[39] Examples of criterion-related validity include:

- **Concurrent validity:** A form of criterion-related validity in which an interpretation is justified by comparing a measurement to a "gold standard" measurement at approximately the same time.[39] For example, heart rate measurements made by palpation of peripheral pulses will have concurrent validity if the heart rate measurements by palpation are associated with the heart rates measured simultaneously from an ECG.

- **Predictive validity:** A form of criterion-related validity in which the measurement is considered to be valid because it is predictive of a future behavior or event.[39] For example, the use of a student's GPA or GRE as admission criteria for graduate school is based on their presumed ability to predict future academic success.

- **Prescriptive validity:** A form of criterion-related validity in which the measurement suggests the form of treatment the person should receive. The prescriptive validity of the measurement is judged based on the successful outcome of the treatment.[39] For example, the measurement of asystole on the ECG could be said to have prescriptive validity if patients with this arrhythmia are successfully revived by cardiopulmonary resuscitation techniques.

Research Subjects and Sampling

Population: The complete collection of elements to be studied. The group to which the results of research are intended to be generalized.[38]

Sample: A subset of elements drawn from a population to draw conclusions or make estimates about the larger population.[36]

Sampling error: The chance difference between the statistic calculated from a sample and the true value of the parameter in the population. Sampling error is inherent in the use of sampling methods.[36]

Probability sampling: A method of sampling that uses some form of random selection. Every member of the population must have the same probability of being selected for the sample, since the sample should be free of bias and representative of the population.[8] Examples of probability sampling methods include:

- **Simple random sampling:** Subjects have an equal chance of being selected for the sample. The sampling method often relies on a table of random numbers or a random number generator on a computer to determine the sample. However, simple random sampling is not the most statistically efficient method of sampling and may not result in a representative sample, since it is the luck of the draw.[36]

- **Systematic sampling:** Subjects are selected by taking every n^{th} subject from the population. The size of the interval is

based on the size of the population and the desired sample size. The greatest advantage associated with this sampling technique is its simplicity.[36]

- **Stratified random sampling:** Also called proportional or quota random sampling, the population is divided into homogenous subgroups (strata) and then a simple random sample is drawn from each. Stratified random sampling assures that the sample will be representative of key subgroups of the population in addition to the overall population.[36]

- **Cluster sampling:** The population is divided into clusters or areas (usually along geographic boundaries) and a random sample of the clusters is selected. Then, all of the units in the selected samples are measured. The sampling technique is less costly and more efficient than simple random sampling, especially when the population is spread across a wide geographic region.[36]

Non-probability sampling: Any method of sampling that does not involve random selection of subjects.[36] Examples of non-probability sampling methods include:

- **Convenience sampling:** As the name suggests, the sample is selected from subjects who are convenient or readily available to the researcher.[36]

- **Purposive sampling:** Subjects are deliberately selected based on predefined criteria chosen by the investigators.[36]

Measures of Center

Values that describe the center of the data.

Mean: The arithmetic average; the sum of all the values divided by number of values.[38]

Median: The point on a distribution at which 50% of the values fall above and below. It is the 50th percentile. The median is identified by first rank ordering the values. If the number of values is odd, the median is the middle value. If the number of values is even, the median is the mean of the two middle values.[38]

Mode: The value that occurs most frequently. A distribution with two modes is termed bimodal. A distribution with more than two modes is termed multimodal.[38]

Measures of Variation

Values that describe how the data vary.

Percentiles: The value below which a certain percent of observations within a distribution will fall. For example, the 20th percentile is the value or score below which 20% of scores are found.[38]

Quartiles: Quartiles divide the data into four equal parts, so that each part represents one fourth of the sampled population. The 25th percentile is also known as the first quartile (Q1), the 50th percentile as the median or second quartile (Q2), and the 75th percentile as the third quartile (Q3).[38]

Range: The difference between the maximum and minimum values.[38]

Standard deviation: A descriptive measure of the spread or dispersion of data; the positive square root of the variance. Describing data by means of standard deviation implies that the data are normally distributed.

Safety and Protection; Professional Responsibilities; Research Essentials

Safety and Protection

1. Standard precautions combine universal precautions and body substance isolation precautions. Standard precautions apply to all blood/body fluids, secretions, and excretions.

2. Transmission-based precautions offer guidelines for the care of specified patients infected with selected pathogens transmitted by airborne, droplet or contact modes.

3. Airborne precautions reduce the risk of airborne transmission of infectious agents through evaporated droplets in air or dust particles.

4. Droplet precautions reduce the risk of droplet transmission of infectious agents through contact of the mucous membranes of the mouth and nose, contact with the conjunctivae, and through coughing, sneezing, talking or suctioning.

5. Contact precautions reduce the risk of transmission of infectious agents through direct or indirect contact. Direct contact involves skin-to-skin transmission; indirect contact involves a contaminated intermediate object, usually within the patient's environment.

6. Personal protective equipment (e.g., gowns, lab coats, masks, gloves, goggles, spill kits, mouthpieces) are used as barriers to protect someone who is assisting a patient with a potentially infectious disease.

7. A sterile field is a designated area that is considered void of all contaminants and microorganisms. Specific protocols are required to develop and maintain the sterile field.

Professional Responsibilities

8. The Americans with Disabilities Act is federal legislation designed to provide a clear and comprehensive national mandate for the elimination of discrimination.

9. A ramp must possess twelve inches of length for each inch of vertical rise (i.e., 8.3% grade).

10. A S.O.A.P. note is a commonly used format for daily notes. The S.O.A.P. acronym stands for: S = Subjective, O = Objective, A = Assessment, P = Plan.

11. Quality improvement refers to a form of objective self-examination designed to improve the quality of services.

12. The Nagi Model describes health status as a product of the relationship between health and function and is defined by four primary concepts: pathology, impairment, functional limitation, and disability.

13. Negligence refers to the failure to do what a reasonable and prudent person would ordinarily have done under the same or similar circumstances for a given situation.

14. Risk management refers to the identification, analysis, and evaluation of risks and the selection of the most advantageous method for treating them.

15. Responsibilities delegated to support personnel by physical therapist assistants must be commensurate with their qualifications. This includes experience, education, and training of the individuals to whom the responsibilities are being assigned.

16. A physical therapist assistant is a technically educated health care provider who assists the physical therapist in the provision of physical therapy. The physical therapist assistant, under the direction and supervision of the physical therapist, is the only paraprofessional who provides physical therapy interventions.

17. A physical therapy aide is a non-licensed worker who is specifically trained under the direction and supervision of a physical therapist. The physical therapy aide may be involved in the provision of physical therapist directed support services.

18. The Physical Therapist Patient/Client Management Model includes examination, evaluation, diagnosis, prognosis (including plan of care), intervention, and outcomes.

19. The Standards of Ethical Conduct for the Physical Therapist Assistant by the American Physical Therapy Association sets forth standards for the published ethical practice of physical therapy. All physical therapist assistants are responsible for maintaining and promoting ethical practice.

Safety and Protection; Professional Responsibilities; Research Essentials

20. Medicare provides health insurance for individuals over 65 years of age and the disabled. Medicaid provides basic medical services for individuals with low income or who qualify for welfare or public assistance benefits in the state of their residence.

21. Workers' Compensation provides protection for employees that are injured on the job. This legislation provides continued income as well as paid medical expenses for employees injured while working.

22. Current Procedural Terminology (CPT) codes are procedure codes used by physical therapists, physical therapist assistants, and other health care professionals to describe the interventions that were provided to a given patient.

23. The International Classification of Diseases (ICD) codes are designed to describe a patient's infirmity through categories based on etiology and affected anatomical systems.

24. Maslow's Hierarchy of Needs includes self-actualization needs, esteem needs, affiliative needs, and physiological needs.

25. Classical conditioning refers to a process where learning occurs when an unconditioned stimulus is repeatedly preceded by a neutral stimulus. The neutral stimulus serves as a conditioned stimulus and the learned reaction that results is termed the conditioned response.

26. Operant conditioning refers to a process where learning occurs when an individual engages in specific behaviors in order to receive certain consequences.

27. Domains of learning are educational terms that describe various aspects of human behavior. The three most commonly recognized domains of learning are the cognitive, psychomotor, and affective domains.

28. The Stages of Dying describe five stages in coming to terms with death. The stages include denial, anger, bargaining, depression, and acceptance.

Research

29. Evidence-based practice refers to a therapist's reliance on patient-centered clinical research, clinical expertise and past experiences, and the patient's values when making clinical decisions about the patient's physical therapy plan of care.

30. There is a hierarchy for the levels of evidence for studies about therapy/intervention, diagnosis, and prognosis. For studies about therapy/interventions, systematic reviews and meta-analyses are considered to be the highest forms of evidence followed by randomized controlled trials.

31. Physical therapists and physical therapist assistants involved in clinical research must adhere to the principles and practices that govern the planning and implementation of research when working with human subjects. These are summarized in the Belmont Report.

32. The three basic ethical principles relevant to research involving human subjects are the principles of respect of persons, beneficence, and justice.

33. Reliability and validity are important properties of measurements. Therapists should select tests and measurements which have been investigated for appropriate forms of reliability and validity.

34. Selecting a representative sample of subjects from the population is an important step in the research process to ensure that the results of the research can be generalized to the population of interest.

35. Probability samples involve some form of random selection; non-probability samples do not.

Safety and Protection; Professional Responsibilities; Research Proficiencies

Safety and Protection; Professional Responsibilities Proficiencies

1. Accessibility Requirements

Determine if each provided measurement is consistent with established accessibility standards. If a given measurement satisfies existing standards, it is considered acceptable. If the measurement fails to satisfy existing standards, it is considered unacceptable.

Determine if each measurement is acceptable or unacceptable, and identify the established accessibility standard for each measurement.

Word Bank: acceptable, unacceptable

Acceptable/Unacceptable	Measurement
a	A ramp with a grade of 9.8%.
Standard:	
b	A ramp that is 20 feet in length with a 24 inch vertical rise.
Standard:	
c	A ramp with a width of 36 inches.
Standard:	
d	A doorway with a width of 34 inches.
Standard:	
e	A hallway with a width of 32 inches.
Standard:	
f	A bathroom sink with 30 inches of height from the floor.
Standard:	
g	A bathroom toilet with 18 inches of height from the floor to the top of the toilet.
Standard:	

Safety and Protection; Professional Responsibilities; Research Proficiencies

Safety and Protection; Professional Responsibilities Proficiencies

2. S.O.A.P. Notes

Identify the appropriate portion of the S.O.A.P. note for each entry. Answers must be selected from the Word Bank.

Word Bank: subjective, objective, assessment, plan

Section	Entry
a	The patient reports hurting the knee after falling down a flight of stairs.
b	Right knee active range of motion is 0-126 degrees.
c	The patient received instructions for shoulder strengthening using elastic tubing.
d	The patient denies pain when coughing.
e	The patient may not have exhibited maximal effort during resistive testing.
f	The patient exhibits 5/5 strength in the left iliopsoas.
g	The patient indicates a desire to return home with her husband after discharge.
h	The patient demonstrated appropriate use of pacing techniques during ambulation.
i	The patient's cardiac status may diminish the patient's rate of recovery.
j	The patient will be referred to a speech-language pathologist.

3. The Nagi Model

Identify the appropriate concept from the Nagi Model based on each description. Answers must be selected from the Word Bank and can be used more than once.

Word Bank: disability, impairment, functional limitation, pathology

Concept	Description
a	lateral collateral ligament sprain
b	diminished knee range of motion
c	difficulty ascending a flight of stairs
d	unable to work as a housekeeper
e	diminished upper extremity sensation
f	unable to propel a wheelchair on level ground

Safety and Protection; Professional Responsibilities; Research Proficiencies

Safety and Protection; Professional Responsibilities Proficiencies

4. Scope of Practice

Determine if each described activity is consistent with the scope of practice for the identified health care provider. Appropriate activities should be labeled acceptable and inappropriate activities should be labeled unacceptable.

Word Bank: acceptable, unacceptable

Acceptable/Unacceptable	Entry
a	A physical therapist assistant completes a discharge summary.
b	A physical therapist instructs a physical therapist assistant to teach an existing patient to utilize axillary crutches.
c	A physical therapist assistant describes a patient's exercise tolerance in the medical record.
d	A physical therapy aide guards a patient ascending stairs.
e	A physical therapist assistant discontinues an existing exercise session due to safety concerns.
f	A physical therapist assistant completes a re-examination on a patient.
g	A physical therapy aide monitors a patient's vital signs during exercise.
h	A physical therapist assistant increases the weight a patient uses on an existing upper extremity progressive resistive exercise.
i	A physical therapy aide returns a previously used hot pack to the hydrocollator unit.

Safety and Protection; Professional Responsibilities; Research Proficiencies

Safety and Protection; Professional Responsibilities Proficiencies

5. Health Care Disciplines

Identify the health care discipline most closely associated with the supplied description. Answers must be selected from the Word Bank and can be used only once.

Word Bank: home health aides, occupational therapists, physical therapist assistants, physical therapists, physical therapy aides, respiratory therapists, social workers, speech-language pathologists

a	These individuals provide health related services to the elderly, disabled, and ill in their homes. Patient care activities include performing housekeeping duties, assisting with ambulation or transfers, and promoting personal hygiene.
b	These individuals are considered support personnel who may be involved in support services directed by physical therapists. They are permitted to function only with continuous on-site supervision by a physical therapist, or in some cases a physical therapist assistant.
c	These individuals evaluate, treat, and care for patients with breathing disorders. Patient care activities include performing postural drainage techniques, measuring lung capacities, administering oxygen and aerosols, and analyzing oxygen and carbon dioxide concentrations.
d	These individuals help people improve their ability to perform activities of daily living, work, and leisure skills. Educational preparation emphasizes the social, emotional, and physiological effects of illness and injury.
e	These individuals provide services to help restore function, improve mobility, relieve pain, and prevent or limit permanent physical disabilities of patients suffering from injuries or disease.
f	These individuals evaluate speech, language, cognitive-communication, and swallowing skills of children and adults.
g	These individuals perform components of physical therapy procedures and related tasks selected and delegated by a supervising physical therapist.
h	These individuals help patients and their families to cope with chronic, acute or terminal illnesses and attempt to resolve problems that stand in the way of recovery or rehabilitation.

Safety and Protection; Professional Responsibilities; Research Proficiencies

Safety and Protection; Professional Responsibilities Proficiencies

6. Safety and Professional Roles Basics

Mark each statement as True or False. If the statement is False, correct the statement in the space provided.

True/False	Statement
a	A computer monitor in a work station should be a minimum of 12 inches away from the eyes.
Correction:	
b	When performing a transfer with a patient that requires assistance, a physical therapist assistant should attempt to be as close to the patient as possible and use a long lever arm.
Correction:	
c	Sterile gowns are only considered sterile in the front from the waist level upwards.
Correction:	
d	If an object on a sterile field becomes contaminated, the entire field is considered non-sterile.
Correction:	
e	A patient with droplet precautions would require a physical therapist assistant to wear a mask if they were within ten feet of the patient.
Correction:	
f	A ramp that is 20 inches in elevation should be a minimum of 20 feet in length.
Correction:	

Safety and Protection; Professional Responsibilities; Research Proficiencies

Safety and Protection; Professional Responsibilities Proficiencies

True/False	Statement
g	A discharge summary should provide a capsule view of the patient's progress during therapy.
Correction:	
h	One inch is equivalent to 3.28 centimeters.
Correction:	
i	Autonomy refers to the moral obligation of health care providers to act for the benefit of others.
Correction:	
j	Prognosis refers to the anticipated level of optimal improvement that may be attained through intervention and the amount of time required to reach that level.
Correction:	
k	The Consolidated Omnibus Budget Reconciliation Act provides protection for employees that are injured on the job.
Correction:	
l	Medicare Part A provides benefits for outpatient care, physician services, and services ordered by physicians such as diagnostic tests, medical equipment, and supplies.
Correction:	
m	International Classification of Diseases Codes are procedure codes used by physical therapists, physical therapist assistants, and other health care professionals to describe specific interventions provided to a given patient.
Correction:	

Safety and Protection; Professional Responsibilities; Research Proficiencies

Safety and Protection; Professional Responsibilities Proficiencies

7. Domains of Learning

Identify the appropriate domain of learning for each described activity. Answers must be selected from the Word Bank and can be used more than once.

Word Bank: affective, cognitive, psychomotor

Domain	Description
a	A patient lists three postoperative contraindications following total hip arthroplasty.
b	A patient reports being fearful that they will reinjure their knee after returning to athletic activities.
c	A patient performs a D2 flexion pattern using the right upper extremity.
d	A patient verbally summarizes the activities included in a home exercise program with their physical therapist assistant.
e	A patient demonstrates a sliding board transfer using the appropriate technique.
f	A patient is extremely cautious when weight bearing on the involved lower extremity.

8. Stages of Dying

Identify the appropriate stage of dying for each description. Answers must be selected from the Word Bank and can be used only once.

Word Bank: acceptance, anger, bargaining, denial, depression

Stage	Description
a	This stage is characterized by an individual trying to negotiate with fate.
b	This stage is characterized by frustration and negative emotional feelings often directed at anyone the individual comes in contact with.
c	This stage is characterized by the individual expressing the depths of their anguish and showing little interest in any form of medical intervention.
d	This stage is characterized by the individual coming to terms with their fate.
e	This stage is characterized by a failure of the individual to believe that their condition is terminal.

Safety and Protection; Professional Responsibilities; Research Proficiencies

Safety and Protection; Professional Responsibilities Proficiencies

9. Teaching and Learning Basics

Mark each statement as True or False. If the statement is False, correct the statement in the space provided.

True/False	Statement
a	According to Maslow's Hierarchy of Needs, esteem needs refer to the need to realize one's full potential as a human being.
Correction:	
b	Therapists should attempt to identify the patient's preferred learning style and available resources.
Correction:	
c	Therapists should attempt to design learning activities that will incorporate the patient's past experiences.
Correction:	

Safety and Protection; Professional Responsibilities; Research Proficiencies

Research Proficiencies

10. Levels of Evidence

Assign a number to each category based on the strength of the design. An assignment of "1" would indicate the most desirable or highest level of evidence from the available options while an assignment of "5" would indicate the least desirable or lowest level of evidence.

Study	Rank
randomized controlled trial	a
case control study	b
systematic review	c
cohort study	d
case report	e

11. Scales of Measurement

Identify the appropriate scale of measurement for each of the following types of data. Answers must be selected from the Word Bank and can be used more than once.

Word Bank: interval, nominal, ordinal, ratio

Data	Scale
range of motion	a
body temperature on the Celsius scale	b
distance walked	c
blood type	d
manual muscle test grades	e
type of breath sounds	f
transfer levels of assistance	g

Safety and Protection; Professional Responsibilities; Research Proficiencies

Research Proficiencies

12. Sampling

Identify the type of sampling most closely associated with the supplied definition. Answers must be selected from the Word Bank and can be used only once.

Word Bank: convenience, purposive, simple random, stratified random, systematic

Type of Sampling	Definition
a	Subjects are selected from those readily available to the researcher.
b	Subjects are selected from a population that has been divided into homogenous subgroups or strata and then a simple random sample is drawn from each.
c	Subjects have an equal chance of being selected for the sample.
d	Subjects are deliberately selected based on predefined criteria chosen by the investigators.
e	Subjects are selected by taking every n^{th} subject from the population.

13. Statistics

Identify the type of statistic most closely associated with the supplied definition. Answers must be selected from the Word Bank and can be used only once.

Word Bank: mean, median, mode, range, standard deviation

Type of Statistic	Definition
a	The arithmetic average; the sum of all the values divided by the number of values.
b	A descriptive measure of the spread or dispersion of data; the positive square root of the variance.
c	The point on a distribution at which 50% of the values fall above and below.
d	The value that occurs most frequently.
e	The difference between the maximum and minimum values.

Safety and Protection; Professional Responsibilities; Research Answer Key

Safety and Protection; Professional Responsibilities

1. Accessibility Requirements

a.   Unacceptable: Guideline - A ramp should have a maximum grade of 8.3%.

b.   Unacceptable: Guideline - A ramp should possess twelve inches of horizontal run for each inch of vertical rise.

c.   Acceptable: Guideline - A ramp should have a minimum width of 36 inches.

d.   Acceptable: Guideline - A doorway should have a minimum width of 32 inches.

e.   Unacceptable: Guideline - A hallway should have a minimum width of 36 inches.

f.   Acceptable: Guideline - A bathroom sink should have a minimum of 29 inches of height from the floor.

g.   Acceptable: Guideline - A bathroom toilet should have 17-19 inches of height from the floor to the top of the toilet.

2. S.O.A.P. Notes

a.   subjective
b.   objective
c.   objective
d.   subjective
e.   assessment
f.   objective
g.   subjective
h.   objective
i.   assessment
j.   plan

3. The Nagi Model

a.   pathology
b.   impairment
c.   functional limitation
d.   disability
e.   impairment
f.   functional limitation

4. Scope of Practice

a.   unacceptable
b.   acceptable
c.   acceptable
d.   unacceptable
e.   acceptable
f.   unacceptable
g.   unacceptable
h.   acceptable
i.   acceptable

5. Health Care Disciplines

a.   home health aides
b.   physical therapy aides
c.   respiratory therapists
d.   occupational therapists
e.   physical therapists
f.   speech-language pathologists
g.   physical therapist assistants
h.   social workers

6. Safety and Professional Roles Basics*

a.   FALSE: Correction: A computer monitor of a work station should be a minimum of 20 inches away from the eyes.

b.   FALSE: Correction: When performing a transfer with a patient that requires assistance, a physical therapist assistant should attempt to be as close to the patient as possible and use a short lever arm.

c.   TRUE

d.   TRUE

e.   FALSE: Correction: A patient with droplet precautions would require a physical therapist assistant to wear a mask if they were within three feet of the patient.

f.   TRUE

g.   TRUE

h.   FALSE: Correction: One inch is equivalent to 2.54 centimeters.

i.   FALSE: Correction: Beneficence refers to the moral obligation to health care providers to act for the benefit of others.

j.   TRUE

k.   FALSE: Correction: The Consolidated Omnibus Budget Reconciliation Act allows an employee to remain under an employer's group plan for a period of time after the loss of a job, death of a spouse, a decrease in hours or a divorce.

l.   FALSE: Correction: Medicare Part B provides benefits for outpatient care, physician services, and services ordered by physicians such as diagnostic tests, medical equipment, and supplies.

m.   FALSE: Correction: Current procedural terminology codes are procedure codes used by physical therapists, physical therapist assistants and other health care professionals to describe specific interventions provided to a given patient.

*The correction presented for each false statement is an example of several possible corrections.

Safety and Protection; Professional Responsibilities; Research Answer Key

7. Domains of Learning
a. cognitive
b. affective
c. psychomotor
d. cognitive
e. psychomotor
f. affective

8. Stages of Dying
a. bargaining
b. anger
c. depression
d. acceptance
e. denial

9. Teaching and Learning Basics*
a. FALSE: Correction: According to Maslow's Hierarchy of Needs, self-actualization refers to the need to realize one's full potential as a human being.
b. TRUE
c. TRUE

*The correction presented for each false statement is an example of several possible corrections.

Research

10. Levels of Evidence
a. 2
b. 4
c. 1
d. 3
e. 5

11. Scales of Measurement
a. ratio
b. interval
c. ratio
d. nominal
e. ordinal
f. nominal
g. ordinal

12. Sampling
a. convenience
b. stratified random
c. simple random
d. purposive
e. systematic

13. Statistics
a. mean
b. standard deviation
c. median
d. mode
e. range

Safety and Protection; Professional Responsibilities; Research References

1. Cameron M, Monroe L. *Physical Rehabilitation: Evidence Based Examination, Evaluation, and Intervention*. W.B. Saunders Company. 2007.

2. Minor M, Minor S. *Patient Care Skills*. Seventh Edition. Pearson Education, Inc. 2014.

3. Fairchild S, O'Shea R, Washington R. *Pierson and Fairchild's Principles and Techniques of Patient Care*. Sixth Edition. Elsevier. 2018.

4. Guide to Infection Prevention for Outpatient Settings: Minimum Expectations for Safe Care version 2.3. Centers for Disease Control and Prevention Web Site. http://www.cdc.gov Updated September 2016. Accessed May 22, 2017.

5. Roy S, Wolf S, Scalzitti D. *The Rehabilitation Specialist's Handbook*. Fourth Edition, F.A. Davis Company. 2013.

6. Kettenbach G. *Writing SOAP Notes*. Second Edition. F.A. Davis Company. 1995

7. Shamus E, Stern D. *Effective Documentation for the Physical Therapy Professional*. Second Edition. McGraw-Hill Inc. 2011.

8. Guidelines: Physical Therapy Documentation of Patient/Client Management. BOD G03-05-16-41, updated 5/19/14. American Physical Therapy Association Web Site. Accessed May 22, 2017.

9. Defensible Documentation Elements. American Physical Therapy Association Web Site. http://www.apta.org/Documentation/DefensibleDocumentation/. Updated 12/8/2015. Accessed May 22, 2017.

10. Davis C. *Patient Practitioner Interaction*. Fourth Edition. Slack Inc. 2006.

11. Scott R. *Promoting Legal and Ethical Awareness*. Mosby Inc. 2009.

12. Nosse L, Friberg D. *Managerial and Supervisory Principles for Physical Therapists*. Third Edition. Lippincott Williams & Wilkins. 2010.

13. Buchbinder S, Shanks N. *Introduction to Health Care Management*. Jones and Bartlett Publishers. 2007.

14. *Guide to Physical Therapist Practice* 3.0. American Physical Therapy Association. 2014.

15. International Classification of Functioning, Disability and Health (ICF). World Health Organization Web Site. http://www.who.int/classifications/icf/en/. Accessed May 22, 2017.

16. Direction and Supervision of the Physical Therapist Assistant. HOD P06-05-18-26, updated 08/07/12. American Physical Therapy Association Web Site. Accessed May 22, 2017.

17. *Mosby's Dictionary of Medicine, Nursing and Health Professions*. Eighth Edition, Mosby. 2009.

18. Criteria for Standards of Practice for Physical Therapy. BOD S01-14-01-01, updated 4/15/14. American Physical Therapy Association Web Site. Accessed May 22, 2017.

19. Code of Ethics for the Physical Therapist. HOD S06-09-07-12, updated June 2009. American Physical Therapy Association Web Site. Accessed May 22, 2017.

20. Curtis K: *The Physical Therapist's Guide to Health Care*. Slack Inc. 1999.

21. Sandstrom R, Lohman H. *Health Services: Policy and Systems for Therapists*. Prentice Hall. 2003.

22. Sadock B, Sadock V. *Kaplan & Sadock's Comprehensive Textbook of Psychiatry*. Ninth Edition. Lippincott Williams & Wilkins. 2009.

23. Edelman C, Mandle C. *Health Promotion Throughout the Lifespan*. Fifth Edition. Mosby. 2002.

24. Purtilo R, Haddad A. *Health Professional and Patient Interaction*. Eighth Edition. Elsevier. 2014.

25. Falvo D. *Effective Patient Education*. Fourth Edition. Jones and Bartlett Publishers. 2011.

26. Haggard A. *Handbook of Patient Education*. Aspen Publishers. 1989.

27. Arends R. *Learning to Teach*. Third Edition, McGraw-Hill Inc. 2005.

Safety and Protection; Professional Responsibilities; Research References

28. Scott R. *Foundations of Physical Therapy: A 21st Century-Focused View of the Profession*. McGraw-Hill Inc. 2002.

29. Sackett DL, Straus SE, Richardson WS, Rosenburg W, Haynes RB. *Evidence-Based Medicine. How to Practice and Teach EBM*. 2nd ed. Edinburgh, Scotland; Churchill Livingstone. 2000.

30. Asking focused questions. Centre for Evidence-Based Medicine Web Site. http://www.cebm.net/index.aspx?o=1036. Updated April 7, 2009. Accessed October 7, 2010.

31. Critical appraisal. Centre for Evidence-Based Medicine Web Site. http://www.cebm.net/index.aspx?o=1157 Updated December 16, 2010. Accessed October 7, 2010.

32. Practice Guidelines. *Physical Therapy* Web Site. http://ptjournal. apta.org/cgi/collection/practice_guidelines Accessed October 3, 2010.

33. Guidelines by Topic. National Guideline Clearinghouse Web Site. http://www.guideline.gov/. Accessed October 3, 2010.

34. Levels of evidence. Centre for Evidence-Based Medicine Web Site. http://www.cebm.net/index.aspx?o=1025. Updated September 16, 2010. Accessed October 3, 2010.

35. Portney L, Watkins MP. *Foundations of Clinical Research: Applications to Practice*. Third Edition. Prentice Hall. 2015.

36. Glossary of Statistical Terms. National Cancer Institute Web Site. http://www.cancer.gov/statistics/glossary. Accessed October 3, 2010.

37. Code of Federal Regulation Title 45. Public Welfare. Part 46. Protection of Human Subjects. US Department of Health and Human Services Web Site. http://www.hhs.gov/ohrp/ humansubjects/guidance/45cfr46.htm. Accessed October 3, 2010.

38. Triola MF. *Elementary Statistics*. 9th ed. Boston, MA: Pearson Addison Wesley. 2004.

39. Rothstein JM, Echternach JL. *Primer on Measurement: An Introductory Guide to Measurement Issues*. Alexandria, VA; American Physical Therapy Association. 1993.

40. Iverson C, Christiansen S, Flanagin A, et al. *AMA Manual of Style: A Guide for Authors and Editors*. 10th ed. New York, NY: Oxford University Press. 2007.

Jumpstart Your Academic Review!

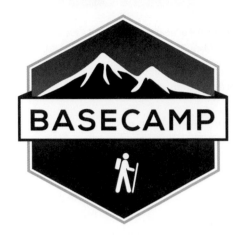

Basecamp

Basecamp offers students a personal guide to navigating through the academic review process. The program is a perfect complement to our best-selling review book **PTAEXAM: The Complete Study Guide**.

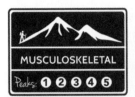
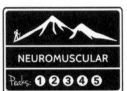
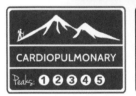
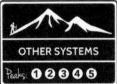
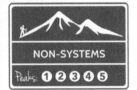

Basecamp - Start Climbing!

We created a completely new learning tool called **Basecamp** that provides you with an incredibly efficient method to review academic content within *PTAEXAM: The Complete Study Guide*. The content is organized in five distinct Mountains (Musculoskeletal, Neuromuscular, Cardiopulmonary, Other Systems, and Non-Systems) and 120 Trails. Each trail has dedicated assignments, video, and exams. A $25 off coupon for **Basecamp** is included within **Insight**. Purchase **Basecamp** today and start climbing!

Enter The Basecamp Arena

Our newest **Basecamp** features, **King of the Mountain** and **Climb**, allow students to challenge one another in real-time. The player to answer the most consecutive questions wins! Our **Basecamp Arena app** provides students with the opportunity to play the competitive games anytime and anywhere. Students can explore their performance data using the **Arena-Scorecard**. See if you have the knowledge to survive in the **Arena**.

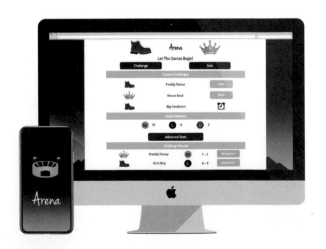

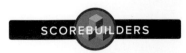

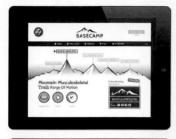
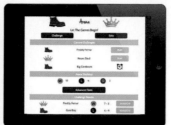
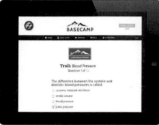
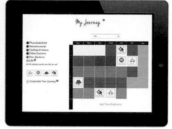

Scalability

Basecamp is designed to fully engage today's students utilizing a variety of forms of media and the latest in eLearning technology. The program is fully accessible on computers, tablets, and mobile devices.

Scorecard

An advanced Scorecard section allows students to monitor their performance in each of the Mountains and the associated Trails. By identifying areas of deficiency students are able to develop appropriate remedial plans and enhance core academic content in needed areas.

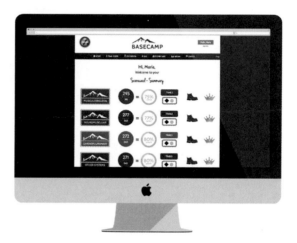

BASECAMP PURCHASING OPTIONS

Basecamp - Standard (30 day access) $55.00

The 30 day option is ideal for students attempting to engage in a meaningful review of core academic content prior to the NPTE-PTA. Various extension options are available.

Basecamp - Annual (One year access) $85.00 (Save up to 20% on class orders)

The one year option provides students and faculty with an ideal method to enhance learning throughout the academic program. Improved content mastery and retention can significantly increase academic performance in the classroom and on the NPTE-PTA.

Basecamp – Lifetime (Forever access) $120.00 (Save up to 20% on class orders)

The forever option allows students and physical therapist assistants to enjoy Basecamp during their academic training and well after they have successfully passed the NPTE-PTA. Take advantage of this tremendous value and let Basecamp assist you to stay in tip-top academic shape throughout your career as a physical therapist assistant.

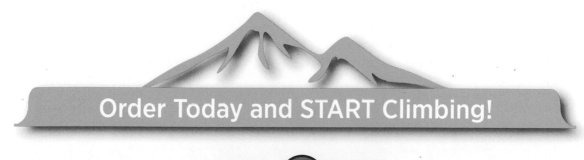

Order Today and START Climbing!

SCOREBUILDERS

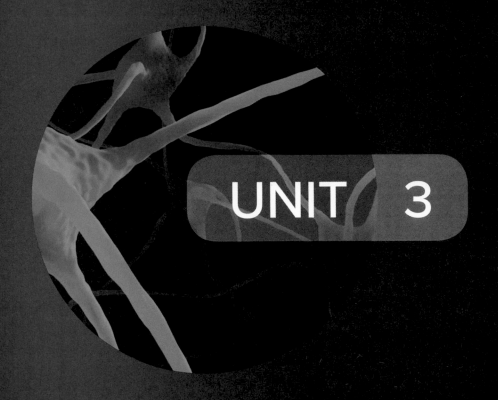

UNIT 3

Examinations Answer Key

Examinations Answer Key

This unit includes an **answer key for the three, 150 question sample examinations** located on our eLearning site called Insight. Candidates should take the examinations using Insight and then consult the answer key. It is important that candidates avoid "browsing" through the answer key prior to taking the sample examinations since any prior exposure to the questions will significantly influence examination scoring.

Candidates who are exposed to numerous sample examinations have several distinct opportunities that otherwise may not be available.

- Candidates have the opportunity to assess their current level of preparedness prior to the actual examination.
- Candidates have the opportunity to refine their test taking skills with sample questions that are similar in design and format to actual examination questions.
- Candidates have the opportunity to build their endurance and stamina when answering multiple-choice questions.

The sample examinations include questions representative of each of the categories and subcategories of the current content outline of the **NPTE-PTA**. A sophisticated performance analysis section offers candidates detailed feedback on their examination performance according to five system areas and five content outline areas.

System Specific Areas	Content Outline Areas
Musculoskeletal System	**Physical Therapy Data Collection**
Neuromuscular and Nervous Systems	**Diseases/Conditions that Impact Effective Treatment**
Cardiovascular and Pulmonary Systems	**Interventions**
Other Systems	**Equipment, Devices, and Technologies; Therapeutic Modalities**
Non-Systems	**Safety and Protection; Professional Responsibilities; Research**

The answer key in **PTAEXAM: The Complete Study Guide** offers a variety of features that can assist students to assess their examination performance and to direct remedial efforts.

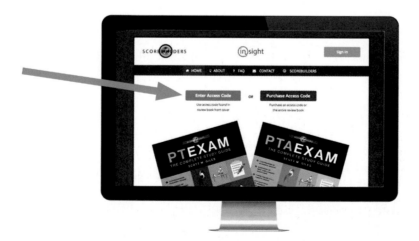

Access the sample examinations included with **PTAEXAM: The Complete Study Guide** by registering your code located on the inside front cover of the book at:

http://insight-sb.com

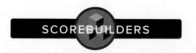

➡ PTAEXAM ONE: QUESTION 84

A physical therapist assistant uses functional electrical stimulation as part of a treatment regimen designed to improve quadriceps strength. Which on:off time ratio would result in the **MOST** rapid onset of muscle fatigue?

1. 3:1
2. 1:4
3. 5:1
4. 1:6

Examinations Answer Key Components

Question

Correct Answer: 3 (Prentice p. 130)

Correct Answer and Resource

Video Explanation

The on:off time ratio is simply a method to show the relative duration of the on time versus the off time. The muscle contracts during the on time and relaxes during the off time. The greater the on time in relation to the off time, the more rapid the onset of muscle fatigue.

General Statement

1. An on:off time ratio of 3:1 indicates that there is three seconds of on time for every one second of off time. This ratio would promote fatigue, however, it is not the best answer.

2. An on:off time ratio of 1:4 indicates that there is one second of on time for every four seconds of off time. This ratio has significantly greater rest periods and therefore fatigue would not tend to be a large factor.

3. **An on:off time ratio of 5:1 indicates that there is five seconds of on time for every one second of off time. This ratio would promote rapid fatigue given the extremely large on time in relation to the short off time.**

4. An on:off time ratio of 1:6 indicates that there is one second of on time for every six seconds of off time. This ratio has the greatest rest period and therefore fatigue would not tend to be a factor.

Explanation of the Correct and Incorrect Options

System: Non-Systems
Content Outline: Equipment, Devices, and Technologies; Therapeutic Modalities

System and Content Outline Assignment

✛ **Test Taking Tip:** Candidates must be extremely careful to answer examination questions in a precise manner. In this particular question, candidates need to identify the on:off time ratio that would result in the most rapid onset of fatigue. The best answer would have the greatest amount of on time in relation to the amount of off time. The correct option must be expressed in the same manner that the ratio is presented, meaning that the on time represents the first number and the off time represents the second number. By reversing these numbers a candidate could possess the requisite academic knowledge to answer the question, but still fail to answer the question correctly.

Test Taking Tip

Level Analysis

◉ Level 2   👓 p. 641-642

Academic Focus Area

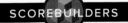

Examinations Answer Key Components Explained

Question

Our questions are designed to replicate the style, format, and difficulty level of the questions on the NPTE-PTA. The questions are located within our eLearning site Insight. All examinations should be taken using Insight to best simulate the actual NPTE-PTA.

Correct Answer and Resource

This section provides the correct answer and the author name and page number that substantiates the correct answer. A bibliography provides complete information on each resource including the edition used.

Video Explanation

Video explanations provide candidates with the opportunity to watch videos that compare and contrast good, better, and best options for selected examination questions.

General Statement

This section introduces relevant subject matter and offers related value added information.

Explanation of the Correct and Incorrect Options

The explanations offer incredibly detailed information supporting why the correct answer is correct and why each incorrect answer is incorrect. This feature is critically important to enhance decision making when choosing between good, better, and best options

System and Content Outline Assignment

This section assigns a system and content outline category to each question allowing candidates to assess examination performance in unique areas.

Test Taking Tip

This section offers unique Test Taking Tips, when possible, to assist candidates to use deductive reasoning strategies when academic knowledge alone is not adequate to correctly answer a question.

Level Analysis

This feature allows candidates to analyze their examination performance according to three different levels of questions.

Level 1 – Questions require candidates to possess basic foundational academic knowledge.

Level 2 – Questions require candidates to integrate numerous pieces of information or to apply knowledge in a given clinical scenario.

Level 3 – Questions require candidates to systematically analyze and often interpret information to determine an appropriate course of action. The questions tend to have some degree of subjectivity and candidates are required to assign varying degrees of importance to different variables.

Candidates have the ability to direct remedial efforts by examining their performance in each of the unique levels.

Academic Focus Area

This feature immediately directs the user to critical pieces in the academic review section related to the particular subject matter. Not all questions will have an academic focus area since some questions are situationally dependent and rely more on decision making than recollection of factual information.

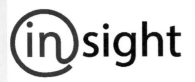

Insight

Insight is a technological marvel that offers candidates an unprecedented look into their sample examination performance.

Performance Analysis

After taking each of the examinations in Insight, candidates utilize the sophisticated performance analysis features to assess their examination performance. A brief description of some of the more prominent performance analysis features is presented.

Candidate Score

A candidate's score reflects the number of questions answered correctly for a given examination.

Mean Score

The mean score allows candidates to compare their score to the average score of thousands of other candidates taking the same examination. The mean score accounts for the relative difficulty of the examination and is a critical piece of data for candidates when assessing examination performance.

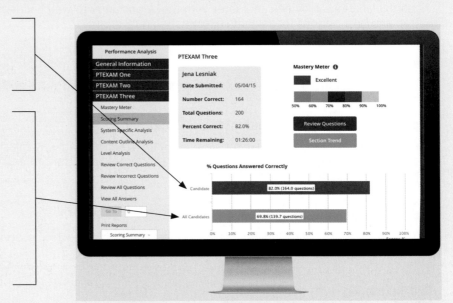

Item Analysis

The item analysis feature allows candidates to identify the percentage of candidates answering the question correctly and the specific percentages of candidates selecting each of the four options. Candidates can utilize this information to critically evaluate their approach to answering questions and improve future decision making. Video explanations provide candidates with a deeper understanding of academic concepts addressed in selected examination questions.

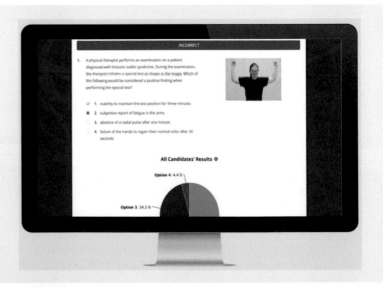

Mastery Meter

The Mastery Meter assigns candidates a level of mastery in each category based on the percentage of questions answered correctly. Candidates should strive to achieve a score of "Superior" or "Excellent" on the Mastery Meter in each category.

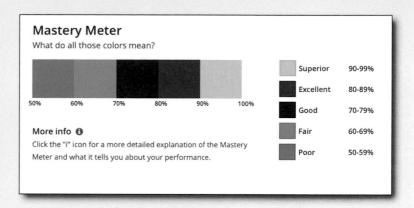

System Analysis

The system analysis offers candidates an immediate analysis in each of the five system areas of the NPTE-PTA. Candidates can click on a given system area and immediately review their performance in relation to the mean score of other users in the same system. They also have the ability to selectively review questions only within that particular system.

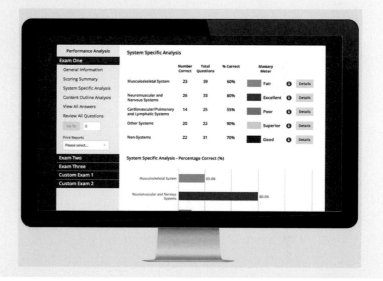

Content Outline Analysis

The content outline analysis offers candidates an immediate analysis in each of the five content outline areas of the NPTE-PTA. Candidates can click on a given content outline area and immediately review their performance in relation to the mean score of other users in the same content outline area. They also have the ability to selectively review questions only within that particular area.

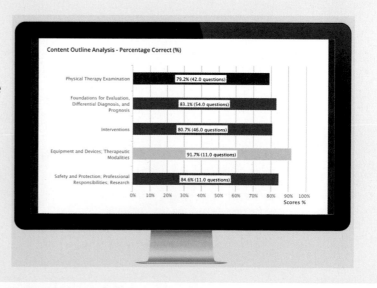

10

PHYSICAL THERAPIST ASSISTANT
EXAM ONE
ANSWER KEY

Scott Giles

PHYSICAL THERAPIST ASSISTANT EXAM ONE ANSWER KEY

STRATEGY

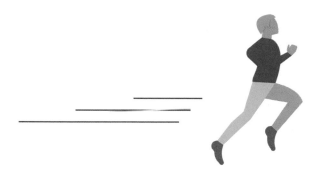

"Good fortune is what happens when opportunity meets preparation."

— Thomas Edison

Candidates need to have a strategy or plan to prepare for the NPTE-PTA. An important component of any comprehensive study plan involves answering multiple-choice questions and carefully analyzing the results. Identifying strengths and weaknesses in the various system and content outline areas can be a useful activity to direct remedial activities.

➡ PTAEXAM ONE: QUESTION 1

A physical therapist assistant presents an in-service to the rehabilitation staff that compares traditional gait terminology with Rancho Los Amigos terminology. Which pair of descriptive terms describes the same general point in the gait cycle?

1. Midstance to heel off and initial swing

2. **Heel strike and initial contact**

3. Foot flat to midstance and loading response

4. Toe off and midswing

Correct Answer: 2 (Roy p. 910)

Traditional gait terminology and Rancho Los Amigos terminology can be used to describe the various components of gait. There are a fair number of similarities between the two classification systems, however, there are also a number of differences. Rancho Los Amigos terminology tends to be more descriptive since it describes intervals of gait, usually with a well defined beginning and end point.

1. Midstance to heel off occurs during stance phase. Initial swing begins when the stance foot lifts from the floor and ends with maximal knee flexion during swing (i.e., swing phase).

2. **Heel strike and initial contact are both terms that describe the moment that the heel contacts the ground and stance phase begins.**

3. The loading response corresponds to the amount of time between initial contact and the beginning of the swing phase for the other leg. This is not the same point in the gait cycle as foot flat to midstance since the loading response does not include the period of time when the other foot is off the floor until the body is directly over the stance limb (i.e., midstance).

4. Toe off is the point in which only the toe of the stance limb remains on the ground, however, midswing occurs during swing phase.

System: Musculoskeletal System
Content Outline: Physical Therapy Data Collection

➡ PTAEXAM ONE: QUESTION 2

A physical therapist assistant monitors the vital signs of a patient running on a treadmill at a series of steadily increasing speeds. A change in which variable would be **MOST** responsible for an observed increase in pulse pressure during the exercise session?

1. Heart rate

2. **Systolic blood pressure**

3. Diastolic blood pressure

4. Cardiac output

Correct Answer: 2 (American College of Sports Medicine p. 502)

Pulse pressure, which is the difference between systolic and diastolic pressure, generally increases in direct proportion to the intensity of exercise since systolic pressure increases with exercise and diastolic pressure tends to stay the same. In a healthy adult, it is common to see a 40-50 mm Hg change in systolic pressure with intense exercise.

1. Heart rate is determined by the number of ventricular contractions per minute. Heart rate increases with an increase in exercise intensity, but would not be directly responsible for the observed increase in pulse pressure.

2. **Systolic blood pressure is the maximum arterial pressure during systole. Systolic pressure initially increases with exertion in a linear progression, often at a rate of 8-12 mm Hg per metabolic equivalent. The relative increase in systolic blood pressure, combined with stable diastolic blood pressure, results in an increase in pulse pressure.**

3. Diastolic blood pressure refers to the arterial pressure during diastole. Diastolic blood pressure remains relatively stable during exercise and therefore would not be responsible for the observed increase in pulse pressure.

4. Cardiac output refers to the amount of blood pumped from the left or right ventricle per minute. It is equal to the product of stroke volume and heart rate. Cardiac output can increase dramatically during exercise, however, is not used as a variable to determine pulse pressure.

System: Cardiovascular and Pulmonary Systems
Content Outline: Diseases/Conditions that Impact Effective Treatment

SCOREBUILDERS

➡ PTAEXAM ONE: QUESTION 3

A physical therapist assistant inspects a patient's wheelchair and identifies that the drive wheel axle is aligned further posterior than it typically would be in a standard wheelchair. This type of alignment would **MOST** likely result in which of the following outcomes?

1. Decreased rolling resistance
2. Increased ability to balance on the rear wheels
3. Decreased turning radius
4. **Increased energy required for propulsion**

Correct Answer: 4 (Tan p. 313)

Posterior alignment of the wheel axle is often utilized for patients with bilateral amputations to increase stability and compensate for the change in the center of gravity. This type of adaptation may also be utilized in a recliner or tilt wheelchair.

1. The posterior alignment of the wheel axle increases the amount of rolling resistance which serves to decrease the mechanical efficiency of the wheelchair.

2. The posterior alignment of the wheel axle decreases the ability of the patient to perform a "wheelie." Patients with spinal cord injuries may have the wheel axle moved forward to make it easier to perform a "wheelie" since this position moves the axle closer to the patient's center of gravity.

3. The posterior alignment of the wheel axle increases the turning radius of the wheelchair since the distance from the wheel axle to the casters increases. An increased turning radius reduces the maneuverability of the wheelchair.

4. **The posterior alignment of the wheel axle increases the amount of energy required for propulsion which serves to decrease the patient's ability to propel the wheelchair.**

System: Non-Systems
Content Outline: Equipment, Devices, and Technologies; Therapeutic Modalities

➡ PTAEXAM ONE: QUESTION 4

A physical therapist assistant works with a patient on gait training using bilateral axillary crutches. The right axillary crutch is modified with a platform attachment. The **MOST** likely reason for this modification is to accommodate a patient with which of the following problems?

1. **A radial nerve injury**
2. A proximal humeral fracture
3. Impaired balance and coordination
4. A transhumeral amputation

Correct Answer: 1 (Fairchild p. 216)

A platform attachment can be added to axillary crutches, forearm crutches or a walker. This modification is used for patients who are unable to bear weight through their wrists and hands, who have deformities of the wrists or fingers, who have an amputation distal to the elbow or who are unable to extend the elbow.

1. **A patient with a radial nerve injury would have significant weakness of the triceps muscle and be unable to extend the elbow. The platform modification would be necessary since the patient would be unable to produce elbow extension and would instead need to bear weight through the elbow and forearm.**

2. A platform attachment would not be appropriate for a patient with a proximal humeral fracture. Whether the weight bearing occurs through the patient's hand or the patient's elbow and forearm, the fracture site would still be experiencing increased weight bearing forces.

3. A patient with impaired balance and coordination would not likely be a good candidate for axillary crutches. In the event a patient with impaired balance and coordination was determined to be an appropriate candidate for axillary crutches, the platform attachment would still not offer any additional compensation for the patient's described impairments.

4. A transhumeral amputation occurs at the level of the mid-humerus. Without an elbow joint and forearm, the patient would have nothing to bear their weight through when using a platform attachment.

System: Non-Systems
Content Outline: Equipment, Devices, and Technologies; Therapeutic Modalities

 Level 2   p. 598-600

 Level 2   p. 603-604

➡ PTAEXAM ONE: QUESTION 5

A physical therapist assistant assesses the posture of a patient from a lateral view using a plumb line. Which of the following medical conditions would be the **LEAST** likely to result in the external auditory meatus being anterior to the plumb line?

1. Ankylosing spondylitis
2. **Graves' disease**
3. Osteoporosis
4. Parkinson's disease

Correct Answer: 2 (Kendall p. 60)

When assessing a patient's posture, a plumb line can be used as a line of reference to determine areas of abnormal posture and the extent of these abnormalities. There are several points of reference along the plumb line that should be assessed including the external auditory meatus, shoulder joint, lumbar vertebrae, hip joint, knee joint, and lateral malleolus. In normal posture, the stationary plumb line runs through the external auditory meatus.

1. Ankylosing spondylitis is a systemic condition that is characterized by inflammation of the spine and larger peripheral joints. Symptoms include recurrent and insidious onset of back pain, morning stiffness, and a flexed posture. This type of posture would result in the external auditory meatus being anterior to the stationary plumb line.

2. **Graves' disease is caused by an autoimmune disease in which certain antibodies produced by the immune system stimulate the thyroid gland causing it to become overactive. Symptoms are consistent with hyperthyroid presentation. Graves' disease is not typically associated with postural changes and therefore would not result in the external auditory meatus being anterior to the stationary plumb line.**

3. Osteoporosis is a metabolic condition that presents with a decrease in bone mass that subsequently increases the risk of fracture. Symptoms include compression and other bone fractures, loss of lumbar lordosis, and postural changes. The tendency of a patient with osteoporosis to exhibit a forward flexed posture would result in the external auditory meatus being anterior to the stationary plumb line.

4. Parkinson's disease is a movement disorder caused by the progressive degeneration of the dopamine-producing cells in the basal ganglia. Symptoms include hypokinesia, poor posture, difficulty initiating movement, festinating, and shuffling gait. The tendency of a patient with Parkinson's disease to exhibit a forward flexed posture would result in the external auditory meatus being anterior to the stationary plumb line.

System: Musculoskeletal System
Content Outline: Diseases/Conditions that Impact Effective Treatment

 Level 3   p. 75, 464, 564

➡ PTAEXAM ONE: QUESTION 6

A patient with cardiovascular pathology is placed on a diuretic. Which type of laboratory test should be the **MOST** essential for the physical therapist assistant to monitor based on the patient's prescribed medication?

1. Cardiac biomarkers
2. Prothrombin time
3. **Serum electrolytes**
4. Serum cholesterol

Correct Answer: 3 (Goodman – Differential Diagnosis p. 258)

A basic understanding of commonly utilized laboratory tests assists in the diagnosis and monitoring of patients with cardiovascular pathology. Failure to effectively interpret the results of relevant laboratory testing can pose a significant risk to patient safety.

1. Cardiac biomarkers are biomarkers measured to evaluate heart function. Cardiac enzyme studies measure the levels of creatine phosphokinase (CK) and the protein troponin in the blood. CK-MB is a relatively specific test for myocardial infarction.

2. Prothrombin time is the amount of time it takes plasma to clot after the addition of tissue factor. Patients on anticoagulants such as Warfarin (i.e., Coumadin) may require frequent monitoring of prothrombin time.

3. **Serum electrolytes are electrically charged minerals that help move nutrients into and wastes out of the body's cells, maintain a healthy water balance, and help stabilize the body's acid level. Serum electrolytes commonly assessed are potassium, sodium, calcium, and magnesium. Diuretics can lead to significantly lowered potassium levels, and to a lesser extent, sodium levels.**

4. A serum cholesterol test (i.e., lipid panel, lipid profile) measures the amount of cholesterol and triglycerides in the blood. A complete lipid profile includes the measurement of four types of lipids in the blood: total cholesterol, high-density lipoprotein (HDL) cholesterol, low-density lipoprotein (LDL) cholesterol, and triglycerides.

System: Cardiovascular and Pulmonary Systems
Content Outline: Diseases/Conditions that Impact Effective Treatment

 Level 2   p. 372

▶ PTAEXAM ONE: QUESTION 7

A patient reports recurrent ankle pain. The physical therapist directs a physical therapist assistant to perform ultrasound over the peroneus longus and brevis tendons. Which of the following locations is the **MOST** appropriate for the application of ultrasound?

1. Inferior to the sustentaculum tali

2. Over the sinus tarsi region

3. **Posterior to the lateral malleolus**

4. Anterior to the lateral malleolus

Correct Answer: 3 (Kendall p. 412)

The peroneus longus and brevis are innervated by the superficial peroneal nerve (L4, L5, S1) and act to evert the foot and assist in plantar flexion of the ankle joint. The peroneus longus also acts to depress the head of the first metatarsal.

1. The sustentaculum tali is a horizontal eminence arising from the medial surface of the calcaneus. The bony prominence serves as the attachment for several ligaments including the plantar calcaneonavicular ligament, also known as the spring ligament.

2. The sinus tarsi is a small osseous canal which runs into the ankle under the talus bone. The structure is at the same approximate level as the lateral malleolus.

3. **The peroneus longus and brevis tendons pass posterior to the lateral malleolus. The peroneus longus inserts on the lateral side of the base of the first metatarsal and first cuneiform, while the peroneus brevis inserts on the tuberosity of the fifth metatarsal.**

4. The tendon of the extensor digitorum longus can be palpated slightly anterior to the lateral malleolus.

System: Musculoskeletal System
Content Outline: Interventions

▶ PTAEXAM ONE: QUESTION 8

A physical therapist assistant prepares to measure medial rotation of a patient's shoulder with a goniometer. Which of the following structures should the assistant use to align the fulcrum?

1. On the lateral midline of the humerus using the lateral epicondyle as a reference

2. Perpendicular to the floor

3. Along the midaxillary line of the thorax

4. **Over the olecranon process**

Correct Answer: 4 (Norkin p. 86)

According to the American Academy of Orthopaedic Surgeons normal shoulder medial rotation is 0-70 degrees.

1. The lateral midline of the humerus using the lateral epicondyle as a reference should be used to align the moveable arm of the goniometer when measuring shoulder flexion and extension.

2. The stationary arm of the goniometer should be aligned parallel or perpendicular to the floor when measuring medial rotation of the shoulder.

3. The midaxillary line of the thorax should be used to align the stationary arm of the goniometer when measuring shoulder flexion and extension.

4. **The fulcrum of the goniometer should be aligned over the olecranon process. The moveable arm of the goniometer should be aligned with the ulna, using the olecranon and ulnar styloid as a reference when measuring medial rotation of the shoulder.**

System: Musculoskeletal System
Content Outline: Physical Therapy Data Collection

⦿ Level 1

⦿ Level 1   p. 87-88

➡ PTAEXAM ONE: QUESTION 9

A physical therapist assistant monitors a patient with a single lead electrocardiogram. After reviewing the obtained data, the rhythm is classified as sinus bradycardia. Which of the following descriptions is the **MOST** indicative of this condition?

1. R-R interval is irregular with a rate between 100 and 200 beats per minute

2. R-R interval is irregular with a rate between 40 and 100 beats per minute

3. R-R interval is regular with a rate greater than 100 beats per minute

4. **R-R interval is regular with a rate less than 60 beats per minute**

Correct Answer: 4 (Hillegass p. 314)

The electrocardiogram is composed of a number of different waves – P, R, T, sometimes U – and the terms "irregular" and "regular" usually refer to the rhythm of the heart rate (i.e., the distance between similar waves). A sinus rhythm indicates that the cardiac impulse originates in the sinoatrial node. Sinus bradycardia is a sinus rhythm with a heart rate of less than 60 beats per minute.

1. Irregular R-R intervals with a heart rate between 100 and 200 beats per minute is characteristic of atrial tachycardia. Atrial tachycardia is defined as three or more consecutive premature atrial complexes, where an ectopic focus in either atrium initiates an impulse before the SA node.

2. Irregular R-R intervals with a heart rate between 40 and 100 beats per minute is characteristic of sinus arrhythmia. Sinus arrhythmia is an irregularity in rhythm where the cardiac impulse is initiated at the SA node, but with a variable quickening and slowing of the impulse formation.

3. Regular R-R intervals with a heart rate greater than 100 beats per minute is sinus tachycardia.

4. **Regular R-R intervals with a heart rate of less than 60 beats per minute is sinus bradycardia.**

System: Cardiovascular and Pulmonary Systems
Content Outline: Diseases/Conditions that Impact Effective Treatment

➡ PTAEXAM ONE: QUESTION 10

A physical therapist assistant reviews the medical record of a patient with an arthritic condition. Which piece of information would be the **MOST** useful to assist in the definitive diagnosis of rheumatoid arthritis?

1. Pain profile

2. Joint symptoms

3. **Blood tests**

4. Age of onset

Correct Answer: 3 (O'Sullivan p. 1033)

Rheumatoid arthritis is a systemic autoimmune disorder of unknown etiology. The disease presents with a chronic inflammatory reaction in the synovial tissues of a joint that results in erosion of cartilage and supporting structures within the capsule. Rheumatoid arthritis is diagnosed based on the clinical presentation of involved joints, the presence of blood rheumatoid factor, and radiographic changes.

1. The pain profile can provide the therapist with information that can assist in the diagnosis of rheumatoid arthritis. Relevant information may include the intensity, duration, symmetry, and location of the pain.

2. A description of the joint symptoms can provide the therapist with information that can assist in the diagnosis of rheumatoid arthritis. Relevant information may include joints affected, stiffness, effusion, pain, size of joint (i.e., small, large), and duration of symptoms (i.e., transient, prolonged).

3. **Blood tests including rheumatoid factor, white blood cell count, erythrocyte sedimentation rate, hemoglobin, and hematocrit values are critically important to confirm the presence of rheumatoid arthritis. For example, rheumatoid factors (RF) are antibodies which may be quantified by a specific blood test referred to as a rheumatoid factor assay. High levels of RF are typically associated with autoimmune diseases such as rheumatoid arthritis, scleroderma, and systemic lupus erythematosus. Although many of the other listed options are useful to assist in the definitive diagnosis of rheumatoid arthritis, blood tests would be the most compelling.**

4. A description of the age of onset can provide the therapist with information that can assist in the diagnosis of rheumatoid arthritis. Although rheumatoid arthritis can begin at any time in life, other types of arthritis such as osteoarthritis typically develop very slowly over a large number of years.

System: Musculoskeletal System
Content Outline: Diseases/Conditions that Impact Effective Treatment

 Level 2   p. 380

 Level 2   p. 116, 540-541

➡ PTAEXAM ONE: QUESTION 11

A physical therapist assistant reads in a patient's medical chart that the patient has been prescribed albuterol. Which of the following conditions would **MOST** likely require the use of this medication?

1. Breast cancer
2. Angina pectoris
3. **Exercise-induced asthma**
4. Spinal cord injury

Correct Answer: 3 (Ciccone p. 405)

Albuterol is a beta-adrenergic agonist, a class of medications that stimulate beta-2 adrenergic receptors. Stimulation of these receptors results in relaxation of the bronchiole smooth muscles leading to bronchodilation.

1. There are several classes of drugs that can be used to treat breast cancer, some of which include alkylating agents, antimetabolites, anticancer antibiotics, antimicrotubule agents, and anticancer hormones. Albuterol would not be used to treat cancer or its associated symptoms.

2. Angina pectoris refers to chest pain that occurs secondary to ischemia of the heart musculature. The most common classes of drugs used to treat this condition include organic nitrates, beta blockers, and calcium channel blockers. Albuterol would not be used to treat angina pectoris.

3. **Exercise-induced asthma occurs when the bronchioles constrict in response to exercise, resulting in shortness of breath and wheezing. Albuterol is a medication that is commonly prescribed for conditions that result from bronchoconstriction, such as asthma or chronic obstructive pulmonary disease.**

4. There are a large variety of medications used to treat the symptoms that occur secondary to a spinal cord injury. Antispasticity medications (e.g., baclofen) are commonly prescribed to help control the spasticity and resultant pain that occur secondary to a spinal cord injury. Albuterol would not be used to treat symptoms of a spinal cord injury.

System: Cardiovascular and Pulmonary Systems
Content Outline: Diseases/Conditions that Impact Effective Treatment

➡ PTAEXAM ONE: QUESTION 12

A physical therapist assistant consults with a teacher regarding a child with autism who has impairments in sensory processing. Which of the following pieces of equipment would be the **MOST** useful to address the child's dyspraxia?

1. Swing
2. **Weighted vest**
3. Sit and spin
4. Rocking chair

Correct Answer: 2 (Long p. 80)

Sensory integration is the process in which the central nervous system accepts, organizes, and modulates afferent sensory information and produces a response. Therapists can provide children with opportunities to experience sensory input in a controlled environment using sensory modulation. Dyspraxia refers to difficulty planning a new motor act and is often caused by difficulty interpreting and modulating tactile input. The condition is common in children with sensory integration dysfunction.

1. Swings are used for children with sensory integration disorders in order to provide vestibular input. The vestibular system plays a role in the development of body posture, muscle tone, ocular-motor control, integration of reflexes, and equilibrium reactions. Addressing the vestibular system would not directly address the child's dyspraxia.

2. **A weighted vest can provide proprioceptive input and can be worn by a child with a sensory processing disorder. The proprioceptive input provides the child with an improved sense of position and understanding of where joints and muscles are in space. Proprioceptive input contributes to the ability to plan movement and would directly address the child's dyspraxia.**

3. A sit and spin can provide vestibular input to a child with a sensory processing disorder. Children with difficulty processing vestibular information may be intolerant to movement. The sit and spin provides the opportunity to experience movement in a controlled environment, however, would not directly address the child's dyspraxia.

4. A rocking chair can provide vestibular input to a child with a sensory processing disorder. Children with sensory integration dysfunction may have difficulty modulating their behavior, presenting with either hypo-arousal or hyper-arousal. Rocking chairs can be used to provide vestibular input to calm a child who is over-aroused. The additional vestibular input would not address the child's dyspraxia.

System: Neuromuscular and Nervous Systems
Content Outline: Interventions

 Level 1   p. 366

Level 2

➡ PTAEXAM ONE: QUESTION 13

A physical therapist assistant instructs a patient in soft tissue mobilization using a foam roller as shown in the image. Which of the following conditions would **MOST** likely benefit from this therapeutic technique?

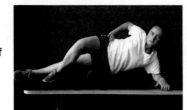

1. Iliolumbar syndrome
2. **Iliotibial band syndrome**
3. Piriformis syndrome
4. Trochanteric bursitis

Correct Answer: 2 (Sarwark p. 678)

There are a multitude of medical diagnoses that affect the hip and lower extremity. Physical therapist assistants should be familiar with the clinical presentation and common interventions employed for each diagnosis.

1. Iliolumbar syndrome, also known as iliac crest pain syndrome, is caused by inflammation or a tear of the iliolumbar ligament. The patient is often tender to palpation over the iliac crest and therefore use of a foam roller would likely exacerbate symptoms. Use of a foam roller on the lateral leg would not specifically address the chief complaints associated with this condition.

2. **Iliotibial band syndrome is characterized by localized pain approximately two centimeters above the knee joint line over the lateral femoral condyle. The syndrome can be caused by activities requiring frequent flexion of the knee such as running or cycling which produce an inflammatory reaction. As a result, use of a foam roller over the lateral leg can be an effective intervention for patients with this condition.**

3. Piriformis syndrome refers to a condition in which the piriformis muscle irritates the sciatic nerve causing pain in the buttocks and referred pain along the course of the sciatic nerve. The primary patient complaint is buttock pain that is made worse by sitting, stair climbing or squatting. Use of a foam roller on the lateral leg would not specifically address the piriformis muscle since the muscle is located in the buttock region.

4. Trochanteric bursitis refers to inflammation of the trochanteric bursa which protects the structures that cross the posterior portion of the greater trochanter. The patient is often extremely sensitive to palpation over the bursa and may experience lateral thigh pain that is exacerbated by use of a foam roller due to the proximity to the bursa.

System: Musculoskeletal System
Content Outline: Interventions

⬤ Level 2

➡ PTAEXAM ONE: QUESTION 14

A physical therapist assistant reads in the medical record that a patient was recently prescribed a thrombolytic agent. Which condition would be considered a contraindication to this type of pharmacological agent?

1. Myocardial infarction
2. **Hemorrhagic stroke**
3. Pulmonary embolism
4. Venous thrombosis

Correct Answer: 2 (Hillegass p. 455)

Thrombolytic agents facilitate clot dissolution through the conversion of plasminogen to plasmin. Plasmin breaks down clots and allows occluded vessels to reopen to restore blood flow. Side effects include hemorrhage and cardiac arrhythmia. Physical therapist assistants must be careful to avoid situations that may cause trauma to the patient due to altered clotting activity.

1. Myocardial infarction (i.e., heart attack) occurs when the blood flow through one or more of the coronary arteries is severely reduced or cut off completely causing tissue death in the portion of the myocardium supplied by the blocked artery. Thrombolytic agents are indicated as a management option for this condition.

2. **Hemorrhagic stroke is characterized by abnormal bleeding in the brain due to a rupture in a blood vessel. Thrombolytic agents are contraindicated for individuals experiencing a hemorrhagic stroke as this can result in increased hemorrhaging. However, thrombolytic agents are indicated for the management of ischemic stroke.**

3. Pulmonary embolism is a condition where one or more arteries in the lungs become blocked. Prompt treatment with anticoagulants and thrombolytic agents is indicated to reduce the risk of death.

4. Venous thrombosis is a condition characterized by the formation of a blood clot (thrombus) within a vein. Thrombolytic agents are indicated as a management option for this condition.

System: Cardiovascular and Pulmonary Systems
Content Outline: Diseases/Conditions that Impact Effective Treatment

⬤ Level 1   👓 p. 251-252, 298-299, 373

➡ PTAEXAM ONE: QUESTION 15

A physical therapist assistant reads a recent entry in a patient's medical record that indicates aspiration was performed in the elbow region. This procedure is **MOST** commonly associated with which of the following conditions?

1. Dorsal ganglion cyst
2. Lateral epicondylitis
3. Medial epicondylitis
4. **Olecranon bursitis**

Correct Answer: 4 (Dutton p. 753)

Aspiration, also known as arthrocentesis, refers to a technique using a sterile needle to remove fluid from a joint. A local anesthetic is typically utilized prior to the needle puncture to minimize discomfort. The obtained fluid is often sent to a laboratory for further analysis.

1. A dorsal ganglion cyst is a benign cyst located on the back of the wrist or hand. Although aspiration may be appropriate, a dorsal ganglion cyst would not be located at the elbow. The primary rationale for aspirating the cyst would be due to cosmesis.

2. Lateral epicondylitis (i.e., tennis elbow) refers to an irritation or inflammation of the common extensor muscles at their origin on the lateral epicondyle of the humerus. Aspiration is not common with lateral epicondylitis, however, if the condition has not responded to conservative treatment an injection of a corticosteroid may be warranted.

3. Medial epicondylitis (i.e., golfer's or swimmer's elbow) results from repeated microtrauma to the flexor carpi radialis and/or the humeral head of the pronator teres during pronation and wrist flexion. Aspiration is not common with medial epicondylitis, however, if the condition has not responded to conservative treatment, an injection of a corticosteroid may be warranted.

4. **Olecranon bursitis is characterized by pain, redness, and swelling around the olecranon caused by inflammation of the elbow's bursa. Aspirating the excess bursa fluid is often performed to relieve the inflammation and prevent further accumulation of fluid. An excessive amount of fluid in this region can inhibit range of motion and functional use of the elbow. The aspirated fluid is often cultured and evaluated for crystals to rule out infection or gout.**

System: Musculoskeletal System
Content Outline: Diseases/Conditions that Impact Effective Treatment

(●) Level 2

➡ PTAEXAM ONE: QUESTION 16

A patient is referred to physical therapy with a diagnosis of left shoulder impingement. During the session, the physical therapist assistant begins to suspect a systemic cause for the patient's pain. Which of the following symptoms would **BEST** support this hypothesis?

1. Pain has been present for years
2. Pain is alleviated with the use of cryotherapy
3. Pain is aggravated by cervical rotation
4. **Pain remains unrelieved with rest**

Correct Answer: 4 (Goodman – Differential Diagnosis p. 104)

In some instances, diagnoses that appear to have a musculo-skeletal origin may actually have a more systemic cause. Asking appropriate questions about pain will assist the physical therapist assistant to delineate between musculoskeletal and systemic causes of pain.

1. Pain caused by a systemic pathology tends to be more recent and sudden in onset. Musculoskeletal pain can have a sudden onset or be present intermittently for years.

2. Pain that is musculoskeletal in origin can typically be relieved with rest, change in position, stretching, heat or cold.

3. Pain that is musculoskeletal in origin is usually aggravated with movement, whereas pain caused by a systemic pathology is difficult to reproduce. Though the site of the movement (i.e., cervical spine) does not match the site of the pain (i.e., shoulder), it is possible that a nerve in the cervical spine is being compressed during rotation and causing radicular pain in the shoulder.

4. **Pain that has a systemic cause is difficult to reproduce. Symptoms are usually unrelieved by rest or a change in position.**

System: Musculoskeletal System
Content Outline: Diseases/Conditions that Impact Effective Treatment

(●) Level 2

➡ PTAEXAM ONE: QUESTION 17

A physical therapist assistant completes a developmental assessment on an infant. At what age should an infant begin to sit with hand support for an extended period of time?

1. **6-7 months**
2. 8-9 months
3. 10-11 months
4. 12-15 months

Correct Answer: 1 (Ratliffe p. 46)

Infants typically develop the stability to sit with hand support in the sixth to seventh month.

1. **Sitting for a prolonged period of time with upper extremity support usually occurs at 6-7 months of age. The infant will also bring objects to midline, hold a bottle with two hands, and roll to prone.**

2. When an infant is 8-9 months of age, they will typically manipulate toys in sitting, raise themselves from supine to sit, pull to stand with support, and transfer objects with a controlled release.

3. When an infant is 10-11 months of age, they will typically stand briefly without support, transition from supine to sitting or quadruped, pull to stand through half kneel, and use a pincer grasp.

4. When an infant is 12-15 months of age, they will typically stand up through quadruped, use a wide array of sitting positions, walk without support, creep up stairs, throw a ball in sitting, and mark paper with crayons.

System: Neuromuscular and Nervous Systems
Content Outline: Physical Therapy Data Collection

➡ PTAEXAM ONE: QUESTION 18

A physical therapist assistant instructs a patient in a self-stretching activity using the FABER test position. This test position should be **MOST** useful to stretch which of the following muscle groups of the hip?

1. Abductors
2. Flexors
3. External rotators
4. **Internal rotators**

Correct Answer: 4 (Kisner p. 752)

The FABER, or figure-4, position occurs with the patient assuming a supine position with the involved leg flexed, abducted, and externally rotated at the hip so that the ankle is resting on the opposite leg. FABER stands for flexion, abduction, and external rotation.

1. The hip abductors are stretched when the hip is positioned in adduction. The FABER position requires the hip to be in abduction.

2. The hip flexors are stretched when the hip is positioned in extension. The FABER position requires the hip to be in flexion.

3. The hip external rotators are stretched when the hip is positioned in internal rotation. The FABER position requires the hip to be in external rotation.

4. **The hip internal rotators are stretched when the hip is positioned in external rotation. The FABER position requires the hip to be in external rotation.**

System: Musculoskeletal System
Content Outline: Interventions

 Level 2   p. 279-281

Level 1   p. 101

➡ PTAEXAM ONE: QUESTION 19

A patient who has a spinal cord injury informs a physical therapist assistant that they will walk again. Which type of injury would make functional ambulation the **MOST** unrealistic?

1. **Complete T9 paraplegia**
2. Posterior cord syndrome
3. Brown-Sequard's syndrome
4. Cauda equina injury

Correct Answer: 1 (O'Sullivan p. 924)

The ability to functionally ambulate following a spinal cord injury is primarily dependent on the patient's available motor and sensory innervation and the associated energy requirements.

1. **A patient with complete T9 paraplegia would possess full upper extremity innervation and would be able to utilize the lower abdominals and intercostals. The patient would not possess any lower extremity innervation and therefore functional ambulation would be unrealistic.**

2. Posterior cord syndrome refers to a relatively rare incomplete lesion caused by compression of the posterior spinal artery. The condition is characterized by loss of proprioception, two-point discrimination, and stereognosis. Motor function is preserved.

3. Brown-Sequard's syndrome refers to an incomplete lesion usually caused by a stab wound, which produces hemisection of the spinal cord. The condition is characterized by paralysis and loss of vibratory and position sense on the same side as the lesion and loss of pain and temperature sense on the opposite side of the lesion.

4. Cauda equina injury occurs below the L1 spinal level where the long nerve roots transcend. Cauda equina injuries can be complete, however, are frequently incomplete due to the large number of nerve roots in the area. The condition is characterized by flaccidity, areflexia, and impairment of bowel and bladder function. Full recovery is not typical due to the distance needed for axonal regeneration.

System: Neuromuscular and Nervous Systems
Content Outline: Diseases/Conditions that Impact Effective
 Treatment

➡ PTAEXAM ONE: QUESTION 20

A physical therapist assistant monitors a patient with a C6 spinal cord injury positioned on a tilt table. After elevating the tilt table to 30 degrees, the patient reports nausea and dizziness. The assistant measures the patient's blood pressure as 70/35 mm Hg. The patient's signs and symptoms are **MOST** indicative of which of the following conditions?

1. Spinal shock
2. Postural hypertension
3. Autonomic dysreflexia
4. **Orthostatic hypotension**

Correct Answer: 4 (Umphred p. 476)

Patients status post spinal cord injury are particularly susceptible to several potentially emergent conditions. Physical therapist assistants must closely monitor patients for signs and symptoms associated with these conditions and, if necessary, provide appropriate and immediate medical management.

1. Spinal shock refers to a physiologic response that occurs between 30 and 60 minutes after trauma to the spinal cord and can last up to several weeks. The patient presents with total flaccid paralysis and loss of all reflexes below the level of injury.

2. Postural hypertension is a term used to describe dizziness caused by a change in position in the presence of high blood pressure. A far more common term is postural hypotension which is synonymous with orthostatic hypotension.

3. Autonomic dysreflexia occurs when a noxious stimulus below the level of the lesion triggers the autonomic nervous system causing a sudden elevation in blood pressure. If not treated, this condition can lead to convulsions, hemorrhage, and death. The condition frequently occurs in patients with lesions at or above T6.

4. **Orthostatic hypotension or postural hypotension occurs due to a loss of sympathetic control of vasoconstriction in combination with absent or severely reduced muscle tone. A decrease in systolic blood pressure greater than 20 mm Hg after moving from supine to sitting is typically indicative of orthostatic hypotension.**

System: Other Systems
Content Outline: Interventions

 Level 2   p. 269-271

 Level 2   p. 267-269, 678

➡ PTAEXAM ONE: QUESTION 21

A physical therapist assistant prepares to treat a patient with continuous ultrasound. Which general rule **BEST** determines the length of treatment when using ultrasound?

1. Two minutes for an area that is two times the size of the transducer face

2. **Five minutes for an area that is two times the size of the transducer face**

3. Five minutes is the maximum treatment time regardless of the treatment area

4. Ten minutes is the maximum treatment time regardless of the treatment area

Correct Answer: 2 (Cameron p. 185)

The duration of ultrasound treatment is based on a number of variables including the treatment goal, the size of the area to be treated, and the effective radiating area of the transducer face.

1. Two minutes would not be enough time to use ultrasound in an area that was two times the size of the transducer face.

2. **An accepted recommendation is that ultrasound can be administered to an area two to three times the size of the effective radiating area of the transducer face in a five minute period. This recommendation equates to roughly twice the size of the transducer face.**

3. There is not a specified maximum amount of time when using ultrasound. Most often ultrasound is used for periods ranging from five to eight minutes in duration.

4. Ten minutes is a relatively long duration for treatment with ultrasound, however, this could be plausible in situations where the size of the area to be treated is large.

System: Non-Systems
Content Outline: Equipment, Devices, and Technologies;
Therapeutic Modalities

➡ PTAEXAM ONE: QUESTION 22

A physical therapist assistant attempts to prevent alveolar collapse in a patient post thoracic surgery. Which of the following breathing devices would be the **MOST** effective for the assistant to utilize in order to achieve the established goal?

1. Inspiratory muscle trainer

2. Mechanical percussors

3. **Incentive spirometer**

4. Flutter valve

Correct Answer: 3 (Frownfelter p. 695)

An incentive spirometer provides visual or in some cases auditory feedback as the patient takes a maximum inspiration. Incentive spirometry increases the amount of air that is inspired and as a result, can be used as a treatment to prevent alveolar collapse after thoracic surgery.

1. Inspiratory muscle trainers are handheld breathing training devices used primarily to increase the strength and endurance of the muscles of inspiration. They are not used to prevent alveolar collapse after thoracic surgery.

2. Mechanical percussors are electronically or pneumatically powered devices employed as a substitute for manual percussion with the hands. They can be used to help mobilize bronchial secretions after thoracic surgery, but only if the patient was retaining secretions.

3. **Incentive spirometers are devices that provide visual or other feedback while the patient performs sustained maximal inspirations. The device is most often used following upper abdominal or thoracic surgery. Indications may include chest wall pain, loss of mobility, weakness of the muscles of inspiration, and the prevention or treatment of atelectasis.**

4. Flutter valves are mucus clearance devices that combine positive expiratory pressure with high frequency oscillations at the airway opening during exhalation.

System: Cardiovascular and Pulmonary Systems
Content Outline: Interventions

 Level 1   p. 623-626

Level 2   p. 391-394

➡ PTAEXAM ONE: QUESTION 23

A physical therapist assistant reviews the surface anatomy of the hand in preparation for a patient post wrist arthrodesis. Which of the following bony structures does **NOT** articulate with the lunate?

1. **Trapezium**
2. Radius
3. Capitate
4. Scaphoid

Correct Answer: 1 (Hoppenfeld p. 66)

The lunate is located in the center of the proximal row of carpal bones between the scaphoid and the triquetrum. The lunate is distinguished by its crescent-like outline. The proximal row of carpal bones from lateral to medial consists of the scaphoid, lunate, triquetrum, and pisiform. The distal row of carpal bones from lateral to medial consists of the trapezium, trapezoid, capitate, and hamate.

1. **The trapezium is located on the lateral side of the carpus between the scaphoid and the first metacarpal. It is distinguished by a deep groove on its palmar surface. The proximal portion of the trapezium articulates with the scaphoid. The distal portion articulates with the bases of the first and second metacarpals.**

2. The radius articulates with the wrist at the radiocarpal joint. The concave surface of the distal end of the radius articulates with the scaphoid and lunate.

3. The capitate is the most central and largest of the carpal bones. The proximal portion of the capitate articulates with the lunate and scaphoid. The distal portion articulates with the base of the third metacarpal.

4. The scaphoid links the proximal and distal carpal rows and helps provide stability to the wrist. Patients who fracture the proximal aspect of the scaphoid are susceptible to avascular necrosis due to disrupted blood supply. The proximal portion of the scaphoid articulates with the radius. The distal portion articulates with the trapezium and trapezoid. The medial surface articulates with the lunate and capitate.

System: Musculoskeletal System
Content Outline: Physical Therapy Data Collection

➡ PTAEXAM ONE: QUESTION 24

A physical therapist assistant concludes that it is necessary to elongate the long head of the triceps brachii as part of a muscle length assessment of the elbow. Which positioning of the upper extremity would be the **MOST** effective for achieving the stated objective?

1. Elbow extension and shoulder extension
2. Elbow extension and shoulder flexion
3. Elbow flexion and shoulder extension
4. **Elbow flexion and shoulder flexion**

Correct Answer: 4 (Kisner p. 67)

The triceps brachii is a two-joint muscle originating on the infraglenoid tubercle of the scapula and inserting on the olecranon process of the ulna. The triceps brachii acts to extend the elbow and assists with shoulder extension. The muscle receives primary innervation from the radial nerve, however, the long head of the triceps is innervated by the axillary nerve.

1. Elongation of a muscle requires the muscle to be positioned opposite of the muscle's action. Elbow extension and shoulder extension are consistent with the action of the triceps brachii and therefore would not result in elongation of the muscle.

2. Elbow extension is consistent with the action of the triceps brachii and therefore would not result in elongation of the muscle. Shoulder flexion is desirable to elongate the triceps brachii, however, the elbow would also need to be flexed since the muscle acts on both the shoulder and elbow.

3. Elbow flexion is opposite the action of the triceps brachii and would therefore promote elongation, however, shoulder extension is not. The most appropriate option would need to elongate the muscle at both the shoulder and elbow.

4. **Elbow flexion and shoulder flexion are both opposite the action of the triceps brachii and therefore would result in elongation of the muscle at both the shoulder and elbow.**

System: Musculoskeletal System
Content Outline: Interventions

 Level 1

 Level 2   p. 107-108

➡ PTAEXAM ONE: QUESTION 25

A patient in the physical therapy gym suddenly grasps their throat and begins to cough. The physical therapist assistant, recognizing the signs of an airway obstruction, should take which of the following actions?

1. Attempt to ventilate
2. Administer abdominal thrusts
3. Perform a quick finger sweep of the mouth
4. **Continue to observe the patient, but do not interfere**

Correct Answer: 4 (Le Baudour p. 150)

Coughing indicates that the airway is not completely obstructed. As a result, the physical therapist assistant should continue to monitor the patient, however, should not formally intervene. Usually a patient that is coughing will independently dislodge the object causing the obstruction.

1. If the patient is not breathing, a rescuer should open the airway and attempt to ventilate. If the rescuer is unable to make the patient's chest rise, the rescuer should reposition and ventilate again. If the chest still does not rise, the rescuer must consider that there is an obstruction. This technique would not be appropriate for a person that is coughing in an attempt to clear an obstruction.

2. If the patient is choking, the rescuer should attempt to perform the Heimlich maneuver while the conscious patient is in sitting or standing. The Heimlich maneuver attempts to remove the obstruction by providing abdominal thrusts. The rescuer would press the fist into the patient's abdomen with a quick inward and upward thrust with the intent of relieving the obstruction. This technique would not be appropriate for a person that is still coughing.

3. A rescuer should use a finger sweep only when they can see solid material obstructing the airway of an unresponsive patient. If the rescuer were to do this without seeing the blockage, it may harm the patient or rescuer. This technique would not be appropriate for a person that is coughing in an attempt to clear an obstruction.

4. **If a mild obstruction is present and the patient is coughing, the rescuer would not interfere with the patient's spontaneous coughing and breathing efforts. The rescuer should attempt to relieve the obstruction only if signs of severe obstruction develop such as the cough becoming silent, respiratory difficulty increasing or the patient becoming unresponsive.**

System: Non-Systems
Content Outline: Safety and Protection; Professional Responsibilities; Research

---

➡ PTAEXAM ONE: QUESTION 26

A physical therapist assistant reviews a patient's medical record prior to beginning treatment. The record indicates the patient was recently placed on amitriptyline (Elavil). Which of the following responses is the **MOST** common side effect associated with this tricyclic antidepressant?

1. **Sedation**
2. Dysarthria
3. Seizures
4. Blood pressure variability

Correct Answer: 1 (Ciccone p. 92)

Antidepressant medications are classified into groups according to function or chemical criteria. As a group, there are a broad range of side effects including sedation, sexual dysfunction, overstimulation, anxiety, seizure activity, arrhythmias, and orthostatic hypotension. Tricyclic antidepressants are particularly inherent to producing sedation.

1. **Sedation is the primary side effect with tricyclic antidepressants, however, other side effects can include confusion and even delirium secondary to the medication's anticholinergic properties. Tricyclic antidepressants have been associated with fatal overdoses and therefore should be used with great caution.**

2. Dysarthria is a motor disorder of speech that is caused by an upper motor neuron lesion that affects the muscles that are used to articulate words and sounds. Speech is often "slurred" due to the muscle weakness. Dysarthria is not a common side effect of tricyclic antidepressants.

3. A variety of antidepressant medications can cause seizure activity, however, this is not a common side effect of tricyclic antidepressants.

4. Selected tricyclic antidepressants can increase the likelihood of orthostatic hypotension, however, this side effect is not nearly as common as sedation.

System: Other Systems
Content Outline: Diseases/Conditions that Impact Effective Treatment

---

 Level 3   👓   p. 676-678

 Level 1   👓   p. 496, 512

➡ PTAEXAM ONE: QUESTION 27

A physical therapist assistant notices significant atrophy of the infraspinatus muscle while treating a patient with shoulder pathology. This finding is **MOST** consistent with an injury to which of the following nerves?

1. Axillary

2. Long thoracic

3. Spinal accessory

4. **Suprascapular**

Correct Answer: 4 (Dutton p. 77)

Injury to motor nerves can result in a variety of symptoms including muscle atrophy, weakness, fasciculation or paralysis. Injury to sensory nerves can result in pain, numbness, sensitivity, tingling or burning.

1. The axillary nerve (C5-C6) originates from the posterior cord of the brachial plexus at the level of the axilla. The nerve innervates the deltoid, teres minor, and long head of the triceps brachii muscles.

2. The long thoracic nerve (C5-C7) descends behind the brachial plexus and the axillary vessels. The nerve innervates the serratus anterior muscle.

3. The spinal accessory nerve (C3-C4) innervates the sternocleidomastoid and trapezius muscles. The nerve is the eleventh of twelve cranial nerves.

4. **The suprascapular nerve (C5-C6) originates from the upper trunk of the brachial plexus. The nerve innervates the infraspinatus and supraspinatus muscles.**

System: Neuromuscular and Nervous Systems
Content Outline: Diseases/Conditions that Impact Effective
   Treatment

➡ PTAEXAM ONE: QUESTION 28

A physical therapist assistant is performing gait training on a patient who has a transtibial amputation. After 15 minutes of training, the patellar tendon-bearing prosthesis is removed for skin inspection. Redness is noted on multiple areas of the residual limb. Which area of redness should be the **GREATEST** concern to the assistant?

1. Patellar tendon

2. Fibular shaft

3. Gastrocnemius muscle

4. **Distal anterior tibia**

Correct Answer: 4 (May p. 25)

Redness is a normal part of wearing a prosthesis, and depending on a patient's medical history and skin tolerance, various degrees of redness will be noted. The prosthetic socket and supporting components (e.g., socks/liners) are designed to spread the forces throughout the residual limb and focus forces on pressure tolerant areas, such as the patellar tendon. Bony prominences are pressure intolerant and a well-designed socket will minimize pressure in these areas.

1. The patellar tendon is pressure tolerant and redness in this area is not a concern as long as it resolves within 10-20 minutes after doffing.

2. The fibular shaft is a pressure tolerant area and should have resolution of redness within 20 minutes after doffing the prosthesis.

3. The gastrocnemius muscle is pressure tolerant, as it can spread the force of weight bearing across a large area.

4. **The distal anterior tibia is not a pressure tolerant area, as it is covered by a thin layer of skin and has little to no adipose tissue to distribute the transmitted forces. If redness is noted in this area, it is necessary to verify that socks and liners are being worn appropriately prior to contacting a prosthetist.**

System: Musculoskeletal System
Content Outline: Interventions

 Level 1   p. 227

Level 3   p. 130-133

➡ PTAEXAM ONE: QUESTION 29

A patient returns from a physician visit and informs a physical therapist assistant that they have decreased their systolic blood pressure by approximately 20 mm Hg over the last two months. Which intervention would **MOST** likely be responsible for the decrease in systolic blood pressure?

1. Dietary changes
2. Limiting alcohol consumption
3. Activity level changes
4. **Pharmacological management**

Correct Answer: 4 (Ciccone p. 318)

Recent revisions in blood pressure guidelines have resulted in more aggressive treatment for hypertension. Treatment often includes lifestyle modifications and pharmacological management.

1. Dietary recommendations include reduced intake of dietary sodium and alcohol and increased consumption of fruits, vegetables, and low-fat dairy products with reduced saturated and total fat content. Following these dietary recommendations would not produce the magnitude of the described blood pressure change.

2. Limiting alcohol intake to two or fewer drinks daily for men and no more than one drink daily for women can assist to reduce blood pressure. Limiting alcohol intake would not produce the magnitude of the described blood pressure change.

3. Activity level recommendations include aerobic physical activity at least 30 minutes a day most days of the week. An increased activity level would not produce the magnitude of the described blood pressure change.

4. **Pharmacological management for high blood pressure includes medications such as diuretics, beta blockers, calcium channel blockers, ACE inhibitors, angiotensin II receptor blockers, and direct vasodilators. Significant changes such as the described change (i.e., 20 mm Hg decrease in systolic blood pressure) typically occur through pharmacological management.**

System: Cardiovascular and Pulmonary Systems
Content Outline: Diseases/Conditions that Impact Effective Treatment

➡ PTAEXAM ONE: QUESTION 30

A patient sustained a non-displaced fracture of the proximal humerus. Which of the following clinical findings would provide the **BEST** support for the patient being cleared to perform active-assisted exercise?

1. Hematoma formation
2. Diminished pain
3. **Callus formation**
4. Remodeling

Correct Answer: 3 (Kaufman p. 143)

Proximal humerus fractures are commonly associated with falls, particularly in older adult females due to decreased bone density. Physical therapist assistants should consider a patient's stage of healing when selecting therapeutic activities.

1. A hematoma occurs in the fracture site soon after injury. This occurs in the inflammatory stage of bone healing and would therefore be too early to initiate active-assisted exercise.

2. Diminished pain often accompanies the initiation of more dynamic therapeutic activities following fracture, however, the finding by itself does not provide the necessary information to determine the patient's current stage of healing.

3. **Callus formation is one of the first indications that healing has occurred. The presence of a callus identified through diagnostic imaging allows the patient to progress to active-assisted exercise.**

4. Remodeling is the final stage of bone healing where the fracture has solidly united with woven bone. A patient would begin active-assisted exercise far earlier in the rehabilitation process.

System: Musculoskeletal System
Content Outline: Interventions

 Level 2   p. 364, 376, 412

 Level 2

➡ PTAEXAM ONE: QUESTION 31

A physical therapist assistant reporting at a team meeting indicates that a patient with a spinal cord injury should be able to perform household ambulation using knee-ankle-foot orthoses (KAFOs) and forearm crutches upon discharge. The patient's quadriceps strength is currently Poor plus (2+/5). What level of spinal cord injury is the **MOST** likely based on the assistant's prediction?

1. L1
2. **L3**
3. L5
4. S1

Correct Answer: 2 (O'Sullivan p. 925)

A patient diagnosed with L3 paraplegia is typically the highest level of injury that may allow for household ambulation using KAFOs or KAFO/AFO combination and an assistive device. Household ambulation would not typically be possible for patients with a lesion above the L3 level due to the lack of quadriceps innervation and the high energy cost associated with household ambulation.

1. Cauda equina injuries occur below the L1 spinal level where the long nerve roots transcend. There is full innervation of the abdominals and intercostals, and minimal hip flexion present at this level. Characteristics include flaccidity, areflexia, and impairment of bowel and bladder function. Full recovery is not typical due to the distance needed for axonal regeneration.

2. **A patient with a lesion at the L3 level has at least partial innervation of the gracilis, iliopsoas, quadratus lumborum, rectus femoris, and sartorius. Patients have full use of their upper extremities and possess hip flexion, adduction, and knee extension. Patients at this level will typically ambulate with KAFOs or KAFO/AFO combination and an assistive device for household and community mobility.**

3. A patient with a lesion at the L5 level has innervation of the extensor digitorum, low back muscles, medial hamstrings, posterior tibialis, quadriceps, and tibialis anterior. Patients at this level will typically use bilateral AFOs for household and community ambulation with an appropriate assistive device.

4. A patient with a lesion at the S1 level has innervation of the upper and lower abdominals, intercostals, and adequate lower extremity strength to use AFOs or modified foot orthotics with ambulation. A patient at this level will also use an assistive device to ambulate in the household and community.

System: Neuromuscular and Nervous Systems
Content Outline: Diseases/Conditions that Impact Effective Treatment

 Level 2   p. 124-125, 267

➡ PTAEXAM ONE: QUESTION 32

A physical therapist treating a patient with a physical therapist assistant decides to discontinue the scheduled physical therapy session due to a suspected pulmonary embolism and requests further consultation from the attending physician. Which of the following clinical findings **BEST** supports the therapist's hypothesis?

1. Partial pressure of oxygen (PaO_2) of 85 mm Hg
2. Resting respiratory rate of 14 breaths per minute
3. Resting heart rate of 100 beats per minute
4. **Increased cough with the presence of hemoptysis**

Correct Answer: 4 (Goodman–Pathology p. 850)

A pulmonary embolism occurs as a result of venous thrombi that have detached and traveled from elsewhere in the body before lodging in a pulmonary artery. Signs and symptoms of pulmonary embolism include a sudden onset of dyspnea, coughing, hypoxia, and chest pain, which may mimic myocardial infarction. Dyspnea presents both at rest and with activity. Complaints of chest pain typically worsen with coughing, eating, deep breathing or bending activities. Coughing may produce blood-tinged sputum (hemoptysis).

1. Since pulmonary embolism causes decreased perfusion, the lung tissue supplied by the blocked vessel becomes ischemic and fails to provide adequate oxygen for the body. PaO_2 is one of the components measured in an arterial blood gas test and shows how well oxygen is moving from the lungs to the blood. Normal PaO_2 is 80-100 mm Hg and therefore a PaO_2 of 85 mm Hg is considered within the normal range.

2. Tachypnea, an elevated respiratory rate, is a common sign of pulmonary embolism. The normal resting respiratory rate for an adult is 12-20 breaths per minute. A resting respiratory rate of 14 breaths per minute is considered within the normal range and therefore would not support the physical therapist's hypothesis.

3. Tachycardia is defined as a resting heart rate greater than 100 beats per minute. Although a resting heart rate of 100 beats per minute is at the upper limit of the normal range, it is not a strong indicator of pulmonary embolism.

4. **Increased cough with the presence of hemoptysis is a common sign associated with pulmonary embolism. This finding would warrant discontinuing a scheduled physical therapy session and consulting with a physician. Other common signs of pulmonary embolism include apprehension, pleuritic chest pain, diaphoresis, lower extremity edema, cyanosis, and fainting.**

System: Cardiovascular and Pulmonary Systems
Content Outline: Diseases/Conditions that Impact Effective Treatment

 Level 3   p. 368, 419, 678

➡ PTAEXAM ONE: QUESTION 33

A physical therapist assistant assesses the functional strength of a patient's hip extensors while observing the patient move from a standing to sitting position. What type of contraction occurs in the hip extensors during this activity?

1. Concentric
2. **Eccentric**
3. Isometric
4. Isokinetic

Correct Answer: 2 (Levangie p. 376)

The gluteus maximus and the hamstring muscles function as primary hip extensors. These muscles contract in an eccentric fashion when moving from standing to sitting.

1. Concentric contractions require a shortening of the involved muscle. The hip extensors would lengthen when moving from standing to sitting and therefore the contraction would not be labeled concentric.

2. **Eccentric contractions require a lengthening of the involved muscle. The contraction generally occurs when there is a need to decelerate a body part. The hip extensors would lengthen when moving from standing to sitting.**

3. Isometric contractions do not change the length of a muscle or produce movement. As a result, the hip extensors cannot contract isometrically when moving from standing to sitting.

4. Isokinetic contractions occur when a muscle contracts and shortens at a constant speed. This can occur only when a muscle's maximal force of contraction exceeds the total load on the muscle. The hip extensors would not lengthen at a constant speed when moving from standing to sitting.

System: Musculoskeletal System
Content Outline: Physical Therapy Data Collection

➡ PTAEXAM ONE: QUESTION 34

A physical therapist assistant prepares to work with a two-month-old infant diagnosed with osteogenesis imperfecta. Which of the following outcomes should the assistant recognize as the **PRIMARY** goal of therapy for this patient?

1. Improve muscle strength and diminish tone
2. Facilitate protected weight bearing
3. **Promote safe handling and positioning**
4. Diminish pulmonary secretions

Correct Answer: 3 (Ratliffe p. 254)

Osteogenesis imperfecta is an autosomal disorder of collagen synthesis that affects bone metabolism. Children with osteogenesis imperfecta often have delayed developmental milestones secondary to ongoing fractures with immobilization, hypermobility of joints, and poorly developed muscles. The disorder is classified into four types that result in diverse clinical presentations ranging from normal appearance with mild symptoms to severe involvement that can be fatal during infancy.

1. The patient would likely have diminished muscle strength due to atrophy, hypermobility of joints, and multiple fractures. Improving strength is therefore desirable, however, would not be the primary goal of therapy for the patient. In addition, tone is not typically altered with osteogenesis imperfecta.

2. Protected weight bearing is desirable in order to reduce the risks associated with fracture and prevent disuse atrophy. Given the patient's age this goal would not be the primary focus of therapy.

3. **A patient with osteogenesis imperfecta is extremely susceptible to fractures during even basic activities such as being carried or bathing. As a result, safe handling and positioning would be the primary goal. This information would be critical to convey to all caregivers, perhaps most notably, the infant's parents.**

4. Osteogenesis imperfecta is a disorder of collagen synthesis that affects bone metabolism. The disorder would not directly influence pulmonary secretions.

System: Musculoskeletal System
Content Outline: Interventions

 Level 2   p. 109

 Level 2   p. 115, 185

➡ PTAEXAM ONE: QUESTION 35

A physical therapist assistant utilizes the Six-Minute Walk Test as a means of quantifying endurance for a patient who has a chronic pulmonary disease. What variable would be the **MOST** appropriate for the assistant to measure when determining the patient's endurance level with this objective test?

1. Perceived exertion
2. Heart rate response
3. Elapsed time
4. **Distance walked**

Correct Answer: 4 (Paz p. 476)

The Six-Minute Walk Test is used to determine a patient's functional exercise capacity. The test is commonly used upon admission, discharge, and to monitor progress or decline throughout physical therapy. This tool is administered to various populations including those with cardiac impairments, pulmonary disease, chronic conditions, and patients recovering from orthopedic surgical procedures.

1. The patient is instructed to walk as quickly as they can and attempt to cover as much ground as possible within the six minute period. The therapist does not attempt to record the patient's perceived exertion, however, the patient must let the therapist know if they experience chest pain or dizziness.

2. The heart rate response will likely increase as the intensity and duration of the test increases, however, the test is not designed to examine the heart rate response. Heart rate, blood pressure, oxygen saturation, and a dyspnea score are typically assessed prior to and after the administration of the test.

3. The elapsed time for the Six-Minute Walk Test is six minutes, as the name implies, and therefore does not vary during the administration of the test.

4. **The test requires the therapist to measure the distance the patient walks within a six minute period with rest periods permitted as necessary.**

System: Cardiovascular and Pulmonary Systems
Content Outline: Physical Therapy Data Collection

➡ PTAEXAM ONE: QUESTION 36

A physical therapist assistant employed in a school setting observes a 10-year-old boy attempt to move from the floor to a standing position. During the activity, the boy has to push on his legs with his hands in order to attain an upright position. This type of finding is **MOST** commonly associated with which of the following diagnoses?

1. Cystic fibrosis
2. Down syndrome
3. **Duchenne muscular dystrophy**
4. Spinal muscular atrophy

Correct Answer: 3 (Palisano p. 400)

Duchenne muscular dystrophy is a sex-linked disorder characterized by progressive muscular weakness beginning between the ages of two and five. Life expectancy with Duchenne muscular dystrophy is late teens to early twenties due to respiratory or cardiac failure. The described method of standing upright is termed Gowers' sign.

1. Cystic fibrosis is a progressive autosomal recessive genetic disorder of the exocrine glands. The primary findings include pancreatic insufficiency, excessive pulmonary secretions within the lungs, and excessive electrolyte secretion of the sweat glands. Life expectancy has increased to 35 years of age.

2. Down syndrome (trisomy 21) is a chromosomal disorder that has an increased incidence in children of older parents. A moderate to severe decrease in cognition is typical, however, the mean life expectancy is 50-60 years of age.

3. **Duchenne muscular dystrophy causes mechanical weakening and cell destruction. Pseudohypertrophy of the calf muscles is often the first observed finding, however, all muscles are eventually affected including respiratory and cardiac muscles.**

4. Spinal muscular atrophy is a progressive autosomal recessive genetic disorder characterized by anterior horn cell degeneration, paralysis, and intact cognition. Spinal muscular atrophy - Type 1 (Werdnig-Hoffman disease) has a life expectancy of less than three years while Type 2 has a slower progression and Type 3 (Kugelberg-Welander) has a normal life expectancy.

System: Neuromuscular and Nervous Systems
Content Outline: Diseases/Conditions that Impact Effective Treatment

 Level 2   p. 385

 Level 2   p. 284, 302-303

SCOREBUILDERS

➡ PTAEXAM ONE: QUESTION 37

A physical therapist assistant uses the proprioceptive neuromuscular facilitation (PNF) technique known as repeated contractions to strengthen the quadriceps of a patient that fails to exhibit the desired muscular response throughout a portion of the range of motion. Which of the following descriptions **BEST** explains how this technique should be applied?

1. With the extremity placed into a shortened range within the pattern

2. **At the point where the desired muscular response begins to diminish**

3. At the end of the available range of motion

4. With a maximal contraction of the antagonistic muscle group

Correct Answer: 2 (Sullivan p. 71)

Repeated contractions should be applied at the point where the contraction begins to diminish. The technique utilizes an isometric contraction followed by subsequent manual stretching and resisted isotonic movement. Repeated contractions assist with enhancing motor neuron recruitment and strengthening of a muscle or group of muscles.

1. Hold-relax active movement is a technique to improve initiation of movement to muscles tested at 1/5 or less. An isometric contraction is performed once the extremity is passively placed into a shortened range within the pattern. Upon relaxation, the extremity is moved into a lengthened position with a quick stretch. The patient then returns the extremity to the shortened position through an isotonic contraction.

2. **Repeated contractions, alternating isometrics, resisted progression, and timing for emphasis are all examples of PNF techniques that are applied with the goal and purpose of increasing strength.**

3. Hold-relax is a technique that applies an isometric contraction at the end of available range to increase range of motion. The contraction is facilitated for all muscle groups at the limiting point in the range. Relaxation occurs and the extremity moves through the newly acquired range to the next point of limitation until there are no further gains in range of motion.

4. Contract-relax is a technique that applies a maximal contraction of the antagonistic muscle group as the extremity reaches the point of limitation. The therapist resists movement for eight to ten seconds with relaxation to follow. The technique is repeated until there are no further gains in range of motion.

System: Neuromuscular and Nervous Systems
Content Outline: Interventions

➡ PTAEXAM ONE: QUESTION 38

A physical therapist assistant instructs a patient positioned in the supine position to bring the left leg toward the chest and maintain the position. Assuming the assistant observes the response shown in the image, what muscle would **MOST** likely have insufficient length?

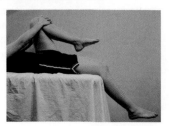

1. Iliopsoas

2. Quadratus lumborum

3. **Rectus femoris**

4. Sartorius

Correct Answer: 3 (Magee p. 728)

The left hip and knee are flexed to the chest to flatten the lumbar spine and stabilize the pelvis. A hip flexion contracture would be denoted by the right leg rising off the table. The length of the rectus femoris can be assessed during the Thomas test by examining the relative position of the knee (i.e., amount of knee flexion).

1. The iliopsoas acts to flex the hip. Tightness in the muscle could be identified using the Thomas test, however, the patient's right leg remains on the table which would be an indication of sufficient length in the one-joint hip flexors.

2. The quadratus lumborum originates on the iliolumbar ligament and the iliac crest. The muscle inserts on the last rib and the transverse processes of the lumbar vertebrae. As a result, the muscle does not act on the hip.

3. **Extension of the right knee is an indication that the patient has tightness in the two-joint rectus femoris muscle. A patient without tightness in the rectus femoris would typically present with the knee in 90 degrees of flexion while maintaining the position.**

4. The sartorius is a two-joint muscle that crosses both the hip and knee. The muscle acts to flex, laterally rotate, and abduct the hip joint. To specifically identify sartorius tightness the therapist would need to identify hip flexion, lateral rotation, and abduction of the hip during the Thomas Test.

System: Musculoskeletal System
Content Outline: Physical Therapy Data Collection

 Level 1   p. 262-263

 Level 2   p. 100-101

▶ PTAEXAM ONE: QUESTION 39

A patient who has vascular intermittent claudication is seen for cardiac rehabilitation. Which ankle-brachial index (ABI) value would be the **MOST** consistent with intermittent claudication symptoms that only occur during fairly intense exercise?

1. 0.35
2. 0.55
3. **0.75**
4. 1.10

Correct Answer: 3 (Hillegass p. 680)

The ankle-brachial index (ABI) is a measure of perfusion of the lower extremities. Abnormal ABI values indicate the presence of peripheral arterial disease, which also indicates a high risk for hypertension, coronary artery disease, and stroke. A patient's ABI can be assessed by comparing the systolic blood pressure in the arm with the systolic blood pressure in the leg. A normal ABI value is typically defined as falling between 1.0 and 1.30.

1. An ABI value of 0.35 indicates that the patient has severe peripheral arterial disease. A patient with severe peripheral arterial disease would have pain both with activity and at rest. There may also be associated tissue necrosis secondary to poor perfusion to the lower extremities.

2. An ABI value of 0.55 indicates that the patient has moderate to severe peripheral arterial disease. A patient with moderate to severe peripheral arterial disease would have pain both with activity and at rest.

3. **An ABI value of 0.75 indicates that the patient has mild to moderate peripheral arterial disease. A patient with mild to moderate peripheral arterial disease would likely only have symptoms with physical activity. Some patients with mild peripheral arterial disease are asymptomatic.**

4. An ABI value of 1.10 is considered to be normal. This patient would not have peripheral arterial disease and would not present with any claudication symptoms.

System: Cardiovascular and Pulmonary Systems
Content Outline: Physical Therapy Data Collection

▶ PTAEXAM ONE: QUESTION 40

A physical therapist assistant treats a patient diagnosed with plantar fasciitis. During the treatment session, the assistant attempts to strengthen the muscles that support the medial longitudinal arch. Which of the following muscles would be **MOST** important to emphasize in the strengthening program?

1. Gastrocnemius, soleus, and plantaris
2. Fibularis (peroneus) longus and brevis
3. Tibialis anterior and extensor hallucis longus
4. **Tibialis posterior and flexor digitorum longus**

Correct Answer: 4 (Dutton p. 1101)

The plantar fascia is a thin layer of tough connective tissue that supports the arch of the foot. Plantar fasciitis is a chronic overuse condition that develops secondary to repetitive stretching of the plantar fascia through excessive foot pronation during the loading phase of gait. Plantar fasciitis is usually unilateral and often presents with tenderness at the insertion of the plantar fascia, extreme morning pain, and difficulty with prolonged standing.

1. The gastrocnemius, soleus, and plantaris muscles form the superficial posterior compartment of the calf and function to plantar flex the ankle. The gastrocnemius and soleus muscles are more likely to need stretching rather than strengthening since tightness in the Achilles tendon is found in the majority of patients with plantar fasciitis.

2. The fibularis (peroneus) longus and brevis muscles form the lateral compartment of the leg with the tendons lying behind the lateral malleolus. Both muscles function to plantar flex the ankle and evert the foot. Although the fibularis longus crosses underneath the foot, the fibularis brevis inserts into the tuberosity of the fifth metatarsal and does not support the medial arch.

3. The tibialis anterior and extensor hallucis longus, along with the extensor digitorum longus, form the anterior compartment of the leg that collectively functions to dorsiflex the ankle. The extensor hallucis longus extends the big toe. The tibialis anterior and extensor digitorum longus also act to invert the foot. The tibialis anterior does support the medial longitudinal arch, however, the extensor hallucis longus does not.

4. **The tibialis posterior and flexor digitorum longus, along with the flexor hallucis longus, form the deep posterior compartment of the calf. These muscles all provide support to the medial longitudinal arch. Strengthening of these muscles, along with the intrinsic muscles of the foot, is essential in managing plantar fasciitis.**

System: Musculoskeletal System
Content Outline: Diseases/Conditions that Impact Effective Treatment

 Level 1   p. 375

 Level 1   p. 55, 65, 116, 158-159

➡ PTAEXAM ONE: QUESTION 41

A physical therapist assistant treats a patient with suspected ulnar nerve palsy. Which of the following clinical findings is **MOST** consistent with this diagnosis?

1. **Wasting of the hypothenar eminence**
2. Wrist drop with increased flexion of the wrist
3. Increased flexion of the metacarpophalangeal joint
4. Proximal interphalangeal joint hyperextension and slight flexion of the distal interphalangeal joint

Correct Answer: 1 (Dutton p. 809)

Nerve palsy is a term used to describe a range of nervous system disorders resulting in weakness or immobility of a nerve. In some cases, the palsy is only temporary and will dissipate with time, however, in other cases, the palsy may be permanent.

1. **The hypothenar eminence consists of the opponens digiti minimi, flexor digiti minimi, and abductor digiti minimi. These muscles are innervated by the ulnar nerve. An ulnar nerve palsy would result in diminished activity in the hypothenar muscles resulting in atrophy.**

2. Wrist drop with increased flexion of the wrist is more characteristic of a radial nerve palsy. The radial nerve innervates the majority of muscles acting to extend the wrist including the extensor carpi radialis longus, extensor carpi radialis brevis, and extensor digitorum.

3. The interossei muscles assist to flex the metacarpophalangeal joint and are innervated by the deep branch of the ulnar nerve. An ulnar nerve palsy would be unlikely to result in increased flexion of the metacarpophalangeal joint since the muscles would be adversely affected by the nerve palsy.

4. Proximal interphalangeal joint hyperextension and slight flexion of the distal interphalangeal joint are often associated with a rupture of the flexor digitorum superficialis. The muscle's primary action is to flex the proximal interphalangeal joint. A rupture of the flexor digitorum superficialis would tend to result in the proximal interphalangeal joint being positioned in extension.

System: Neuromuscular and Nervous Systems
Content Outline: Diseases/Conditions that Impact Effective Treatment

➡ PTAEXAM ONE: QUESTION 42

Which of the following degenerative central nervous system disorders should the physical therapist assistant recognize as consisting primarily of destruction of the motor neurons in the anterior horn cells of the spinal cord?

1. Parkinson's disease
2. Huntington's disease
3. **Amyotrophic lateral sclerosis**
4. Multiple sclerosis

Correct Answer: 3 (Goodman – Pathology p. 1455)

Degenerative diseases of the central nervous system can affect gray matter and/or white matter and are characterized by the slow deterioration of body functions that are controlled by the brain and spinal cord. Knowledge of the pathology of a specific disease can assist the therapist to identify relevant clinical symptoms.

1. The pathology of Parkinson's disease consists of destruction of the dopamine-producing cells within the basal ganglia.

2. The pathology of Huntington's disease is not definitive, however, often consists of tissue changes within the brain including atrophy of the basal ganglia and enlargement of the ventricles.

3. **The pathology of amyotrophic lateral sclerosis primarily consists of destruction of the motor neurons in the anterior horn cells of the spinal cord. Degeneration of motor cells may also be present in the brainstem and cerebral cortex.**

4. The pathology of multiple sclerosis consists of axonal demyelination and sclerotic plaques found throughout the brain and spinal cord.

System: Neuromuscular and Nervous Systems
Content Outline: Diseases/Conditions that Impact Effective Treatment

 Level 2   p. 227, 236

Level 2   p. 247, 292-293

➡ PTAEXAM ONE: QUESTION 43

A physical therapist assistant prepares a patient who has global aphasia post CVA for discharge from a rehabilitation hospital. The patient will be returning home with her husband and daughter. Which of the following methods of education is the **MOST** appropriate for the assistant to use to facilitate a safe discharge?

1. **Perform hands-on training sessions with the patient and family members**

2. Videotape the patient performing transfers and activities of daily living

3. Provide written instructions on all activities of daily living and functional tasks

4. Meet with family members to discuss the patient's present status and abilities

Correct Answer: 1 (O'Sullivan p. 703)

In order to facilitate a safe discharge, it is imperative that the physical therapist assistant is certain that the patient and family are aware of and can perform the necessary activities of daily living (ADLs) and functional tasks that will be required. The most effective manner in which to ascertain the family's readiness is to have them perform the required tasks and observe their competence.

1. **Hands-on training sessions provide unique opportunities for the physical therapist assistant to assess the competence of family members in a structured environment.**

2. Videotaping the necessary transfers and ADLs will provide the family with a visual aid, however, it does not ensure that they are able to safely perform the tasks with the patient.

3. Providing written instructions on all ADLs and functional tasks is an important part of a home exercise program and should be included in all discharge plans. This action, however, does not ensure that family members are able to safely perform the tasks with the patient.

4. Meeting with the family member to discuss the patient's present status and abilities is an important part of any discharge planning, however, it does not ensure that family members are able to safely perform the tasks with the patient.

System: Neuromuscular and Nervous Systems
Content Outline: Interventions

➡ PTAEXAM ONE: QUESTION 44

A patient is scheduled to undergo a transtibial amputation of the left lower extremity. In addition, the patient is one month post right total knee arthroplasty. Given the patient's past and current surgical history, the physical therapist assistant should expect which of the following activities to be the **MOST** difficult for the patient following their amputation?

1. Rolling from supine to sidelying

2. Moving from supine to sitting

3. **Moving from sitting to standing**

4. Ambulating in the parallel bars

Correct Answer: 3 (O'Sullivan p. 1006)

All of the listed tasks are reasonable expectations for the patient, however, moving from sitting to standing would be the most difficult due to the required lower extremity strength and the necessary balance required to complete the activity.

1. Rolling from supine to sidelying should be a relatively easy task for the patient since they can utilize upper extremity strength to initiate the movement.

2. Transferring from supine to sitting should be a relatively easy task for the patient since it is a non-weight bearing activity. The patient's sitting balance should not be impaired and the patient should be able to transfer to sitting using upper extremity support.

3. **Transferring from sitting to standing would be the most difficult for the patient since the activity requires adequate strength and dynamic balance. The patient's strength will be decreased in the right lower extremity secondary to the recent total knee arthroplasty and balance will be altered due to the left transtibial amputation.**

4. Ambulating in the parallel bars requires greater strength and balance than performing bed mobility, however, the patient is able to use the parallel bars to provide a stable base of support. The patient can use upper extremity strength to decrease some of the demand on the right lower extremity and to maintain balance during the activity.

System: Other Systems
Content Outline: Interventions

 Level 3   p. 700-703

 Level 2

➡ PTAEXAM ONE: QUESTION 45

A physical therapist assistant prepares to use an intermittent compression device to treat a patient who has lower extremity edema. The assistant would like to carefully monitor the patient during the session due to a history of mixed arterial and venous disease. Which of the following assessment procedures would be the **LEAST** beneficial to ensure that the patient is safely tolerating compression treatment?

1. Observation of lower extremity skin color
2. **Figure eight measurement at the ankle**
3. Capillary refill time of the great toe
4. Palpation of the dorsalis pedis artery

Correct Answer: 2 (Sussman p. 486)

Patients with venous insufficiency are often candidates for compression therapy to help reduce the edema that is associated with the disease. However, caution must be taken when using compression therapy on patients with arterial insufficiency since lower extremity circulation is already diminished and compression can further occlude blood flow.

1. Observing for changes in skin color would be an appropriate method for determining if circulation is impaired. When circulation becomes impaired, the skin typically becomes pale and cyanotic. This method, though acceptable, would not be the primary choice for assessing circulation since it is more of an indirect assessment.

2. **A figure eight measurement is a specific girth measurement for the ankle that is used to quantify edema. This measurement may be used to assess the effectiveness of compression therapy (i.e., reduction in edema). However, it would not be used to assess the relative safety of the intervention since it is not an assessment of circulation.**

3. Capillary refill is an assessment procedure in which the nail bed is compressed and then released. The time that it takes for color to return to the nail bed is recorded. Decreased capillary refill time is indicative of poor circulation and may signify that the intervention is unsafe.

4. Palpation of peripheral pulses is an appropriate method for assessing circulation in the distal lower extremities. The dorsalis pedis and posterior tibial arteries are the two most commonly assessed arteries in the lower leg. A diminished or absent pulse is indicative of poor circulation and may signify that the intervention is unsafe.

System: Cardiovascular and Pulmonary Systems
Content Outline: Physical Therapy Data Collection

➡ PTAEXAM ONE: QUESTION 46

A physical therapist assistant attempts to assess the extent of ataxia in a patient's upper extremities. Which of the following tests is **BEST** for assessing ataxia?

1. Manual muscle test
2. Sensory test for light touch
3. Functional assessment of bed mobility
4. **Finger to nose test**

Correct Answer: 4 (O'Sullivan p. 218)

Ataxia refers to the inability to perform coordinated movements usually as a result of cerebellar pathology. Ataxia can affect gait, patterns of movement, and posture. The condition increases the incidence of errors in the rate, rhythm, and timing of responses.

1. A manual muscle test is utilized to assess the strength of a muscle or muscle group. Ataxia is not necessarily due to weakness, rather the loss of muscular coordination.

2. A sensory test for light touch determines perception of tactile touch input. The test area is lightly touched or stroked using a brush, cotton ball or tissue. Sensory testing assesses the ascending pathways of the spinal cord.

3. Functional assessment of rolling in bed tests the overall mobility and strength of a patient, but is not a specific test for ataxia.

4. **A finger to nose test requires the patient to perform coordinated and controlled voluntary movement. A patient with ataxia may have difficulty completing the activity in an accurate and fluid manner.**

System: Neuromuscular and Nervous Systems
Content Outline: Physical Therapy Data Collection

⦿ Level 2

⦿ Level 2   p. 238

➡ PTAEXAM ONE: QUESTION 47

An 11-month-old patient who has cerebral palsy attempts to maintain a quadruped position. Which of the following primitive reflexes would **MOST** interfere with this activity if it was not integrated?

1. Galant
2. **Symmetrical tonic neck**
3. Plantar grasp
4. Positive support

Correct Answer: 2 (Ratliffe p. 26)

Primitive reflexes are reflexes which begin in utero or in early infancy. Most of these reflexes become integrated as the infant ages. Integration denotes that the reflex is no longer present when the stimulus is provided. Failure to integrate primitive reflexes can lead to impaired movement.

1. The Galant reflex is stimulated by stroking lateral to the spine. The response is lateral sidebending to the same side as the side of the stimulus. An infant would typically be able to maintain the quadruped position if this reflex was stimulated.

2. **Head positioning is the stimulus for the symmetrical tonic neck reflex. When the head is flexed, the upper extremities flex and the lower extremities extend. When the head extends the upper extremities extend and the lower extremities flex. The reaction of the extremities would not allow the infant to maintain a quadruped position.**

3. The plantar grasp reflex is stimulated by placing pressure on the ball of the foot, generally in standing. The response is for the toes to curl or flex. The reflex will have no impact on an infant's ability to maintain quadruped since the balls of the feet are not in contact with the floor.

4. The positive support reflex is stimulated by bearing weight through the feet. The response is for the lower extremities to extend, thereby allowing the infant to bear weight through the lower extremities. The reflex will have no impact on an infant's ability to maintain quadruped since they are not bearing weight through the feet.

System: Neuromuscular and Nervous Systems
Content Outline: Interventions

➡ PTAEXAM ONE: QUESTION 48

A physical therapist assistant attempts to assess the temperature of a patient's skin in an area susceptible to a pressure ulcer. Which area of the assistant's body would be the **MOST** appropriate to utilize when assessing the patient's skin temperature?

1. **Dorsum of the hand**
2. Hypothenar eminence
3. Thenar eminence
4. Second and third finger pads

Correct Answer: 1 (Goodman – Differential Diagnosis p. 162)

Physical therapist assistants routinely assess the temperature of a patient's skin. Altered skin temperature can be indicative of impaired circulation or an active disease process. Typically, the assistant will compare and contrast symmetrical body parts.

1. **The dorsum of the hand is most sensitive to temperature changes in the body. The relative superficial nature of the area and the available cutaneous receptors allow even subtle temperature changes to be detected.**

2. The hypothenar eminence consists of the opponens digiti minimi, flexor digiti minimi, and abductor digiti minimi muscles. The hypothenar eminence would not typically be used to assess skin temperature.

3. The thenar eminence consists of the abductor pollicis brevis, flexor pollicis brevis, and opponens pollicis. The thenar eminence would not typically be used to assess skin temperature.

4. The second and third finger pads are the most common area of the hand used for palpation, but are not as sensitive to temperature change as the dorsum of the hand. The finger pads are useful in assessing fine tactile discrimination, skin moisture, and texture.

System: Other Systems
Content Outline: Physical Therapy Data Collection

 Level 1   p. 277-278

● Level 1   p. 268-269, 442, 444, 538-539

 SCOREBUILDERS

➡ PTAEXAM ONE: QUESTION 49

A physical therapist assistant asks a patient to raise one hand to indicate that they felt a Semmes-Weinstein monofilament contacting their skin. Which situation would **BEST** support this type of testing procedure?

1. The patient does not speak English
2. The patient has ideomotor apraxia
3. The patient has diabetes mellitus
4. **The patient has Broca's aphasia**

Correct Answer: 4 (O'Sullivan p. 1272)

Sensory testing is commonly performed using Semmes-Weinstein monofilaments in order to gather objective data regarding protective sensation. The testing protocol involves touching the monofilament to designated points on the bottom of the foot. Traditionally, the patient is instructed to respond "yes" when they feel the monofilament touching their skin.

1. If a patient does not speak English, a translator should be provided to explain the testing procedure. If the patient does not understand the test, then the data gathered cannot be considered accurate. Asking the patient to raise one hand to indicate that they have felt the monofilament contact their skin is not the best option, as it is unlikely that the patient understands the request.

2. Ideomotor apraxia is a condition where a person plans a movement or task, but cannot volitionally perform it. Automatic movement may occur, however, a person cannot impose additional movement on command. Asking a patient to raise one hand to indicate that they have felt the monofilament contacting their skin is not the best option, as the patient will likely have difficulty executing this motor task.

3. A Semmes-Weinstein monofilament test can be utilized to screen for peripheral polyneuropathy in patients with diabetes mellitus. However, diabetes mellitus does not typically prevent patients from responding verbally to indicate that they have felt the monofilament contacting their skin.

4. **Broca's aphasia is a form of non-fluent aphasia that is also known as "expressive aphasia." Individuals with this condition have intact auditory and reading comprehension, but have impaired repetition and naming skills. Individuals with Broca's aphasia commonly become frustrated when making language errors. Asking an individual with Broca's aphasia to indicate they have felt the monofilament touching their skin by raising one hand is appropriate because it eliminates the need for a verbal response.**

System: Neuromuscular and Nervous Systems
Content Outline: Physical Therapy Data Collection

 Level 2   p. 232, 243-244, 442

➡ PTAEXAM ONE: QUESTION 50

A physical therapist assistant instructs a patient post fractured left hip in gait training activities. The patient is weight bearing as tolerated and uses a large base quad cane. Which of the following techniques would be the **MOST** appropriate?

1. Using the quad cane on the left with the longer legs positioned away from the patient
2. **Using the quad cane on the right with the longer legs positioned away from the patient**
3. Using the quad cane on the left with the longer legs positioned toward the patient
4. Using the quad cane on the right with the longer legs positioned toward the patient

Correct Answer: 2 (Minor p. 295)

A quad cane should be utilized in the hand opposite from the affected lower extremity. The device is designed so that the longer legs are positioned away from the patient.

1. The quad cane should be used in the hand opposite the affected lower extremity.

2. **The quad cane, positioned in the right hand with the longer legs pointing away from the patient, will allow for proper distribution of the weight during gait and as a result, the patient will be less likely to trip over the longer legs of the cane.**

3. The quad cane should be used in the hand opposite the affected lower extremity with the longer legs of the quad cane positioned away from the patient.

4. The quad cane should be used with the longer legs positioned away from the patient so that the patient does not trip over them.

System: Non-Systems
Content Outline: Equipment, Devices, and Technologies; Therapeutic Modalities

 Level 2   p. 603-604

➡ PTAEXAM ONE: QUESTION 51

A physical therapist assistant uses ultrasound to heat tissues at a depth of approximately four centimeters. Which parameter of ultrasound would **MOST** influence the depth of tissue heating?

1. Intensity
2. **Frequency**
3. Effective radiating area
4. Beam nonuniformity ratio

Correct Answer: 2 (Cameron p. 184)

Physical therapist assistants must utilize ultrasound treatment parameters that are consistent with the desired therapeutic outcome. Four centimeters is a significant amount of tissue depth and would therefore require a frequency of 1 MHz.

1. Intensity is a measure of the rate at which energy is being delivered per unit of area. Intensity for continuous ultrasound is normally set between .5 to 2.0 W/cm^2 for thermal effects. Pulsed ultrasound is normally set between .5 to .75 W/cm^2 with a 20% duty cycle for nonthermal effects.

2. **Frequency should be selected according to the depth of tissues to be treated. The most common frequency settings are 1 MHz and 3 MHz. A frequency setting of 1 MHz is used for heating of deeper tissues (up to five centimeters) where a setting of 3 MHz is used for heating superficial tissues with a depth of penetration of less than two centimeters.**

3. Effective radiating area refers to the portion of the surface of the transducer that produces the sound wave. The effective radiating area is dependent on the surface area of the crystal. An area two to three times the size of the transducer typically requires a duration of five minutes of treatment. Ideally, the effective radiating area nearly matches the size of the faceplate of the ultrasound soundhead.

4. Beam nonuniformity ratio (BNR) refers to the ratio of intensity of the highest peak to the average intensity of all peaks. The BNR is determined by the intrinsic biophysical properties of the piezoelectric transducer.

System: Non-Systems
Content Outline: Equipment, Devices, and Technologies; Therapeutic Modalities

➡ PTAEXAM ONE: QUESTION 52

A patient sustained a superficial wound that appears as a moderate abrasion on the anterior surface of their thigh approximately four inches above the superior pole of the patella. Which type of wound dressing would **MOST** likely be utilized?

1. Calcium alginate dressing
2. Hydrocolloid dressing
3. Hydrogel dressing
4. **Transparent film dressing**

Correct Answer: 4 (Sussman p. 504)

Physical therapist assistants utilize particular wound dressings based on the established therapeutic objectives. General indications for utilizing a dressing include protecting a wound, managing exudate, preventing infection, reducing pain, and promoting healing.

1. A calcium alginate dressing is highly absorptive and typically utilized with wounds that produce moderate to heavy exudate. A superficial wound such as an abrasion would produce minimal exudate and therefore is unlikely to saturate the alginate to the extent necessary for it to form a beneficial hydrophilic gel.

2. Hydrocolloid dressings consist of gel-forming polymers (e.g., carboxymethylcellulose, gelatin, pectin) backed by a strong film or foam adhesive. The dressings absorb exudate by swelling into a gel-like mass and vary in permeability, thickness, and transparency. A hydrocolloid dressing is not used for a superficial wound, however, is often used on partial and full-thickness wounds.

3. Hydrogel dressings are moisture-retentive primary dressings that are commonly used on superficial and partial-thickness wounds (e.g., abrasions, blisters, pressure ulcers) with minimal drainage. This type of dressing is typically used to prevent a wound from dehydrating and impeding the healing process. Small superficial abrasions with minimal to no drainage are much more commonly treated with transparent film dressings than hydrogel dressings because the transparent nature of the dressing allows for quick and easy inspection of the wound.

4. **Transparent film dressings consist of thin membranes coated with a layer of acrylic adhesive. Since the film is transparent, it allows for frequent assessment of the wound and offers some level of protection. The films are oxygen permeable, however, are impermeable to microorganisms and moisture. The relatively superficial nature and clinical presentation (i.e., abrasion) of the wound result in a transparent film dressing serving as the most appropriate choice.**

System: Other Systems
Content Outline: Interventions

 Level 1   p. 623-626

Level 3   p. 441, 443, 448-449

➡ PTAEXAM ONE: QUESTION 53

A physical therapist assistant notices two prominent tendons visible on the posterior surface of the left knee while a patient completes a leg curl exercise. As shown in the image, the visible medial and lateral tendons are **MOST** likely associated with which of the following muscles?

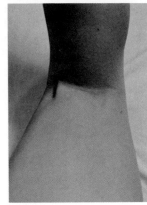

1. Semimembranosus and semitendinosus
2. **Semitendinosus and biceps femoris**
3. Popliteus and semitendinosus
4. Semimembranosus and biceps femoris

Correct Answer: 2 (Magee p. 857)

The hamstring muscles include the semitendinosus, semi-membranosus, and biceps femoris. The muscles' primary action is to flex the knee. As a result, the tendons of each of the hamstring muscles become more prominent with resisted knee flexion.

1. The semimembranosus and semitendinosus are hamstring muscles that act to flex the knee joint, however, they are both located on the medial aspect of the posterior knee joint. The image shows two tendons, one that is located on the medial aspect of the posterior surface of the knee joint and the other on the lateral aspect.

2. **The semitendinosus and biceps femoris are hamstring muscles whose tendons become prominent when performing a leg curl. The biceps femoris is the lateral tendon, while the semitendinosus is the medial tendon.**

3. The popliteus muscle is located deep within the posterior surface of the knee joint and would not appear as a tendinous cord-like structure. The semitendinosus is a medial hamstrings muscle that would be prominent on the medial aspect of the posterior surface of the knee joint.

4. The semimembranosus muscle is a medial hamstrings muscle, however, the muscle's tendon is not nearly as prominent as the semitendinosus. The biceps femoris is a lateral hamstrings muscle that would be prominent on the lateral aspect of the posterior surface of the knee joint.

System: Musculoskeletal System
Content Outline: Physical Therapy Data Collection

➡ PTAEXAM ONE: QUESTION 54

A physical therapist assistant would like to monitor a patient with a history of recurrent dysrhythmias during selected formal exercise activities. Which of the following monitoring devices would be the **MOST** beneficial?

1. Pulmonary artery catheter
2. **Electrocardiogram**
3. Intracranial pressure monitor
4. Pulse oximeter

Correct Answer: 2 (Hillegass p. 310)

An electrocardiogram (ECG) is a recording of the electrical activity of the heart over time produced by an electrocardiograph, usually via skin electrodes. It is a common monitoring device for patients with known or suspected cardiac abnormalities.

1. A pulmonary artery catheter monitors cardiovascular pressures in the pulmonary artery.

2. **The electrocardiogram provides a graphic record of the electrical activity of the heart at rest or during exercise. Dysrhythmia is a general term used to denote disturbances in the heart's rhythm, which are best monitored by an electrocardiogram.**

3. An intracranial pressure monitor consists of a small plastic tube usually inserted in the left or right anterior portion of the brain. The monitor is often used to assess the pressure surrounding the brain of patients in the intensive care unit who have sustained head trauma, brain hemorrhage, brain surgery or conditions in which the brain may swell.

4. A pulse oximeter is an instrument that uses a light-emitting diode, a photodiode signal detector, and a microprocessor to determine the percentage of oxygen saturation of arterial blood.

System: Cardiovascular and Pulmonary Systems
Content Outline: Interventions

⦿ Level 1

⦿ Level 1   👓 p. 380

➡ PTAEXAM ONE: QUESTION 55

A physical therapist assistant repeats several clinical tests on a patient with a C6 nerve root injury. Which of the following clinical findings should the assistant **LEAST** expect with this type of injury?

1. Diminished sensation on the anterior arm and the index finger

2. Weakness in the biceps and supinator muscles

3. Diminished deep tendon reflex response of the brachioradialis

4. **Paresthesias of the long and ring fingers**

Correct Answer: 4 (Magee p. 24)

Involvement of a specific nerve root often results in predictable impairments including diminished sensation, muscle weakness, impaired reflexes, and paresthesias.

1. Diminished sensation on the anterior arm and index finger is characteristic of a C6 nerve root injury and is assessed using light touch from a cotton ball.

2. Weakness in the biceps and supinator muscles is characteristic of a C6 nerve root injury and is assessed through resistive testing as part of an upper quarter screening and/or specific manual muscle testing.

3. A diminished brachioradialis reflex is characteristic of a C6 nerve root injury and is assessed by striking the blunt end of a reflex hammer at the distal end of the radius with the patient's elbow flexed to 90 degrees and the upper extremity supported by the physical therapist assistant.

4. **Paresthesias of the long and ring fingers are commonly associated with the C7 nerve root. Other findings of a C7 nerve root injury include weakness of the triceps and wrist flexors, and a diminished triceps reflex.**

System: Neuromuscular and Nervous Systems
Content Outline: Diseases/Conditions that Impact Effective Treatment

➡ PTAEXAM ONE: QUESTION 56

A recent entry in the medical record indicates a patient exhibits dysdiadochokinesia. Based on the patient's documented deficit, which activity should the physical therapist assistant expect to be the **MOST** difficult for the patient?

1. **Alternate supination and pronation of the forearms**

2. Perform a standing squat

3. March in place

4. Walk along a straight line

Correct Answer: 1 (Umphred p. 638)

Dysdiadochokinesia refers to the inability to perform rapid, alternating movements. This condition results in inappropriate timing of muscle firing and difficulty with cessation of ongoing movement.

1. **When the patient attempts pronation and supination of the forearms, the movement is slow and will lose range and rhythm quickly. The presence of dysdiadochokinesia is commonly associated with a cerebellar lesion.**

2. Performing a standing squat is not a velocity-based activity requiring alternating movement and therefore does not assess dysdiadochokinesia. The activity requires concentric and eccentric muscle control of the trunk and lower extremities.

3. Marching in place to a specific cadence is sometimes used to test for a cerebellar movement disorder. A positive test occurs when a patient is unable to follow the rhythm of the cadence.

4. Walking along a straight line is often used to identify signs of cerebellar pathology such as ataxia. Characteristics of an ataxic gait include uneven step length, increased base of support, inability to walk a straight line without lurching, impaired rhythm, and a high stepping pattern.

System: Neuromuscular and Nervous Systems
Content Outline: Interventions

⦿ Level 1   p. 222-223

⦿ Level 2   p. 239

SCOREBUILDERS

➡ PTAEXAM ONE: QUESTION 57

A physical therapist assistant is treating a patient diagnosed with leukemia who is currently receiving chemotherapy. The patient has been referred to physical therapy to improve their functional mobility and endurance. Which activity would be the **LEAST** desirable to accomplish the stated goal?

1. Yoga
2. Bike riding
3. **Jumping rope**
4. Swimming

Correct Answer: 3 (Palisano p. 394)

Leukemia is a cancer of the blood that occurs when leukocytes change into malignant cells. These immature cells proliferate, accumulate in bone marrow, and ultimately cease the production of normal cells. This process can spread to the lymph nodes, liver, spleen, and other areas of the body. Treatment will vary based on the type and degree of leukemia, but may include immunotherapy, cytotoxic agents, chemotherapy or radiation, and bone marrow transplant.

1. Yoga is an appropriate low-impact activity that focuses on stretching. Patients undergoing medical treatment for leukemia must work to maintain range of motion and muscle length. Yoga will allow for improvement in range of motion, strength, and cardiovascular endurance.

2. Bike riding is an appropriate endurance activity for a patient undergoing medical treatment for leukemia. This activity will allow for improvement in strength, balance, and cardiovascular endurance.

3. **Patients with leukemia are at risk for osteonecrosis, which can occur at the hips, knees, and ankles. Patients may or may not present with symptoms related to osteonecrosis and therefore therapists must be aware of potential risk factors. High-impact activities such as jumping rope should be avoided as an intervention to improve endurance since these types of activities place the patient at risk for further injury.**

4. Swimming is an appropriate low-impact endurance activity that uses buoyancy and the properties of water to minimize weight bearing forces through the lower extremities.

System: Other Systems
Content Outline: Interventions

➡ PTAEXAM ONE: QUESTION 58

A physical therapist assistant observes a patient utilize a suspensory strategy to regain their balance. Which active movement would be **MOST** characteristic of this postural strategy?

1. Trunk extension
2. Hip extension
3. **Knee flexion**
4. Ankle plantar flexion

Correct Answer: 3 (O'Sullivan p. 232)

The suspensory strategy is used to lower the center of gravity during standing or ambulation in order to improve balance and stability. Examples of this strategy include knee flexion, crouching or squatting. This strategy is often used when both mobility and stability are required during a task (e.g., surfing).

1. Trunk extension would not be effective to lower the center of gravity and is therefore not consistent with the suspensory strategy.

2. Hip extension would not be effective to lower the center of gravity and is therefore not consistent with the suspensory strategy. Hip flexion, however, would be consistent with this strategy.

3. **Knee flexion is often the immediate action utilized in standing to lower the center of gravity following a significant perturbation. This action often provides the individual with the ability to regain their balance.**

4. Ankle plantar flexion would not be effective to lower the center of gravity and is therefore not consistent with the suspensory strategy.

System: Neuromuscular and Nervous Systems
Content Outline: Interventions

Level 3

Level 1   p. 241

➡ PTAEXAM ONE: QUESTION 59

A physical therapist assistant performs an upper extremity manual muscle test on a patient. Assuming the patient has the ability to move the upper extremities against gravity, which of the following muscles should the assistant test with the patient in the prone position?

1. Pronator teres
2. Pectoralis major
3. Biceps brachii
4. **Middle trapezius**

Correct Answer: 4 (Kendall p. 329)

The middle fibers of the trapezius originate on the spinous processes of the first through fifth thoracic vertebrae and insert on the medial margin of the acromion and superior lip of the spine of the scapula. The muscle is innervated by the spinal accessory nerve and ventral rami C2, C3, C4.

1. The pronator teres is tested in a supine position. The test arm is positioned with forearm pronation and partial elbow flexion. The therapist provides pressure at the lower forearm in the direction of forearm supination.

2. The pectoralis major is tested with the patient in a supine position. The test arm is flexed to 90 degrees at the shoulder with slight medial rotation and elbow extension. Pressure is applied against the forearm in the direction of horizontal abduction.

3. The biceps brachii is tested with the patient in a supine position. The test arm is flexed at the elbow to 90 degrees with supination of the forearm. The therapist provides pressure at the distal end of the forearm in the direction of extension.

4. **The middle trapezius is tested with the patient in a prone position. The test arm is abducted at the shoulder to 90 degrees with lateral rotation and elbow extension. The therapist provides pressure against the forearm in a downward direction.**

System: Musculoskeletal System
Content Outline: Physical Therapy Data Collection

➡ PTAEXAM ONE: QUESTION 60

A physical therapist assistant prepares a patient education program for a patient with chronic venous insufficiency. Which of the following instructions would be the **LEAST** appropriate to include in the patient education program?

1. Wear shoes that accommodate to the size and shape of your feet
2. Observe your skin daily for breakdown
3. **Wear your compression stockings only at night**
4. Keep your feet elevated as much as possible throughout the day

Correct Answer: 3 (Cameron p. 420)

Chronic venous insufficiency is a common disorder of the lower extremity veins in which the veins do not work properly and blood pools in the lower extremities, leading to increased pressure within the veins. If uncontrolled, fluid may leak into the surrounding tissues in the ankles and feet and may eventually cause skin breakdown and ulceration.

1. Wearing shoes that accommodate to the size and shape of the foot is an important component of an education program for a patient with venous insufficiency. Successful implementation of the program reduces the risk of skin abrasions, ulcerations, and wound infections.

2. Swelling, cellulitis, and chronic lower extremity ulcers are common complications of venous insufficiency. Daily observation of the skin is a necessary component of an education program for a patient with venous insufficiency.

3. **Patients with chronic venous insufficiency often wear graduated compression stockings which attempt to improve circulation by preventing backward flow through the veins of the lower extremities. It is recommended that compression stockings are applied in the morning since swelling is usually minimal. The stockings should be left on during the day for activity such as ambulation to promote blood flow to the heart and avoid venous stasis.**

4. Elevating the feet throughout the day reduces pressure in the lower extremity veins and helps to improve blood flow. Positioning guidelines would be part of an education program for a patient with venous insufficiency.

System: Cardiovascular and Pulmonary Systems
Content Outline: Interventions

 Level 1   p. 78

 Level 2   p. 417

▶ PTAEXAM ONE: QUESTION 61

A physical therapist assistant prepares to measure the blood pressure of a patient who has a history of cardiac disease. Which of the following values describes the **MOST** appropriate rate to release the pressure when obtaining the blood pressure measurement?

1. **2-3 mm Hg per second**
2. 3-5 mm Hg per second
3. 5-7 mm Hg per second
4. 8-10 mm Hg per second

Correct Answer: 1 (Fairchild p. 60)

Deflating the cuff at a rate of 2-3 mm Hg per second is recommended to identify normal Korotkoff's sounds and obtain a valid measure of the patient's blood pressure. Rates faster than 2-3 mm Hg per second will tend to increase the measurement error.

1. **After inflating the cuff to 20 mm Hg above the estimated systolic pressure, the physical therapist assistant should carefully unscrew (open) the valve and deflate the bladder no more than 2-3 mm Hg per second while listening for the Korotkoff sounds.**

2. 3-5 mm Hg per second is faster than the recommended rate of 2-3 mm Hg per second.

3. 5-7 mm Hg per second is more than twice as fast as the recommended rate of 2-3 mm Hg per second.

4. 8-10 mm Hg per second is more than three times as fast as the recommended rate of 2-3 mm Hg per second.

System: Cardiovascular and Pulmonary Systems
Content Outline: Physical Therapy Data Collection

▶ PTAEXAM ONE: QUESTION 62

A physical therapist assistant performs a gross range of motion screening and determines a patient has excessive medial rotation and limited lateral rotation of the hip. Which alignment of the hip would be the **MOST** consistent with the identified findings?

1. 10 degrees of anteversion
2. **18 degrees of anteversion**
3. 5 degrees of retroversion
4. 8 degrees of retroversion

Correct Answer: 2 (Magee p. 710)

Femoral anteversion or forward torsion of the femoral neck is measured by the angle of the femoral neck in relation to the femoral condyles. The mean angle of anteversion in an adult is 8-15 degrees. The amount of femoral anteversion present can be quantified using Craig's test.

1. 10 degrees of anteversion is within the normal range and therefore would not serve as an indicator that the patient possesses excessive medial rotation and limited lateral rotation of the hip.

2. **18 degrees of anteversion is considered to be excessive and therefore would make the patient more likely to exhibit excessive medial rotation and limited lateral rotation of the hip.**

3. Retroversion occurs when the plane of the femoral neck rotates backward in relation to the coronal condylar plane. This finding would not result in excessive medial rotation and limited lateral rotation of the hip.

4. Retroversion or less than the mean angle of anteversion (i.e., 8-15 degrees) would not typically be associated with excessive medial rotation and limited lateral rotation of the hip.

System: Musculoskeletal System
Content Outline: Physical Therapy Data Collection

 Level 1   p. 376

 Level 2   p. 100

➡ PTAEXAM ONE: QUESTION 63

A patient sustains a chemical burn on the cubital area of the elbow. What position would be the **MOST** appropriate for splinting of the involved upper extremity?

1. Elbow flexion and forearm pronation

2. Elbow flexion and forearm supination

3. Elbow extension and forearm pronation

4. **Elbow extension and forearm supination**

Correct Answer: 4 (O'Sullivan p. 1111)

A burn in the cubital area of the elbow would impact the motions at the elbow and the forearm. The general rule for positioning is to place the affected area in a position that is opposite from the impending contracture. The elbow is most susceptible to a flexion contracture and the forearm is most susceptible to a pronation contracture. Physical therapist assistants must be aware of patient positioning following a burn in order to avoid potential contractures. Daily monitoring of the patient's medical status, range of motion, and skin condition will assist health care providers to determine how long specific positions should be maintained and what other modifications may be necessary.

1. Splinting in the position of elbow flexion and forearm pronation would result in the patient being susceptible to elbow flexion and forearm pronation contractures.

2. Splinting in the position of elbow flexion and forearm supination would result in the patient being susceptible to an elbow flexion contracture.

3. Splinting in the position of elbow extension and forearm pronation would result in the patient being susceptible to a forearm pronation contracture.

4. **Splinting in the position of elbow extension and forearm supination will effectively limit contractures and maximize functional use of the upper extremity.**

System: Other Systems
Content Outline: Interventions

➡ PTAEXAM ONE: QUESTION 64

A physical therapist assistant documents gait training performed during a treatment session. Which descriptive term is only associated with the swing phase of the gait cycle?

1. Heel strike

2. **Deceleration**

3. Loading response

4. Midstance

Correct Answer: 2 (O'Sullivan p. 255)

The phases of gait are classified based on either points in time (traditional terminology) or periods of time (Rancho Los Amigos terminology). Stance phase represents approximately 60 percent of the gait cycle, while swing phase represents approximately 40 percent.

1. Heel strike is traditional terminology that refers to the instant that the heel touches the ground to begin stance phase. Heel strike is a component of stance phase.

2. **Deceleration is traditional terminology that begins directly after midswing as the swing limb begins to extend and ends just prior to heel strike. Deceleration is a component of swing phase.**

3. Loading response is Rancho Los Amigos terminology that corresponds to the amount of time between initial contact and the beginning of the swing phase for the other leg. Loading response is a component of stance phase.

4. Midstance is a term utilized in traditional terminology and Rancho Los Amigos terminology. In traditional terminology, midstance refers to the point during the stance phase when the entire body weight is directly over the stance limb. In Rancho Los Amigos terminology, midstance corresponds to the point in the stance phase when the other foot is off the floor until the body is directly over the stance limb. Midstance is a component of stance phase.

System: Musculoskeletal System
Content Outline: Physical Therapy Data Collection

 Level 2   p. 453

Level 1   p. 81-82

➡ PTAEXAM ONE: QUESTION 65

A physical therapist assistant initiates an exercise program for a patient who has a lower extremity injury. Which of the following parameters is the single **MOST** important factor in an exercise program designed to increase muscular strength?

1. Recovery time between exercise sets

2. Number of repetitions per set

3. Duration of the exercise session

4. **Intensity of the exercise**

Correct Answer: 4 (Kisner p. 179)

Gains in strength are greatest when a muscle is exercised against resistance at maximal intensity.

1. The recovery time between sets is determined based on the specific parameters of the strengthening activities (e.g., intensity, sets, repetitions) and the unique patient needs. Although an important variable to consider, recovery time would not be the most important factor.

2. The number of repetitions per set refers to the number of times a particular movement is repeated. The number of repetitions selected is usually dependent on whether the goal of the resistive exercise is to improve strength or endurance. The actual number of repetitions per set is important, however, would not be as critical as intensity when the established goal is to increase strength.

3. Duration is the total timeframe in which the resistive program is carried out. The duration will be highly dependent on the patient's current status and the established therapeutic goals.

4. **The intensity of exercise refers to the amount of resistance imposed on the contracting muscle during each repetition of an exercise. The overload principle specifies that if muscle performance is to improve, a load must be selected that exceeds the metabolic capacity of the muscle. Muscle strength will not increase without adequate intensity.**

System: Musculoskeletal System
Content Outline: Interventions

➡ PTAEXAM ONE: QUESTION 66

A physical therapist assistant works on wheelchair mobility with a patient who has right-sided hemiparesis. Which of the following wheelchair adaptations would be the **MOST** beneficial for the patient to ensure safety during stand pivot transfers?

1. Anti-tip tubes

2. **Pull-to wheel lock with brake extensions**

3. Elevating leg rests

4. Removable full-length armrests

Correct Answer: 2 (Tan p. 323)

Performing transfer training with a patient who has had a cerebrovascular accident is an important component of the physical therapy plan of care to maximize the patient's functional independence. Impairments that are present following a left hemisphere cerebrovascular accident that may affect a patient's ability to safely transfer include weakness, paralysis of the right side, increased frustration, decreased processing, possible motor apraxia, and right hemianopsia.

1. Anti-tip tubes attach to the posterior of the wheelchair to prevent tipping in the event of a posterior loss of balance. Patients who would benefit from anti-tip tubes have impairments in or absence of trunk control. Anti-tip tubes can also be used when mastering wheelchair mobility on steep inclines until the patient gains enough strength and postural control to master the technique.

2. **A pull-to wheel lock allows for closer access to surfaces during transfers. Brake extensions on the right side allow the patient to reach with the uninvolved upper extremity to lock the wheelchair prior to transferring. The patient's ability to use the right hand to lock the brakes is most likely limited due to the right-sided hemiparesis.**

3. Elevating leg rests are indicated for patients who need support of the lower extremity. Elevating leg rests can prevent dependent edema and may assist in redistributing weight bearing forces, however, would not be the most essential wheelchair adaptation to ensure safety during a stand pivot transfer.

4. Removable full-length armrests allow for a squat pivot or sliding board transfer, however, would not be necessary for a stand pivot transfer.

System: Non-Systems
Content Outline: Equipment, Devices, and Technologies;
    Therapeutic Modalities

 Level 2   p. 109-110

 Level 2   p. 598-600

➡ PTAEXAM ONE: QUESTION 67

A physical therapist assistant performs gait training using crutches on a patient post total hip arthroplasty. The patient has orders for partial weight bearing. Which of the following gait patterns would be the **MOST** appropriate for this patient?

1. Four-point

2. Two-point

3. **Three-point**

4. Swing-to

Correct Answer: 3 (Minor p. 297)

Gait training often includes the introduction of an assistive device such as a cane, crutches or a walker. The most appropriate gait pattern for the patient following total hip arthroplasty depends on the patient's weight bearing status, as well as their strength, balance, and cognitive abilities.

1. A four-point gait pattern is performed with two crutches or canes. The patient advances the crutch/cane on the left followed by the right leg, then advances the crutch/cane on the right followed by the left leg. This gait pattern does not allow for partial weight bearing status and is most often utilized when a patient has poor balance, incoordination or muscle weakness.

2. With a two-point gait pattern, the patient advances one assistive device and the opposite lower extremity simultaneously. During the beginning of the stance phase of one limb, the assistive device on the opposite side provides support. Each step is one point. This gait pattern requires the patient to have good balance as only two points of floor contact are maintained at any one time. This gait pattern most closely resembles normal gait and would be inappropriate for a patient that is partial weight bearing.

3. **A three-point gait pattern is used when one limb is affected, such as after joint arthroplasty. This pattern is used when the weight bearing orders are for non-weight bearing or partial weight bearing. Three points of support contact the floor with weight borne through each crutch and the uninvolved lower extremity. The crutches are advanced followed by the affected lower extremity, then the unaffected lower extremity.**

4. In a swing-to gait pattern the patient advances the lower extremities simultaneously to the point of the crutches. This gait pattern is used when a patient has trunk and/or bilateral lower extremity weakness, paresis or paralysis. This gait pattern would be inappropriate for a patient following total hip arthroplasty.

System: Non-Systems
Content Outline: Equipment, Devices, and Technologies; Therapeutic Modalities

 Level 1   p. 603-605

➡ PTAEXAM ONE: QUESTION 68

A physical therapist assistant performs gait training with a patient outdoors to simulate the uneven terrain that the patient will encounter upon discharge. The assistant monitors the patient closely due to extreme heat and humidity. What is the **PRIMARY** mode of heat loss during exercise?

1. Conduction

2. Convection

3. **Evaporation**

4. Radiation

Correct Answer: 3 (American College of Sports Medicine p. 68)

As an individual starts to exercise and produce more heat, sweating provides compensatory heat loss through evaporation. The effectiveness of sweating to cool the body is affected by humidity. A humid environment, where there is a high level of water vapor in the air, limits evaporation of sweat. As a result, physical therapist assistants must closely monitor patients when exercising in extreme heat and humidity to avoid a substantial increase in core temperature.

1. Conduction refers to the gain or loss of heat as a result of direct contact between two materials at different temperatures.

2. Convection refers to the gain or loss of heat as a result of air or water moving in a constant motion across the body. Convection can be useful to dissipate heat, however, in extreme heat and humidity this method is less effective than evaporation. The rate of convection increases with air movement from the wind.

3. **Evaporation refers to the transfer of heat as a liquid absorbs energy and changes form to a vapor.**

4. Radiation refers to the direct transfer of heat from an energy source of higher temperature to one of cooler temperature. Heat energy is directly absorbed without the need for a medium. An example is an infrared lamp.

System: Other Systems
Content Outline: Diseases/Conditions that Impact Effective Treatment

 Level 1   p. 614

➡ PTAEXAM ONE: QUESTION 69

A physical therapist assistant performs resisted isometric testing on a patient. The patient reports feeling pain during the test, however, strength is normal. Which of the following conclusions regarding this test is the **MOST** likely?

1. A severe lesion such as a fracture
2. **A minor lesion of a muscle or tendon**
3. A complete rupture of a muscle or tendon
4. Intermittent claudication may be present

Correct Answer: 2 (Magee p. 38)

Resisted isometric testing attempts to identify the status of contractile tissue (i.e., muscles, tendons, associated attachments) and the nervous tissue supplying the contractile tissue.

1. A severe lesion such as a fracture would tend to result in resisted movement that is classified as weak and painful.

2. **A minor lesion of a muscle or tendon would tend to result in resisted movement that is classified as strong and painful.**

3. A complete rupture of a muscle or tendon would tend to result in resisted movement that is classified as weak and pain free.

4. Intermittent claudication occurs as a result of insufficient blood supply and ischemia in active muscles. Resisted movement tends to produce or exacerbate pain and cramping in muscles distal to the occluded vessel. Strength could be negatively impacted depending on the severity of the pain.

System: Musculoskeletal System
Content Outline: Physical Therapy Data Collection

➡ PTAEXAM ONE: QUESTION 70

A physical therapist assistant observes the standing posture of a patient from a lateral view. If the patient has normal postural alignment, which of the following anatomical reference points would be **MOST** appropriate for where the plumb line would fall?

1. Posterior to the lobe of the ear
2. Slightly anterior to the center of the hip joint
3. **Slightly anterior to a midline through the knee**
4. Slightly posterior to the lateral malleolus

Correct Answer: 3 (Kendall p. 60)

A plumb line refers to a cord with a plumb bob attached which creates a vertical line. When properly positioned, a physical therapist assistant can use the line to determine if selected anatomical reference points are consistent with corresponding points in standard posture.

1. Assuming normal posture, the plumb line should fall directly through the lobe of the ear (i.e., external auditory meatus).

2. Assuming normal posture, the plumb line should fall slightly posterior to the center of the hip joint.

3. **Assuming normal posture, the plumb line should fall anterior to a midline through the knee. This would be consistent with standard posture.**

4. Assuming normal posture, the plumb line should fall slightly anterior to the lateral malleolus.

System: Musculoskeletal System
Content Outline: Physical Therapy Data Collection

⦿ Level 2

⦿ Level 1   p. 75

➡ PTAEXAM ONE: QUESTION 71

A patient who has shoulder pain of unknown etiology is referred by their physician for magnetic resonance imaging. Results of the test reveal a partial tear of the infraspinatus muscle. Which muscle group would be the **MOST** affected by this finding?

1. **Shoulder lateral rotators**
2. Shoulder medial rotators
3. Shoulder abductors
4. Shoulder adductors

Correct Answer: 1 (Kendall p. 321)

The infraspinatus muscle originates on the medial two-thirds of the infraspinous fossa of the scapula and inserts on the greater tubercle of the humerus. The muscle is innervated by the supra-scapular nerve.

1. **The primary action of the infraspinatus is lateral rotation of the shoulder joint. The muscle also plays an important role in stabilizing the head of the humerus in the glenoid cavity. Other muscles that function as shoulder lateral rotators include the teres minor and posterior deltoid.**
2. The shoulder medial rotators include the subscapularis, teres major, pectoralis major, latissimus dorsi, and anterior deltoid muscles.
3. The shoulder abductors include the middle deltoid and su-praspinatus muscles.
4. The shoulder adductors include the pectoralis major, latissi-mus dorsi, and teres major muscles.

System: Musculoskeletal System
Content Outline: Diseases/Conditions that Impact Effective Treatment

➡ PTAEXAM ONE: QUESTION 72

A patient uses a fixed support strategy to control backward sway when in a standing position. Which muscle would **MOST** likely be activated first in this scenario?

1. **Tibialis anterior**
2. Gastrocnemius
3. Hamstrings
4. Paraspinals

Correct Answer: 1 (O'Sullivan p. 231)

A fixed support strategy refers to specific strategies employed to control the center of mass over a fixed base of support. The center of mass is the average position of all parts of the system, weighted according to their masses. The base of support refers to the area beneath the person that is inclusive of every point of contact between the person and the supporting surface.

1. **The tibialis anterior would be the first muscle activated with backward sway in standing, followed by the quadriceps, and then the abdominals. The ankle strategy relies on muscle activation in a distal to proximal sequence.**
2. The gastrocnemius would be the first muscle activated with forward sway (not backward sway).
3. The hamstrings would be more active with forward sway than backward sway. The typical activation sequence with forward sway would be the gastrocnemius, followed by the hamstrings, and then the paraspinals.
4. The paraspinals would be more active with forward sway than backward sway. The typical activation sequence with forward sway would be the gastrocnemius, followed by the hamstrings, and then the paraspinals.

System: Neuromuscular and Nervous Systems
Content Outline: Diseases/Conditions that Impact Effective Treatment

 Level 1   p. 53-55

 Level 1   p. 55, 65, 240-241

➡ PTAEXAM ONE: QUESTION 73

A patient completing a resistive exercise program following an ankle injury reports to the physical therapist assistant that lifting weights often causes them to void small amounts of urine. Which of the following actions is the **MOST** appropriate for the assistant to take?

1. Refer the patient to a support group

2. Instruct the patient in pelvic floor muscle strengthening exercises

3. Discontinue resistive exercises as part of the established plan of care

4. **Educate the patient about incontinence**

Correct Answer: 4 (Kisner p. 990)

Incontinence refers to an inability to control the release of urine, feces or gas and is a common occurrence for many men and women. The causes of incontinence may include weak pelvic floor muscles or medical conditions such as an enlarged prostate, prostatitis, cancer, neurological disorders or obstruction. Proper diagnosis is necessary in order to effectively treat this condition.

1. The use of a support group would be a potential adjunct activity for the patient, however, at this time, education is the appropriate action.

2. It would be inappropriate to begin pelvic floor exercises without a referral from a physician since the cause of the incontinence is unknown.

3. The physical therapist assistant should not discontinue resistive exercises since strengthening is often a necessary component of a rehabilitation program following an ankle injury. In addition, discontinuing the resistive exercises would be considered a change in the established plan of care and would not be considered an appropriate assistant action without more compelling information. This action also does not directly address the current issue of uncontrolled voiding of urine.

4. **The patient may significantly benefit from formal education about incontinence. The action would provide the patient with necessary information and make the patient more likely to see a physician about this issue. A vast majority of patients with incontinence can be successfully treated with non-invasive measures such as pelvic floor exercises.**

System: Other Systems
Content Outline: Interventions

➡ PTAEXAM ONE: QUESTION 74

A patient who has complete C7 tetraplegia presents with a problem list that includes inability to complete an independent bed to wheelchair transfer, decreased passive lower extremity range of motion, tissue breakdown over the ischial tuberosities, and decreased upper extremity strength. Which of the following treatment activities should be given the **HIGHEST** priority?

1. **Pressure relief activities**

2. Transfer training using a sliding board

3. Self-range of motion activities

4. Upper extremity strengthening exercises

Correct Answer: 1 (O'Sullivan p. 906)

The highest priority should be given to educating the patient on appropriate skin care including pressure relief activities. A patient with C7 tetraplegia can perform lateral and forward weight shifting in the wheelchair to assist with pressure relief.

1. **Education and instruction in pressure relief activities is the highest priority for a patient that has compromised sensation. The patient can perform independent relief through weight shifting each two-hour period to avoid further skin breakdown and infection.**

2. Transfer training using a sliding board will be a component of the treatment plan, but would not be the highest priority. Weight shifting is a precursor to performing a sliding board transfer.

3. Self-range of motion will be a component of the treatment plan. Patients must maintain an expected length in each muscle group in order to function at maximum potential. Pressure relief must be given the highest priority, however, so that the patient can progress through rehabilitation without skin breakdown.

4. Upper extremity strengthening will be a component of the treatment plan and focuses on maximizing strength in the available muscles. Although strengthening is desirable, failure to prevent tissue breakdown will place the patient at considerable risk for serious medical complications.

System: Neuromuscular and Nervous Systems
Content Outline: Interventions

 Level 3   p. 480-481

● Level 3   p. 268-271, 538-539

➡ PTAEXAM ONE: QUESTION 75

A physical therapist assistant assesses the strength of selected lower extremity muscles on a patient post knee injury. The test pictured in the image would be **MOST** effective to examine the strength of which of the following muscles of the hip?

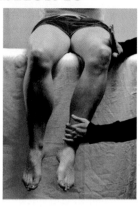

1. Abductors
2. Adductors
3. Medial rotators
4. **Lateral rotators**

Correct Answer: 4 (Kendall p. 430)

The hip lateral rotators include the gluteus maximus, obturator internus, obturator externus, piriformis, gemelli, and sartorius. Weakness of the lateral rotators usually results in medial rotation of the femur accompanied by pronation of the foot and a tendency toward a valgus position at the knee.

1. The strength of the hip abductors is assessed with the patient in sidelying with the test leg raised. The physical therapist assistant should apply pressure to the distal aspect of the femur, pushing the leg downward in an attempt to adduct the thigh. The hip abductors include the gluteus medius, gluteus minimus, piriformis, obturator internus, and tensor fasciae latae.

2. The strength of the hip adductors is assessed with the patient in sidelying with the test leg closest to the surface adducted. The physical therapist assistant should apply pressure to the distal aspect of the femur, pushing the leg downward in an attempt to abduct the thigh. The hip adductors include the adductor longus, adductor brevis, adductor magnus, and gracilis.

3. The strength of the hip medial rotators is assessed with the patient in sitting. The physical therapist assistant should apply pressure to the lateral side of the leg above the ankle, pushing the leg inward in an attempt to rotate the thigh laterally. The hip medial rotators include the pectineus, adductor longus, tensor fasciae latae, gluteus minimus, and gluteus medius.

4. **The strength of the hip lateral rotators is assessed with the patient in sitting. The physical therapist assistant should apply pressure to the medial side of the leg above the ankle, pushing the leg outward in an attempt to rotate the thigh medially.**

System: Musculoskeletal System
Content Outline: Physical Therapy Data Collection

➡ PTAEXAM ONE: QUESTION 76

A physical therapist assistant identifies the presence of epibole in a pressure injury. With which pressure injury stage is this observation **MOST** visible?

1. Stage 1
2. Stage 2
3. **Stage 3**
4. Unstageable

Correct Answer: 3 (Sussman p. 234)

Pressure injuries, also referred to as decubitus ulcers, result from sustained or prolonged pressure on tissue at levels greater than that of capillary pressure. Skin covering bony prominences is particularly susceptible to localized ischemia and tissue necrosis due to pressure. Factors contributing to pressure injuries include shearing forces, moisture, heat, friction, medications, muscle atrophy, malnutrition, and debilitating medical conditions. Epibole refers to skin that is rolled or curled under wound edges and may be dry, callused or hyperkeratotic.

1. A stage 1 pressure injury is characterized by intact skin with a localized area of non-blanchable erythema. Epibole is associated with full-thickness skin loss and therefore would not be present in a stage 1 pressure injury.

2. A stage 2 pressure injury is characterized by partial-thickness skin loss with exposed dermis. Epibole is associated with full-thickness skin loss and therefore would not be present in a stage 2 pressure injury.

3. **A stage 3 pressure injury is characterized by full-thickness skin loss in which adipose tissue is visible in the ulcer. The depth of tissue change varies by anatomical location and may include undermining and tunneling. Granulation tissue and epibole are often also present in a stage 3 pressure injury.**

4. An unstageable pressure injury is characterized by full-thickness skin and tissue loss in which the extent of tissue damage within the pressure injury cannot be determined because it is obscured by slough or eschar. Although epibole may be present in an unstageable pressure injury, the presentation is highly variable making this finding less obvious (i.e., visible) than with a stage 3 pressure injury.

System: Other Systems
Content Outline: Diseases/Conditions that Impact Effective Treatment

● Level 1   👓 p. 78-79

● Level 1   👓 p. 442, 444, 538-539

➡ PTAEXAM ONE: QUESTION 77

During a treatment session, a patient makes a culturally insensitive remark that the physical therapist assistant feels is offensive. Which of the following actions is the **MOST** appropriate for the assistant to take?

1. Document the incident in the medical record
2. Transfer the patient to another therapist's schedule
3. Recommend discharging the patient from physical therapy
4. **Inform the patient that the remark was offensive and continue with treatment**

Correct Answer: 4 (O'Sullivan p. 34)

A physical therapist assistant must make a patient aware of behavior that is unacceptable. Failure to address the issue directly with the patient may serve to reinforce the behavior.

1. Documentation would be more appropriate in instances such as a patient's refusal of physical therapy services, a fall or injury, or to provide a status update for various members of the health care team.

2. The patient should not be transferred to another therapist's schedule due to a culturally insensitive remark. A physical therapist assistant must be able to provide direct feedback to patients regarding their status, progress, and behaviors when necessary.

3. Discharge from physical therapy should only occur when all attainable goals are met or when a patient makes a decision to cease physical therapy services. It would be inappropriate for a physical therapist assistant to recommend discharging a patient from physical therapy for making a culturally insensitive remark, particularly since there is no indication that a similar incident has occurred previously.

4. **The physical therapist assistant should provide immediate feedback to the patient when an inappropriate behavior is witnessed. A culturally insensitive remark would not warrant the interruption or cessation of the existing plan of care.**

System: Non-Systems
Content Outline: Safety and Protection; Professional
    Responsibilities; Research

Level 3

➡ PTAEXAM ONE: QUESTION 78

A physical therapist assistant treats a patient post right CVA who exhibits "pusher syndrome." When observing the patient's posture in the sitting position, which of the following findings should the assistant **MOST** likely expect to detect?

1. **Increased lean to the left along with increased weight bearing through the left buttocks**
2. Increased lean to the right along with increased weight bearing through the right buttocks
3. Increased weight bearing through the right buttocks and the head rotated to the right; unresponsive to stimuli on the left
4. Unequal weight bearing and the head rotated to the left; unresponsive to stimuli on the right

Correct Answer: 1 (O'Sullivan p. 695)

Pusher syndrome is characterized by a significant lateral deviation toward the hemiplegic side. Pusher syndrome most commonly occurs in patients that have sustained a right CVA. Therapeutic intervention for a patient that exhibits pusher syndrome may include the use of a mirror, a small wedge placed under the left lateral thigh, weight shifting across midline, and facilitation techniques for trunk control.

1. **A patient with right CVA (left hemiplegia) with pusher syndrome would typically exhibit a lateral lean to the left in sitting with increased weight bearing on the left buttocks.**

2. A patient with right CVA (left hemiplegia) without pusher syndrome would typically exhibit less weight bearing through the left side due to the existing sensory and motor deficits. Intervention would include midline orientation and weight shifting in sitting.

3. A patient with right CVA (left hemiplegia) who demonstrates the inability to interpret stimuli on the left side of the body is exhibiting unilateral neglect. Neglect is most often associated with a lesion of the right frontal lobe of the brain.

4. A patient with right CVA (left hemiplegia) would not typically rotate the head towards the affected (left) side, but rather away from it secondary to neglect. The patient would be more responsive to stimuli on the right.

System: Neuromuscular and Nervous Systems
Content Outline: Diseases/Conditions that Impact Effective
    Treatment

Level 2

➡ PTAEXAM ONE: QUESTION 79

A two-year-old who has T10 spina bifida receives physical therapy for gait training. Which of the following assistive devices should the physical therapist assistant use to teach a child how to maintain standing in the **INITIAL** stages of gait training?

1. Bilateral hip-knee-ankle-foot orthoses (HKAFO) and forearm crutches
2. **Parapodium and the parallel bars**
3. Bilateral knee-ankle-foot orthoses (KAFO) and the parallel bars
4. Bilateral ankle-foot orthoses (AFO) and the parallel bars

Correct Answer: 2 (O'Sullivan p. 1339)

The parapodium provides the necessary amount of support and is optimal to assist with standing activities for children with thoracic and high level lumbar lesions. The parallel bars are the most stable assistive device to initiate standing and gait training.

1. HKAFOs would require a swing-through or reciprocal gait pattern. Using HKAFOs with forearm (Lofstrand) crutches requires a high level of balance and energy expenditure and is not appropriate for initial standing activities.
2. **The parapodium is a HKAFO with a thoracolumbar orthosis that supports the trunk and lower extremities. It has a large base of support and is used with or without an assistive device. This would be ideal for a patient with T10 spina bifida to initiate standing within the parallel bars.**
3. A patient with T10 spina bifida would not initially use KAFOs in the parallel bars when working on standing activities due to the deficits in strength and sensation below the T10 level.
4. A patient with T10 spina bifida would not possess the necessary motor function to use bilateral AFOs.

System: Neuromuscular and Nervous Systems
Content Outline: Interventions

➡ PTAEXAM ONE: QUESTION 80

A physical therapist assistant notices a small area of skin irritation under the chin of a patient wearing a rigid cervical orthosis. The patient reports that the area is not painful, but it is becoming increasingly itchy. Which of the following actions is the **MOST** appropriate for the assistant to take?

1. Instruct the patient to apply 1% hydrocortisone cream to the area twice daily
2. Apply powder to the area and instruct the patient to avoid scratching
3. **Provide the patient with a liner to use as a barrier between the skin and the orthosis**
4. Discontinue use of the orthosis until the skin has become less irritated

Correct Answer: 3 (Seymour p. 393)

Patients can experience itching or skin irritation when using a cervical orthosis. Since an orthosis is applied directly over the skin, it is imperative to utilize a liner that maximizes comfort, promotes cleanliness, limits moisture, and reduces skin irritation. Failure to select an appropriate liner may result in skin breakdown.

1. Hydrocortisone may be used to treat an existing area of irritation, however, it does not address the primary cause of irritation.
2. Powder may assist to temporarily reduce friction over a particular area, but it does not address the primary cause of irritation.
3. **Liners made from lambs' wool are commonly utilized and prevent chafing and irritation of the patient's skin. This liner is easily donned and provides an adequate barrier between the skin and orthosis.**
4. Discontinuing the use of the cervical orthosis would be undesirable since it is prescribed based on medical necessity.

System: Non-Systems
Content Outline: Equipment, Devices, and Technologies; Therapeutic Modalities

 Level 2   p. 124-125

 Level 3

➡ PTA EXAM ONE: QUESTION 81

A patient who has a spinal cord injury develops a respiratory infection. Which of the following diagnoses would make the patient the **MOST** susceptible to respiratory problems?

1. **Complete C4 tetraplegia**
2. Cauda equina lesion
3. Brown-Sequard's syndrome
4. Posterior cord syndrome

Correct Answer: 1 (Umphred p. 481)

A patient with complete C4 tetraplegia will present with a loss of motor and sensory function secondary to damage to the spinal cord. Since the primary muscle of respiration, the diaphragm, is impaired the patient will be unable to voluntarily or effectively ventilate.

1. **A patient with complete C4 tetraplegia will have a reduced ventilatory capacity due to muscle paralysis. The patient will exhibit limited ability to clear secretions, impaired chest mobility, and alveolar hypoventilation.**

2. A cauda equina lesion is an injury that occurs below the L1 spinal level where the long nerve roots transcend. Cauda equina injuries are frequently incomplete due to the large number of nerve roots in the area and as a result are often considered to be peripheral nerve injuries. Characteristics include flaccidity, areflexia, and impairment of bowel and bladder function.

3. Brown-Sequard's syndrome is an incomplete lesion usually caused by a stab wound, which produces hemisection of the spinal cord. There is paralysis and loss of vibratory and position sense on the same side as the lesion due to the damage to the corticospinal tract and dorsal columns. There is a loss of pain and temperature sense on the opposite side of the lesion from damage to the lateral spinothalamic tract.

4. Posterior cord syndrome is an extremely rare condition that presents with a loss of proprioception, two-point discrimination, graphesthesia, and stereognosis below the level of the lesion. Patients typically present with a wide based steppage gait.

System: Neuromuscular and Nervous Systems
Content Outline: Diseases/Conditions that Impact Effective
  Treatment

➡ PTA EXAM ONE: QUESTION 82

A patient with a spinal cord injury exercising on a treatment table in the supine position begins to experience signs and symptoms of autonomic dysreflexia, including a dramatic increase in blood pressure. Which of the following actions should be the **MOST** immediate to address the patient's blood pressure response?

1. Elevate the patient's legs
2. Call for assistance
3. **Sit the patient upright**
4. Check the urinary drainage system

Correct Answer: 3 (Fairchild p. 338)

Autonomic dysreflexia is caused by a noxious stimulus below the level of the lesion that triggers the autonomic nervous system causing a sudden elevation in blood pressure. If untreated, this condition can lead to convulsions, hemorrhage, and death.

1. Elevation of the patient's legs would be contraindicated since the position would serve to increase the return of circulation and further increase blood pressure.

2. Calling for assistance is an acceptable option given the seriousness of autonomic dysreflexia, however, the action would not be the most immediate action to address the patient's blood pressure response.

3. **The physical therapist assistant should immediately position the patient in sitting to address the autonomic nervous system response and reduce the patient's elevated blood pressure. After the patient has been positioned in sitting, the urinary drainage system should be checked since a blocked catheter is a common noxious stimulus that triggers the sympathetic response.**

4. The common causes of autonomic dysreflexia include distended or full bladder, kink or blockage in the catheter, bladder infections, pressure ulcers, extreme temperature changes, tight clothing or an ingrown toenail. A physical therapist assistant should check the urinary drainage system immediately after moving the patient into a sitting position.

System: Neuromuscular and Nervous Systems
Content Outline: Interventions

 Level 2   p. 266-267

 Level 3   p. 44, 268, 676

➡ PTAEXAM ONE: QUESTION 83

A patient is currently one week post transtibial amputation and has a post-operative rigid dressing. Which of the following goals is **NOT** a benefit of the rigid dressing?

1. Limits the development of post-operative edema in the residual limb

2. Allows for earlier ambulation with the attachment of a pylon and foot

3. Allows for earlier fitting of a definitive prosthesis

4. **Allows for daily wound inspection and dressing changes**

Correct Answer: 4 (Seymour p. 126)

A rigid dressing, usually made from plaster of Paris or fiberglass, does not allow for wound inspection or dressing changes. The rigid dressing is applied in the operating room and remains on the residual limb approximately 7-14 days until the sutures are removed and proper shaping occurs.

1. The rigid dressing limits the development of post-operative edema by maintaining total contact with the surface of the residual limb.

2. The rigid dressing allows for earlier ambulation since the rigid construction of the cast allows for pylon attachment and weight bearing.

3. The rigid dressing allows for earlier fitting of a definitive prosthesis since healing occurs more rapidly. The limb also receives better protection and is less likely to develop a flexion contracture since the rigid dressing limits knee motion.

4. **A rigid dressing does not allow for wound inspection and dressing changes since the rigid dressing remains on the residual limb for an extended period of time. An elastic bandage or a shrinker would be examples of soft dressings that allow for frequent wound inspection and dressing changes.**

System: Other Systems
Content Outline: Diseases/Conditions that Impact Effective Treatment

➡ PTAEXAM ONE: QUESTION 84

A physical therapist assistant uses functional electrical stimulation as part of a treatment regimen designed to improve quadriceps strength. Which of the following ratios for on:off time would result in the **MOST** rapid onset of muscle fatigue?

1. 3:1

2. 1:4

3. **5:1**

4. 1:6

Correct Answer: 3 (Prentice p. 130)

The on:off time ratio is simply a method to show the relative duration of the on time versus the off time. The muscle contracts during the on time and relaxes during the off time. The greater the on time in relation to the off time, the more rapid the onset of muscle fatigue.

1. An on:off time ratio of 3:1 indicates that there is three seconds of on time for every one second of off time. This ratio would promote fatigue, however, it is not the best answer.

2. An on:off time ratio of 1:4 indicates that there is one second of on time for every four seconds of off time. This ratio has significantly greater rest periods and therefore fatigue would not tend to be a large factor.

3. **An on:off time ratio of 5:1 indicates that there is five seconds of on time for every one second of off time. This ratio would promote rapid fatigue given the extremely large on time in relation to the short off time.**

4. An on:off time ratio of 1:6 indicates that there is one second of on time for every six seconds of off time. This ratio has the greatest rest period and therefore fatigue would not tend to be a factor.

System: Non-Systems
Content Outline: Equipment, Devices, and Technologies; Therapeutic Modalities

⊕ **Test Taking Tip:** Candidates must be extremely careful to answer examination questions in a precise manner. In this particular question, candidates need to identify the on:off time ratio that would result in the most rapid onset of fatigue. The best answer would have the greatest amount of on time in relation to the amount of off time. The correct option must be expressed in the same manner that the ratio is presented, meaning that the on time represents the first number and the off time represents the second number. By reversing these numbers a candidate could possess the requisite academic knowledge to answer the question, but still fail to answer the question correctly.

▶ PTAEXAM ONE: QUESTION 85

A patient post radial head fracture has developed an elbow flexion contracture. Which of the following interventions is considered a passive exercise technique to increase range of motion?

1. Contract-relax
2. Hold-relax
3. **Maintained pressure**
4. Rhythmic stabilization

Correct Answer: 3 (Sullivan p. 64)

Maintained pressure is an effective passive technique that can be used to increase range of motion by facilitating local muscle relaxation.

1. Contract-relax is a technique used to increase range of motion. As the extremity reaches the point of limitation, the patient performs a maximal contraction of the antagonistic muscle group. The therapist resists movement for eight to ten seconds with relaxation to follow. The technique should be repeated until no further gains in range of motion are noted.

2. Hold-relax is an isometric contraction used to increase range of motion. The contraction is facilitated at the limiting point in the range of motion. Relaxation occurs and the extremity moves through the newly acquired range to the next point of limitation until no further increases in range of motion occur.

3. **Maintained pressure over the belly or tendon of a muscle can produce a calming effect and create relaxation of the musculotendinous unit. The effects of pressure are immediate, with little evidence of long-term effects.**

4. Rhythmic stabilization is a technique used to increase range of motion and coordinate isometric contractions. The technique requires isometric contractions of all muscles around a joint against progressive resistance. The patient should relax and move into the newly acquired range and repeat the technique.

System: Neuromuscular and Nervous Systems
Content Outline: Interventions

▶ PTAEXAM ONE: QUESTION 86

A physician instructs a patient to utilize a knee derotation brace for all athletic activities. Which of the following conditions would **MOST** warrant the use of this type of brace?

1. Medial meniscus repair
2. Anterior cruciate ligament reconstruction
3. **Anterior cruciate ligament insufficiency**
4. Posterior cruciate ligament reconstruction

Correct Answer: 3 (Kisner p. 809)

Derotation braces are most effective in patients with ligamentous instability, usually involving the anterior and posterior cruciate ligaments. The literature is inconclusive on the efficacy of functional bracing following reconstruction.

1. A patient with a medial meniscus repair would not tend to experience functional instability unless there were other structures involved such as the anterior cruciate ligament. Meniscal repairs are most often performed when the lesion is in the vascular outer third of the medial or lateral meniscus.

2. Anterior cruciate ligament reconstruction is typically performed due to disabling instability or frequent episodes of the knee giving way. The purpose of the surgical procedure is to reduce functional instability. Full return to vigorous activities following ACL reconstruction often takes four to six months.

3. **A patient with anterior cruciate ligament insufficiency would be far more likely to experience functional instability than a patient who had anterior cruciate ligament reconstruction. As a result, the patient with the insufficiency would be a better candidate for the derotation brace.**

4. Posterior cruciate ligament reconstruction is considerably less common than anterior cruciate ligament reconstruction. The purpose of the surgical procedure is to reduce functional instability. Full return to vigorous activities following PCL reconstruction often takes nine months to one year.

System: Non-Systems
Content Outline: Equipment, Devices, and Technologies;
   Therapeutic Modalities

 Level 2   p. 264

 Level 2   p. 112-113, 146-147

➡ PTAEXAM ONE: QUESTION 87

A patient is treated using pulsed wave ultrasound at 1.2 W/cm^2 for 7 minutes. The specific parameters of the pulsed wave are 2 msec on time and 8 msec off time for one pulse period. What duty cycle should the physical therapist assistant document?

1. 10%
2. 20%
3. 25%
4. 50%

Correct Answer: 2 (Cameron p. 185)

Duty cycle is defined as the ratio of the on time to the total time. When ultrasound is used in a pulsed mode with a 20% or lower duty cycle, the heat produced during the on time of the cycle is dispersed during the off time and as a result, there is no measurable net increase in temperature. Ultrasound using a 20% or lower duty cycle would typically be used for nonthermal effects.

1. A 10% duty cycle would result if the parameters of the pulsed wave were 1 msec on time and 9 msec off time. Duty cycle = 1 msec / (1 msec + 9 msec) = .10 (100) = 10%.

2. **The question indicates that the parameters of the pulsed wave are 2 msec on time and 8 msec off time for one pulse period. As a result, duty cycle = 2 msec / (2 msec + 8 msec) = .20 (100) = 20%.**

3. This option may have been a common response for candidates who incorrectly answered the question since it is intuitive to take the on time and divide it by the off time. This calculation would be as follows: 2 msec / 8 msec = .25 (100) = 25%. Although the math is correct, the option remains incorrect since by definition duty cycle is defined as the ratio of the on time to the total time (not only the off time).

4. A 50% duty cycle would result any time the on time was the same as the off time (e.g., if the parameters of the pulsed wave were 2 msec on time and 2 msec off time). In this scenario, duty cycle equals 2 msec / (2 msec + 2 msec) = .50 (100) = 50%.

System: Non-Systems
Content Outline: Equipment, Devices, and Technologies; Therapeutic Modalities

➡ PTAEXAM ONE: QUESTION 88

A patient with Alzheimer's disease is referred to physical therapy for instruction in an exercise program. Which of the following steps should the physical therapist assistant perform **FIRST**?

1. Provide verbal and written instructions
2. Frequently repeat multiple step directions
3. Assess the patient's cognitive status
4. Avoid using medical terminology

Correct Answer: 3 (O'Sullivan p. 165)

Physical therapist assistants should attempt to provide exercise instructions that are consistent with the abilities and limitations of the target audience. This is particularly important with Alzheimer's disease since cognitive status can vary greatly from patient to patient.

1. Providing verbal and written instructions is an effective method to improve patient understanding and can be particularly important in the case of a home exercise program. The breadth and depth of the instructions would be heavily influenced by the patient's cognitive status.

2. Repetition is an effective technique to enhance learning and memory. The appropriate amount of repetition will be dictated in part by the patient's cognitive status.

3. **It is essential for the physical therapist assistant to determine the patient's cognitive status prior to providing formal exercise instruction. The patient's cognitive status will have a significant impact on a variety of factors including the ability to interpret instructions, the ability to perform exercises correctly, and the ability to recall elements of the exercise program.**

4. Physical therapist assistants should avoid using medical terminology whenever possible. Although this is good advice, it would not be as important as assessing the patient's cognitive status.

System: Neuromuscular and Nervous Systems
Content Outline: Interventions

➡ PTAEXAM ONE: QUESTION 89

A physical therapist assistant instructs a patient to close their eyes and hold out one hand. The assistant places a series of different weights in the patient's hand one at a time. The patient is then asked to identify the comparative weight of the objects. What sensory test has the assistant performed?

1. **Barognosis**
2. Graphesthesia
3. Recognition of texture
4. Stereognosis

Correct Answer: 1 (O'Sullivan p. 111)

Barognosis, graphesthesia, recognition of texture, and stereognosis are considered combined cortical sensations.

1. **Barognosis refers to the ability of a patient to identify the comparative weight of objects in a series. This can be done by placing a series of different weights in the same hand or by placing different weights in each hand simultaneously.**

2. Graphesthesia refers to the ability of a patient to verbally identify letters or numbers traced on the palm of the hand typically with a fingertip or the eraser of a pencil.

3. Recognition of texture refers to the ability to differentiate among various textures such as cotton, wool or silk. Items may be identified by name or texture such as rough or smooth.

4. Stereognosis refers to the ability to identify an object without sight. Objects used are typically easily obtainable and familiar objects such as a coin, key or comb. Patients are asked to verbally identify the object by name.

System: Neuromuscular and Nervous Systems
Content Outline: Physical Therapy Data Collection

➡ PTAEXAM ONE: QUESTION 90

A physical therapist assistant instructs a patient with a low back injury in a series of five pelvic stabilization exercises. The patient indicates that they understand the exercises, however, frequently becomes confused and is unable to perform them correctly. Which of the following actions is the **MOST** appropriate for the assistant to take?

1. Repeat the exercise instructions
2. **Reduce the number of exercises in the series**
3. Select a different treatment option
4. Conclude the patient is not a candidate for physical therapy

Correct Answer: 2 (Kisner p. 27)

A physical therapist assistant should attempt to simplify the exercise session in order to reduce the patient's confusion.

1. Repeating the exercise instructions can be valuable, however, given that the patient "frequently becomes confused" this action is unlikely to resolve the patient's problem.

2. **Reducing the number of exercises in the series serves to simplify the program. Five pelvic stabilization exercises is a significant number for the patient to learn and as a result it is reasonable to hypothesize that the number of exercises may be the primary reason for the patient's difficulty.**

3. There is not enough evidence available to suggest that the patient is unable to learn the exercises or that the exercises, if performed appropriately, are not of value. As a result, selecting a different treatment option is not justified.

4. A therapist should attempt to alter the learning environment or the method of providing patient instruction prior to concluding that a patient is not a candidate for physical therapy.

System: Non-Systems
Content Outline: Safety and Protection; Professional Responsibilities; Research

▶ PTAEXAM ONE: QUESTION 91

A physical therapist assistant works with a four-month-old infant. During mat activities the infant suddenly becomes unconscious. Which of the following arteries is the **MOST** appropriate for the assistant to palpate to assess the infant's pulse?

1. Radial

2. **Brachial**

3. Popliteal

4. Carotid

Correct Answer: 2 (Fairchild p. 53)

An infant's pulse is often palpated at the brachial artery, while the femoral artery can be used as an alternate site.

1. The radial and carotid arteries are the most commonly assessed arteries in the adult patient due to the relative ease of access. The radial artery is located at the wrist on the volar surface, medial to the styloid process of the radius, however, it is not easily palpated in an infant.

2. **The brachial artery is the most appropriate artery to assess on the infant. The artery can be easily palpated on the medial aspect of the midshaft of the humerus and therefore provides the physical therapist assistant with a timely and accurate method to assess the patient's pulse.**

3. The popliteal artery is the continuation of the femoral artery in the popliteal space, bifurcating into the anterior and posterior tibial arteries. The artery is often difficult to palpate and would, therefore, not be the best choice with an infant.

4. The carotid artery lies inferior to the angle of the mandible and anterior to the sternocleidomastoid muscle. The infant's typical stature, small and chubby neck, make locating the carotid artery difficult especially in an emergent situation.

System: Cardiovascular and Pulmonary Systems
Content Outline: Interventions

▶ PTAEXAM ONE: QUESTION 92

A physical therapist assistant performs ice massage on a patient who has infrapatellar tendonitis. The **MOST** appropriate treatment time for this procedure is typically how many minutes?

1. 3-5

2. **5-10**

3. 10-15

4. 15-20

Correct Answer: 2 (Cameron p. 138)

Ice massage is typically performed by freezing water in paper cups and applying the ice directly to the treatment area. Ice massage tends to create a more intense cooling since the ice is applied directly to a localized target area.

1. Sufficient cooling with ice massage would not occur with a 3-5 minute treatment time.

2. **Ice massage requires a treatment time of 5-10 minutes due to the intensity of the cooling.**

3. A treatment time of 10-15 minutes would be excessive with ice massage and could result in signs and symptoms of cold intolerance.

4. A treatment time of 15-20 minutes would be within the established range for an ice pack, but would not be acceptable for ice massage.

System: Non-Systems
Content Outline: Equipment, Devices, and Technologies; Therapeutic Modalities

 Level 1   p. 381-382

Level 1   p. 615-616

 SCOREBUILDERS

➡ PTAEXAM ONE: QUESTION 93

A physical therapist assistant observes a patient's gait and identifies a lack of toe off. Which finding in the patient's medical history would be **MOST** likely to contribute to this observation?

1. Vertigo

2. Lymphedema

3. **Type 2 diabetes mellitus**

4. Raynaud's phenomenon

Correct Answer: 3 (O'Sullivan p. 592)

A physical therapist assistant must consider a patient's entire medical history as a relevant factor when assessing any identified gait impairment. According to traditional gait terminology, toe off is the point in which only the toe of the stance limb remains on the ground.

1. Vertigo is used to describe a sense of movement and rotation of oneself or the surrounding environment. It typically is a sensation of spinning, but can also present as linear motion or falling. Vertigo may have a peripheral or central origin. While an acute episode of vertigo can contribute to gait deviations, a history of this condition is not likely to have an impact specifically on toe off given the episodic nature of this condition.

2. Lymphedema is a chronic, incurable condition that is characterized by an accumulation of protein-rich fluid (i.e., lymph) in the body. The result is edema that typically presents in the extremities, but can occur anywhere in the body including the face, neck, abdomen, genitalia, and trunk. While lymphedema may contribute to gait deviations by affecting the extremities, it is not likely to specifically impact toe off.

3. **Type 2 diabetes mellitus is a chronic metabolic disease characterized by an inappropriate cellular response to insulin. Patients with diabetes commonly develop neuropathy which can affect gait mechanics, particularly in the distal lower extremities. Additionally, diminished sensation can lead to wounds on the feet that go undetected by the individual. Gait deviations in an individual with a history of type 2 diabetes should prompt the assistant to examine skin integrity and sensation of the feet, as well as motor control, to determine any potential diabetic influence.**

4. Raynaud's phenomenon is characterized by changes in temperature and pallor in the digits when changes in environmental temperature are experienced. While this condition may impair the patient's gait during a significant exacerbation, gait deviations are not commonly associated with this condition.

System: Other Systems
Content Outline: Diseases/Conditions that Impact Effective Treatment

 Level 3   p. 81, 248, 466-467, 528-529

➡ PTAEXAM ONE: QUESTION 94

A physical therapist assistant works with a patient post total knee arthroplasty who presents with increased knee flexion during the stance phase of gait. Which of the following interventions would **BEST** address this gait deviation?

1. **Isometric quadriceps setting exercises in supine with the leg positioned in extension and the heel on a towel roll**

2. Isometric quadriceps setting exercises in supine with a pillow under the knee

3. Active knee flexion exercises in sitting

4. Isometric gluteal setting exercises performed in supine

Correct Answer: 1 (Kisner p. 785)

A total knee arthroplasty is a procedure performed for patients with progressive and disabling pain in the knee joint, such as severe osteoarthritis. Regaining normal joint range of motion is important following a total knee arthroplasty in order to normalize the gait pattern.

1. **Following a total knee arthroplasty the quadriceps muscles can be inhibited by pain, joint edema, and muscle weakness. Quadriceps inhibition can contribute to increased knee flexion during the stance phase of gait. Quadriceps strengthening is an important aspect of the physical therapy plan of care following total knee arthroplasty. This option promotes improved knee extension range of motion through passive extension, strengthens the knee extensors, and improves knee extension during gait.**

2. Placing a pillow under the knee following a total knee arthroplasty should be avoided. This position shortens the knee flexors and inhibits achievement of full range of motion into knee extension.

3. Active knee flexion exercises in sitting are indicated to improve knee flexion strength and range of motion, however, it will not address the quadriceps strengthening and knee extension range of motion that is needed to improve the patient's gait.

4. Isometric gluteal setting exercises strengthen the hip extensor musculature and may be indicated for this patient, however, they will not directly influence the amount of knee flexion present during the stance phase of gait.

System: Musculoskeletal System
Content Outline: Interventions

 Level 2   p. 118-119, 170-171

➡ PTA EXAM ONE: QUESTION 95

A patient with a compensated rearfoot varus deformity prepares to utilize a set of rigid orthoses. Which recommendation would be the **MOST** appropriate when wearing the orthoses the first day?

1. No break-in period is necessary

2. **Wear the orthoses for 1-2 hours**

3. Wear the orthoses for 2-4 hours

4. Wear the orthoses for 6-8 hours

Correct Answer: 2 (Higgins p. 342)

Rigid orthoses are used in individuals requiring a great deal of mechanical control. Semirigid orthoses offer less control, however, they are more durable for patients involved in high impact activities.

1. Rigid and semirigid orthoses both require a break-in period. Failure to utilize an appropriate break-in period may cause significant discomfort and can potentially lead to more severe complications such as tissue breakdown.

2. **Wearing the orthoses 1-2 hours initially would be an appropriate wearing schedule for rigid orthoses. The break-in period for rigid orthoses can be as brief as two weeks or as long as six weeks.**

3. Wearing the orthoses 2-4 hours initially would be a more appropriate wearing schedule for semirigid or temporary orthoses (e.g., Spenco).

4. Wearing the orthoses 6-8 hours initially would potentially be excessive for any type of orthosis. Individuals should be able to comfortably wear orthoses for a full day before attempting to use the orthoses during higher level functional activities such as running.

System: Musculoskeletal System
Content Outline: Interventions

➡ PTA EXAM ONE: QUESTION 96

A physical therapist assistant observes a patient complete a standing arm curl with a dumbbell using the starting and ending positions as shown in the image. Which of the following scenarios would produce the **MOST** power?

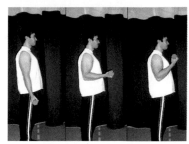

1. Lifting a two pound dumbbell in two seconds

2. Lifting a two pound dumbbell in three seconds

3. **Lifting a four pound dumbbell in one second**

4. Lifting a four pound dumbbell in four seconds

Correct Answer: 3 (Coburn p. 52)

Power is calculated as the amount of work divided by the time needed to perform the work. Work is defined as the product of force and distance. Each of the presented options involve the same amount of distance, therefore the relevant variables to consider are the weight of the dumbbell and the time to complete the repetition.

1. A 2 pound dumbbell lifted in two seconds would produce more power than the same weight lifted over a longer period of time, however, it would not be as great as a heavier weight (i.e., 4 pounds) lifted over a shorter period of time (i.e., one second).

2. A 2 pound dumbbell lifted in three seconds would produce the smallest amount of power of the presented options since the weight is relatively light (i.e., 2 pounds) and the amount of time to complete the repetition is relatively long (i.e., three seconds).

3. **A 4 pound dumbbell lifted in one second would produce the greatest amount of power since the weight lifted is the heaviest of the presented options and the amount of time to complete the repetition (i.e., one second) is the shortest.**

4. A 4 pound dumbbell lifted in four seconds would produce less power than the same amount of weight lifted over a shorter period of time.

System: Musculoskeletal System
Content Outline: Interventions

⦿ Level 2

⦿ Level 1   👓   p. 109-110

⬤ PTAEXAM ONE: QUESTION 97

A physical therapist assistant works with a patient who sustained a lesion to the long thoracic nerve. Which of the following objective findings should the assistant **MOST** expect as a result of this injury?

1. Decreased sensation on the lateral forearm
2. Atrophy of the deltoid muscle
3. **Inability to elevate the arm overhead**
4. Fair strength with shoulder extension

Correct Answer: 3 (Dutton p. 75)

The long thoracic nerve is a motor nerve that originates from the C5-C7 nerve roots and innervates the serratus anterior muscle. Due to the nerve's long and superficial course, it is susceptible to injury through entrapment, compression or traction.

1. The long thoracic nerve is purely a motor nerve, therefore, a lesion to this nerve would not result in sensory disturbances. Decreased sensation on the lateral forearm is commonly found with an injury to the musculocutaneous nerve (C5-C6).

2. The deltoid muscle is innervated by the axillary nerve (C5-C6). Atrophy may result when an injury to the axillary nerve occurs.

3. **Injury to the long thoracic nerve results in weakness of the serratus anterior muscle. The serratus anterior works in combination with the trapezius muscle to upwardly rotate the scapula during elevation of the arm. Weakness of the serratus anterior muscle would make it difficult for a patient to elevate their arm overhead.**

4. The serratus anterior does not contribute to the movement of shoulder extension. Weakness in shoulder extension would likely be the result of a thoracodorsal nerve lesion since the latissimus dorsi is the primary shoulder extensor.

System: Neuromuscular and Nervous Systems
Content Outline: Diseases/Conditions that Impact Effective Treatment

⬤ PTAEXAM ONE: QUESTION 98

A physical therapist assistant suspects that a patient's chronic lower extremity swelling is due to lymphedema. Which of the following symptoms is the **MOST** consistent with the later stages of this condition?

1. Swelling that is relieved by elevation
2. Swelling proximal to the site of lymph dysfunction
3. **Fibrotic changes of the dermis**
4. Pitting edema

Correct Answer: 3 (O'Sullivan p. 588)

Lymphedema is a chronic condition characterized by an abnormal accumulation of lymph fluid caused by a mechanical insufficiency of the lymphatic system. Primary lymphedema is caused by a congenital or hereditary condition in which lymph node formation is abnormal. Secondary lymphedema is caused by injury to the lymphatic system (e.g., blockage, dissection, fibrosis).

1. In the early stages of the condition, swelling may be relieved by elevation of the lower extremities. In the later stages, swelling becomes irreversible and is no longer relieved with elevation.

2. Regardless of the stage, lymphedema is characterized by swelling adjacent and distal to the site of lymph dysfunction.

3. **In the later stages of the condition, fibrotic changes occur within the dermal layer of the skin. Fibrosis results in hardening of the limbs which eventually leads to increasing size of the limbs.**

4. Pitting edema is common in the early stages of the condition. However, as fibrotic changes occur in the later stages, the pitting edema evolves into non-pitting edema.

System: Cardiovascular and Pulmonary Systems
Content Outline: Diseases/Conditions that Impact Effective Treatment

---

⬤ Level 2

⬤ Level 2   👓   p. 486-487

➡ PTAEXAM ONE: QUESTION 99

A physical therapist assistant notes that a newborn has extremely limited dorsiflexion. Which positional foot deformity would be the **MOST** likely with this range of motion limitation?

1. Calcaneovalgus
2. Metatarsus adductus
3. Syndactyly
4. **Talipes equinovarus**

Correct Answer: 4 (Sarwark p. 1025)

Positional deformities are abnormalities that are mechanically produced by the fetal environment. The deformities are most often caused by restrictions in fetal movement or fetal compression. Early identification of the deformities is critical to minimize the impact of the deformities on the developing newborn.

1. Calcaneovalgus is a foot deformity characterized by the forefoot being curved out laterally, the hindfoot positioned in valgus, and full or even excessive dorsiflexion range of motion. Calcaneovalgus is an extremely common positional deformity in newborns most often caused by intrauterine positioning.

2. Metatarsus adductus is a foot deformity characterized by a medially curved forefoot while the hindfoot remains in normal alignment. The condition is believed to be caused by intrauterine positioning. The presence of metatarsus adductus would not impact a patient's dorsiflexion range of motion.

3. Syndactyly refers to the presence of webbed toes or fingers. The genetic condition is most commonly observed between the second and third toes. The presence of syndactyly would not impact a patient's dorsiflexion range of motion.

4. **Talipes equinovarus, also known as "clubfoot," is a deformity characterized by adduction of the forefoot, varus positioning of the hindfoot, and plantar flexion at the ankle. The positioning associated with talipes equinovarus would likely result in a limitation in dorsiflexion range of motion. Medical management for the condition begins shortly after birth and includes splinting and serial casting with the goal of restoring proper positioning of the foot and ankle.**

System: Musculoskeletal System
Content Outline: Diseases/Conditions that Impact Effective Treatment

➡ PTAEXAM ONE: QUESTION 100

An older adult patient has difficulty communicating in physical therapy due to presbycusis. What intervention is the **MOST** appropriate to improve communication with the patient?

1. Speak with a louder voice
2. Speak in a higher tone
3. Speak with a lower voice
4. **Speak in a lower tone**

Correct Answer: 4 (Kaufman p. 392)

Presbycusis is the normal loss of auditory acuity that occurs in older age. The lower frequencies are preserved to a greater extent than the higher frequencies. A hearing aid may be used to improve the receptive abilities of the older adult.

1. Speaking with a louder voice will help transmit the communication over any background noise, however, with presbycusis the most relevant variable to alter is related to frequency. As a result, lowering your speaking tone would be the best option.

2. Speaking in a higher tone would not be beneficial, as the hair cells in the ear capable of receiving higher frequencies are compromised.

3. Speaking with a lower voice would not be beneficial, as background noise would likely diminish the ability to transmit the communication.

4. **Speaking in a lower tone or register is the best option. The hair cells that can receive this frequency are mostly preserved, therefore are capable of effectively transmitting the communication.**

System: Non-Systems
Content Outline: Safety and Protection; Professional Responsibilities; Research

 Level 1   p. 117

 Level 2   p. 500-501

➥ PTAEXAM ONE: QUESTION 101

A physical therapist assistant inspects a wound over a patient's sacrum. Based on the wound shown in the image, which classification would the assistant **MOST** likely use to document this pressure ulcer?

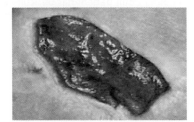

1. Stage 1
2. Stage 2
3. **Stage 3**
4. Stage 4

Correct Answer: 3 (Sussman p. 236)

The National Pressure Ulcer Advisory Panel pressure ulcer staging criteria was developed for use with pressure injuries. The staging criteria range from stage 1–4.

1. A stage 1 pressure injury is characterized by an observable pressure related alteration of intact skin whose indicators, as compared to an adjacent or opposite area on the body, may include changes in skin color, skin temperature, skin stiffness or sensation.

2. A stage 2 pressure injury is characterized by partial-thickness skin loss that involves the epidermis and/or dermis. The ulcer is superficial and presents clinically as an abrasion, a blister or a shallow crater.

3. **A stage 3 pressure injury is characterized by full-thickness skin loss that involves damage or necrosis of subcutaneous tissue that may extend down to, but not through, underlying fascia. The ulcer presents clinically as a deep crater with or without undermining adjacent tissue.**

4. A stage 4 pressure injury is characterized by full-thickness skin loss with extensive destruction, tissue necrosis or damage to muscle, bone or supporting structures (e.g., tendon, joint capsule).

System: Other Systems
Content Outline: Physical Therapy Data Collection

➥ PTAEXAM ONE: QUESTION 102

A patient who has diabetes mellitus is scheduled to walk approximately one half mile as part of a community fitness initiative. The physical therapist assistant checks the patient's blood glucose level before initiating the activity and finds it is 100 mg/dL. The assistant should advise the patient with which of the following recommendations?

1. **Proceed with performing the activity**
2. Increase food intake with a fruit or bread exchange
3. Increase food intake with a half sandwich with fruit or milk
4. Do not exercise until the blood glucose is under better control

Correct Answer: 1 (Hillegass p. 237)

Physical therapist assistants must be aware of the impact of exercise on a patient's glucose level. Therapists must also be able to discern the intensity of an activity and the glucose level required for successful completion. Low intensity exercise can be completed with a blood glucose level of 100 mg/dL without further food supplementation. If the intensity of the exercise increases, the patient would require an increase in food to sustain a safe blood glucose level during exercise.

1. **The patient is safe to perform the activity (low intensity exercise) if the blood glucose is 100 mg/dL. If the blood glucose value was less than 100 mg/dL, the patient would increase food intake prior to performing the activity. Supplementing additional carbohydrates is not needed for this intensity of exercise.**

2. Low intensity exercise, such as ambulating one half mile, would not require further food intake since the patient's blood glucose was measured as 100 mg/dL. Exercise of moderate intensity, such as an hour of golfing or swimming, would require an additional 10 to 15 grams of carbohydrates (i.e., a fruit or bread exchange) if blood glucose was measured between 100-180 mg/dL prior to exercise.

3. Low intensity exercise, such as ambulating one half mile, would not require further food intake since the patient's blood glucose was measured as 100 mg/dL. Strenuous exercise, such as one to two hours of hockey or basketball, would require an additional 25 to 50 grams of carbohydrates (i.e., half sandwich with fruit or milk) if blood glucose was measured between 100-180 mg/dL prior to exercise.

4. Typically, a patient is advised not to exercise if blood glucose is greater than 300 mg/dL. A patient at this blood glucose level would be at risk for diabetic ketoacidosis and should consult a physician prior to initiating any form of exercise.

System: Other Systems
Content Outline: Interventions

 Level 1   p. 444

Level 3   p. 466-467

➡ PTAEXAM ONE: QUESTION 103

A physical therapist assistant supervises an aerobic exercise program for a nine-year-old patient. Which statement **BEST** describes the heart rate and stroke volume of the child compared to an adult during aerobic exercise?

1. Increased heart rate and increased stroke volume
2. **Increased heart rate and decreased stroke volume**
3. Decreased heart rate and increased stroke volume
4. Decreased heart rate and decreased stroke volume

Correct Answer: 2 (Nyland p. 159)

Physical therapist assistants must consider the physiological, metabolic, and anatomical differences in children compared to adults when implementing an aerobic exercise program. Applying adult standards to children without careful consideration places children at an unnecessary safety risk.

1. As a person moves from infancy to adulthood, heart rate values will generally decrease. Therefore, a child's heart rate will typically be higher than an adult's heart rate. Stroke volume refers to the volume of blood ejected by each contraction of the left ventricle. Stroke volume increases from infancy to adulthood. This is expected since stroke volume has been found to be closely related to height, body surface area, and weight.

2. **A child would be expected to have an increased heart rate and a decreased stroke volume.**

3. A child would not be expected to have a decreased heart rate or an increased stroke volume.

4. A child would not be expected to have a decreased heart rate, however, would be expected to have a decreased stroke volume.

System: Cardiovascular and Pulmonary Systems
Content Outline: Interventions

➡ PTAEXAM ONE: QUESTION 104

A physical therapist assistant works on transfer training with a patient who is currently taking a diuretic medication. Which side effect is **MOST** likely to occur during the session secondary to the use of this type of medication?

1. **Postural hypotension**
2. Bleeding
3. Sedation
4. Headache

Correct Answer: 1 (Ciccone p. 318)

Diuretics are a group of medications that are commonly used to treat edema associated with heart failure, kidney disease or liver disease. Diuretics work by increasing the excretion of urine by the kidneys, thereby reducing the volume of fluid that is retained within the body.

1. **Postural hypotension (lightheadedness or dizziness associated with a change in position) is a common side effect associated with the use of diuretics due to a reduction in blood volume. Postural hypotension could occur during transfer training since the activity requires frequent position changes.**

2. Though there is a risk for bleeding to occur while performing transfers, bleeding is not a side effect associated with the use of diuretics. Bleeding is a side effect more commonly associated with thrombolytic medications.

3. Though sedation may affect a patient's ability to perform transfers, it is not a side effect associated with the use of diuretics. Sedation is a side effect more commonly associated with narcotic or antidepressant medications.

4. Headache is a side effect that is associated with the use of some diuretic medications. However, this side effect is less common than postural hypotension and would not necessarily be associated with transfer training.

System: Cardiovascular and Pulmonary Systems
Content Outline: Diseases/Conditions that Impact Effective Treatment

 Level 2   p. 382

Level 2   p. 372, 678

➡ PTAEXAM ONE: QUESTION 105

A physical therapist assistant treats a patient who sustained a right lateral ankle sprain less than six hours ago. The assistant contemplates the use of cold water immersion as a cryotherapeutic agent. What would be the **PRIMARY** limitation of this type of intervention?

1. Decreased cell metabolism
2. Excessive vasoconstriction of blood vessels
3. **The involved extremity cannot be elevated**
4. Decreased nerve conduction velocity

Correct Answer: 3 (Cameron p. 131)

There are a wide range of cryotherapeutic agents commonly used in physical therapy including cold whirlpool, ice packs, ice massage, cold sprays, and contrast baths. Physical therapist assistants should be aware of the advantages and limitations of each of the identified cryotherapeutic agents.

1. Cryotherapy decreases metabolic reactions including those involved in the inflammatory process.

2. Cryotherapy initially causes local vasoconstriction of smooth muscles in an attempt to conserve heat. Vasoconstriction is responsible for decreasing the formation and accumulation of edema.

3. **Cold water immersion is an acceptable form of cryotherapy, however, is not ideal when treating an acute lower extremity injury since the injured limb cannot be elevated. Inflammation is most effectively controlled if the cryotherapeutic agent is applied in conjunction with elevation and compression. Several other cryotherapeutic agents such as ice packs or Cryo Cuff may be more desirable interventions.**

4. Cryotherapy decreases the nerve conduction velocity of both sensory and motor nerves. Cryotherapy has the greatest effect on the conduction velocity of myelinated and small fibers, and the least effect on the conduction velocity of unmyelinated and large fibers.

System: Non-Systems
Content Outline: Equipment, Devices, and Technologies; Therapeutic Modalities

➡ PTAEXAM ONE: QUESTION 106

A physical therapist assistant reviews the results of a pulmonary function test for a patient recently admitted to the hospital. The assistant notes that the patient's total lung capacity is significantly increased when compared to established norms. Which of the following medical conditions would **MOST** likely produce this type of result?

1. Chronic bronchitis
2. **Emphysema**
3. Spinal cord injury
4. Pulmonary fibrosis

Correct Answer: 2 (Frownfelter p. 86)

Emphysema is a chronic obstructive pulmonary disease characterized by an abnormal and permanent enlargement of the air spaces distal to the terminal bronchiole, accompanied by destructive changes in their walls. Changes in lung tissue resulting from these anatomic changes include loss of elastic recoil, collapse of airways during exhalation, and airflow obstruction.

1. In chronic bronchitis there is hypertrophy of the submucosal glands in the large and small bronchi and trachea with hypersecretion of mucus. sufficient to cause a productive cough. Pulmonary function tests demonstrate a forced expiratory volume in one second (FEV_1) of < 65% of the predicted value. Total lung capacity is not increased in true chronic bronchitis.

2. **As a result of the pathologic changes to the lung tissue in emphysema, the lungs become hyperinflated. Due to the loss of elastic recoil, obstruction to airflow is seen as an increase in total lung capacity, residual volume, and functional residual capacity.**

3. Spinal cord injury is a neuromuscular cause of restrictive lung dysfunction. Characteristic changes in pulmonary function tests may include decreases in total lung capacity, vital capacity, and inspiratory capacity.

4. Pulmonary fibrosis is an inflammatory process affecting the alveoli that grossly distorts the architecture of the lung. These changes cause a decrease in lung compliance and a decrease in lung volumes including total lung capacity, vital capacity, functional residual capacity, and residual volume.

System: Cardiovascular and Pulmonary Systems
Content Outline: Diseases/Conditions that Impact Effective Treatment

 Level 2   p. 617-618

 Level 2   p. 366-367, 402-403

➡ PTAEXAM ONE: QUESTION 107

A physical therapist assistant treating a patient who has rheumatoid arthritis identifies the presence of hallux valgus. The patient reports pain and tenderness in the area of the great toe. Which of the following actions would be the **MOST** beneficial to address this condition?

1. **Recommend a shoe with a wide toe box**
2. Improve alignment of the great toe by using a metatarsal bar
3. Increase flexion range of motion of the great toe
4. Use a heel cup to redistribute forces

Correct Answer: 1 (O'Sullivan p. 1073)

Hallux valgus is an abnormal medial deviation of the first metatarsal with or without rotation of the hallux. This is a common finding with rheumatoid arthritis and can lead to painful motion of the joint as well as difficulty wearing specific footwear.

1. **A patient with hallux valgus demonstrates lateral deviation of the great toe, swelling of the metatarsophalangeal (MTP) joint, shortening of the flexor hallucis brevis, and pain and tenderness of the great toe. The most effective intervention would be the use of a shoe with a wide toe box in order to reduce pressure and better accommodate the MTP joint and great toe.**

2. Hallux valgus cannot be realigned through conservative management. A metatarsal bar would be more appropriately used to redistribute pressure with MTP joint dislocation or improve alignment of the toes as part of treatment for hammer or claw toes.

3. Increasing flexion of the great toe is not an intervention that is used to improve hallux valgus. The typical shortening of the flexor hallucis brevis found with hallux valgus would require stretching in order to increase extension of the great toe.

4. A heel cup would not serve to redistribute the weight bearing stresses found with hallux valgus. A heel cup would be more appropriately used to diminish pressure with a painful heel, particularly in the presence of a bone spur.

System: Other Systems
Content Outline: Interventions

➡ PTAEXAM ONE: QUESTION 108

A physical therapist assistant prepares to use phonophoresis as a component of a patient's plan of care, but is concerned about the potential of the intervention to exacerbate the patient's current inflammation. Which of the following actions would be the **MOST** effective to address the assistant's concern?

1. Utilize ultrasound with a frequency of 1 MHz
2. Limit treatment time to five minutes
3. **Incorporate a pulsed 20% duty cycle**
4. Select an ultrasound intensity less than 1.5 W/cm²

Correct Answer: 3 (Cameron p. 185)

Physical therapist assistants must select ultrasound treatment parameters that are consistent with the desired therapeutic outcome. Failure to select appropriate parameters can lead to poor outcomes and potentially jeopardize patient safety.

1. The frequency of ultrasound selected primarily determines the depth of penetration. A frequency setting of 1 MHz is used for heating of deeper tissues (up to five centimeters).

2. Limiting the treatment time to five minutes does effectively control the duration of ultrasound, but it does not address several other critical factors that significantly influence changes in tissue temperature (e.g., duty cycle, intensity).

3. **When ultrasound is used in a pulsed mode with a 20% or lower duty cycle, the heat produced during the on time of the cycle is dispersed during the off time and as a result there is no measurable net increase in temperature. Ultrasound using a 20% or lower duty cycle would typically be used for nonthermal effects.**

4. Limiting the intensity of ultrasound to less than 1.5 W/cm² is helpful to avoid exacerbating the patient's current inflammation, however, the patient's condition could still be exacerbated at many intensity levels below 1.5 W/cm².

System: Non-Systems
Content Outline: Equipment, Devices, and Technologies;
   Therapeutic Modalities

 Level 2   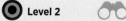   p. 73

 Level 2   p. 623-626

▶ PTAEXAM ONE: QUESTION 109

A physical therapist assistant attempts to assess the integrity of the first cranial nerve. Which action should the assistant ask the patient to perform to complete this assessment?

1. Protrude the tongue
2. Complete a vision test
3. Perform a shoulder shrug
4. **Identify familiar odors with the eyes closed**

Correct Answer: 4 (Tan p. 14)

Lesions affecting the cranial nerves often produce specific and predictable alterations. As a result, it is often desirable to perform cranial nerve testing.

1. The hypoglossal nerve (cranial nerve XII) is assessed by asking the patient to protrude the tongue. A positive test may be indicated by an inability to fully protrude the tongue or the tongue deviating to one side during protrusion.

2. The optic nerve (cranial nerve II) is assessed by asking the patient to identify objects or read selected items from a chart or diagram. A positive test may be indicated by an inability to identify objects at a reasonable distance.

3. The accessory nerve (cranial nerve XI) is assessed by asking a patient, positioned in sitting with the arms at their side, to shrug their shoulders and maintain the position while the physical therapist assistant applies resistance through the shoulders in the direction of shoulder depression. A positive test may be indicated by an inability to maintain the test position against resistance.

4. **The olfactory nerve (cranial nerve I) is assessed by placing an item with a familiar odor under the patient's nostril and the patient is then asked to identify the odor. A positive test may be indicated by an inability to identify familiar odors.**

System: Neuromuscular and Nervous Systems
Content Outline: Physical Therapy Data Collection

▶ PTAEXAM ONE: QUESTION 110

A patient eight days post anterior cruciate ligament reconstruction using a patellar tendon autograft is treated in physical therapy. Which of the following exercises would be the **MOST** appropriate based on the patient's post-operative status?

1. Limited range isokinetics at 30 degrees per second
2. Unilateral leg press
3. **Mini-squats in standing**
4. Active knee extension in short sitting

Correct Answer: 3 (Kisner p. 815)

Anterior cruciate ligament reconstruction refers to the use of a graft to replace a damaged anterior cruciate ligament. The graft is placed through drilled holes in the femoral and tibial tunnels and then anchored with a fixation device. The focus of the early post-operative period is to protect the healing graft and donor site, and at the same time avoid post-operative complications such as adhesions, contractures, and articular degeneration.

1. Performing isokinetics at 30 degrees per second on a patient eight days status post anterior cruciate ligament reconstruction could potentially jeopardize the integrity of the graft.

2. A unilateral leg press is similar to a squat, however, it is usually performed in a supine position. The exercise is not as desirable as the mini-squat given the patient's post-operative status since the leg press activity is unilateral and therefore the patient would not have the benefit of using the uninvolved lower extremity to assist, if necessary. In addition, the mini-squat implies limited range where the unilateral leg press does not.

3. **A mini-squat is a closed-chain exercise typically performed in standing that enables the patient to vary the force through the involved extremity by simply shifting their weight. This exercise significantly limits the amount of knee flexion and as a result does not place a great deal of stress through the reconstructed knee. When completing mini-squats in standing it is important that the knees do not move anterior to the toes as the hips descend since this will increase the shear forces of the tibia and could unnecessarily stress the graft.**

4. Active knee extension in short sitting is an open-chain activity that places a significant amount of force on the anterior surface of the knee and in particular, the patellar tendon donor area.

System: Musculoskeletal System
Content Outline: Interventions

 Level 1   p. 224-226

 Level 2   p. 121, 146-147

▶ PTAEXAM ONE: QUESTION 111

A physical therapist assistant collects data as part of a research project that requires direct observation of children performing selected gross motor activities. The assistant is concerned about the influence of an observer on the children's performance. Which of the following strategies would be the **MOST** effective to control for this source of error?

1. Provide initial and refresher observer training
2. Increase observer awareness of the influence of their background
3. **Have an observer spend time with the children before direct observation**
4. Ask the children to ignore the presence of the observer

Correct Answer: 3 (Portney p. 310)

A research project should be designed to eliminate as many extraneous variables as possible. Failure to eliminate or at least reduce the potential impact of an observer on the children's performance would be a significant limitation of the study.

1. Observer training would be beneficial in order to provide the observers with a better sense of their purpose, role, and actions. This action would be desirable, but would not address the nuance of the observer for the children.

2. An individual's background can influence their observations particularly when the data collected is open for interpretation. This option also focuses on the observer and not the children.

3. **Spending time with the children prior to direct observation will allow the children to feel more at ease and as a result their performance may be more reflective of their current abilities.**

4. Asking the children to ignore the presence of the observer would likely serve to bring additional attention to the observer and therefore influence behavior.

System: Non-Systems
Content Outline: Safety and Protection; Professional Responsibilities; Research

▶ PTAEXAM ONE: QUESTION 112

A physical therapist assistant prepares to treat a patient who has impingement syndrome with iontophoresis. The assistant applies iontophoresis directly over the insertion of the supraspinatus muscle. What bony landmark should the assistant use to **BEST** find a point of reference to locate this tendon?

1. Lesser tubercle of the humerus
2. **Greater tubercle of the humerus**
3. Supraspinous fossa of the scapula
4. Deltoid tuberosity of the humerus

Correct Answer: 2 (Kendall p. 314)

Impingement syndrome is a commonly used term describing mechanical impingement of the rotator cuff tendon beneath the anteroinferior portion of the acromion. Symptoms of impingement syndrome include difficulty reaching up behind the back, pain with overhead use of the arm, and weakness of the shoulder muscles.

1. The subscapularis muscle originates on the subscapular fossa of the scapula and inserts on the lesser tubercle of the humerus. The muscle is innervated by the subscapular nerve.

2. **The supraspinatus muscle inserts on the greater tubercle of the humerus. The muscle is innervated by the suprascapular nerve.**

3. The supraspinatus muscle originates on the supraspinous fossa of the scapula. The question asks about the insertion of the muscle.

4. The deltoid tuberosity is the insertion point for the three heads of the deltoid. The anterior deltoid originates on the lateral third of the clavicle, the middle deltoid originates on the acromion process, and the posterior deltoid originates on the spine of the scapula. The deltoid is innervated by the axillary nerve.

System: Musculoskeletal System
Content Outline: Interventions

 Level 3

 Level 1

SCOREBUILDERS

▶ PTAEXAM ONE: QUESTION 113

A physical therapist assistant participates in a study that examines the effect of goniometer size on the reliability of passive shoulder joint measurements. The assistant concludes that goniometric measurements of passive shoulder range of motion can be highly reliable when taken by a single therapist, regardless of the size of the goniometer. This finding is **BEST** described by which of the following terms?

1. Interrater reliability
2. **Intrarater reliability**
3. Internal validity
4. External validity

Correct Answer: 2 (Norkin p. 45)

Reliability, or the extent to which a measurement is consistent and free from error, is a prerequisite of any measurement. There are a number of types of reliability that may be estimated: test-retest, rater (intrarater and interrater), alternate forms, and internal consistency.

1. Interrater reliability refers to the reproducibility of measurements made by two or more raters who measure the same group of subjects.

2. **Intrarater reliability refers to the reproducibility of measurements made by one individual across two or more trials.**

3. Internal validity focuses on cause and effect relationships. Specifically, is there evidence that, given a statistical relationship between the independent variable and dependent variable in an experiment, one causes the other.

4. External validity refers to the extent to which the results of a study can be generalized beyond the study sample to persons, settings, and times that are different from those employed in the experimental situation. External validity is concerned with the usefulness of the information outside the experimental situation.

System: Non-Systems
Content Outline: Safety and Protection; Professional Responsibilities; Research

▶ PTAEXAM ONE: QUESTION 114

A patient who sustained an injury to the superficial peroneal nerve is treated by a physical therapist assistant. In which area of the body should the assistant **MOST** likely expect to find altered sensation?

1. Sole of the foot
2. Plantar surface of the toes
3. **Lateral aspect of the leg and dorsum of the foot**
4. Triangular area between the first and second toes

Correct Answer: 3 (Kendall p. 369)

The superficial peroneal nerve innervates the peroneus longus and brevis. It is a branch of the sciatic nerve.

1. The sole of the foot receives cutaneous innervation from the medial and lateral plantar nerves, which are branches of the tibial nerve. The tibial nerve is a branch of the sciatic nerve.

2. The plantar surface of the toes is innervated by the medial and lateral plantar nerves, which are branches of the tibial nerve. The tibial nerve is a branch of the sciatic nerve.

3. **A peripheral nerve injury affecting the superficial peroneal nerve often results in sensory alterations along the lateral aspect of the leg and dorsum of the foot.**

4. The triangular area between the first and second toes is innervated by the deep peroneal nerve. It is a branch of the sciatic nerve.

System: Neuromuscular and Nervous Systems
Content Outline: Physical Therapy Data Collection

 Level 1   p. 706

Level 1

➡ PTAEXAM ONE: QUESTION 115

A physician orders a nasogastric tube for a patient admitted to the hospital. Which of the following indications does **NOT** accurately describe a potential use of the nasogastric tube?

1. Administer medications directly into the gastrointestinal tract
2. Obtain gastric specimens
3. Remove fluid or gas from the stomach
4. **Obtain venous blood samples from the stomach**

Correct Answer: 4 (Fairchild p. 278)

A nasogastric tube is a plastic tube that enters the body through a nostril and terminates in a patient's stomach. As a result, the tube is not used for obtaining venous samples.

1. A nasogastric tube can administer medications directly into the gastrointestinal tract. The patient can also be fed nutrients directly through the nasogastric tube if they are unable to take in adequate nutrition orally. Oral feeding or drinking is contraindicated when the nasogastric tube is in place, but exercise is permitted with caution. Head and neck movements should be closely monitored.

2. A nasogastric tube can be used to obtain gastric specimens. The tube is taped to the patient's face so that it does not easily become dislodged.

3. A nasogastric tube can be used to remove fluid or gas from the stomach and may be utilized to keep the stomach empty after surgery. This would also allow the bowels to rest if needed.

4. **An intravenous line can be used to obtain venous blood samples (but not from the stomach). Intravenous lines also infuse fluids, nutrients, medications, and electrolytes. A nasogastric tube does not obtain venous samples.**

System: Other Systems
Content Outline: Interventions

➡ PTAEXAM ONE: QUESTION 116

A physical therapist assistant applies a dressing to an area of skin on a patient's heel as a prophylactic measure to reduce the risk of skin breakdown in an area that was determined to be particularly susceptible. Which of the following types of dressings is the assistant **MOST** likely applying?

1. Calcium alginate
2. Hydrocolloid
3. Hydrogel
4. **Transparent film**

Correct Answer: 4 (Sussman p. 504)

A physical therapist assistant selects a particular wound dressing based on the established therapeutic objectives. Possible indications for utilizing a dressing include protecting the wound, managing exudate, preventing infection, reducing pain, and promoting healing.

1. A calcium alginate dressing is highly absorptive and typically utilized with wounds that produce moderate to heavy exudate. A wound producing minimal exudate is unlikely to saturate the alginate to the extent necessary for it to form a beneficial hydrophilic gel.

2. Hydrocolloid dressings consist of gel-forming polymers (e.g., carboxymethylcellulose, gelatin, pectin) backed by a strong film or foam adhesive. The dressings absorb exudate by swelling into a gel-like mass and vary in permeability, thickness, and transparency. A hydrocolloid dressing is not used for a superficial wound, however, is often used on partial and full-thickness wounds.

3. Hydrogel dressings are moisture-retentive primary dressings that provide a moist environment for wound healing. A hydrogel dressing is not typically used as a prophylactic measure and is instead used to prevent a wound from dehydrating and impeding the healing process.

4. **Transparent film dressings consist of thin membranes coated with a layer of acrylic adhesive. Since the film is transparent it allows for frequent assessment of the wound and offers some level of protection. The films are oxygen permeable, however, are impermeable to microorganisms and moisture.**

System: Other Systems
Content Outline: Interventions

  Level 2   p. 43, 607

  Level 2   p. 447-449

➡ PTAEXAM ONE: QUESTION 117

A physical therapist assistant works on mat activities to improve bed mobility and dressing independence with a patient diagnosed with C7 complete tetraplegia. Preserving tightness of which muscle groups would **MOST** benefit the patient's functional potential?

1. Finger extensors and hamstrings
2. **Finger flexors and low back**
3. Wrist flexors and hamstrings
4. Wrist extensors and low back

Correct Answer: 2 (Fell p. 866)

A patient with complete C7 tetraplegia may benefit from maintaining tightness in certain muscle groups in order to assist with function. Patients without finger innervation will be able to simulate grasp using shortened long finger flexors to perform a tenodesis grip. Patients without trunk innervation may also be able to derive benefit during transfers and bed mobility through the use of tightness within the low back muscles.

1. Patients should avoid simultaneous wrist and finger extension as it places the flexor muscles on maximum stretch. Finger extensors are not a target muscle group in terms of maintaining a shortened length. Hamstring muscles must have adequate length in order to maintain long sitting and assist with bed mobility and dressing skills. Therefore, stretching these muscles is essential to prevent tightness.

2. **Both finger flexors and low back muscles would benefit from maintaining some tightness of the muscles. When the long finger flexors are tight, the patient can use a tenodesis grasp (wrist extension assists with finger flexion to produce a grasp). Tightness of the low back muscles allows for movement of the head and upper extremities while in long sitting which can assist with functional mobility and activities of daily living.**

3. Patients should avoid tightness of both the wrist flexors and hamstrings muscle groups. The wrist flexors should have adequate length so that the patient can perform wrist extension to use a tenodesis grasp. The hamstrings also require adequate length in order to allow long sitting and functional mobility in bed.

4. Patients should avoid tightness of the wrist extensors muscle group. Wrist extensors require full range of motion so that the patient can perform wrist extension and enhance the capacity to grasp objects through tenodesis. The low back muscles will benefit from mild tightness which can improve the patient's overall function.

System: Neuromuscular and Nervous Systems
Content Outline: Diseases/Conditions that Impact Effective Treatment

➡ PTAEXAM ONE: QUESTION 118

A physical therapist assistant listens to the lung sounds of a patient with chronic bronchitis. The patient was admitted to the hospital two days ago after complaining of shortness of breath and difficulty breathing. While performing auscultation, the assistant identifies distinct lung sounds with a high constant pitch during exhalation. This finding is **MOST** consistent with which type of breath sound?

1. Crackles
2. Rales
3. Rhonchi
4. **Wheezes**

Correct Answer: 4 (Frownfelter p. 206)

Wheezes are described as high-pitched, musical sounds made by air passing through narrowed tracheobronchial airways.

1. Crackles are discontinuous, adventitious breath sounds heard during auscultation of the lungs due to fluid accumulation in the distal airways or when collapsed alveoli reopen during inspiration.

2. Rales are synonymous with crackles.

3. Rhonchi are lower-pitched, continuous, adventitious breath sounds occurring during inspiration or expiration and are caused by the turbulence of air passing through secretions in large and mid-sized bronchi.

4. **Wheezes are continuous, high-pitched, adventitious breath sounds that are most frequently heard on exhalation and are associated with airway obstruction or bronchospasm. There can also be inspiratory wheezing caused by movement of air through secretions. Wheezes are commonly associated with asthma and bronchitis.**

System: Cardiovascular and Pulmonary Systems
Content Outline: Physical Therapy Data Collection

 Level 2   p. 269-272, 312-313

 Level 3   p. 378-379

PTAEXAM ONE: QUESTION 119

A physical therapist assistant attempts to identify a patient's risk factors for coronary artery disease as part of a health screening. The patient's heart rate is recorded as 78 beats per minute and blood pressure as 110/70 mm Hg. A recent laboratory report indicates a total cholesterol level of 170 mg/dL with high-density lipoproteins reported as 20 mg/dL and low-density lipoproteins as 110 mg/dL. Which of the following values would be considered atypical?

1. Heart rate

2. Blood pressure

3. **High-density lipoproteins (HDL)**

4. Low-density lipoproteins (LDL)

Correct Answer: 3 (Paz p. 26)

A value less than 40 mg/dL is considered low for HDL cholesterol. Values of 60 mg/dL or greater are considered high. A low HDL value is strongly associated with an increased risk for coronary artery disease.

1. 78 beats per minute is a normal resting heart rate. The range of normal is 60-100 beats per minute.

2. A systolic blood pressure of 110 mm Hg and a diastolic blood pressure of 70 mm Hg are considered within normal limits.

3. **An HDL cholesterol level of 20 mg/dL is very low and is associated with an increased risk of coronary artery disease. The patient would likely be treated by their physician with pharmacological and non-pharmacological therapies to raise the HDL cholesterol level.**

4. The optimal level of LDL cholesterol is less than 100 mg/dL. A value of 110 mg/dL is considered near optimal. High levels of LDL cholesterol increase the risk of coronary artery disease.

System: Other Systems
Content Outline: Diseases/Conditions that Impact Effective
   Treatment

PTAEXAM ONE: QUESTION 120

A physical therapist assistant measures a patient's shoulder medial rotation as 0–70 degrees and classifies the end-feel as firm. Which portion of the joint capsule is primarily responsible for the firm end-feel?

1. Anterior

2. **Posterior**

3. Inferior

4. Superior

Correct Answer: 2 (Norkin p. 86)

The glenohumeral joint is a synovial ball and socket joint, in which the round head of the humerus (convex) articulates with the shallow glenoid cavity (concave) of the scapula. The glenohumeral joint has three degrees of freedom. The capsule of the glenohumeral joint is reinforced by the superior glenohumeral ligament, middle glenohumeral ligament, inferior glenohumeral ligament, and the coracohumeral ligament.

1. A firm end-feel caused by the anterior joint capsule would most often be associated with lateral rotation of the glenohumeral joint as the humeral head slides anteriorly on the glenoid fossa.

2. **A firm end-feel caused by the posterior joint capsule would most often be associated with medial rotation of the gleno-humeral joint as the humeral head slides posteriorly on the glenoid fossa.**

3. A firm end-feel caused by the inferior joint capsule would most often be associated with flexion and abduction of the glenohumeral joint. In flexion, the humeral head moves posteriorly and inferiorly, and in abduction the humeral head moves inferiorly.

4. A firm end-feel caused by the superior joint capsule would most often be associated with extension and adduction of the glenohumeral joint. In extension, the humeral head moves anteriorly and superiorly, and in adduction the humeral head moves superiorly.

System: Musculoskeletal System
Content Outline: Physical Therapy Data Collection

 Level 1   p. 368-370

Level 2

➡ PTAEXAM ONE: QUESTION 121

A physical therapist assistant positions a patient in prone to measure passive knee flexion. Which of the following rationales is the **MOST** likely cause of limited range of motion in this position?

1. Active insufficiency of the knee extensors
2. Active insufficiency of the knee flexors
3. **Passive insufficiency of the knee extensors**
4. Passive insufficiency of the knee flexors

Correct Answer: 3 (Kisner p. 61)

Passive insufficiency occurs when a two-joint muscle cannot lengthen to the extent required to allow full range of motion of all joints it crosses simultaneously. When the muscle is in a lengthened position, the actin filaments are pulled away from the myosin heads so that they cannot create as many cross-bridges. Active insufficiency occurs when a two-joint muscle is incapable of shortening to the extent necessary to produce full range of motion at all joints crossed simultaneously. When the muscle is in a shortened position the overlap of actin and myosin reduces the number of sites available for cross-bridge formation.

1. Active insufficiency occurs with active movement and not passive movement. The question specifically asks about passive knee flexion.

2. Active insufficiency occurs with active movement and not passive movement.

3. **Passive insufficiency refers to a lack of muscle length. When performing passive knee flexion the two-joint knee extensors are placed on stretch and therefore in the presence of insufficient length, may contribute to a limitation in knee flexion.**

4. When performing passive knee flexion, the knee flexors would shorten and therefore would not limit knee flexion range of motion.

System: Musculoskeletal System
Content Outline: Physical Therapy Data Collection

➡ PTAEXAM ONE: QUESTION 122

A physical therapist assistant implements a training program for a patient without cardiovascular pathology. The assistant calculates the patient's age-predicted maximal heart rate as 175 bpm. Which of the following values would be the **MOST** appropriate target heart rate for the patient during cardiovascular exercise?

1. 93 beats per minute
2. **135 beats per minute**
3. 169 beats per minute
4. 195 beats per minute

Correct Answer: 2 (American College of Sports Medicine p. 473)

The target heart rate for exercise can be approximated using a percentage of the maximum heart rate, which can be estimated as 220 – age. With this approach, 70-85% of maximum heart rate or 50-70% of maximum oxygen uptake (VO_{2max}) is the recommended exercise intensity according to the American College of Sports Medicine. If the maximal heart rate is 175 beats per minute, the target heart rate range is (70% x 175) to (85% x 175), or 123 to 149 beats per minute. Some sources recommend a more broadly defined target heart rate range of 60-90%. In either case, the correct answer would be option 2.

1. 93 beats per minute is below the recommended range for exercise intensity. 93 beats per minute corresponds to 53% of the maximum heart rate.

2. **135 beats per minute is within the recommended range for exercise intensity. 135 beats per minute corresponds to 77% of the maximum heart rate.**

3. 169 beats per minute is above the recommended range for exercise intensity. 169 beats per minute corresponds to 97% of the maximum heart rate.

4. 195 beats per minute is above the recommended range for exercise intensity. 195 beats per minute corresponds to 111% of the maximum heart rate.

System: Cardiovascular and Pulmonary Systems
Content Outline: Interventions

➡ PTAEXAM ONE: QUESTION 123

A patient who has complete C5 tetraplegia works on a forward raise for pressure relief. The patient utilizes loops that are attached to the back of the wheelchair to assist with the forward raise. Which of the following muscles would the patient **MOST** likely need to be particularly strong in order to be successful with this technique?

1. Brachioradialis and brachialis
2. Rhomboids and levator scapulae
3. **Biceps and deltoids**
4. Triceps and flexor digitorum profundus

Correct Answer: 3 (Roy p. 363)

A patient with C5 tetraplegia would not have muscles innervated below the C5 level. Primary innervations and actions for each of the muscles are listed.

1. The brachioradialis (C5-C6) and brachialis (C5-C6) would both be innervated. The primary action of the brachioradialis and brachialis is to flex the elbow.
2. The rhomboids (C4-C5) and levator scapulae (C3-C5) would both be innervated. The rhomboids adduct and rotate the scapula downward. The levator scapulae elevate and rotate the scapula downward.
3. **The biceps (C5-C6) and deltoids (C5-C6) would both be innervated. The deltoids (anterior, middle, posterior) assist with all shoulder motions with the exception of adduction. The biceps act to flex the shoulder, flex the elbow, and supinate the forearm.**
4. The triceps (C7-C8) and flexor digitorum profundus (C8-T1) would not be innervated in a patient with C5 tetraplegia.

System: Neuromuscular and Nervous Systems
Content Outline: Interventions

➡ PTAEXAM ONE: QUESTION 124

A physical therapist assistant instructs a patient to change their wound dressing daily between weekly visits to the wound center. At the next visit, the patient reports that they instead changed the dressing only when it was soaked through in an effort to conserve supplies. As a result, which of the following terms would the assistant **MOST** likely use to describe the periwound area?

1. Infected
2. Gangrenous
3. **Macerated**
4. Indurated

Correct Answer: 3 (Sussman p. 376)

When providing self-care patient education, it is vital to include information on the impact of not adhering to therapy recommendations. Patients are more likely to be compliant if rationale, goals, and risk factors are understood.

1. There are no identifiable signs of infection with the presented information.
2. Gangrene refers to tissue death and may be described as wet or dry. Dry gangrene develops slowly in response to decreased blood flow and has a characteristic blue-black appearance. Wet gangrene frequently develops in response to tissue injury or burns and can be life-threatening if untreated.
3. **Macerated tissue is the result of prolonged exposure to excessive moisture. The appearance is initially blanched and somewhat swollen. If not addressed, epithelial cells will become disrupted and begin to separate from the underlying dermis, leaving the area with a raw, red, and wet appearance. Macerated tissue is prone to infection and additional injury.**
4. Induration refers to an abnormal firmness or hardening of the skin which is typically indicative of pathology. Induration is often due to increased exudate or fibrous tissue in an area.

System: Other Systems
Content Outline: Interventions

 Level 2   p. 267, 269-271

 Level 2 p. 450-451

SCOREBUILDERS

▶ PTAEXAM ONE: QUESTION 125

A patient two weeks post transtibial amputation is instructed by their physician to remain at rest for two days after contracting bronchitis. Which of the following positions is the **MOST** appropriate for the patient while in bed?

1. Supine with a pillow under the patient's knees
2. Supine with a pillow under the patient's thighs and knees
3. **Supine with the legs extended**
4. Sidelying in the fetal position

Correct Answer: 3 (Seymour p. 145)

It is important for a patient with a transtibial amputation to keep the knee extended in order to prevent shortening of the hamstring muscles and avoid developing a flexion contracture at the knee.

1. Lying in supine with a pillow under the knees is a comfortable position for the patient after transtibial amputation. However, placing a pillow under the knee puts the knee in a partially flexed position. This promotes the development of hamstrings muscle tightness, which may lead to a flexion contracture at the knee.

2. Lying in supine with a pillow under the thighs and knees puts the hip and knee in a flexed position. This promotes the development of hip flexor and hamstrings muscle tightness, which may lead to flexion contractures at the hip or knee.

3. **The supine position with the legs extended is the most appropriate position since it promotes lengthening of the hip flexors and hamstring muscles and prevents the development of flexion contractures.**

4. Sidelying in the fetal position places the hips and knees in a flexed position. This promotes the development of hip flexor and hamstrings muscle tightness, which may lead to flexion contractures at the hip or knee.

System: Musculoskeletal System
Content Outline: Interventions

▶ PTAEXAM ONE: QUESTION 126

A patient uses patient-controlled analgesia with a lockout interval following an inpatient surgical procedure. Which medication would be **MOST** consistent with this delivery model?

1. Atorvastatin (Lipitor)
2. Baclofen (Lioresal)
3. **Meperidine (Demerol)**
4. Methotrexate (Trexall)

Correct Answer: 3 (Roy p. 1137)

Patient-controlled analgesia allows the patient to manage their pain by delivering an intravenous analgesic dose with preset parameters. Opioids are often the medication of choice for patient-controlled analgesia to manage severe acute pain. A lockout interval refers to the period of time in which a patient-controlled analgesia system will not allow the patient to receive medication.

1. Atorvastatin (Lipitor) is a commonly used antihyperlipidemia agent. This class of pharmacological agents consists of five categories of lipid-modifying agents. The most commonly used drugs, the statins, inhibit enzyme action in cholesterol synthesis, break down low-density lipoproteins, decrease triglyceride levels, and increase high-density lipoprotein levels. This medication is not utilized for patient-controlled analgesia.

2. Baclofen (Lioresal) is a commonly used antispasticity agent. This class of pharmacological agents promotes relaxation in spastic muscles by binding selectively within the central nervous system or within the skeletal muscle cells. This medication is not utilized for patient-controlled analgesia.

3. **Meperidine (Demerol) is a commonly used opioid agent. This class of pharmacological agents provides analgesia for acute severe pain management. The medication stimulates opioid receptors within the central nervous system to prevent pain impulses from reaching their destination. The potential serious side effects (e.g., sedation, respiratory depression) and the potential for physical dependence result in the medication often being administered with a lockout interval.**

4. Methotrexate (Trexall) is a commonly used disease-modifying antirheumatic drug that functions by slowing or halting the progression of rheumatic disease. It is used early during the disease process to slow the progression prior to widespread damage of the affected joints. It acts to induce remission by modifying the pathology and inhibiting the immune response responsible for rheumatic disease. This medication is also used to treat various types of cancers, but is not utilized for patient-controlled analgesia.

System: Musculoskeletal System
Content Outline: Diseases/Conditions that Impact Effective Treatment

 Level 2   p. 130-133

 Level 2   p. 122-123

➡ PTAEXAM ONE: QUESTION 127

A physical therapist assistant treats a patient three days post shoulder surgery. The patient reports general malaise and a slightly elevated body temperature during the last 24 hours. The assistant notes that the patient's shoulder is edematous, warm to touch, and observes a small amount of yellow fluid seeping from the incision. Which of the following actions is the **MOST** appropriate for the assistant to take?

1. Send the patient to the emergency room
2. **Communicate the information to the referring physician**
3. Document the findings in the medical record
4. Ask the patient to make an appointment with the referring physician

Correct Answer: 2 (Goodman – Pathology p. 319)

Physical therapist assistants must be aware of any signs or symptoms of infection, particularly in patients following surgery. Common signs of infection include elevated body temperature, purulent exudate, swelling, edema, and redness.

1. The patient's presentation requires the physical therapist assistant to take formal action, but would not be indicative of an emergent condition that requires the patient to be seen in the emergency room.

2. **The possibility of infection in a patient three days status post surgery warrants immediate consultation with the referring physician. It would also be necessary to communicate the information immediately to the supervising physical therapist.**

3. The subjective and objective information gathered by the physical therapist assistant should be documented in the medical record, however, this action would not address the primary issue which is the possibility of an infection.

4. Asking the patient to make an appointment with the physician is not an appropriate action since it places the burden solely on the patient. The physical therapist assistant is responsible for communicating any potential change in a patient's medical status to the supervising physical therapist and/or physician in a timely manner.

System: Other Systems
Content Outline: Diseases/Conditions that Impact Effective Treatment

➡ PTAEXAM ONE: QUESTION 128

A physical therapist assistant instructs a patient how to fall safely to the floor when using axillary crutches. Which of the following strategies should be the **FIRST** to occur in the case of a forward fall?

1. Reach towards the floor
2. Turn the face towards one side
3. **Release the crutches**
4. Flex the trunk and head

Correct Answer: 3 (Fairchild p. 259)

Physical therapist assistants are responsible for instructing patients how to properly use various assistive devices. The instructions typically include training in fall prevention and strategies to minimize injury in the event of a fall.

1. Reaching forward toward the floor would be a desirable action in the event of a forward fall, however, the question specifically asks for the "first" action.

2. Turning the face towards one side would be a desirable action in the event of a forward fall to minimize the relative trauma to the face, however, this would not be the "first" action.

3. **A patient should release the crutches in the event of a forward fall in order to utilize the upper extremities to minimize the impact of the fall.**

4. Flexing the trunk and head are instructions that are necessary when teaching a patient to properly fall backward. The coupled motions are used to facilitate the patient to fall on their buttocks instead of directly landing on their head.

System: Non-Systems
Content Outline: Safety and Protection; Professional Responsibilities; Research

 Level 3

 Level 2

➡ PTAEXAM ONE: QUESTION 129

A physical therapist assistant reviews the past medical history of a patient who has recently been diagnosed with adhesive capsulitis. Which of the following medical conditions is **MOST** associated with an increased incidence of adhesive capsulitis?

1. **Diabetes mellitus**

2. Hemophilia

3. Peripheral vascular disease

4. Osteomalacia

Correct Answer: 1 (Goodman – Pathology p. 513)

Adhesive capsulitis refers to an inflammation and adherence of the articular capsule resulting in limited joint play and restricted active and passive movement. The condition is more common in women than in men and tends to appear in the fourth, fifth, and sixth decades of life.

1. **Diabetes mellitus is a group of metabolic diseases characterized by high blood sugar levels that result from defects in insulin secretion, the actions of insulin or both. Patients with diabetes mellitus have an increased incidence of adhesive capsulitis and often experience a longer duration of symptoms and greater limitation of motion.**

2. Hemophilia is a bleeding disorder of genetic etiology. It is a sex-linked autosomal recessive trait. Patients with hemophilia are prone to hemarthrosis, intramuscular hemorrhage, and secondary complications from hematomas. The condition is not associated with an increased incidence of adhesive capsulitis.

3. Peripheral vascular disease refers to any disease or pathology of the circulatory system outside of the brain and heart. The disease is characterized by narrowing of the arteries, and reduced blood flow to the legs, arms, brain and other organs. The cause, in most cases, is atherosclerosis. The condition is not associated with an increased incidence of adhesive capsulitis.

4. Osteomalacia refers to softening of the bone without loss of bone matrix. There is insufficient mineralization of the bone matrix normally caused by insufficient calcium absorption and increased renal phosphorus losses. Symptoms include bone pain, aching, fatigue, and periarticular tenderness. The condition is not associated with an increased incidence of adhesive capsulitis.

System: Other Systems
Content Outline: Diseases/Conditions that Impact Effective Treatment

➡ PTAEXAM ONE: QUESTION 130

A patient exhibits a compensatory contralateral step-to gait pattern and persistent left knee pain. Which of the following conditions would **MOST** likely result in this type of long-term compensatory gait pattern?

1. **Degenerative joint disease**

2. Anterior cruciate ligament sprain

3. Osgood-Schlatter disease

4. Patellofemoral syndrome

Correct Answer: 1 (Dunleavy p. 79)

A compensatory contralateral step-to gait pattern for a patient with left knee pain refers to a shortened swing phase on the right when the left limb is in the stance phase of gait. Protective gait patterns (e.g., antalgic gait) are often the result of disease (usually bone or joint), joint inflammation or injuries to muscles, tendons, and/or ligaments.

1. **Osteoarthritis is a chronic disease that causes degeneration of articular cartilage, primarily in weight bearing joints (e.g., knee, hip). Subsequent deformity and thickening of subchondral bone occur resulting in impaired functional status. As the disease progresses in severity, the patient may present with a deviated gait pattern, atypical movement patterns, and muscle atrophy. The described gait deviation would most likely occur over time with the progression of degenerative joint disease.**

2. An anterior cruciate ligament sprain is characterized by knee pain, effusion, and edema that limit range of motion. The patient may be unable to bear weight on the involved extremity resulting in dependence on an assistive device. Although a patient may exhibit an antalgic gait with a contralateral step-to gait pattern in the early stages of an anterior cruciate ligament sprain, this compensatory gait pattern would not be expected over the long term.

3. Osgood-Schlatter disease refers to traction apophysitis occurring at the tibial tuberosity. It typically affects adolescents involved in sports that require running, jumping, directional changes, and repeated knee flexion (e.g., soccer, ballet). Although an antalgic gait pattern may likely occur with Osgood-Schlatter disease, it is a self-limiting condition that typically has an excellent prognosis.

4. Patellofemoral syndrome is caused by an abnormal tracking of the patella (usually laterally) between the femoral condyles. Prognosis for a full recovery is good with successful conservative management of patellofemoral syndrome. Long-term gait compensation is more likely to occur with degenerative joint disease.

System: Musculoskeletal System
Content Outline: Diseases/Conditions that Impact Effective Treatment

 Level 2   p. 112, 142-143

Level 2   p. 115, 154-155

➡ PTAEXAM ONE: QUESTION 131

A physical therapist assistant works with a patient who has post-polio syndrome. Which of the following examination components is the **LEAST** likely to be affected based on the patient's diagnosis?

1. Strength
2. **Sensation**
3. Endurance
4. Functional mobility

Correct Answer: 2 (Goodman – Pathology p. 1690)

Post-polio syndrome is a term used to describe symptoms that occur years after the onset of poliomyelitis. The condition is characterized by a weakening of the muscles that were originally affected by polio. Symptoms include progressive muscle weakness, fatigue, and muscle atrophy.

1. Patients with post-polio syndrome experience a decrease in strength. This finding may be related to the degeneration of individual nerve terminals in the motor units that remain after the initial illness.

2. **The polio virus attacks specific neurons in the brainstem and anterior horn cells of the spinal cord. As a result, sensation is not typically affected.**

3. Endurance is compromised in patients with post-polio syndrome secondary to the loss of strength, vasomotor abnormalities, joint pain, and myalgias.

4. Functional mobility will decrease as a result of the patient's loss of strength and endurance. Pain will also often increase with physical activity which may result in the patient becoming less active.

System: Neuromuscular and Nervous Systems
Content Outline: Diseases/Conditions that Impact Effective Treatment

➡ PTAEXAM ONE: QUESTION 132

A physical therapist assistant completes an upper quarter screening on a patient who has a suspected cervical spine lesion. Which of the following findings would **NOT** be expected with involvement of the C5 nerve root?

1. **Muscle weakness in the supinator and wrist extensors**
2. Diminished sensation in the deltoid area
3. Muscle weakness in the deltoid and biceps
4. Diminished biceps and brachioradialis reflexes

Correct Answer: 1 (Magee p. 24)

Involvement of a specific nerve root often results in predictable impairments including diminished sensation, muscle weakness, impaired reflexes, and paresthesias.

1. **Muscle weakness of the supinator (C5, C6, C7) and the extensor digitorum (C6, C7, C8) is associated with C6 involvement.**

2. Diminished sensation in the deltoid area and the anterior aspect of the entire arm to the base of the thumb is associated with the C5 dermatome.

3. Muscle weakness of the deltoid (C5, C6) and the biceps (C5, C6) is associated with the C5 myotome.

4. Diminished biceps (C5, C6) and brachioradialis (C5, C6) reflexes are associated with C5 involvement.

System: Neuromuscular and Nervous Systems
Content Outline: Diseases/Conditions that Impact Effective Treatment

➡ PTAEXAM ONE: QUESTION 133

Prior to working with a patient in the hospital setting, which of the following methods is **BEST** for a health care provider to use to verify the identity of the patient?

1. Checking the patient's chart

2. Asking the patient's caregiver

3. Confirming with the patient's physician

4. **Checking the patient's wrist band**

Correct Answer: 4 (Fairchild p. 3)

Prior to working with a patient in the hospital setting, a health care provider should verify the identity of the patient. Failure to accurately determine the identity of the patient could lead to severe consequences for the patient and the health care provider.

1. Checking the patient's chart allows the health care provider to access updated patient medical information, but would not definitively verify the patient's identity.

2. Asking the patient's caregiver about the patient's identity is an appropriate action, however, it relies solely on the accuracy of the information communicated by the caregiver. Although this would be accurate in the vast majority of instances, using a wrist band would be the most accurate method.

3. Confirming with the patient's physician can be useful to verify the identity of the patient, however, this method relies solely on the recollection of the physician. Given the numbers of patients that a physician encounters on a daily basis, it is distinctly possible that the physician could be mistaken.

4. **Checking the patient's wrist band is the most reliable method of verifying patient identity in the hospital. In addition, the health care provider should ask the patient to recite their first and last name, along with their date of birth. A wrist band is routinely applied in any hospital setting upon admission and is not removed until discharge.**

System: Non-Systems
Content Outline: Equipment, Devices, and Technologies;
  Therapeutic Modalities

➡ PTAEXAM ONE: QUESTION 134

A physical therapist assistant uses a floor scale to educate a patient on their current weight bearing status post lower extremity injury. Assuming the patient weighs 250 pounds and has been cleared for 30 percent weight bearing, what would be the **MOST** appropriate amount of weight in pounds transmitted through the involved lower extremity?

1. 50

2. **75**

3. 100

4. 175

Correct Answer: 2 (Fairchild p. 220)

The amount of weight bearing is often expressed as allowable pounds of pressure or as a percentage of total weight. A physical therapist assistant can assist patients to gain an awareness of the amount of weight transmitted through an extremity using a floor scale.

1. 50 pounds of weight transmitted through the involved lower extremity would correspond to 20% of the patient's body weight (50 pounds / 250 pounds x 100 = 20% weight bearing).

2. **75 pounds of weight transmitted through the involved lower extremity would correspond to 30% of the patient's body weight (75 pounds / 250 pounds x 100 = 30% weight bearing).**

3. 100 pounds of weight transmitted through the involved lower extremity would correspond to 40% of the patient's body weight (100 pounds / 250 pounds x 100 = 40% weight bearing).

4. 175 pounds of weight transmitted through the involved lower extremity would correspond to 70% of the patient's body weight (175 pounds / 250 pounds x 100 = 70% weight bearing).

System: Non-Systems
Content Outline: Equipment, Devices, and Technologies;
  Therapeutic Modalities

⬤ Level 1

⬤ Level 1   p. 604

➡ PTAEXAM ONE: QUESTION 135

A physical therapist assistant observes an electrocardiogram of a patient who is taking beta-blockers. Which of the following electrocardiogram changes would **MOST** likely be caused by beta-blockers?

1. **Sinus bradycardia**
2. Sinus tachycardia
3. Premature ventricular contractions
4. ST segment sagging

Correct Answer: 1 (Hillegass p. 314)

Beta-adrenergic blocking agents (beta-blockers) decrease heart rate, blood pressure, and myocardial contractility.

1. **Sinus bradycardia is a slow sinus rhythm of less than 60 beats per minute. It may occur from beta-blocker medication, during sleep, in physically fit individuals, acute myocardial infarction, carotid sinus pressure, and in response to increased vagal tone due to pain.**

2. Sinus tachycardia is a rapid sinus rhythm of greater than 100 beats per minute. It is usually caused by something that increases sympathetic activity, such as excitement, pain, fever, hypoxia, exercise, and stimulants. Beta-blockers have the opposite effect on heart rate.

3. A premature ventricular contraction (PVC) is a premature beat arising from an ectopic focus in the ventricle. PVCs may be precipitated by anxiety, tobacco, alcohol, caffeine, and any condition causing myocardial ischemia. PVCs are not caused by beta-blockers.

4. ST segment sagging or depression is indicative of myocardial ischemia and is not caused by beta-blockers.

System: Cardiovascular and Pulmonary Systems
Content Outline: Diseases/Conditions that Impact Effective Treatment

➡ PTAEXAM ONE: QUESTION 136

A physical therapist assistant uses neuromuscular electrical stimulation on a patient post open knee meniscectomy. What frequency of treatment is the **MOST** beneficial for the assistant to utilize when the goal is to promote strengthening?

1. Two times per day
2. One time per week
3. **Three times per week**
4. Once every two weeks

Correct Answer: 3 (Prentice p. 134)

The question indicates that the focus of the intervention is to increase strength and therefore it is necessary for the intervention to be performed multiple times each week. Frequency is also influenced by variables such as intensity, repetitions, and sets.

1. Two times per day would be excessive since the intensity of the strengthening activity would require more recovery time. Failure to have sufficient recovery time may lead to delayed onset muscle soreness, excessive microtrauma, and possible injury.

2. One time per week is insufficient based on the stated goal of promoting strength. This frequency may be more appropriate for a maintenance program.

3. **Three times per week is a general guideline for strengthening activities. The frequency allows for adequate intensity and sufficient rest time to minimize microtrauma and avoid delayed onset muscle soreness.**

4. Once every two weeks is insufficient for virtually any therapeutic purpose, most notably strengthening.

System: Non-Systems
Content Outline: Equipment, Devices, and Technologies; Therapeutic Modalities

 Level 2   p. 380, 511

Level 2   p. 641-642

➡ PTAEXAM ONE: QUESTION 137

A physical therapist assistant assesses a patient's present pain level and concludes that the current patient-controlled analgesia protocol is not adequate. Which of the following actions is the MOST appropriate for the assistant to take?

1. Modify the allowable medication dosage
2. Eliminate the lockout interval
3. **Contact the patient's nurse**
4. Page the patient's referring physician

Correct Answer: 3 (Fairchild p. 285)

Patient-controlled analgesia allows the patient to manage their pain by delivering an intravenous analgesic dose with preset parameters. Opioids are often the self-administered medication used with patient-controlled analgesia.

1. Modifying the allowable medication dosage is the responsibility of the medical team which is led by the physician. Engaging in this type of activity would be outside the scope of practice of a physical therapist assistant.

2. A lockout interval refers to the period of time where a patient-controlled analgesia system will not allow the patient to receive medication. Eliminating the lockout interval would alter the patient's established medication schedule and would therefore be outside the scope of practice of a physical therapist assistant.

3. **A nurse is the health care professional responsible for assessing the overall effectiveness of patient-controlled analgesia and adjusting settings based on the standard orders. The amount of contact time the nurse spends with the patient would allow them to better assess if the patient's present pain level is an isolated event or a recurring theme. If needed, the nurse would then be able to contact the referring physician and discuss the most appropriate action.**

4. Paging the patient's referring physician would be more appropriate in the event of an emergent situation. The nurse would be the more logical choice in this instance given the stated findings. If necessary, the physician could later be consulted by the nurse or the physical therapist assistant.

System: Non-Systems
Content Outline: Equipment, Devices, and Technologies;
    Therapeutic Modalities

➡ PTAEXAM ONE: QUESTION 138

A physical therapist assistant inserts a heel lift into a patient's shoe. Which of the following conditions would MOST warrant this type of modification?

1. **Equinus contracture**
2. Sesamoiditis
3. Metatarsalgia
4. Pes cavus deformity

Correct Answer: 1 (Brody p. 652)

A heel lift is a wedge-shaped shoe insert which places the foot in a relatively plantar flexed position. It is indicated for patients with a fixed equinus deformity, Achilles tendonitis, and plantar fasciitis.

1. **An equinus contracture refers to the inability to bring the foot up to a neutral position due to either tightness of the muscles and/or tendons in the calf, scarring of the ankle joint capsule or spurring that restricts normal ankle motion. The name originates from horses (equine) who essentially walk on their toes. A heel lift may be used with an equinus contracture in an attempt to improve the fluidity and efficiency of movement.**

2. Sesamoiditis refers to the inflammation surrounding the sesamoid bones under the first metatarsal head. Shoe prescription would include a transverse metatarsal bar to redistribute pressure from the metatarsal heads to the metatarsal shafts. A rocker sole can be used to reduce motion of the painful joint. A heel lift may serve to exacerbate pressure on the sesamoid bones.

3. Metatarsalgia refers to pain around the metatarsal heads secondary to compression of the plantar digital nerve. Shoe prescription would be similar to the description provided for sesamoiditis. A heel lift may serve to exacerbate pressure on the metatarsals.

4. A pes cavus deformity refers to an exaggerated longitudinal arch that results in a plantar flexed forefoot, retracted toes, and increased weight bearing stress to the metatarsal heads and heel. Shoe prescription would include a cushion sole to absorb shock, a metatarsal bar to shift weight from the metatarsal heads, and a lateral flare to increase overall stability. A heel lift may serve to exacerbate pressure on the metatarsals.

System: Non-Systems
Content Outline: Equipment, Devices, and Technologies;
    Therapeutic Modalities

⏺ Level 3

⏺ Level 2   p. 125

► PTAEXAM ONE: QUESTION 139

An entry in the medical record indicates that a patient experienced hypovolemic shock. Which of the following conditions would **MOST** likely be associated with the development of hypovolemic shock?

1. **Burns**
2. Compartment syndrome
3. Myocardial infarction
4. Cardiac tamponade

Correct Answer: 1 (Goodman – Pathology p. 706)

Hypovolemic shock refers to a life-threatening condition caused by insufficient circulating blood volume. Symptoms of this condition include hypotension due to lack of circulating blood volume, anxiety, altered mental state, cool and clammy skin, rapid and thready pulse, thirst, and fatigue due to inadequate oxygenation.

1. **The most common causes of hypovolemic shock include hemorrhage (i.e., blood loss) or severe burns (i.e., fluid loss) which can dramatically reduce tissue perfusion. Hypovolemia due to damaged blood vessels is a common complication of burns and can result in the heart being unable to pump a sufficient amount of blood to the body.**

2. Compartment syndrome is a serious medical condition that causes compression of nerves and blood vessels in an enclosed body space. The result is a dangerous disruption of nerve conduction and blood flow that can threaten the viability of body structures. Anterior compartment syndrome is an example of a compartment syndrome affecting the anterior compartment of the lower leg.

3. Myocardial infarction occurs when there is poor coronary artery perfusion, ischemia, and subsequent necrosis of the cardiac tissue usually due to thrombus, arterial blockage or atherosclerosis. Symptoms of this condition include deep pain or pressure in the substernal area with or without pain radiating to the jaw or into the left arm or the back.

4. Cardiac tamponade occurs when fluid in the pericardium creates pressure on the heart, preventing the heart from properly filling with blood. As a result, less blood leaves the heart, which causes a sharp drop in blood pressure. If left untreated, cardiac tamponade can be fatal.

System: Non-Systems
Content Outline: Safety and Protection; Professional
    Responsibilities; Research

► PTAEXAM ONE: QUESTION 140

A patient sustains a deep laceration on the anterior surface of the forearm. The physical therapist assistant attempts to stop the bleeding by applying direct pressure over the wound, but is unsuccessful. The **MOST** appropriate action is for the assistant to attempt to apply compression over the pressure point of which of the following arteries?

1. **Brachial**
2. Femoral
3. Radial
4. Ulnar

Correct Answer: 1 (Fairchild p. 332)

When direct pressure and elevation fail to stop severe bleeding from an open wound, physical therapist assistants may attempt to use the pressure point of a major artery. This technique is most often employed when the wound is located on an upper or lower extremity. The use of a pressure point not only stops circulation to the injured extremity, but also stops circulation within the arterial distribution. As a result, this technique should be employed only when it is absolutely necessary.

1. **The brachial artery can be compressed against the medial aspect of the humerus in an attempt to control the bleeding. The pressure point is located on the inside of the arm in the groove between the triceps and biceps, approximately midway between the axilla and the elbow. The brachial artery's location, proximal to the forearm, makes it possible to control bleeding.**

2. The femoral artery can be compressed against the pelvic bone. The pressure point is on the front of the thigh immediately below the middle of the crease of the groin where the artery crosses over the pelvic bone as it moves to the leg. Applying pressure to an artery in the lower extremity would not be helpful to control bleeding in the forearm.

3. The radial artery is covered by only fascia and skin at the distal end of the radius and is therefore extremely accessible. The artery is located at the wrist on the volar surface, medial to the styloid process of the radius. The distal location of the artery would not effectively stop bleeding caused by a laceration in the forearm.

4. The radial and ulnar arteries are the two main arteries of the forearm. The ulnar artery lies lateral to the tendon of the flexor carpi ulnaris. Applying pressure to the ulnar artery would not be an effective technique to stop the bleeding.

System: Non-Systems
Content Outline: Safety and Protection; Professional
    Responsibilities; Research

  Level 2   p. 44, 678

  Level 2   p. 676-678

➡ PTAEXAM ONE: QUESTION 141

A physical therapist assistant attempts to enhance a patient's shoulder stability through the use of approximation. Which of the following neurodevelopmental positions would be the **MOST** appropriate to accomplish the stated objective?

1. Bridging
2. Half-kneeling
3. **Prone on elbows**
4. Sitting

Correct Answer: 3 (O'Sullivan p. 415)

Approximation is a therapeutic exercise technique designed to facilitate contraction and stability through joint compression. The compression force is most often applied to joints through gravity acting on body weight, manual contacts or weight belts.

1. Bridging occurs when a patient positioned in hooklying lifts their buttocks and low back from a fixed surface. The position can be used to facilitate pelvic motion and for strengthening the hip extensors. Bridging does not require the involvement of the upper extremities.

2. A half-kneeling position refers to a position where the body is supported by a single knee and the foot of the forward lower extremity. The position can be used to enhance trunk and lower extremity control as well as to improve balance reactions. Half-kneeling does not require the involvement of the upper extremities.

3. **Prone on elbows is characterized by prone positioning with weight bearing on the elbows and through the forearms. Approximation occurs in prone on elbows due to the force of gravity and body weight combined with the distal component being fixed (i.e., elbow in direct contact with the surface). The technique is commonly used to enhance shoulder stability.**

4. A sitting position would not necessarily permit weight bearing through the upper extremities. Approximation would not occur unless the upper extremity was in direct contact with a surface (i.e., closed-chain).

System: Neuromuscular and Nervous Systems
Content Outline: Interventions

➡ PTAEXAM ONE: QUESTION 142

A physical therapist assistant instructs a patient to perform a standing stretch as shown in the image. Which of the following structures is on the **MOST** stretch with this technique?

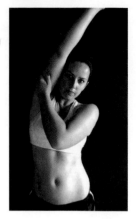

1. Horizontal abductors
2. **Inferior capsule**
3. Pectoralis major
4. Pectoralis minor

Correct Answer: 2 (Dutton p. 694)

Physical therapist assistants routinely instruct patients in a variety of self-stretching activities. Specific stretching exercises should be prescribed based on the established therapeutic objectives.

1. The horizontal abductors would be stretched by moving the arm into horizontal adduction. Horizontal adduction requires the upper arm to move toward the chest in a transverse plane with the shoulder flexed at 90 degrees.

2. **The capsule encompasses the glenohumeral joint and attaches to the scapula, humerus, and head of the biceps. The inferior portion of the capsule is tightened when the arm is raised overhead. A restriction in the inferior capsule often accompanies prolonged periods of immobilization and results in difficulty lifting the arm overhead.**

3. The pectoralis major consists of a sternocostal head and a clavicular head. Collectively, the muscle horizontally adducts and medially rotates the humerus. As a result, the muscle is stretched by placing the arms in horizontal abduction and lateral rotation. An example of a pectoralis major stretch would be a corner wall stretch.

4. The pectoralis minor stabilizes the scapula by drawing it inferiorly and anteriorly against the thoracic wall. The pectoralis minor is stretched in a manner similar to the various methods used to stretch the pectoralis major (e.g., corner wall stretch).

System: Musculoskeletal System
Content Outline: Interventions

 Level 2   p. 264

Level 1

▶ PTAEXAM ONE: QUESTION 143

A physical therapist assistant observes a patient standing in a pool immersed in water to the level of the neck performing a number of upper extremity exercises. Which active movement would be the **MOST** resisted by buoyancy with the patient starting with the upper extremity positioned at the side and the elbow in 90 degrees of flexion?

1. Elbow flexion
2. **Elbow extension**
3. Shoulder abduction
4. Shoulder medial rotation

Correct Answer: 2 (Coburn p. 67)

Archimedes' principle of buoyancy states that there is an upward force on the body when immersed in water equal to the amount of water that has been displaced by the body. When an individual exercises in water, the buoyant force works in opposition to the gravitational force.

1. Elbow flexion is a sagittal plane motion that would best be classified as buoyancy assisted since the motion occurs in the same direction as the buoyant force. As a result, the buoyant force would make performing elbow flexion significantly easier for the patient.

2. **Elbow extension is a sagittal plane motion that would best be classified as buoyancy resisted since the motion occurs in the opposite direction as the buoyant force. As a result, the buoyant force would make performing elbow extension more difficult for the patient.**

3. Shoulder abduction is a frontal plane motion that would best be classified as buoyancy assisted since the motion occurs in the same direction as the buoyant force. As a result, the buoyant force would make performing shoulder abduction easier for the patient.

4. Shoulder medial rotation is a transverse plane motion that would best be classified as buoyancy supported since the motion occurs parallel to the bottom of the pool. The buoyant force would assist to support the arm, but would not be resisted by buoyancy.

System: Musculoskeletal System
Content Outline: Interventions

▶ PTAEXAM ONE: QUESTION 144

A physical therapist assistant treats a patient who has epilepsy and is five days post total hip arthroplasty. Which of the following treatment environments would initially be the **MOST** desirable when treating this patient?

1. Therapeutic pool
2. Physical therapy gym
3. Hallway adjacent to the patient's room
4. **Private treatment room**

Correct Answer: 4 (Goodman - Differential Diagnosis p. 30)

Physical therapist assistants must be cognizant of side effects that may influence treatment when working with patients with epilepsy. General side effects of antiepileptic drugs that can affect therapy include headache, fatigue, dizziness, vomiting, and cerebellar dysfunction.

1. A therapeutic pool would not be ideal for a patient that is five days status post hip arthroplasty due to the lack of integrity of the incision. The therapeutic pool may have bright lights, vary in noise level, and present with other environmental risk factors that could precipitate a seizure.

2. The physical therapy gym is often a loud and busy setting that can serve as an environmental stimulus to precipitate a seizure. Although a gym is a desirable setting to work on many facets of rehabilitation after total hip arthroplasty, a private treatment room would be a more desirable initial setting given the presence of epilepsy.

3. The hallway may be loud, busy or contain bright lights. Although the setting allows for a variety of functional activities (e.g., gait training, mobility training), the presence of the environmental stimuli increases the risk of seizure activity.

4. **Treatment in a private treatment room is the most ideal option for this patient initially secondary to the diagnosis of epilepsy. When possible, it is desirable to avoid environmental stimuli that facilitate seizure activity. The risk of seizure activity associated with environmental stimuli increases significantly if the epilepsy is poorly controlled with drug therapy.**

System: Other Systems
Content Outline: Interventions

 Level 2   p. 630

Level 2   p. 248-249

SCOREBUILDERS

▶ PTAEXAM ONE: QUESTION 145

A physical therapist assistant treats a patient with a diagnosis of gouty arthritis. The assistant should **MOST** likely expect the patient's subjective reports of pain to be in which area of the body?

1. Hip
2. Knee
3. Ankle
4. **Toe**

Correct Answer: 4 (Goodman – Differential Diagnosis p. 413)

Gouty arthritis is a condition characterized by excess uric acid in the blood that results in the formation of crystals within the joints, which triggers a painful inflammatory response. Gouty arthritis can affect any of the joints in the body, though it commonly affects the peripheral joints of the lower extremities.

1. Though any joint can be affected by gouty arthritis, the hip is not a joint that is typically affected.

2. Though the knee can be affected by gouty arthritis, it makes up a relatively small percentage of the cases.

3. Though the ankle can be affected by gouty arthritis, it makes up a relatively small percentage of the cases.

4. **The peripheral joints of the feet are the sites most commonly affected by gouty arthritis. The metatarsophalangeal joint of the great toe is affected in 90% of the cases of gouty arthritis.**

System: Other Systems
Content Outline: Diseases/Conditions that Impact Effective Treatment

▶ PTAEXAM ONE: QUESTION 146

A group of physical therapists and physical therapist assistants develop a research project that examines the effect of increased abdominal muscle strength on forced vital capacity and forced expiratory volume. In order to conduct the study, the therapists are required to have the approval of the hospital Institutional Review Board. What is the **PRIMARY** purpose of this committee?

1. Protect the hospital from unnecessary litigation
2. **Ensure the rights of research subjects are protected**
3. Examine the design of the research project
4. Assess the financial ramifications of the research project

Correct Answer: 2 (Portney p. 52)

Federal regulations require an Institutional Review Board (IRB) review all research proposals prior to implementation to ensure that the rights of research subjects are protected.

1. By ensuring the rights of research subjects, the IRB may protect the hospital from litigation, however, protection from litigation is not the primary purpose of the committee.

2. **Ensuring the rights of research subjects is the primary purpose of the IRB. To do this, the IRB evaluates the scientific merit of the project, the competence of the investigators, the risk to subjects, and the feasibility of the project based on available resources.**

3. In evaluating the scientific merit of the project, the IRB will examine the research design. This is done to ensure that the rights of research subjects are protected since if the project is not scientifically sound, there can be no benefit.

4. In evaluating the research proposal, the IRB will consider the feasibility of the project based on the identified resources. The financial impact, however, is not the primary purpose of the IRB committee.

System: Non-Systems
Content Outline: Safety and Protection; Professional Responsibilities; Research

 Level 1   p. 564

 Level 1   p. 705

➡ PTAEXAM ONE: QUESTION 147

A patient sustained a patella fracture in a motor vehicle accident and the knee is maintained in extension using a straight leg knee immobilizer. Which of the following gait deviations would **MOST** likely be caused by the use of this type of immobilizer?

1. **Vaulting**
2. Antalgic gait
3. Increased plantar flexion
4. Trendelenburg gait

Correct Answer: 1 (Magee p. 1013)

The patella is a sesamoid bone attached to the tendon of the quadriceps femoris muscle. It plays a large role in the knee extensor mechanism functioning as an anatomical pulley. Following a patella fracture, the knee is typically immobilized in extension to prevent excessive force on the patella from the quadriceps tendon.

1. **Vaulting is characterized by heel elevation during stance in combination with hip and knee extension. Vaulting is performed to raise the pelvis in order to clear the contralateral limb during the swing phase. When the knee is locked in extension, the normal degree of knee flexion required during the swing phase does not occur resulting in difficulty clearing the foot. Vaulting can be an effective compensatory strategy when the knee is unable to flex.**

2. An antalgic gait is a protective gait pattern where the stance time is decreased to avoid weight bearing on the involved side due to pain. This is typically associated with a rapid and shorter swing phase of the uninvolved limb. Causes of antalgic gait include disease (usually bone or joint), joint inflammation, or injuries to muscles, tendons, and/or ligaments.

3. Increased plantar flexion is unlikely since the patient will have difficulty advancing the limb through the swing phase due to the lack of knee flexion. Exaggerated dorsiflexion is more likely to occur in order to clear the foot.

4. A Trendelenburg gait pattern is a compensatory pattern that occurs primarily as a result of gluteus medius weakness. As a result of this weakness, the gluteus medius does not stabilize the pelvis during stance. A drop of the contralateral pelvis is observed with a trunk lean ipsilateral to the side of the weakness.

System: Musculoskeletal System
Content Outline: Diseases/Conditions that Impact Effective Treatment

➡ PTAEXAM ONE: QUESTION 148

A physical therapist assistant observes a patient who sustained an injury to the musculocutaneous nerve complete a number of activities of daily living and functional skills. Which of the following tasks would be the **MOST** difficult for the patient to perform based on the stated injury?

1. Picking up marbles from the floor
2. Push-ups against a wall
3. **Drinking from a gallon of milk**
4. Holding the arm out to the side

Correct Answer: 3 (Kendall p. 253)

Peripheral nerves, which supply sensory and motor functions to the entire body, are commonly injured due to compression or shear forces, such as entrapment or sudden stretch. The musculocutaneous nerve innervates the brachialis, biceps brachii, and coracobrachialis muscles. Since the brachialis and biceps are two of the three primary elbow flexors, loss of motor function of these two muscles would dramatically weaken elbow flexion.

1. Picking up marbles from the floor requires a pincer grasp. Since the thenar muscles and muscles that oppose the thumb are innervated by the median nerve, activities that require fine motor skills would be most impacted by an injury to the median nerve rather than the musculocutaneous nerve.

2. Push-ups involve multiple joints and require the contribution of numerous muscles including the pectoralis major, anterior deltoid, and triceps. The muscles primarily involved in a push-up are not innervated by the musculocutaneous nerve.

3. **Drinking a gallon of milk requires elbow flexion range of motion and good strength of the elbow flexors. Since the musculocutaneous nerve supplies both the biceps brachii and brachialis muscles, this action would likely be the most difficult for the patient.**

4. Holding the arm out to the side requires activation of primarily the deltoid and supraspinatus muscles. The deltoid muscle is innervated by the axillary nerve and the supraspinatus is innervated by the suprascapular nerve. Injury to the musculocutaneous nerve would not impact the ability to hold the arm out to the side.

System: Neuromuscular and Nervous Systems
Content Outline: Diseases/Conditions that Impact Effective Treatment

➡ PTAEXAM ONE: QUESTION 149

A physical therapist assistant initiates an exercise program for a patient rehabilitating from cardiac surgery. During the treatment session, the assistant monitors the patient's oxygen saturation rate. Which of the following would be **MOST** representative of a normal oxygen saturation rate?

1. 82%
2. 87%
3. 92%
4. **97%**

Correct Answer: 4 (Hillegass p. 558)

Oxygen saturation (SaO$_2$) measures the percentage of hemoglobin saturated with oxygen. The normal range for oxygen saturation is between 95-98% in healthy individuals.

1. A value of 82% SaO$_2$ demonstrates significant hypoxemia resulting in the patient requiring continuous use of supplemental oxygen. Exercise would be contraindicated at this level.

2. A value of 87% SaO$_2$ is below the range for acceptable oxygen saturation. The patient would likely use supplemental oxygen at rest and with exercise. The patient should maintain 90% SaO$_2$ or better with supplemental oxygen use.

3. A value of 92% SaO$_2$ is not within normal limits for oxygen saturation. In most cases, the patient would be monitored to ensure that SaO$_2$ does not fall below 90% during exertion or exercise.

4. **A value of 97% SaO$_2$ is within the specified range of 95-98% for normal arterial oxygen saturation.**

System: Cardiovascular and Pulmonary Systems
Content Outline: Physical Therapy Data Collection

➡ PTAEXAM ONE: QUESTION 150

A physical therapist assistant attempts to educate a patient by using their hands to demonstrate facet movement in the cervical spine. The assistant indicates that the upper facets move bilaterally up and forward on the lower facets. This type of movement is characteristic of which of the following cervical motions?

1. **Flexion**
2. Extension
3. Sidebending
4. Rotation

Correct Answer: 1 (Magee p. 165)

The zygapophyseal joints are synovial joints covered with hyaline cartilage between the superior articular process of one vertebra and the inferior articular process of the vertebra directly above it. There are two facet joints involved in each spinal segment.

1. **Cervical flexion is characterized by the upper facets sliding up and anteriorly on the lower facets. This action serves to "open the joint."**

2. Cervical extension is characterized by the upper facets sliding down and posteriorly on the lower facets. This action serves to "close the joint."

3. Cervical sidebending is characterized by the upper facet sliding down and posteriorly on the side towards the movement. The facet on the side opposite the movement moves up and anteriorly.

4. Cervical rotation is characterized by the upper facet sliding down and posteriorly on the side towards the movement. The facet on the side opposite the movement moves up and anteriorly.

System: Musculoskeletal System
Content Outline: Physical Therapy Data Collection

  Level 2   p. 383

  Level 1   p. 68-69

NOTES

11

PHYSICAL THERAPIST ASSISTANT
EXAM TWO
ANSWER KEY

Scott Giles

PHYSICAL THERAPIST ASSISTANT EXAM TWO ANSWER KEY

DIRECTION

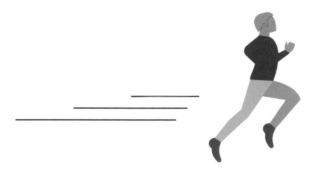

"If you don't know where you are going you could wind up some place else."

— Yogi Berra

Candidates must be proactive throughout the study process and avoid relying on their past accomplishments. Candidates that assess their progress throughout the study plan and make appropriate modifications often outperform candidates that prepare for the NPTE-PTA in a more random fashion.

➡ PTAEXAM TWO: QUESTION 1

A physical therapist assistant instructs a patient post thoracic surgery how to produce an effective cough. Which position would be the **MOST** appropriate to initiate treatment?

1. Standing
2. **Sitting**
3. Sidelying
4. Hooklying

Correct Answer: 2 (Hillegass p. 544)

An effective cough requires an inspiration greater than tidal volume, followed by closure of the glottis, abdominal muscle contraction, and sudden opening of the glottis for the forceful expulsion of the inspired air.

1. Although it is possible to perform a maximal inhalation needed for an effective cough, the standing position would not be the most appropriate position to initiate treatment after thoracic surgery.

2. **Sitting upright will maximize all of the steps needed to produce an effective cough.**

3. The sidelying position does not promote the maximal inhalation needed for an effective cough.

4. Hooklying refers to a position where the patient is lying in supine with their hips and knees bent and the feet flat on the floor with the arms positioned at their side. The hooklying position does not promote the maximal inhalation needed for an effective cough.

System: Cardiovascular and Pulmonary Systems
Content Outline: Interventions

➡ PTAEXAM TWO: QUESTION 2

A physical therapist assistant focuses on increasing range of motion through stretching and the use of proprioceptive neuromuscular facilitation (PNF) techniques. The patient in the image is performing an isotonic contraction of the hamstrings against resistance followed by passive stretching of the hamstrings by the assistant. Which of the following PNF techniques is being used on this patient?

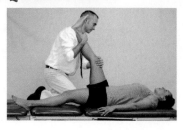

1. Alternating isometrics
2. Resisted progression
3. Agonistic reversal
4. **Contract-relax**

Correct Answer: 4 (Sullivan p. 66)

Proprioceptive neuromuscular facilitation techniques can assist with improving range of motion, stability, and coordination of movement. Hold-relax, contract-relax, and rhythmic stabilization can all be used to increase range of motion when immobility is due to muscle tightness.

1. Alternating isometrics consists of isometric contractions that are performed alternating from muscles on one side of the joint to the other side without rest. Alternating isometrics emphasizes endurance or strengthening.

2. Resisted progression is a technique used to improve coordination of proximal components during gait. Resistance is applied to an area such as the pelvis, hips or extremity during the gait cycle in order to enhance coordination, strength or endurance.

3. Agonistic reversal consists of a concentric contraction that is performed against resistance followed by alternating concentric and eccentric contractions with resistance. Agonistic reversal is used in a slow and sequential manner and may be used incrementally throughout the range to attain maximum control.

4. **Contract-relax is a technique used specifically to increase range of motion. As the extremity reaches the point of limitation, the patient performs a maximal contraction of the antagonistic muscle group. The therapist resists movement for eight to ten seconds with relaxation to follow and movement into the shortened range. The technique is repeated until no further gains in range of motion are noted.**

System: Neuromuscular and Nervous Systems
Content Outline: Interventions

 Level 2

 Level 1   p. 262-263

➡ PTAEXAM TWO: QUESTION 3

While performing gait analysis on a patient, a physical therapist assistant observes a posterior trunk lean during heel strike (initial contact) to foot flat (loading response). Which of the following interventions would be the **MOST** appropriate to address the observed gait pattern?

1. Strengthening exercises for the quadriceps
2. **Strengthening exercises for the gluteus maximus**
3. Stretching exercises for the hip extensors
4. Stretching exercises for the hip internal rotators

Correct Answer: 2 (Dutton p. 313)

The gluteus maximus gait, which is a compensation for weakness of the gluteus maximus muscle, is characterized by a posterior trunk lean between heel strike (initial contact) and foot flat (loading response) in an attempt to maintain hip extension. In normal gait, the hip extensors should act concentrically to extend the hip during the early stance phase of the gait cycle.

1. The quadriceps should be activating eccentrically during the early stance phase. Hyperextension of the knee often occurs as a compensation to keep the knee from buckling, which is accomplished by an anterior trunk lean during early stance. Strengthening of the quadriceps would not address the weak hip extensors, primarily the gluteus maximus, that led to the described gait deviation.

2. **Strengthening exercises for the gluteus maximus would be the most appropriate intervention since the gait deviation described is typically a compensation for weak hip extensors, primarily the gluteus maximus. An emphasis on the concentric phase would also be useful due to the role of the hip extensors during this phase of the gait cycle.**

3. Stretching exercises for the hip extensors would not be indicated since the gait deviation is associated with weakness of the hip extensors, not shortening. Stretching may also further weaken these muscles.

4. Stretching exercises for the hip internal rotators would be appropriate if the internal rotators were tight. Tightness in the internal rotators often results in a toe-in gait pattern.

System: Musculoskeletal System
Content Outline: Interventions

➡ PTAEXAM TWO: QUESTION 4

A patient post CVA scores 39/56 on the Berg Balance Scale prior to discharge home from a rehabilitation facility. The physical therapist assistant should be able to make which of the following conclusions from the results of the assessment?

1. The patient will require a low burden of care once discharged home
2. The patient will have difficulty independently reaching for objects
3. **The patient is at significant risk for multiple or recurrent falls**
4. The patient will require assistance during ambulation

Correct Answer: 3 (O'Sullivan p. 234)

The Berg Balance Scale is a tool designed to assess a patient's risk for falling. There are fourteen tasks, each scored on an ordinal scale from 0-4. These tasks include static activities, transitional movements, and dynamic activities in sitting and standing positions. The maximum score is a 56 with a score less than 45 indicating an increased risk for falling. This tool can be used as a one-time examination or as an ongoing tool to monitor a patient who may be at risk for falls.

1. The Functional Independence Measure (FIM) provides a level of burden through assessment of mobility and ADL management. This interdisciplinary tool assesses 18 specific activities within six major categories to assess overall level of function and burden of care during mobility and ADLs. The Berg Balance Scale does not measure the burden of care.

2. The Functional Reach Test is a single task screening tool used to assess standing balance and risk of falling. A person is required to stand upright with a static base of support. A yardstick is positioned to measure the forward distance that a patient can reach without moving the feet. A patient that falls below the age appropriate range for functional reach has an increased risk for falling. The Berg Balance Scale does not measure functional reach.

3. **A Berg Balance Scale score of less than 40 indicates significant increased risk for recurrent or multiple falls. A person scoring a 39 would not be a candidate for returning home alone without assistance and would likely require assistance for all mobility in order to ensure patient safety.**

4. The Barthel Index is designed to measure the amount of assistance needed to perform ten different ADL and mobility activities with a total maximum score of 100. The index consists of 10 categories that includes ambulation on level surfaces. The Berg Balance Scale does not measure balance during ambulation or the required level of assistance during functional activities and instead looks at the risk of falling.

System: Neuromuscular and Nervous Systems
Content Outline: Physical Therapy Data Collection

 Level 2   p. 81-85

 Level 2   p. 241

➡ PTAEXAM TWO: QUESTION 5

A physical therapist assistant uses a subjective pain scale to assess pain intensity that consists of a 10 cm line with each end anchored by one extreme of perceived pain intensity. The patient is asked to mark on the line the point that best describes their present pain level. Which pain scale is being used here?

1. Descriptor Differential Scale
2. Verbal Rating Scale
3. **Visual Analogue Scale**
4. Numerical Rating Scale

Correct Answer: 3 (Umphred p. 990)

There are a variety of commonly used pain scales in physical therapy. Physical therapist assistants should have familiarity with the various scales and be able to select an appropriate scale based on the breadth and depth of information they are attempting to collect.

1. The Descriptor Differential Scale consists of 12 descriptor items each centered over 21 horizontal dashes. At the extreme left dash is a minus sign and at the extreme right dash is a plus sign. Patients are asked to rate the magnitude of their pain in terms of each descriptor.

2. A Verbal Rating Scale is most often used to assess pain affect. The scale typically consists of a series of adjectives describing increasing levels of unpleasantness such as "distracting," "oppressive" or "agonizing."

3. **A Visual Analogue Scale is a tool used to assess pain intensity using a 10-15 centimeter line with the left anchor indicating "no pain" and the right anchor indicating "the worst pain you can have." The level of perceived pain is indicated on the line and is reassessed frequently over the course of physical therapy to qualify changes in the pain level and to assess progress.**

4. A Numerical Rating Scale asks patients to rate their perceived level of pain intensity on a numerical scale from 0-10 or 0-100. The 0 represents "no pain" and the 10 or 100 represents "pain as bad as it could be."

System: Other Systems
Content Outline: Physical Therapy Data Collection

➡ PTAEXAM TWO: QUESTION 6

A physical therapist assistant works with a patient diagnosed with Duchenne muscular dystrophy less than one year ago. Assuming a normal progression, which of the following findings should the assistant expect to occur **FIRST**?

1. Distal muscle weakness
2. **Proximal muscle weakness**
3. Impaired respiratory function
4. Inability to perform activities of daily living

Correct Answer: 2 (Ratliffe p. 241)

Duchenne muscular dystrophy is an inherited disorder, characterized by rapidly worsening muscle weakness that starts in the proximal muscles of the lower extremities and pelvis, and later affects all voluntary muscles.

1. Distal muscles are affected later in the course of the disease process.

2. **Muscle weakness and atrophy begin in the proximal muscles of the lower extremities and pelvis, then progress to the muscles of the shoulders and neck, followed by loss of upper extremity muscles and respiratory muscles.**

3. The muscles of respiration are not initially affected in patients with Duchenne muscular dystrophy.

4. As the condition progresses, weakness begins to interfere with activities of daily living.

System: Neuromuscular and Nervous Systems
Content Outline: Diseases/Conditions that Impact Effective Treatment

 Level 1   p. 72-73

 Level 2   p. 284, 302-303

➡ PTAEXAM TWO: QUESTION 7

A patient reports experiencing an increase in low back pain following ballistic activities. The patient previously participated in competitive gymnastics, however, reports that her back was unable to tolerate the intensity of training. Based on the presented x-ray, which of the following medical conditions should the physical therapist assistant **MOST** suspect?

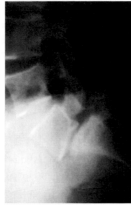

1. Spondylitis

2. Spondylolysis

3. **Spondylolisthesis**

4. Spondyloptosis

Correct Answer: 3 (Magee p. 569)

There are a variety of commonly encountered medical conditions that significantly impact the lumbar spine. Physical therapist assistants should be familiar with the clinical presentation and management of these medical conditions.

1. Spondylitis refers to inflammation of a vertebra.

2. Spondylolysis refers to a defect in the pars interarticularis or the arch of the vertebra. This is most common in the L5 vertebra, but can also occur in other lumbar or thoracic vertebrae.

3. **Spondylolisthesis refers to the forward displacement of one vertebra over another. The x-ray involves spondylolisthesis at the L5-S1 level. Individuals involved in physical activities such as weight lifting, gymnastics or football are particularly susceptible to this condition. The severity of the spondylolisthesis is classified on a scale of 1-5 based on how much a given vertebral body has slipped forward over the vertebral body beneath it.**

4. Spondyloptosis refers to the condition where a vertebral body has shifted completely off of the adjacent vertebral body (grade 5).

System: Musculoskeletal System
Content Outline: Diseases/Conditions that Impact Effective
    Treatment

➡ PTAEXAM TWO: QUESTION 8

A patient recently diagnosed with anemia asks the physical therapist assistant what effect this condition will have on their ability to participate in an exercise program. Which of the following responses is the **MOST** appropriate for the assistant to give to the patient?

1. You may feel as though your muscles are weak

2. You may experience frequent nausea

3. Your aerobic capacity may be reduced

4. **You may have a tendency to become fatigued**

Correct Answer: 4 (Goodman – Pathology p. 713)

Anemia refers to a reduction in the number of circulating red blood cells or reduction in hemoglobin. Symptoms of anemia include pallor of the skin, vertigo, and general malaise.

1. Although a patient may sense that their muscles are weak, fatigue will have a greater impact on the patient's ability to complete a formal exercise program.

2. Nausea refers to the sensation of unease and discomfort in the stomach with an urge to vomit. Nausea is a common side effect of many medications and is commonly associated with chemotherapy, pregnancy, and general anesthesia. Nausea is not typically associated with anemia.

3. Anemia may adversely affect aerobic capacity. However, this is not a term that most patients would readily understand.

4. **Anemia is a common cause of fatigue. Fatigue often results since there are an inadequate number of red blood cells available to transport oxygen to the tissues of the body.**

System: Cardiovascular and Pulmonary Systems
Content Outline: Diseases/Conditions that Impact Effective
    Treatment

⦿ Level 2   p. 166-167

⦿ Level 2   p. 358, 369-370

➡ PTAEXAM TWO: QUESTION 9

A physical therapist assistant working with a pediatric population suspects a patient's allergic reaction to latex is associated with their medical condition. Which of the following medical diagnoses would be the **MOST** likely to have latex allergies?

1. **Myelomeningocele**
2. Cerebral palsy
3. Down syndrome
4. Muscular dystrophy

Correct Answer: 1 (Palisano p. 555)

Latex allergies are common in approximately 70% of children with myelomeningocele. Latex is common in the environment and can be life-threatening for children with latex allergies.

1. **Myelomeningocele is a severe form of spina bifida characterized by herniation of meninges, cerebrospinal fluid, and the spinal cord extending through the defect in the vertebrae. Some children with myelomeningocele may have life-threatening anaphylaxis when exposed to certain types of latex. Most health care organizations including children's hospitals have precaution policies related to latex exposure. Physical therapist assistants should ask if a child with myelomeningocele specifically has latex allergies.**

2. Cerebral palsy is an umbrella term used to describe a group of non-progressive movement disorders that result from brain damage. Latex allergies are not as prevalent in the population of children with cerebral palsy, however, physical therapist assistants should always ask about allergies (e.g., foods, medications, products) during an examination. This is especially important when working in a school or community organization.

3. Down syndrome is a genetic abnormality consisting of an extra twenty-first chromosome, termed trisomy 21. Latex allergies are not as prevalent in the population of children with Down syndrome, however, physical therapist assistants should always ask about allergies (e.g., foods, medications, products) during an examination. This is especially important when working in a school or community organization.

4. Muscular dystrophy is a sex-linked disorder characterized by progressive muscular weakness. Latex allergies are not as prevalent in the population of children with muscular dystrophy, however, physical therapist assistants should always ask about allergies (e.g., foods, medications, products) during an examination. This is especially important when working in a school or community organization.

System: Neuromuscular and Nervous Systems
Content Outline: Diseases/Conditions that Impact Effective Treatment

➡ PTAEXAM TWO: QUESTION 10

A patient informs a physical therapist assistant how frustrated they feel after being examined by their physician, reporting that they become so nervous that they cannot ask any questions during scheduled office visits. Which of the following responses is the **MOST** appropriate if the desired outcome is for the patient to be a more active participant?

1. Offer to go with the patient to their next scheduled physician visit
2. Offer to call the physician and ask any relevant questions
3. **Suggest that the patient write down questions for the physician and bring them to the next scheduled visit**
4. Tell the patient it is a very normal response to be nervous in the presence of a physician

Correct Answer: 3 (Purtilo p. 90)

The physical therapist assistant should attempt to identify a strategy or strategies that the patient can use to take a more active role during visits with the physician.

1. It is probably not realistic for the physical therapist assistant to go with the patient to their next scheduled visit. In addition, the action places the burden on the physical therapist assistant and does not promote a long-term change in the patient's current behavior.

2. Offering to call the physician and ask any relevant questions is similar to the previous option, however, may be slightly more practical. The action, however, does not require the patient to take a more active role and instead uses the physical therapist assistant as an intermediary.

3. **Writing down questions allows the patient to reflect on the information they would like to gather in advance and provides the structure necessary to reduce the influence of the patient's anxiety during office visits.**

4. Acknowledging that many people are nervous in the presence of a physician may make the patient momentarily feel better, however, it does not provide the patient with a viable method to change their current behavior.

System: Non-Systems
Content Outline: Safety and Protection; Professional Responsibilities; Research

 Level 2   p. 284, 330-331

● Level 3

⟹ PTAEXAM TWO: QUESTION 11

A physical therapist assistant treating a patient rehabilitating from spinal surgery four days ago observes the patient's incision. What type of healing is **BEST** depicted in the image?

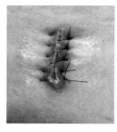

1. **Primary intention**
2. Delayed primary intention
3. Secondary intention
4. Tertiary intention

Correct Answer: 1 (Sussman p. 215)

Healing by intention refers to the method by which a wound heals. Wound characteristics such as etiology, depth, border integrity, and wound bed contamination are typically considered when determining which closure method is most appropriate.

1. **Healing by primary intention is most commonly associated with acute wounds that have minimal associated tissue loss (e.g., surgical wound, laceration, puncture wound). In these wounds, clean edges are reapproximated and closed with sutures, staples or adhesives to facilitate re-epithelialization.**

2. Healing by delayed primary intention is most commonly associated with acute wounds that have minimal associated tissue loss, but are at high risk for developing complications (e.g., infection, dehiscence). These wounds are temporarily left open until risk factors have been alleviated and then are closed by usual primary intention methods.

3. Healing by secondary intention is most commonly associated with wounds which have significant tissue loss, necrosis or borders that cannot be reapproximated (e.g., full-thickness wound, pressure ulcer). These wounds are left open and typically require specialized dressings and ongoing wound care to facilitate healing.

4. Healing by tertiary intention is synonymous with healing by delayed primary intention. Risk factors such as wound bed contamination, infection, and significant local edema increase the risk of healing complications and must be addressed before the wound can be appropriately closed by usual primary intention methods.

System: Other Systems
Content Outline: Diseases/Conditions that Impact Effective
    Treatment

⟹ PTAEXAM TWO: QUESTION 12

Which of the following components of balance would be **MOST** impacted by a patient using the suspensory strategy to control their balance?

1. Line of gravity
2. **Center of mass**
3. Base of support
4. Limits of stability

Correct Answer: 2 (Kisner p. 268)

The suspensory strategy is used to lower the center of mass during standing or ambulation in order to control balance. Examples of this strategy include knee flexion, crouching or squatting.

1. The line of gravity refers to a vertical line through the center of gravity. The center of gravity refers to the vertical projection of the center of mass to the ground. The line of gravity would not necessarily be dramatically altered using the suspensory strategy.

2. **The center of mass refers to the point that corresponds to the center of the total body mass. This point is where the body is in perfect equilibrium. The center of mass would be dramatically lowered using the suspensory strategy as the body assumes a crouching or squatting position.**

3. The base of support is defined as the perimeter of the contact area between the body and its support surface. Foot placement is the primary determinant of base of support. The suspensory strategy involves assuming a crouching or squatting position, however, not necessarily increasing the base of support.

4. Limits of stability refers to the sway boundaries in which an individual can maintain equilibrium without changing their base of support. Limits of stability would not be significantly altered using the suspensory strategy.

System: Neuromuscular and Nervous Systems
Content Outline: Interventions

⦿ Level 2   👓 p. 440

⦿ Level 2   👓 p. 240-241

➡ PTAEXAM TWO: QUESTION 13

A physical therapist assistant positions a patient as shown in the image to assess the patient's report of complete paresis of the right lower extremity. The assistant instructs the patient to perform a rapid straight leg raise with their left lower extremity. Which of the following findings would **BEST** dispute the patient's assertion?

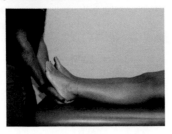

1. The patient is unable to lift their left heel from the assistant's hand.

2. The patient experiences radiating pain into the right lower extremity.

3. **The patient exerts a downward force into the assistant's hand with their right heel.**

4. The patient reports severe pain while performing the straight leg raise.

Correct Answer: 3 (Magee p. 612)

The Hoover test is often employed as a gross test for malingering. The therapist places one hand underneath each calcaneus with the patient lying in supine. The patient is then asked to perform a straight leg raise on the uninvolved extremity while the therapist simultaneously assesses motor output on the involved side.

1. The Hoover test relies on assessing the reaction of the contralateral limb rather than the quality of the straight leg raise.

2. The Hoover test is designed to provide insight on potential malingering rather than serving as a provocative test intended to create radiating pain or other signs or symptoms.

3. **A rapid straight leg raise of the left (uninvolved) lower extremity should result in the patient exerting a downward force into the therapist's hand with the right (involved) heel. This action would be considered a normal response due to the effort associated with performing the straight leg raise, therefore disputing the patient's claim of complete paresis of the right lower extremity.**

4. The Hoover test is not influenced by the presence or absence of pain.

System: Neuromuscular and Nervous Systems
Content Outline: Physical Therapy Data Collection

➡ PTAEXAM TWO: QUESTION 14

A patient diagnosed with ankylosing spondylitis exhibits a forward stooped posture. Which upper extremity proprioceptive neuromuscular facilitation (PNF) pattern should the physical therapist assistant **BEST** utilize in order to achieve the goal of improving this patient's posture?

1. D1 extension

2. D1 flexion

3. D2 extension

4. **D2 flexion**

Correct Answer: 4 (Sullivan p. 300)

A proprioceptive neuromuscular facilitation approach utilizes methods that promote or hasten the response of the neuromuscular mechanism through stimulation of the proprioceptors. The two diagonal patterns are commonly referred to as D1 and D2 where "D" stands for diagonal and "1" and "2" refer to specific patterns of movement. To improve the patient's standing posture the physical therapist assistant should use a pattern that requires the patient to move the arms upward and away from the body (D2 flexion).

1. The command for D1 extension would be to open your hand and push down and away from your body.

2. The command for D1 flexion would be to close your hand and pull up and across your body.

3. The command for D2 extension would be to close your hand and pull down and across your body.

4. **The command for D2 flexion would be to open your hand and pull up and away from your body. The pattern emphasizes shoulder flexion, abduction, and lateral rotation which would facilitate improved standing posture.**

System: Neuromuscular and Nervous Systems
Content Outline: Interventions

Level 1

Level 2   p. 261

➡ PTAEXAM TWO: QUESTION 15

A physical therapist assistant attempts to examine a wound with full-thickness skin loss that is obscured by eschar. Which pressure injury stage is **BEST** depicted by this scenario?

1. Stage 2
2. Stage 3
3. Stage 4
4. **Unstageable**

Correct Answer: 4 (Sussman p. 235)

Pressure injuries, also referred to as decubitus ulcers, result from sustained or prolonged pressure on tissue at levels greater than that of capillary pressure. Skin covering bony prominences is particularly susceptible to localized ischemia and tissue necrosis due to pressure. Factors contributing to pressure injuries include shearing forces, moisture, heat, friction, medications, muscle atrophy, malnutrition, and debilitating medical conditions.

1. A stage 2 pressure injury describes partial-thickness loss of skin with exposed dermis. The wound bed is viable, pink or red, moist, and may also present as an intact or ruptured serum-filled blister. Adipose and deeper tissues are not visible. Granulation tissue, slough, and eschar are not present. These injuries commonly result from shear over the pelvis and shear in the heel. This stage should not be used to describe moisture-associated skin damage including incontinence-associated dermatitis, intertriginous dermatitis, medical adhesive-related skin injury or traumatic wounds.

2. A stage 3 pressure injury describes full-thickness loss of skin in which adipose is visible in the ulcer and granulation tissue and epibole are often present. Slough and/or eschar may be visible, but they do not obscure the extent of tissue loss. Fascia, muscle, tendon, ligament, cartilage, and/or bone are not exposed.

3. A stage 4 pressure injury describes full-thickness skin and tissue loss with exposed or directly palpable fascia, muscle, tendon, ligament, cartilage or bone in the ulcer. Slough and/or eschar may be visible, but they do not obscure the extent of tissue loss.

4. **An unstageable pressure injury is characterized by full-thickness skin and tissue loss in which the extent of tissue damage within the ulcer cannot be confirmed because it is obscured by slough or eschar. If slough or eschar is removed, a stage 3 or stage 4 pressure injury will be revealed.**

System: Other Systems
Content Outline: Physical Therapy Data Collection

➡ PTAEXAM TWO: QUESTION 16

Which of the following objective findings would **MOST** severely limit a patient who has peripheral arterial disease from participating in an ambulation exercise program?

1. **Signs of resting claudication**
2. Decreased peripheral pulses
3. Cool skin upon palpation
4. Blood pressure of 165/90 mm Hg

Correct Answer: 1 (Hillegass p. 63)

Peripheral arterial disease refers to a condition involving the arterial system that results in compromised circulation to the extremities. Resting claudication is typically considered a contraindication to active exercise in patients with peripheral arterial disease.

1. **Claudication pain is a symptom of ischemia of the lower extremity muscles caused by peripheral arterial disease. Resting claudication pain is typically considered a contraindication to exercise with peripheral arterial disease and may be an indication that the disease process is more advanced.**

2. Decreased peripheral pulses are a common sign associated with peripheral arterial disease, but would only severely limit ambulation if blood flow was markedly diminished or absent. Decreased peripheral pulses are a result of plaque buildup in the arteries which decreases blood flow and subsequently oxygen to the extremities.

3. Cool skin may be a sign of peripheral arterial disease, but would only severely limit ambulation if blood flow was markedly diminished or absent. Cool skin results from the diminished circulation, particularly in the extremities.

4. A blood pressure of 165/90 mm Hg can occur during rest or exercise and does not severely limit ambulation.

System: Cardiovascular and Pulmonary Systems
Content Outline: Interventions

 Level 2   p. 444, 538-539

 Level 2

➡ PTAEXAM TWO: QUESTION 17

A physical therapist assistant assesses a pressure injury and identifies the presence of tunneling. With which pressure injury stage is this observation **MOST** likely to be identified?

1. Stage 1 and 3
2. Stage 2 and 4
3. **Stage 3 and 4**
4. Stage 2 and unstageable

Correct Answer: 3 (Sussman p. 79)

Pressure injuries, also referred to as decubitus ulcers, result from sustained or prolonged pressure on tissue at levels greater than that of capillary pressure. Skin covering bony prominences is particularly susceptible to localized ischemia and tissue necrosis due to pressure. Factors contributing to pressure injuries include shearing forces, moisture, heat, friction, medications, muscle atrophy, malnutrition, and debilitating medical conditions. Tunneling refers to channels that extend from a wound into and through subcutaneous tissue or muscle.

1. A stage 1 pressure injury is characterized by intact skin with a localized area of non-blanchable erythema. As a result, this type of ulcer would not present with tunneling due to the lack of depth of the tissue injury. Tunneling may occur in stage 3 pressure injuries since they are characterized by full-thickness skin loss.

2. A stage 2 pressure injury is characterized by partial-thickness skin loss with exposed dermis. As a result, this type of ulcer would not present with tunneling due to the lack of depth of the tissue injury. Tunneling may occur in stage 4 pressure injuries since they are characterized by full-thickness skin loss.

3. **Stage 3 and 4 pressure injuries both may exhibit tunneling since they are characterized by full-thickness skin loss. The incidence of tunneling is greater in stage 4 pressure injuries.**

4. A stage 2 pressure injury is characterized by partial-thickness skin loss with exposed dermis. As a result, this type of ulcer would not present with tunneling due to the lack of depth of the tissue injury. An unstageable pressure injury is characterized by full-thickness skin and tissue loss in which the extent of tissue damage within the ulcer cannot be confirmed because it is obscured by slough or eschar. Since this type of pressure injury is characterized by full-thickness skin loss, tunneling often occurs.

System: Other Systems
Content Outline: Diseases/Conditions that Impact Effective Treatment

➡ PTAEXAM TWO: QUESTION 18

As shown in the image, a physical therapist assistant is performing surface palpation on a patient with an acromioclavicular injury. Which anatomical landmark is **MOST** consistent with the location of the assistant's finger?

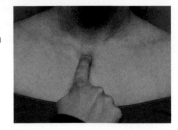

1. Manubrium
2. Sternoclavicular joint
3. **Suprasternal notch**
4. Xiphoid process

Correct Answer: 3 (Dutton p. 1387)

Physical therapist assistants must possess knowledge of surface anatomy and be able to identify anatomical structures through observation or palpation. It is often important to inspect the integrity of selected structures within a reasonable proximity of the primary injury.

1. The manubrium refers to the broad upper portion of the sternum. The manubrium has a quadrangular shape and articulates with the clavicles and the first two ribs.

2. The sternoclavicular joint consists of the clavicle articulating with the manubrium of the sternum.

3. **The anatomical landmark consistent with the therapist's finger is the suprasternal notch. The suprasternal notch refers to the "V" shaped notch at the top of the sternum.**

4. The xiphoid process refers to the small extension of the lower portion of the sternum. The xiphoid process is cartilaginous at birth and usually ossifies and unites with the body of the sternum by 40 years of age.

System: Musculoskeletal System
Content Outline: Physical Therapy Data Collection

 Level 1   p. 442, 444, 538-539

Level 1

➡ PTAEXAM TWO: QUESTION 19

A patient post total hip arthroplasty (posterolateral approach) has been instructed to wear a knee immobilizer due to the surgeon's concern that the patient is a high risk for hip dislocation. Which of the following rationales for the use of a knee immobilizer is the **MOST** plausible to address the surgeon's concern?

1. It serves as a constant reminder to the patient that the hip is susceptible to injury
2. **It reduces hip flexion by maintaining knee extension**
3. It facilitates quadriceps contraction during weight bearing activities
4. It limits post-operative edema and promotes lower extremity stability

Correct Answer: 2 (Paz p. 101)

Hip flexion greater than 90 degrees is often considered a contraindication following total hip arthroplasty surgery using a posterolateral surgical approach. Other contraindications in the early post-operative phase include restricting adduction and medial rotation.

1. A knee immobilizer can serve as an external feedback mechanism to remind the patient that the hip is vulnerable to injury, however, this would not be the primary rationale to use the device.
2. **A knee immobilizer limits hip flexion by maintaining the knee in an extended position. The immobilizer can be particularly helpful in patients who are unable to maintain posterior hip precautions independently.**
3. A knee immobilizer is commonly used following knee surgery to provide stability to the lower extremity. The immobilizer is most often prescribed in the presence of quadriceps weakness to prevent "buckling" or "giving way" of the knee. The knee immobilizer, however, would not improve stability of the hip following total hip arthroplasty.
4. The knee immobilizer offers some compression to the knee, however, would have little impact on the patient's post-operative edema particularly since the surgery involved the hip. In addition, limiting post-operative edema would play a relatively minor role in promoting lower extremity stability.

System: Musculoskeletal System
Content Outline: Interventions

➡ PTAEXAM TWO: QUESTION 20

A patient has been experiencing recurrent angina and completed an exercise stress test that was positive. The physical therapist assistant should understand that a positive exercise stress test is **MOST** indicative of the presence of which of the following findings?

1. Balanced oxygen demand and supply
2. **Ischemia**
3. Normal vital signs
4. Cardiac arrhythmias

Correct Answer: 2 (O'Sullivan p. 556)

An exercise stress test is used to determine the ability of the cardiovascular system to accommodate for increasing metabolic demand. Patients are typically tested using a bicycle ergometer, treadmill or upper extremity ergometer. This form of testing provides a general link between a patient's impairment and overall functional capacity.

1. A patient that performs an exercise stress test and demonstrates a balanced oxygen supply and demand would typically have a negative stress test. A negative stress test shows that a patient's cardiovascular system was able to handle the expected increasing metabolic demands without any form of ischemia present.
2. **An exercise stress test is used to determine the presence of ischemia and evaluate the overall functional capacity of a patient. The patient is typically monitored through a 12-lead electrocardiogram and vital signs. An echocardiogram is often used to further assess perfusion. Determination of the presence of ischemia is the goal of the exercise stress test.**
3. Since an exercise stress test attempts to determine the presence of ischemia, a positive test would typically be characterized by abnormal vital signs appearing at some point during the testing procedure.
4. Cardiac arrhythmias are not necessary to have a positive stress test. The exercise stress test is designed to determine the presence of ischemia.

System: Cardiovascular and Pulmonary Systems
Content Outline: Physical Therapy Data Collection

⦿ Level 2

⦿ Level 2   p. 380-381

➡ PTAEXAM TWO: QUESTION 21

A patient sustained a traumatic injury to the right shoulder less than one week ago and presents with pain, inflammation, and muscle spasm globally in the shoulder. Which of the following interventions is the **MOST** appropriate for the physical therapist assistant to use at this stage?

1. Grade I and II joint mobilizations
2. Bent over rows with a light hand weight
3. Doorway stretches for the pectoralis major
4. Proprioceptive neuromuscular facilitation patterns without resistance

Correct Answer: 1 (Kisner p. 325)

The acute stage of healing is characterized by inflammation, pain, edema, muscle spasm, impaired movement, joint effusion, and decreased use of affected areas. The plan of care for this stage of healing should include patient education, control of pain, reduction of muscle spasm, maintenance of joint mobility, and reduction of swelling.

1. **The patient presents with pain, inflammation, and muscle spasm. The most appropriate intervention would be grade I and II joint mobilizations to help control pain by stimulating mechanoreceptors.**

2. Bent over rows with a light hand weight would be more appropriate for the subacute stage of healing. Strengthening exercises used during the acute stage will likely exacerbate the patient's symptoms.

3. Doorway stretches for the pectoralis major would be more appropriate for the subacute stage of healing. Stretching exercises used during the acute stage will likely exacerbate the patient's symptoms. More conservative activities such as pain-free passive range of motion would be more appropriate for the acute stage.

4. Proprioceptive neuromuscular facilitation patterns would be more appropriate for the subacute stage of healing. Active range of motion (AROM) exercises at the site of injury during the acute stage will likely exacerbate the patient's symptoms. AROM exercises used at adjacent joints would be an acceptable intervention for the acute stage.

System: Musculoskeletal System
Content Outline: Interventions

➡ PTAEXAM TWO: QUESTION 22

During gait training of a patient with a transtibial prosthesis, the physical therapist assistant observes excessive knee flexion during foot flat (loading response) on the prosthetic side. Which of the following rationales is the **MOST** likely cause of this gait deviation?

1. Weakness of the hip flexors
2. **Alignment of the foot into excessive dorsiflexion**
3. Pistoning of the residual limb within the prosthesis
4. Excessive softness of the SACH (solid ankle, cushion heel) foot

Correct Answer: 2 (Lusardi p. 678)

A physical therapist assistant must discern patient-centered and prosthetic causative factors for biomechanical issues that result in gait deviations. Knee instability can primarily result from malalignment, weakness, and contracture.

1. Knee instability that occurs during initial contact through midstance is often associated with weakness of the hip extensors. Hip flexor weakness would not directly influence instability of the knee.

2. **If the prosthetic foot is aligned into excessive dorsiflexion, there is potential for knee instability during the loading response. The excessive dorsiflexion creates a flexion moment at the knee upon loading on the prosthetic side.**

3. Pistoning of the residual limb within a socket can result from inadequate suspension. The prosthesis will typically become longer and the patient will experience difficulty with toe clearance during the swing phase.

4. Knee instability can occur due to a SACH foot that is too stiff, thus creating a greater flexion moment at the knee upon contact. A soft SACH foot results in plantar flexion at the ankle and a subsequent extension moment at the knee.

System: Musculoskeletal System
Content Outline: Interventions

 Level 2   p. 104-105

 Level 2   p. 134-135

➡ PTAEXAM TWO: QUESTION 23

A physical therapist assistant treats a patient with a tibial plateau fracture that is currently partial weight bearing. During the treatment session, the physical therapist directs the assistant to instruct the patient to ascend and descend stairs using bilateral canes. Assuming the patient falls during the training session, which individual would be **MOST** liable for the incident?

1. **Physical therapist**
2. Physical therapist assistant
3. Patient
4. Referring physician

Correct Answer: 1 (Code of Ethics)

The Code of Ethics for the Physical Therapist indicates that "Physical therapists shall demonstrate professional judgment informed by professional standards, evidence (including current literature and established best practice), practitioner experience, and patient/client values." The described scenario clearly indicates that the physical therapist did not demonstrate professional judgment by having a patient that is partial weight bearing use bilateral canes.

1. **The physical therapist would be most liable for the incident since bilateral canes do not permit partial weight bearing and this action likely contributed to the adverse event during the training session. Although the physical therapist was not directly involved at the time of the incident, the delegation of an inappropriate intervention results in the physical therapist assuming primary liability.**

2. A physical therapist assistant is a technically educated health care provider who assists the physical therapist in the provision of physical therapy services. Physical therapist assistants are able to instruct patients in ascending and descending stairs with an appropriate assistive device, however, based on the patient's current weight bearing status, the use of bilateral canes is inappropriate. Although the physical therapist assistant will share in the liability, the physical therapist would remain the most liable based on the inappropriate delegation.

3. The patient would not be liable for the incident since it is unreasonable to expect that a patient would possess the requisite knowledge to recognize that bilateral canes were an inappropriate assistive device for their prescribed weight bearing status.

4. There is no evidence to support the belief that the patient was inappropriately referred to physical therapy by the referring physician or that the patient's weight bearing status was not clearly communicated in the referral.

System: Non-Systems
Content Outline: Safety and Protection; Professional
  Responsibilities; Research

 Level 3   **p. 689-692**

➡ PTAEXAM TWO: QUESTION 24

A patient has patellofemoral pain syndrome which has been aggravated by some of the exercises prescribed by their personal trainer. Which of the following exercises would be the **MOST** likely to exacerbate the patient's patellofemoral pain?

1. Terminal knee extension in standing
2. Mini-squats from 0-30 degrees of knee flexion
3. **Resisted long arc quads from 0-45 degrees of knee flexion**
4. Quadriceps setting in terminal knee extension in supine

Correct Answer: 3 (Dutton p. 986)

Patellofemoral pain syndrome is characterized by pain in the region of the patella caused by abnormal contact and/or tracking between the patella and trochlear groove of the femur. Patellofemoral pain typically increases with increasing patellofemoral joint reaction forces.

1. This exercise is a closed-chain activity that occurs near the end-range of extension. With closed-chain activities, the patellofemoral joint reaction forces are relatively low from 0-30 degrees of flexion. Exercises performed within this range are unlikely to exacerbate patellofemoral symptoms.

2. This exercise is similar to terminal knee extension in standing, though it uses more knee flexion range of motion. However, the range of motion used (i.e., 0-30 degrees) is still within the acceptable range for avoiding an exacerbation of patellofemoral symptoms.

3. **In contrast to closed-chain activities, the patellofemoral joint reaction forces for open-chain activities are their lowest at 90 degrees of flexion. The joint reaction forces increase as the knee moves closer to full extension. Therefore, open-chain resisted exercises between 0 and 45 degrees of knee flexion are not recommended.**

4. Though quadriceps setting in supine is technically an open-chain exercise performed in terminal extension, this exercise is unlikely to exacerbate the patient's condition. Quadriceps setting is a relatively low-level exercise that involves minimal movement of the patella within the trochlear groove.

System: Musculoskeletal System
Content Outline: Interventions

 Level 2   **p. 115-116, 156-157**

SCOREBUILDERS

➡ PTAEXAM TWO: QUESTION 25

A physical therapist assistant works on improving the range of motion of a patient post total hip arthroplasty using a posterolateral approach. The patient is having difficulty reaching their feet to don and doff their shoes independently. Which of the following motions should be emphasized to achieve improved independence with this skill?

1. Hip flexion

2. Hip medial rotation

3. Knee extension

4. **Hip lateral rotation**

Correct Answer: 4 (Kisner p. 727)

A total hip arthroplasty using a posterolateral approach leaves the abductor muscles intact, however, it penetrates the posterior capsule resulting in post-operative joint instability. In order to prevent dislocation of the femoral head component, the patient should avoid excessive hip flexion greater than 90 degrees, hip adduction, and hip medial rotation.

1. Hip flexion should be avoided at angles greater than 90 degrees since this results in stress on the weakened posterior capsule of the hip joint and increases the risk for hip dislocation. This patient should not bend over in a sitting position to don and doff their shoes since this would increase hip flexion past 90 degrees.

2. Hip medial rotation should be avoided since this motion places stress on the weakened posterior capsule and results in the femoral head component assuming a position where it may dislocate.

3. Knee extension is not a precaution for this patient, however, if the knee was extended the patient would have to flex the hip greater than 90 degrees to reach their feet.

4. **Hip lateral rotation places the femoral head component in a stable position following a posterolateral approach. Improved range of motion into lateral rotation should be emphasized in order to maximize function for this patient. The patient can laterally rotate the hip and place their foot on the opposite knee to don and doff their shoes as long as hip flexion does not exceed 90 degrees.**

System: Musculoskeletal System
Content Outline: Interventions

➡ PTAEXAM TWO: QUESTION 26

A physical therapist assistant instructs a patient to perform a stretch as shown in the image. Which of the following muscles would **MOST** likely be stretched here?

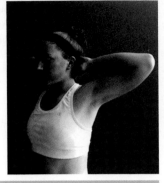

1. **Pectoralis minor**

2. Triceps

3. Middle trapezius

4. Upper trapezius

Correct Answer: 1 (Dutton p. 694)

Physical therapist assistants routinely instruct patients in self stretching activities. Specific stretching exercises should be prescribed based on the established therapeutic objectives.

1. **The pectoralis minor muscle originates on ribs three to five and inserts on the coracoid process of the scapula. The muscle acts to stabilize the scapula by drawing it inferiorly and anteriorly against the thoracic wall. The pectoralis minor is stretched in a manner similar to the various methods used to stretch the pectoralis major (e.g., corner wall stretch).**

2. The triceps muscle originates on the lateral and medial surface of the humerus and the infraglenoid tubercle of the scapula. The muscle inserts on the olecranon process of the ulna. The triceps muscle acts to extend the elbow and assists in shoulder extension. The triceps can be stretched by placing both arms over the head and bending one elbow so it points toward the ceiling. The patient then grasps the elbow pointing toward the ceiling with the contralateral hand and gently pulls the arm backwards.

3. The middle fibers of the trapezius muscle originate on the spinous processes of the first through fifth thoracic vertebrae and insert on the spine of the scapula. The middle fibers act to adduct the scapula. The middle fibers of the trapezius can be stretched by clasping the hands in front of the body at chest height with the shoulders and upper back rounded forward. The patient should then be instructed to pull the shoulder blades apart.

4. The upper fibers of the trapezius muscle originate from the external occipital protuberance, superior nuchal line, and the ligamentum nuchae. The muscle inserts on the lateral third of the clavicle and acts to assist with scapular elevation. The upper fibers of the trapezius can be stretched by bringing the contralateral arm to the opposite ear and pulling the head towards the contralateral shoulder while keeping the opposite shoulder depressed.

System: Musculoskeletal System
Content Outline: Interventions

Level 2   👓 p. 117-119, 168-169

Level 1

▶ PTAEXAM TWO: QUESTION 27

A physical therapist assistant intends to use compression therapy as part of a patient's plan of care. The use of compression therapy would be contraindicated in which of the following impairments?

1. **Lower extremity edema due to congestive heart failure**

2. Decreased mobility following total knee arthroplasty

3. Hypertrophic scarring following a burn to the lower extremities

4. Residual limb edema following transfemoral amputation

Correct Answer: 1 (Cameron p. 414)

Compression therapy is the use of external pressure on the body to improve fluid balance and circulation or modify scar tissue formation. Indications for the use of compression include control of edema, prevention of deep venous thrombosis, treatment of venous stasis ulcers, residual limb shaping after amputation, and control of hypertrophic scarring.

1. **Edema of the limbs is an indication for compression therapy. However, in patients with congestive heart failure, compression therapy should not be used since the movement of fluid from the periphery back to the heart may further increase the stress on an already failing heart.**

2. Compression therapy may be used after total knee arthroplasty to decrease the risk for deep venous thrombosis (DVT). The risk for DVT increases when local blood flow is decreased as is seen in immobilized patients who have undergone major surgery. Specifically, compression therapy can help reduce the risk of DVT by increasing circulation.

3. Hypertrophic scarring is a common complication of burn injuries. Compression therapy is the most common treatment used to control hypertrophic scar formation. Compression garments have been shown to decrease the height and increase the pliability of hypertrophic scars.

4. Compression therapy is commonly used after amputation to help shape the residual limb in preparation for proper fit of the prosthesis. Compression helps with residual limb shaping by controlling edema.

System: Cardiovascular and Pulmonary Systems
Content Outline: Interventions

▶ PTAEXAM TWO: QUESTION 28

A physical therapist assistant works with a patient diagnosed with congestive heart failure who presents with dyspnea during ambulation. The patient has an ejection fraction of less than 55 percent. Which of the following interventions would be the **MOST** appropriate?

1. Instruction in pursed-lip breathing

2. Progressive resistive exercises

3. **Education on energy conservation**

4. Instruction in diaphragmatic breathing

Correct Answer: 3 (O'Sullivan p. 568)

The ejection fraction is a measure of left ventricular contractility. It is determined by dividing stroke volume by left ventricular end-diastolic volume. Normal ejection fraction is approximately 55-70 percent. Anything less than 55 percent of the blood pumped out of the ventricles with each heart beat is abnormal and indicates impairment in left ventricular function. Ejection fraction is decreased in patients with left-sided congestive heart failure.

1. Pursed-lip breathing is a breathing exercise used most often with patients who have chronic obstructive pulmonary disease. The goals of pursed-lip breathing are to reduce respiratory rate, reduce dyspnea, and maintain a small positive pressure in the bronchioles which may help prevent airway collapse. Pursed-lip breathing is not the most appropriate intervention for this patient since the underlying cause is not pulmonary.

2. Progressive resistive exercises are not the most appropriate intervention for this patient since resistive exercises do not directly address the patient's dyspnea during ambulation.

3. **The primary goals of treating a patient with congestive heart failure include improving exercise tolerance and increasing knowledge of the disease process. Since the heart is unable to meet the metabolic demands of the body, pacing and energy conservation techniques are necessary for the patient to improve their tolerance for activities of daily living and potentially exercise.**

4. Diaphragmatic breathing is a technique used to improve the patient's ability to enlist the diaphragm for breathing and to minimize the action of the accessory muscles. Diaphragmatic breathing is not the most appropriate intervention for this patient since their dyspnea is not the result of inefficient use of the diaphragm.

System: Cardiovascular and Pulmonary Systems
Content Outline: Interventions

 Level 2   p. 635-636

Level 2   p. 364, 398-399

➡ PTAEXAM TWO: QUESTION 29

A physical therapist assistant uses metabolic equivalents (METs) as a method to establish exercise intensity for a 36-year-old patient. The patient is recreationally active and has no relevant past medical history. Which MET level would be the **MOST** appropriate for the assistant to use given the patient's anticipated maximal aerobic capacity?

1. 3
2. 6
3. **10**
4. 15

Correct Answer: 3 (Nyland p. 127)

One metabolic equivalent is the amount of oxygen consumed at rest and is equal to approximately 3.5 milliliters of oxygen per kilogram of body weight per minute. This measure allows therapists to describe the energy requirements of an activity as a multiple of the metabolic rate.

1. Maximal aerobic capacity of 3 METs is extremely low regardless of age and gender. For example, walking three miles per hour on a level, firm surface is approximately 3.5 METs. A maximal aerobic capacity of 3 METs is likely associated with significant pathology or illness.

2. Maximal aerobic capacity for older men and women typically ranges from 5-8 METs. The patient's age and activity level make it likely that the patient's maximal aerobic capacity is significantly greater than 6 METs.

3. **Maximal aerobic capacity for men and women typically ranges from 8-12 METs. The patient's age and activity level make it likely that the individual's anticipated maximal aerobic capacity would fall within this range.**

4. Maximal aerobic capacity for highly trained men and women has been shown to reach 15-20 METs. This is unlikely for the described patient given the available information.

System: Cardiovascular and Pulmonary Systems
Content Outline: Interventions

➡ PTAEXAM TWO: QUESTION 30

A physical therapist assistant works with a patient who has type 2 diabetes and bilateral lower extremity neuropathy. Which of the following instructions is the **MOST** appropriate for the assistant to use to educate the patient about appropriate foot care?

1. Soak the feet in warm water daily, then apply petroleum jelly to retain skin moisture

2. Wear shoes which are snug on the toes to prevent blister formation

3. Use alcohol-based creams and lotions to ensure that the foot is thoroughly cleaned

4. **Choose socks without seams to avoid irritating the skin on the foot**

Correct Answer: 4 (Sussman p. 363)

There are several precautions that the patient with a neuropathic limb must take. A neuropathic limb is very susceptible to damage and infection. Failure to take necessary precautions could result in an ulcer developing.

1. Patients with a neuropathic limb should not soak their feet in water since prolonged soaking can remove the natural protective barrier from the skin and result in more fragile skin that becomes prone to infection. However, after washing and drying the feet, application of a petroleum jelly would be appropriate to help the skin retain natural moisture.

2. While patients with a neuropathic limb should not wear shoes that are too loose, they should also avoid buying shoes that are too snug in the toe box. Since neuropathy results in insensate skin, excessive contact between the toes and shoes can result in skin breakdown. It is recommended that the patient buy shoes which allow for 0.5-0.75 inches of space beyond the longest toe.

3. Patients with a neuropathic limb should not use alcohol-based creams and lotions since the alcohol will dehydrate the skin, which results in skin that is more susceptible to trauma and infection.

4. **Patients with a neuropathic limb should choose socks that are seamless and have no holes or repairs. Folds or irregularities in the socks can lead to skin irritation and eventually skin breakdown.**

System: Other Systems
Content Outline: Interventions

 Level 2   p. 386, 394

Level 2   p. 442-443

➡ PTAEXAM TWO: QUESTION 31

A physical therapist assistant performs postural drainage on a patient with bronchiectasis. The patient's medical history includes diabetes and hypertension, both of which are poorly controlled. Which lung segment would **MOST** likely require the assistant to modify the standard treatment procedure?

1. Apical segment of right upper lobe
2. **Posterior segment of left lower lobe**
3. Anterior segment of right upper lobe
4. Superior segment of left lower lobe

Correct Answer: 2 (Frownfelter p. 315)

Postural drainage is a passive technique in which the patient is placed in positions that allow gravity to help drain retained secretions from the lungs. The goal of treatment is to mobilize the secretions from the smaller, peripheral segments to the larger, more central airways. Several of the techniques require Trendelenburg (head down) positioning, which may be contraindicated in certain patient populations (e.g., patients with uncontrolled hypertension).

1. The patient is positioned in sitting to treat the apical segments of the upper lobes.

2. **The patient is positioned in prone using the Trendelenburg position to treat the posterior segments of the lower lobes. Due to the patient's uncontrolled hypertension, the treatment position would have to be modified. Leaving the head of the bed flat would be an appropriate modification to the standard treatment procedure.**

3. The patient is positioned in supine, flat on the table, to treat the anterior segment of the right upper lobe.

4. The patient is positioned in prone, flat on the table, to treat the superior segment of the lower lobes.

System: Other Systems
Content Outline: Interventions

➡ PTAEXAM TWO: QUESTION 32

A physical therapist assistant discusses the use of a topical moisturizer with a patient to combat dryness and itching of the skin in the area of a healed burn. Which type of burn would **MOST** likely require the use of a moisturizer for an indefinite period?

1. Superficial burn on the palm of the hand caused by steam
2. Superficial partial-thickness burn on the dorsum of the hand caused by chemical exposure
3. Deep partial-thickness burn on the anterior thigh caused by contact with boiling water
4. **Full-thickness burn on the volar surface of the forearm caused by fire**

Correct Answer: 4 (Sussman p. 406)

The sebaceous glands are microscopic glands in the skin that produce oil to lubricate and moisten the skin. The sebaceous glands are destroyed in full-thickness burns making it necessary to use moisturizers to limit dryness and itching. The depth of the burn is a better predictor of the need for a topical moisturizer than the cause of the burn.

1. A superficial burn involves only the outer epidermis. The involved area would likely be red with slight edema, however, the sebaceous glands would be minimally impacted.

2. A superficial partial-thickness burn involves the epidermis and the upper portion of the dermis. The sebaceous glands are located in the dermis and are connected to hair follicles that move sebum to the surface of the skin using the hair shaft. Although impacted initially, the sebaceous glands will eventually recover the ability to produce oil to lubricate and moisten the skin.

3. A deep partial-thickness burn involves complete destruction of the epidermis and the majority of the dermis. The sebaceous glands would be impacted to a larger extent than in a superficial partial-thickness burn since the majority of the dermis would be affected. However, since the burn is not full-thickness, there will eventually be some recovery of the sebaceous glands.

4. **A full-thickness burn involves complete destruction of the epidermis and dermis along with partial damage to the subcutaneous fat layer. The magnitude of the tissue damage destroys the sebaceous glands and creates a permanent need for topical moisturizers.**

System: Other Systems
Content Outline: Interventions

 Level 2   p. 389-390, 412

 Level 2   p. 451-452

➡ PTAEXAM TWO: QUESTION 33

A physical therapist assistant works with a patient who is six weeks post total hip arthroplasty (posterolateral approach). The patient's medical history includes Graves' disease. Which intervention should the assistant avoid when treating the patient?

1. Resisted hip lateral rotation in a supine position
2. Hip abduction with an ankle weight in a standing position
3. Ascending and descending stairs
4. **Ambulation in a warm therapy pool**

Correct Answer: 4 (Goodman – Differential Diagnosis p. 396)

Caution must be taken when prescribing exercises for a patient with recent total hip arthroplasty. Typical precautions for a total hip arthroplasty with a posterolateral approach include medial rotation, adduction, and flexion greater than 90 degrees. Physical therapist assistants must also consider other relevant co-morbidities when determining appropriate interventions.

1. A patient with total hip arthroplasty with a posterolateral approach should not perform resisted hip medial rotation. However, resisted hip lateral rotation would be an appropriate exercise.

2. A patient with total hip arthroplasty with a posterolateral approach should not perform resisted hip adduction. However, resisted hip abduction would be an appropriate exercise.

3. Ascending and descending stairs may be difficult for a patient after total hip arthroplasty. However, this intervention would not cause the patient to violate any of the typically established hip precautions with a posterolateral approach.

4. **Ambulation in a pool or on land would be an appropriate intervention for this patient. However, the warm therapy pool would make this intervention inappropriate since patients with Graves' disease have an accelerated metabolic rate and are often intolerant of warm environments.**

System: Other Systems
Content Outline: Interventions

➡ PTAEXAM TWO: QUESTION 34

A physical therapist assistant suspects that a patient being treated for shin splints may actually have chronic exertional compartment syndrome. Where should the assistant palpate to assess if perfusion to the foot has been affected?

1. Anterior to the lateral malleolus
2. Posterior to the lateral malleolus
3. Anterior to the medial malleolus
4. **Posterior to the medial malleolus**

Correct Answer: 4 (Hoppenfeld p. 212)

Chronic exertional compartment syndrome is a condition characterized by pain and swelling within the muscular compartments of the lower leg that is often precipitated by exercise. The swelling can be so excessive that it affects blood flow to the structures within the lower leg and foot. The dorsalis pedis artery and posterior tibial artery are the two main sources of blood supply to the foot.

1. There are no major blood vessels that run near the lateral malleolus, though tendons and ligaments can be palpated in this area. The anterior talofibular ligament can be palpated anterior to the lateral malleolus.

2. There are no major blood vessels that run near the lateral malleolus, though tendons and ligaments can be palpated in this area. The fibularis longus and brevis tendons can be palpated posterior to the lateral malleolus.

3. The posterior tibial artery can be found and palpated in the medial ankle, however, it cannot be palpated in the area anterior to the medial malleolus. The tendon of the tibialis anterior can be palpated anterior to the medial malleolus.

4. **The posterior tibial artery is one of the two major arteries that supply blood to the foot. It can be palpated in the space between the flexor digitorum longus and the flexor hallucis longus tendons which run posterior to the medial malleolus.**

System: Cardiovascular and Pulmonary Systems
Content Outline: Physical Therapy Data Collection

 Level 2   p. 118, 464-465, 564

 Level 2

➡ PTAEXAM TWO: QUESTION 35

A patient has been diagnosed with median nerve entrapment. The patient reports experiencing paresthesias and progressive weakness in the hand. Which muscle would **MOST** likely contribute to the entrapment?

1. Abductor pollicis longus
2. Flexor digiti minimi
3. Flexor digitorum profundus
4. **Pronator teres**

Correct Answer: 4 (Dutton p. 763)

Median nerve entrapment is often associated with racquet sports or with activities requiring repetitive gripping with pronation of the forearm and extension of the elbow. Patients with median nerve entrapment often experience sensory alterations in the lateral aspect of the hand and lateral three and a half fingers. Motor alterations may be found in the anterior forearm or the hand.

1. The abductor pollicis longus is innervated by the radial nerve and therefore would not contribute to median nerve entrapment.

2. The flexor digiti minimi is innervated by the ulnar nerve and therefore would not contribute to median nerve entrapment.

3. The medial aspect of the flexor digitorum profundus is innervated by the ulnar nerve while the lateral aspect is innervated by the median nerve. Although the lateral aspect of the flexor digitorum profundus is innervated by the median nerve, the muscle would not contribute to median nerve entrapment.

4. **The median nerve arises from the cubital fossa and passes between the two heads of the pronator teres. As a result, the pronator teres can be a possible source of median nerve entrapment.**

System: Neuromuscular and Nervous Systems
Content Outline: Diseases/Conditions that Impact Effective Treatment

➡ PTAEXAM TWO: QUESTION 36

A 13-year-old girl sustained a grade III anterior cruciate ligament sprain while playing soccer and is concerned about the future impact of the injury on her athletic career. As she considers the possibility of having anterior cruciate reconstruction, which of the following factors would have the **GREATEST** influence on her candidacy for surgery?

1. Anthropometric measurements
2. Hamstrings/quadriceps strength ratio
3. **Skeletal maturity**
4. Somatotype

Correct Answer: 3 (Hertling p. 501)

Physical therapist assistants should possess a general idea of how specific factors such as normal growth and development influence a candidate's eligibility for selected medical and surgical procedures.

1. Common anthropometric measurements used for adults include height, weight, body mass index (BMI), waist-to-hip ratio, and percentage of body fat. These measures are then compared to reference standards to assess items such as weight status and the risk for various diseases.

2. Hamstrings/quadriceps strength ratio is a general measure of the relative strength of the hamstrings compared to the relative strength of the quadriceps. Strength is an important factor both prior to and post surgery, however, it is unlikely that this would influence candidacy for surgery.

3. **Due to the potential impact on future bone growth, lack of skeletal maturity can be a contraindication to anterior cruciate ligament reconstruction surgery.**

4. Somatotype is a term used to classify a system of body typing. The most common classifications of somatotype include endomorph, mesomorph, and ectomorph.

System: Musculoskeletal System
Content Outline: Diseases/Conditions that Impact Effective Treatment

 Level 2   p. 236

 Level 2

➡ PTAEXAM TWO: QUESTION 37

An athlete sustained a grade III lateral ankle sprain while playing basketball and plans to return to full participation in athletic activities. Which component of the rehabilitation process is **MOST** important to address the concern of chronic functional instability?

1. Use of ice and compression to rapidly reduce the inflammation and swelling

2. High-voltage pulsed current to promote tissue healing

3. **Single-leg support proprioception exercises with dynamic strengthening**

4. Isometric stabilization exercises and isokinetic ankle strengthening exercises

Correct Answer: 3 (Dutton p. 1154)

The vast majority of ankle sprains occur due to significant inversion and plantar flexion and involve the lateral ligament complex. A grade III sprain involves complete rupture of the ligament with profound instability and laxity. Functional treatment is often considered the most critical intervention to prevent chronic ankle instability.

1. Use of ice and compression is part of the early intervention of lateral ankle sprains to assist in the reduction of pain and swelling. Since chronic symptoms of weakness, pain, and joint instability may occur after significant inversion sprains, dynamic muscular support, functional closed-chain activities, and proprioception exercises are critical to prevent recurrent ankle sprains and chronic instability.

2. High-voltage pulsed current can be used to help reduce pain and swelling and promote tissue healing. Protecting the torn ligaments from unwanted stress is the cornerstone of the acute phase of healing. Early progression to closed-chain activities and proprioceptive exercises is a vital component of rehabilitation following lateral ankle sprains.

3. **Single-leg support proprioception exercises with dynamic strengthening can be provided with the use of elastic cords or manual perturbations. This provides the dynamic support and balance training needed to stimulate and encourage strength in a weight bearing, closed-chain functional position.**

4. Isometric stabilization exercises and isometric strengthening can be utilized based on the patient's pain tolerance in the early stages of recovery following a lateral ankle sprain. Isokinetic strengthening exercises may be used in the moderate to minimal protection phases of healing, however, they require specialized equipment and would not be as beneficial as the other presented options.

System: Musculoskeletal System
Content Outline: Interventions

➡ PTAEXAM TWO: QUESTION 38

As part of the plan of care, a physical therapist assistant elects to use mechanical lumbar traction for a patient who sustained a back injury. If the primary goal of the treatment is to decrease the patient's muscle spasm, which of the following percentages of body weight is the **MOST** appropriate for the assistant to use?

1. 10%

2. 15%

3. **25%**

4. 50%

Correct Answer: 3 (Cameron p. 385)

The optimal amount of force when using traction depends on the patient's clinical presentation, the goals of the treatment, and the position selected. There are, however, some general guidelines that therapists can use. Guidelines are often expressed in percentages of total body weight instead of strictly an amount of force in pounds or kilograms since this method accommodates for patients of varying sizes.

1. Ten percent of the patient's body weight would be far less than the amount of force needed to accomplish the identified goal of decreasing the patient's muscle spasm.

2. Fifteen percent of the patient's body weight would be less than the amount of force needed, although it is possible that this amount of force could be used as a trial to determine how the patient will tolerate traction. Assuming the patient tolerates fifteen percent, the therapist could then move to twenty-five percent.

3. **Twenty-five percent of the patient's body weight is generally recommended when the goal of treatment is to decrease muscle spasm or stretch soft tissue in the lumbar spine.**

4. Fifty percent of the patient's body weight is required for mechanical separation of the lumbar spine, however, the amount of force would be excessive to diminish muscle spasm.

System: Non-Systems
Content Outline: Equipment, Devices, and Technologies; Therapeutic Modalities

 Level 2   p. 144-145

Level 2   p. 633-634

➡ PTAEXAM TWO: QUESTION 39

A physical therapist assistant reviews the results of laboratory testing on a patient reported to be dehydrated at the time the blood sample was taken. Which of the following findings would be the **MOST** likely based on the patient's hydration status?

1. Increased coagulation time
2. Decreased hematocrit level
3. **Increased blood urea nitrogen level**
4. Decreased hemoglobin level

Correct Answer: 3 (Goodman – Pathology p. 1707)

A blood urea nitrogen (BUN) test measures the amount of nitrogen in the blood that comes from the waste product urea. Urea is made when protein is broken down in the body.

1. Prothrombin time and partial thromboplastin time measure the coagulation of the blood. Increased coagulation time indicates an increased time to form a clot. Neither test is affected by hydration status.

2. Hematocrit measures the percentage of red blood cells in a volume of blood. Hematocrit may be increased when the body's water content is decreased from dehydration, diarrhea, vomiting, excessive sweating, severe burns, and the use of diuretics.

3. **A blood urea nitrogen test is performed to assess kidney function. An increased blood urea nitrogen level can be indicative of dehydration, renal failure or heart failure. Normal blood urea nitrogen levels for adults are 10-20 mg/dL.**

4. Hemoglobin is the iron-containing molecule of red blood cells that binds with oxygen. A low hemoglobin level is indicative of anemia and suggests the oxygen-carrying capacity of the blood is decreased. Hemoglobin may be increased when the body's water content is decreased from dehydration, diarrhea, vomiting, excessive sweating, severe burns, and the use of diuretics.

System: Other Systems
Content Outline: Diseases/Conditions that Impact Effective Treatment

➡ PTAEXAM TWO: QUESTION 40

A physical therapist assistant performs measurements on a patient for the fit of a wheelchair and determines the seat width is too excessive for this patient. Which of the following adverse effects would **MOST** likely result from this finding?

1. Difficulty changing position within the wheelchair
2. Insufficient trunk support
3. **Difficulty propelling the wheelchair**
4. Increased pressure to the distal posterior thighs

Correct Answer: 3 (O'Sullivan p. 1417)

Seat width is determined by measuring the widest aspect of the user's buttocks, hips or thighs and adding approximately two inches. This provides space for bulky clothing, orthoses or clearance of the trochanters from the armrest side panel. The standard seat width for an adult wheelchair is 18 inches.

1. Difficulty changing position within the wheelchair may be due to a wheelchair that is too small and constricts movement. A seat with excess width would not prohibit the patient from moving within the wheelchair.

2. Insufficient trunk support may be due to a wheelchair that has less back support than is recommended. Back support is measured from the seat of the chair to the floor of the axilla with the patient's shoulder flexed to 90 degrees. Subtracting approximately four inches will allow the back height to be below the inferior angles of the scapulae. The standard back height is 16–16.5 inches.

3. **Difficulty propelling a wheelchair may be due to excessive seat width. This will require the patient to stabilize at the shoulders and excessively abduct the upper extremities to reach the wheels. This produces a less functional push and increases the difficulty maneuvering through tight spaces.**

4. Increased pressure to the distal posterior thighs typically results from excessive seat depth. Seat depth is measured from the patient's posterior buttocks, along the lateral thigh to the popliteal fold; then subtract approximately two inches to avoid pressure from the front edge of the seat against the popliteal space. The standard seat depth for an adult wheelchair is 16 inches.

System: Non-Systems
Content Outline: Equipment, Devices, and Technologies; Therapeutic Modalities

⦿ Level 2

⦿ Level 2   p. 596-597

➡ PTAEXAM TWO: QUESTION 41

A physical therapist assistant discusses the process of learning to drive an adapted van with a patient who sustained a spinal cord injury. What is the **HIGHEST** spinal cord injury level where this activity would be a realistic independent functional outcome?

1. C4
2. **C6**
3. T1
4. T3

Correct Answer: 2 (Umphred p. 473)

A patient with a spinal cord injury would need to have adequate upper extremity active movement to manipulate the hand controls. Prior to driving, an individual would have several unique tests that determine range of motion, strength, vision, and reaction time. The test is usually performed by a physical therapist, occupational therapist or a certified driving instructor.

1. A patient with a C4 spinal cord injury would not have adequate upper extremity movement to independently manipulate hand controls. The diaphragm and trapezius would be innervated.

2. **A patient with a C6 spinal cord injury would possess the requisite upper extremity movement to drive an adapted van with hand controls and use a lift to get the wheelchair in and out of the vehicle. The extensor carpi radialis, infraspinatus, latissimus dorsi, pectoralis major, pronator teres, serratus anterior, and teres minor would be innervated.**

3. A patient with a T1 spinal cord injury would be able to drive an adapted van. The patient would have full upper extremity innervation including a strong grasp. The option is not the correct response since the question asks the highest spinal cord injury level where driving is a realistic functional outcome.

4. A patient with a T3 spinal cord injury would also be able to drive an adapted van. The patient's clinical presentation would be consistent with the description of the patient at the T1 level.

System: Neuromuscular and Nervous Systems
Content Outline: Diseases/Conditions that Impact Effective Treatment

➡ PTAEXAM TWO: QUESTION 42

A physical therapist assistant reviews the results of a pulmonary function test. Assuming normal values, which of the following measurements should the assistant expect to be the **GREATEST**?

1. **Vital capacity**
2. Tidal volume
3. Residual volume
4. Inspiratory reserve volume

Correct Answer: 1 (Frownfelter p. 139)

Lung volumes and lung capacities refer to the volume of air in the lungs at different phases of the respiratory cycle. Vital capacity is defined as the amount of air that can be exhaled following a maximal inspiratory effort.

1. **Vital capacity is comprised of inspiratory reserve volume (IRV), tidal volume (TV), and expiratory reserve volume (ERV). Vital capacity is approximately 4,000–5,000 mL, but varies directly with height and indirectly with age.**

2. Tidal volume is the amount of air inspired and expired during normal resting ventilation. This volume is approximately 500 mL.

3. The lungs are not emptied of air even after maximal exhalation. The residual volume is the amount of air remaining in the lungs after the expiratory reserve volume has been exhaled. This volume is approximately 900–1,200 mL.

4. Inspiratory reserve volume is the volume that can be inhaled in excess of tidal breathing. This volume is approximately 2,300–3,000 mL.

System: Cardiovascular and Pulmonary Systems
Content Outline: Physical Therapy Data Collection

Level 2   👓   p. 269-271   Level 1   👓   p. 361-362

➡ PTAEXAM TWO: QUESTION 43

A physical therapist assistant completing a lower quarter screening attempts to palpate the tendon of the tibialis anterior. Which of the following actions is the **MOST** appropriate to facilitate palpation of the tendon by the assistant?

1. Ask the patient to actively move the foot into dorsiflexion and eversion

2. **Ask the patient to actively move the foot into dorsiflexion and inversion**

3. Passively move the patient's foot into dorsiflexion and eversion

4. Passively move the patient's foot into dorsiflexion and inversion

Correct Answer: 2 (Kendall p. 410)

The tibialis anterior acts to dorsiflex the ankle joint and assists in inversion of the foot. The muscle is innervated by the deep peroneal nerve.

1. Active movement would be helpful to facilitate palpation of the tendon, however, the tibialis anterior assists to invert the foot and not evert.

2. **The action of the tibialis anterior is to dorsiflex the ankle and invert the foot. To facilitate palpation of the tendon the patient must actively move in the direction of the muscle's action.**

3. Passive movement would not be as useful as active movement to assist with facilitation of a contractile structure.

4. Dorsiflexion of the ankle and inversion of the foot is consistent with the action of the tibialis anterior, however, passive movement would not be as desirable as active movement to facilitate palpation of the tendon.

System: Musculoskeletal System
Content Outline: Physical Therapy Data Collection

➡ PTAEXAM TWO: QUESTION 44

A physical therapist assistant treats a patient with Parkinson's disease who has been receiving levodopa therapy for two years. Which of the following side effects should the assistant **MOST** likely expect given the long-term use of this medication?

1. Bradykinesia

2. **Choreoathetosis**

3. Shuffling gait

4. Rigidity

Correct Answer: 2 (Ciccone p. 137)

Parkinson's disease is a movement disorder caused by the progressive degeneration of the dopamine-producing cells in the basal ganglia. The disease is characterized by difficulties in planning, initiation, and execution of movement. Levodopa is a medication commonly used to improve motor function and general mobility in patients with Parkinson's disease.

1. Bradykinesia (i.e., slowness of movement) is a common characteristic of Parkinson's disease which would improve with the administration of levodopa.

2. **Choreoathetosis is a type of dyskinesia characterized by uncontrolled, involuntary movements. The onset of dyskinesias can occur as soon as three months after first receiving levodopa therapy.**

3. Shuffling gait is a common characteristic of Parkinson's disease which would improve with the administration of levodopa.

4. Rigidity is a common characteristic of Parkinson's disease which would improve with the administration of levodopa.

System: Neuromuscular and Nervous Systems
Content Outline: Diseases/Conditions that Impact Effective Treatment

 Level 1

 Level 2   p. 246, 250, 309-310

➡ PTAEXAM TWO: QUESTION 45

A physical therapist assistant treats a patient who has multiple myeloma. Which of the following systems should the assistant expect to be targeted once symptoms of the disease begin?

1. **Musculoskeletal**
2. Cardiovascular
3. Integumentary
4. Neurologic

Correct Answer: 1 (Goodman – Pathology p. 1273)

Multiple myeloma is a primary malignant cancer of plasma cells within the bone marrow. Initially, the cancer affects the bones and marrow of the vertebrae, ribs, skull, pelvis, and femur. The median age of diagnosis is approximately 70 years of age. Although it affects multiple systems with its progression, it initially affects the musculoskeletal system and has potential for severe and devastating effects.

1. **A patient recently diagnosed with multiple myeloma will typically experience a variety of symptoms affecting the musculoskeletal system such as skeletal muscle wasting, fatigue, and bone pain. Low-level exercise, fall prevention, and weight bearing activities as tolerated can assist the patient to manage the symptoms of this disease process.**

2. The cardiovascular system is not typically a primary target of multiple myeloma. The patient will often experience fatigue, but this is secondary to the effects of the disease process rather than a compromised cardiovascular system.

3. The integumentary system is not typically a primary target of multiple myeloma. The patient may have subsequent skin breakdown in later stages of the disease process, especially if the patient becomes immobile.

4. The neurologic system is not typically a primary target of multiple myeloma. Neurologic complications can occur with progression of the cancer. The excessive bone loss can result in nerve compression as well as instability and damage to the spinal cord.

System: Other Systems
Content Outline: Diseases/Conditions that Impact Effective Treatment

➡ PTAEXAM TWO: QUESTION 46

A physical therapist assistant reviews the pulmonary function tests on a healthy patient. Assuming the patient ages normally, which of the following pulmonary values should the assistant expect to remain **MOST** stable over the patient's lifespan?

1. **Tidal volume**
2. Residual volume
3. Forced vital capacity
4. Inspiratory capacity

Correct Answer: 1 (Lusardi p. 19)

Physical therapist assistants must possess knowledge surrounding the effects of aging on exercise tolerance. With normal aging, there is typically greater air space within the alveoli, decreased surface area for oxygen exchange, decreased force during inspiration, and an overall diminished exercise tolerance.

1. **Tidal volume, or the amount of air in a normal resting breath, tends to remain stable over time. Typically, tidal volume is 500 mL (i.e., half of a liter).**

2. As a result of the aging process, residual volume can increase by 30-50% due to the loss of alveoli and increasing stiffness of the rib cage.

3. As a result of the aging process, forced vital capacity can decrease by 40-50% due to the loss of alveoli and increasing stiffness of the rib cage. Forced vital capacity includes the inspiratory reserve volume, expiratory reserve volume, and tidal volume.

4. Inspiratory capacity is the combination of inspiratory reserve volume and tidal volume. As a result of the aging process, there is a decrease in the inspiratory reserve volume resulting in a decreased inspiratory capacity.

System: Cardiovascular and Pulmonary Systems
Content Outline: Diseases/Conditions that Impact Effective Treatment

⦿ Level 2

⦿ Level 2   👓 p. 361-362

➡ PTAEXAM TWO: QUESTION 47

A patient sustained a fracture of the acetabulum that was treated with open reduction and internal fixation seven weeks ago. Which of the following objective measures would be the **MOST** influential variable when determining the patient's weight bearing status?

1. Visual analogue pain scale rating
2. **Radiographic confirmation of bone healing**
3. Lower extremity manual muscle testing
4. Balance and coordination assessment

Correct Answer: 2 (Magee p. 64)

The primary determinant of weight bearing status following a fracture is based on the relative stability of the fracture. The amount of time since the injury (i.e., seven weeks) should allow for bone healing to be visible using diagnostic imaging.

1. The pain level following a fracture is not directly correlated with the relative stability of the fracture.

2. **An x-ray is a radiographic photograph commonly used to assist with the diagnosis of musculoskeletal problems such as fractures, dislocations, and bone loss. The diagnostic tool provides the physician with the best indicator of the relative stability of the fracture and therefore would be the most influential variable when determining weight bearing status.**

3. A manual muscle test would assess the relative strength of selected muscles, but would not provide information on the relative stability of the fracture.

4. A balance and coordination assessment may be useful when determining an appropriate assistive device or the level of assistance needed, however, this is not directly related to the relative stability of the fracture.

System: Musculoskeletal System
Content Outline: Diseases/Conditions that Impact Effective Treatment

➡ PTAEXAM TWO: QUESTION 48

A 74-year-old patient reports experiencing increased urinary incontinence over the past year. What physiological change is **MOST** commonly associated with this condition in older adults?

1. Reduced kidney filtration capacity
2. Increased reservoir capacity of the bladder
3. Spasm of the detrusor muscle
4. **Decreased urge sensation**

Correct Answer: 4 (Kaufman p. 387)

Urinary incontinence occurs frequently in older adults due to a combination of physiological changes that may be exacerbated by underlying medical conditions. Commonly, a combination of reduced sensitivity to needing to urinate, along with reduced bladder capacity creates this condition.

1. Kidney function decreases with age, however, it is not the primary reason for incontinence. Decreased kidney function is directly responsible for incomplete excretion of waste products.

2. The bladder capacity does not increase with age, rather it becomes diminished leading to more frequent bouts of urination. However, with proper voiding this is not a major contributing factor in the development of incontinence.

3. The detrusor muscle can become spastic in the company of neurological trauma, however, it is not a common reason for incontinence associated with aging.

4. **Decreased urge sensation is one of the leading reasons for incontinence in older adults. The bladder becomes full, but due to decreased bladder sensitivity the older adult may not recognize this and as a result experiences episodes of incontinence.**

System: Other Systems
Content Outline: Diseases/Conditions that Impact Effective Treatment

 Level 2   p. 609-613

 Level 2   p. 480-481

➡ PTAEXAM TWO: QUESTION 49

A physical therapist assistant prepares to implement an exercise program aimed at improving a patient's core and lower extremity strength. The assistant would like to avoid exercises that may elevate the patient's blood pressure. Which exercise would be the **MOST** likely to increase the patient's blood pressure?

1. **Wall sits for 15 seconds for 10 repetitions**
2. Leg press for 10 repetitions
3. Walking at 2.0 miles per hour on a treadmill for 10 minutes
4. Standing hip abduction using an elastic band for 10 repetitions

Correct Answer: 1 (American College of Sports Medicine p. 626)

Physical therapist assistants often need to carefully consider relevant aspects of a patient's medical history when designing an exercise program. Resistive activities in general can be potentially dangerous for patients with high blood pressure if they are likely to result in the patient holding their breath during the activity (i.e., Valsalva maneuver). The Valsalva maneuver produces increased intrathoracic pressure, increased central venous pressure, and decreased venous return and therefore should be avoided, especially by patients with heart, blood vessel or lung disease.

1. **A wall sit is an isometric exercise targeting the lower extremities and core. This exercise requires isometric control which increases the likelihood of the Valsalva maneuver being used. This action would increase the patient's already elevated blood pressure and may create an unnecessary safety risk.**

2. A leg press is similar to a squat, however, is usually performed in a supine position. A patient is less likely to perform the Valsalva maneuver when performing a leg press than during a wall sit since the exercise requires continuous movement which is more conducive to a synchronized breathing pattern.

3. Walking on a treadmill at a relatively slow rate of speed (i.e., 2.0 miles per hour) for 10 minutes is a low intensity exercise and is therefore unlikely to significantly exacerbate the patient's blood pressure.

4. Standing hip abduction using an elastic band requires significantly less muscular activity than the wall sit or the leg press and is therefore not likely to significantly exacerbate the patient's blood pressure. In addition, the exercise requires continuous movement making use of the Valsalva maneuver less likely.

System: Cardiovascular and Pulmonary Systems
Content Outline: Interventions

➡ PTAEXAM TWO: QUESTION 50

A physical therapist assistant observes a patient having difficulty controlling the involved lower extremity during foot flat (loading response). Which of the following statements **BEST** describes the muscle activation at the knee during this phase of the gait cycle?

1. Increased quadriceps activity and increased hamstrings activity
2. **Increased quadriceps activity and decreased hamstrings activity**
3. Decreased quadriceps activity and increased hamstrings activity
4. Decreased quadriceps activity and decreased hamstrings activity

Correct Answer: 2 (Dutton p. 299)

Rancho Los Amigos stages of gait include initial contact, loading response, midstance, terminal stance, pre-swing, initial swing, midswing, and terminal swing. Loading response corresponds to the period between initial contact and the beginning of the swing phase for the opposite leg.

1. The goal of the loading response phase is to accept body weight onto the stance limb in a manner that ensures limb stability and permits forward progression. The acceptance of body weight relies heavily on the quadriceps while the hamstrings are less active.

2. **The loading response phase requires increased quadriceps activity to limit the rate of knee flexion. Hamstrings activity, particularly of the semimembranosus and semitendinosus, is decreased since the muscles are no longer needed to prevent knee hyperextension.**

3. Decreased quadriceps activity during the loading response phase could result in an excessive rate of knee flexion causing buckling or instability at the knee. The hamstrings are less active in the loading response phase than in other phases of the gait cycle such as during terminal swing.

4. Quadriceps activity is increased as the limb accepts body weight during the loading response phase, however, hamstrings activity is diminished.

System: Musculoskeletal System
Content Outline: Physical Therapy Data Collection

 Level 3   🔭 p. 108-109, 111

 Level 2   🔭 p. 81-83

➡ PTAEXAM TWO: QUESTION 51

A patient in a rehabilitation hospital reports experiencing feelings of uselessness of life and the possibility of committing suicide to a physical therapist assistant. Which of the following actions would be **MOST** appropriate for the assistant to take?

1. Suggest the patient be placed on a locked unit

2. Ask nursing to check on the patient every 15 minutes

3. **Discuss the situation with the patient's case manager**

4. Review the patient's past medical history for signs and symptoms of mental illness

Correct Answer: 3 (O'Sullivan p. 1206)

Any formal or informal indication that a patient may be suicidal should be taken seriously. The case manager communicates with all of the members of the rehabilitation team and is therefore an appropriate individual for the physical therapist assistant to contact.

1. The physical therapist assistant is not trained or qualified to determine a course of action for a patient that is potentially suicidal.

2. A nurse can frequently check on a patient, however, this action does not ensure the patient's safety given their tenuous mental state.

3. **The case manager would likely contact the attending physician or appropriate mental health provider for direct intervention.**

4. The patient's past medical history may or may not have any bearing on the patient's current status. In addition, the action does not address the patient's expressed suicidal intent.

System: Non-Systems
Content Outline: Safety and Protection; Professional
    Responsibilities; Research

➡ PTAEXAM TWO: QUESTION 52

A physical therapist assistant positions a patient as shown in the image prior to testing for clonus. Which of the following actions is the **MOST** appropriate for the assistant to perform in order to complete the test?

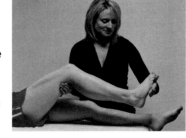

1. **Provide a quick stretch to the plantar flexors**

2. Provide a quick stretch to the dorsiflexors

3. Provide a quick stretch to the plantar flexors while extending the knee

4. Provide a quick stretch to the dorsiflexors while extending the knee

Correct Answer: 1 (O'Sullivan p. 169)

Clonus refers to rhythmic oscillation of a body part resulting from a quick stretch. The test is ideally performed by providing a stretch to the plantar flexors with the gastrocnemius in a relaxed position.

1. **Clonus is evaluated by supporting the knee in a partially flexed position, encouraging the patient to relax, and passively moving the foot. The therapist provides a quick stretch into dorsiflexion and observes any rhythmic oscillations between plantar flexion and dorsiflexion.**

2. When assessing clonus, the therapist provides a quick stretch to the plantar flexor muscle group, not the dorsiflexor muscle group.

3. When assessing clonus, the therapist provides a quick stretch to the plantar flexor muscle group, however, the knee should be partially flexed rather than extended in order to successfully place the gastrocnemius on slack and elicit the response.

4. When assessing clonus, the therapist should provide a quick stretch to the plantar flexor muscle group and maintain the knee in slight flexion. This option is completely opposite (i.e., quick stretch to the dorsiflexors while extending the knee).

System: Neuromuscular and Nervous Systems
Content Outline: Physical Therapy Data Collection

⦿ Level 3

⦿ Level 1   👓   p. 239

PTAEXAM TWO: QUESTION 53

A patient who has ankylosing spondylitis reports progressive stiffening of the spine and associated pain for more than five years. A physical therapist assistant observes the patient's posture in the standing position. Which of the following postures should the assistant **MOST** expect to observe?

1. Posterior thoracic rib hump
2. **Flattened lumbar curve, exaggerated thoracic curve**
3. Excessive lumbar curve, flattened thoracic curve
4. Lateral curvature of the spine with fixed rotation of the vertebrae

Correct Answer: 2 (Goodman – Differential Diagnosis p. 447)

Ankylosing spondylitis is a form of systemic rheumatic arthritis that is associated with an increase in thoracic kyphosis and loss of the lumbar curve. Ankylosing spondylitis occurs three times more often in males than females with a typical age of onset of 20-40 years.

1. A posterior thoracic rib hump is characteristic of scoliosis. The rotated vertebrae cause a rotation in the corresponding rib segments and result in posterior displacement of the rib cage.

2. **The clinical presentation of ankylosing spondylitis initially includes recurrent and insidious onset of back pain, morning stiffness, and impaired spinal extension. Chronic inflammation causes destruction of the ligamentous-osseous junction with subsequent fibrosis and ossification. The patient may exhibit flexion at the hips, spinal kyphosis, fatigue, weight loss, and peripheral joint involvement. If the costovertebral joints are affected there may be impaired chest mobility, compromised breathing, and decreased vital capacity.**

3. Excessive lumbar curve with a flattened thoracic curve is opposite from the typical clinical presentation of ankylosing spondylitis.

4. Lateral curvature of the spine with fixed rotation of the vertebrae is descriptive of scoliosis.

System: Musculoskeletal System
Content Outline: Diseases/Conditions that Impact Effective Treatment

PTAEXAM TWO: QUESTION 54

A physical therapist assistant prepares to assess the balance of a patient who has a neurological disorder. Which of the following methods is the **MOST** appropriate to assess the vestibular component of balance?

1. Assess cutaneous sensation
2. **Apply a perturbation to alter the body's center of gravity**
3. Assess proprioception in a weight bearing posture
4. Quantify visual acuity and depth perception

Correct Answer: 2 (Goodman – Pathology p. 1631)

Balance requires complex integration of the vestibular, visual, and somatosensory systems. Each system is responsive to specific stimuli and therefore can be assessed individually or collectively.

1. Cutaneous sensation is commonly assessed as part of a neurological assessment, however, would not be directly associated with the vestibular system. Cutaneous sensory receptors include free nerve endings, Ruffini endings, hair follicle endings, and Meissner's corpuscles.

2. **The vestibular system reports information to the brain regarding the position and movement of the head with respect to gravity and movement. Assessment of the vestibular system often includes perturbations that require the body to make automatic adjustments that restore normal alignment.**

3. The somatosensory system provides information about the relative orientation and movement of the body in relation to the support surface. Examining proprioception in a weight bearing posture would be a common method used for assessment of the somatosensory system.

4. The visual system allows individuals to perceive movement and detect the relative orientation of the body in space. Visual receptors allow for perceptual acuity regarding verticality, motion of objects and self, environmental orientation, postural sway, and movements of the head and neck. Visual acuity and depth perception contribute to the feedback gathered by the visual system.

System: Neuromuscular and Nervous Systems
Content Outline: Physical Therapy Data Collection

 Level 2   p. 550

 Level 2   p. 239-240

➡ PTAEXAM TWO: QUESTION 55

A patient slightly lowers their gown to reveal a burn as depicted in the image. This should be classified in the medical record as what type of burn?

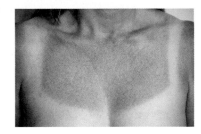

1. **Superficial**
2. Superficial partial-thickness
3. Deep partial-thickness
4. Full-thickness

Correct Answer: 1 (Goodman – Pathology p. 454)

The burn classification system most commonly utilized uses the terms superficial, partial-thickness (superficial and deep), and full-thickness. The system provides a general description of the most common clinical findings associated with each type of burn.

1. **A superficial burn involves only the outer epidermis. The involved area may be red with slight edema and often presents as a sunburn similar to what is shown in the associated image. Healing occurs without evidence of scarring in 2-5 days.**

2. A superficial partial-thickness burn involves the epidermis and the upper portion of the dermis. The involved area may be extremely painful and exhibit blisters. Healing occurs with minimal to no scarring in 5-21 days.

3. A deep partial-thickness burn involves complete destruction of the epidermis and the majority of the dermis. The involved area may appear to be discolored with broken blisters and edema. Damage to nerve endings may result in only moderate levels of pain. Healing occurs with the potential for hypertrophic scars and keloids in 21-35 days.

4. A full-thickness burn involves complete destruction of the epidermis and dermis along with partial damage of the subcutaneous fat layer. The involved area often presents with eschar formation and minimal to no pain. Patients with full-thickness burns require grafts and may be susceptible to infection.

System: Other Systems
Content Outline: Diseases/Conditions that Impact Effective Treatment

➡ PTAEXAM TWO: QUESTION 56

A physical therapist assistant observes a patient during gait training. The patient has normal strength and equal leg length. While passing midstance, the patient slightly vaults and exhibits early heel off. Which of the following impairments is the **MOST** likely cause of this gait deviation?

1. Weakness of the dorsiflexors
2. Weakness of the hip abductors
3. Limited plantar flexion
4. **Limited dorsiflexion**

Correct Answer: 4 (Magee p. 1007)

A patient with limited dorsiflexion may compensate with a vault or bounce through mid to late stance. Approximately ten degrees of dorsiflexion is required for late stance through toe off.

1. Weakness of the dorsiflexors will typically create a "steppage gait pattern." The patient will present with foot slap at initial contact and compensate by lifting the knee higher than normal to clear the foot and avoid dragging the toe.

2. Weakness of the hip abductors (gluteus medius and minimus) will typically create a contralateral dip of the pelvis during the stance phase of the weak side, also known as a Trendelenburg gait pattern. The patient will typically compensate with excessive lateral trunk flexion and weight shifting over the stance leg.

3. Limited plantar flexion would not result in a vaulting gait pattern. The patient would require plantar flexion to vault (ascend onto the toes) during gait. Plantar flexion of 0-20 degrees is required for normal gait biomechanics with approximately 15 degrees during the loading response and 20 degrees during the pre-swing phase.

4. **Limited dorsiflexion will typically result in premature elevation of the heel during midstance. The patient will appear to have a bounce during gait secondary to the gastrocnemius-soleus tightness.**

System: Musculoskeletal System
Content Outline: Physical Therapy Data Collection

⦿ Level 1   p. 451-452

⦿ Level 2   p. 84-85

➡ PTAEXAM TWO: QUESTION 57

A physical therapist assistant inspects the abdomen of a patient with an ascending colostomy. What description **BEST** delineates the location of this colostomy?

1. Upper portion of the abdomen

2. Lower portion of the abdomen

3. Left side of the abdomen

4. **Right side of the abdomen**

Correct Answer: 4 (Smeltzer p. 1104)

A colostomy is a surgical opening in the colon created for the elimination of feces. This type of procedure can be required when an injury or pathology prohibits the colon from functioning properly. Examples of conditions associated with the potential need for a colostomy include cancer, inflammatory bowel disease, congenital anomalies, and trauma to the abdomen.

1. The transverse colon, located across the upper portion of the abdomen, follows the ascending colon and the hepatic flexure. The transverse colon ends with a bend in the colon called the splenic flexure.

2. The sigmoid colon is a portion of the large intestine and serves as a connection to the rectum. This structure is located in the lower portion of the abdomen.

3. The descending colon, located on the left side of the abdomen, follows the transverse colon and the splenic flexure.

4. **The ascending colon is the beginning portion of the large intestine located on the right side of the abdomen. The ascending colon extends upward to a bend in the colon called the hepatic flexure.**

System: Other Systems
Content Outline: Diseases/Conditions that Impact Effective Treatment

➡ PTAEXAM TWO: QUESTION 58

A patient sustains burns to the anterior surface of the right upper extremity and to the anterior surface of the trunk. According to the rule of nines, the patient has burns over what percentage of the total body surface area?

1. 13.5%

2. **22.5%**

3. 27.0%

4. 36.0%

Correct Answer: 2 (Roy p. 551)

The rule of nines is commonly utilized to assess the percentage of the body surface affected by a burn. Each area of the body has a specific percentage allocated to it in order to approximate the total percentage of the body surface affected. The values are as follows: head (9%), each upper extremity (9%), the trunk (36%), each lower extremity (18%), and the genital area (1%).

1. A value of 13.5% is less than the percentage of body surface affected. A candidate may have generated an answer of 13.5% by allocating only 9% for the anterior trunk instead of 18% and then adding 4.5% for the anterior surface of the upper extremity.

2. **The anterior surface of the right upper extremity equals 4.5% and the anterior surface of the trunk equals 18% (4.5% + 18% = 22.5%).**

3. A value of 27% is greater than the percentage of body surface affected in the described scenario. A candidate may have generated an answer of 27% by incorrectly allocating 9% for the anterior surface of the right upper extremity and then adding 18% for the anterior surface of the trunk.

4. The entire trunk is valued at 36% of the body using the rule of nines.

System: Other Systems
Content Outline: Physical Therapy Data Collection

⬤ Level 1

⬤ Level 1   👓   p. 452

➡ PTA EXAM TWO: QUESTION 59

A physical therapist assistant reviews the evaluation of a patient that indicates diminished sensation in the L3 dermatome. What location is the **MOST** appropriate for the assistant to use to confirm this finding?

1. Dorsum of the foot
2. **Anterior thigh**
3. Groin
4. Lateral calf

Correct Answer: 2 (Magee p. 24)

A dermatome refers to an area of skin supplied by a dorsal root of a spinal nerve.

1. Sensation in the dorsum of the foot is supplied by the L5 and S1 spinal nerves. The L5 dermatome corresponds to the medial portion of the dorsum of the foot and the S1 dermatome corresponds to the lateral portion of the dorsum of the foot.

2. **Sensation in the anterior thigh is supplied by the L2 and L3 spinal nerves.**

3. Sensation in the groin is supplied by the S3 and S4 spinal nerves. The S3 dermatome corresponds to the groin and medial thigh and the S4 dermatome corresponds to the perineum, genitals, and lower sacrum.

4. Sensation in the lateral calf is supplied by the L5 spinal nerve.

System: Neuromuscular and Nervous Systems
Content Outline: Physical Therapy Data Collection

➡ PTA EXAM TWO: QUESTION 60

A physical therapist assistant attempts to obtain a history from a patient who recently immigrated to the United States. The patient does not speak English and seems to be intimidated by the hospital environment. Which of the following actions is the **MOST** appropriate for the assistant to take?

1. Ask the patient to communicate in writing
2. Ask another assistant or physical therapist to obtain the history
3. Move the patient to a private treatment room
4. **Request an interpreter**

Correct Answer: 4 (Goodman – Differential Diagnosis p. 33)

Health care providers must utilize available resources to ensure that all patients receive quality health care. Title VI of the Civil Rights Act of 1964 prohibits exclusion from services and discrimination on grounds of race, color or national origin. This extends to people with non-English or limited English proficiency. Failure to request an interpreter given the patient's obvious need would be a violation of the patient's rights.

1. Communicating in writing is not desirable in this situation since it is unlikely that the patient would be able to communicate in a written form that would be understood by the physical therapist assistant. In addition, writing alone does not provide the patient with an effective method of communication especially in the hospital environment.

2. This option may be more desirable if it was clear that another physical therapist or physical therapist assistant possessed the necessary language skills to communicate effectively with the patient.

3. Moving the patient to a private treatment room may address the patient's intimidation with the hospital environment, however, it does not address the more critical communication element.

4. **An interpreter would provide the patient and physical therapist assistant with an effective method to communicate with each other. This action would ensure that the patient can actively participate in their care and that the physical therapist assistant can appropriately direct future sessions.**

System: Non-Systems
Content Outline: Safety and Protection; Professional Responsibilities; Research

 Level 1   p. 71, 222-223

 Level 3   p. 702

➡ PTAEXAM TWO: QUESTION 61

A patient presents to the emergency room with multiple burns on the upper extremity and chest. The wounds all appear dry, but vary in size and are poorly defined. Examination reveals significant irregularity in the patient's cardiac rhythm. What type of burn was the **MOST** likely source of the patient's injury?

1. Friction
2. Chemical
3. **Electrical**
4. Radiation

Correct Answer: 3 (Sussman p. 403)

A burn injury can be caused by heat, chemicals, radiation, friction or electricity and results in damage to the skin and underlying structures. The characteristics of the wound (e.g., pattern, moisture level) can be important indicators as to the source or cause of the burn.

1. A friction burn results from the skin rubbing against a surface and causing an abrasive wound. A friction burn would likely be a single, well-defined wound and would not typically be scattered throughout the entire arm and chest. Additionally, a friction burn would not be associated with an alteration in the patient's cardiac rhythm.

2. A chemical burn is caused by direct contact between the skin and a chemical agent, which can be either acidic or basic. It is possible that a chemical burn could be scattered throughout a large area and be poorly defined. Additionally, a chemical burn could be described as dry, especially if it were caused by an acidic agent. However, a chemical burn would not be associated with an alteration in the patient's cardiac rhythm.

3. **An electrical burn occurs when an electrical current passes through the body. These burns are often spread over a larger area since they contain an entrance wound (i.e., at the site of contact) and several poorly defined exit wounds (i.e., where the current leaves the body). Electrical burns often appear dry, which likely occurs secondary to the electrical cauterization of the blood vessels. If the electrical current passes through the heart, it can also result in the development of cardiac arrhythmias.**

4. A radiation burn occurs as a result of excessive exposure to ionizing radiation (e.g., ultraviolet radiation from the sun). A radiation burn would likely be more uniform in its pattern instead of appearing as multiple scattered burn sites. Additionally, a radiation burn would not be associated with an alteration in the patient's cardiac rhythm.

System: Other Systems
Content Outline: Diseases/Conditions that Impact Effective Treatment

➡ PTAEXAM TWO: QUESTION 62

A physician analyzes the results of a magnetic resonance imaging study to determine the extent of a patient's lung cancer. When staging the patient's cancer using the TNM system, which of the following factors would **NOT** be considered?

1. Size of the tumor
2. Involvement of the lymphatic system
3. **Rate of growth of the cancer cells**
4. Presence of metastasis

Correct Answer: 3 (Goodman – Pathology p. 368)

The TNM system is one of the most commonly used methods for staging cancer. The system describes a malignancy based on the size and extent of the primary tumor, lymph node involvement, and presence of metastasis. For most cancers, the TNM combination will correspond to a stage designation that further defines the severity of the disease.

1. The "T" in the TNM system refers to the size and extent of the primary tumor. Tumors that are larger in size will generally result in a poorer prognosis for the patient.

2. The "N" in the TNM system refers to the extent of lymph node involvement. Cancer that involves the lymph nodes generally results in a poorer prognosis for the patient.

3. **The rate of growth of cancer cells is highly variable depending on the actual type of cancer. This variable is determined by examining cancer cells using a microscope. The rate of growth of cancer cells, although extremely relevant, is not considered when using the TNM system to stage a patient's cancer.**

4. The "M" in the TNM system refers to the presence of metastasis of the cancer cells. Cancer that involves metastasis to other areas of the body generally results in a poorer prognosis for the patient.

System: Other Systems
Content Outline: Diseases/Conditions that Impact Effective Treatment

● Level 2   👓   p. 451

● Level 1   👓   p. 490

➡ PTAEXAM TWO: QUESTION 63

A patient two days post arthrotomy of the knee completes a quadriceps setting exercise while in the supine position. During the exercise, the patient begins to experience severe pain. Which of the following actions is the **MOST** appropriate for the physical therapist assistant to take?

1. Have the patient perform the exercise in sidelying

2. Have the patient flex the knee prior to initiating the exercise

3. Place a pillow under the ankle

4. **Discontinue the exercise**

Correct Answer: 4 (Brody p. 25)

A quadriceps setting exercise requires the patient to perform an isometric contraction of the quadriceps muscle. The resistive activity places minimal stress on the knee compared to many other resistive activities and as a result is often utilized early in a post-operative program.

1. Sidelying is often used to diminish the influence of gravity, however, in the described scenario the patient is performing an isometric activity with the lower extremity supported. As a result, it is possible that the patient would have more difficulty and associated pain completing the activity in sidelying.

2. Flexing the knee prior to initiating the exercise may decrease the patient's discomfort, however, the severity of the pain makes it critical that the exercise is discontinued.

3. Placing a pillow under the ankle would result in further extension of the knee. Given the patient's relative acuity secondary to their post-operative status, this position would likely increase the patient's pain.

4. **Severe pain in a patient rehabilitating from a surgical procedure is an acceptable reason to immediately discontinue an exercise. It is reasonable to attempt to modify an activity in the presence of pain, however, given the severity of the pain and the absence of information on the cause of the pain, discontinuing the exercise is a more desirable option.**

System: Musculoskeletal System
Content Outline: Interventions

➡ PTAEXAM TWO: QUESTION 64

A physical therapist assistant working in a wound clinic presents an in-service on the aging process and its effect on the skin. Which of the following skin changes is **MOST** likely to occur as a person ages?

1. Increase in skin elasticity

2. **Decrease in skin turgor**

3. Increase in sebaceous gland activity

4. Decrease in skin dryness

Correct Answer: 2 (Sussman p. 63)

There are several changes that occur within the integumentary system as patients age. These changes combine to create skin that is more fragile and prone to tearing. Physical therapist assistants can use observation and palpation to evaluate a patient's skin texture.

1. As a person ages, skin elasticity will decrease, not increase. Collagen and elastin fibers shrink, leading to a reduction in the elastic response of the skin. These changes result in skin that is more fragile and prone to damage.

2. **As a person ages, skin turgor will decrease. Turgor refers to the resistance of skin to deformation. This can be assessed by pinching the skin and observing how quickly it returns to its resting position. The aging process results in thinning of the epithelial layers and results in a loss of turgor.**

3. As a person ages, the secretions of the sebaceous gland decrease, not increase. A decrease in sebaceous gland activity results in skin that is dry and therefore more easily damaged.

4. As a person ages, skin dryness increases, not decreases. This increase in dryness is a direct result of decreased activity of the sebaceous glands. Dry skin increases the risk that the skin will become damaged.

System: Other Systems
Content Outline: Diseases/Conditions that Impact Effective Treatment

 Level 3

 Level 1   p. 500

➡ PTAEXAM TWO: QUESTION 65

A middle-aged patient who sustained a fractured femur asks questions about their expected functional level following rehabilitation. Assuming an uncomplicated recovery, which of the following factors would provide the **MOST** accurate prediction of the patient's functional level?

1. Frequency of physical therapy visits

2. Previous medical history

3. **Previous functional level**

4. Adherence with a home exercise program

Correct Answer: 3 (Hertling p. 101)

A variety of factors can be useful when attempting to predict a patient's future functional level. Which variable is the most important is often determined by the unique characteristics of the patient's current disease or medical condition.

1. The frequency of physical therapy visits may be associated with the patient's rate of progress, however, it is not as strong of a predictor of functional level as the other options.

2. The previous medical history of a patient is often valuable information when predicting a patient's functional level, however, the option is more limited in scope than the patient's previous functional level. If the patient's previous medical history was significant, there is a reasonable chance that it would already be reflected in the patient's previous functional level.

3. **A middle-aged patient rehabilitating from a fractured femur should have a near complete recovery. As a result, the patient's previous functional level would serve as the best predictor of the patient's future functional level.**

4. A patient that is adherent with a home exercise program may have fewer complications than a patient who is less adherent, however, this variable alone remains a poor predictor of functional level.

System: Musculoskeletal System
Content Outline: Diseases/Conditions that Impact Effective Treatment

➡ PTAEXAM TWO: QUESTION 66

A physical therapist assistant attempts to strengthen the lumbricals on a patient who has a low metatarsal arch. Which of the following exercises would be the **MOST** appropriate?

1. Resisted extension of the metatarsophalangeal joint

2. **Resisted flexion of the metatarsophalangeal joint**

3. Resisted abduction of the metatarsophalangeal joint

4. Resisted adduction of the metatarsophalangeal joint

Correct Answer: 2 (Kendall p. 404)

The lumbricals act to flex the metatarsophalangeal joints and assist in extension of the interphalangeal joints of the second through fifth digits. The lumbricals are innervated by the tibial nerve.

1. The extensor digitorum longus extends the metatarsophalangeal joints of the second through fifth digits. The extensor digitorum brevis extends the metatarsophalangeal joints of the first through fourth digits.

2. **Resisted flexion of the metatarsophalangeal joint can be used to strengthen the lumbricals. This can be performed with manual resistance or by gathering a towel or another similar object placed on the floor.**

3. The dorsal interossei abduct the second through fourth digits from the axial line through the second digit and assist in flexion of the metatarsophalangeal joints.

4. The plantar interossei adduct the third, fourth, and fifth digits toward the axial line through the second digit and assist in flexion of the metatarsophalangeal joints.

System: Musculoskeletal System
Content Outline: Interventions

 Level 2

 Level 1

➡ PTAEXAM TWO: QUESTION 67

A physical therapist assistant treats a patient who has low back pain with a hot pack draped over the lower back while the patient lies in the prone position. Which of the following actions is the **MOST** effective method to monitor the patient while using the hot pack?

1. Check on the patient at least every ten minutes

2. **Supply the patient with a bell to ring if the hot pack becomes too hot**

3. Instruct the patient to remove the hot pack if it becomes too hot

4. Select an alternate superficial heating modality

Correct Answer: 2 (Bellew p. 70)

Given the potential for burns, formal measures must be adopted to ensure safe use throughout the treatment session.

1. Checking on a patient on a frequent basis is desirable, however, ten minutes is not frequent enough, particularly when considering that the duration of treatment with a hot pack may only be 15-20 minutes.

2. **Supplying the patient with a bell to ring if the hot pack becomes too intense provides a form of instant communication with the physical therapist assistant. The use of a bell does not negate the need for the physical therapist assistant to formally check on the patient frequently.**

3. It may be challenging for the patient to independently remove the hot pack based on the selected positioning. In addition, this option places the burden solely on the patient to make a decision on whether or not to continue using the hot pack. This decision should be made by the physical therapist assistant with feedback from the patient.

4. There is no need to discontinue a selected intervention in the absence of data to support this decision. Hot packs can be a safe and effective form of superficial heat when applied with the necessary precautions.

System: Non-Systems
Content Outline: Equipment, Devices, and Technologies; Therapeutic Modalities

⊕ **Test Taking Tip:** A candidate may like option 1 since it indicates that the physical therapist assistant would check on the patient using a regular interval even if the patient does not ring the bell. They may also be attracted to option 2 since the bell provides the patient with a formal method to contact the physical therapist assistant. Candidates must carefully reflect on which of the viable options best meets the intended objective of the question. In this particular question, the primary objective is to maintain patient safety and as a result the best option is to supply the patient with a bell.

➡ PTAEXAM TWO: QUESTION 68

A physical therapist assistant works with a patient diagnosed with Parkinson's disease. Which of the following clinical findings should the assistant **MOST** expect to identify?

1. Aphasia

2. Ballistic movements

3. Severe muscle atrophy

4. **Cogwheel rigidity**

Correct Answer: 4 (O'Sullivan p. 810)

Parkinson's disease is a degenerative disorder characterized by a decrease in production of dopamine (neurotransmitter) within the corpus striatum portion of the basal ganglia. Clinical presentation may include hypokinesia, difficulty initiating movement, festinating and shuffling gait, bradykinesia, poor posture, and "cogwheel" or "lead pipe" rigidity.

1. Aphasia is an acquired neurological communication impairment caused by damage to the brain. The condition is most commonly associated with brain injury, head trauma, CVA, tumor or infection.

2. Ballistic movements refer to large amplitude involuntary movements affecting the proximal limb musculature, manifested in jerking, flinging movements of the extremity. Ballismus usually results from a lesion in the subthalamic nucleus. Often only one side of the body is involved, resulting in hemiballismus.

3. Severe muscle atrophy is an expected clinical finding in diseases that affect the nerves that control muscles (e.g., poliomyelitis, amyotrophic lateral sclerosis, Guillain-Barre syndrome) and diseases affecting the muscles directly (e.g., muscular dystrophy, myotonia congenita).

4. **Cogwheel rigidity refers to a jerky, ratchet-like resistance to passive movement as muscles sequentially tense and relax. The condition is most often associated with Parkinson's disease.**

System: Neuromuscular and Nervous Systems
Content Outline: Diseases/Conditions that Impact Effective Treatment

 Level 3   p. 619-620

 Level 2   p. 250, 308-309

⏵ PTAEXAM TWO: QUESTION 69

An 80-year-old female patient falls and fractures her femur. Her surgeon performs surgery to fixate the fracture, but warns the patient that she is at risk for delayed union at the fracture site. Which of the following fracture sites would have the **GREATEST** risk for this complication?

1. **Femoral neck**
2. Intertrochanteric region
3. Subtrochanteric region
4. Femoral shaft

Correct Answer: 1 (Dutton p. 50)

Femoral fractures can occur in various locations along the femur including the femoral neck, intertrochanteric region, subtrochanteric region, and femoral shaft. The type of fixation used during surgery and the resulting complications following surgery will vary depending on the location of the fracture.

1. **Femoral neck fractures are intracapsular and may lead to a disruption of the blood supply to the femoral head. Because of this, nonunion (or delayed union) and osteonecrosis are more common with these fractures.**

2. Intertrochanteric hip fractures are extracapsular and therefore do not affect the blood supply. Though nonunion is less of an issue, implant failure is more likely with these fractures since the fixation needed to stabilize the break is greater.

3. Subtrochanteric hip fractures occur in the region distal to the trochanters. Because this region is extracapsular, fractures in this area will not affect blood supply and are therefore not at high risk for nonunion or delayed union.

4. Femoral shaft fractures can occur anywhere distal to the subtrochanteric region along the shaft of the femur. Because the femoral shaft is extracapsular, fractures in this area will not affect blood supply and are therefore not at high risk for nonunion or delayed union.

System: Musculoskeletal System
Content Outline: Diseases/Conditions that Impact Effective Treatment

⏵ PTAEXAM TWO: QUESTION 70

A physical therapist assistant reads in the medical record that a patient requires a gluten free diet. Which of the following medical conditions is **MOST** likely associated with this dietary restriction?

1. Diverticulitis
2. Crohn's disease
3. **Celiac disease**
4. Irritable bowel syndrome

Correct Answer: 3 (Goodman – Pathology p. 882)

Physical therapist assistants must possess an understanding of dietary choices based on specific medical conditions. Patients with diagnoses or comorbidities that relate to the gastrointestinal system may require modification of particular interventions such as positioning, treatment environment, and timing of physical therapy sessions.

1. Diverticulitis refers to inflamed or infected diverticula which are pouch-like protrusions within the colon. The exact etiology of diverticulitis is unknown, however, it may be associated with a low fiber diet. Treatment includes an increased amount of daily dietary fiber. Some patients with diverticulitis may develop complications including intestinal fistula, malnutrition, and bowel obstruction.

2. Crohn's disease is a form of inflammatory bowel disease in which the lining of the gastrointestinal tract becomes abnormally inflamed. The etiology of Crohn's disease is idiopathic, but likely the result of an imbalance between anti-inflammatory and pro-inflammatory mediators within the gastrointestinal tract. Symptoms are typically associated with the inflammatory process or associated complications.

3. **Celiac disease results from the body's intolerance of gluten, a protein component of wheat. The condition is characterized by poor nutritional absorption. Signs and symptoms include recurrent diarrhea, abdominal cramping, gas, and signs of malnutrition. Once diagnosed, treatment includes a gluten free diet and vitamin supplements in order to receive adequate nutrition.**

4. Irritable bowel syndrome consists of recurrent symptoms of the gastrointestinal system that interfere with the normal functioning of the colon. Possible etiologies include food sensitivities, stress, immune system dysfunction or bacterial infections. Symptoms can include abdominal pain, bloating, nausea, vomiting, and changes in the consistency of stool. Irritable bowel syndrome can typically be controlled by diet, pharmacological intervention, and stress management.

System: Other Systems
Content Outline: Diseases/Conditions that Impact Effective Treatment

 Level 1   p. 121-122

 Level 2

➡ PTAEXAM TWO: QUESTION 71

A physical therapist assistant administers ultrasound over a patient's anterior thigh. After one minute of treatment, the patient reports feeling a slight burning sensation under the sound head. Which of the following actions is the **MOST** appropriate for the assistant to take?

1. Explain to the patient that what they feel is not out of the ordinary when using ultrasound
2. **Temporarily discontinue treatment and examine the amount of coupling agent utilized**
3. Discontinue treatment and contact the referring physician
4. Continue with treatment utilizing the current parameters

Correct Answer: 2 (Bellew p. 98)

A patient report of a slight burning sensation under the soundhead can be due to inadequate coupling, loosening of the crystal or hot spots due to a high beam nonuniformity ratio.

1. A complaint of a slight burning sensation would be an abnormal response when using ultrasound. As a result, it would be inappropriate to inform the patient that what they feel is "not out of the ordinary." It may be normal to feel a dull warming, however, a slight burning sensation would require an immediate response.

2. **The complaint of a slight burning sensation may indicate improper coupling. By temporarily discontinuing the treatment and examining the amount of coupling agent used, the physical therapist assistant may be able to continue with treatment. If the physical therapist assistant adds coupling agent and the patient reports a similar sensation, the intervention should be discontinued and the ultrasound unit should be formally inspected by a qualified technician.**

3. Discontinuing treatment would be an acceptable option, however, there is not presently a need to contact the referring physician. A physical therapist assistant may elect to contact the physician in situations where the patient has been injured by a physical therapy intervention or if there has been a change in the patient's medical status.

4. Continuing with treatment utilizing the current parameters is not appropriate since the patient has already reported a slight burning sensation. Failure to respond specifically to the patient's subjective report creates an unnecessary safety risk.

System: Non-Systems
Content Outline: Equipment, Devices, and Technologies; Therapeutic Modalities

➡ PTAEXAM TWO: QUESTION 72

During palpation, a physical therapist assistant determines that the spine of a patient's scapula is level with the spinous process of T2. Which postural deformity is **MOST** likely to be associated with this clinical finding?

1. Forward head
2. **Shoulder elevation**
3. Rounded shoulders
4. Scapular winging

Correct Answer: 2 (Dutton p. 604)

Palpation can be used to determine postural abnormalities. The spine of the scapula typically aligns with the spinous process of the T3 vertebra. Variation from the ideal position can indicate muscle imbalances that often correlate with postural abnormalities.

1. Forward head posture is characterized by lengthening of the neck flexors and shortening of the neck extensors, resulting in anterior displacement of the head relative to the shoulders. Forward head posture is not likely to cause significant elevation of the scapula from its normal position.

2. **Shoulder elevation is characterized by a shortening of muscles that cause the scapula to elevate, including the upper trapezius and levator scapulae. Elevation of the scapula commonly results in the spine of the scapula appearing to be level with a spinous process above its normal position at T3.**

3. Palpation of an individual demonstrating a rounded shoulder postural deformity is more likely to reveal scapular protraction. This movement is not likely to cause the spine of the scapula to move cranially.

4. Scapular winging, characterized by the inability to maintain the scapula against the thorax, is more consistent with impairment of the long thoracic nerve or weakness of the serratus anterior muscle. Palpation of an individual with this condition would reveal that although the spine of the scapula is still level with T3, the medial border of the scapula is lifted off of the thorax.

System: Musculoskeletal System
Content Outline: Physical Therapy Data Collection

 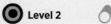

➡ PTAEXAM TWO: QUESTION 73

A physical therapist assistant reviews the medical record of a patient who recently had a "long" spinal fusion. Which medical condition would **MOST** likely require this type of surgical procedure?

1. Ankylosing spondylitis

2. **Scoliosis**

3. Spinal disk herniation

4. Spinal segment instability

Correct Answer: 2 (Goodman – Pathology p. 1166)

Spinal fusion is a surgical procedure that creates a solid bridge of bone between two or more adjacent vertebrae. Spinal fusions are classified as long if they occur across many spinal levels and short if they occur across few, most often one, spinal levels.

1. Ankylosing spondylitis is a systemic condition that is characterized by inflammation of the spine and larger peripheral joints. The goals of medical management for this condition are to reduce inflammation, maintain functional mobility, and relieve pain, typically through conservative interventions and pharmacological management.

2. **Scoliosis is characterized by a lateral curvature of the spine. A patient with a primary curve greater than 40 degrees usually requires surgical spinal stabilization. This most often occurs using posterior spinal fusion and stabilization with instrumentation (e.g., Harrington rod). Given the number of spinal segments impacted by the scoliotic curve, the fusion to correct this issue typically involves a large number of spinal segments (i.e., long fusion).**

3. Spinal disk herniation occurs when the nucleus pulposus bulges through the exterior wall of the annulus fibrosus. When the disk herniates, it often results in the compression of nearby nerve roots and causes pain, numbness, and/or weakness into the extremities. The large majority of disk herniations occur at the L4-L5 or L5-S1 vertebral level. When spinal fusion is necessary due to disk herniation, the procedure most often involves only one or two spinal segments.

4. Spinal segment instability describes abnormal movement between adjacent vertebrae. There are a number of possible causes of spinal segment instability including disk degeneration that produces a loss of tension "turgor" and disk bulging that eventually results in abnormal movements between vertebrae. Spinal segment instability may necessitate spinal fusion, however, it would only involve a few vertebrae and therefore would not be considered a long spinal fusion.

System: Musculoskeletal System
Content Outline: Diseases/Conditions that Impact Effective Treatment

 Level 1   p. 117, 119-120, 164-165

➡ PTAEXAM TWO: QUESTION 74

A physical therapist assistant recommends a wheelchair for a patient with both handrims mounted on one side. Which of the following diagnoses would be the **MOST** likely to benefit from this type of wheelchair?

1. Guillain-Barre syndrome

2. Multiple sclerosis

3. **Stroke**

4. Transtibial amputation

Correct answer: 3 (Tan p. 323)

A one-arm drive wheelchair utilizes two handrims fabricated on one drive wheel. The wheelchair is capable of being propelled with one arm since the drive wheels are connected by a linkage bar.

1. Guillain-Barre syndrome refers to a temporary inflammation and demyelination of the peripheral nerves' myelin sheaths, potentially resulting in axonal degeneration. A patient with Guillain-Barre syndrome often presents with symmetrical motor weakness in a distal to proximal progression, however, would be unlikely to utilize a wheelchair with a one-arm drive.

2. Multiple sclerosis produces patches of demyelination of the myelin sheaths that decreases the efficiency of nerve impulse transmission. A patient with multiple sclerosis would typically present with symptoms such as clumsiness, weakness, ataxia, and balance issues, however, would be unlikely to utilize a wheelchair with a one-arm drive.

3. **A stroke occurs when there is an interruption of cerebral circulation that results in cerebral insufficiency, destruction of surrounding brain tissue, and subsequent neurological deficit. A patient with a stroke would most likely benefit from a wheelchair with a one-arm drive since the clinical presentation often includes an inability to utilize one upper extremity due to flaccidity.**

4. A transtibial amputation refers to the surgical removal of the lower extremity below the knee joint. A patient with a transtibial amputation would typically have full upper extremity function making a wheelchair with a one-arm drive unnecessary.

System: Non-Systems
Content Outline: Equipment, Devices, and Technologies; Therapeutic Modalities

 Level 2   p. 252, 598-600

➡ PTAEXAM TWO: QUESTION 75

A physical therapist assistant documents the gait of a patient with hemiplegia as equinus. Which of the following findings would **MOST** likely contribute to this type of gait pattern?

1. **Excessive activity of the gastrocnemius**
2. Weakness of the tibialis posterior
3. Excessive activity of the tibialis anterior
4. Weakness of the flexor digitorum longus

Correct Answer: 1 (Roy p. 335)

An equinus gait pattern is characterized by excessive plantar flexion of the ankle. This type of gait pattern is most often caused by excessive activity of the gastrocnemius, a plantar flexion contracture or weak dorsiflexors.

1. **The gastrocnemius acts to plantar flex the ankle and therefore excessive activity of the muscle would contribute to an equinus gait. The gastrocnemius is innervated by the tibial nerve (S1-S2).**

2. The tibialis posterior acts to plantar flex the ankle and invert the foot, however, weakness of the muscle would tend to promote a dorsiflexed position of the ankle. The tibialis posterior is innervated by the tibial nerve (L5-S1).

3. The tibialis anterior acts to dorsiflex the ankle and therefore excessive activity of the muscle would promote a dorsiflexed position of the ankle. The tibialis anterior is innervated by the deep peroneal nerve (L4-S1).

4. Similar to the tibialis posterior, the flexor digitorum longus acts to plantar flex the ankle, therefore, weakness of the muscle would tend to promote a dorsiflexed position of the ankle. Additionally, the flexor digitorum longus flexes the phalanges of digits 2-5. The flexor digitorum longus is innervated by the tibial nerve (L5-S1).

System: Neuromuscular and Nervous Systems
Content Outline: Diseases/Conditions that Impact Effective
   Treatment

➡ PTAEXAM TWO: QUESTION 76

A physical therapist assistant informs a patient that a ramp needed to access their house with a wheelchair will require two separate sections with a landing area. What variable of the ramp would have **MOST** likely influenced this decision?

1. Slope
2. Angle of inclination
3. **Length**
4. Width

Correct Answer: 3 (Minor p. 19)

Physical therapist assistants often participate in home visits to determine accessibility needs. During a home visit a variety of standard measurements are taken and then compared to acceptable accessibility guidelines established by the Americans with Disabilities Act. Although the guidelines established by the Americans with Disabilities Act are not enforced in a patient's home, they are nonetheless useful when attempting to determine obstacles to accessibility.

1. The slope of the ramp describes the relative relationship of rise to run. The slope should be no greater than one inch of rise for every 12 inches of run. Slope is a critical factor in ramp design, but is not directly linked to the number of sections of a ramp.

2. The angle of inclination of the ramp is an alternate method for expressing slope. The angle of inclination is expressed as a percent grade. A percent grade of 100% would be completely vertical while a percent grade of 0% would be completely horizontal. The percent grade is determined by taking the rise, dividing the value by the run, and then multiplying the number by 100 to convert the value to a percentage.

3. **The length of the ramp is the most critical variable to consider when determining the number of sections of a ramp. Any ramp with more than 30 consecutive feet of horizontal run would require more than one section and a transitional landing area.**

4. The width of the ramp would not be a relevant variable when determining the necessary sections of a ramp. A ramp should be a minimum of 36 inches wide according to the Americans with Disabilities Act.

System: Non-Systems
Content Outline: Safety and Protection; Professional
   Responsibilities; Research

Level 1

Level 2   p. 682

➡ PTAEXAM TWO: QUESTION 77

A physical therapist assistant observes a five-month-old infant in the supine position with the legs elevated and the hips positioned in flexion, abduction, and lateral rotation. Which observation would represent the **MOST** advanced volitional movement in this position?

1. Reaching of the hand to the ipsilateral knee
2. Reaching of the hand to the ipsilateral foot
3. Reaching of the hand to the contralateral knee
4. **Reaching of the hand to the contralateral foot**

Correct Answer: 4 (Tecklin p. 40)

An infant often is able to lift their lower extremities from the surface when positioned in supine as they gain increasing control of their antigravity flexors. The progression of the hands to knees followed by the hands to feet is the precursor to the infant bringing their feet to their mouth. This action facilitates cognitive development by touch.

1. Reaching of the hand to the ipsilateral knee would be the least difficult of the options since the knee is in closer proximity to the infant's hand than the foot. In addition, the movement does not require the infant to cross midline.

2. Reaching of the hand to the ipsilateral foot is more complex than reaching to the ipsilateral knee, however, the movement is not as complex as reaching for the contralateral foot.

3. Reaching of the hand to the contralateral knee is more complex than reaching to the ipsilateral knee, however, the movement is not as complex as reaching for the contralateral foot.

4. **Reaching of the hand to the contralateral foot is the most complex of the options since the foot is further away from the infant's hand than the knee. In addition, the movement requires the infant to cross midline.**

System: Neuromuscular and Nervous Systems
Content Outline: Interventions

➡ PTAEXAM TWO: QUESTION 78

A physical therapist assistant wearing sterile protective clothing establishes a sterile field prior to changing a wound dressing. What part of the protective clothing would **NOT** be considered sterile even before coming in contact with a non-sterile object?

1. Gloves
2. Sleeves of the gown
3. Front of the gown above waist level
4. **Front of the gown below waist level**

Correct Answer: 4 (Fairchild p. 38)

Once a sterile field has been established a physical therapist assistant must be careful to maintain the sterile field and minimize any chance of contamination. The four rules of asepsis that a physical therapist assistant should follow are: 1) know which items are sterile, 2) know which items are not sterile, 3) separate sterile items from non-sterile items, 4) if a sterile item becomes contaminated, the situation must be remedied immediately.

1. Gloves offer protection to the physical therapist assistant's hands to reduce the likelihood of becoming infected with microorganisms and decrease the risk of the patient receiving microorganisms from the physical therapist assistant. Sterile gloves are considered to be sterile after they are applied.

2. A gown is used to protect the physical therapist assistant's clothing from being contaminated or soiled by a contaminant. The gown also reduces the probability of the physical therapist assistant transmitting a microorganism from their clothing to the patient. The sleeves of a sterile gown are considered to be sterile after they are applied.

3. The front of the gown above the waist level is considered to be sterile after the gown is applied.

4. **The front of the gown below the waist level is not considered to be sterile after the gown is applied since there is an increased chance of incidental contact with a non-sterile object without the physical therapist assistant's knowledge.**

System: Non-Systems
Content Outline: Safety and Protection; Professional
    Responsibilities; Research

⦿ Level 2

⦿ Level 1   p. 675

➡ PTAEXAM TWO: QUESTION 79

A patient experiences visible swelling and morning stiffness in their hands that often diminishes with activity. The physical therapist assistant should recognize the patient's signs and symptoms as being **MOST** associated with which of the following conditions?

1. Carpal tunnel syndrome
2. Osteoporosis
3. **Rheumatoid arthritis**
4. Osteoarthritis

Correct Answer: 3 (Paz p. 333)

Rheumatoid arthritis is a chronic systemic autoimmune disorder of unknown etiology characterized by inflammatory changes in joints and related structures. The disease is two to three times more common in women than men.

1. Carpal tunnel syndrome is a medical condition caused by compression of the median nerve resulting in paresthesias, numbness, and muscle weakness in the hand. Symptoms include night pain, muscle atrophy, decreased grip strength, and decreased wrist mobility.

2. Osteoporosis is a metabolic condition that presents with a decrease in bone mass resulting in a greater risk of fracture. Symptoms include compression and other fractures, low thoracic or lumbar pain, loss of lumbar lordosis, kyphosis, decrease in height, Dowager's hump, and postural changes.

3. **Symptoms of rheumatoid arthritis include morning stiffness, limited range of motion, effusion, pain with movement, and low grade fever. Smaller peripheral joints are initially affected, however, symptoms may progress to larger synovial joints.**

4. Osteoarthritis is a chronic disease that is characterized by degeneration of articular cartilage typically in weight bearing joints. Patients with osteoarthritis typically experience an increase in pain and stiffness with activity, rather than a decrease. Subsequent deformity and thickening of subchondral bone results in impaired functional status. The most commonly affected sites include the hands, spine, hips, and knees.

System: Musculoskeletal System
Content Outline: Diseases/Conditions that Impact Effective Treatment

➡ PTAEXAM TWO: QUESTION 80

A physical therapist assistant instructs a patient who has C6 tetraplegia in functional activities. Which of the following activities would be the **LEAST** appropriate?

1. Independent raises for skin protection
2. Manual wheelchair propulsion
3. Assisted to independent transfers with a sliding board
4. **Independent self-range of motion of the lower extremities**

Correct Answer: 4 (Umphred p. 472)

A patient with C6 tetraplegia does not have sufficient motor innervation to consistently perform independent self-range of motion of the lower extremities. The lowest motor innervation at the C6 level includes extensor carpi radialis, infraspinatus, latissimus dorsi, pectoralis major, teres minor, pronator teres, and serratus anterior.

1. A patient with C6 tetraplegia can provide pressure relief using a wheelchair with push handles or loops attached.

2. A patient with C6 tetraplegia can perform manual wheelchair propulsion with friction surface handrims or rim projections.

3. A patient with C6 tetraplegia can perform assisted to independent transfers using a sliding board. A patient with C7 tetraplegia is typically independent with transfers with or without a sliding board.

4. **A patient with C6 tetraplegia cannot typically perform self-range of motion of the lower extremities. The activity is more appropriate for a patient with C7 tetraplegia.**

System: Neuromuscular and Nervous Systems
Content Outline: Interventions

 Level 2   p. 116, 540-541

Level 2   p. 269-271

► PTA EXAM TWO: QUESTION 81

A patient at the confused-appropriate level of cognitive functioning post traumatic brain injury is progressing well in therapy, however, has been experiencing diplopia. Which of the following treatment strategies would be the **MOST** appropriate to address diplopia?

1. Provide non-verbal instructions within the patient's direct line of sight

2. **Place a patch over one of the patient's eyes**

3. Ask the patient to turn the head to one side when experiencing diplopia

4. Instruct the patient to carefully focus on a single object

Correct Answer: 2 (O'Sullivan p. 1231)

Diplopia refers to double vision resulting from defective function of the extraocular muscles that is typically caused by damage to the brain. A patient with diplopia is often instructed to wear a patch alternately over one of their eyes. Specific strengthening exercises of the extraocular muscles can serve to improve the patient's vision.

1. Verbal instruction is often more desirable than non-verbal instruction since double vision would tend to minimize the effectiveness of non-verbal instruction.

2. **A patient with diplopia will actually see two sets of the environment. If wearing the patch over the alternate eye does not resolve the problem, the patient may require prism glasses.**

3. The patient will not alleviate diplopia through positioning of the head. Double vision can result from damage to the brain and requires strengthening and the use of an eye patch.

4. A patient with diplopia can use the extraocular muscles of each eye, but they are not in focus. Verbal cueing to "focus" on a single object will not alleviate diplopia since strengthening is required.

System: Neuromuscular and Nervous Systems
Content Outline: Interventions

● Level 2

► PTA EXAM TWO: QUESTION 82

A physical therapist assistant strongly suspects a patient is intoxicated upon arrival for a treatment session. When asked about drinking, the patient reports consuming six or seven alcoholic beverages before driving to therapy. Which of the following actions is the **MOST** appropriate for the assistant to take?

1. Continue to treat the patient, assuming he can remain inoffensive to other patients

2. Modify the patient's present treatment program to minimize the effects of alcohol

3. **Contact a member of the patient's family to take the patient home**

4. Instruct the patient to leave the clinic

Correct Answer: 3 (Guide for Professional Conduct)

A physical therapist assistant should never treat a patient under the influence of alcohol. Therapists should be aware of signs and symptoms associated with intoxication and be willing to take necessary action to avoid harm to the patient and others when this situation is identified.

1. The amount of alcohol consumed would make it unsafe for the patient to participate in physical therapy. Effects of alcohol include impaired judgment, delayed reactions, impaired memory, and poor coordination.

2. Modifying the program to minimize the effects of alcohol condones the patient's behavior and makes it likely the same behavior would occur in the future.

3. **Contacting a member of the patient's family allows the physical therapist assistant to discontinue the session and at the same time provides the patient with a safe method to return home.**

4. Instructing the patient to leave the clinic could create a safety issue for the patient and possibly others, particularly if the patient is driving a motor vehicle.

System: Non-Systems
Content Outline: Safety and Protection; Professional Responsibilities; Research

● Level 3

► PTAEXAM TWO: QUESTION 83

A physical therapist assistant instructs a patient's spouse to remove and reapply a bandage. Which of the following instructional methods would be the **MOST** effective to ensure the task is performed appropriately?

1. Have the patient instruct the spouse how to remove and reapply the bandage

2. Provide written instructions on how to remove and reapply the bandage

3. **Instruct the spouse to remove and reapply the bandage and observe their performance**

4. Instruct the spouse to contact the physical therapy department if they have specific questions on how to remove or reapply the bandage

Correct Answer: 3 (Brody p. 41)

The physical therapist assistant should observe the removal and reapplication of the bandage in order to determine if the spouse is capable of performing the task. Although this will not ensure the task is done appropriately in the future, it will provide the patient with the opportunity for feedback based on their current performance.

1. If the patient instructs the spouse how to remove and reapply the bandage, the physical therapist assistant can conclude that the patient can explain the task, but this does not ensure that the spouse can independently perform the task.

2. Written instructions are helpful for the patient and spouse as a resource, but will not ensure independence. Demonstration is the best instructional method to ensure proper technique and independence.

3. **Patient and family education is a critical component of a comprehensive plan of care. Direct observation of the spouse's performance is the best method to increase the probability that the activity will be performed correctly.**

4. The physical therapist assistant would be exercising poor judgment if they requested the patient to call the department with questions on bandaging without providing additional instruction. The physical therapist assistant must provide instruction and observe the family members' performance to ensure competence.

System: Other Systems
Content Outline: Interventions

► PTAEXAM TWO: QUESTION 84

A physical therapist assistant would like to minimize the likelihood of a burn when using iontophoresis. Which of the following actions would be the **MOST** effective to achieve the assistant's objective?

1. **Increase the size of the cathode relative to the anode**

2. Decrease the space between the electrodes

3. Increase the current intensity

4. Decrease the moisture of the electrodes

Correct Answer: 1 (Prentice p. 185)

Current density (mA/cm^2) is calculated by taking the current amplitude (mA) and dividing by the surface area (cm^2). Greater current density will result in an increased risk of an electrochemical burn.

1. **Increasing the size of the cathode relative to the anode serves to decrease current density and therefore reduces the probability of a burn when using iontophoresis. The cathode refers to the negatively charged electrode in a direct current system and the anode refers to the positively charged electrode. The accumulation of positively charged ions in a small area creates an alkaline reaction that is more likely to create tissue damage. As a result, it is desirable to increase the size of the cathode.**

2. Decreasing the space between the electrodes decreases the surface area and therefore increases current density resulting in an increased risk of an electrochemical burn.

3. Increasing the current intensity will increase the force and speed of propulsion of the ions and increase ion uptake. The result of this is increased current density and an increased risk of an electrochemical burn.

4. Commercially produced electrodes most commonly used with iontophoresis have a small chamber covered by a semipermeable membrane which houses the ionized solution. This type of electrode eliminates the need to soak a more traditional electrode in water or saline and instead is simply self-adherent.

System: Non-Systems
Content Outline: Equipment, Devices, and Technologies; Therapeutic Modalities

 Level 3   p. 700-703

Level 2   p. 644-646

➡ PTAEXAM TWO: QUESTION 85

A physical therapist assistant performs ultrasound treatment to the right anterior shoulder of a patient at 1.5 W/cm², pulsed 20%, 1 MHz, for 6 minutes. If the goal of the treatment is to increase tissue temperature, which parameter would be the **MOST** critical for the assistant to alter?

1. Treatment time

2. **Duty cycle**

3. Frequency

4. Intensity

Correct Answer: 2 (Cameron p. 185)

Physical therapist assistants must utilize specific parameters when using ultrasound based on the desired physiological effect. Failure to utilize the correct parameters will minimize the effectiveness of the session and could potentially jeopardize patient safety in extreme cases.

1. The duration of the ultrasound is an important parameter, however, it is typically determined based on the size of the area to be treated and not by the desired increase in tissue temperature.

2. **Duty cycle is defined as the ratio of the on time to the total time. When ultrasound is used in a pulsed mode with a 20% or lower duty cycle, the heat produced during the on time of the cycle is dispersed during the off time and as a result there is no measurable net increase in temperature. To increase tissue temperature it would be necessary to significantly increase the duty cycle or use a continuous mode.**

3. The frequency of ultrasound selected primarily determines the depth of penetration. A frequency setting of 1 MHz is used for heating of deeper tissues (up to five centimeters). A frequency setting of 3 MHz produces a more rapid heating with a depth of penetration of less than two centimeters.

4. Intensity for continuous ultrasound is normally set between .5 to 2.0 W/cm² for thermal effects. Pulsed ultrasound is normally set between .5 to .75 W/cm² with a 20% duty cycle for nonthermal effects.

System: Non-Systems
Content Outline: Equipment, Devices, and Technologies; Therapeutic Modalities

 Level 2   p. 623-626

➡ PTAEXAM TWO: QUESTION 86

A physical therapist assistant assesses the integrity of the vestibulocochlear nerve by administering the Rinne test on a patient. After striking the tine of the tuning fork to begin vibration, what bony prominence should the assistant utilize to position the stem of the tuning fork?

1. Midline of the skull

2. Occipital protuberance

3. Inion

4. **Mastoid process**

Correct Answer: 4 (Magee p. 133)

The Rinne test is designed to compare bone conduction hearing with air conduction hearing. A vibrating tuning fork is placed on the mastoid process and then placed next to the ear. Air conducted sound should be approximately twice as long as bone conducted sound.

1. The Weber test is another commonly used hearing test that requires placing a tuning fork on the midline of the skull on the patient's forehead.

2. The occipital protuberance refers to a prominence on the outer surface of the occipital bone.

3. The inion refers to the most prominent projecting point of the occipital bone at the midline of the base of the skull. The inion marks the center of the superior nuchal line.

4. **The mastoid process refers to a protruding bony area in the lower part of the skull situated behind the ear. This structure is used while performing the Rinne test.**

System: Neuromuscular and Nervous Systems
Content Outline: Physical Therapy Data Collection

 Level 1

➡ PTAEXAM TWO: QUESTION 87

A patient who sustained a common peroneal nerve injury post motor vehicle accident presents with ankle dorsiflexion and eversion strength of Poor (2/5). Which of the following interventions would provide the **MOST** immediate assistance to the patient with activities of daily living?

1. Electrical stimulation
2. **Orthosis**
3. Exercise program
4. Aquatic program

Correct Answer: 2 (Seymour p. 31)

There are a variety of interventions that can assist patients to perform activities of daily living following a peripheral nerve injury. In this particular question, the candidate is asked to identify the most appropriate intervention to assist the patient with activities of daily living.

1. Electrical stimulation can be used to facilitate motor activity within the affected muscle, however, the effectiveness of this intervention may be limited depending on the severity of the damage to the nerve. In addition, the intervention would not immediately assist the patient with activities of daily living.

2. **The use of an orthosis would ensure adequate foot clearance and stability during activities of daily living. This form of intervention would have an immediate impact on the patient's ability to perform activities of daily living.**

3. An exercise program would be beneficial for the patient for a variety of reasons. The patient will need to perform selected movements in a different manner since the lower extremity musculature has been affected. Exercise will also be necessary to strengthen the surrounding musculature to provide additional stability. Despite the stated benefits, the intervention would not provide the same magnitude of benefit as the orthosis when performing activities of daily living.

4. An aquatic program allows the patient to exercise in a decreased weight bearing environment, however, the intervention is unlikely to have an immediate impact on the patient's ability to perform activities of daily living.

System: Other Systems
Content Outline: Interventions

➡ PTAEXAM TWO: QUESTION 88

A physical therapist assistant discusses the importance of a proper diet with a patient who has congestive heart failure. Which of the following substances would **MOST** likely be restricted in the patient's diet?

1. High-density lipoproteins
2. Low-density lipoproteins
3. **Sodium**
4. Triglycerides

Correct Answer: 3 (Goodman – Pathology p. 595)

Patients with congestive heart failure often present with excessive fluid retention in the pulmonary and systemic circulation. As a result, a diet high in potassium is prescribed, while items high in sodium are restricted.

1. High-density lipoproteins (HDL) are the smallest particles in the classes of lipoproteins. They are composed of proteins, cholesterol, and a small amount of triglycerides. HDL plays an important role in lipid metabolism by transporting cholesterol back to the liver from the cells. High levels of HDL reduce the incidence of coronary artery disease. There is no association between HDL and congestive heart failure.

2. Low-density lipoproteins (LDL) are the major carriers of cholesterol in plasma. Elevated LDL is a cause of coronary artery disease. There is no association between LDL and congestive heart failure.

3. **Due to poor cardiac output in congestive heart failure, renal and extrarenal sensors initiate a process to retain fluid to increase arterial blood flow. Retention of sodium is part of that process. By controlling sodium intake and water retention, congestive heart failure can be more effectively controlled.**

4. Triglycerides are a combination of glycerol and fatty acids. Elevated triglycerides are not independently predictive of coronary artery disease, but are associated with known risk factors for atherosclerosis, including low HDL cholesterol level and uncontrolled diabetes. There is no association between triglycerides and congestive heart failure.

System: Cardiovascular and Pulmonary Systems
Content Outline: Interventions

 Level 2   p. 124-125

Level 2   p. 364

➧ PTAEXAM TWO: QUESTION 89

A physical therapist assistant suspects that a patient's upper extremity range of motion limitation may be the result of a fear-based psychological response. Which of the following examination findings would be **MOST** consistent with the assistant's hypothesis?

1. Decreased passive range of motion; weak but pain-free resistive testing

2. Decreased active range of motion; strong but painful resistive testing

3. Decreased active and passive range of motion; strong and pain-free resistive testing

4. **Decreased active range of motion; decreased effort with resistive testing**

Correct Answer: 4 (Dunleavy p. 84)

Although pain is certainly related to physiological processes, pain is a subjective experience. The experience of pain is often shaped by a host of psychological factors. Fear-based psychological responses during movement testing typically result in a voluntary limitation of active and resisted motion. Physical therapist assistants should be aware of the potential ability of psychological factors to influence a patient's clinical presentation.

1. Decreased passive range of motion would be unlikely with a fear-based psychological response since the patient does not have to participate. Weak but pain-free resistive testing would more likely be expected with a grade III muscle strain due to the complete rupture of the muscle. Although severe pain is expected when the injury initially occurs, a lack of pain often exists following the acute phase of the injury.

2. Although decreased active range of motion is likely with a fear-based psychological response, a decreased effort with resistive testing would also be expected. Strong but painful resistive testing would be expected with a grade I strain or minor lesion of the musculotendinous unit. Grade I strains present with localized pain, minimal swelling, and tenderness.

3. Although decreased active range of motion would be expected in a fear-based psychological response, decreased passive range of motion would not be expected. A decreased effort with resistive testing would also be expected with a fear-based psychological response rather than strong and pain-free resistive testing.

4. **Decreased active range of motion and decreased effort with resistive testing would be expected with a fear-based psychological response during clinical examination. The voluntary limitation of active motion and the lack of effort with resistive testing are often associated with the fear of pain.**

System: Musculoskeletal System
Content Outline: Physical Therapy Data Collection

➧ PTAEXAM TWO: QUESTION 90

A patient post total hip arthroplasty is placed on anticoagulant medication. Which of the following laboratory values would be the **MOST** affected based on the patient's current medication?

1. Hematocrit

2. Hemoglobin

3. **Prothrombin time**

4. White blood cell count

Correct Answer: 3 (Paz p. 171)

Anticoagulant drugs are often prescribed post-operatively for patients at risk for acquiring deep vein thrombosis.

1. Hematocrit is used in the identification of abnormal states of hydration, polycythemia, and anemia. A low hematocrit may result in a feeling of weakness, chills or dyspnea. A high hematocrit may result in an increased risk of thrombus.

2. Hemoglobin is used to assess blood loss, anemia, and bone marrow suppression. Low hemoglobin may indicate anemia or recent hemorrhage, while elevated hemoglobin suggests hemoconcentration caused by polycythemia or dehydration.

3. **Prothrombin time is often used as a screening procedure to examine extrinsic coagulation factors (V, VII, X, prothrombin, and fibrinogen) and to determine the effectiveness of oral anticoagulant therapy. An abnormal prothrombin time is most often caused by liver disease, injury or by treatment with blood thinners. Abnormal values can place patients at risk for side effects ranging from a high likelihood of bleeding to a high likelihood of developing a clot.**

4. White blood cell count is commonly used to identify the presence of infection, allergens, bone marrow integrity or the degree of immunosuppression. An increase in white blood cell count can occur after hemorrhage, surgery, coronary occlusion or malignant growth.

System: Other Systems
Content Outline: Diseases/Conditions that Impact Effective Treatment

 Level 2   p. 70-71

Level 2   p. 369-370

➡ PTAEXAM TWO: QUESTION 91

During a discussion about a patient who has spinal stenosis, a physician shows a physical therapist assistant an image of the patient's spine obtained through computed tomography. What color would vertebrae appear when using this imaging technique?

1. Black
2. Light gray
3. Dark gray
4. **White**

Correct Answer: 4 (Magee p. 69)

Computed tomography produces cross-sectional images based on x-ray attenuation. The test is commonly used to diagnose spinal lesions and in diagnostic studies of the brain. The relative color of each item using computed tomography is dependent on the relative density. The greater the density, the less penetration of x-rays and the whiter the image will appear. Specific structures listed in descending degree of density are metal, bone, soft tissue, water, fat, and air.

1. Cerebrospinal fluid would appear as black using computed tomography since it is radiolucent.

2. Soft tissue structures would appear as various shades of gray depending on their relative density.

3. A structure that is darker gray has less relative density than a structure that appears as a lighter shade of gray.

4. **Vertebrae are composed of extremely dense bone and therefore appear to be white.**

System: Musculoskeletal Systems
Content Outline: Diseases/Conditions that Impact Effective Treatment

➡ PTAEXAM TWO: QUESTION 92

A physical therapist assistant attempts to provide exercise instructions to a 16-year-old patient who is accompanied by her mother. During the treatment session, the mother makes several comments to the patient that appear to be extremely upsetting and result in the patient losing concentration. Which of the following actions is the **MOST** appropriate for the assistant to take?

1. Document the mother's comments in the medical record
2. Ask the patient if her mother is verbally abusive
3. **Ask the mother to return to the waiting area**
4. Discontinue the treatment session

Correct Answer: 3 (Goodman - Differential Diagnosis p. 35)

The physical therapist assistant's primary concern should be to establish an environment that is conducive to instructing the patient in the exercise program. Failure to address the negative interaction between the mother and daughter may limit the effectiveness of the session.

1. Documentation may be an appropriate option, however, it does not address the primary objective which is to allow the patient to receive exercise instructions in an appropriate learning environment.

2. It would be inappropriate to ask the child a question about this topic, particularly in the presence of the mother.

3. **The physical therapist assistant increases the likelihood that the child will be able to concentrate on the exercise instructions by asking the mother to return to the waiting area. The question provides ample information to hypothesize that the mother's actions may be the reason the child is upset.**

4. The child appears to be upset and is losing concentration, however, there is no indication that the session is hopeless. Discontinuing the treatment session would be a premature decision without first trying to modify the current learning environment.

System: Non-Systems
Content Outline: Safety and Protection; Professional Responsibilities; Research

 Level 1   p. 609-613

 Level 3

➡ PTAEXAM TWO: QUESTION 93

A physical therapist assistant attempts to determine a schedule for calibration and maintenance of an ultrasound unit. Which of the following factors is the **MOST** important for the assistant to consider when determining an appropriate schedule?

1. Beam nonuniformity ratio
2. **Frequency of use**
3. Cost associated with calibration and maintenance
4. Availability of qualified personnel to inspect the unit

Correct Answer: 2 (Prentice p. 419)

Electrical equipment must be calibrated and maintained by qualified personnel on a regular schedule consistent with the manufacturer's recommendations. The regular schedule, once established, can be modified based on variables such as increased frequency of use or reports of faulty performance.

1. Beam nonuniformity ratio (BNR) refers to the ratio of intensity of the highest peak to the average intensity of all peaks. The BNR is determined by the intrinsic biophysical properties of the piezoelectric transducer. The BNR of an ultrasound device would not be a factor in determining a calibration and maintenance schedule.

2. **The frequency of use of an ultrasound device is extremely important when determining a schedule for calibration and maintenance. Ultrasound units used frequently may be calibrated several times a year, while a unit used sparingly would likely warrant a longer interval.**

3. The cost associated with calibration and maintenance of the ultrasound unit should not be a factor in establishing a calibration and maintenance schedule. Relying on a variable such as cost implies that when there are ample resources available calibration and maintenance take place and when resources are not available calibration and maintenance can be deferred.

4. The availability of qualified personnel to inspect the ultrasound unit would not be a factor in determining a calibration and maintenance schedule. If appropriate personnel are not available within the health care organization, there are a variety of external companies who can provide the necessary service.

System: Non-Systems
Content Outline: Equipment, Devices, and Technologies; Therapeutic Modalities

● **Level 3**

➡ PTAEXAM TWO: QUESTION 94

A physical therapist assistant works with a patient on fall prevention training. The assistant determines that the patient has difficulty adapting their vision from low lighting to bright environments. What home modification recommendation would be the **MOST** appropriate based on this information?

1. Use unfiltered direct lighting
2. Replace bathroom light bulbs with red bulbs
3. **Use diffuse lighting**
4. Use only dim lighting

Correct Answer: 3 (Kaufman p. 361)

Glare sensitivity is a common visual impairment experienced by aging adults. This makes transitioning between bright and dark areas more difficult, and can result in loss of balance or falling if not accommodated for.

1. Unfiltered direct light would provoke glare sensitivity, therefore the use of filtered light (e.g., diffused through a lampshade or blinds) is preferable.

2. The color of the light is not an issue, however, the directness is. Therefore, standard bulbs are most appropriate, as long as the light is well diffused.

3. **Diffuse (filtered) lighting decreases sensitivity to glare and reduces the home adaptations that an individual needs to make when transitioning between rooms. It is recommended to use blinds and lampshades to help filter light in the home.**

4. Dim lighting would create its own fall hazard as objects would not be fully visualized. Instead, diffuse lighting should be used uniformly throughout the house.

System: Non-Systems
Content Outline: Safety and Protection; Professional Responsibilities; Research

● **Level 3**   p. 501

➡ PTA EXAM TWO: QUESTION 95

A physical therapist assistant works on standing balance activities with a patient following a right transtibial amputation. Assuming the patient is not yet utilizing a prosthesis, what impact would the amputation have on the location of the patient's center of mass?

1. Move inferior and to the right of midline
2. Move inferior and to the left of midline
3. Move superior and to the right of midline
4. **Move superior and to the left of midline**

Correct Answer: 4 (Johansson p. 46)

The center of mass is the average position of all parts of the system, weighted according to their masses. In a standing position, the normal center of mass is located just anterior to the second sacral vertebra.

1. The center of mass moving inferior and to the right of midline would occur if weight was added to the right lower extremity, such as through a cast or orthosis, or if weight was removed from the left upper extremity.

2. The center of mass moving inferior and to the left of midline would occur if weight was added to the left lower extremity, such as through a cast or orthosis, or if weight was removed from the right upper extremity.

3. The center of mass moving superior and to the right of midline would occur if weight was added to the right side of the abdomen or the right upper extremity. This scenario could also occur if weight was removed from the left lower extremity.

4. **The center of mass moving superior and to the left of midline would occur if weight was added to the left side of the abdomen or the left upper extremity. This scenario could also occur if weight was removed from the right lower extremity. A right transtibial amputation is consistent with weight being removed from the right lower extremity.**

System: Musculoskeletal System
Content Outline: Diseases/Conditions that Impact Effective
   Treatment

➡ PTA EXAM TWO: QUESTION 96

A physical therapist assistant observes the gait pattern of a patient with a right hip flexion contracture. Which gait deviation would be **MOST** likely based on the contracture?

1. **Diminished step length on the left**
2. Diminished step length on the right
3. Steppage gait on the left
4. Steppage gait on the right

Correct Answer: 1 (Dutton p. 313)

A hip flexion contracture is a common cause of gait abnormalities often associated with pathology or immobility. A hip flexion contracture can result in a variety of compensatory findings including reduced contralateral step length, excessive knee flexion, decreased hip extension, increased anterior pelvic tilt, and increased lumbar lordosis. Prone lying is a common positional activity to stretch the shortened hip flexors.

1. **A right hip flexion contracture would decrease hip extension during gait due to diminished muscle length and passive tension of the iliopsoas. Decreased hip extension during terminal stance causes a decrease in single limb support time on the affected limb which results in shorter step length on the unaffected side.**

2. Diminished step length on the right would be more likely to occur if the patient had a left hip flexion contracture.

3. A steppage gait primarily occurs in an attempt to clear the foot in the presence of dorsiflexor weakness. The foot will slap at initial contact with the ground secondary to the decreased control. A hip flexion contracture would not produce a steppage gait.

4. A steppage gait primarily occurs in an attempt to clear the foot in the presence of dorsiflexor weakness. A hip flexion contracture would not produce a steppage gait.

System: Musculoskeletal System
Content Outline: Diseases/Conditions that Impact Effective
   Treatment

 Level 1   p. 126-127

 Level 2   p. 81-85

➡ PTAEXAM TWO: QUESTION 97

A physical therapist assistant reviewing a patient's medical record identifies an order for Doppler ultrasonography. Which of the following conditions would this test **MOST** likely be used to assess?

1. Peripheral neuropathy
2. **Intermittent claudication**
3. Cardiac arrhythmias
4. Bursitis

Correct Answer: 2 (Hillegass p. 295)

Doppler ultrasound is a non-invasive instrument used to assess arterial blood flow. Doppler ultrasonography measures how sound waves are reflected off of moving blood cells. As the velocity of the blood flow changes, the pitch of the sound waves changes. This change in pitch gives the therapist important information about the blood flow through a vessel.

1. A patient with peripheral neuropathy would not be assessed with Doppler ultrasonography. Nerve conduction velocity testing may be used to assess the extent of nerve damage in a patient with peripheral neuropathy.

2. **Intermittent claudication is characterized by painful cramping or aching of the lower extremities during physical activity. The condition is associated with impaired blood flow in the lower extremities and thus decreased perfusion to the lower extremity muscles. Doppler ultrasonography can be used in a patient with intermittent claudication to determine the extent of impaired arterial blood flow.**

3. A patient with cardiac arrhythmias would not be assessed with Doppler ultrasonography. An electrocardiogram may be used to assess the presence of cardiac arrhythmias.

4. Therapeutic ultrasound is a common modality used to treat inflammatory conditions like bursitis. However, Doppler ultrasonography is an assessment tool that would not be used to diagnose bursitis. Bursitis is typically diagnosed through signs and symptoms and occasionally through radiography.

System: Cardiovascular and Pulmonary Systems
Content Outline: Diseases/Conditions that Impact Effective Treatment

➡ PTAEXAM TWO: QUESTION 98

A physical therapist assistant completes a cognitive function test on a patient post CVA. As part of the test, the assistant assesses the patient's abstract thinking ability. Which of the following tasks would be the **MOST** appropriate?

1. Orientation to time, person, and place
2. Copy drawn figures of varying size and shape
3. **Discuss how two objects are similar**
4. Identify letters or numbers traced on the skin

Correct Answer: 3 (O'Sullivan p. 165)

A patient with impaired abstract thinking may have involvement of the frontal lobe, diffuse encephalopathy or psychiatric illness.

1. Orientation can be assessed by asking a person to identify time (e.g., day, month, season), person (e.g., name), and place (e.g., city, state). Disorientation is most commonly associated with traumatic brain injury, delirium, and advanced dementia.

2. Copying drawn figures of varying size and shape assesses constructional ability. Impairments in constructional ability are often associated with damage to the parietal lobe or stroke.

3. **Abstract ability is commonly tested using two specific methods. The first method is by asking a patient to describe how two items such as a cat and a mouse are similar. The other method is by asking a patient to interpret the meaning of a proverb such as "a rolling stone gathers no moss." Patients with difficulty in abstract thinking may provide answers that tend to be literal or concrete.**

4. The ability to recognize symbols, letters or numbers traced on the skin refers to graphesthesia. Patients with language or speech disorders secondary to stroke can identify the correct figure by pointing at an image located in a chart instead of through verbal identification.

System: Neuromuscular and Nervous Systems
Content Outline: Physical Therapy Data Collection

 Level 2   👓 p. 609-613

 Level 1

▶ PTAEXAM TWO: QUESTION 99

A physical therapist assistant documents in the medical record that a patient has moved from Stage 5 to Stage 6 of the Brunnstrom Stages of Recovery. Which of the following progressions is the MOST typical of this transition?

1. Absence of associated reactions

2. **Disappearance of spasticity**

3. Voluntary movement begins outside of synergy patterns

4. Normal motor function

Correct Answer: 2 (Brunnstrom p. 47)

Brunnstrom separates neurological recovery into seven separate stages based on progression through abnormal tone and spasticity. The seven stages of recovery describe tone, reflex activity, and volitional movement.

1. In stage 2, movement occurs primarily in the form of associated reactions and spasticity begins to develop. In stage 3, voluntary movement begins within basic limb synergies.

2. **In stage 5, spasticity is still present although it continues to decrease. Stage 6 is characterized by the disappearance of spasticity and the ability to complete isolated joint movements in a coordinated fashion.**

3. In stage 4, movement patterns are not dictated solely by limb synergies and voluntary movement patterns begin outside of limb synergies.

4. In stage 7, normal motor function is restored.

System: Neuromuscular and Nervous Systems
Content Outline: Physical Therapy Data Collection

▶ PTAEXAM TWO: QUESTION 100

A physical therapist assistant chooses a 3.0 MHz ultrasound beam to treat a patient who has carpal tunnel syndrome. The majority of ultrasound energy will be absorbed within a depth of how many centimeters?

1. **1-2**

2. 2-3

3. 4-5

4. 5-6

Correct Answer: 1 (Cameron p. 184)

Frequency should be selected according to the depth of tissues to be treated. The most common frequency settings are 1.0 MHz and 3.0 MHz. A frequency setting of 1.0 MHz is used for heating of deeper tissues (up to five centimeters) where a setting of 3.0 MHz is used for heating superficial tissues with a depth of penetration of less than two centimeters.

1. **Tissues 1-2 centimeters in depth can be effectively treated with ultrasound using a frequency of 3.0 MHz.**

2. Tissues 2-3 centimeters in depth require ultrasound using a frequency of 1.0 MHz since a frequency of 3.0 MHz would not provide sufficient depth.

3. Tissues up to 5 centimeters in depth can be treated with ultrasound using a frequency of 1.0 MHz.

4. Tissues greater than 5 centimeters in depth are not effectively treated with ultrasound.

System: Non-Systems
Content Outline: Equipment, Devices, and Technologies;
    Therapeutic Modalities

 Level 1   p. 258

 Level 1   p. 623-626

SCOREBUILDERS

➡ PTA EXAM TWO: QUESTION 101

As part of the medical history, a patient reports a sudden onset of pain. Which medical condition is **MOST** consistent with this clinical presentation?

1. Bicipital tendonitis
2. **Hamstrings strain**
3. Osgood-Schlatter disease
4. Peripheral vascular disease

Correct Answer: 2 (Dutton p. 942)

The patient interview provides therapists with an opportunity to identify specific characteristics of pain. Subjective pain descriptors can provide valuable information related to a patient's medical condition. Characteristics to explore may include location, intensity, description, duration, and pattern.

1. Bicipital tendonitis is an inflammatory process of the tendon of the long head of the biceps. The condition is characterized by subjective reports of a deep ache directly in front and on top of the shoulder, made worse with overhead activities or lifting. Pain tends to come on gradually over time and can be heavily influenced by activity.

2. **The hamstrings consist of the semimembranosus, semitendinosus, and biceps femoris muscles. A hamstrings strain is typically caused by muscle overload that occurs when one or more of the muscles is stretched beyond its capacity or challenged with a sudden load. Pain varies based on the severity of the injury, but is usually described as a sudden, sharp pain in the back of the thigh.**

3. Osgood-Schlatter disease, also known as traction apophysitis, is a self-limiting condition that results from repetitive traction on the tibial tuberosity apophysis. The condition is caused by repetitive tension to the patellar tendon and commonly occurs in young athletes. Pain often occurs in the form of point tenderness over the patella tendon at the insertion on the tibial tubercle. Pain tends to come on gradually and is typically made worse with increasing activity.

4. Peripheral vascular disease (PVD) is a condition where there is narrowing of the lumen of blood vessels causing a reduction in circulation usually secondary to atherosclerosis. Symptoms will differ depending on which blood vessel has been compromised. During the early stages of PVD, intermittent claudication may be the only manifestation. In later stages, the patient may experience tingling and numbness of the affected extremities along with pain at rest and during sleep.

System: Musculoskeletal System
Content Outline: Diseases/Conditions that Impact Effective Treatment

Level 1

➡ PTA EXAM TWO: QUESTION 102

A physical therapist assistant reads in the medical record that a patient exhibits asthenia. Which of the following tests would be the **MOST** useful to identify the presence of this condition?

1. **Manual resistance to assess muscle strength**
2. Marching in place
3. Alternating finger to nose
4. Placing the feet on floor markers while walking

Correct Answer: 1 (Roy p. 329)

There are a variety of tests designed to identify unique coordination deficits. The tests are often included as part of a neurological assessment. Physical therapist assistants should be familiar with how to perform these tests and how to interpret the associated results.

1. **Manual resistance to assess muscle strength is often used to test for asthenia. Asthenia refers to generalized weakness, typically secondary to cerebellar pathology.**

2. Marching in place is often used to test for a cerebellar movement disorder. A positive test occurs when a patient is unable to follow the rhythm of the cadence.

3. Alternating finger to nose is often used to test for dysdiadochokinesia. Dysdiadochokinesia refers to the inability to perform rapid alternating movements. This condition is a result of damage to the cerebellum.

4. Placing the feet on floor markers while walking is often used to test for dysmetria. Dysmetria refers to the inability to control the range of a movement and the force of muscular activity. This condition is a result of damage to the cerebellum.

System: Neuromuscular and Nervous Systems
Content Outline: Physical Therapy Data Collection

Level 2   p. 239

➡ PTAEXAM TWO: QUESTION 103

A physical therapist assistant works with a patient post CVA who has right hemiplegia. Which of the following therapeutic positions should the assistant anticipate to be the **MOST** difficult for the patient to maintain based on their diagnosis?

1. Half-kneel with involved leg anterior
2. **Half-kneel with involved leg posterior**
3. Bilateral tall kneeling
4. Bilateral lower extremity bridge

Correct Answer: 2 (Sullivan p. 50)

Kneeling and half-kneeling are upright postures where the knees are flexed and the weight bearing occurs through the hips and lower trunk onto the patella tendon and proximal tibia. Half-kneeling also incorporates weight bearing through the anterior foot. Physical therapist assistants must understand the required base of support as well as the center of mass for each position.

1. Half-kneel with the involved leg anterior provides a base of support that is angled between the anterior flexed leg and the posterior supporting leg. There is some stretch to the one-joint quadriceps in this position, however, the quadriceps are not as inhibited as they are in tall kneeling and can therefore assist the patient to maintain this position. This position is relatively easy to maintain with respect to the other options provided.

2. **Half-kneel with the involved leg posterior is the most difficult position for the patient to maintain since the posterior leg is responsible for increased body weight as compared to tall kneeling. The overall increased stability demands placed on the affected posterior limb provides additional challenge to all of the supporting muscles in order to maintain hip extension and lower trunk control.**

3. Bilateral tall kneeling is an activity that is typically mastered after half-kneeling with the involved leg anterior, but before half-kneeling with the involved leg posterior. The prolonged stretch and maintained pressure on the quadriceps tendons in bilateral tall kneeling will tend to increase the inhibitory influence and limit the effectiveness of the quadriceps. Although the posture is challenging, the ability to assist the involved extremity with the uninvolved extremity in a symmetrical posture makes this slightly less difficult than half-kneel with the involved leg posterior.

4. A bilateral lower extremity bridge would be the easiest activity since there is a large base of support while lying supine on a mat table compared to upright kneeling. The patient also has the ability to utilize the uninvolved lower extremity to assist the weaker extremity. Bridging promotes static and dynamic control in the lower trunk.

System: Neuromuscular and Nervous Systems
Content Outline: Interventions

 Level 3

➡ PTAEXAM TWO: QUESTION 104

A physical therapist assistant treats a patient diagnosed with chronic arterial disease who is experiencing signs and symptoms of intermittent claudication with activity. The primary treatment goal is to increase the patient's ambulation distance. Which of the following ambulation parameters are the **MOST** appropriate to facilitate achievement of the goal?

1. **Short duration, frequent intervals**
2. Short duration, infrequent intervals
3. Long duration, frequent intervals
4. Long duration, infrequent intervals

Correct Answer: 1 (Hillegass p. 593)

Intermittent claudication occurs as a result of insufficient blood supply and ischemia in active muscles. The condition occurs with activity, subsides during periods of rest, and as a result can limit the duration of exercise activities. Symptoms most commonly include pain and cramping in muscles distal to the occluded vessel.

1. **Treadmill and track walking are the most effective modes of exercise to reduce claudication. The initial workloads are set to elicit claudication symptoms within three to five minutes. This is followed by a period of standing or sitting to allow symptoms to resolve. The exercise-rest-exercise pattern is repeated throughout the exercise session. Due to the short duration of each bout of exercise before the onset of symptoms, frequent exercise bouts are indicated.**

2. Since the patient can only exercise for shorter durations before the onset of symptoms, exercising at infrequent intervals would not allow the patient to progress toward the goal of increasing ambulation distance.

3. Patients who experience claudication from chronic arterial disease usually can only walk for short periods before the onset of pain limits their ability to continue exercise. Therefore, long duration of exercise with frequent intervals is not a realistic plan to progress toward the goal of increasing ambulation distance.

4. Although the infrequent intervals may provide the patient with less total activity, the long duration of the exercise remains problematic.

System: Cardiovascular and Pulmonary Systems
Content Outline: Interventions

 Level 2

➡ PTAEXAM TWO: QUESTION 105

A patient post bone marrow transplant is referred to physical therapy for instruction in an exercise program. The physical therapist assistant plans to use oxygen saturation measurements to monitor the patient's exercise tolerance. Assuming the patient's oxygen saturation was measured as 95 percent at rest, which of the following guidelines would be the **MOST** appropriate for determining when to discontinue the exercise?

1. When the patient's oxygen saturation is below 95%
2. **When the patient's oxygen saturation is below 90%**
3. When the patient's oxygen saturation is below 85%
4. When the patient's oxygen saturation is below 80%

Correct Answer: 2 (Paz p. 371)

An oxygen saturation at rest greater than 95% is considered to be within normal limits. A rate of 90% or less is often used as a guideline to discontinue exercise activities. Supplemental oxygen may be indicated if oxygen saturation is 90% or less.

1. An oxygen saturation of 95% is within normal limits.
2. **When oxygen saturation falls below 90% exercise should be discontinued and the patient should rest. This corresponds to a partial pressure of oxygen (PaO_2) of approximately 60 mm Hg, which represents a state of arterial hypoxemia. This is the most common indication for supplemental oxygen therapy.**
3. A patient with an oxygen saturation of 85% is in a state of hypoxemia. Exercise should have been terminated before this level of hypoxemia was reached.
4. A patient with an oxygen saturation of 80% is in a severe hypoxemic state. Exercise should have been terminated before this level of hypoxemia was reached.

System: Other Systems
Content Outline: Interventions

➡ PTAEXAM TWO: QUESTION 106

A physical therapist assistant attempts to select an assistive device for a patient post traumatic brain injury. The patient is occasionally impulsive, however, has fair standing balance and good upper and lower extremity strength. Which of the following assistive devices would be the **MOST** appropriate for the assistant to select for the patient?

1. Cane
2. Axillary crutches
3. Lofstrand crutches
4. **Walker**

Correct Answer: 4 (Fairchild p. 216)

A walker would be the most appropriate assistive device to use since the patient can stand without support, however, has only fair standing balance and is impulsive at times. A walker does not require a great deal of coordination.

1. A cane is appropriate to assist with balance and stability, however, it does not provide a large amount of assistance due to the small base of support. A cane would not be appropriate for a patient that presents with impulsivity and only fair standing balance.
2. Axillary crutches are appropriate for patients of all weight bearing levels, however, require a higher level of coordination. Injury can occur to axillary vessels and nerves if used improperly. The device would not be appropriate for the patient based on their present balance and the medical diagnosis.
3. Lofstrand crutches are an option for patients that need more support than a cane. The crutches provide minimal stability and require functional standing balance and coordination for use. Lofstrand crutches would not be appropriate for a patient with fair balance and impulsivity.
4. **A walker is appropriate for patients of varying weight bearing levels. The device offers the greatest amount of stability due to its large base of support. The stability offered by the walker is necessary due to the patient's fair standing balance and impulsivity. Proper supervision would be necessary based on the patient's diagnosis.**

System: Non-Systems
Content Outline: Equipment, Devices, and Technologies;
   Therapeutic Modalities

 Level 2   p. 368, 383

 Level 2   p. 602-603

➡ PTAEXAM TWO: QUESTION 107

A patient is two days post surgical insertion of a urinary catheter. This procedure is **MOST** commonly performed with which of the following types of catheters?

1. Condom

2. Foley

3. **Suprapubic**

4. Swan-Ganz

Correct Answer: 3 (Fairchild p. 281)

An internal or indwelling catheter is inserted through the urethra and into the bladder. Females can utilize internal catheters, while males can use internal or external catheters.

1. An external catheter is applied over the shaft of the penis and is held in place by a padded strap or adhesive tape. The catheter has no practical application for females.

2. A Foley catheter is an indwelling urinary tract catheter that has a balloon attachment at one end. The balloon, which is filled with air or sterile water, must be deflated before the catheter can be removed. The catheter does not require surgical insertion.

3. **A suprapubic catheter is an indwelling urinary catheter that is surgically inserted directly into the patient's bladder. Insertion of a suprapubic catheter is performed under general anesthesia.**

4. A Swan-Ganz catheter is a soft, flexible catheter that is inserted through a vein into the pulmonary artery. The device is used to provide continuous measurements of pulmonary artery pressure.

System: Other Systems
Content Outline: Diseases/Conditions that Impact Effective Treatment

➡ PTAEXAM TWO: QUESTION 108

A physical therapist assistant completes documentation after administering an ultrasound treatment. Which of the following treatment parameters would be the **LEAST** important to document?

1. **Patient position**

2. Treatment time

3. Intensity

4. Duty cycle

Correct Answer: 1 (Cameron p. 186)

The following items are typically documented when using ultrasound: area of the body treated, duration, frequency, intensity, duty cycle, and patient response to treatment.

1. **Patient position is primarily determined based on accessibility to the body surface being treated and patient comfort. Although this is an important item to consider when using ultrasound, it is not as critical as the specific parameters of the ultrasound treatment.**

2. The treatment time refers to the period of time that ultrasound is being emitted. The treatment time when using ultrasound is primarily determined based on the size of the surface area to be treated. Given the variability in treatment times when using ultrasound, it is a necessary parameter to document.

3. Intensity is a measure of the rate at which energy is being delivered per unit of area. Intensity levels vary considerably based on the desired physiologic effects and therefore, it is a necessary parameter to document.

4. Duty cycle is defined as the ratio of the on time to the total time. The duty cycle selected will significantly influence changes in tissue temperature and therefore, it is a necessary parameter to document.

System: Non-Systems
Content Outline: Equipment, Devices, and Technologies; Therapeutic Modalities

---

 Level 1   p. 609

● Level 2   p. 623-626

➡ PTA EXAM TWO: QUESTION 109

A physical therapist assistant treats a patient who has Alzheimer's disease. Which of the following treatments would be recommended as a **PRIMARY** intervention for this patient population?

1. **Physical activity**
2. Stretching
3. Coordination training
4. Pulmonary therapy

Correct Answer: 1 (Goodman – Pathology p. 1472)

Alzheimer's disease is a progressive neurodegenerative disorder that results in deterioration within the brain. Amyloid plaques and neurofibrillary tangles result in further damage to the nervous system. Alzheimer's disease is initially noted by a change in higher cortical functions with subtle changes in memory, impaired concentration, and difficulty with new learning. There is compelling evidence that physical activity can improve memory and delay overall decline.

1. **During the early stages of Alzheimer's disease a patient should continue with daily physical activity. As the disease progresses, a patient will rely on caregiver support to assist with a daily exercise program. Physical activity and structured exercise can assist with memory as well as decrease the effects of Alzheimer's disease including restlessness and wandering.**

2. Stretching is typically most appropriate for patients that exhibit contractures or present with hypertonicity. This type of clinical presentation is not consistent with Alzheimer's disease.

3. Coordination training is most appropriate for patients that present with ataxia, nystagmus, impaired balance and equilibrium deficits typically due to a lesion within the cerebellum. This type of clinical presentation is not consistent with Alzheimer's disease.

4. Pulmonary therapy is most appropriate for patients that present with a compromised pulmonary system and may include airway clearance, breathing techniques, assisted cough, and ventilatory muscle training. Patients with Alzheimer's disease do not typically exhibit a compromised pulmonary system.

System: Neuromuscular and Nervous Systems
Content Outline: Interventions

➡ PTA EXAM TWO: QUESTION 110

A physical therapist assistant discusses pain management for a patient post total hip arthroplasty with the patient's nurse. Which objective finding would make the use of patient-controlled analgesia the **MOST** unrealistic?

1. **Altered cognitive status**
2. Elevated respiratory rate
3. Advanced age
4. History of substance abuse

Correct Answer: 1 (Fairchild p. 285)

Patient-controlled analgesia allows the patient to manage their pain by delivering an intravenous analgesic dose with preset parameters. The medication is self-administered by pressing a button to receive a preset dose of medicine.

1. **Altered cognitive status would make it problematic for the patient to understand the rationale for the use of patient controlled analgesia and to follow the supplied instructions. Patient controlled analgesia is an ineffective form of pain management for patients with altered cognition.**

2. An elevated respiratory rate would not necessarily prohibit the use of patient controlled analgesia. The use of intravenous narcotics through patient controlled analgesia is likely to produce sedation and a decreased respiratory rate.

3. Advanced age would not necessarily prohibit the use of patient controlled analgesia since the ability to follow instructions and physically push the button is not age dependent. Infants and very young children are typically poor candidates for patient controlled analgesia since they are likely to have difficulty conceptualizing the purpose and required routine.

4. A history of substance abuse may make the use of patient controlled analgesia undesirable. However, the ability to control the type of medication, demand dose, and dose interval makes this option remain a possibility depending on the unique circumstances associated with the patient's history of substance abuse.

System: Musculoskeletal System
Content Outline: Diseases/Conditions that Impact Effective Treatment

● Level 2   ◠◠ p. 246, 290-291

● Level 2

➡ PTAEXAM TWO: QUESTION 111

The presence of which of the following findings may assist a child with cerebral palsy during a stand pivot transfer?

1. Primitive reflexes
2. **Spasticity**
3. Athetosis
4. Equinovarus contracture

Correct Answer: 2 (Palisano p. 451)

Cerebral palsy is a disorder of the development of movement and posture as a result of brain lesions occurring in the fetal or infant brain. Common impairments related to cerebral palsy include persistence of primitive reflexes, spasticity, ataxia, and equinovarus.

1. Persistence of primitive reflexes such as the asymmetrical tonic neck reflex may limit a child's gross motor development such as rolling or independent sitting. Primitive reflexes would interfere with completion of a stand pivot transfer.

2. **Spasticity may assist a child with cerebral palsy to stand because of lack of reciprocal inhibition of antagonist muscle groups causing simultaneous activation of muscles (i.e., cocontraction).**

3. Athetosis or athetoid movement may be observed with cerebral palsy. Athetoid movement is characterized by slow, continuous, writhing movements that interfere with stable upright positions such as sitting and standing. Athetoid movement would interfere with completion of a stand pivot transfer.

4. Equinovarus contractures may be observed in children with cerebral palsy usually as a result of spasticity and improper positioning. An equinovarus contracture would interfere with weight bearing and would therefore interfere with completion of a stand pivot transfer.

System: Neuromuscular and Nervous Systems
Content Outline: Interventions

➡ PTAEXAM TWO: QUESTION 112

During a patient interview, a physical therapist assistant asks the patient about any feelings of dependency on coffee, tea or soft drinks. Which of the following clinical scenarios would **MOST** appropriately warrant this type of question?

1. A patient following arthroscopic medial meniscectomy
2. **A patient with premature ventricular contractions**
3. A patient with restrictive pulmonary disease
4. A patient with respiratory alkalosis

Correct Answer: 2 (Hillegass p. 325)

Premature ventricular contractions (PVCs) are premature beats arising from an ectopic focus in one of the ventricles of the heart. Coffee, tea, and soft drinks may contain caffeine, a stimulant that may precipitate premature ventricular contractions. Other causes of PVCs are nicotine, stress, alcohol, and certain electrolyte imbalances.

1. It would not be important to know if a patient who is post arthroscopic medial meniscectomy has a dependence on coffee, tea, and soft drinks, since these drinks would not influence their condition or course of physical therapy.

2. **It would be important to know if a patient known to have PVCs has a dependence on coffee, tea, and soft drinks since these drinks may contain caffeine, a stimulant that can precipitate PVCs. The physical therapist assistant should inform the patient about the possible connection between these drinks and the occurrence of PVCs.**

3. It would not be important to know if a patient who has restrictive pulmonary disease has a dependence on coffee, tea, and soft drinks, since these drinks would not influence their condition or course of physical therapy.

4. It would not be important to know if a patient with respiratory alkalosis has a dependence on coffee, tea, and soft drinks, since these drinks would not influence their condition or course of physical therapy.

System: Cardiovascular and Pulmonary Systems
Content Outline: Diseases/Conditions that Impact Effective Treatment

 Level 2   p. 297-298, 595-596

 Level 2

➡ PTAEXAM TWO: QUESTION 113

A physical therapist assistant instructs a patient in a traditional bench press exercise using free weights. Which modification would be the **MOST** beneficial to limit the amount of stress placed on the anterior capsule of the shoulder?

1. Grasp the bar with a supinated grip with the hands slightly wider than shoulder width apart

2. Ensure that the elbows are fully extended at the conclusion of the upward movement

3. **Ensure that the bar does not contact the chest during the downward movement**

4. Attempt to slightly raise the head off of the bench during the upward movement

Correct Answer: 3 (Coburn p. 550)

The bench press is a commonly used exercise that functions to strengthen the pectoralis major, anterior deltoid, serratus anterior, pectoralis minor, and triceps brachii. Physical therapist assistants must be able to adapt specific exercises to the unique needs of each patient.

1. The bench press should be performed with a pronated grip rather than a supinated grip. The patient should grasp the bar with the hands slightly wider than shoulder width apart.

2. The elbows are typically fully extended at the conclusion of the upward movement of the bench press. As a result, this action does not serve to limit the amount of stress on the anterior capsule of the shoulder.

3. **In a typical bench press, the patient is instructed to lower the bar until it touches the chest at approximately nipple level. As a result, ensuring that the bar does not contact the chest serves to reduce the amount of stress on the anterior capsule of the shoulder. Therapists should attempt to avoid instructing patients with known or suspected shoulder pathology in exercises that place the arms and hands behind the plane of the shoulder.**

4. The head should remain in contact with the bench at all times during a bench press. Attempting to lift the head is a common substitution pattern that should be avoided since it has the potential to jeopardize patient safety.

System: Musculoskeletal System
Content Outline: Interventions

➡ PTAEXAM TWO: QUESTION 114

A physical therapist assistant works with a patient with C7 tetraplegia on transferring from a manual wheelchair to a mat table with a sliding board. According to the head-hips relationship principle, which direction should the patient move their head to initiate the transfer?

1. **Down and away from the mat**

2. Up and towards the mat

3. Down and towards the mat

4. Up and away from the mat

Correct Answer: 1 (Fell p. 1093)

The head-hips principle is a compensatory movement strategy used to perform transfers and bed mobility in patients with complete and incomplete spinal cord injuries. When using the head-hips principle, the patient utilizes momentum through voluntary head movement in one direction to produce movement of the buttocks in the opposite direction.

1. **In order to best perform a sliding board transfer, a patient with C7 tetraplegia would lock the elbows using muscle substitution or stabilize using the triceps. The patient would then lean forward onto the bilateral upper extremities, while tucking the chin into the chest. The patient quickly and forcefully moves the head and shoulders down and away from the destination surface in order to lift and move the buttocks to perform a transfer in the direction of the destination.**

2. A patient with a spinal cord injury would not be successful if the patient moved their head towards the mat surface to initiate the transfer since they would not possess adequate muscle strength to pull themselves onto the destination surface. Moving the head up and towards the mat results in the hips staying on the initial surface with momentum away from the destination surface.

3. A patient with a spinal cord injury would not be successful if the patient moved their head down and towards the destination surface since this would result in the hips moving up and away from the destination surface, not towards it.

4. A patient with a spinal cord injury would not be successful if the patient moved their head up and away from the destination surface since the hips would not rise from the wheelchair seat. This motion would not allow the patient to effectively utilize the sliding board.

System: Neuromuscular and Nervous Systems
Content Outline: Interventions

⦿ Level 2

⦿ Level 2   p. 269-272, 312-313, 595

➡ PTAEXAM TWO: QUESTION 115

After performing a manual muscle test of the tibialis anterior, a physical therapist assistant assigns a numerical scale grade of 4 to patient A and a grade of 2 to patient B. Which of the following statements is the **BEST** interpretation of the patients' strength?

1. Patients A and B have equal strength
2. **Patient A is stronger than patient B**
3. Patient A is twice as strong as patient B
4. Patient B is twice as strong as patient A

Correct Answer: 2 (Portney p. 68)

Manual muscle test grades are examples of ordinal measurements, which in essence represent labels specifying relative rank or position. Ordinal measurements are rank-ordered into categories that have a "greater than – less than" relationship. The intervals between ranks on an ordinal scale may not be consistent and may not be known.

1. The numerical scale used in manual muscle testing ranks the strength by strongest (equivalent to the grade of 5) and weakest (equivalent to the grade of 0). In this situation, the grades are not equal, 4 does not equal 2, therefore, they cannot have equal strength.

2. **Based on the traditional 0–5 manual muscle grading scale, a grade of 4 represents more muscle strength than a grade of 2.**

3. The numerical scale does not provide an "absolute" value, therefore, it is impossible to say that a grade of 4 is two times stronger than a grade of 2. Furthermore, the testing positions of these grades are not the same and as a result they cannot be compared in this manner.

4. The numerical order of the manual muscle testing scale indicates that a grade of 5 is the strongest and a grade of 0 is the weakest. Therefore, a grade of 2 cannot indicate greater strength than a grade of 4.

System: Musculoskeletal System
Content Outline: Physical Therapy Data Collection

➡ PTAEXAM TWO: QUESTION 116

After performing a wound inspection, a physical therapist assistant documents the exudate from a patient's wound as serous. Based on the documentation, which color **BEST** describes this type of exudate?

1. **Clear**
2. Pink
3. Red
4. Yellow

Correct Answer: 1 (Sussman p. 458)

It is normal during the stages of healing to observe exudate from a wound. The physical therapist assistant should inspect the exudate and determine whether it is a normal response to healing or an abnormal response that needs to be reported.

1. **Serous exudate is described as a clear or light color fluid with a thin, watery consistency. This particular type of exudate is normal during the inflammatory and proliferative phases of healing.**

2. Serosanguineous (pink) exudate can be a normal exudate in a healthy healing wound.

3. Sanguineous (red) exudate indicates a bloody discharge which may be indicative of either new blood vessel growth (normal healing tissue) or a disruption of blood vessels (abnormal).

4. Purulent (yellow) exudate is generally indicative of infection.

System: Other Systems
Content Outline: Physical Therapy Data Collection

 Level 2   p. 705-706

 Level 1   p. 445

 SCOREBUILDERS

➡ PTAEXAM TWO: QUESTION 117

A physical therapist assistant performs a muscle length test for the long head of the triceps. Which of the following findings is the **MOST** consistent with shortening of this muscle?

1. Limitation of elbow flexion with the shoulder maintained at the end range of extension

2. Limitation of elbow extension with the shoulder maintained at the end range of extension

3. Limitation of elbow extension with the shoulder maintained at the end range of flexion

4. **Limitation of elbow flexion with the shoulder maintained at the end range of flexion**

Correct Answer: 4 (Kisner p. 115)

Muscle length testing involves elongating the muscle in the direction opposite of its actions while assessing resistance to passive movement. Although all three heads of the triceps extend the elbow, the long head originates from the infraglenoid tubercle of the scapula and extends the shoulder as well.

1. Although assessing elbow flexion is appropriate for muscle length testing of the triceps, placing the shoulder at the end range of extension would give slack to the long head of the triceps.

2. A limitation of elbow extension with the shoulder maintained at the end range of extension would be a sign of shortening of the biceps brachii, especially if the forearm is maintained in a pronated position, since the biceps muscle is also a supinator.

3. Although assessing the end range of shoulder flexion is part of muscle length testing for the long head of the triceps, elbow extension places this muscle on slack.

4. **A limitation of elbow flexion while the shoulder is maintained at the end range of flexion is indicative of shortening of the long head of the triceps.**

System: Musculoskeletal System
Content Outline: Physical Therapy Data Collection

➡ PTAEXAM TWO: QUESTION 118

A physical therapist assistant observes that a patient appears to have recently gained weight. Which of the following medical conditions would **MOST** likely be associated with weight gain?

1. Addison's disease

2. Crohn's disease

3. **Congestive heart failure**

4. Graves' disease

Correct Answer: 3 (Hillegass p. 100)

Weight gain typically occurs when the calories from food consumed exceed the calories that are burned off. Weight gain can also be associated with a variety of medical conditions such as hypothyroidism, Cushing's syndrome, organ disease, congestive heart failure, essential fatty acid deficiencies, and blood sugar imbalance.

1. Addison's disease is a form of adrenal dysfunction that presents with hypofunction of the adrenal cortex. Subsequently, there is decreased production of both cortisol and aldosterone. Symptoms may include hypotension, weakness, anorexia, and altered pigmentation. Weight loss often results from loss of appetite and chronic diarrhea.

2. Crohn's disease is a form of inflammatory bowel disease that usually affects the intestines. The condition causes inflammation of the lining of the digestive tract. Individuals with Crohn's disease often have a decreased appetite, however, at the same time, the chronic nature of the disease increases an individual's caloric needs. The combination of decreased appetite and increased caloric need often leads to significant weight loss.

3. **Congestive heart failure occurs when the heart can no longer meet the metabolic demands of the body. The impairment in cardiac output causes the body to compensate for this deficit and results in a variety of symptoms including tachycardia, weight gain, cyanotic extremities, and shortness of breath. Weight gain primarily results from an increase in the amount of fluid in the body. Pharmacological management, such as diuretics, helps to reduce the amount of fluid in the body.**

4. Graves' disease is caused by an autoimmune disease in which certain antibodies produced by the immune system stimulate the thyroid gland causing it to become overactive. Symptoms are consistent with hyperthyroid presentation including mild enlargement of the thyroid gland (goiter), heat intolerance, nervousness, tremor, and palpitations. Hyperthyroidism increases metabolism which often results in weight loss.

System: Other Systems
Content Outline: Diseases/Conditions that Impact Effective Treatment

 Level 2   p. 106-108

 Level 2   p. 364, 398-399

➡ PTA EXAM TWO: QUESTION 119

A physical therapist assistant is treating a patient that has been prescribed levodopa. The patient has been taking the drug as directed for two weeks. Which physical therapy intervention would be **MOST** affected secondary to the potential negative side effects of the prescribed medication?

1. **Balance activities**
2. Strengthening activities
3. Range of motion activities
4. Endurance activities

Correct Answer: 1 (Ciccone p. 135)

Dopamine replacement therapy (e.g., levodopa) is the most effective treatment to reduce the symptoms of Parkinson's disease. Symptoms often include bradykinesia, rigidity, tremor, and movement disorders. The medical management of Parkinson's disease relies heavily on pharmacological intervention.

1. **During the initial use of levodopa, patients regularly experience lightheadedness and orthostatic hypotension. Balance activities would pose the greatest challenge for this patient during this period with the newly prescribed medication. The patient should be monitored closely to ensure safety with activities that challenge their balance.**

2. Strengthening activities increase the patient's overall strength and can include isometric, concentric, and eccentric strengthening. Levodopa does not typically negatively influence a patient's strength and therefore strengthening activities should not increase in difficulty due to the prescribed medication.

3. Range of motion activities promote adequate mobility at each joint. Levodopa does not typically negatively influence a patient's range of motion and therefore range of motion activities should not increase in difficulty due to the prescribed medication.

4. Endurance activities improve the aerobic system in order to meet oxygen demands. Levodopa can initially cause orthostatic hypotension which can impact the cardiovascular system, however, the patient should still be able to perform endurance activities. Endurance activities can be performed without significantly challenging the patient's balance.

System: Neuromuscular and Nervous Systems
Content Outline: Diseases/Conditions that Impact Effective Treatment

➡ PTA EXAM TWO: QUESTION 120

A physical therapist assistant attempts to assess a patient's relative risk for developing coronary artery disease. Which of the following scenarios would result in the patient being at the **GREATEST** risk?

1. A 51-year-old female with a sedentary lifestyle
2. A 53-year-old female with a high-density lipoprotein level of 60 mg/dL
3. **A 48-year old male with total serum cholesterol of 224 mg/dL**
4. A 55-year-old male with a body mass index of 26 kg/m²

Correct Answer: 3 (Coburn p. 152)

Coronary artery disease is a condition characterized by a narrowing or blockage of the coronary arteries. Risk factors for coronary artery disease include age, cigarette smoking, sedentary lifestyle, obesity, hypertension, dyslipidemia, and prediabetes.

1. The probability of developing coronary artery disease increases with age, however, females are at less relative risk than males. A sedentary lifestyle increases the relative risk of developing coronary artery disease.

2. Females are at less relative risk than males for developing coronary artery disease. The established risk threshold for women is equal to or greater than 55 years. Individuals with high-density lipoprotein levels less than 40 mg/dL increases the relative risk of developing coronary artery disease.

3. **Males are at more relative risk than females for developing coronary artery disease. The established risk threshold for males is equal to or greater than 45 years. Individuals with a total serum cholesterol of greater than 200 mg/dL increases the relative risk of developing coronary artery disease.**

4. Males are at more relative risk than females for developing coronary artery disease. Obesity increases the relative risk for developing coronary artery disease, however, a body mass index of 26 kg/m² is considered overweight, not obese.

System: Cardiovascular and Pulmonary Systems
Content Outline: Diseases/Conditions that Impact Effective Treatment

 Level 3   p. 246, 511

 Level 1   p. 363-364, 411

➡ PTAEXAM TWO: QUESTION 121

A physical therapist assistant instructs a patient in the use of a transcutaneous electrical nerve stimulation unit as part of a home program. The assistant provides detailed instructions on the care and use of the unit. Which of the following activities is **NOT** the responsibility of the patient?

1. Modulate the current intensity
2. Application of new electrodes
3. Change the battery
4. **Alter the pulse rate and width**

Correct Answer: 4 (Cameron p. 246)

Physical therapist assistants routinely educate patients on how to use various portable electrical devices such as a transcutaneous electrical nerve stimulation (TENS) unit at home. Physical therapist assistants must be sure that patients understand which parameters they are independently able to modify and which parameters should be modified only by the therapist.

1. Patients need to adjust the current intensity of the TENS unit with each use. Current intensity refers to the movement of charged particles and is most often measured in amperes.

2. Applying new electrodes is a relatively easy task that does not require changing any of the specified treatment parameters.

3. Changing the battery of a TENS unit is a relatively easy task that does not require changing any of the specified treatment parameters.

4. **Specific pulse rates and widths are selected by the therapist based on the TENS technique selected. Common techniques include conventional TENS, acupuncture-like TENS, brief-intense TENS, and noxious TENS. Pulse rate and width should not be altered by the patient throughout the duration of treatment, unless specified by the therapist.**

System: Non-Systems
Content Outline: Equipment, Devices, and Technologies; Therapeutic Modalities

➡ PTAEXAM TWO: QUESTION 122

A patient post right radial head fracture is treated in physical therapy. The patient's involved elbow range of motion begins at 15 degrees of flexion and ends at 90 degrees of flexion. Which of the following formats **BEST** reflects how the physical therapist assistant should record the patient's elbow range of motion in the medical record?

1. 0-15-90 degrees
2. 15-0-90 degrees
3. **15-90 degrees**
4. 0-90 degrees

Correct Answer: 3 (Norkin p. 35)

Physical therapist assistants must accurately record the results of goniometric measurements in a manner that is easily interpreted by all health care providers. Any recording of range of motion must include the beginning of the range as well as the end of the range.

1. This style of recording is not acceptable since it is not possible to have two distinct values to the right of the "0".

2. The use of "0" between the starting and ending values indicates the patient has 15 degrees of elbow hyperextension. The total available degrees of movement would be 105 degrees.

3. **The recording depicts a patient who begins in 15 degrees of elbow flexion and ends in 90 degrees of elbow flexion. The total available degrees of movement would be 75 degrees.**

4. The recording depicts a patient who is able to fully extend the elbow and flex the elbow to 90 degrees. The total available degrees of movement would be 90 degrees.

System: Musculoskeletal System
Content Outline: Physical Therapy Data Collection

 Level 2   p. 642-643

Level 1   p. 86-87, 94

➡ PTAEXAM TWO: QUESTION 123

A health care provider is struck in the face with a sudden involuntary movement of a patient's upper extremity. This incident would **MOST** likely be associated with which of the following conditions?

1. Athetosis
2. Chorea
3. **Hemiballism**
4. Rigidity

Correct Answer: 3 (O' Sullivan p. 213)

An involuntary movement is defined as a movement that the person does not start or stop at the person's own command or with an observer's command. Muscle fiber contractions of either central or peripheral origin can create small or large scale responses that produce distinctive movement patterns.

1. Athetosis is a movement disorder that presents with slow, twisting, and writhing movements that are large in amplitude. Athetoid movement is primarily seen in the face, tongue, trunk, and extremities and is a common finding in several forms of cerebral palsy. Athetosis would not likely be responsible for the health care provider being struck in the face due to the slowness of the movement.

2. Chorea is a form of hyperkinesia that presents with brief, irregular contractions that are rapid, but not to the degree of myoclonic jerks. Chorea is typically secondary to damage of the caudate nucleus. The condition is often equated to "fidgeting" and therefore would be unlikely to contribute to the described scenario.

3. **Hemiballismus is a movement disorder characterized by large amplitude, sudden, violent, flailing motions of the arm and leg on one side of the body. The condition is an impairment associated with a lesion of the basal ganglia. The rapidity and extent of the movement associated with hemiballismus makes it likely that the condition contributed to the health care provider being struck in the face.**

4. Rigidity refers to a state of severe hypertonicity where a sustained muscle contraction does not allow for any movement at a specified joint. The relative absence of movement associated with rigidity would not allow the shoulder range of motion necessary to strike the health care provider.

System: Neuromuscular and Nervous Systems
Content Outline: Interventions

➡ PTAEXAM TWO: QUESTION 124

A patient who has a history of falls due to age-related attention deficits participates in balance training. Which of the following activities would be the **MOST** difficult for the patient to perform given the age-related attention deficits?

1. Maintaining a posture while focusing on a distant object
2. **Ambulating while performing mental arithmetic**
3. Holding a specific posture while listening to music
4. Ambulating in a narrow, uncrowded hallway

Correct Answer: 2 (Robnett p. 103)

Older adults demonstrate significant loss of divided attention, which is the ability to process two or more sources of information at the same time. This is known as dual-tasking and a deficit in this ability can be associated with a greater risk for falls in older adults.

1. Maintaining a posture while maintaining focus on a distant object is an example of single focus or single task activity. This is not affected as a result of normal aging.

2. **Ambulating while performing a demanding activity, like mental math, is an example of dual tasking and challenges the older adult's attention to a greater extent than the other options.**

3. An older adult's ability to maintain selective attention (i.e., disregard irrelevant information) is diminished to a lesser extent than their ability to dual task, therefore this activity would not be the most difficult for the patient.

4. Ambulation in a narrow, uncrowded hallway would not challenge the older adult's ability to dual task, therefore it would not be as impaired as having to navigate a crowded hallway.

System: Neuromuscular and Nervous Systems
Content Outline: Interventions

 Level 1   p. 239

 Level 3

➡ PTAEXAM TWO: QUESTION 125

A physical therapist assistant instructs a patient in a home stretching program that includes the stretch shown in the image. Which of the following structures is **MOST** likely targeted with this technique?

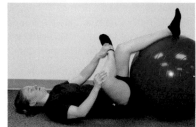

1. Gluteus medius
2. Iliotibial band
3. **Piriformis**
4. Rectus femoris

Correct Answer: 3 (Brody p. 576)

The image shows a patient stretching the right piriformis. The patient uses the left leg to assist with lateral rotation of the right hip. The patient will perceive tension in the right buttock when performing the stretch.

1. The gluteus medius originates on the ilium and inserts on the greater trochanter. The primary action of the muscle is abduction of the hip. As a result, the hip would not be abducted when stretching the gluteus medius.

2. The iliotibial band is a thick tendon-like reinforcement of the tensor fasciae latae that runs from the iliac crest to the lateral condyle of the tibia. The iliotibial band acts to flex and abduct the hip. As a result, the hip would not be in a flexed and laterally rotated position when stretching the iliotibial band.

3. **The piriformis muscle originates on the sacrum and inserts on the greater trochanter. The muscle acts to laterally rotate the femur, however, with the hip flexed more than 60 degrees, the piriformis medially rotates the femur.**

4. The rectus femoris originates on the anterior inferior iliac spine and inserts into the patellar tendon. The muscle acts to flex the hip and extend the knee. As a result, the hip would not be in a flexed position when stretching the rectus femoris.

System: Musculoskeletal System
Content Outline: Interventions

➡ PTAEXAM TWO: QUESTION 126

A terminally ill patient completes a formal document that names his daughter as the individual to make health care decisions in the event that he is unable. Which term is **MOST** consistent with this type of advanced directive?

1. Living will
2. Physician's directive
3. **Durable power of attorney**
4. Euthanasia

Correct Answer: 3 (Scott – Promoting Legal and Ethical Awareness p. 194)

Durable power of attorney for health care decisions refers to a legal document that delegates decision making to a specified individual in the event another individual is found to be incompetent to make a medical decision.

1. A living will is a legal document that a person uses to make known his or her wishes regarding life prolonging medical treatments. It can also be referred to as an advance directive, health care directive or physician's directive.

2. The term "physician's directive" is synonymous with a living will.

3. **The power associated with the durable power of attorney becomes operative when and if the patient becomes legally incompetent to make decisions. The patient often designates a spouse, relative, friend or attorney to act on their behalf.**

4. Euthanasia is the act of ending a person's life and usually pertains to patients in either vegetative states or that are terminally ill. Passive euthanasia is the practice of withholding or withdrawing life-sustaining devices and measures. Active euthanasia involves the deliberate intervention in order to facilitate a person's death.

System: Non-Systems
Content Outline: Safety and Protection; Professional Responsibilities; Research

 Level 1

 Level 2   p. 502-503

➡ PTAEXAM TWO: QUESTION 127

A patient rehabilitating from a left shoulder injury performs a resistive exercise as shown in the image. Which muscle would be the **MOST** emphasized when performing the pictured exercise?

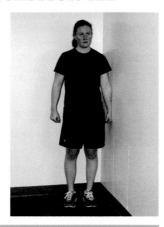

1. Pectoralis major

2. **Supraspinatus**

3. Teres major

4. Teres minor

Correct Answer: 2 (Magee p. 287)

The image shows a patient performing an isometric shoulder exercise emphasizing shoulder abduction. An isometric exercise utilizes isometric contractions that occur when tension develops, but there is no change in the length of the muscle.

1. The clavicular head of the pectoralis major originates on the anterior surface of the medial half of the clavicle. The sternocostal head originates on the anterior surface of the sternum and six costal cartilages and the aponeurosis of the external oblique muscle. The muscles insert on the lateral lip of the intertubercular groove of the humerus. The clavicular head acts to flex the humerus while the sternocostal head extends the humerus. Collectively, the muscle adducts and medially rotates the humerus.

2. **The supraspinatus originates on the middle two-thirds of the supraspinous fossa of the scapula and inserts on the greater tubercle of the humerus. The muscle acts to abduct the shoulder and stabilize the head of the humerus in the glenoid fossa.**

3. The teres major originates on the dorsal surface of the inferior angle of the scapula and the lower third of the border of the scapula. The muscle inserts on the lesser tubercle of the humerus. The muscle acts to medially rotate, adduct, and extend the shoulder.

4. The teres minor originates on the upper two-thirds of the dorsal surface of the lateral border of the scapula and inserts on the greater tubercle of the humerus. The muscle acts primarily to laterally rotate the shoulder.

System: Musculoskeletal System
Content Outline: Interventions

➡ PTAEXAM TWO: QUESTION 128

A physical therapist assistant treating a four-year-old child with cerebral palsy decides to utilize sustained positioning through lower extremity casting. What is the **PRIMARY** goal of this intervention?

1. Increased standing tolerance

2. Increased core stability

3. **Decreased hypertonicity**

4. Decreased dependent edema

Correct Answer: 3 (Fell p. 639)

Sustained positioning is a therapeutic technique often utilized with patients with cerebral palsy. Inhibitive casting is a specific type of sustained positioning that incorporates a series of static casts to decrease hypertonicity, increase range of motion, and improve overall function. Patients are often encouraged to trial inhibitive casting as a prerequisite to a custom molded orthosis. The orthosis utilizes tone reducing properties in order to normalize tone and maintain range of motion.

1. Casting of the lower extremity would not be an intervention used to increase a patient's standing tolerance. Standing while utilizing a standing frame would be an example of an intervention used to increase standing tolerance.

2. Casting of the lower extremity would not be an intervention used to increase a patient's core stability. Therapeutic techniques such as approximation, weight bearing, and rotational activities would be effective interventions to increase core stability.

3. **Casting of the lower extremity allows for sustained positioning at the ankle in a predetermined position. This process is closely monitored and casting is repeated at set intervals to further improve range and decrease the hypertonicity that is often associated with cerebral palsy. The design of the cast integrates pressure points to decrease tone and diminish the influence of spasticity.**

4. Casting of the lower extremity would not be an intervention used to decrease dependent edema. Custom compression stockings to assist with venous return would be an example of an intervention used to decrease dependent edema.

System: Neuromuscular and Nervous Systems
Content Outline: Interventions

⦿ Level 1

⦿ Level 2   👓   p. 283, 296-297

➡ PTAEXAM TWO: QUESTION 129

A physical therapist assistant completes a developmental assessment on an infant. Which position would typically be the **LAST** to occur assuming normal development?

1. **Modified plantigrade**
2. Quadruped
3. Ring sitting
4. Bridging

Correct Answer: 1 (O'Sullivan p. 415)

Physical therapist assistants can use existing neurodevelopmental postures to assess normal development and to accomplish a variety of specific therapeutic objectives. These objectives include, but are not limited to, influencing tone, balance reactions, stability, and weight bearing.

1. **Modified plantigrade typically occurs at 10 months with an age range of 10-12 months. Modified plantigrade is characterized by lower extremity weight bearing in supported standing while leaning with upper extremity support on a table or weight bearing surface.**

2. Quadruped typically occurs at 8 months with an age range of 7-9 months. Quadruped describes a position where body weight is supported by both upper extremities as well as both lower extremities (i.e., hands and knees).

3. Ring sitting typically occurs at 6 months with an age range of 5-7 months. Ring sitting refers to an independent sitting position where the lower extremities form the shape of a ring. The position allows the infant to use their upper extremities for reaching or grasping objects.

4. Bridging typically occurs at 5 months with an age range of 5-7 months. Bridging occurs when a patient positioned in hooklying lifts their buttocks and low back from a fixed surface.

System: Neuromuscular and Nervous Systems
Content Outline: Physical Therapy Data Collection

➡ PTAEXAM TWO: QUESTION 130

A physical therapist assistant reviews the medical record of a patient with known cardiopulmonary pathology. The patient's past medical history includes gastroesophageal reflux disease. Which activity would potentially be the **MOST** problematic for the patient?

1. Performing diaphragmatic breathing exercises in a semi-Fowler position
2. Initiating a progressive ambulation program on a treadmill
3. **Administering percussion to the anterior basal segments of the lower lobes**
4. Assessing tactile fremitus while palpating the chest wall in sitting

Correct Answer: 3 (Goodman – Pathology p. 871)

Gastroesophageal reflux disease (GERD) is the result of an incompetent lower esophageal sphincter that allows reflux of gastric contents. The backwards movement of stomach acids and contents can cause esophageal tissue injury over time as well as other pathology. Positioning with the head lower than the body significantly increases the likelihood of reflux and therefore should be avoided whenever possible.

1. Diaphragmatic breathing is a breathing technique that can decrease the work of breathing by lowering respiratory rate, increasing tidal volume, and decreasing the use of accessory muscles of respiration by facilitating use of the diaphragm. The semi-Fowler position places a patient in supine with the head of the bed elevated to 45 degrees and pillows under the knees for support and maintenance of a proper lumbar curve. The position would not be problematic for a patient with GERD since the patient is relatively upright.

2. Ambulation on a treadmill is an appropriate activity for a patient with GERD. The activity is rhythmic, occurs in an upright position, and does not involve excessive movement of the stomach.

3. **To administer percussion to the anterior basal segments of the lower lobes, the patient is positioned in supine with the foot of the bed elevated 18 inches. Percussion is applied over the lower ribs on the left and right side. Positioning with the head lower than the feet would significantly increase the likelihood of reflux.**

4. Tactile fremitus refers to the vibration of spoken words felt through the chest wall. The assessment procedure provides information about the density of the lungs and the thoracic cavity. Tactile fremitus is assessed using the ulnar border of the hand or the palmar surface of one or both hands. The option indicates that tactile fremitus is being assessed in an upright position (i.e., sitting) and therefore would not be problematic for a patient with GERD.

System: Cardiovascular and Pulmonary Systems
Content Outline: Interventions

 Level 1   p. 262

Level 2   p. 470, 563

➡ PTAEXAM TWO: QUESTION 131

A physical therapist assistant is treating a patient in an acute care setting who has a hematologic disorder. Which of the following measures would be the **MOST** appropriate for the assistant to monitor on a daily basis in order to ensure patient safety during treatment?

1. Hemoglobin
2. **Complete blood count**
3. Arterial blood gas
4. Blood glucose

Correct Answer: 2 (Paz p. 195)

When treating a patient with a hematologic disorder, a physical therapist assistant should monitor a patient's complete blood count (CBC) along with the coagulation profile in order to determine the potential risk for bruising, decreased oxygen carrying capacity at rest or with exercise, or thrombus formation. This information will allow a therapist to modify or defer physical therapy intervention if warranted secondary to abnormal lab values.

1. Hemoglobin is the iron containing pigment in red blood cells that functions to carry oxygen in the blood. Low hemoglobin may indicate anemia or blood loss; elevated hemoglobin suggests polycythemia or dehydration. Hemoglobin is important to monitor, but not in isolation. A patient with a hematologic disorder requires monitoring of all components of a CBC in order to assess the patient's status.

2. **A CBC measures red blood cell count, total white blood cell count, white blood cell differential, platelets, hemoglobin, and hematocrit. A CBC is performed to assess health, to diagnose and monitor a medical condition, and to monitor the effects of medical treatment. A patient with a hematologic disorder requires daily monitoring of a CBC to allow the therapist to determine trends and to recognize abnormal lab values that may require modification or deferment of services.**

3. Arterial blood gases are collected to evaluate acid–base status (pH), ventilation ($PaCO_2$), and oxygenation of arterial blood (PaO_2). This profile is typically not affected by a hematologic disorder and therefore, would not require daily monitoring in this scenario.

4. Blood glucose refers to sugar that is transported through the bloodstream to supply energy to all the cells. Daily monitoring of blood glucose is most appropriate for a patient diagnosed with diabetes mellitus. This is imperative to prevent the effects of hyper or hypoglycemia. This profile is typically not affected by a hematologic disorder and therefore, would not require daily monitoring in this scenario.

System: Other Systems
Content Outline: Physical Therapy Data Collection

➡ PTAEXAM TWO: QUESTION 132

A physical therapist assistant administers the Six-Minute Walk Test to a patient with reduced aerobic capacity. Which of the following statements **BEST** describes a limitation of the selected test?

1. Offers a limited number of rest periods
2. Requires a face mask to be worn for the collection of air samples
3. Utilizes a minimum required walking speed
4. **Fails to provide insight into the mechanism of exercise limitation**

Correct Answer: 4 (Frownfelter p. 280)

The Six-Minute Walk Test is used to determine a patient's functional exercise capacity. The test is commonly used upon admission, at discharge, and to monitor progress or decline throughout physical therapy. This tool is administered to various populations including those with cardiac impairments, pulmonary disease, chronic conditions, and patients recovering from orthopedic surgical procedures.

1. The individual is allowed to stop and rest as needed during the Six-Minute Walk Test. If the individual does stop, they are asked to remain where they are until they can resume walking.

2. The Six-Minute Walk Test does not require the collection of inspired and expired air samples through the use of a face mask. This would, however, be necessary when completing a maximal exercise test.

3. The individual is instructed to walk as quickly as they can and attempt to cover as much ground as possible during the Six-Minute Walk Test. The test does not utilize predetermined rates of speed or specific stages.

4. **The Six-Minute Walk Test is used to quantify a patient's functional exercise capacity, however, it does not offer the therapist any insight into the mechanism of exercise limitation.**

System: Cardiovascular and Pulmonary Systems
Content Outline: Physical Therapy Data Collection

 Level 2   p. 368-370

 Level 2   p. 385

SCOREBUILDERS

➡ PTA EXAM TWO: QUESTION 133

A physical therapist assistant observes the gait of a patient post lateral ankle sprain. The patient walks without crutches, but the assistant notices an antalgic gait. Which description is the **MOST** accurate when describing the unaffected extremity during walking?

1. **Shorter swing phase and shorter step length**
2. Shorter swing phase and longer step length
3. Longer swing phase and shorter step length
4. Longer swing phase and longer step length

Correct Answer: 1 (Dutton p. 307)

An injury to one extremity will invariably alter the movement pattern in both extremities. Physical therapist assistants must carefully assess the impact of an injury on the entire body.

1. **When an injury occurs to a single extremity, an individual typically attempts to spend less time weight bearing on the affected extremity. This results in a shortening of the stance time on the affected extremity which requires the unaffected extremity to contact the ground sooner (i.e., shorter swing phase). A shorter swing phase on the unaffected extremity typically produces a shorter step length.**

2. A shorter swing phase on the unaffected extremity tends to shorten step length.

3. A longer swing phase on the unaffected extremity is unlikely since this would require the stance phase to be longer on the affected extremity. The amount of pain the patient is experiencing makes this unlikely.

4. A longer swing phase on the unaffected extremity typically produces a longer step length, however, the longer swing phase on the unaffected extremity is unlikely for the reasons discussed in option 3.

System: Musculoskeletal System
Content Outline: Physical Therapy Data Collection

➡ PTA EXAM TWO: QUESTION 134

A physical therapist assistant guards a patient who is descending a step with axillary crutches. Based on the image, which of the following scenarios is the **MOST** likely?

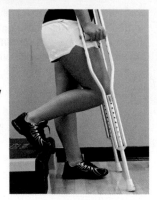

1. **Partial weight bearing secondary to a left lateral ankle sprain**
2. Partial weight bearing secondary to a right lateral ankle sprain
3. Toe touch weight bearing secondary to a left lateral ankle sprain
4. Toe touch weight bearing secondary to a right lateral ankle sprain

Correct Answer: 1 (Fairchild p. 248)

When descending a step with axillary crutches the involved lower extremity and crutches are moved from the step to the ground, while the upper extremities and the uninvolved lower extremity are used to slowly lower the body.

1. **The patient should use the upper extremities and the uninvolved lower extremity to slowly lower the body when descending a step. As a result, the patient's left ankle would be the involved ankle. Partial weight bearing occurs when a patient is allowed to put a particular amount of weight through the involved extremity.**

2. If the right ankle was the involved ankle, the patient would use the upper extremities and the left lower extremity to slowly lower the body when descending a step.

3. The patient's left ankle is the involved ankle, however, the picture does not depict toe touch weight bearing. Toe touch weight bearing occurs when a patient is unable to place any weight through the involved extremity, however, can place the toes on the ground to assist with balance.

4. The right ankle is not the involved ankle and the depicted weight bearing status is better described as partial weight bearing.

System: Musculoskeletal System
Content Outline: Diseases/Conditions that Impact Effective Treatment

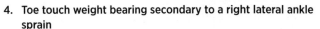

⦿ Level 2   👓 p. 84

⦿ Level 2   👓 p. 605-607

➡ PTAEXAM TWO: QUESTION 135

A physical therapist assistant conducts an inservice on exercise guidelines for a group of senior citizens. During the inservice, the assistant discusses the benefits of improving cardiovascular status through a low intensity activity such as a walking program. What frequency of exercise would be the **MOST** desirable to achieve the stated objective?

1. Twice per day

2. One time per week

3. Three times per week

4. **Five times per week**

Correct Answer: 4 (American College of Sports Medicine p. 175)

To minimize medical problems and promote long-term compliance with this population, exercise intensity should start low and progress gradually according to individual tolerance and preference. Exercise performed at a moderate intensity should be performed for 30 minutes on most days of the week. If exercise is at a vigorous level, it should be performed at least three times per week. Since the cited exercise is low intensity, five times per week is the most appropriate option.

1. The physical therapist assistant can recommend that individuals who have difficulty sustaining exercise for 30 minutes continuously, or who prefer shorter bouts of exercise, should exercise for shorter periods (e.g., 10 minutes) several times each day. This is not the most desirable combination of exercise intensity and frequency, however, to improve cardiovascular status.

2. One time per week is an inadequate frequency to improve cardiovascular fitness when exercising at low intensity.

3. Three times per week is an appropriate frequency if the exercise is at a vigorous level. It would not be the most desirable frequency for low intensity exercise.

4. **Since walking is a low intensity activity, more frequent exercise sessions are needed to improve cardiovascular status. Five times per week is the most desirable option.**

System: Cardiovascular and Pulmonary Systems
Content Outline: Interventions

➡ PTAEXAM TWO: QUESTION 136

A physical therapist assistant reviews the medical record of a patient who has congestive heart failure. The assistant would like to implement a formal exercise program, but is concerned about the patient's exercise tolerance. Which of the following responses is the **MOST** likely reason for the patient's limited exercise tolerance?

1. Diminished lung volumes

2. Arterial oxygen desaturation

3. **Insufficient stroke volume during ventricular systole**

4. Excessive rise in blood pressure

Correct Answer: 3 (Hillegass p. 88)

Congestive heart failure refers to the heart's inability to maintain a cardiac output that is adequate to meet the demands of the tissues secondary to an abnormality in the pumping ability of the heart muscle.

1. Diminished lung volumes are more commonly associated with obstructive or restrictive lung conditions and are not typically associated with congestive heart failure.

2. The level of arterial oxygenation is not significantly impacted with congestive heart failure, rather the primary issue is that a smaller volume of blood is pumped with each contraction of the ventricles.

3. **Congestive heart failure may be due to a diminished pumping ability of the ventricles secondary to muscle weakening (systolic dysfunction) or to stiffening of the heart muscle that impairs the ventricles' capacity to relax and fill (diastolic dysfunction). With systolic dysfunction, the weak heart pumps a smaller volume of blood for each contraction of the ventricles (stroke volume), reducing cardiac output. The resultant decrease in the delivery of oxygenated blood to the active tissues limits the patient's ability to exercise.**

4. Most patients with congestive heart failure take multiple medications including diuretics, vasodilators, ACE inhibitors, and beta-blockers. The medications serve to reduce the hemodynamic response to exercise. An excessive increase in blood pressure is therefore unlikely.

System: Cardiovascular and Pulmonary Systems
Content Outline: Diseases/Conditions that Impact Effective Treatment

  Level 2   p. 386

  Level 2   p. 364, 398-399

➡ PTAEXAM TWO: QUESTION 137

A physical therapist assistant measures a patient for a wheelchair. When measuring back height, which method is the **MOST** accurate?

1. Measure from the seat of the chair to the base of the axilla and subtract two inches

2. **Measure from the seat of the chair to the base of the axilla and subtract four inches**

3. Measure from the seat of the chair to the acromion process and subtract two inches

4. Measure from the seat of the chair to the acromion process and subtract four inches

Correct Answer: 2 (Fairchild p. 137)

There are a variety of specific measurements that must be performed when fitting a patient for a wheelchair. Failure to obtain accurate measurements can result in a wheelchair that is not appropriately sized. An improperly fit wheelchair can result in increased difficulty with mobility and potential complications such as pressure sores or skin breakdown.

1. Measuring from the seat of the chair to the base of the axilla and subtracting two inches would result in the back height being at the mid-scapular level. This back height would be too high to allow for optimal mobility.

2. **Back height should be determined by measuring from the seat of the chair to the base of the axilla and subtracting four inches. This method will allow the back height to fall below the inferior angle of the scapula. The height of the seat cushion used, if applicable, must be added to the obtained measurement.**

3. Measuring from the seat of the chair to the acromion process and subtracting two inches would result in a back height that is excessive and would significantly restrict the patient's movement.

4. Measuring from the seat of the chair to the acromion process and subtracting four inches is more desirable than option 3, but would still not allow the back height to fall below the inferior angle of the scapula.

System: Non-Systems
Content Outline: Equipment, Devices, and Technologies; Therapeutic Modalities

➡ PTAEXAM TWO: QUESTION 138

A patient exercising in an outpatient facility informs their physical therapist assistant that they are experiencing chest pain. After resting for 20 minutes the patient's condition is unchanged, however, they insist it is something that they can work through. Which of the following actions is the **MOST** appropriate for the assistant to take?

1. Allow the patient to resume exercise and continue to monitor the patient

2. Reduce the intensity of the exercise and continue to monitor the patient

3. Discontinue the treatment session and encourage the patient to make an appointment with their physician

4. **Discontinue the treatment session and call an ambulance**

Correct Answer: 4 (Hillegass p. 535)

Changes in anginal symptoms may reflect a change in coronary status. Any increase or change in anginal symptoms should be recorded and receive immediate medical attention.

1. Continued angina after 20 minutes of rest is cause for concern since it may indicate a serious change in the patient's coronary status. The patient should not be allowed to exercise, even if the patient indicates they can work through it.

2. Reducing the intensity of exercise does not negate the fact that the patient has continued angina after 20 minutes of rest.

3. Discontinuing the treatment session is necessary, however, encouraging the patient to make an appointment with their physician does not ensure that the patient will receive immediate medical attention.

4. **If anginal symptoms are not relieved by cessation of exercise and rest, the patient should be transported to the nearest hospital emergency center.**

System: Cardiovascular and Pulmonary Systems
Content Outline: Interventions

 Level 1   p. 596-597

 Level 3   p. 365

➡ PTAEXAM TWO: QUESTION 139

A patient being treated in an acute care hospital reports excessive thirst on multiple occasions during a treatment session. Which electrolyte imbalance would **MOST** likely be associated with this scenario?

1. Hypercalcemia

2. Hyperkalemia

3. Hypermagnesemia

4. **Hypernatremia**

Correct Answer: 4 (Paz p. 358)

Electrolytes play a critical role in maintaining homeostasis within the body. Examples of critical roles played by electrolytes include regulating cardiac function, fluid balance, acid-base balance, and neurologic activity. The most serious electrolyte imbalances involve abnormalities in the level of calcium, potassium, and sodium.

1. Hypercalcemia refers to an excessive level of calcium in the blood. Normal serum calcium is 8.4-10.2 mg/dL. The condition is most commonly associated with hyperparathyroidism since excessive parathyroid hormone raises the level of circulating calcium above normal. Symptoms typically include constipation, pain, nausea, and vomiting.

2. Hyperkalemia refers to an excessive level of potassium in the blood. Normal serum potassium is 3.5-5.0 mEq/L. Levels higher than 7 mEq/L can have significant hemodynamic and neurologic consequences, while levels exceeding 8.5 mEq/L can cause respiratory paralysis or cardiac arrest. Symptoms typically are related to abnormalities in muscular or cardiac function.

3. Hypermagnesemia refers to an excessive level of magnesium in the blood. Normal serum magnesium is 1.5-2.0 mEq/L. This condition is relatively rare since the kidneys are able to eliminate excess magnesium by rapidly reducing its tubular absorption. Hypermagnesemia is most often caused by renal failure. Symptoms typically include hypotension and respiratory depression.

4. **Hypernatremia refers to an excessive level of sodium in the blood. Normal serum sodium is 135-145 mEq/L. The condition results when there is a net water loss or a sodium gain and reflects too little water in relation to total body sodium and potassium. Hypernatremia is most often caused by impaired thirst or restricted access to water and can be facilitated by pathologic conditions with increased fluid loss. The primary symptom of this condition is thirst.**

System: Other Systems
Content Outline: Diseases/Conditions that Impact Effective Treatment

➡ PTAEXAM TWO: QUESTION 140

A patient was administered a narcotic medication one hour prior to the onset of a physical therapy session. Which form of administration ensures that the medication will be 100 percent bioavailable?

1. **Intravenous**

2. Oral

3. Inhalation

4. Sublingual

Correct Answer: 1 (Ciccone p. 19)

Bioavailability refers to the percentage of a drug that ultimately reaches the systemic circulation. The method of drug administration affects bioavailability since the drug must diffuse across cell membrane barriers and may also experience liver metabolism.

1. **Intravenous injection is the only method of drug administration that ensures 100% bioavailability. By injecting the drug directly into the systemic circulation, the drug is fully available to the bloodstream and thus the target tissues.**

2. A drug administered orally would not be 100% bioavailable. The drug will travel down the gastrointestinal tract and must be absorbed through the intestines to reach the bloodstream. The total dose of the drug may not pass through the intestinal wall. Even if the drug does pass through the intestinal wall, it then must travel through the liver (known as the first-pass effect). In the liver, the drug may experience significant metabolization before reaching the systemic circulation.

3. A drug administered via inhalation must diffuse across the alveoli where it then enters the pulmonary circulation. From the pulmonary circulation, it is transported directly to the heart and enters the systemic circulation. Though this form of administration avoids the first-pass effect of the liver, the drug still needs to be absorbed across the alveolar membrane and therefore is not 100% bioavailable. Additionally, drug particles may be trapped by cilia and mucus within the respiratory tract and not even reach the alveoli.

4. A drug administered sublingually is absorbed through the oral mucosa into the venous system. The veins carry the drug to the heart where it can then enter the systemic circulation. Though sublingual administration avoids the first-pass effect of the liver, it still needs to be absorbed through the oral mucosa and is therefore not considered to be 100% bioavailable.

System: Other Systems
Content Outline: Diseases/Conditions that Impact Effective Treatment

Level 2

Level 1   p. 509

➡ PTAEXAM TWO: QUESTION 141

A physical therapist assistant inspects the progress of a partial-thickness wound on a patient's anterior forearm. The assistant notes evidence of resurfacing of the wound with notable changes in the edges of the wound. This observation is **MOST** consistent with which of the following conditions?

1. Maceration
2. Granulation
3. **Epithelialization**
4. Infection

Correct Answer: 3 (Sussman p. 25)

A partial-thickness wound extends through the epidermis and possibly into, but not through, the dermis. Examples include abrasions, blisters, and skin tears. A partial-thickness wound will typically heal by re-epithelialization or epidermal resurfacing depending on the depth of injury.

1. Maceration refers to a softening of connective tissue fibers due to excessive moisture. The result is a loss of pigmentation and a wound that is highly susceptible to breakdown or enlargement.

2. Granulation refers to perfused, fibrous connective tissue that replaces a fibrin clot in a healing wound. The tissue is highly vascular and fills the defects of full-thickness wounds.

3. **Epithelialization refers to the process of epidermal resurfacing and appears as pink or red skin. This process is a function of keratinocytes, which make up the layers of the dermis and epidermis as well as the linings of various body organs.**

4. Signs and symptoms of infection include the production of pus, redness, pain, and swelling. More generalized symptoms of infection may include fever, chills, and an increased pulse rate. Laboratory values associated with infection include an increased erythrocyte sedimentation rate and white blood cell count.

System: Other Systems
Content Outline: Physical Therapy Data Collection

➡ PTAEXAM TWO: QUESTION 142

A patient refuses physical therapy services after being transported to the gym. The physical therapist assistant explains the potential consequences of refusing treatment, however, the patient does not reconsider. Which of the following actions is the **MOST** appropriate for the assistant to take initially?

1. Continue with the patient treatment
2. Convince the patient to have therapy
3. Contact the referring physician
4. **Document the incident in the medical record**

Correct Answer: 4 (Scott – Promoting Legal and Ethical Awareness p. 231)

The Guide for Professional Conduct published by the American Physical Therapy Association states that "A therapist shall respect the patient's/client's right to make decisions regarding the recommended plan of care, including consent, modification or refusal."

1. A therapist does not have the right to treat a patient against their wishes.

2. The therapist is obligated to inform the patient of the potential consequences of refusing treatment, however, the purpose of this action is to allow the patient to make an informed decision and not to "convince" them to have therapy.

3. Contacting the referring physician when a patient refuses treatment is appropriate and necessary, however, it would not be the "initial" therapist action.

4. **The therapist must document that the patient refused treatment and was informed of the potential consequences associated with this decision. Failure to document this important information in a timely manner could place the therapist at unnecessary legal risk.**

System: Non-Systems
Content Outline: Safety and Protection; Professional Responsibilities; Research

---

 Level 2   p. 439, 443

Level 3

➡ PTAEXAM TWO: QUESTION 143

A patient sustained a grade I ankle sprain two days ago during a marching band competition. The patient's description of the mechanism of injury is consistent with inversion and plantar flexion. Which of the following ligaments would **MOST** likely be affected?

1. **Anterior talofibular ligament**
2. Calcaneofibular ligament
3. Anterior tibiofibular ligament
4. Deltoid ligament

Correct Answer: 1 (Magee p. 893)

A grade I ankle sprain is a minor injury that involves stretching of the ligament or perhaps a small partial tear of the ligament. Treatment consists of rest, ice, compression, and elevation.

1. **The anterior talofibular ligament is a thickening of the anterior joint capsule that extends from the anterior surface of the lateral malleolus to the lateral facet of the talus and the lateral surface of the talar neck. The ligament functions to resist ankle inversion with the foot in plantar flexion. Regardless of the position of the foot, the anterior talofibular ligament is the most likely ligament torn with an inversion injury.**

2. The calcaneofibular ligament is a round cord that passes posteroinferiorly from the tip of the lateral malleolus to the lateral surface of the calcaneus. The ligament functions to resist ankle inversion and dorsiflexion.

3. The anterior tibiofibular ligament provides support to the distal tibiofibular joint. The ligament resists distal and posterior glide of the fibula.

4. The deltoid ligament refers to the collective medial ligaments of the ankle. The ligament as a whole attaches proximally to the medial aspect of the medial malleolus and fans out to the various distal attachments. The ligament provides medial ligamentous support by resisting eversion of the talus.

System: Musculoskeletal System
Content Outline: Diseases/Conditions that Impact Effective Treatment

➡ PTAEXAM TWO: QUESTION 144

A physical therapist assistant prepares to administer iontophoresis over the anterior surface of a patient's knee. The assistant would like to keep the current density low in order to avoid skin irritation. Which of the listed parameters would **BEST** accomplish the stated objective?

1. **Current amplitude of 4 mA; electrode with an area of 12 cm²**
2. Current amplitude of 4 mA; electrode with an area of 4 cm²
3. Current amplitude of 3 mA; electrode with an area of 6 cm²
4. Current amplitude of 3 mA; electrode with an area of 4 cm²

Correct Answer: 1 (Cameron p. 280)

The current density may be altered either by increasing or decreasing current intensity or by changing the size of the electrode. Current density with iontophoresis equals current amplitude (mA) divided by electrode size (cm²). Failure to utilize appropriate treatment parameters or failure to monitor the patient's response to treatment creates an unnecessary safety risk.

1. **Current density = 4 mA / 12 cm² = .33 mA/cm²**
2. Current density = 4 mA / 4 cm² = 1.0 mA/cm²
3. Current density = 3 mA / 6 cm² = .50 mA/cm²
4. Current density = 3 mA / 4 cm² = .75 mA/cm²

System: Non-Systems
Content Outline: Equipment, Devices, and Technologies; Therapeutic Modalities

 Level 1   p. 65, 144-145

 Level 2   p. 644-646

➡ PTAEXAM TWO: QUESTION 145

A physical therapist assistant performs a goniometric measurement on a patient's wrist. Based on the motion measured in the image, which value would be **MOST** anticipated assuming the patient has normal wrist range of motion?

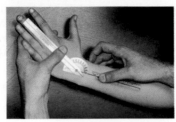

1. **0-20 degrees**
2. 0-30 degrees
3. 0-40 degrees
4. 0-70 degrees

Correct Answer: 1 (Norkin p. 159)

The presented image depicts a physical therapist assistant measuring radial deviation of the wrist. The measurement is performed with the axis of the goniometer aligned over the middle of the dorsal aspect of the wrist over the capitate. The stationary arm is aligned along the dorsal midline of the forearm using the lateral epicondyle of the humerus for reference. The moving arm is positioned over the dorsal midline of the third metacarpal.

1. **A measurement of 0-20 degrees is consistent with normal wrist radial deviation.**

2. A measurement of 0-30 degrees is consistent with normal wrist ulnar deviation.

3. A measurement of 0-40 degrees would be greater than the normal values of wrist radial or ulnar deviation.

4. A measurement of 0-70 degrees is consistent with normal wrist extension.

System: Musculoskeletal System
Content Outline: Physical Therapy Data Collection

➡ PTAEXAM TWO: QUESTION 146

A physical therapist assistant treats a patient with Parkinson's disease using whole-body vibration. Which symptom associated with Parkinson's disease would this intervention **MOST** influence?

1. Dysphagia
2. **Tremor**
3. Akinesia
4. Cognitive impairment

Correct Answer: 2 (Fell p. 664)

Whole-body vibration consists of transferring vibration of varying frequencies to the body as a whole in one or multiple planes. Vibration training can be utilized as an intervention to improve muscle strength, power, flexibility, and coordination. Common medical conditions treated with whole-body vibration include osteoporosis, balance disorders, and Parkinson's disease.

1. Dysphagia refers to the inability to swallow properly. Treatment of dysphagia does not include whole-body vibration, but rather focuses on proper body positioning and compensatory strategies to avoid aspiration when swallowing. Educational topics include the use of thick liquids and conscious swallowing.

2. **Whole-body vibration has been found to effectively decrease tremors and rigidity in patients with Parkinson's disease. Vibratory input to the muscle spindle biases information about muscle length, resulting in more fluid and purposeful movement during memory-guided activity.**

3. Akinesia refers to the inability to initiate movement. The decrease in tremor and rigidity associated with vibration can allow for improved gait and increased step length, however, the actual inability to initiate movement is not directly affected by this intervention.

4. Cognitive, memory, and language impairments can be associated with Parkinson's disease. These impairments most often involve executive functioning within the brain. Cognitive impairments are not affected with the use of whole-body vibration. Adaptive strategies are most commonly utilized to assist with cognitive deficits.

System: Neuromuscular and Nervous Systems
Content Outline: Interventions

Level 2   p. 86

Level 1   p. 238-239, 250, 308-309

➡ PTAEXAM TWO: QUESTION 147

A physical therapist assistant tests a small area of skin for hypersensitivity prior to using a cold immersion bath. The patient begins to demonstrate evidence of cold intolerance within 60 seconds after cold application. Which of the following responses should the assistant take?

1. Limit cold exposure to ten minutes or less
2. Select an alternate cryotherapeutic agent
3. Continue with the cold immersion bath
4. **Discontinue cold application and document the findings**

Correct Answer: 4 (Cameron p. 133)

Signs of cold intolerance include pain, cyanosis, wheals, mottling, increased pulse rate, and a significant drop in blood pressure.

1. Limiting cold exposure to ten minutes or less would still place the patient at significant risk for an adverse reaction to the cold since the patient exhibited evidence of cold intolerance in 60 seconds.

2. Selecting an alternate cryotherapeutic agent would minimally decrease the likelihood of cold intolerance since the magnitude of tissue cooling is relatively uniform across different cryotherapeutic agents.

3. Continuing with the cold immersion bath after observing evidence of cold intolerance would place the patient at significant risk for experiencing a more severe reaction to the cold.

4. **A physical therapist assistant should immediately stop the application of cold when any sign of cold intolerance is observed.**

System: Non-Systems
Content Outline: Equipment, Devices, and Technologies; Therapeutic Modalities

➡ PTAEXAM TWO: QUESTION 148

A patient who has T10 paraplegia is working with a physical therapist assistant on how to react in the event of a backward fall. The patient is instructed to place one hand behind the head and the other across their lap as seen in the image. Placing the hand across the lap is important for which of the following reasons?

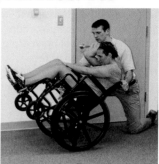

1. Allows the patient to remain within the chair upon landing
2. Allows the patient to hold onto one armrest to stabilize the wheelchair
3. **Prevents the lower extremities from hitting the patient's face**
4. Allows the patient to secure the brake to slow the fall

Correct Answer: 3 (Fairchild p. 166)

Patients that use wheelchairs as their primary mode of mobility should be proficient with all aspects of wheelchair mobility, including a backward fall. Patients with tetraplegia and paraplegia must stabilize their lower extremities during a backward fall to avoid injury secondary to the backward momentum. Patients can also learn how to return the wheelchair to an upright position, however, this is unrealistic for the majority of patients with a complete spinal cord injury.

1. The patient will likely not remain completely within the chair after a backward fall secondary to limited trunk control and lower extremity paralysis.

2. Holding the armrest is a preventative measure to decrease the movement of the lower extremities, not to stabilize the wheelchair.

3. **The primary goal of placing one arm across the lap is to limit the movement of the lower extremities with the forearm so that they do not fall into the patient's face during the backward fall.**

4. Even if the patient is able to reach the brake with the hand placed across the lap, this would not slow the progression of the fall and is not the primary purpose of placing one arm across the lap.

System: Non-Systems
Content Outline: Equipment, Devices, and Technologies; Therapeutic Modalities

⦿ Level 3   👓 p. 615-619

⦿ Level 2

➡ PTAEXAM TWO: QUESTION 149

A physical therapist assistant elects to use a communication board with a patient in an acute care setting. Which of the following patients would **MOST** likely benefit from the use of this image?

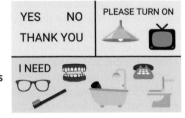

1. A 45-year-old male who speaks limited English
2. A 60-year-old female with hemianopsia
3. **A 75-year-old male with Broca's aphasia**
4. An 88-year-old female with end-stage dementia

Correct Answer: 3 (O'Sullivan p. 656)

Communication boards are often used to communicate with patients that are nonverbal or have impairments in verbal expression. The boards typically use pictures, symbols, and simple words to facilitate communication with individuals who have limited expressive language ability.

1. A 45-year-old male who speaks limited English would most benefit from the use of an interpreter. Although a communication board might provide limited help, the use of an interpreter would be the best choice to maximize communication with the patient.

2. A 60-year-old female with hemianopsia experiences a loss of vision in half of the visual field. Similar to patients with unilateral neglect, patients with hemianopsia may also exhibit a lack of awareness of the side contralateral to the lesion. Use of active visual scanning or tracking movements by turning the head toward the involved side is typically a useful strategy for patients with hemianopsia.

3. **A 75-year-old male with Broca's aphasia would most likely benefit from the use of a communication board. Broca's aphasia is also known as expressive aphasia in which auditory and reading comprehension are intact, but the patient has impaired naming skills and difficulty with language production.**

4. In end-stage dementia, there is typically severe cognitive and physical decline. Individuals lose the ability to communicate or respond to their environment and need constant supervision and assistance with all activities of daily living. A patient in the earlier stages of dementia would be more likely to benefit from the use of a communication board.

System: Neuromuscular and Nervous Systems
Content Outline: Interventions

➡ PTAEXAM TWO: QUESTION 150

A physical therapist assistant works with a patient who has patellofemoral syndrome. The physical therapist directs the assistant to measure the patient's Q angle. Which three bony landmarks should the assistant use to measure the Q angle?

1. Anterior superior iliac spine, superior border of the patella, tibial tubercle
2. **Anterior superior iliac spine, midpoint of the patella, tibial tubercle**
3. Anterior superior iliac spine, inferior border of the patella, midpoint of the patella tendon
4. Greater trochanter, midpoint of the patella, tibial tubercle

Correct Answer: 2 (Hertling p. 499)

The Q angle refers to the angle between the quadriceps muscles and the patella tendon. The angle represents the angle of quadriceps muscle force. Normal Q angle values are 13 degrees for males and 18 degrees for females. An increased Q angle above 18 degrees may be associated with patellar tracking dysfunction, subluxing patella, increased femoral anteversion or increased lateral tibial torsion.

1. The anterior superior iliac spine and tibial tubercle are landmarks used when measuring Q angle, however, the midpoint of the patella should be used as the axis instead of the superior border of the patella.

2. **The most accurate measure of the angle of quadriceps muscular force (i.e., Q angle) utilizes the origin and insertion of the quadriceps muscle and the midpoint of the patella.**

3. The inferior border of the patella is located too far distally to use as the axis when measuring Q angle. The midpoint of the patella tendon is relatively close to the axis and may be difficult to accurately locate compared to a bony landmark such as the tibial tubercle.

4. The greater trochanter is not associated with the origin of the quadriceps muscle and is located too far laterally to use as a landmark when measuring Q angle.

System: Musculoskeletal System
Content Outline: Physical Therapy Data Collection

 Level 2   p. 243-244

 Level 1   p. 123-124, 156-157

NOTES

12

PHYSICAL THERAPIST ASSISTANT
EXAM THREE
ANSWER KEY

Scott Giles

PHYSICAL THERAPIST ASSISTANT
EXAM THREE ANSWER KEY

EXCELLENCE

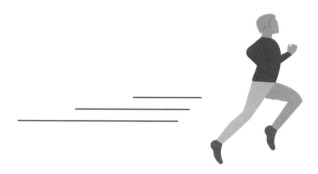

"Aiming for perfection is always a goal in progress."

— Thomas J. Watson Jr.

Candidates do not have to be perfect to pass the NPTE-PTA, however, should attempt to strive for perfection. The relative importance of the examination makes it imperative that candidates become intolerant of any risk of failure.

➡ PTAEXAM THREE: QUESTION 1

A patient who has greater trochanteric bursitis completes an active range of motion exercise for hip flexion. What direction does the femoral head slide on the acetabulum during hip flexion?

1. Slides superiorly on the acetabulum

2. Slides inferiorly on the acetabulum

3. Slides anteriorly and superiorly on the acetabulum

4. **Slides posteriorly and inferiorly on the acetabulum**

Correct Answer: 4 (Norkin p. 255)

The hip joint consists of a convex femoral head within a concave acetabulum, therefore, roll and slide occur in opposite directions.

1. The femoral head slides superiorly on the acetabulum during hip adduction. Normal hip adduction range of motion is 0-30 degrees.

2. The femoral head slides inferiorly on the acetabulum during hip abduction. Normal hip abduction range of motion is 0-45 degrees.

3. The femoral head slides anteriorly and superiorly on the acetabulum during hip extension. Normal hip extension range of motion is 0-30 degrees.

4. **The femoral head slides posteriorly and inferiorly on the acetabulum during hip flexion. Normal hip flexion range of motion is 0-120 degrees.**

System: Musculoskeletal System
Content Outline: Interventions

➡ PTAEXAM THREE: QUESTION 2

A physical therapist assistant completes a two-point discrimination sensory assessment on the right hand of a patient who has a peripheral nerve injury. Which of the following instructions is the **MOST** appropriate for the assistant to ask the patient to indicate during the test?

1. The specific location where the stimulus is felt

2. When two points are felt

3. When the stimulus is first felt

4. **If one or two points are felt**

Correct Answer: 4 (O'Sullivan p. 110)

Two-point discrimination is a testing procedure that quantifies the smallest distance between two stimuli where the patient is able to identify two distinct points. To prevent the patient from anticipating the stimulus, the physical therapist assistant should periodically stimulate with a single point. The distance between the two points is measured with a ruler.

1. If a patient only identifies the location of the stimulus, the therapist cannot discern if there is two-point discrimination or not. The therapist can only surmise that the patient has light touch sensation in the areas assessed.

2. A therapist must ask the patient to identify each touch as one or two points to assess two-point discrimination.

3. If the patient only identifies when they feel a stimulus, the therapist cannot discern if there is two-point discrimination or not. The therapist can only surmise that the patient has light touch sensation in the areas assessed.

4. **Typical two-point discrimination values for the hand include 2 to 4 mm on the fingertips, 4 to 6 mm on the dorsum of the fingers, 8 to 12 mm on the palm, and 20-30 mm on the dorsum of the hand. Two-point discrimination is often impaired with a peripheral nerve injury, parietal lobe lesion or central pathway lesion. Testing is reliable with children older than seven years of age.**

System: Neuromuscular and Nervous Systems
Content Outline: Physical Therapy Data Collection

 Level 1   p. 103-104

 Level 1   p. 233-234

➡ PTAEXAM THREE: QUESTION 3

A physical therapist assistant prepares to initiate an exercise program for a patient who has diabetes mellitus. Which of the following objective measures should the assistant find the **MOST** useful to monitor in order to avoid significant complications from exercise?

1. Systolic blood pressure
2. Respiratory rate
3. **Blood glucose value**
4. Oxygen saturation rate

Correct Answer: 3 (Goodman – Pathology p. 1707)

Decreased blood glucose levels result from inadequate food intake, intense or prolonged exercise or excessive insulin levels. Symptoms include confusion, weakness, clammy skin, and increased pulse rate. Increased blood glucose levels indicate that there is inadequate circulating insulin. Symptoms include polydipsia, polyuria, blurred vision, and dehydration.

1. Systolic blood pressure is the maximum arterial pressure during systole (i.e., contraction of the left ventricle). Normal systolic blood pressure is less than or equal to 120 mm Hg. The physical therapist assistant may monitor the patient's blood pressure response to exercise, however, this is not the most useful measure to avoid significant complications from exercise in a patient with diabetes mellitus (DM).

2. Typical respiration rate is 12-20 breaths per minute. The physical therapist assistant may monitor respiration in response to exercise, however, this is not the most useful measure to avoid significant complications from exercise in a patient with DM.

3. **A patient with DM must check their blood glucose level prior to exercise and must monitor themselves for signs and symptoms of hypoglycemia. A patient with DM will have both benefits and potential risks with exercise. Exercise is contraindicated in patients with poor control of blood glucose levels, dehydration, extreme environmental temperatures, hypertension, and other factors that would precipitate significant changes in blood glucose levels. Severe hypoglycemia can be life-threatening if left untreated.**

4. Oxygen saturation measures the percentage of hemoglobin binding sites in the blood that are bound to oxygen. The physical therapist assistant may monitor oxygen saturation in response to exercise, however, this is not the most useful measure to avoid significant complications from exercise in a patient with DM.

System: Other Systems
Content Outline: Interventions

➡ PTAEXAM THREE: QUESTION 4

A physical therapist assistant utilizes a variety of transfer techniques to move patients of various functional abilities. Which of the following types of transfers would be classified as assisted rather than dependent?

1. Sliding transfer
2. Hydraulic lift
3. **Sliding board transfer**
4. Two-person lift

Correct Answer: 3 (Minor p. 190)

Physical therapist assistants should select transfers for patients based on their unique abilities and limitations. Types of transfers range from completely dependent to independent.

1. The sliding transfer is considered a dependent transfer most often used when transferring a patient in supine from a treatment table or bed to a similar surface. When performing the transfer, therapists often use a "draw" sheet to move the patient from one surface to the other.

2. The hydraulic lift is a device required for dependent transfers when a patient is obese, there is only one therapist available to assist with the transfer or the patient is totally dependent.

3. **The sliding board transfer is used for a patient that possesses sitting balance, upper extremity strength, and can adequately follow directions. The transfer is used when patients can assist or are independent.**

4. The two-person lift is considered a dependent transfer used to transfer a patient between two surfaces of different heights or when transferring a patient to the floor.

System: Non-Systems
Content Outline: Equipment, Devices, and Technologies; Therapeutic Modalities

---

 Level 2   p. 466-467

 Level 1   p. 594-596

SCOREBUILDERS

➡ PTAEXAM THREE: QUESTION 5

A physical therapist assistant treats a patient post Achilles tendon repair using cryotherapy. What cryotherapeutic agent would provide the **GREATEST** magnitude of tissue cooling?

1. Frozen gel packs
2. **Ice massage**
3. Vapocoolant spray
4. Cold water bath

Correct Answer: 2 (Cameron p. 137)

Cryotherapy is a commonly used therapeutic intervention in rehabilitation. Primary uses of cryotherapy include reducing inflammation, pain control, and spasticity management. Physical therapist assistants must be aware of contraindications and precautions of cryotherapy as well as signs or symptoms of cold intolerance.

1. Frozen gel packs contain silica gel and are available in a variety of shapes and sizes. The packs are stored in a refrigeration unit and are usually applied with a moist towel. Cold packs may not maintain uniform contact with the treatment surface and require a treatment time of approximately 20 minutes.

2. **Ice massage is typically performed by freezing water in paper cups and applying the ice directly to the treatment area. Ice massage tends to create a more intense cooling since the ice is applied directly to a localized target area. The treatment time is 5-10 minutes using ice massage due to the intensity of the cooling.**

3. Fluori-Methane is a commonly used vapocoolant spray. Vapocoolant sprays allow for a brief cooling to a very localized area of application. The vapocoolant spray is applied in parallel strokes along the skin in the area of trigger points. Stretching immediately follows the application of the vapocoolant spray.

4. A cold water bath is commonly used for immersion of the distal extremities. A basin or whirlpool is most often used to hold the cold water. A cold bath requires water temperature ranging from 55 to 64 degrees Fahrenheit (13 to 18 degrees Celsius). The body part typically requires a treatment time of 15 to 20 minutes to attain the desired therapeutic effects.

System: Non-Systems
Content Outline: Equipment, Devices, and Technologies; Therapeutic Modalities

➡ PTAEXAM THREE: QUESTION 6

A physical therapist assistant performs a circulatory screening. In order to assess the pulse of the posterior tibial artery, where should the assistant palpate?

1. Medial aspect of the arm midway between the shoulder and elbow
2. **Posterior aspect of the medial malleolus**
3. Posterior aspect of the knee
4. Dorsal aspect of the foot between the first and second metatarsals

Correct Answer: 2 (Fairchild p. 54)

Physical therapist assistants must be aware of common upper and lower extremity circulatory pulse locations. Pulses should be evaluated for rhythm, strength, and circulatory efficiency.

1. The brachial artery is found in the upper extremity and is assessed by palpating the medial aspect of the arm between the shoulder and elbow. It is a major artery of the upper extremity supplying the majority of blood flow and is closely positioned to the median nerve. The brachial artery is also used frequently to obtain blood pressure due to its superficial and palpable pulse.

2. **The posterior tibial artery is found in the lower extremity and is assessed by palpating the posterior aspect of the medial malleolus. This artery provides approximately 75% of the blood flow to the foot and may be difficult to assess with obesity, significant swelling or synovial thickening.**

3. The popliteal artery is found in the lower extremity and is assessed by palpating the posterior aspect of the knee. This pulse can be found deep within the popliteal fossa and is generally difficult to palpate. Weakness of this pulse may indicate femoral artery occlusion since the popliteal artery is a continuation of the femoral artery.

4. The dorsalis pedis artery is found in the lower extremity and is assessed by palpating over the dorsal aspect of the foot between the first and second metatarsal bones. If anterior compartment syndrome is suspected, this pulse should be assessed and compared to the uninvolved foot, however, this pulse is normally absent in approximately 10% of the population.

System: Cardiovascular and Pulmonary Systems
Content Outline: Physical Therapy Data Collection

 Level 2   p. 615-619

Level 1   p. 381-382

➡ PTAEXAM THREE: QUESTION 7

A patient four weeks post anterior cruciate ligament reconstruction using a patellar tendon autograft informs a physical therapist assistant that they are going on vacation for a week in a tropical location. What advice should the assistant give to the patient that would be the **MOST** beneficial to protect their scar from the sun?

1. **Keep the scar covered when outside in the sun**
2. Apply sunscreen with a minimum of 15 SPF directly to the scar
3. Apply sunscreen with a minimum of 30 SPF directly to the scar
4. Apply sunscreen with a minimum of 50 SPF directly to the scar

Correct Answer: 1 (Sussman p. 421)

An anterior cruciate ligament reconstruction using a patellar tendon autograft is a common surgical procedure that requires a 3-4 inch vertical incision over the anterior surface of the knee. It is imperative for the patient to protect the sensitive scar tissue from the sun since exposure can result in thickening and discoloration of the healing tissue.

1. **Keeping the scar covered when outside in the sun provides the best form of protection. This is particularly important in the presented scenario since it has only been four weeks since surgery and the scar is still maturing. Scars should be covered with clothing or a bandage that allows air to circulate. Plastic or other bandages that allow moisture to build up should not be used. As scars mature, they typically fade in color and become softer, flatter, and less sensitive. Scars are considered to be mature in 12-18 months.**

2. Applying sunscreen with a minimum of 15 SPF directly to the scar provides limited protection from the potentially harmful effects of the sun. SPF stands for sun protection factor and refers to the theoretical amount of time an individual can stay in the sun without being sunburned. An SPF of 15 would allow an individual to stay in the sun 15 times longer than they would be able to without protection. Although the sunscreen is beneficial, it is not as protective as keeping the scar covered.

3. Applying sunscreen with a minimum of 30 SPF directly to the scar is typically the minimum SPF recommended when protecting a scar from the sun. This recommendation, however, would be more appropriate for a scar that is more mature. It is important to remember that ultraviolet rays are also present on cloudy days.

4. Applying sunscreen with a minimum of 50 SPF directly to the scar offers greater protection than the other listed SPF options, however, it is not as desirable as covering the four-week-old scar when outside in the sun.

System: Other Systems
Content Outline: Diseases/Conditions that Impact Effective
   Treatment

➡ PTAEXAM THREE: QUESTION 8

A patient being treated for low back pain indicates that they recently were diagnosed with benign prostatic hyperplasia. Which of the following symptoms is **MOST** commonly associated with this condition?

1. Epigastric pain
2. Painful urination
3. Painful ejaculation
4. **Urge to urinate frequently**

Correct Answer: 4 (Goodman – Differential
   Diagnosis p. 369)

Benign prostatic hyperplasia (BPH) is an enlargement of the prostate that commonly occurs in men over 50 years old. The enlargement of the prostate squeezes the urethra and interferes with urinary function and, less frequently, sexual function.

1. BPH is more commonly associated with lower abdominal, low back or thigh pain, not epigastric pain.

2. Though a patient with BPH may experience urinary problems, painful urination is not typically one of the symptoms. Painful urination is more likely with conditions such as prostatitis.

3. Though a patient with BPH may experience sexual dysfunction (e.g., difficulty attaining an erection), painful ejaculation is not typically one of the symptoms. Painful ejaculation is more likely with conditions such as prostatitis.

4. **Patients with BPH typically have issues passing urine due to the enlargement of the prostate and its position next to the urethra. Symptoms include hesitancy of urination, small amounts of urine when voiding, dribbling at the end of urination, urge to urinate frequently, and nocturia.**

System: Other Systems
Content Outline: Diseases/Conditions that Impact Effective
   Treatment

⦿ Level 2

⦿ Level 1

➡ PTAEXAM THREE: QUESTION 9

A physical therapist assistant monitors a patient completing a submaximal exercise test on a treadmill. Which of the following measurement methods would provide the assistant with an objective measurement of endurance?

1. Facial color

2. Facial expression

3. Rating on a perceived exertion scale

4. **Respiration rate**

Correct Answer: 4 (Fairchild p. 62)

Each of the presented options provides a physical therapist assistant with information that can be used to gain insight on endurance, however, only respiration rate is considered to be an objective measure.

1. Facial color is a subjective measure that can be easily assessed through observation. Prolonged exercise often results in a gradual reddening or flushing of the face.

2. Facial expression is a subjective measure that can be used effectively by physical therapist assistants to gain insight on a patient's endurance and activity tolerance. As patients become more fatigued, it is often apparent by simply watching for changes in facial expression.

3. Rating on a perceived exertion scale is a subjective measure that attempts to quantify exercise intensity. One of the most common scales used in physical therapy is Borg's Rating of Perceived Exertion Scale (RPE). The 20-point RPE scale ranges from a minimum value of 6 to a maximum value of 20. The scale is designed to assess intensity and not necessarily endurance.

4. **Respiration rate is an objective measure that can be used as a gross method to assess endurance. Normal respiration in an adult is 12-20 breaths per minute. Respiration rate tends to increase proportionately with increases in exercise intensity.**

System: Cardiovascular and Pulmonary Systems
Content Outline: Physical Therapy Data Collection

➡ PTAEXAM THREE: QUESTION 10

A physical therapist assistant prepares to instruct a patient in a home exercise program designed to increase lower extremity flexibility. The assistant is somewhat concerned since the patient has difficulty following multi-step instructions and tends to be overly aggressive on prescribed exercises. Which type of stretching would be the **MOST** appropriate?

1. Ballistic

2. Dynamic

3. Proprioceptive neuromuscular facilitation

4. **Static**

Correct Answer: 4 (Kisner p. 87)

Stretching refers to the lengthening of muscles and their associated structures. Stretching helps muscles stay flexible and strong and serves as a form of injury prevention. Common forms of stretching include static, dynamic, ballistic, and proprioceptive neuromuscular facilitation (PNF).

1. Ballistic stretching is characterized by quick, jerky movements that result in a rapid change in muscle length. Because ballistic stretching occurs quickly, it activates the muscle spindles and results in greater resistance to stretch. This type of stretching would likely be problematic for the described patient based on their tendency to be overly aggressive with exercise.

2. Dynamic stretching involves the patient actively moving a body segment to the end of range (but not beyond this limit) while the antagonist muscle relaxes and stretches. Unlike static stretching, the end-range movement is held only briefly and is performed repeatedly. Dynamic stretching is most commonly used as a "warm-up." The patient's difficulty following multi-step directions and aggressiveness make static stretching a more desirable form of stretching.

3. PNF incorporates active muscle contractions into stretching techniques. Muscular contraction is thought to lead to muscle relaxation through the principles of autogenic or reciprocal inhibition. Because these techniques exert their effects on muscle fibers, they are more effective at treating range of motion limitations due to muscle spasm as opposed to connective tissue tightness. The patient's inability to follow multi-step directions makes this form of stretching impractical.

4. **Static stretching involves placing the muscle at its maximal length and holding the position against an external force for a prolonged period of time. It is considered to be the safest form of stretching and results in the greatest gains in tissue extensibility. The relative simplicity of static stretching combined with being the most conservative stretching technique makes this the most appropriate option for the patient.**

System: Musculoskeletal System
Content Outline: Interventions

 Level 1   p. 384-385

 Level 3   p. 106-108

➡ PTAEXAM THREE: QUESTION 11

A physical therapist assistant selects a frequency of 3.0 MHz to perform therapeutic ultrasound on a patient. Which of the following conditions would **MOST** warrant the use of this frequency?

1. Lumbar paravertebral muscle spasm

2. Hip flexion contracture

3. Quadriceps strain

4. **Anterior talofibular ligament sprain**

Correct Answer: 4 (Cameron p. 184)

A higher frequency results in greater attenuation of energy in superficial structures. As a result, an ultrasound generator with a frequency of 3.0 MHz may be more desirable than a generator with a frequency of 1.0 MHz when treating a superficial structure.

1. The lumbar paravertebral muscles refer to a relatively diverse group of muscles next to the spine. The muscles collectively support the spine and produce movement. The relative depth of the muscles would make it necessary to utilize a frequency of 1.0 MHz to reach the target area.

2. A hip flexion contracture typically results from shortening of the iliopsoas muscle. The iliopsoas is formed by the iliacus and psoas major muscles and is considered to be the most powerful flexor of the hip. Ultrasound in this area would require a frequency of 1.0 MHz due to the depth of the iliopsoas.

3. The quadriceps muscles are a large muscle group consisting of the rectus femoris, vastus lateralis, vastus medialis, and vastus intermedius. A strain in this area would require a frequency of 1.0 MHz due to the depth of the quadriceps muscles.

4. **The anterior talofibular ligament is a thickening of the anterior joint capsule that extends from the anterior surface of the lateral malleolus to the lateral facet of the talus and the lateral surface of the talar neck. The relatively superficial ligament is only two to five millimeters thick and therefore a frequency of 3.0 MHz would be adequate.**

System: Non-Systems
Content Outline: Equipment, Devices, and Technologies; Therapeutic Modalities

➡ PTAEXAM THREE: QUESTION 12

A physical therapist assistant performs prosthetic training with a patient post transfemoral amputation. What initial instruction would be the **MOST** appropriate when ascending the stairs?

1. Utilize the handrail to propel your legs to the next step simultaneously

2. **Place your body weight on the prosthetic side and lead with your uninvolved leg**

3. Place your body weight on the uninvolved side and lead with your prosthesis

4. Avoid using stairs with your prosthesis

Correct Answer: 2 (Seymour p. 168)

A patient with a unilateral transfemoral amputation will ascend stairs leading with the uninvolved lower extremity. This allows for greater stability as the uninvolved lower extremity uses its strength to lift the patient to the next step with the prosthetic side to follow.

1. A handrail will assist a patient when ascending and descending the stairs, however, the patient should not rely on a handrail and upper extremity strength to advance up or down a step or flight of stairs.

2. **This sequence of ascending with the uninvolved lower extremity is used for any unilateral weakness in order to have the uninvolved lower extremity lift the body weight against gravity to the next step.**

3. The patient would not effectively ascend the stairs with the prosthetic side secondary to lack of proprioception, sensation, strength, and control of the knee joint of the prosthesis.

4. A patient should not have to avoid stairs secondary to having a prosthetic limb. A patient with a transfemoral prosthesis should be able to ambulate on all surfaces with or without an assistive device.

System: Musculoskeletal System
Content Outline: Interventions

 Level 2   p. 623-626

 Level 2   p. 605-606

➡ PTAEXAM THREE: QUESTION 13

A physical therapist assistant is performing transfer training with a patient four days post transtibial amputation. Assuming an uncomplicated recovery, which of the following transfers is the **MOST** appropriate for the assistant to utilize from a wheelchair to a mat table?

1. Two-person lift
2. Hydraulic lift
3. **Stand pivot**
4. Sliding board

Correct Answer: 3 (Seymour p. 160)

Physical therapist assistants should select transfers for patients based on their unique abilities and limitations. A patient status post transtibial amputation should be able to utilize their uninvolved lower extremity during the transfer and as a result, the physical therapist assistant would not need to utilize a dependent transfer.

1. A two-person lift is used to transfer a patient between two surfaces of different heights or when transferring a patient to the floor.

2. A hydraulic lift is a device required for dependent transfers when a patient is obese, when there is only one therapist available to assist with the transfer or when the patient is totally dependent.

3. **A stand pivot transfer is used when a patient is able to stand and bear weight through one or both of the lower extremities. The patient must possess functional balance and the ability to pivot.**

4. A sliding board transfer is used for a patient who has sitting balance, some upper extremity strength, and can adequately follow directions.

System: Musculoskeletal System
Content Outline: Interventions

➡ PTAEXAM THREE: QUESTION 14

A physical therapist assistant positions a patient to perform a manual muscle test of the supinator. To isolate the supinator and minimize the action of the biceps, the assistant should place the patient's elbow in which of the following positions?

1. 30 degrees of elbow flexion
2. 60 degrees of elbow flexion
3. 90 degrees of elbow flexion
4. **Terminal elbow flexion**

Correct Answer: 4 (Kendall p. 289)

The supinator is innervated by the radial nerve (C5, C6, C7) and acts to supinate the forearm. The biceps is innervated by the musculocutaneous nerve (C5-C6) and acts to flex the elbow and supinate the forearm. A therapist can isolate one muscle from another muscle with a similar action by placing the de-emphasized muscle in a shortened position during the testing procedure. This finding is based on the length-tension relationship which specifies that a muscle can generate the greatest tension at its resting length.

1. The biceps is significantly lengthened in this position, however, 30 degrees of elbow flexion allows the biceps to generate a reasonable amount of force.

2. The biceps is slightly lengthened in 60 degrees of elbow flexion, however, the muscle is able to generate a significant amount of force since the position is relatively close to the muscle's resting length.

3. The biceps is typically tested with the elbow in 90 degrees of flexion and therefore this is an undesirable position to minimize the action of the muscle.

4. **Placing the biceps in a maximally shortened position significantly limits the muscle's ability to function as a supinator. Therapists should avoid maximum pressure in this position since the shortened position of the biceps can result in significant cramping.**

System: Musculoskeletal System
Content Outline: Physical Therapy Data Collection

 Level 2   p. 594-596

● Level 1

➡ PTAEXAM THREE: QUESTION 15

While measuring a patient's resting heart rate, the physical therapist assistant palpates the patient's radial pulse and counts the pulse for 15 seconds. After 15 seconds, the assistant records the patient's resting heart rate in the hospital chart as 73 beats per minute. Which description **BEST** summarizes the described measurement?

1. Valid measurement of resting heart rate
2. Reliable measurement of resting heart rate
3. Measurement on the interval scale of measurement
4. **Measurement error of resting heart rate**

Correct Answer: 4 (Portney p. 79)

Resting heart rate is measured as a whole number. To convert pulse rate in 15 seconds to pulse rate per minute, multiply the 15 second rate by four. 73 is not a multiple of four, and therefore is a measurement error.

1. Validity refers to the degree to which a test or measurement accurately reflects or assesses the specific concept the clinician is attempting to measure. Validity is concerned with the success at measuring what was set out to measure. The error made by the physical therapist assistant compromises the validity of the measurement.

2. Reliability refers to the extent to which a test or measurement is consistent or yields the same result on repeated trials. Reliability cannot be assessed in the example since there is only a single measurement.

3. The interval scale is characterized by known and equal distances or intervals between the units of measurement. Heart rate would be more representative of a ratio scale measure since, in addition to known and equal distances or intervals, there is an absolute zero point representing a total absence of the property being measured.

4. **Sources of measurement error can be attributed to three parts of the measurement system: 1) the tester or rater making the measurement, 2) the instrument used, and 3) variability in the attribute being measured. In this particular case, the source of measurement error was the physical therapist assistant.**

System: Non-Systems
Content Outline: Safety and Protection; Professional
    Responsibilities; Research

➡ PTAEXAM THREE: QUESTION 16

A physical therapist directs a physical therapist assistant to measure the seat depth for a patient as part of the assessment for appropriate fit of a wheelchair. How many inches should the assistant subtract from the standard measurement taken for wheelchair depth?

1. 1
2. **2**
3. 4
4. 6

Correct Answer: 2 (Fairchild p. 137)

Seat depth is determined by measuring from the patient's posterior buttock, along the lateral thigh to the popliteal fold, then subtracting approximately two inches to avoid pressure from the front edge of the seat against the popliteal space. Normal seat depth in an adult size wheelchair is 16 inches.

1. One inch of space may result in the patient experiencing increased pressure in the popliteal area or even potentially compromised circulation since the amount of space between the front edge of the seat and the popliteal space is less than the recommended amount of two inches.

2. **Two inches of space between the front edge of the seat and the popliteal space is the recommended amount of space. This distance corresponds to the width of three or four fingers.**

3. Four inches of space may result in the patient experiencing decreased trunk stability, increased weight bearing on the ischial tuberosities due to the body weight being shifted posteriorly secondary to the lack of support to the thighs, and poor balance since the base of support has been reduced.

4. Six inches of space would serve to exacerbate the difficulties discussed in option 3.

System: Non-Systems
Content Outline: Equipment, Devices, and Technologies;
    Therapeutic Modalities

 Level 2   p. 705-707

 Level 1   p. 596-597

➡ PTAEXAM THREE: QUESTION 17

A patient with atrial flutter suddenly becomes extremely lightheaded while exercising and appears to lose consciousness. Which of the following physiologic responses **BEST** explains the change in the patient's status?

1. Increased filling of the ventricles

2. Increased system congestion

3. Decreased atrial depolarization

4. **Decreased blood traveling to the brain**

Correct answer: 4 (Hillegass p. 320)

Atrial flutter is a common abnormal heart rhythm characterized by rapid atrial tachycardia. This rapid rate creates decreased filling time of the ventricles resulting in diminished amounts of blood being ejected from the heart. This form of arrhythmia produces sawtooth shaped P waves.

1. The rapid rate of atrial contraction (i.e., 250-350 beats per minute) associated with atrial flutter results in decreased filling time of the ventricles and diminished amounts of blood being ejected from the heart.

2. Increased system congestion is more characteristic of congestive heart failure than a supraventricular arrhythmia such as atrial flutter. Congestive heart failure is often caused by diminished pumping ability of the ventricles due to muscle weakening (systolic dysfunction) or to stiffening of the heart muscle that impairs the ventricles' capacity to relax and fill (diastolic dysfunction).

3. Atrial flutter is characterized by an extremely rapid rate of atrial depolarization (i.e., 250-350 beats per minute). This rapid rate creates decreased filling time of the ventricles resulting in diminished amounts of blood being ejected from the heart.

4. **Atrial flutter results in decreased blood traveling to the brain as well as other areas of the body. As a result, vital organs such as the heart muscles and brain may not receive enough blood causing mild symptoms (e.g., palpitations, lightheadedness, weakness) or more serious symptoms (e.g., fainting, angina, organ failure).**

System: Cardiovascular and Pulmonary Systems
Content Outline: Diseases/Conditions that Impact Effective Treatment

 Level 2

➡ PTAEXAM THREE: QUESTION 18

A physical therapist assistant prepares to work on standing balance with a patient who has been on extended bed rest following abdominal surgery. The patient has only been out of bed a few times with the assistance of the nursing staff. Which of the following measures is the **MOST** important for the assistant to assess after assisting the patient from a supine to sitting position?

1. **Systolic blood pressure**

2. Diastolic blood pressure

3. Rating of perceived exertion

4. Oxygen saturation rate

Correct Answer: 1 (Fairchild p. 333)

Orthostatic hypotension results from an inability to compensate quickly for changes in blood pressure. When a person stands up suddenly, gravity tends to cause blood to pool in the veins of the legs and lower body. As a result, the amount of blood returned to the heart is reduced and blood pressure falls. Dizziness or lightheadedness is the most common symptom. Normally, the body quickly responds to a decrease in blood pressure, however, compensatory mechanisms may malfunction or function too slowly in patients who have been on extended bed rest.

1. **During bed rest, when the leg muscles are not used regularly, blood pools in the leg veins and is not pumped back to the heart. This results in diminished blood volume which serves to reduce blood pressure. Systolic blood pressure is the maximum arterial pressure during systole or contraction of the left ventricle. It is the most important measure to assess after prolonged bed rest due to the risk of orthostatic hypotension. A decrease in systolic blood pressure of 20 mm Hg or greater with vertical positioning is indicative of orthostatic hypotension.**

2. Diastolic blood pressure refers to the arterial pressure during diastole (between ventricular contractions), therefore, it is not as useful a measure to assess the patient's response to vertical positioning.

3. Rating of perceived exertion is a subjective measure of how hard the body is working. It is based on the sensations experienced during physical activity including increased heart rate, respiration rate, sweating, and muscle fatigue. It is not a useful measure to assess the patient's response to vertical positioning.

4. Oxygen saturation measures the percentage of hemoglobin binding sites in the blood bound to oxygen. It is not affected by changing positions.

System: Other Systems
Content Outline: Interventions

 Level 3   p. 376

➡ PTAEXAM THREE: QUESTION 19

A physician indicates that a patient post CVA has significant perceptual deficits. What anatomical region would **MOST** likely be affected by the stroke?

1. Primary motor cortex
2. **Somatosensory cortex**
3. Basal ganglia
4. Cerebellum

Correct Answer: 2 (O'Sullivan p. 100)

A lesion affecting the somatosensory cortex often results in numerous impairments including loss of sensation, perception, proprioception, and diminished motor control.

1. The primary motor cortex is located in the precentral gyrus within the frontal lobe and contains the largest concentration of corticospinal neurons. This area lies directly in front of the central sulcus and primarily controls contralateral voluntary movements.

2. **The somatosensory cortex occupies the postcentral gyrus which is directly behind the central sulcus. The structure is responsible for complex processing of sensory information and damage can cause severely impaired perception. The somatosensory cortex receives information regarding touch, temperature, pain, and discriminative senses including stereognosis and position sense.**

3. The basal ganglia are a group of nuclei (putamen, caudate nucleus, substantia nigra, subthalamic nuclei, globus pallidus) that are located at the base of the cerebral cortex. The basal ganglia influence movement and postural control.

4. The cerebellum regulates movement, muscle tone, and postural control. Symptoms of a cerebellar lesion include ataxia, tremor, hypotonia, and asthenia.

System: Neuromuscular and Nervous Systems
Content Outline: Diseases/Conditions that Impact Effective Treatment

➡ PTAEXAM THREE: QUESTION 20

A physical therapist assistant reviews the parameters for using transcutaneous electrical nerve stimulation (TENS). When comparing sensory to motor stimulation, the assistant should recognize that sensory stimulation requires which of the following parameters?

1. Greater phase duration
2. **Greater frequency**
3. Stronger amplitude
4. Shorter treatment time

Correct Answer: 2 (Cameron p. 263)

Motor stimulation requires sufficient phase charge to elicit a muscle contraction. This is accomplished by using a low frequency and long phase duration. Sensory stimulation, also called conventional TENS, requires a sufficient phase charge to achieve a sensory response, but is below the motor threshold. This is accomplished by using a high frequency and short phase duration.

1. Phase duration is shorter with sensory level stimulation compared to motor level stimulation.

2. **Frequency is significantly greater with sensory level stimulation compared to motor level stimulation.**

3. Sensory level stimulation requires lower amplitude than motor level stimulation.

4. Treatment time is highly variable with sensory and motor stimulation TENS.

System: Non-Systems
Content Outline: Equipment, Devices, and Technologies; Therapeutic Modalities

---

 Level 2

 Level 1   p. 642-643

➧ PTAEXAM THREE: QUESTION 21

A physical therapist assistant performs gait training with a child who has cerebral palsy. The assistant would like to utilize a reverse walker to help with the patient's gait impairments. Which of the following impairments best illustrates the **PRIMARY** rationale for prescribing a reverse walker instead of a traditional walker?

1. Displays a Trendelenburg gait pattern
2. Exhibits excessive upper extremity weakness
3. **Displays a forward trunk lean with gait**
4. Demonstrates excessive extensor tone

Correct Answer: 3 (Tan p. 298)

Reverse walkers, also known as posterior walkers, are designed differently from traditional walkers in that the support system is behind the patient. As a result, the patient tends to hold the device with the shoulders in more extension and the scapulae in more depression and retraction, which leads to improved thoracic extension. Reverse walkers have also proven to be more energy efficient than traditional walkers.

1. A Trendelenburg gait pattern is characterized by contralateral hip drop and ipsilateral trunk lean and is caused by weak hip abductor musculature. A reverse walker would not be any more effective at correcting a Trendelenburg gait pattern than would a traditional walker.

2. Upper extremity weakness could affect a patient's ability to use an assistive device. Depending on the area of weakness, modifications to the assistive device may need to be made (e.g., platform attachment). However, a reverse walker would not be any easier to use than a traditional walker for a patient with upper extremity weakness.

3. **Patients with cerebral palsy may demonstrate a crouched gait pattern where they walk with a forward trunk lean and the lower extremity joints are held in flexion. A reverse walker would potentially be effective for a patient with cerebral palsy to help increase thoracic extension and therefore improve upright posture.**

4. A patient with excessive extensor tone would not benefit from a reverse walker, as this device would facilitate extension and lead to a further increase in their tone. A traditional walker may be more beneficial for patients with excessive extensor tone.

System: Non-Systems
Content Outline: Equipment, Devices, and Technologies; Therapeutic Modalities

⬤ **Level 3**

➧ PTAEXAM THREE: QUESTION 22

A patient who has ankylosing spondylitis is referred to physical therapy for instruction in a home exercise program. Strengthening of which of the following muscles would be the **MOST** beneficial for the patient?

1. Rectus abdominis
2. Internal and external obliques
3. Quadratus lumborum
4. **Erector spinae**

Correct Answer: 4 (Dutton p. 226)

Ankylosing spondylitis is a form of systemic rheumatic arthritis that results in inflammation of the axial skeleton with subsequent back pain. The condition is associated with an increase in thoracic kyphosis and loss of the lumbar curve. The patient often develops a forward stooped posture observed in standing.

1. Strengthening of the rectus abdominis will produce a flexion moment in the trunk. This will further accentuate the thoracic kyphosis and decrease the lumbar lordosis.

2. Strengthening of the internal and external obliques when contracting bilaterally will produce a flexion moment of the trunk and when contracting unilaterally, will produce a rotary moment of the trunk. General core strengthening is desirable, however, the emphasis would be on strengthening the back extensors.

3. Strengthening of the quadratus lumborum will produce a lateral bending of the trunk when performed in a closed-chain activity and a hip hiking movement when performed in an open-chain activity. These motions would not be the emphasis of a strengthening program for a patient with ankylosing spondylitis. The quadratus lumborum also assists with extension, however, the muscle is just one of many muscles that serve this function.

4. **Extension exercises are often an important component of a comprehensive plan of care to assist patients with ankylosing spondylitis to maintain the normal curves of the spine while at the same time limiting the forward bending nature of the disease process.**

System: Musculoskeletal System
Content Outline: Interventions

⬤ **Level 1**   p. 550

➡ PTAEXAM THREE: QUESTION 23

A patient begins to experience acute angina and reports using nitroglycerin to alleviate the angina. What mode of administration is the **MOST** appropriate for this medication?

1. Oral
2. Buccal
3. **Sublingual**
4. Topical

Correct Answer: 3 (Ciccone p. 336)

Drugs can be administered through the alimentary canal or through nonalimentary routes. Each route has distinct advantages and disadvantages.

1. Oral administration is the most common method of administration. It is considered the easiest form of taking medication when self-medication is required and is relatively safe since drugs enter the system in a fairly controlled manner.

2. Buccal administration occurs when the drug is placed between the cheeks and gums. Drugs administered in this manner are absorbed through the oral mucosa.

3. **Sublingual administration occurs when placing drugs under the tongue. Sublingual administration of nitroglycerin is the most appropriate mode of administration with acute angina due to the rapid absorption into the systemic circulation.**

4. Topical administration refers to the application of drugs topically to the surface of the skin or mucous membranes. Topical administration is used most often to treat the outer layer of the skin and not other areas since most medications are absorbed poorly through the epidermis and into the systemic circulation.

System: Cardiovascular and Pulmonary Systems
Content Outline: Diseases/Conditions that Impact Effective
  Treatment

➡ PTAEXAM THREE: QUESTION 24

A physical therapist assistant prepares to conduct a manual muscle test of the hip flexors. Assuming a grade of Poor (2/5), what position is the **MOST** appropriate for the assistant to utilize?

1. Prone
2. **Sidelying**
3. Supine
4. Standing

Correct Answer: 2 (Kendall p. 422)

A grade of poor indicates that the hip flexors can produce movement with gravity eliminated, but cannot function against gravity. Muscles acting to flex the hip include the iliopsoas, sartorius, rectus femoris, and pectineus.

1. A prone position would place the hip flexors in an elongated position and make it impossible for the physical therapist assistant to offer resistance in a direction opposite of the muscle's action.

2. **The hip flexors would need to be tested in sidelying due to the grade of "poor." If the hip flexors were given a grade of "good" or "normal" the recommended testing position would be sitting upright with the knees bent over the side of the table.**

3. A supine position would not be considered gravity-eliminated and therefore would not be appropriate given the muscle's current grade. A supine position is sometimes employed as a substitute for sitting upright, most often in situations where the muscle's strength is "good" or "normal."

4. Testing the hip flexors in standing would be problematic since the muscles would need to work against gravity and it would be impossible to adequately stabilize the patient during the testing.

System: Musculoskeletal System
Content Outline: Physical Therapy Data Collection

Level 2 p. 509

Level 2 p. 77-79

➡ PTAEXAM THREE: QUESTION 25

A physical therapist assistant observes the postural strategies of a patient following a series of manual perturbations. What strategy is **BEST** illustrated in the image?

1. Ankle
2. **Hip**
3. Suspensory
4. Stepping

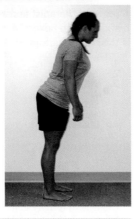

Correct Answer: 2 (O'Sullivan p. 232)

Automatic postural strategies are automatic motor responses that are used to maintain the center of gravity over the base of support. These responses occur in a predictable pattern based on the magnitude of the perturbation.

1. The ankle strategy is the first strategy to be elicited by a small range and slow velocity perturbation when the feet are on the ground. Muscle groups contract in a distal to proximal progression to control postural sway from the ankle joint.

2. **The presented image is an example of the hip strategy which is elicited by a greater force, challenge or perturbation. The hips will move (in the opposite direction from the head) in order to maintain balance. Muscle groups contract in a proximal to distal progression in order to counteract the loss of balance.**

3. The suspensory strategy is used to lower the center of gravity during standing or ambulation in order to better control the center of gravity. Examples of this strategy include knee flexion, crouching or squatting. This strategy is often used when both mobility and stability are required during a task (e.g., surfing).

4. The stepping strategy is elicited through unexpected challenges or perturbations during static standing or when the perturbation produces a movement that displaces the center of gravity beyond the base of support. The lower extremities step and/or upper extremities reach to regain a new base of support.

System: Neuromuscular and Nervous Systems
Content Outline: Physical Therapy Data Collection

➡ PTAEXAM THREE: QUESTION 26

A physical therapist assistant attempts to stabilize the scapula while performing a goniometric measurement of isolated glenohumeral abduction on a patient. Failure to stabilize the scapula will lead to which of the following motions occurring at the scapula?

1. Downward rotation and elevation
2. Downward rotation and depression
3. **Upward rotation and elevation**
4. Upward rotation and depression

Correct Answer: 3 (Norkin p. 80)

Normal glenohumeral abduction is 0-120 degrees. When measuring glenohumeral abduction, the axis of the goniometer should be placed over the anterior aspect of the acromial process. The stationary arm should be positioned parallel to the midline of the anterior aspect of the sternum and the moveable arm should be positioned on the medial midline of the humerus. Failure to stabilize the scapula will result in the obtained range of motion value being greater than the actual amount of glenohumeral abduction available.

1. Glenohumeral abduction requires upward rotation of the scapula and not downward rotation.

2. Glenohumeral abduction requires upward rotation and elevation of the scapula and not downward rotation and depression.

3. **Failure to stabilize the scapula when measuring glenohumeral abduction will result in upward rotation and elevation of the scapula. When measuring shoulder complex abduction, the thorax should be stabilized to prevent lateral flexion of the trunk.**

4. Glenohumeral abduction requires elevation of the scapula and not depression.

System: Musculoskeletal System
Content Outline: Physical Therapy Data Collection

● Level 1   p. 240-241

● Level 2   p. 87-88

▶ PTAEXAM THREE: QUESTION 27

A physical therapist assistant prepares to work with a patient who has a dorsal scapular nerve injury. What muscles should the assistant expect to be **MOST** affected by this injury?

1. Serratus anterior and pectoralis minor
2. **Levator scapulae and rhomboids**
3. Latissimus dorsi and teres major
4. Supraspinatus and infraspinatus

Correct Answer: 2 (Kendall p. 348)

Damage to a peripheral nerve can significantly impair muscle function. The severity of the impact ranges from a mild disturbance to denervation.

1. The serratus anterior is innervated by the long thoracic nerve and the pectoralis minor is innervated by the medial pectoral nerve.

2. **The levator scapulae and rhomboids are innervated by the dorsal scapular nerve.**

3. The latissimus dorsi is innervated by the thoracodorsal nerve and the teres major is innervated by the lower subscapular nerve.

4. The supraspinatus and infraspinatus are innervated by the suprascapular nerve.

System: Neuromuscular and Nervous Systems
Content Outline: Diseases/Conditions that Impact Effective Treatment

⊕ Test Taking Tip: In some cases, a candidate may not have a full complement of academic information available to answer a given question, however, may still be able to identify the correct option or at least eliminate one or more of the incorrect options. For example, in option 1 the physical therapist assistant may know that the serratus anterior is innervated by the long thoracic nerve, but may not know the innervation of the pectoralis minor. By recognizing that at least one of the muscles listed in option 1 is not associated with the dorsal scapular nerve, the physical therapist assistant can safely eliminate this option. Candidates should not become anxious or unsettled when they identify information that they are not familiar with on the NPTE-PTA and instead attempt to answer the question based on their existing academic knowledge. Candidates can use this strategy to enhance their examination score.

▶ PTAEXAM THREE: QUESTION 28

A patient who has cerebral palsy exhibits slow, involuntary, continuous writhing movements of the upper and lower extremities. Which of the following motor impairments is **MOST** representative of this type of motor disturbance?

1. Spasticity
2. Ataxia
3. Hypotonia
4. **Athetosis**

Correct Answer: 4 (Tecklin p. 193)

Cerebral palsy is an umbrella term used to describe a group of non-progressive movement disorders that result from brain damage. Athetoid cerebral palsy involves damage to the basal ganglia.

1. Spasticity refers to an increased resistance to passive stretch. Spasticity is commonly observed with patients diagnosed with cerebral palsy due to upper motor neuron damage.

2. Ataxia is a generalized term used to describe motor impairments of cerebellar origin. It is characterized by the inability to perform coordinated movement and may affect gait, posture, and patterns of movements.

3. Hypotonia refers to decreased or absent tone where resistance to passive movement is decreased, stretch reflexes are diminished, and limbs are easily moved. Hypotonicity in children is often associated with motor delays.

4. **Athetosis refers to involuntary movements characterized as slow, irregular, and twisting. Peripheral movements occur without central stability. This type of motor disturbance makes it extremely difficult to maintain a static body position.**

System: Neuromuscular and Nervous Systems
Content Outline: Diseases/Conditions that Impact Effective Treatment

 Level 1   p. 227

 Level 1   p. 238-239

➡ PTAEXAM THREE: QUESTION 29

A note in the medical record indicates that a patient was recently prescribed Lasix (furosemide). Which of the following conditions is **MOST** commonly associated with the use of this medication?

1. Atrial flutter
2. Deep vein thrombosis
3. Hyperlipidemia
4. **Chronic heart failure**

Correct Answer: 4 (Goodman – Pathology p. 599)

Lasix (furosemide) is a loop diuretic that is often used in the treatment of edema or hypertension. Lasix increases the excretion of sodium and chloride in the kidneys, thereby increasing urination and decreasing the volume of fluid that is retained within the body.

1. Atrial flutter is a type of cardiac arrhythmia characterized by a rapid contraction rate of the atria. Digoxin is an example of a medication that may be used to treat atrial flutter.

2. Deep vein thrombosis is a condition where a blood clot forms in a vein, most commonly in the lower extremities. Thrombolytic drugs would be administered to help break up an already existing blood clot.

3. Hyperlipidemia is a condition characterized by high levels of lipids (i.e., triglycerides, cholesterol) within the blood. Atorvastatin (Lipitor) is an example of a medication that may be used to treat hyperlipidemia.

4. **Chronic heart failure is a condition characterized by an inability of the heart to effectively pump blood to meet the metabolic demands of the body. Chronic heart failure can result in pulmonary edema or peripheral edema, depending on the side of the heart that is affected. Lasix is a medication that is commonly prescribed to help lessen the edema associated with chronic heart failure.**

System: Cardiovascular and Pulmonary Systems
Content Outline: Diseases/Conditions that Impact Effective
    Treatment

➡ PTAEXAM THREE: QUESTION 30

A physical therapist assistant instructs a patient to make a fist. The patient is able to make a fist, but is unable to flex the distal phalanx of the ring finger. What tendon has **MOST** likely been ruptured?

1. Flexor carpi radialis
2. Flexor digitorum superficialis
3. **Flexor digitorum profundus**
4. Extensor digitorum communis

Correct Answer: 3 (Dutton p. 792)

The flexor digitorum profundus muscle originates on the anterior and medial surfaces of the proximal portion of the ulna, interosseous membrane, and deep antebrachial fascia. The muscle inserts via four tendons into the anterior surface of the bases of the distal phalanges.

1. The flexor carpi radialis muscle acts to flex and abduct the wrist and may assist in pronation of the forearm and in flexion of the elbow.

2. The flexor digitorum superficialis muscle acts to flex the proximal interphalangeal joints of the second through fifth digits, and assists in flexion of the metacarpophalangeal joints and flexion of the wrist.

3. **The flexor digitorum profundus muscle acts to flex the distal interphalangeal joints of the index, middle, ring, and little fingers, and assists in flexion of the proximal interphalangeal and metacarpophalangeal joints. A ruptured flexor digitorum profundus tendon would, therefore, make it impossible to flex the distal phalanx.**

4. The extensor digitorum communis muscle acts to extend the metacarpophalangeal joints and in conjunction with the lumbricals and interossei, extends the interphalangeal joints of the second through fifth digits. The muscle assists in abduction of the index, ring, and little fingers and in extension and abduction of the wrist.

System: Musculoskeletal System
Content Outline: Diseases/Conditions that Impact Effective
    Treatment

 Level 2   p. 364, 372

 Level 1

➡ PTAEXAM THREE: QUESTION 31

A physical therapist assistant implements an aquatic program for a patient who has a lower extremity injury. The program requires the patient to run in place using a flotation device while tethered to the side of the pool using an elastic cord. Which of the following actions would be the **MOST** appropriate to increase resistance?

1. Increase the water temperature
2. **Increase the speed of movement**
3. Increase the depth of the water
4. Remove the flotation device

Correct Answer: 2 (Kisner p. 298)

The therapeutic effects of immersion in water relate to the principles of hydrodynamics and thermodynamics. Some of the more relevant concepts associated with these principles include density, specific gravity, hydrostatic pressure, buoyancy, and viscosity.

1. Changes in the water temperature can influence variables such as oxygen uptake, but would not significantly influence resistance.

2. **The viscosity of water provides resistance to a body in motion. Viscosity refers to the thickness or resistance to the flow of a liquid. The faster the relative speed of the body, the greater the magnitude of resistance.**

3. Increasing the depth of the water would not result in a significant change in resistance since the patient is using a flotation device and therefore their level of immersion would remain relatively constant.

4. Removal of the flotation device would likely increase resistance since the patient may tend to move faster without the flotation device, however, it remains less desirable than simply continuing to use the belt and increasing the speed of movement.

System: Other Systems
Content Outline: Interventions

➡ PTAEXAM THREE: QUESTION 32

A patient reports feeling lightheaded and dizzy while exercising. The physical therapist assistant immediately moves the patient to a nearby chair and begins to assess vital signs. The assistant measures the patient's respiration rate as 10 breaths per minute, pulse rate as 45 beats per minute, and blood pressure as 115/80 mm Hg. Which of the following statements is the **MOST** accurate regarding the patient's vital signs?

1. **Pulse rate and respiration rate are below normal levels**
2. Pulse rate and blood pressure are above normal levels
3. Blood pressure and respiration rate are above normal levels
4. The patient's vital signs are within normal limits

Correct Answer: 1 (Fairchild p. 52)

Normal range for pulse rate is 60-100 beats per minute for an adult, while respiration rate is 12-20 breaths per minute. Normal blood pressure is less than or equal to 120 mm Hg systolic and 80 mm Hg diastolic.

1. **A pulse of 45 beats per minute and a respiration rate of 10 breaths per minute are below the normal range and can contribute to the patient's complaints.**

2. A pulse of 45 beats per minute is below the normal range and a blood pressure of 115/80 mm Hg is within the normal range.

3. A blood pressure of 115/80 mm Hg is within the normal range and a respiration rate of 10 breaths per minute is below the normal range.

4. Blood pressure is the only vital sign that is within normal limits. Pulse rate and respiration rate are below the normal range.

System: Cardiovascular and Pulmonary Systems
Content Outline: Interventions

 Level 2   p. 630

 Level 2   p. 376, 381-382, 384-385

➠ PTAEXAM THREE: QUESTION 33

A physical therapist directs a physical therapist assistant to perform only closed kinetic chain exercises with a patient. Which of the following exercises would **NOT** be appropriate based on the therapist's directive?

1. Exercise on a stair machine

2. Limited squats to 45 degrees

3. Walking backwards on a treadmill

4. **Isokinetic knee extension and flexion**

Correct Answer: 4 (Dutton p. 1031)

Closed-chain activities involve the body moving over a fixed distal segment. Closed-chain activities are often integrated into lower extremity strengthening programs. Open-chain activities involve the distal segment, usually the hand or foot, moving freely in space.

1. Exercising on a stair machine requires the patient to maintain contact with the stair mechanism with their feet which would maintain the lower extremity in a fixed position.

2. Limited squats to 45 degrees require the feet to stay in contact with the ground while the hips and knees are gradually flexed and the trunk remains erect.

3. Walking backwards on a treadmill, or retro-walking, requires the lower extremity to be in contact with the treadmill for the majority of the activity. As a result, the activity would be considered a form of closed-chain exercise.

4. **Isokinetic knee extension and flexion requires the distal segment to move freely in space. As a result, the exercise is considered to be a form of open-chain exercise. Isokinetic contractions occur when a muscle is contracting at the same speed throughout the entire available range.**

System: Musculoskeletal System
Content Outline: Interventions

➠ PTAEXAM THREE: QUESTION 34

A patient who has anterior compartment syndrome presents with an inability to dorsiflex the foot and a mild sensory disturbance between the first and second toes. What nerve has **MOST** likely been injured?

1. **Deep peroneal nerve**

2. Medial plantar nerve

3. Tibial nerve

4. Lateral plantar nerve

Correct Answer: 1 (Magee p. 942)

Anterior compartment syndrome often affects the deep peroneal nerve as it passes under the extensor retinaculum. The result of nerve compression ranges from a mild sensory disturbance to an inability to dorsiflex the foot.

1. **The deep peroneal nerve innervates the tibialis anterior, extensor hallucis longus, extensor digitorum longus, extensor digitorum brevis, and peroneus tertius muscles.**

2. The medial plantar nerve is the larger of the two branches of the tibial nerve. The nerve supplies cutaneous branches to the medial three and a half digits, and motor branches to the abductor hallucis, flexor digitorum brevis, flexor hallucis brevis, and lumbrical I.

3. The tibial nerve innervates the tibialis posterior, flexor hallucis longus, flexor digitorum longus, soleus, gastrocnemius, plantaris, and popliteus muscles.

4. The lateral plantar nerve is the smaller of the two branches of the tibial nerve. The nerve supplies cutaneous branches to the lateral one and a half toes and motor branches to muscles of the sole of the foot that are not supplied by the medial plantar nerve. These include abductor digit minimi, flexor digiti minimi, opponens digiti minimi, dorsal interossei, quadratus plantae, adductor hallucis, lumbrical II, III, IV, and plantar interossei.

System: Neuromuscular and Nervous Systems
Content Outline: Diseases/Conditions that Impact Effective Treatment

 Level 2   p. 109-110

 Level 1   p. 228

➡ PTAEXAM THREE: QUESTION 35

A patient is admitted to the hospital following a recent illness. Laboratory testing reveals a markedly high platelet count. This finding is **MOST** commonly associated with which of the following conditions?

1. Emphysema

2. Metabolic acidosis

3. Renal failure

4. **Malignancy**

Correct Answer: 4 (Goodman – Differential Diagnosis p. 218)

Thrombocytosis refers to an increased number of blood platelets. This condition is usually temporary and can occur as a compensatory measure after severe hemorrhage, surgery, iron deficiency, and as a manifestation of certain cancers.

1. Emphysema is defined as an abnormal permanent enlargement of air spaces distal to the terminal bronchioles. Blood values will include an increase in red blood cells to carry the oxygen and abnormal carbon dioxide and carbon monoxide levels. Pulmonary function tests will show an increase in total lung capacity, functional residual capacity, and residual volume. The vital capacity is decreased.

2. Metabolic acidosis is an acid-base disorder defined as an accumulation of acids or a deficit of bases within the blood. Causes may include renal failure, starvation, diabetic or alcoholic ketoacidosis. Blood values will show a decrease in serum pH due to a decrease in HCO_{3-} or an increase in H+ ions. An arterial pH < 7.35 in the absence of an elevated $PaCO_2$ is considered metabolic acidosis.

3. Renal failure is defined as an abrupt or rapid decline in renal filtration and function. There are three categories: prerenal, intrinsic, and post renal failure. Typical causes include hypovolemia, congestive heart failure, dehydration, sepsis, and autoimmune diseases. Blood values include hypocalcemia, hyperkalemia, elevated blood urea nitrogen, creatinine, magnesium, and uric acid.

4. **Malignancy is defined as cells that have the ability to spread, invade, and destroy tissue. A tumor that is malignant may or may not respond to treatment or may return after removal. Blood values vary based on type, degree, and location of the malignancy, however, are often increased as a manifestation of an occult neoplasm such as lung cancer.**

System: Other Systems
Content Outline: Diseases/Conditions that Impact Effective Treatment

➡ PTAEXAM THREE: QUESTION 36

A patient begins to cry in the middle of a treatment session. The physical therapist assistant attempts to comfort the patient, however, eventually has to discontinue treatment. What section of the S.O.A.P. note would be the **MOST** appropriate to document the incident?

1. Subjective

2. Objective

3. **Assessment**

4. Plan

Correct Answer: 3 (Quinn p. 134)

Inability to continue treatment due to a patient's emotional state should be documented in the assessment section of the S.O.A.P. note. This type of entry serves to justify the decision to terminate treatment.

1. The subjective section refers to information the patient communicates directly to the physical therapist assistant. This could include patient statements, social history, medical history or patient complaints.

2. The objective section refers to information the physical therapist assistant observes. Common examples include range of motion measurements, muscle strength, and functional abilities.

3. **The assessment section allows the physical therapist assistant to express their opinion. Short and long-term goals are often expressed in this section as well as changes in the treatment program.**

4. The plan section includes ideas for future physical therapy sessions. Frequency and expected duration of physical therapy services can also be incorporated into this section.

System: Non-Systems
Content Outline: Safety and Protection; Professional Responsibilities; Research

---

 Level 2   p. 369-370

 Level 1   p. 684

➡ PTAEXAM THREE: QUESTION 37

A physical therapist assistant performs autolytic debridement in an attempt to remove nonviable tissue from a Stage 4 pressure injury. Autolytic debridement removes necrotic tissue by using which of the following methods?

1. A sharp instrument

2. An externally applied force

3. **The body's own mechanisms**

4. A commercially prepared enzyme

Correct Answer: 3 (Sussman p. 445)

Autolytic debridement is typically performed using a moisture-retentive dressing. The dressing maintains a moist wound environment which promotes rehydration of viable tissue and allows the body's enzymes to digest necrotic tissue.

1. Sharp debridement requires the use of scalpel, scissors, and/or forceps to selectively remove nonviable tissue, foreign material or debris from a wound.

2. Wound irrigation removes nonviable tissue from the wound bed using pressurized fluid which serves as an externally applied force. Pulsatile lavage is an example of a specific wound irrigation technique.

3. **Autolytic debridement refers to using the body's own mechanisms to remove nonviable tissue. Common methods of autolytic debridement include transparent films, hydrocolloids, hydrogels, and alginates.**

4. Enzymatic debridement requires the application of a commercially prepared enzyme to the surface of nonviable tissue. The applied enzyme attempts to degrade the nonviable tissue through gradual digestion.

System: Other Systems
Content Outline: Interventions

➡ PTAEXAM THREE: QUESTION 38

A physical therapist is responsible for supervising a physical therapist assistant at an off-site location. Which of the following scenarios would **NOT** necessitate a supervisory visit by the physical therapist?

1. A change in the patient's medical status

2. A modification in the patient's plan of care

3. A request by the physical therapist assistant

4. **An alteration in the patient's level of motivation**

Correct Answer: 4 (Guide to Physical Therapist Practice)

When a physical therapist delegates patient care responsibilities to physical therapist assistants or other supportive personnel, the physical therapist remains responsible for overseeing the physical therapy program.

1. A change in the patient's medical status requires reassessment and possibly a change in the established plan of care.

2. A physical therapist is solely responsible for modifying an established plan of care. A physical therapist assistant may be able to modify a parameter of an existing intervention within an established plan of care (i.e., changing the weight of a progressive resistive exercise).

3. The physical therapist is required to provide patient-related consultation at the request of another practitioner.

4. **Physical therapist assistants often deal with changes in patients' level of motivation. This observation in isolation would not warrant a supervisory visit by the physical therapist.**

System: Non-Systems
Content Outline: Safety and Protection; Professional Responsibilities; Research

---

● Level 1   👓   p. 446-447   ● Level 2   👓   p. 691-692

➡ PTAEXAM THREE: QUESTION 39

A physical therapist assistant performs a gross muscle length test of the hamstrings with a patient in a short sitting position. Which of the following patient responses is the **MOST** common substitution to exaggerate the length of the hamstrings?

1. Weight shift to the contralateral side
2. Anterior rotation of the pelvis
3. **Posterior rotation of the pelvis**
4. Hiking of the contralateral hip

Correct Answer: 3 (Magee p. 674)

The hamstring muscles consist of the semitendinosus, semimembranosus, and biceps femoris. The semitendinosus and semimembranosus are considered the medial hamstrings since they insert on the medial surface of the tibia. The biceps femoris is considered the lateral hamstrings since the muscle inserts on the lateral surface of the tibia and the lateral surface of the head of the fibula.

1. Weight shifting to the contralateral side in short sitting without other compensatory movement would have minimal impact on measured hamstrings length.

2. Anterior rotation of the pelvis would tend to make the apparent hamstrings length shorter than the actual length due to the hamstrings origin on the tuberosity of the ischium.

3. **Posterior rotation of the pelvis would tend to make the apparent hamstrings length longer than the actual length due to the hamstrings origin on the tuberosity of the ischium. Patients often attempt to posteriorly rotate the pelvis in short sitting by leaning backwards.**

4. Hip hiking of the contralateral limb may cause the patient to weight shift toward the involved side. This adaptation would have minimal impact on measured hamstrings length.

System: Musculoskeletal System
Content Outline: Physical Therapy Data Collection

➡ PTAEXAM THREE: QUESTION 40

An entry in the medical record indicates that a patient has tricuspid valve regurgitation. This condition would **MOST** likely result in an increased volume of blood in which of the following chambers of the heart?

1. Left atrium
2. **Right atrium**
3. Left ventricle
4. Right ventricle

Correct Answer: 2 (Hillegass p. 18)

During systole of the right and left atria, blood passes through the tricuspid valve and the mitral valve respectively. During ventricular systole, the valves close to prevent blood from flowing backwards into the atria. Tricuspid valve regurgitation refers to leakage of blood backwards through the tricuspid valve each time the right ventricle contracts.

1. An increased volume of blood in the left atrium is often associated with mitral valve regurgitation. The mitral valve is located between the left atrium and left ventricle. As the left ventricle contracts some blood leaks backwards into the left atrium which increases the volume of blood in the left atrium and diminishes blood flow to the rest of the body. The increased blood pressure in the left atrium can increase pressure in the pulmonary veins and may also lead to atrial fibrillation.

2. **An increased volume of blood in the right atrium is often associated with tricuspid valve regurgitation. The tricuspid valve is located between the right atrium and right ventricle. As the right ventricle contracts some blood leaks backwards into the right atrium which increases the volume of blood in the right atrium. This increase in volume enlarges the right atrium which can change the pressure in the nearby chambers and blood vessels.**

3. An increased volume of blood in the left ventricle is often associated with aortic valve regurgitation. The aortic valve is located between the left ventricle and the aorta. As the volume and pressure of the blood in the left ventricle increases, the ventricular walls often show evidence of hypertrophy and become less efficient.

4. An increased volume of blood in the right ventricle is often associated with pulmonary valve regurgitation. The pulmonary valve is located between the right ventricle and pulmonary artery. The condition is most often associated with pulmonary hypertension or tetralogy of Fallot.

System: Cardiovascular and Pulmonary Systems
Content Outline: Diseases/Conditions that Impact Effective Treatment

 Level 1

 Level 1

SCOREBUILDERS

➡ PTAEXAM THREE: QUESTION 41

A physical therapist assistant performs ice massage on a patient post lateral ankle sprain. Which of the following hypertension medications would have a direct antagonistic effect with the current treatment?

1. Beta-adrenergic blockers

2. Diuretics

3. Digitalis

4. **Vasodilators**

Correct Answer: 4 (Ciccone p. 324)

There are a variety of different medications that can be used to treat hypertension. The major categories include diuretics, sympatholytic drugs, vasodilators, renin-angiotensin system inhibitors, and calcium-channel blockers. Therapists should be aware of these medications and how they may affect current therapy treatments.

1. Beta-adrenergic blockers decrease blood pressure by decreasing heart rate and decreasing myocardial contraction force, which in turn reduces cardiac output. They do not exert a direct effect on the peripheral vasculature.

2. Diuretics decrease blood pressure by increasing the excretion of water and sodium, thereby decreasing the volume of blood within the circulatory system. They do not exert a direct effect on the peripheral vasculature.

3. Digitalis is more commonly used to treat congestive heart failure. Digitalis improves cardiac pumping ability by increasing the concentration of intracellular calcium. Digitalis does not have a direct effect on the peripheral vasculature.

4. **Vasodilators decrease blood pressure by dilating the peripheral vasculature and thus decreasing peripheral resistance. They exert their effect directly on the smooth muscle cells of the peripheral vessels. The dilation that results from use of vasodilators may work as an antagonist to cryotherapy since cryotherapy works by constricting peripheral blood vessels to help reduce blood flow to a swollen body part.**

System: Cardiovascular and Pulmonary Systems
Content Outline: Diseases/Conditions that Impact Effective Treatment

➡ PTAEXAM THREE: QUESTION 42

A physical therapist assistant prepares to assess a deep tendon reflex response on a patient's triceps. What is the **MOST** appropriate positioning of the patient's upper extremity during this testing procedure?

1. **Shoulder extension and elbow flexion**

2. Shoulder flexion and elbow extension

3. Shoulder extension and elbow extension

4. Shoulder flexion and elbow flexion

Correct Answer: 1 (Magee p. 201)

Deep tendon reflexes are performed to test the integrity of the spinal reflex. A physical therapist assistant should assess a deep tendon reflex by placing the tendon on slight stretch. A reflex hammer is used to sharply tap over the tendon. Reflexes can be graded as normal, exaggerated (hyper) or depressed (hypo) or can be graded on a scale of 0-4.

1. **Shoulder extension and elbow flexion would be the most appropriate position to test the triceps reflex. The reflex is best elicited with the patient in sitting or standing with the arm supported by the therapist. The therapist strikes the triceps tendon with a reflex hammer where it crosses the olecranon fossa. Stimulation of the triceps reflex elicits involuntary contraction of the triceps. An acceptable alternate position to test the triceps reflex would be shoulder abduction and elbow flexion.**

2. Shoulder flexion and elbow extension would not place the triceps tendon on adequate stretch to elicit the triceps reflex.

3. Shoulder extension and elbow extension would result in an ineffective position to elicit the triceps reflex since the triceps is already in a maximally shortened position.

4. Shoulder flexion and elbow flexion place the triceps on total stretch secondary to the origin and insertion of the triceps muscle. A deep tendon reflex should be tested with the tendon on slight stretch.

System: Neuromuscular and Nervous Systems
Content Outline: Physical Therapy Data Collection

 Level 2   p. 511-512

 Level 1   p. 229-231

➡ PTAEXAM THREE: QUESTION 43

A patient ambulating in the physical therapy gym suddenly grabs the forearm of the physical therapist assistant and reports feeling faint. Which of the following actions should the assistant take **FIRST**?

1. Assess the patient's pulse rate

2. Ask the patient if they have ever previously fainted

3. Loosen any tight clothing

4. **Assist the patient to a sitting position**

Correct Answer: 4 (Code of Ethics)

The physical therapist assistant must take immediate action to ensure patient safety. By assisting the patient to a chair, the physical therapist assistant can adequately assess the patient without compromising patient safety.

1. Assessing the patient's pulse rate may provide the physical therapist assistant with additional information on the patient's current medical status, however, the more immediate concern would be to assist the patient to a stable and secure position to minimize the risk of a fall.

2. Gathering additional information on the patient's past medical history will eventually be warranted, however, the action does not specifically address the immediate safety concern.

3. Loosening tight clothing may assist the patient to be more comfortable, however, this action would not be appropriate until the patient is in a secure position.

4. **The physical therapist assistant's primary responsibility is to preserve patient safety. Assisting the patient to a sitting position takes the patient out of immediate danger. Each of the remaining options is viable, however, only after patient safety has been preserved.**

System: Cardiovascular and Pulmonary Systems
Content Outline: Interventions

Level 3

➡ PTAEXAM THREE: QUESTION 44

A physical therapist assistant provides pre-operative instructions to a patient scheduled for a lower extremity amputation. Which of the following conditions is the **MOST** common cause of lower extremity amputation?

1. Tumor

2. Trauma

3. **Peripheral vascular disease**

4. Cardiac disease

Correct Answer: 3 (Seymour p. 10)

Peripheral vascular disease refers to diseases of blood vessels outside the heart and brain. The condition is often caused by narrowing of vessels that carry blood to the legs, arms, stomach or kidneys.

1. Certain tumors will require extremity amputation, however, this is not the most common causative factor for lower extremity amputation. Sarcomas are the most common type of malignant tumor that require amputation.

2. Trauma may result in the need for amputation, however, this is not the most common causative factor for lower extremity amputation. Trauma remains the most common cause of upper extremity amputation.

3. **Peripheral vascular disease is caused by atherosclerotic or inflammatory processes causing lumen narrowing (stenosis), embolism, vasospasm, trauma or thrombus formation. Initially, symptoms may include intermittent claudication and in severe cases, the condition can progress to amputation. The relative risk of limb amputation is largely dependent on the number and severity of cardiovascular risk factors (i.e., smoking, hypertension, diabetes).**

4. Cardiac disease itself is not a common causative factor for lower extremity amputation.

System: Other Systems
Content Outline: Diseases/Conditions that Impact Effective Treatment

Level 1 p. 125, 406-407

▶ PTAEXAM THREE: QUESTION 45

A physical therapist assistant uses the rule of nines on a three-year-old patient to determine the approximate percentage of the body affected by a burn. When using this assessment tool, what area of the child's body would be given a higher percentage value compared to an adult?

1. **The head**
2. The trunk
3. The legs
4. The genitalia

Correct Answer: 1 (Sussman p. 407)

The rule of nines is an assessment tool used to determine the total surface area of the body that is affected by a burn. The body is divided into 11 areas, with each area representing 9% of the total surface area, and the genitalia representing the additional 1%. When using the rule of nines, the surface area percentages must be altered if the patient is an infant or child.

1. **The head of an infant makes up a larger percentage of the total surface area as compared to an adult. For an adult, the front and the back of the head each comprise 4.5% of the total surface area.**
2. The trunk of an infant is similar in percentage value to that of an adult. For an adult, the front and the back of the trunk each comprise 18% of the total surface area (36% total for the entire trunk).
3. The legs of an infant make up a smaller percentage of the total surface area as compared to an adult. For an adult, the front and the back of a leg each comprise 9% (18% total for an entire leg) of the total surface area.
4. The genitalia of an infant are similar in percentage value to that of an adult. For an adult, the genitalia comprise 1% of the total surface area.

System: Other Systems
Content Outline: Physical Therapy Data Collection

▶ PTAEXAM THREE: QUESTION 46

A physical therapist assistant instructs a patient in pelvic floor muscle strengthening exercises. Which of the following instructions would be the **MOST** effective to assist the patient to perform a pelvic floor contraction?

1. Tighten your muscles like you were trying to expel a large amount of urine in a very short amount of time
2. **Pull your muscles upward and inward as if attempting to stop the flow of urine**
3. Tighten your abdominal muscles and anteriorly rotate your pelvis
4. Gently push out as if you had to pass gas

Correct Answer: 2 (Brody p. 500)

The pelvic floor muscles support the pelvic organs against intra-abdominal pressure, provide closure of the urethra and rectum for continence, and support sexual function. Pelvic floor exercises, also known as Kegel exercises, assist to maintain the strength and function of the pelvic floor muscles.

1. Placing a downward pressure on the pelvic floor serves to increase intra-abdominal pressure and encourages protrusion or prolapse of the pelvic organs.
2. **The correct technique for pelvic floor exercises includes pulling the pelvic floor muscles up and in. Isometric contractions should be held for five to ten seconds with complete relaxation after each contraction. Five to ten contractions should be performed in a series and three to four series should be performed each day.**
3. Tightening the abdominal muscles will trigger reflexive contraction of the pelvic floor, however, anteriorly rotating the pelvis will lengthen the abdominal muscles. Performing both actions simultaneously will reduce the strength of any pelvic floor contraction.
4. The act of "gently pushing out as if you had to pass gas" places a downward pressure on the pelvic floor muscles. This action is opposite of the necessary action for pelvic floor strengthening.

System: Other Systems
Content Outline: Interventions

 Level 1   p. 452

 Level 2   p. 476, 478, 544-545

➡ PTAEXAM THREE: QUESTION 47

The physical therapy department sponsors a community education program on diabetes mellitus. Which of the following characteristics is **NOT** typical of type 1 diabetes?

1. Age of onset less than 25 years of age

2. **Gradual onset**

3. Controlled through insulin and diet

4. Islet cell antibodies present at onset

Correct Answer: 2 (Goodman – Pathology p. 509)

Diabetes mellitus (DM) is a multi-system disease with both biochemical and anatomical consequences. There is persistent hyperglycemia due to diminished or absent production of insulin. Type 1 DM occurs when the pancreas fails to produce enough or any insulin. Symptoms include weight loss, polyuria, polydipsia, blurred vision, and dehydration. Type 2 DM occurs when the body cannot properly respond to insulin. Symptoms are relatively the same as with type 1, however, ketoacidosis does not occur since insulin is still produced.

1. A patient with type 1 DM is typically younger than 25 years at the age of onset. A patient with type 2 DM is typically older than 40 years at the age of onset.

2. **Type 1 DM typically has an abrupt onset and accounts for 5-10 percent of all cases. This type of diabetes requires insulin injections and is more common in children and young adults. Type 2 DM typically occurs in patients over 40 years of age, has a gradual onset, and can usually be controlled with diet, exercise, and oral insulin medication.**

3. A patient with type 1 DM requires insulin injections and proper diet to control blood sugar levels. A patient with type 2 DM will typically manage their medical condition with proper diet, exercise, and oral hypoglycemic medication, although sometimes insulin injections are required.

4. The exact etiology of type 1 DM is unknown, however, some theories suggest that the destruction of islet of Langerhans cells within the pancreas is secondary to possible autoimmune or viral causative factors.

System: Other Systems
Content Outline: Diseases/Conditions that Impact Effective Treatment

➡ PTAEXAM THREE: QUESTION 48

A physical therapist assistant treats a patient who has a pressure injury over the left ischial tuberosity. The patient's stage 3 pressure injury has healed over time and currently shows characteristics of a stage 1 pressure injury. What pressure injury stage should be assigned?

1. Stage 1 pressure injury

2. Modified stage 1 pressure injury

3. **Stage 3 pressure injury**

4. Modified stage 3 pressure injury

Correct Answer: 3 (Fairchild p. 296)

A pressure injury describes a localized injury to the skin and/or underlying tissue, usually over a bony prominence, as a result of pressure or pressure in combination with shear and/or friction forces. The National Pressure Ulcer Advisory Panel pressure ulcer staging criteria was developed for use with pressure injuries. The staging criteria range from 1–4.

1. A stage 1 pressure injury is characterized by an observable pressure related alteration of intact skin whose indicators, as compared to an adjacent or opposite area on the body, may include changes in skin color, skin temperature, skin stiffness or sensation. Pressure ulcers cannot be classified regressively as they heal. Therefore, an ulcer that had been graded as a stage 3 would still be known as a stage 3 pressure injury as it heals.

2. Terms such as "modified" would not be used to describe the healing status of a wound. Instead the percentage of the wound that has healed is often reported.

3. **A stage 3 pressure injury is characterized by full-thickness skin loss that involves damage or necrosis of subcutaneous tissue that may extend down to, but not through, underlying fascia. The ulcer presents clinically as a deep crater with or without undermining adjacent tissue.**

4. The ulcer would remain a stage 3 pressure injury, however, terms such as "modified" would not be used to describe the healing status of the wound. Instead the percentage of the wound that has healed is often reported.

System: Other Systems
Content Outline: Physical Therapy Data Collection

 Level 2   p. 466-467, 526-527

 Level 3   p. 444

➡ PTAEXAM THREE: QUESTION 49

A physical therapist assistant plans to apply ultrasound over an extremely irregular body surface area. Which method of ultrasound administration would be the **MOST** appropriate?

1. Direct contact with a gel coupling agent
2. Direct contact without a gel coupling agent
3. Water immersion with a gel coupling agent
4. **Water immersion without a gel coupling agent**

Correct Answer: 4 (Bellew p. 98)

Ultrasound waves do not travel through air and, as a result, a coupling agent is required. Coupling agents are designed to decrease acoustical impedance by eliminating as much air as possible between the transducer and the target area. Coupling agents can be direct or indirect and include gels, gel pads, mineral oil, water, and lotions.

1. Direct contact requires the face of the transducer to be parallel with the surface of the skin so that ultrasound waves will be introduced at a 90 degree angle. This method of administration requires a coupling agent, however, is potentially problematic with extremely irregular body surface areas.

2. Direct contact requires the face of the transducer to be parallel with the surface of the skin so that ultrasound waves will be introduced at a 90 degree angle. This method of administration requires a coupling agent.

3. Water immersion is an indirect coupling method requiring the treatment area to be immersed in water. This method of administration is ideal for irregular surfaces since the transducer does not need to be in direct contact with the treatment area. A gel coupling agent is not required since water serves as the coupling agent. A coupling agent would be more appropriate when using direct contact.

4. **Water immersion is an indirect coupling method requiring the treatment area to be immersed in water. This method of administration is ideal for irregular surfaces since the transducer does not need to be in direct contact with the treatment area. A gel coupling agent is not required with water immersion since water serves as the coupling agent.**

System: Non-Systems
Content Outline: Equipment, Devices, and Technologies;
  Therapeutic Modalities

➡ PTAEXAM THREE: QUESTION 50

A physical therapist assistant completes a manual muscle test where resistance is applied toward plantar flexion and eversion. This description **BEST** describes a manual muscle test of which of the following muscles?

1. **Tibialis anterior**
2. Tibialis posterior
3. Peroneus longus
4. Peroneus brevis

Correct Answer: 1 (Kendall p. 410)

The tibialis anterior acts to dorsiflex the ankle joint and assists with inversion of the foot. The muscle is innervated by the deep peroneal nerve.

1. **When testing the tibialis anterior, pressure should be applied against the medial side of the dorsal surface of the foot, in the direction of plantar flexion of the ankle joint and eversion of the foot.**

2. When testing the tibialis posterior, pressure should be applied against the medial side and plantar surface of the foot, in the direction of dorsiflexion of the ankle joint and eversion of the foot.

3. When testing the peroneus longus, pressure should be applied against the lateral border and sole of the foot, in the direction of dorsiflexion of the ankle joint and inversion of the foot.

4. When testing the peroneus brevis, pressure should be applied in the same manner as described for the peroneus longus.

System: Musculoskeletal System
Content Outline: Physical Therapy Data Collection

 Level 2   p. 623-626

Level 1

➡ PTAEXAM THREE: QUESTION 51

A physical therapist assistant considers using functional electrical stimulation as part of a patient's care plan. Which patient would be the **MOST** appropriate for this type of intervention?

1. A patient with chronic low back pain secondary to a motor vehicle accident

2. A patient having difficulty performing a straight leg raise after an ACL repair

3. A patient with a slowly healing wound on their medial lower leg

4. **A patient that acquired foot drop after a total knee arthroplasty**

Correct Answer: 4 (Cameron p. 239)

Functional electrical stimulation (FES) is a specific type of neuromuscular electrical stimulation (NMES) that is used during the performance of a functional activity. An FES device can stimulate a contraction of the desired muscle group during a functional activity resulting in improved performance of the activity. FES is most commonly used to improve a patient's gait.

1. A patient with low back pain would be an appropriate candidate for electrical stimulation, especially if they are experiencing chronic pain. However, this patient would more likely benefit from transcutaneous electrical nerve stimulation (TENS), which is a specific type of electrical stimulation that decreases the perception of pain by blocking pain signals to the brain.

2. A patient that has difficulty contracting a specific muscle group would be an appropriate candidate for electrical stimulation. However, this patient would more likely benefit from NMES, which is a specific type of electrical stimulation that improves the strength of weak or denervated muscles. NMES is only considered to be FES if it is used in conjunction with a functional activity. A straight leg raise is not an example of a functional activity.

3. A patient with a slowly healing wound would be an appropriate candidate for electrical stimulation. High-voltage pulsed current electrical stimulation has been shown to help improve wound healing through a variety of mechanisms, including attraction of cells to the wound site, edema reduction, and promotion of circulation. Using electrical stimulation for wound healing is not an example of FES.

4. **A patient with foot drop would be an appropriate candidate for electrical stimulation, specifically for the use of FES. FES devices are used to stimulate the contraction of a specific muscle group during a functional activity. In this scenario, the device would be used to stimulate the ankle dorsiflexors to lessen the patient's foot drop and thereby improve their gait.**

System: Non-Systems
Content Outline: Equipment, Devices, and Technologies; Therapeutic Modalities

➡ PTAEXAM THREE: QUESTION 52

When performing a goniometric measurement of elbow flexion with a patient in the supine position, which of the following structures should the physical therapist assistant stabilize in order to isolate elbow flexion?

1. **Distal end of the humerus**

2. Proximal end of the humerus

3. Distal end of the ulna

4. Proximal end of the radius

Correct Answer: 1 (Norkin p. 120)

When measuring elbow flexion, the physical therapist assistant should align the fulcrum of the goniometer over the lateral epicondyle of the humerus. The stationary arm should be aligned with the lateral midline of the humerus using the center of the acromial process as a reference. The moveable arm should be aligned with the lateral midline of the radius using the radial head and radial styloid process as references. Normal elbow flexion is 0-150 degrees.

1. **The distal end of the humerus should be stabilized when measuring elbow flexion to prevent flexion of the shoulder. The therapist should place a pad (i.e., folded towel) between the table and the distal humerus to prevent extension of the shoulder.**

2. Stabilization of the proximal end of the humerus is too far away from the elbow to adequately stabilize the joint during elbow flexion.

3. The distal end of the radius and ulna would be stabilized when measuring wrist flexion and extension or wrist radial and ulnar deviation.

4. Any attempt to stabilize the proximal end of the radius would interfere with elbow flexion range of motion.

System: Musculoskeletal System
Content Outline: Physical Therapy Data Collection

  Level 2   p. 641-642

  Level 1   p. 88

SCOREBUILDERS

➡ PTAEXAM THREE: QUESTION 53

A patient that required a mechanical ventilator for two weeks following a near drowning incident is cleared to gradually decrease use of the device. Which measured cardiopulmonary value would indicate a sign of distress during the weaning process?

1. **Respiratory rate of 38 breaths per minute**
2. Tidal volume of 350 milliliters
3. Pulse oximetry measured at 91 percent
4. Heart rate change of 10 beats per minute over baseline

Correct Answer: 1 (Paz p. 396)

The process of decreasing or discontinuing mechanical ventilation is termed the weaning process. There are expected criteria that need to be satisfied in order to attempt weaning. Physical therapist assistants should be aware of signs of distress during this process.

1. **A significantly elevated respiratory rate (e.g., 38 breaths per minute) is a cardinal sign of distress during the weaning process. Persistent tachypnea may result in failure to wean from the mechanical ventilator.**
2. A tidal volume of 350 milliliters would not be considered a sign of distress during the weaning process. A tidal volume value less than 325 milliliters would be considered a sign of distress.
3. A pulse oximetry value of 91 percent would not be considered a sign of distress during the weaning process. A pulse oximetry value less than 90 percent would be considered a sign of distress.
4. A heart rate change of 10 beats per minute over baseline would not be considered a sign of distress during the weaning process. A heart rate change of greater than 20 beats per minute would be considered a sign of distress.

System: Non-Systems
Content Outline: Safety and Protection; Professional Responsibilities; Research

➡ PTAEXAM THREE: QUESTION 54

Which of the following scenarios would be the **BEST** example of an individual's right to autonomy being violated?

1. An adult who refuses surgery
2. **An adult coerced to have surgery**
3. An infant whose parents elect for surgery
4. An athlete who seeks a second opinion

Correct Answer: 2 (Portney p. 49)

Individual autonomy is a principle that refers to the capacity to be one's own person and to live one's life according to reasons and motives that are taken as one's own, and not the product of manipulative or distorting external forces.

1. An adult who refuses surgery is an example of a patient exhibiting autonomy since they are making an independent decision without any evidence of external influence.
2. **An adult coerced to have surgery is a clear violation of an individual's right to autonomy. Coercion is defined as the practice of persuading an individual to do something using force or threats. This type of persuasion often results in patients selecting a different course of action than would have been selected if the patient was able to make an independent decision.**
3. An infant does not possess the mental capacity to make an informed decision that is in their best interest. As a result, decisions are made by a legally qualified surrogate such as a parent, legal guardian or court appointed advocate. A parental decision for an infant to have surgery would therefore not be considered a violation of the patient's autonomy.
4. An athlete electing to have a second opinion is an example of a patient exhibiting autonomy since they are making an independent decision without any evidence of external influence. Many patients obtain a second opinion in order to receive an independent medical assessment.

System: Non-Systems
Content Outline: Safety and Protection; Professional Responsibilities; Research

 Level 3   p. 374-375

 Level 2   p. 689

➡ PTAEXAM THREE: QUESTION 55

A physical therapist assistant monitors the blood pressure response of a patient during aerobic exercise on a stationary bicycle. The assistant notes a relatively linear increase in systolic blood pressure with increasing exercise intensity. Which of the following reasons **BEST** explains the patient's blood pressure response?

1. **Increased cardiac output**
2. Decreased peripheral resistance
3. Increased oxygen saturation
4. Decreased myocardial oxygen consumption

Correct Answer: 1 (American College of Sports Medicine p. 478)

Cardiac output is the volume of blood pumped into the systemic circulation per minute and is equal to the product of heart rate and stroke volume.

1. **The trend towards lower blood pressure during exercise brought about by a decrease in peripheral resistance is negated by an increase in cardiac output. The increased heart rate and force of contraction of the myocardium (stroke volume) has the net effect of increasing systolic blood pressure in a normal population.**

2. A decrease in peripheral resistance to blood flow tends to cause a decrease in blood pressure due to dilation of blood vessels in the exercising muscles.

3. Oxygen saturation is not affected by exercise in individuals with healthy lungs. Oxygen saturation may decrease during exercise in patients with chronic lung disease.

4. An increase in heart rate while cycling will increase myocardial oxygen consumption as the heart muscle utilizes more oxygen. Cardiac output increases to supply oxygenated blood to the exercising muscles.

System: Cardiovascular and Pulmonary Systems
Content Outline: Interventions

➡ PTAEXAM THREE: QUESTION 56

A patient is admitted to the hospital with a stage 3 pressure injury over the right ischial tuberosity. The patient's past medical history includes severe chronic obstructive pulmonary disease. Which of the following positions is the **MOST** appropriate for this patient?

1. Supine with pillows under the knees
2. Prone with pillows under the knees
3. **Left sidelying with pillows between the knees**
4. Right sidelying with pillows between the knees

Correct Answer: 3 (Frownfelter p. 515)

Left sidelying would be the position of choice in order to relieve pressure on the ulcer and maximize the patient's respiration. Recognizing contraindications for chronic obstructive pulmonary disease as well as positioning for pressure relief will allow for safe and effective positioning to enhance recovery.

1. Although the supine position with pillows under the knees is a comfortable position that reduces lumbar lordosis and strain, there would be pressure directly over the right ischial tuberosity and this would hinder progress or worsen the pressure injury.

2. A prone position would allow for pressure relief over the right ischial tuberosity, however, the patient has severe chronic obstructive pulmonary disease and should not lie in prone as breathing would be very difficult. Pillows are also not typically placed under the knees when a patient is in prone.

3. **Left sidelying does not compromise respiration and avoids placing stress on the right ischial tuberosity.**

4. A right sidelying position would assist the patient with breathing and would not compromise overall respiration, however, there would be significant pressure over the right ischial tuberosity.

System: Other Systems
Content Outline: Interventions

 Level 2   p. 42, 358

 Level 2   p. 366, 444

➡ PTAEXAM THREE: QUESTION 57

A physical therapist assistant performs a manual muscle test on the medial rotators of a patient's shoulder. Which of the following muscles would **NOT** be involved in this specific test?

1. Pectoralis major

2. Teres major

3. Latissimus dorsi

4. **Teres minor**

Correct Answer: 4 (Kendall p. 321)

The primary muscles being assessed while testing the shoulder medial rotators include the pectoralis major, latissimus dorsi, subscapularis, and teres major. The test is performed with the patient in supine and resistance is applied to the forearm in the direction of laterally rotating the humerus. The test can alternately be performed with the patient in prone.

1. The pectoralis major–upper fibers act to flex and medially rotate the shoulder joint, and horizontally adduct the humerus. The upper fibers are innervated by the lateral pectoral nerve. The pectoralis major–lower fibers act to depress the shoulder girdle and obliquely adduct the humerus. The lower fibers are innervated by the lateral and medial pectoral nerves.

2. The teres major acts to medially rotate, adduct, and extend the shoulder joint. The muscle is innervated by the lower subscapular nerve (C5, C6, C7).

3. The latissimus dorsi with the origin fixed acts to medially rotate, adduct, and extend the shoulder joint. The muscle is innervated by the thoracodorsal nerve (C6, C7, C8).

4. **The teres minor acts to laterally rotate the shoulder joint and stabilize the head of the humerus in the glenoid cavity. The muscle is innervated by the axillary nerve (C5, C6).**

System: Musculoskeletal System
Content Outline: Physical Therapy Data Collection

➡ PTAEXAM THREE: QUESTION 58

A patient with a unilateral transfemoral prosthesis places the prosthetic foot either medially or laterally during the heel strike (initial contact) phase of gait. The patient reports it is difficult to control the placement of the prosthesis. Which of the following activities is **MOST** likely to correct the problem?

1. Standing on the prosthesis and tapping the contralateral foot on a step

2. Side stepping to the side of the prosthesis with a resistance band

3. **Controlled tapping of the prosthesis on a colored circle while standing**

4. Repeated sit to stand transfers from a normal height chair

Correct Answer: 3 (May p. 138)

Controlling the prosthesis is a difficult task experienced by most patients following amputation. The patient must learn how to coordinate the proximal musculature (gluteals/hip flexors) in order to place the limb correctly. Initially, this can be facilitated using visual feedback, such as colored markers or a mirror.

1. Standing on the prosthesis promotes hip abduction strength and balance, however, this would be more helpful for controlling the placement of the contralateral limb during heel strike.

2. Side stepping is a functional exercise that will help develop hip abduction strength and balance on the prosthetic limb, however, it is not the most appropriate option to improve placement of the prosthesis.

3. **Simulating the movement is the most appropriate as it focuses directly on the issue the patient is experiencing and utilizes visual feedback to improve coordination.**

4. Sit to stand motions are helpful in developing the strength of the lower extremities, however, they will not influence coordination, which is the primary identified deficit.

System: Musculoskeletal System
Content Outline: Interventions

 Level 1   p. 53-55

 Level 3

➡ PTAEXAM THREE: QUESTION 59

A patient informs a physical therapist assistant that she noticed a small lump on her right breast while dressing. The patient was referred to physical therapy with lateral epicondylitis and has no significant past medical history. Which of the following actions is the MOST appropriate for the assistant to take?

1. Inspect the breast to assess the lump

2. **Instruct the patient to make an immediate appointment with her physician**

3. Inform the patient she may have cancer

4. Document the patient's comment in the medical record

Correct Answer: 2 (Goodman – Pathology p. 1060)

Ninety percent of breast cancer is discovered through self-identification. Research has demonstrated that in the United States one in nine women may be affected by breast cancer over the course of their life. As a result, it is imperative that the physical therapist assistant impress upon the patient the importance of consulting with her physician.

1. Inspecting the lump would be inappropriate, especially when considering the patient's medical diagnosis. Physical therapist assistants must refer patients to appropriate medical personnel when warranted based on the results of subjective and objective data.

2. **The patient's statement makes it imperative that the patient contact the physician. The physical therapist assistant should be careful not to alarm the patient, however, must stress the importance of an appointment with the physician.**

3. It would be inappropriate for the physical therapist assistant to suggest that the patient may have cancer. Physical therapists and physical therapist assistants cannot medically diagnose and should avoid suggestive comments related to a given diagnosis.

4. It is acceptable to document the patient's comments in the medical record, however, the priority needs to be related to follow-up with the physician.

System: Other Systems
Content Outline: Diseases/Conditions that Impact Effective Treatment

➡ PTAEXAM THREE: QUESTION 60

An exercise program designed for a patient emphasizes large amplitude movements as depicted in the image. For which of the following conditions would this type of exercise program be MOST beneficial?

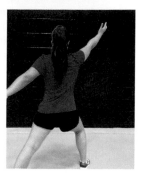

1. Juvenile rheumatoid arthritis

2. Huntington's disease

3. Peripheral vascular disease

4. **Parkinson's disease**

Correct Answer: 4 (O'Sullivan p. 833)

Amplitude-based intervention or "training big" is a theoretical framework based on using repetitive high-amplitude movements to improve motor performance. These large body and extremity movements are performed to counter the paucity of movement typically associated with Parkinson's disease.

1. Juvenile rheumatoid arthritis is a form of arthritis found in children less than 16 years of age that presents with inflammation and stiffness to multiple joints. Functional mobility, strengthening, and endurance training will assist a patient in overall function. Modalities, splints, and orthoses optimize the quality of life. Large amplitude movements would not improve overall motor outcomes for these patients.

2. Huntington's disease is a neurological disorder characterized by degeneration of the basal ganglia. Initial symptoms include involuntary choreic movements. Physical therapy should maximize endurance, strength, and functional mobility with focus on motor control and coactivation of core muscles. Large amplitude movements would not improve overall motor outcomes for these patients.

3. Peripheral vascular disease is the narrowing of the lumen of blood vessels. Physical therapy should include a progressive walking program where the patient walks until the pain is not tolerated followed by a period of rest. Large amplitude movements would not improve overall motor outcomes for these patients.

4. **Parkinson's disease is characterized by a decrease in dopamine within the basal ganglia. Impairments include difficulty with initiating and stopping movement, festinating gait, poor posture, and "cogwheel" or "lead pipe" rigidity. Physical therapy intervention should include maximizing endurance and functional mobility. Verbal cueing, oral/visual feedback, and large amplitude movements are often utilized.**

System: Neuromuscular and Nervous Systems
Content Outline: Interventions

 Level 3   p. 488-490, 520-521

 Level 2   p. 250, 308-309

▶ PTAEXAM THREE: QUESTION 61

A patient is directed to reach for an object beyond arm's length during therapeutic activities emphasizing core training and balance activities as depicted in the image. Which response would be **MOST** desirable when performing this activity?

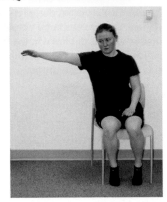

1. Left trunk elongation, left weight shift, right hip hiking

2. Right trunk elongation, right weight shift, right hip hiking

3. Left trunk elongation, left weight shift, left hip hiking

4. **Right trunk elongation, right weight shift, left hip hiking**

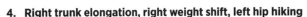

Correct Answer: 4 (O'Sullivan p. 426)

When treating patients, physical therapist assistants must be cognizant of the goals of specific activities and use therapeutic interventions that relate to the goal. For example, reaching above shoulder level will produce trunk elongation and weight shift ipsilaterally and reaching towards the floor will produce trunk elongation and weight shift contralaterally.

1. A patient that presents with left trunk elongation, left weight shift, and right hip hiking is likely reaching for an object just beyond their reach at shoulder height or higher on their left side.

2. A patient that presents with right trunk elongation and right weight shift would typically be reaching for an object beyond arm's length at shoulder level or higher on their right side. They would, however, present with left hip hiking, not right hip hiking.

3. A patient that presents with left trunk elongation and left weight shift would typically be reaching for an object beyond arm's length at shoulder level or higher on their left side. They would, however, present with right hip hiking, not left hip hiking.

4. **A patient that presents with right trunk elongation, right weight shift, and left hip hiking is likely reaching for an object just beyond reach at shoulder height or higher on their right side.**

System: Neuromuscular and Nervous Systems
Content Outline: Interventions

▶ PTAEXAM THREE: QUESTION 62

A patient who has T10 paraplegia is discharged from a rehabilitation hospital following 12 weeks of intense rehabilitation. Which of the following pieces of equipment would be the **MOST** essential to assist the patient with functional mobility?

1. Lofstrand crutches

2. Lofstrand crutches and ankle-foot orthoses

3. Lofstrand crutches and knee-ankle-foot orthoses

4. **Wheelchair with pressure relieving cushion**

Correct Answer: 4 (Roy p. 369)

A patient with a lesion above T12 would not be a functional ambulator due to the extreme energy demands and therefore would utilize a wheelchair as their primary mode of mobility.

1. A patient with an incomplete lesion may ambulate without an orthotic using Lofstrand crutches, however, this would not be an option for a complete spinal cord lesion.

2. A patient with a complete lesion at L4 or L5 would typically ambulate with crutches or canes and bilateral AFOs. The extensor digitorum, medial hamstrings, posterior tibialis, quadriceps, tibialis anterior, and low back muscles would be the lowest innervated muscles.

3. A patient with a complete lesion at L2 or L3 would typically ambulate with crutches and bilateral KAFOs. Patients at this level of injury may also use a manual wheelchair for energy conservation and convenience. The gracilis, iliopsoas, quadratus lumborum, rectus femoris, and sartorius would be the lowest innervated muscles.

4. **A patient with T10 paraplegia will require a wheelchair for community ambulation due to the increased energy expenditure associated with ambulation. The lower abdominals and intercostals would be the lowest innervated muscles.**

System: Neuromuscular and Nervous Systems
Content Outline: Interventions

◉ Level 1

◉ Level 2   👓 p. 269-271

➡ PTAEXAM THREE: QUESTION 63

A physical therapist assistant instructs a patient in an exercise designed to increase pelvic floor awareness and strength. The exercise requires the patient to perform isometric contractions of the pelvic floor muscles. Which of the following positions is the most appropriate **INITIAL** position for this exercise?

1. Supine
2. Sitting
3. Tall kneeling
4. Standing

Correct Answer: 1 (Kisner p. 992)

The pelvic floor muscles follow the same general strengthening principles as other muscles of the body. As a result, the initial position for the pelvic floor exercise should remove or minimize the influence of gravity. As the patient demonstrates mastery of the initial position, the physical therapist assistant can select positions that will provide the patient with a greater challenge.

1. **Kegel exercises or isometric contractions of the pelvic floor are often utilized as part of a treatment program for incontinence. Supine and sidelying are the typical gravity-eliminated positions to initiate strengthening. A patient may also use a gravity-assisted position where the hips are above the level of the heart such as supported bridging or on elbows and knees in order to have gravity assist the contraction.**

2. A patient would progress to sitting once there is adequate strength and awareness of the pelvic floor muscles. Sitting requires exercise against gravity and therefore would not be the most appropriate initial position.

3. A patient would progress to tall kneeling once there is adequate strength and awareness of the pelvic floor in a sitting position. Tall kneeling requires proximal control and balance to maintain the position.

4. Standing is the highest level in the general progression of pelvic floor strengthening. The normal sequence is supine or sidelying followed by quadruped, sitting, tall kneeling, and standing.

System: Other Systems
Content Outline: Interventions

➡ PTAEXAM THREE: QUESTION 64

A physical therapist assistant reviews risk factors for the development of a pressure injury. Which of the following patients would be the **MOST** at risk for this type of injury?

1. 55-year-old Caucasian male with diabetes
2. **60-year-old African American female with a C7 spinal cord injury**
3. 80-year-old African American male with chronic obstructive pulmonary disease
4. 65-year-old Caucasian female status post total knee arthroplasty

Correct Answer: 2 (Sussman p. 247)

Pressure injuries are areas of local tissue damage, usually developing where soft tissues become compressed between a bony prominence and an external surface for prolonged periods of time. Risk factors for the development of pressure injuries include female gender, African American race, advanced age, and conditions that cause immobility.

1. A patient with diabetes is at risk for developing an ulcer, though it would more likely be a neuropathic ulcer, not a pressure injury. The other patient demographics are not consistent with the risk factors for pressure injuries.

2. **This patient would be at the greatest risk for the development of a pressure injury due to her race (i.e., African American), gender (i.e., female), and medical condition (i.e., spinal cord injury). Patients with spinal cord injuries are often immobile, which places them at high risk for developing pressure injuries.**

3. While the patient's age and race would place him at increased risk for pressure injury development, chronic obstructive pulmonary disease is not a condition that would significantly limit the patient's mobility.

4. While a patient status post total knee arthroplasty may be immobile immediately after surgery, they will not experience the same level of immobility as a patient with a spinal cord injury. The patient is also at less risk due to her race.

System: Other Systems
Content Outline: Diseases/Conditions that Impact Effective Treatment

---

 Level 2   p. 476, 478, 483

Level 2   p. 538-539

➡ PTAEXAM THREE: QUESTION 65

A physical therapist assistant performs a patient chart review and finds the patient is positive for the Helicobacter pylori bacterium. The assistant should recognize this bacterium as being **MOST** associated with which of the following conditions?

1. Meningitis
2. Pneumonia
3. **Gastric ulcer disease**
4. Tetanus

Correct Answer: 3 (Ciccone p. 425)

Bacterial infections can be harmful and potentially life-threatening if left untreated. Bacteria will multiply and utilize nutrients of its host, produce direct tissue damage, and produce an immune response that can ultimately harm the host.

1. Meningitis is the inflammation of the membranes surrounding the brain and spinal cord. There are multiple forms of meningitis and multiple bacteria that can produce this condition. Neisseria meningitidis is one of the bacterium that is a leading cause of bacterial meningitis. It is treated primarily with penicillin G.

2. Pneumonia refers to inflammation of the lungs due to bacterial, viral, fungal or parasitic infection. The common bacterium in most cases of community-acquired pneumonia is Streptococcus pneumoniae. It is treated primarily with penicillin, ampicillin, or if penicillin-resistant, vancomycin.

3. **Gastric ulcer disease is often caused by the Gram-negative bacterium Helicobacter pylori that is found in the upper gastrointestinal tract. This infection is believed to be a potential cause of gastroduodenal ulcers and must be treated with antibiotics.**

4. Tetanus is an acute and often fatal disease if left untreated marked by a continuous state of muscular contraction and rigidity of voluntary muscles. The bacterium Clostridium tetani is a common cause of tetanus and it is treated with penicillin and vancomycin.

System: Other Systems
Content Outline: Diseases/Conditions that Impact Effective Treatment

➡ PTAEXAM THREE: QUESTION 66

Following an acute myocardial infarction, a patient continues to experience frequent arrhythmias. A physical therapist assistant should recognize an abnormality in which of the following lab values as being the **MOST** likely to contribute to the arrhythmias?

1. **Potassium**
2. Hemoglobin
3. Hematocrit
4. Platelet count

Correct Answer: 1 (Goodman – Pathology p. 1705)

A cardiac arrhythmia is a disturbance in heart rate and rhythm as a result of an abnormality in the electrical conduction system in the heart. Dysrhythmias are common complications of a myocardial infarction because of the interruption to the cardiac conduction system and imbalance of autonomic regulation. The severity and type of arrhythmia is dependent on the location and extent of damage to the myocardium.

1. **Potassium plays a role in the generation of the cardiac action potential, specifically affecting the duration and repolarization. Both hypokalemia and hyperkalemia can result in the interruption of the action potential and cardiac dysrhythmias. Patients with hypokalemia may report dizziness and/or palpitations.**

2. Hemoglobin is the oxygen carrying protein in red blood cells. Normal hemoglobin values for adult males are 13.3-16.2 gm/dL and for females are 12.0-15.8 gm/dL. Abnormalities in hemoglobin are associated with impaired aerobic capacity, diminished exercise tolerance, increased fatigue, and tachycardia. Therapeutic intervention is contraindicated with hemoglobin levels less than 8 gm/dL.

3. Hematocrit is the percentage of red blood cells in total blood volume. An elevated hematocrit level can occur with dehydration, polycythemia vera or an overproduction of red blood cells. Low hematocrit levels can indicate anemia or blood loss. Exercise is contraindicated with levels less than 25%.

4. The role of platelets is to initiate the clotting sequence to repair damaged blood vessels. Bleeding can occur with platelet levels less than 15,000-20,000 cells/mm³. With levels below 20,000 cells/mm³ activity should be limited to activities of daily living.

System: Cardiovascular and Pulmonary Systems
Content Outline: Diseases/Conditions that Impact Effective Treatment

 Level 2   p. 471

 Level 2   p. 507, 638

➡ PTAEXAM THREE: QUESTION 67

A patient who has a grade II lumbar spondylolisthesis experiences symptoms of neurogenic claudication. Which of the following exercises would **MOST** likely exacerbate the patient's symptoms?

1. **Walking on a treadmill with zero incline**
2. Cycling with varying resistance
3. Abdominal crunches on an exercise ball
4. Contraction of the multifidi in a flexed position

Correct Answer: 1 (Dutton p. 1488)

Spondylolisthesis is the forward slippage of one vertebra on the vertebra below, most commonly occurring at the L4-L5 level or the L5-S1 level. There are several grades of spondylolisthesis (i.e., grade I-IV) classified by the extent of the forward slippage. Degenerative spondylolisthesis is caused by weakening of the facet joints allowing for the forward slippage due to degenerative changes. These changes include segmental ligamentous instability and subluxation of the hypertrophic facet joints, which can result in stenosis of the spinal canal. This may cause leg pain in a radicular-type pattern or, more commonly, can manifest as neurogenic claudication.

1. **Walking on a treadmill with zero incline will most likely exacerbate the patient's symptoms due to the extension of the spine that occurs when walking upright. Extension decreases the anteroposterior diameter of the canal causing even more compression on the neural tissues and worsening the patient's symptoms. Patients with neurogenic claudication are typically more comfortable leaning forward or sitting, which flexes the spine, thereby widening the anteroposterior diameter of the canal.**

2. Cycling with varying resistance should be easier for the patient since the lumbar spine is in a more flexed position when cycling. Lumbar flexion increases the anteroposterior diameter of the canal, allowing more room for the neural tissues and improving the microcirculation.

3. Abdominal crunches on an exercise ball are appropriate in the management of spondylolisthesis as a means of abdominal strengthening and reduction of the lumbar lordosis. This would be considered part of the progression of abdominal strengthening.

4. Contraction of the multifidi in a flexed position is an appropriate spinal stabilization activity in the management of spondylolisthesis. The required flexed position would also be appropriate to reduce the risk of exacerbating the symptoms of neurogenic claudication.

System: Musculoskeletal System
Content Outline: Interventions

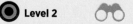 Level 2   p. 166-167

➡ PTAEXAM THREE: QUESTION 68

A physical therapist assistant is asked by the clinic manager to help develop a fall prevention program. What would be the **FIRST** step when developing this type of program?

1. Set goals and objectives for the program
2. **Identify the intended audience**
3. Identify valid and reliable screening tools
4. Develop a plan for each class

Correct Answer: 2 (Kisner p. 55)

Primary prevention is aimed at preventing a target problem or condition in individuals that do not currently have the condition, but are at risk. Secondary prevention is aimed at decreasing the duration and/or severity of the target problem or condition. The goal of tertiary prevention is to decrease the degree of disability for individuals with chronic diseases or conditions. There are typically five steps to follow when developing and implementing prevention programs.

1. Setting goals and objectives is the second step to developing and implementing a prevention program. Once the intended audience is identified, the purpose of the program along with the goals and objectives should be clearly established.

2. **The first step in developing and implementing a prevention program is to identify the need for the program, which involves identifying the intended audience. Once the audience is established, the next step is to set the goals and objectives of the program.**

3. Identifying valid and reliable screening tools is part of step number three: develop the intervention. This step involves identifying the appropriate screening tools, developing a plan for each class, including handouts for the participants, as well as establishing the logistics for implementing the program.

4. Developing a plan for each class is also part of step three: develop the intervention. Step four is to implement the intervention and step five (final step) involves evaluating the results or outcomes.

System: Non-Systems
Content Outline: Safety and Protection; Professional Responsibilities; Research

 Level 2

SCOREBUILDERS

➡ PTAEXAM THREE: QUESTION 69

A physical therapist assistant performs goniometric measurements on a patient post knee surgery to quantify the extent of the patient's extension lag. Which of the following rationales is the **LEAST** plausible cause of the extension lag?

1. Muscle weakness
2. **Bony obstruction**
3. Inhibition by pain
4. Patient apprehension

Correct Answer: 2 (Kisner p. 776)

Patients that demonstrate an extension lag have greater passive extension than active extension. The difference in the passive and active extension range of motion is used to quantify the amount of the lag.

1. Muscle weakness would provide a plausible rationale for an extension lag since force production is necessary to produce active motion. Inability to produce adequate force to move the tibia on the femur while performing active extension would produce the lag.

2. **A bony obstruction would not produce an extension lag since passive range of motion and active range of motion would be equal. In essence, the obstruction would interfere with the ability to perform both passive and active knee extension.**

3. Inhibition by pain would provide a plausible rationale for an extension lag. The amount of pain produced during an active muscle contraction may make it impossible for the muscle to generate the required amount of force to actively extend the tibia on the femur. The difference in the passive extension versus the active extension would determine the amount of the extension lag.

4. Patient apprehension would provide a plausible rationale for an extension lag since the patient may be unwilling to actively move the knee through the available active range of motion due to fear or anxiety.

System: Musculoskeletal System
Content Outline: Physical Therapy Data Collection

➡ PTAEXAM THREE: QUESTION 70

A physical therapist assistant instructs a patient in the supine position to posteriorly rotate the pelvis. The patient has full active and passive range of motion in the upper extremities, but is unable to achieve full shoulder flexion while maintaining a posterior pelvic tilt. Which of the following restrictions **BEST** explains this finding?

1. Capsular adhesions
2. **Latissimus dorsi tightness**
3. Pectoralis minor tightness
4. Quadratus lumborum tightness

Correct Answer: 2 (Kendall p. 325)

A posterior pelvic tilt results in the posterior superior iliac spines of the pelvis moving posteriorly and inferiorly. This motion results in hip extension and lumbar spine flexion.

1. The capsular pattern at the glenohumeral joint is lateral rotation, abduction, and medial rotation. A capsular pattern of restriction at the glenohumeral joint would limit range of motion, however, would not be influenced by the position of the pelvis.

2. **Shortening of the latissimus dorsi often results in a limitation of shoulder flexion or abduction due to the muscle's origin on the external lip of the iliac crest and its insertion on the intertubercular groove of the humerus.**

3. Pectoralis minor tightness may have a direct effect on shoulder range of motion, however, would not be influenced by the position of the pelvis. Pectoralis minor tightness is often best identified by positioning a patient in supine with the arms at their side and the palms facing upward. The relative tightness of the muscle is determined by the extent to which the shoulder is raised from the table and the amount of resistance felt to downward pressure on the shoulder.

4. Quadratus lumborum tightness may affect the ability of the pelvis to achieve the posterior pelvic tilt position required in the question, however, would not affect shoulder range of motion since the muscle does not directly attach to the shoulder joint.

System: Musculoskeletal System
Content Outline: Interventions

Level 2

Level 2

➡ PTAEXAM THREE: QUESTION 71

A physical therapist assistant observes a burn on the dorsal surface of a patient's arm that presents as mottled red with a number of blisters. The assistant informs the patient that healing should occur in less than three weeks. This description is **MOST** indicative of which type of burn?

1. Superficial
2. **Superficial partial-thickness**
3. Deep partial-thickness
4. Full-thickness

Correct Answer: 2 (Goodman – Pathology p. 454)

The burn classification system most commonly utilized uses the terms superficial, partial-thickness (superficial and deep), and full-thickness. The system provides a general description of the most common clinical findings associated with each type of burn.

1. A superficial burn involves only the outer epidermis. The involved area may be red with slight edema. Healing occurs without evidence of scarring in 2-5 days.

2. **A superficial partial-thickness burn involves the epidermis and the upper portion of the dermis. The involved area may be extremely painful and exhibit blisters. Healing occurs with minimal to no scarring in 5-21 days.**

3. A deep partial-thickness burn involves complete destruction of the epidermis and the majority of the dermis. The involved area may appear to be discolored with broken blisters and edema. Damage to nerve endings may result in only moderate levels of pain. Healing occurs with the potential for hypertrophic scars and keloids in 21-35 days.

4. A full-thickness burn involves complete destruction of the epidermis and dermis along with partial damage of the subcutaneous fat layer. The involved area often presents with eschar formation and minimal to no pain. Patients with full-thickness burns require grafts and may be susceptible to infection.

System: Other Systems
Content Outline: Diseases/Conditions that Impact Effective Treatment

➡ PTAEXAM THREE: QUESTION 72

A physical therapist assistant prepares to complete a sensory assessment on a patient with a lower extremity burn. Which of the following findings would serve as the **BEST** predictor of altered sensation?

1. Presence of a skin graft
2. **Depth of burn injury**
3. Percentage of body surface affected
4. Extent of hypertrophic scarring

Correct Answer: 2 (Sussman p. 405)

Patients with burns often experience a number of sensory changes. These changes can include impaired sensation or increased sensitivity. Although many factors contribute to sensory alteration, the depth of the burn appears to be the best predictor.

1. Skin grafts are typically used with full-thickness burns and although there is a predictable pattern of sensory alteration with full-thickness burns, the absence of a skin graft would not be useful to predict sensory changes in less severe burns (i.e., superficial and partial-thickness).

2. **It is possible to predict the relative extent of sensory alteration based on the depth of the burn. For example, a superficial partial-thickness burn is characterized by extreme pain and significant sensitivity to temperature change, while a full-thickness burn is characterized by an absence of pain and inability to identify temperature change.**

3. The percentage of body surface affected provides information on the size or extent of the burn, but does not provide information on other important variables such as the depth or severity of the burn.

4. Hypertrophic scarring refers to an overgrowth of dermal constituents that remain within the boundaries of the wound. This occurs as a result of scar formation when the burn extends into the dermis. Hypertrophic scarring results in poor cosmesis and the development of contractures that may limit function. The presence of hypertrophic scarring provides only limited information regarding the extent of altered sensation.

System: Other Systems
Content Outline: Diseases/Conditions that Impact Effective Treatment

 Level 1   p. 451-452, 524-525

 Level 2   p. 451-452

➡ PTAEXAM THREE: QUESTION 73

A patient has a history of a transient ischemic attack. Which variable should the physical therapist assistant recognize as **MOST** differentiating a transient ischemic attack from a cerebrovascular accident?

1. Presence of an aura
2. Magnitude of the initial symptoms
3. **Time for resolution of symptoms**
4. Extent of speech and vision problems

Correct Answer: 3 (Nichols – Larsen p. 151)

A transient ischemic attack (TIA) is usually linked to an atherosclerotic thrombosis which causes a temporary interruption of blood supply to an area of the brain. A TIA most often occurs in the carotid and vertebrobasilar arteries. A TIA does not cause permanent residual neurological deficits, however, is often an indication of future risk for a stroke. Both TIA and stroke require formal medical attention.

1. An aura typically refers to a feeling and symptoms that are experienced before a specific event. In medicine, an aura is most often associated with a migraine. An aura is not typically associated with a TIA or stroke.

2. The initial symptoms of a TIA and stroke are similar and often include drooping or numbness on one side of the face, numbness or weakness of one arm, slurred speech, vision problems, headache, dizziness, lack of coordination, confusion, and loss of consciousness.

3. **The effects of a TIA may be similar to a stroke, but symptoms associated with a TIA resolve quickly, sometimes within minutes or possibly lasting as long as 24 to 48 hours. Symptoms of stroke may resolve over time, however, in some instances residual deficits are permanent.**

4. Speech and vision problems are often associated with a TIA and stroke, however, the resolution of the symptoms is what differentiates these conditions. Speech and vision problems associated with a TIA, if present, should resolve within 24 to 48 hours.

System: Neuromuscular and Nervous Systems
Content Outline: Diseases/Conditions that Impact Effective Treatment

➡ PTAEXAM THREE: QUESTION 74

A physical therapist assistant monitors the vital signs of a patient during a graded exercise test. When interpreting the data collected during the exercise test, which finding serves as the **BEST** indicator that the patient exerted a maximal effort?

1. **Failure of the heart rate to increase with further increases in intensity**
2. Rise in systolic blood pressure of 50 mm Hg when compared to the resting value
3. Rating of 12/20 on a perceived exertion scale
4. Rating of 2/4 on the dyspnea scale

Correct Answer: 1 (American College of Sports Medicine p. 375)

Failure of the heart rate to increase with further increases in intensity occurs when the patient can no longer meet the demands imposed by the exercise, signifying the patient has produced a maximal effort.

1. **Failure of the heart rate to increase with further increases in exercise intensity is an objective indicator that the patient made a maximal effort during graded exercise testing.**

2. The normal response to exercise is a progressive increase in systolic blood pressure, typically 10 mm Hg per MET, with a possible plateau at peak exercise. A rise in systolic blood pressure of 50 mm Hg over the resting rate is common during graded exercise testing, however, it is not necessarily an indication of a maximal effort.

3. A rating of 12 on the 6-20 perceived exertion scale corresponds only to a perception of "fairly light" to "somewhat hard." A rating of > 17 ("very hard") is an indicator of a maximal effort.

4. A rating of 2 out of 4 on the dyspnea scale corresponds to a perception of "moderate, bothersome" degree of breathlessness. This level does not indicate a maximal effort.

System: Cardiovascular and Pulmonary Systems
Content Outline: Interventions

 Level 2   p. 251-252

Level 2

➡ PTAEXAM THREE: QUESTION 75

During a gait analysis on a patient rehabilitating from a lower extremity injury, the physical therapist assistant measures the number of steps taken by the patient in a 30 second period. The assistant has measured which of the following gait parameters?

1. Acceleration
2. **Cadence**
3. Velocity
4. Speed

Correct Answer: 2 (Levangie p. 528)

Time and distance parameters are often used to provide a basic description of gait. Commonly used temporal variables include stance time, single limb and double support time, cadence, and speed. Commonly used distance variables include stride length, step length, width of base of support, and degrees of toe-out.

1. Acceleration is the rate of change of velocity with respect to time.

2. **Cadence is defined as the number of steps taken by a person per unit of time. Walking with increased cadence decreases the duration of double support time. A cadence of 110 steps per minute is typical in a male, while 116 steps per minute is typical in a female.**

3. Velocity is the rate of linear forward motion of the body which is measured most often in centimeters per second, meters per second or miles per hour. Walking velocity equals distance walked divided by time.

4. Speed is usually classified as slow, free or fast. Free speed of gait refers to a person's normal walking speed.

System: Musculoskeletal System
Content Outline: Physical Therapy Data Collection

➡ PTAEXAM THREE: QUESTION 76

A physical therapist assistant works with a patient with hemiparesis who uses a hemiplegic chair for mobility. Which activity would become more challenging for the patient based on the prescribed wheelchair?

1. Reaching for objects outside the base of support
2. **Performing a standing transfer**
3. Performing independent pressure relief
4. Propelling the wheelchair

Correct Answer: 2 (Tan p. 323)

A hemiplegic chair incorporates a seat that is approximately two inches lower than a standard chair to enable the user to use the lower extremities to propel the chair. The patient typically uses one handrim and one or both feet to help propel and steer the wheelchair. One or both front riggings on the wheelchair are removed to provide the feet with necessary space for propulsion.

1. Reaching for objects outside the base of support may be challenging for the patient depending on the level of involvement, however, a hemiplegic chair would not increase the complexity of the task.

2. **Performing a standing transfer would be more challenging with a hemiplegic chair since the lower seat would require significantly more upper and lower extremity strength to attain a standing position.**

3. Performing independent pressure relief may be challenging for the patient depending on the level of involvement, however, a hemiplegic chair would not increase the complexity of the task.

4. Propelling a wheelchair would be enhanced by using a hemiplegic chair since the lower seat allows the patient's feet to contact the ground and assist with propulsion.

System: Non-Systems
Content Outline: Equipment, Devices, and Technologies; Therapeutic Modalities

---

 Level 1   p. 84

 Level 3   p. 598-600

➡ PTAEXAM THREE: QUESTION 77

A patient who has a posterolateral lumbar disk herniation reports centralization of all symptoms while lying in a prone position on a treatment table. Which of the following exercises should the patient perform **LAST** as part of the typical treatment progression?

1. Propping up in prone on elbows (forearms)
2. **Extension in a standing position**
3. Prone press-ups into full extension
4. Pelvic tilting in a quadruped position

Correct Answer: 2 (Dutton p. 1485)

A disk herniation occurs when the nucleus pulposus bulges through the exterior wall of the annulus fibrosus. Herniations occur most commonly on the posterolateral portion of the disk. Once tolerated, McKenzie extension exercises are often incorporated into the exercise program. Certain motions produce or increase the symptoms and cause what is referred to as peripheralization (symptoms move away from the spine or more distally), whereas other motions decrease or eliminate the symptoms and cause what is referred to as centralization (symptoms move toward the spine or more proximally toward the source of the symptoms). The goal of any exercise or position is to centralize the patient's symptoms.

1. Propping up in prone on elbows (forearms) is typically the next progression once the patient tolerates (with centralization of symptoms) lying in prone. If this is not well tolerated, another alternative is to place a pillow under the patient's chest to encourage lumbar extension without the patient having to prop up on the elbows (forearms) in prone.

2. **Extension in a standing position would be the last progression of the options listed, as standing requires more lumbar compression (loading) than any of the other positions. Once tolerated, it is desirable to teach the patient to perform extension in standing after sitting or being in positions of lumbar flexion. This action should help encourage the nucleus pulposus to move from posterior to anterior or more centrally.**

3. Prone press-ups into full extension would be the next progression after the patient tolerates (with centralization) propping up on elbows (forearms) in the prone position. It would not, however, be the last progression.

4. Pelvic tilting in a quadruped position allows the patient to perform isolated lumbar flexion and extension while monitoring the patient response. The quadruped position does not involve the compression (loading) that lumbar extension does in the standing position.

System: Musculoskeletal System
Content Outline: Interventions

➡ PTAEXAM THREE: QUESTION 78

When selecting an assistive device for a patient with a lower extremity injury, which of the following patient characteristics should be the **LEAST** critical for the physical therapist assistant to consider?

1. Cognitive ability
2. **Height and weight**
3. Upper and lower extremity strength
4. Level of coordination

Correct Answer: 2 (Fairchild p. 214)

A physical therapist assistant must select an assistive device for patients based on their weight bearing status as well as their current abilities and limitations.

1. The patient must possess the cognitive ability to comprehend the supplied instructions and use the assistive device in a manner consistent with the physical therapist assistant's instructions.

2. **The majority of assistive devices are appropriate for patients of varying weight and can be readily adjusted (e.g., raised or lowered) to accommodate for different heights. As a result, these variables would be the least critical when selecting an assistive device.**

3. A patient's upper and lower extremity strength are critical to assess when selecting an appropriate assistive device. For example, a patient using a swing-through gait pattern would need significant upper extremity strength, but would be less dependent on lower extremity strength. Conversely, a patient using a single cane would need significant lower extremity strength, but would be less dependent on upper extremity strength.

4. Patients must possess a requisite amount of coordination to use specific assistive devices. For example, a patient with poor coordination would likely be able to use a walker, but would have significant difficulty using bilateral canes.

System: Non-Systems
Content Outline: Equipment, Devices, and Technologies; Therapeutic Modalities

 Level 2

 Level 1

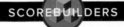

▶ PTAEXAM THREE: QUESTION 79

A physical therapist assistant completes a posture screening and muscle length test of the hip flexors on a patient. The assistant determines that the patient has extremely tight hip flexors bilaterally. What common structural deformity is **MOST** often associated with tight hip flexors?

1. Scoliosis
2. Kyphosis
3. **Lordosis**
4. Spondylolysis

Correct Answer: 3 (Kendall p. 70)

Patients with tight hip flexors frequently exhibit increased lordosis. Shortness of the hip flexors is often observed in standing as lumbar lordosis or identified through special tests such as the Thomas test.

1. Scoliosis refers to a lateral curvature of the spine. Scoliosis can occur in the cervical, thoracic or lumbar spine. Classifications of scoliosis include idiopathic, non-structural, and structural. Scoliosis is not necessarily associated with tight hip flexors.

2. Kyphosis refers to excessive curvature of the spine in a posterior direction usually identified in the thoracic spine. A structural change in the thoracic spine would not necessarily be associated with tight hip flexors.

3. **Lordosis refers to an excessive curvature of the spine in an anterior direction, usually identified in the cervical or lumbar spine. Tight hip flexors are often associated with excessive lordosis (anterior pelvic tilt) due to the origin and insertion of the hip flexors.**

4. Spondylolysis refers to a defect in the pars interarticularis or the arch of the vertebra. This is most common in the L5 vertebra, but can also occur in other lumbar or thoracic vertebra.

System: Musculoskeletal System
Content Outline: Physical Therapy Data Collection

▶ PTAEXAM THREE: QUESTION 80

A physical therapist assistant reviews the medical record of a patient admitted to the hospital with suspected renal involvement. Which laboratory test would be the **MOST** useful to assess the patient's present renal function?

1. Platelet count
2. Hemoglobin
3. **Blood urea nitrogen**
4. Hematocrit

Correct Answer: 3 (Goodman – Pathology p. 1707)

Blood urea nitrogen is a common measure used to assess renal function. The normal blood urea nitrogen level for adults is 10-20 mg/dL.

1. Platelet count identifies the number of platelets present in whole blood. If the platelet level is high, it indicates increased risk of thrombosis and if the level is low, it indicates increased risk of bruising and bleeding.

2. Hemoglobin is the iron containing pigment in red blood cells that functions to carry oxygen in the blood. Low hemoglobin may indicate anemia or blood loss. Elevated hemoglobin suggests polycythemia or dehydration.

3. **Blood urea nitrogen is used to assess kidney function. An increased blood urea nitrogen level can be indicative of dehydration, renal failure or heart failure. A decreased blood urea nitrogen level can be indicative of malnourishment, hepatic failure or pregnancy.**

4. Hematocrit measures the percentage of red blood cells in a volume of blood. Hematocrit may be decreased with anemia, nutritional deficiency, and leukemia. Hematocrit may be increased with dehydration, polycythemia, and burns.

System: Other Systems
Content Outline: Diseases/Conditions that Impact Effective Treatment

 Level 2   p. 123

 Level 2

➡ PTAEXAM THREE: QUESTION 81

A patient sustained a grade II strain to the iliopsoas muscle. Which of the following phases of the gait cycle should the physical therapist assistant expect to be the **MOST** impacted by this injury?

1. Toe off (pre-swing) and acceleration (initial swing)
2. Heel strike (initial contact) and acceleration (initial swing)
3. Foot flat (loading response) and deceleration (terminal swing)
4. Midstance and deceleration (terminal swing)

Correct Answer: 1 (Dutton p. 298)

A strain is an injury involving the musculotendinous unit that involves a muscle, tendon or their attachments to the bone. Signs and symptoms associated with a grade II strain include localized pain, moderate swelling, tenderness, and impaired motor function. A grade II strain is likely to negatively influence a patient's gait at the point in the gait cycle where the affected muscle is most active.

1. **The iliopsoas contracts eccentrically beginning at midstance and continues through to toe off (pre-swing). The iliopsoas then switches quickly to a concentric contraction to advance the limb forward at acceleration (initial swing). Therefore, weakness of the hip flexors is best observed during the toe off (pre-swing) and acceleration (initial swing) phases.**

2. During heel strike (initial contact), the hip extensors are active to resist the flexion moment at the hip. The iliopsoas is not active during this phase, but is active during acceleration (initial swing).

3. During foot flat (loading response), the hip extensors work concentrically to extend the hip and then eccentrically during deceleration (terminal swing) to slow the rate of both hip flexion (gluteus maximus) and knee extension (hamstrings). The iliopsoas is not active during either of these phases of gait.

4. The hip abductors are most active at midstance to stabilize the pelvis and prevent contralateral hip drop. The iliopsoas begins to contract eccentrically at midstance to control the rate of hip extension, but is not active during deceleration (terminal swing).

System: Musculoskeletal System
Content Outline: Diseases/Conditions that Impact Effective Treatment

➡ PTAEXAM THREE: QUESTION 82

A physical therapist assistant attempts to assess the motor component of the axillary nerve by conducting a manual muscle test. Which of the following muscles would be the **MOST** appropriate to utilize?

1. Teres minor
2. Teres major
3. Subscapularis
4. Supraspinatus

Correct Answer: 1 (Kendall p. 321)

The teres minor and deltoid muscles are innervated by the axillary nerve.

1. **The teres minor is innervated by the axillary nerve (C5, C6). The muscle acts to laterally rotate the shoulder joint and stabilize the head of the humerus in the glenoid cavity.**

2. The teres major is innervated by the lower subscapular nerve (C5, C6, C7). The muscle acts to medially rotate, adduct, and extend the shoulder joint.

3. The subscapularis is innervated by the upper (C5, C6) and lower subscapular nerve (C5, C6, C7) which extends from the all three trunks of the brachial plexus via the posterior cord. The muscle acts to medially rotate the shoulder joint and stabilize the head of the humerus in the glenoid cavity.

4. The supraspinatus is innervated by the suprascapular nerve (C4, C5, C6). The muscle acts to abduct the shoulder joint and stabilize the head of the humerus in the glenoid cavity.

System: Musculoskeletal System
Content Outline: Physical Therapy Data Collection

 Level 2   p. 55, 62, 81-85

 Level 1   p. 227

➡ PTAEXAM THREE: QUESTION 83

A physical therapist assistant is asked by a nurse to perform a transfer on a patient recently admitted to the hospital. Which of the following methods is the **MOST** appropriate to confirm the patient's identity prior to completing the transfer?

1. Contact the attending physician

2. Check the patient's medical record

3. Ask the patient their name

4. **Examine the patient's identification bracelet**

Correct Answer: 4 (Fairchild p. 3)

Physical therapist assistants must be extremely careful to accurately determine the identity of a given patient prior to initiating physical therapy services. Failure to take adequate steps to ensure patient identity can result in unnecessary risk for both the patient and the physical therapist assistant.

1. Contacting the attending physician would not be a practical response and would rely solely on the physician's ability to accurately identify the patient.

2. Checking the patient's medical record may not allow the physical therapist assistant to definitively link the medical record to a specific patient.

3. Asking the patient their name may be a useful strategy, however, the relative value of the option is dependent on whether the patient is able to recall and verbalize their actual name.

4. **Examining the patient's identification bracelet allows the physical therapist assistant to definitively determine the patient's identity. The bracelet is typically applied immediately upon admission to the hospital and is not removed until discharge.**

System: Non-Systems
Content Outline: Safety and Protection; Professional
   Responsibilities; Research

➡ PTAEXAM THREE: QUESTION 84

A physical therapist assistant applies silver sulfadiazine to an open wound on a patient's forearm. What type of aseptic equipment is necessary when applying the topical agent?

1. Gloves

2. **Sterile gloves**

3. Gloves, gown

4. Sterile gloves, gown

Correct Answer: 2 (Paz p. 306)

Silver sulfadiazine is an antimicrobial drug used for the prevention and treatment of wound sepsis.

1. Gloves offer protection to the physical therapist assistant's hands to reduce the likelihood of becoming infected with microorganisms and decrease the risk of the patient receiving microorganisms from the physical therapist assistant. Non-sterile gloves would pose an unnecessary risk given the patient's current status.

2. **The presence of an open wound and the direct application of a topical agent necessitates the use of sterile gloves.**

3. Gloves (i.e., non-sterile) would not be appropriate and a gown would not be warranted since there is not a risk of splash given the method of topical agent application and the location of the wound.

4. Sterile gloves would be required, however, additional aseptic equipment would not be necessary.

System: Other Systems
Content Outline: Interventions

⦿ **Level 2**

⦿ **Level 2**

▶ PTAEXAM THREE: QUESTION 85

A physical therapist assistant works with a patient that is sitting on the edge of a mat surface with their feet on the floor and asks the patient to reach for an object placed two feet in front of them on the floor. Which pattern of muscle activity is **MOST** responsible for the modulation of movement during this task?

1. Concentric contraction of the spinal flexors
2. Eccentric contraction of the spinal flexors
3. Concentric contraction of the spinal extensors
4. **Eccentric contraction of the spinal extensors**

Correct Answer: 4 (Umphred p. 732)

Trunk movements in sitting are initiated by either the upper trunk or lower trunk depending on the demands of the task. Reaching forward towards the floor while in a sitting position would be an upper trunk initiated movement that results in an anterior weight shift. The lower trunk and body provide stability that allows the arms to reach towards the floor.

1. Reaching forward anterior to the base of support would likely elicit concentric contraction of the spinal flexors, however, the modulation of the forward movement would be most influenced by eccentric contraction of the spinal extensors.

2. An eccentric contraction of the spinal flexors would more likely be associated with spinal extension when moving outside of the base of support in a posterior direction.

3. Reaching forward anterior to the base of support would not elicit concentric contraction of the spinal extensors, but rather eccentric contraction. Concentric contraction of the extensors would typically occur when attempting to sit upright during unsupported sitting within the base of support.

4. **When a patient reaches forward anterior to the base of support, the forward spinal flexion is controlled primarily through eccentric contraction of the spinal extensors. The extensors control the deceleration and modulation of the forward motion.**

System: Neuromuscular and Nervous Systems
Content Outline: Interventions

▶ PTAEXAM THREE: QUESTION 86

A physical therapist assistant orders a wheelchair for a patient who has C4 tetraplegia. Which wheelchair would be the **MOST** appropriate for this patient?

1. Manual wheelchair with friction surface handrims
2. Manual wheelchair with handrim projections
3. **Power wheelchair with sip and puff controls**
4. Power wheelchair with joystick controls

Correct Answer: 3 (O'Sullivan p. 921)

A patient with C4 tetraplegia would require a power wheelchair with a sip and puff, head, mouth or chin controls. The wheelchair would also require a tilt-in-space frame to allow for pressure relief.

1. Friction surface handrims are used when patients do not have a functional grip or the strength necessary to adequately propel a wheelchair. Patients with C6-C7 tetraplegia commonly rely on this feature.

2. Handrim projections add depth to the wheel and allow the patient to more easily propel the wheelchair. This is indicated at C5 where the lowest innervation includes the biceps, brachialis, brachioradialis, deltoids, rhomboids, and supinator. Although a patient with C5 tetraplegia may utilize handrim projections, the necessary energy expenditure may necessitate the use of a power wheelchair for mobility.

3. **A patient with C4 tetraplegia will have innervation of the face and neck, diaphragm, and trapezius muscles. The patient should be able to verbally direct all aspects of wheelchair management and would be a candidate for a power wheelchair with head or mouth controls.**

4. A patient with C5 tetraplegia is appropriate for a power wheelchair with joystick control. Patients utilize a power wheelchair for community mobility secondary to the high energy expenditure of using a manual wheelchair with handrim projections.

System: Neuromuscular and Nervous Systems
Content Outline: Interventions

 Level 2   p. 109

 Level 2   p. 269-270

➡ PTAEXAM THREE: QUESTION 87

A patient post CVA involving the right hemisphere exhibits figure-ground discrimination dysfunction. Which of the following activities would likely be the **MOST** difficult for the patient based on the reported perceptual deficit?

1. Navigating the hospital using written directions or a map

2. Attempting to identify a familiar object when it is placed on its side

3. **Picking forks out of a drawer of disorganized silverware**

4. Pointing to left and right body parts after receiving verbal instructions

Correct Answer: 3 (O'Sullivan p. 1250)

Perception is the mechanism by which the brain interprets sensory information received from the environment. Perception is commonly altered in patients sustaining a stroke involving the right hemisphere.

1. Topographical disorientation involves difficulty comprehending the relationship of one location to another. Navigating in the hospital using written directions or a map would be an appropriate method to screen for this condition.

2. Form-constancy dysfunction involves difficulty attending to subtle variations or changes in form such as a size variation of the same object. Having a patient attempt to identify a familiar object when it is placed on its side would be an appropriate method to screen for this condition.

3. **Figure-ground discrimination dysfunction involves difficulty distinguishing the foreground from the background in a complex visual array. Having the patient pick forks out of a drawer of disorganized silverware would be an appropriate method to screen for this condition.**

4. Right-left discrimination dysfunction involves difficulty understanding and using the concepts of right and left. Having the patient point to left and right body parts after receiving verbal instruction would be an appropriate method to screen for this condition.

System: Neuromuscular and Nervous Systems
Content Outline: Interventions

 Level 2

➡ PTAEXAM THREE: QUESTION 88

A physical therapist assistant assesses selected characteristics of a patient's peripheral pulse. For which of the following medical conditions would the type of assessment shown in the image be **MOST** essential?

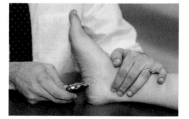

1. Cor pulmonale

2. Hypertension

3. **Intermittent claudication**

4. Pulmonary embolism

Correct Answer: 3 (Goodman – Pathology p. 633)

A peripheral pulse refers to a periodic fluctuation in the flow of blood through a peripheral artery caused by the ejection of blood with each heartbeat. The image shows the physical therapist assistant assessing the posterior tibial artery by palpating in the space between the medial malleolus and the Achilles tendon.

1. Cor pulmonale is right-sided heart failure arising from disease of the lungs. Signs of right ventricular failure include elevated central venous pressure with distension of the neck veins, ascites, and peripheral edema. Patients with cor pulmonale often experience significant shortness of breath with exertion.

2. Hypertension refers to a condition in which blood pressure is persistently elevated. Stages of hypertension include Stage 1 hypertension, Stage 2 hypertension, and hypertensive crisis. The presence of hypertension would necessitate the need for formal measurements of blood pressure using a pneumatic cuff and sphygmomanometer.

3. **Intermittent claudication is characterized by lower extremity cramps which develop during activity and disappear after rest. The peripheral pulses are often absent or markedly diminished when a patient complains of cramping. The cramps develop during activity since the narrowed arteries and collateral circulation to the muscles are unable to supply the extra blood required by the actively contracting lower extremity muscles.**

4. Pulmonary embolism is a condition where one or more arteries in the lungs become blocked. In most cases, pulmonary embolism is caused by blood clots from the lower extremities. Symptoms can vary greatly, but may include shortness of breath, chest pain that worsens with deep breathing, coughing up bloody or blood-streaked sputum, and a rapid or irregular pulse.

System: Cardiovascular and Pulmonary Systems
Content Outline: Diseases/Conditions that Impact Effective Treatment

 Level 2   p. 381

⮕ PTAEXAM THREE: QUESTION 89

A physical therapist assistant attempts to obtain informed consent from a 17-year-old patient prior to initiating a formal exercise test. The patient signs the informed consent form, however, the patient's parents dropped him off at the outpatient clinic and are now unavailable to sign the form. Which of the following actions should the assistant take?

1. Complete the exercise test

2. Secure another physical therapist assistant or physical therapist to witness the exercise test

3. Contact the referring physician to obtain approval to complete the exercise test

4. **Reschedule the exercise test**

Correct Answer: 4 (Scott – Promoting Legal and Ethical Awareness p. 222)

Obtaining informed consent from patients before exercise testing is an important ethical and legal consideration. Therapists have an obligation to obtain informed consent from patients prior to initiating intervention activities. If a patient is under the age of 18, the therapist is required to obtain informed consent from the patient and a parent or legal guardian.

1. The physical therapist assistant should have a valid consent form before performing the exercise test.

2. Having another physical therapist assistant or physical therapist witness the test is not a substitute for legal informed consent.

3. Having the physician approve the test is not a substitute for legal informed consent.

4. **A patient's status as a minor makes it necessary that a parent or legal guardian sign the consent form. The physical therapist assistant should reschedule the test to a time when a parent can sign the consent form.**

System: Non-Systems
Content Outline: Safety and Protection; Professional Responsibilities; Research

⮕ PTAEXAM THREE: QUESTION 90

When documenting the parameters of an electrical stimulation treatment using alternating current, which of the following standard units of measure should the physical therapist assistant use when recording current frequency?

1. Volt

2. **Hertz**

3. Coulomb

4. Pulses per second

Correct Answer: 2 (Bellew p. 260)

Frequency controls, often labeled rate, determine the type of response or muscle contraction that electrical stimulation will produce. As the frequency of any waveform is increased, the amplitude tends to increase and decrease more rapidly.

1. Voltage refers to the electrical force capable of moving charged particles through a conductor between two regions or points.

2. **Hertz is a unit of measure which describes the number of cycles per second when using alternating current.**

3. A coulomb is the amount of electrical charge transported in one second by a steady current of one ampere.

4. Pulses per second is utilized to describe the frequency of pulsed current.

System: Non-Systems
Content Outline: Equipment, Devices, and Technologies; Therapeutic Modalities

---

 Level 3   p. 690, 706

 Level 1   p. 638-641

SCOREBUILDERS

➡ PTAEXAM THREE: QUESTION 91

Which of the following medical conditions should a physical therapist assistant consider as being contraindicated to the application of intermittent compression?

1. Venous stasis ulcer
2. **Acute pulmonary edema**
3. Intermittent claudication
4. Lymphedema

Correct Answer: 2 (Prentice p. 579)

Intermittent compression is effective in controlling edema since it increases the extravascular hydrostatic pressure and circulation. Intermittent compression is most commonly used to control edema due to venous insufficiency or lymphatic dysfunction.

1. Venous stasis ulcers occur secondary to inadequate functioning of the venous system resulting in inadequate circulation and eventual tissue damage and ulceration. Intermittent compression improves venous circulation and facilitates the healing of previously formed ulcers.

2. **Acute pulmonary edema should not be treated with intermittent compression since the shift of fluid from the peripheral to the central circulation may significantly increase stress on the heart.**

3. Intermittent claudication occurs when blood flow is not adequate to meet the demand of the peripheral tissue, most often during activity. The result is ischemia which produces symptoms such as muscle pain, numbness, tingling, and fatigue. Caution should be used when applying compression in the presence of peripheral artery disease, however, intermittent claudication itself would not be a contraindication to intermittent compression.

4. Lymphedema refers to an abnormal accumulation of tissue fluid in the interstitial spaces. Stagnation of the tissue fluid promotes the inflammatory response and increases the probability of infection. Intermittent compression is commonly used to treat lymphedema.

System: Non-Systems
Content Outline: Equipment, Devices, and Technologies; Therapeutic Modalities

➡ PTAEXAM THREE: QUESTION 92

A patient with cerebellar dysfunction exhibits signs of dysmetria. Which of the following activities should be the **MOST** difficult for the patient?

1. Rapid alternating pronation and supination of the forearms
2. **Placing feet on floor markers while walking**
3. Walking at varying speeds
4. Marching in place

Correct Answer: 2 (Umphred p. 637)

Dysmetria refers to an inability to modulate movement where patients will either overestimate or underestimate their targets. The cerebellum is normally responsible for the timing, force, extent, and direction of the limb movement in order to correctly reach a target.

1. Dysdiadochokinesia refers to the inability to perform rapid alternating movements such as pronation and supination of the forearms. As speed increases there is typically a rapid loss of range of movement and rhythm of movement. This condition is a result of damage to the cerebellum.

2. **Dysmetria occurs with cerebellar lesions and is defined as the inability to appropriately reach a target. An example of dysmetria would be the inability of a patient to place their feet on floor markers successfully while walking.**

3. Difficulty walking at varying speeds is common with cerebellar pathology, however, the activity is not associated with dysmetria.

4. Patients with cerebellar lesions often have difficulty modulating movement. As a result, irregular stepping patterns and poor upright stance make activities such as marching in place difficult.

System: Neuromuscular and Nervous Systems
Content Outline: Interventions

 Level 2   p. 367, 636

 Level 2   p. 239

➡ PTAEXAM THREE: QUESTION 93

A physical therapist assistant works with a patient who has a knee sprain. During the initial treatment session, the patient appears to be relaxed and comfortable, however, is extremely withdrawn. Which of the following questions would be the **MOST** appropriate to further engage the patient?

1. Is this the first time you have injured your knee?

2. Have you ever been to physical therapy before?

3. How long after your injury did you see a physician?

4. **What do you hope to achieve in physical therapy?**

Correct Answer: 4 (Goodman – Differential Diagnosis p. 35)

Physical therapist assistants often use a variety of strategies to increase the level of patient participation in treatment sessions. Open-ended questions allow patients to answer with a myriad of responses, while closed-ended questions can often be answered with a yes or no response.

1. The question can be answered with a simple "yes or no" and therefore would be unlikely to increase patient participation.

2. The question would also require a simple "yes or no" response.

3. The question requires the patient to respond with an amount of time. The response, although not a "yes or no," would be equally unlikely to further engage the patient.

4. **The question requires the patient to provide some level of insight towards their physical therapy goals and may provide a foundation for a meaningful exchange between the patient and physical therapist assistant. The information obtained by the physical therapist assistant can be valuable when assisting a physical therapist to design an appropriate plan of care.**

System: Musculoskeletal System
Content Outline: Physical Therapy Data Collection

➡ PTAEXAM THREE: QUESTION 94

A physical therapist assistant determines a patient's heart rate by counting the number of QRS complexes in a six second electrocardiogram strip. Assuming the assistant identifies eight QRS complexes in the strip, the patient's heart rate should be recorded as how many beats per minute?

1. 40

2. 60

3. **80**

4. 100

Correct Answer: 3 (Hillegass p. 310)

The QRS complex reflects the depolarization of the ventricles during the cardiac cycle. If the heart rhythm is regular, the minute heart rate can be determined by counting the number of QRS complexes in six seconds on the electrocardiogram paper, then multiplying this number by 10 to get the heart rate for one minute.

1. For a heart rate of 40 beats per minute, there would be four QRS complexes in six seconds.

2. For a heart rate of 60 beats per minute, there would be six QRS complexes in six seconds.

3. **For a heart rate of 80 beats per minute, there would be 8 QRS complexes in six seconds. Eight QRS complexes per six second interval x 10 six second intervals per minute = 80 QRS complexes per minute.**

4. For a heart rate of 100 beats per minute, there would be 10 QRS complexes in six seconds.

System: Cardiovascular and Pulmonary Systems
Content Outline: Physical Therapy Data Collection

● Level 3

● Level 1   👓 p. 380

➡ PTAEXAM THREE: QUESTION 95

A physical therapist assistant prepares to apply a sterile dressing to a wound after debridement. The assistant begins the process by drying the wound using a towel, applies medication to the wound using a gauze pad, and then applies a series of dressings that are secured using a bandage. The application of which of these steps would **NOT** warrant the use of sterile technique?

1. **Bandage**
2. Dressings
3. Medication
4. Towel

Correct Answer: 1 (Fairchild p. 304)

Application of a bandage does not require sterile technique since the bandage does not come in direct contact with the wound. All other aspects of the scenario require sterile technique to protect the wound and surrounding area, the patient, and the caregiver from contamination.

1. **A bandage is applied over a dressing. The function of a bandage is to keep the dressing in position, provide a barrier between the dressing and the environment, provide pressure, and protect the wound. Since the bandage does not come in direct contact with the area surrounding the wound, sterile technique is not required.**

2. A dressing for a wound is usually comprised of several layers. The function of a dressing is to prevent contamination to the wound, prevent microorganisms within the wound from infecting other areas, assist with healing, apply pressure, absorb drainage, and prevent further injury to the wound. Application of all layers of a dressing requires sterile technique.

3. The application of medication is part of the dressing in this scenario and should be applied using sterile technique.

4. If the patient is using the towel directly on the area of the wound, the towel must be sterile and the physical therapist assistant must use sterile technique to avoid contamination.

System: Other Systems
Content Outline: Interventions

➡ PTAEXAM THREE: QUESTION 96

A physical therapist assistant attempts to explain to a patient how electrical stimulation can help decrease the perception of pain. Which of the following descriptions **BEST** explains the gate control theory of pain?

1. The threshold for stimulating peripheral nociceptors is decreased
2. The threshold for stimulating peripheral nociceptors is increased
3. **Pain signals are inhibited by stimulating non-nociceptive sensory nerves**
4. Pain signals are inhibited when endorphins bind to opiate receptors

Correct Answer: 3 (Cameron p. 51)

The gate control theory of pain modulation explains how pain signals to the brain can be overridden by the stimulation of other sensory nerves. Pain sensation is determined by input to T cells within the spinal cord. The T cells receive excitatory input from nociceptors (e.g., A-delta and C fibers) and inhibitory input from non-nociceptor sensory nerves (e.g., A-beta fibers).

1. The peripheral sensitization theory explains why individuals experience chronic pain. The peripheral nociceptors become more responsive since the threshold for stimulating them becomes decreased over time. This theory would explain an increase, not a decrease, in the patient's pain.

2. An increase in the threshold for stimulating peripheral nociceptors would result in less pain since it would take a larger amount of input to stimulate the nerve fibers. However, this is not the explanation that the gate control theory is based on.

3. **The gate control theory states that pain signals to the brain are inhibited through the stimulation of non-nociceptive sensory nerves. Massage, electrical stimulation, and traction are interventions that stimulate non-nociceptive sensory nerves, thereby reducing the transmission of pain signals to the brain.**

4. Pain signals can be inhibited by the release of endogenous endorphins, which bind to opiate receptors in the nervous system and block the transmission of pain signals. However, this is not the explanation that the gate control theory is based on.

System: Neuromuscular and Nervous Systems
Content Outline: Diseases/Conditions that Impact Effective Treatment

 Level 2

 Level 2   p. 72, 642-643

➡ PTAEXAM THREE: QUESTION 97

A physical therapist assistant performs postural drainage to the anterior basal segments of the lower lobes. During the treatment session, the patient suddenly reports dizziness and mild dyspnea. Which of the following actions should the assistant do **FIRST**?

1. Reassure the patient that the response is normal
2. Assess the patient's vital signs
3. **Elevate the patient's head**
4. Call for assistance

Correct Answer: 3 (Hillegass p. 541)

Postural drainage is the assumption of one or more body positions that allow gravity to drain secretions from each of the patient's lung segments. In each position, the segmental bronchus of the area to be drained is positioned perpendicular to the floor. Postural drainage to the anterior basal segment of the lower lobes would require the bottom of the bed to be elevated 18 inches.

1. A subjective complaint of dizziness and mild dyspnea would exceed a "normal" patient response. The physical therapist assistant must act based on the patient's comment even though it would not be entirely unexpected given the necessary patient position for postural drainage of the anterior basal segment of the lower lobes.

2. Assessing the patient's vital signs is a desirable option, however, only after the patient is repositioned with the head elevated.

3. **Dizziness and dyspnea are signs of intolerance to the head down postural drainage position required to drain the anterior basal segments of the lower lobes. Elevating the patient's head will likely relieve the symptoms.**

4. Calling for assistance is not necessary since the patient's symptoms should subside once the head is elevated.

System: Cardiovascular and Pulmonary Systems
Content Outline: Interventions

➡ PTAEXAM THREE: QUESTION 98

A patient recently diagnosed with deep venous thrombophlebitis is placed on heparin. Which of the following adverse signs is the **PRIMARY** side effect associated with heparin?

1. Hypotension
2. Depression
3. **Excessive anticoagulation**
4. Thrombocytopenia

Correct Answer: 3 (Ciccone p. 380)

Anticoagulant agents delay or prevent blood coagulation (clotting). Heparin is an anticoagulant used to prevent and treat disorders such as pulmonary embolism, which result from vascular thrombosis. Heparin inhibits coagulation by preventing the conversion of prothrombin to thrombin and by preventing the release of thromboplastin from platelets.

1. Hypotension, a lower than normal systolic or diastolic blood pressure, is not a side effect of heparin.

2. Depression, a mood disorder characterized by loss of interest or pleasure in living, is not a side effect associated with heparin.

3. **The most common side effect of heparin is abnormal bleeding. A physical therapist assistant should be careful to avoid excessive contact or bumping of the limbs of a patient taking heparin since this may cause bruising or bleeding.**

4. Thrombocytopenia, or an abnormal decrease in the number of blood platelets, has been associated with heparin use, but is not the primary side effect.

System: Cardiovascular and Pulmonary Systems
Content Outline: Diseases/Conditions that Impact Effective Treatment

 Level 3   p. 388

Level 1   p. 371

➡ PTAEXAM THREE: QUESTION 99

While completing a pain questionnaire, a patient selects words such as cramping, dull, and aching to describe their pain. What related structure is **MOST** consistent with this pain description?

1. Nerve root
2. **Muscle**
3. Bone
4. Vascular

Correct Answer: 2 (Magee p. 8)

The patient interview provides a physical therapist assistant with an opportunity to identify specific characteristics of pain. Subjective pain descriptors can provide valuable information related to a patient's condition. Characteristics to explore may include location, intensity, description, duration, and pattern.

1. Nerve root pain is often characterized as sharp, shooting, and burning. The pain tends to travel in the distribution of the specific nerve root.

2. **Muscle pain is often characterized as cramping, dull, and aching. The pain tends to worsen when the involved muscle contracts or is lengthened.**

3. Bone pain is often characterized as deep, intolerable, boring, and highly localized.

4. Vascular pain is often characterized as diffuse, throbbing, aching, and poorly localized. The pain is often referred to other parts of the body.

System: Musculoskeletal System
Content Outline: Physical Therapy Data Collection

➡ PTAEXAM THREE: QUESTION 100

A patient post Colles' fracture has moderate edema in their fingers and the dorsum of their hand and reports pain during active range of motion. Which of the following measurements is the **MOST** appropriate to accurately quantify the patient's edema?

1. **Volumetric**
2. Circumferential
3. Girth
4. Anthropometric

Correct Answer: 1 (Magee p. 478)

Volumetric measurements are often used to quantify the presence of edema in the wrist and hand by examining the amount of water displaced following immersion.

1. **A patient with moderate edema in the fingers and dorsum of the hand would displace more water than the contralateral extremity due to the involved limb's increased volume. Although the contralateral extremity serves as an effective baseline measure, it is important to recognize that there may normally be a small difference between the dominant and non-dominant hand.**

2. Circumferential measurements using a flexible tape measure are most commonly used to obtain a gross estimate of edema or muscle atrophy. The test would not commonly be used for the hand due to the difficulty associated with obtaining an accurate measurement because of the relative nonuniformity of the hand.

3. Girth measurements are synonymous with circumferential measurements.

4. Common anthropometric measurements used for adults include height, weight, body mass index (BMI), waist-to hip ratio, and percentage of body fat. These measures are then compared to reference standards to assess items such as weight status and the risk for various diseases.

System: Other Systems
Content Outline: Physical Therapy Data Collection

 Level 2   p. 111

 Level 2

➡ PTAEXAM THREE: QUESTION 101

A patient post CVA presents with paralysis and numbness on the side of the body contralateral to the vascular accident. What descending pathway is **MOST** likely damaged based on the patient's clinical presentation?

1. **Corticospinal tract**
2. Vestibulospinal tract
3. Tectospinal tract
4. Rubrospinal tract

Correct Answer: 1 (O'Sullivan p. 209)

The corticospinal tract is the largest descending pathway where 80% of the fibers decussate and descend on the opposite side; 20% continue to descend ipsilaterally. The corticospinal tract carries information from the motor cortex directly to the spinal cord.

1. **The corticospinal tract is concerned with skilled fine motor control primarily of the distal limbs.**

2. The vestibulospinal tract is responsible for gross postural adjustments subsequent to head movements and acceleration.

3. The tectospinal tract is responsible for visual information related to spatial awareness. The tract ends at the cervical spine and controls the musculature of the neck as well as head position.

4. The rubrospinal tract communicates with the thalamus and cerebellum and plays an important role in the coordination of movement.

System: Neuromuscular and Nervous Systems
Content Outline: Diseases/Conditions that Impact Effective
    Treatment

➡ PTAEXAM THREE: QUESTION 102

A physical therapist assistant works with a patient who sustained an injury to the thoracodorsal nerve. Which of the following clinical findings would be the **MOST** consistent with this injury?

1. Shoulder medial rotation weakness
2. **Shoulder extension weakness**
3. Paralysis of the rhomboids
4. Paralysis of the diaphragm

Correct Answer: 2 (Kendall p. 324)

The thoracodorsal nerve (C6, C7, C8) is a branch of the posterior cord of the brachial plexus. The nerve follows the course of the subscapular artery along the posterior wall of the axilla to the latissimus dorsi.

1. The medial rotators of the shoulder include the subscapularis, teres major, pectoralis major, latissimus dorsi, and anterior deltoid. The latissimus dorsi would be affected by an injury to the thoracodorsal nerve, however, the presence of a number of other muscles which act to medially rotate the humerus would be adequate to compensate for any impairment in the latissimus dorsi.

2. **The latissimus dorsi is innervated by the thoracodorsal nerve (C6, C7, C8). Weakness of the latissimus dorsi would produce impaired strength during shoulder extension resistive testing despite the fact that several other muscles also function to extend the shoulder. These muscles include the posterior deltoid and teres major.**

3. The rhomboids are innervated by the dorsal scapular nerve (C4, C5).

4. The diaphragm is innervated by the phrenic nerve (C3, C4, C5).

System: Neuromuscular and Nervous Systems
Content Outline: Diseases/Conditions that Impact Effective
    Treatment

 Level 2   p. 220

 Level 2   p. 227

➡ PTAEXAM THREE: QUESTION 103

A physical therapist assistant prepares to treat a patient for trigger points in their right upper trapezius muscle using a vapocoolant spray. Which of the following actions would be the correct procedure for positioning the patient before applying the spray?

1. Have the patient actively side bend their neck to the left
2. Have the patient actively side bend their neck to the right
3. **Passively move the patient's head into left side bending**
4. Passively move the patient's head into right side bending

Correct Answer: 3 (Cameron p. 140)

A vapocoolant spray produces rapid cooling through evaporation, with temperature changes occurring superficially in the epidermis. This therapeutic modality is most commonly used in the treatment of trigger points. When applying a vapocoolant spray, the target muscle should be on stretch during the application.

1. When treating the right upper trapezius muscle, the neck should be in left side bending so that the muscle is in a stretched position. However, the assistant should passively move the neck into this position. The patient should not actively side bend to the left.

2. It would be inappropriate to have the patient side bend their neck to the right when treating the right upper trapezius muscle as this would put the muscle into a shortened position. The neck should be in left side bending so that the muscle is in a stretched position.

3. **When positioning the patient to treat the right upper trapezius muscle, the assistant should move the patient's neck into left side bending and hold it there while applying the spray. This will place the target muscle on stretch and ensure that the patient can stay relaxed during the application.**

4. It would be appropriate to passively move the patient's neck to ensure that they can stay relaxed. However, the patient should be moved into left side bending to stretch the right upper trapezius muscle. The patient would be moved into right side bending if the assistant were treating the left upper trapezius muscle.

System: Non-Systems
Content Outline: Equipment, Devices, and Technologies;
   Therapeutic Modalities

➡ PTAEXAM THREE: QUESTION 104

A patient performing a prone knee hang as shown in the image reports direct pressure and discomfort on the patellofemoral region. Which of the following actions would be the **MOST** appropriate to address the patient's comment and still maintain the goal of this exercise?

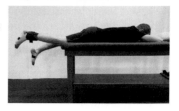

1. **Place a folded towel under the patient's distal femur**
2. Scoot the patient's body further up on the treatment table
3. Decrease the amount of weight in the ankle cuff weight
4. Apply ice to alleviate any discomfort during the stretch

Correct Answer: 1 (Dunleavy p. 126)

A prone knee hang exercise is a commonly used sustained passive stretching technique for an individual with limited knee extension. The body should be fully supported in the prone position on the treatment table with the end of the table supporting the distal thighs, proximal to the patella to avoid compression on the patellofemoral joint. A cuff weight placed around the ankle creates a sustained passive stretch on the hamstrings as the muscle relaxes, which increases knee extension.

1. **Placing a folded towel under the patient's distal femur would further ensure there is no pressure on the patella and may be more comfortable to the distal femur area. This modification may provide further stabilization to the distal femur as gravity is used to increase knee extension.**

2. Having the patient scoot the body further up on the treatment table would likely result in greater compressive forces on the patella. Use of a folded towel placed under the patient's distal femur is the most appropriate choice to make this technique more comfortable for the patient and limit compressive forces on the patella while still maintaining the sustained stretch into knee extension.

3. Decreasing the amount of weight used in the ankle cuff weight may potentially make the exercise more comfortable by reducing the intensity of the stretch, however, it may also reduce the effectiveness of the exercise. In addition, the patient's report of "direct pressure and discomfort" on the patellofemoral region combined with the proximity of the patella to the end of the plinth in the image result in placement of the towel under the distal femur being the best option.

4. Although applying ice may temporarily alleviate any discomfort, this should not be necessary since the technique can easily be modified to increase patient comfort and limit compressive forces on the patella.

System: Musculoskeletal System
Content Outline: Interventions

  Level 2   p. 619

 Level 2   p. 106-108

➡ PTAEXAM THREE: QUESTION 105

A physical therapist assistant reads in the medical chart that a patient is taking digitalis. The patient is **MOST** likely taking this medication to treat which of the following conditions?

1. Angina
2. **Atrial fibrillation**
3. Hypertension
4. Thrombus formation

Correct Answer: 2 (Hillegass p. 468)

Digitalis is a cardiac glycoside that is generally used in the management of arrhythmias, though it is also commonly used to treat congestive heart failure. Digitalis works by either enhancing parasympathetic activity or depressing sympathetic activity, thus slowing the heart rate and depressing electrical conductivity.

1. Angina is chest pain due to ischemia of the heart musculature, thus it is generally treated with anti-ischemic drugs (e.g., beta-blockers, nitrates). Acute angina attacks are often treated with sublingual nitroglycerin.

2. **Atrial fibrillation is an arrhythmia characterized by erratic electrical conductivity within the atria. By depressing electrical conductivity, digitalis can effectively prevent the conduction of atrial arrhythmias into the ventricles.**

3. Hypertension (i.e., high blood pressure) can be treated by several different classes of medications. Diuretics reduce overall blood volume to decrease blood pressure. Vasodilators decrease peripheral resistance or venous return to decrease blood pressure. Other classes of medications affect the sympathetic nervous system directly to inhibit its activity or act on the kidneys to decrease the production of renin, both of which result in decreases in blood pressure.

4. Thrombi (i.e., blood clots) can form in the lumen of arteries and result in reduced blood flow which may eventually lead to myocardial ischemia or infarction. Thrombi are treated with thrombolytic agents which act to break up the thrombus and maintain normal blood flow.

System: Cardiovascular and Pulmonary Systems
Content Outline: Diseases/Conditions that Impact Effective Treatment

➡ PTAEXAM THREE: QUESTION 106

A physical therapist assistant attempts to determine if a patient with known heart disease is an appropriate candidate for an exercise program. Which of the following findings would **MOST** likely exclude the patient from participating?

1. An ejection fraction of 45%
2. History of an uncomplicated myocardial infarction two months ago
3. Electrocardiogram shows ST segment depression of one millimeter
4. **Presence of ventricular arrhythmias at rest**

Correct Answer: 4 (O'Sullivan p. 560)

The American Association of Cardiovascular and Pulmonary Rehabilitation (AACVPR) and the American College of Physicians (ACP) have provided a framework for determining a patient's risk of increased morbidity and mortality. Patients are classified as low, moderate or high risk based on a number of factors.

1. Normal ejection fraction is between 55% and 70%. A patient with an ejection fraction of 45% would be considered at moderate risk for increased morbidity and mortality. Though this patient may have decreased exercise tolerance due to a reduced ejection fraction, they still would be allowed to engage in an exercise program.

2. A patient with a history of an uncomplicated myocardial infarction and/or cardiac surgery (e.g., angioplasty, coronary artery bypass graft surgery) would be classified as low risk for increased morbidity and mortality. Patients commonly engage in exercise following myocardial infarction.

3. A patient with ST segment depression of one millimeter on their electrocardiogram would be classified as moderate risk for increased morbidity and mortality. A patient with marked ST segment depression (i.e., greater than two millimeters) would be classified as high risk, however, would not be excluded from exercise.

4. **A patient with ventricular arrhythmias at rest would be classified as high risk for increased morbidity and mortality. Additionally, the AACVPR recommends that patients with uncontrolled arrhythmias be excluded from exercise. Other conditions that meet these guidelines include unstable angina, symptomatic heart failure, moderate to severe aortic stenosis, uncontrolled diabetes, acute systemic illness or fever, uncontrolled tachycardia, resting systolic blood pressure greater than 200 mm Hg, resting diastolic blood pressure greater than 110 mm Hg, and thrombophlebitis.**

System: Cardiovascular and Pulmonary Systems
Content Outline: Diseases/Conditions that Impact Effective Treatment

 Level 2

 p. 380-381

Level 2

➡ PTAEXAM THREE: QUESTION 107

A patient who has Parkinson's disease presents with Good (4/5) strength in the lower extremities, 10 degree flexion contracture at the hips, and exaggerated forward posture in the standing position. Which of the following activities would be the **MOST** appropriate to incorporate into a home program?

1. Lying in a prone position
2. Progressive relaxation exercises
3. Lower extremity resistive exercises with ankle weights
4. Postural awareness exercises in standing

Correct Answer: 1 (Umphred p. 613)

Prone lying is a commonly employed positional technique designed to stretch the hip flexors in patients with Parkinson's disease. Increased flexibility of the hip muscles will improve standing posture and enable the body's center of gravity to remain within the base of support. Although some of the other options are appropriate, they would not provide the same degree of benefit for the patient based on the described clinical presentation.

1. **Prone lying is a static positioning activity designed to stretch the hip flexors. If the patient was unable to tolerate prone lying, the physical therapist assistant could place one or more pillows under the patient's hips and gradually remove pillows over time as the patient improves their flexibility.**

2. Progressive relaxation exercises can be incorporated using gentle rocking or segmental trunk rotation, however, the patient needs to have adequate range of motion in the hip flexors to optimize their functional status.

3. Strengthening is a restorative intervention used with patients with Parkinson's disease, however, the patient's strength in the lower extremities is already good (i.e., 4/5) and therefore would not be an immediate treatment priority.

4. Postural awareness exercises in standing are an appropriate intervention, however, the relative benefit of the activity is limited without adequate muscle length. By improving the patient's hip flexibility, the patient would be able to exhibit improved standing posture.

System: Other Systems
Content Outline: Interventions

➡ PTAEXAM THREE: QUESTION 108

A physical therapist assistant measures the strength of the iliopsoas in sitting, however, after performing the test the assistant realizes that the hamstrings were not placed on slack. Which of the following changes in range of motion would the assistant have **MOST** likely observed during the testing?

1. Increased hip flexion
2. **Decreased hip flexion**
3. Increased hip extension
4. Decreased hip extension

Correct Answer: 2 (Kendall p. 422)

The iliopsoas is formed by the iliacus and psoas major muscles and is considered to be the most powerful flexor of the hip. When testing the iliopsoas, the two-joint hamstring muscles must be placed on sufficient slack in order to avoid passive insufficiency. Passive insufficiency occurs when a two-joint muscle is lengthened over both joints simultaneously. Placing the hamstrings in midrange is typically sufficient to avoid passive insufficiency when testing the hip flexors.

1. Increased hip flexion range of motion would not be likely when testing the iliopsoas since the hamstrings were not placed on sufficient slack to allow for the hip to move through the full available flexion range of motion.

2. **Decreased hip flexion range of motion when testing the iliopsoas would be likely due to the hamstrings being lengthened over the hip and knee simultaneously resulting in passive insufficiency.**

3. Increased hip extension range of motion when testing the iliopsoas would not occur since the testing procedure does not require hip extension. In addition, hamstrings tightness (i.e., not placed on slack) would not contribute to increased hip extension.

4. Decreased hip extension range of motion when testing the iliopsoas would not be likely since the testing procedure does not require hip extension. In addition, hamstrings tightness (i.e., not placed on slack) would not limit hip extension range of motion.

System: Musculoskeletal System
Content Outline: Physical Therapy Data Collection

◉ Level 3

◉ Level 3

➡ PTAEXAM THREE: QUESTION 109

An entry in a patient's medical record indicates that the patient has recently received viscosupplementation. This type of procedure is **MOST** commonly performed to treat which of the following conditions?

1. Arrhythmias

2. Bursitis

3. **Osteoarthritis**

4. Spasticity

Correct Answer: 3 (Ciccone p. 251)

Viscosupplementation is a technique in which hyaluronan is injected into a patient's joint. Hyaluronan is a polysaccharide that restores the normal viscosity of the synovial fluid and helps to restore the lubricating properties of synovial fluid within that joint.

1. An arrhythmia is a cardiac condition characterized by the cardiac cycle being irregular in either rate or rhythm. Arrhythmias are typically treated with the use of antiarrhythmic agents (e.g., beta blockers, calcium channel blockers).

2. Bursitis is a condition characterized by the inflammation of a bursa, commonly in the hip, knee, shoulder or elbow. Bursitis is typically treated conservatively with rest, ice, physical therapy, and anti-inflammatory drugs. In cases that do not respond to conservative treatment, a steroid injection may be necessary.

3. **Osteoarthritis is a condition characterized by the loss of articular cartilage within a joint secondary to mechanical stresses. Viscosupplementation is commonly used in the treatment of osteoarthritis as the improved lubrication within the joint can help reduce joint stresses and reduce the progression of cartilaginous destruction. The benefits of viscosupplementation are relatively transient.**

4. Spasticity is a symptom characterized by resistance of a muscle to passive stretch and often occurs secondary to damage to the central nervous system. Spasticity is often treated with the use of baclofen, a medication which reduces the effects of spasticity through muscle relaxation.

System: Musculoskeletal System
Content Outline: Interventions

➡ PTAEXAM THREE: QUESTION 110

A physical therapist assistant reviews the medical record of a patient recently involved in a motor vehicle accident. A note in the medical record indicates that the patient uses a halo-vest cervicothoracic orthosis. Use of this type of orthosis is **MOST** likely associated with which of the following diagnoses?

1. **Spinal fracture**

2. Acute myofascial pain syndrome

3. Traumatic brain injury

4. Herniated nucleus pulposus

Correct Answer: 1 (Tan p. 236)

The halo-vest cervicothoracic orthosis consists of a rigid halo secured to the skull with four external fixation pins. The halo supports four posts which attach to the front and back of the vest.

1. **A halo-vest cervicothoracic orthosis is often used in the management of spinal fractures affecting the cervical spine. The device limits approximately 95% of cervical motion and is most often used in patients with high cervical fractures.**

2. A patient with acute myofascial pain syndrome may use a cervical orthosis to aid in the healing of tissues. A soft cervical collar would be the most appropriate orthosis used for this patient. The collar limits the least amount of cervical motion, but does serve as a reminder to the patient to restrict their motion so that soft tissues can be allowed to heal.

3. A patient with a traumatic brain injury is unlikely to have restrictions on their cervical range of motion, unless the injury also resulted in significant damage to cervical structures.

4. A patient with a herniated nucleus pulposus may or may not require a cervical orthosis depending on their prescribed level of motion restriction. Even if a patient did require a cervical orthosis, a halo-vest cervicothoracic orthosis would not be an appropriate option since it restricts 95% of cervical motion.

System: Musculoskeletal System
Content Outline: Interventions

 Level 2   p. 115, 154-155

 Level 2   p. 124-125

➡ PTAEXAM THREE: QUESTION 111

A physical therapist assistant monitors a patient's vital signs while completing 20 minutes of jogging at 5 mph on a treadmill. As the session approaches its conclusion, the assistant incorporates a cool down period. Which of the following responses should the assistant anticipate during the post-exercise period?

1. A progressive increase in systolic blood pressure
2. **A progressive decrease in systolic blood pressure**
3. A progressive increase in diastolic blood pressure
4. A progressive increase in rate pressure product

Correct Answer: 2 (American College of Sports Medicine p. 55)

Incorporating a cool down period provides a gradual recovery and a return of the heart rate and blood pressure to near resting values. Additional benefits of cool down include enhanced venous return, increased dissipation of body heat, increased removal of lactic acid, and reduced likelihood of ventricular arrhythmias.

1. A progressive increase in systolic blood pressure is the normal response to an increase in workload and therefore would not be associated with the post-exercise period.
2. **A progressive decrease in systolic blood pressure is the normal post-exercise response.**
3. A progressive increase in diastolic blood pressure would be considered an abnormal response since it should not occur during an increase in work or during the post-exercise period.
4. Rate pressure product or double-product is the product of heart rate and systolic blood pressure. Both heart rate and systolic blood pressure are expected to decrease during the post-exercise period. Rate pressure product is an indicator of myocardial oxygen consumption.

System: Cardiovascular and Pulmonary Systems
Content Outline: Interventions

➡ PTAEXAM THREE: QUESTION 112

A patient post stroke ambulates with a large base quad cane. The patient presents with left neglect and diminished proprioception. Which of the following methods is the **MOST** appropriate to ensure patient safety?

1. Provide continuous verbal cues
2. Provide visual cues and demonstration
3. **Provide manual assistance on the left side**
4. Provide manual assistance on the right side

Correct Answer: 3 (O'Sullivan p. 1242)

A physical therapist assistant must carefully consider a patient's current limitations and identify remedial strategies to assist the patient to achieve established goals. The presence of left neglect and diminished proprioception requires the physical therapist assistant to take formal action to avoid jeopardizing patient safety.

1. Verbal cues may be beneficial for the patient, however, without concurrent manual assistance the patient would likely still have increased difficulty with ambulation and may be at increased risk for a fall.
2. Demonstration prior to practice is important, however, this type of educational strategy would not directly address the left neglect and diminished proprioception.
3. **The physical therapist assistant should offer manual assistance on the patient's left side during ambulation activities. The manual assistance can facilitate motor activity and weight bearing, as well as proprioception on the affected side. Manual contact significantly reduces the risk for fall or injury.**
4. The patient presents with left neglect and as a result manual assistance would not typically be necessary on the right side of the body.

System: Neuromuscular and Nervous Systems
Content Outline: Interventions

 Level 2   p. 42

Level 3

➡ PTAEXAM THREE: QUESTION 113

A physical therapist assistant assesses the deep tendon reflexes of a patient as part of a lower quarter screening. The assistant determines all lower extremity deep tendon reflex responses to be 2+, except the right Achilles reflex response is 0. Which of the following clinical conditions would be the **MOST** consistent with this finding?

1. Cerebral palsy
2. Multiple sclerosis
3. **Peripheral neuropathy**
4. Intermittent claudication

Correct Answer: 3 (Goodman – Differential Diagnosis p. 623)

Deep tendon reflexes (DTR) elicit a muscle contraction when the muscle's tendon is stimulated. A grade of 2+ would be a normal response.

1. Cerebral palsy is a neuromuscular disorder of posture and controlled movement, however, the clinical presentation is highly variable based on the area and extent of central nervous system damage. It is not uncommon to see bilateral differences in reflexes, however, it is unlikely that a reflex would be absent in an upper motor neuron disorder such as cerebral palsy.

2. Multiple sclerosis is a chronic autoimmune inflammatory disease of the central nervous system characterized by demyelination of the myelin sheaths that surround nerves within the brain and spinal cord. Symptoms can include visual problems, paresthesias and sensory changes, clumsiness, weakness, ataxia, balance dysfunction, and fatigue. Deep tendon reflexes would not typically be absent with multiple sclerosis since it is an upper motor neuron disorder.

3. **Peripheral neuropathy is a broad term that describes a lesion to a peripheral nerve. Patients with peripheral neuropathy may exhibit motor, sensory, and autonomic changes including extreme sensitivity to touch, loss of sensation, muscle weakness, and loss of vasomotor tone. Deep tendon reflexes may be asymmetrical based on the location of the involved peripheral nerve and usually present as diminished or absent.**

4. Intermittent claudication occurs as a result of insufficient blood supply and ischemia in active muscles. The condition occurs with activity, subsides during periods of rest, and often limits the duration of exercise activities. Symptoms most commonly include pain and cramping in muscles distal to the occluded vessel. Deep tendon reflexes would not typically be affected.

System: Neuromuscular and Nervous Systems
Content Outline: Diseases/Conditions that Impact Effective Treatment

➡ PTAEXAM THREE: QUESTION 114

An employee with a disclosed disability informs their employer that they are unable to perform an essential function of their job unless their workstation is modified. Which of the following reasons would provide the employer with justification for **NOT** granting this request?

1. The accommodation would cost hundreds of dollars
2. The accommodation would require an expansion of the present workstation
3. **The accommodation would fundamentally alter the operation of the business**
4. The accommodation would not address the needs of other employees

Correct Answer: 3 (Fairchild p. 349)

Employers are required to make reasonable accommodations for qualified individuals with a disability who satisfy the job related requirements of a position held or desired and who can perform the "essential functions" of such position with or without reasonable accommodations.

1. An accommodation that costs hundreds of dollars does not necessarily indicate that the accommodation is unreasonable or creates an "undue hardship" for the employer.

2. Workstation modifications are common and are most often designed to allow a qualified employee or applicant to perform an essential job function.

3. **An accommodation that fundamentally alters the operation of a business would be considered an "undue hardship." Additional examples of situations where an accommodation would not necessarily be granted would be the elimination of a primary job responsibility or lowering established productivity standards.**

4. The Americans with Disabilities Act applies primarily, but not exclusively, to "disabled" individuals. It is not necessary to ensure that an accommodation made for a qualified individual addresses the needs of other employees.

System: Non-Systems
Content Outline: Safety and Protection; Professional Responsibilities; Research

---

 Level 2   p. 231, 442

Level 1   p. 682

➡ PTAEXAM THREE: QUESTION 115

A physical therapist assistant works with a patient who sustained a torn anterior cruciate ligament (ACL) and a medial meniscus tear. Which scenario would result in the **GREATEST** likelihood of a successful surgical meniscus repair?

1. A tear involving the inner third of the meniscus with reconstruction of the ACL

2. A tear involving the inner third of the meniscus with conservative management of the ACL

3. **A tear involving the outer third of the meniscus with reconstruction of the ACL**

4. A tear involving the outer third of the meniscus with conservative management of the ACL

Correct Answer: 3 (Dutton p. 972)

Meniscal tears often occur in conjunction with anterior cruciate ligament injuries. In athletic-related ACL injuries, the incidence of meniscal tears approaches fifty percent. The medial and lateral menisci are firmly attached to the proximal surface of the tibia. The menisci are thick at the periphery and thinner at their internal unattached edges. Menisci function to deepen the articular surfaces of the tibia where they articulate with the femoral condyles.

1. A surgically repaired tear involving the inner third of the medial meniscus is less likely to be successful since the inner third of the meniscus is avascular. Although ACL reconstruction increases success rates, the avascularity of the inner third of the meniscus remains a limiting factor.

2. A surgically repaired tear involving the inner third of the medial meniscus is less likely to be successful since the inner third of the meniscus is avascular. In addition, conservative management (i.e., nonoperative) of the ACL increases the failure rate of the surgically repaired meniscus.

3. **A surgically repaired tear involving the outer third of the medial meniscus is more likely to be successful since the outer third of the meniscus is vascular. In addition, ACL reconstruction increases success rates.**

4. A surgically repaired tear involving the outer third of the medial meniscus is more likely to be successful since the outer third of the meniscus is vascular, however, conservative management (i.e., nonoperative) of the ACL increases the failure rate of the surgically repaired meniscus.

System: Musculoskeletal System
Content Outline: Diseases/Conditions that Impact Effective Treatment

➡ PTAEXAM THREE: QUESTION 116

A patient who has adhesive capsulitis of the shoulder is asked to perform several tasks. Which of the following functional activities would the patient have the **MOST** difficulty performing?

1. Reaching across the body

2. Reaching into the back hip pocket

3. Performing a push-up

4. **Combing their hair**

Correct Answer: 4 (Dutton p. 585)

Patients with adhesive capsulitis (i.e., frozen shoulder) will typically demonstrate range of motion restrictions consistent with the capsular pattern of the affected joint. For the shoulder, the capsular pattern involves maximal loss of lateral rotation, moderate loss of abduction, and minimal loss of medial rotation.

1. Reaching across the body is a functional activity that involves shoulder horizontal adduction. Horizontal adduction is not a motion included in the capsular pattern of the shoulder.

2. Reaching into the back hip pocket is a functional activity that involves shoulder medial rotation, extension, and adduction. Shoulder extension and adduction are not motions included in the capsular pattern of the shoulder. Shoulder medial rotation is part of the capsular pattern, but it is typically only minimally affected.

3. Impairment in the ability to perform a push-up is usually secondary to a strength deficit, not a range of motion limitation. The push-up position generally requires approximately 90 degrees of flexion at the shoulder. A patient with adhesive capsulitis would likely possess the necessary range of motion to perform a push-up.

4. **Combing the hair is a functional activity that involves shoulder abduction and lateral rotation. These two motions are the most limited in patients with adhesive capsulitis of the shoulder.**

System: Musculoskeletal System
Content Outline: Diseases/Conditions that Impact Effective Treatment

---

 Level 2   p. 121-122

 Level 2   p. 76, 112, 142-143

➡ PTAEXAM THREE: QUESTION 117

A three-year-old child with osteogenesis imperfecta participates in an aquatic therapy program. What is the **PRIMARY** goal of aquatic therapy for a patient diagnosed with this condition?

1. Decrease abnormal tone

2. Decrease bone density

3. Increase range of motion

4. **Increase strength**

Correct Answer: 4 (Palisano p. 236)

Osteogenesis imperfecta is an autosomal disorder of collagen synthesis that affects bone metabolism. Children with osteogenesis imperfecta often have delayed developmental milestones secondary to ongoing fractures that result in immobilization, hypermobility of joints, and poorly developed muscles. This disorder is classified into four types with diverse clinical presentations ranging from normal appearance with mild symptoms to severe involvement that can be fatal during infancy. Bisphosphonate medication has been reported to reduce the occurrence of fractures, strengthen skeletal structures, and improve bone density with this population.

1. The elevated temperature in certain therapeutic pools would be beneficial to decrease hypertonicity/spasticity, however, children with osteogenesis imperfecta do not exhibit tonal abnormalities. As a result, decreasing abnormal tone would not be the primary goal of aquatic therapy for this patient.

2. Aquatic therapy can have a positive effect on increasing bone density (not decreasing) through weight bearing and resistance exercise. A goal of decreasing bone density would not be appropriate with osteogenesis imperfecta since the associated collagen synthesis disorder already negatively affects bone density.

3. The elevated temperature and properties of buoyancy within therapeutic pools would be beneficial to increase range of motion, however, children with osteogenesis imperfecta do not typically present with decreased range of motion or contractures. As a result, increasing range of motion would not be the primary goal of aquatic therapy for this patient.

4. **Aquatic therapy is an appropriate intervention for a child with osteogenesis imperfecta. It is a safe method of protected strengthening of the muscles due to buoyancy and the physical properties of water. Strengthening in a pool can occur safely in a supported weight bearing position and can be finely graded in terms of exercise intensity. Cardiovascular training and balance training are other benefits of this intervention.**

System: Musculoskeletal System
Content Outline: Interventions

➡ PTAEXAM THREE: QUESTION 118

A physical therapist assistant uses the Modified Ashworth Scale when assessing a patient post stroke. Which of the following procedures is the **MOST** appropriate for the assistant to perform when using this assessment scale?

1. Manual muscle testing

2. Deep tendon reflex testing

3. Active range of motion

4. **Passive range of motion**

Correct Answer: 4 (O'Sullivan p. 172)

The Modified Ashworth Scale (MAS) is an instrument that is used to assess muscle spasticity. The MAS uses ordinal scoring, with a grade of "0" indicating the absence of spasticity and a grade of "4" indicating the presence of rigidity.

1. Strength testing may be used for patients who have had a stroke to determine which muscles have been affected as a result of the neurological damage. However, strength testing would not provide valuable information when using the MAS since the instrument is used to assess spasticity.

2. Deep tendon reflex testing may be used for patients who have had a stroke to determine if the patient has hyporeflexia or hyperreflexia as a result of the neurological damage. However, deep tendon reflex testing would not provide valuable information when using the MAS since the instrument is used to assess spasticity.

3. Active range of motion may be used for patients who have had a stroke to determine the patient's functional use of their extremities. However, active range of motion would not provide valuable information when using the MAS since the instrument is used to assess spasticity, which requires a passive assessment.

4. **The MAS is an assessment tool that is used to grade spasticity. Spasticity is defined as increased resistance to passive stretch that is velocity-dependent, therefore, passive range of motion would be the most appropriate method for measuring spasticity.**

System: Neuromuscular and Nervous Systems
Content Outline: Physical Therapy Data Collection

 Level 2   p. 115, 185

 Level 1

▶ PTAEXAM THREE: QUESTION 119

The goals for a patient post total knee arthroplasty include general conditioning and independent household mobility. Which component of the patient's treatment would be the **MOST** appropriate to delegate to a physical therapy aide?

1. Stair training

2. Progressive gait training with a straight cane

3. Patient education regarding the surgical procedure

4. **Ambulation with a walker for endurance**

Correct Answer: 4 (Guide to Physical Therapist Practice)

A physical therapy aide is a non-licensed worker, trained under the direction of a physical therapist, who requires continuous on-site supervision. A physical therapist, and in some jurisdictions a physical therapist assistant, are required, before delegating any component of a treatment plan, to have an understanding of the physical therapy aide's level of training as well as the patient's current abilities.

1. Stair training is a skilled activity that requires the constant supervision of a licensed physical therapist or physical therapist assistant. The term "training" implies that the patient is being taught a new skill. Delegating this type of skilled activity to a physical therapy aide is inappropriate and would potentially jeopardize patient safety.

2. Progressive gait training implies that there will be some progression within the activity based on the patient's performance. The decision to progress a patient during an activity is the responsibility of the physical therapist or physical therapist assistant and would be inappropriate for a physical therapy aide.

3. Patient education regarding the surgical procedure requires an individual to possess specific knowledge of the actual surgical procedure performed by the surgeon. A physical therapy aide does not possess the educational background to provide the patient with this information.

4. **A physical therapist, and in some jurisdictions a physical therapist assistant, may delegate ambulation activities to a physical therapy aide if they feel the aide's training is adequate to complete the activity. This decision would be heavily influenced by the patient's current status and competence with ambulation. Ambulation for endurance implies that the patient already possesses basic competence with the activity.**

System: Non-Systems
Content Outline: Safety and Protection; Professional Responsibilities; Research

▶ PTAEXAM THREE: QUESTION 120

A physical therapist assistant is treating a patient with an acquired brain injury who begins to perseverate. In order to refocus the patient and achieve the desired therapeutic outcome, the assistant should utilize which of the following techniques?

1. Focus on the topic of perseveration for a short period of time in order to appease the patient

2. **Guide the patient into an interesting new activity and reward successful completion of the task**

3. Take the patient back to their room for quiet time and attempt to resume therapy once they have stopped perseverating

4. Continue with repetitive verbal cues to cease perseveration

Correct Answer: 2 (O'Sullivan p. 657)

Perseveration is the continued repetition of a word, phrase or movement. Initiating a new activity during therapy may allow the patient to redirect attention and subsequently receive positive reinforcement for attending to the selected task.

1. It is not necessary to attempt to appease the patient since the patient cannot independently move beyond whatever they are perseverating on. Staying with the topic will not assist in moving forward.

2. **Patients with a lesion in the premotor or prefrontal cortex often exhibit perseveration. Since the patient typically continues the repetition of a word, phrase or movement after the cessation of the original stimulus, the best intervention would be to redirect the patient away from the current activity.**

3. The patient will not benefit from "quiet time" since the patient is not perseverating due to a behavioral issue. Redirecting the patient may successfully allow the patient to move forward and continue with therapy without interruption.

4. Verbal cueing is not an effective technique to cease perseveration. The patient typically requires a redirection of their attention to another activity or environment.

System: Neuromuscular and Nervous Systems
Content Outline: Interventions

 Level 2   p. 692-693

 Level 3   p. 265, 274-276

SCOREBUILDERS

➡ PTAEXAM THREE: QUESTION 121

A patient reports experiencing pain during testing of active shoulder range of motion. The physical therapist assistant hypothesizes that the pain may be associated with anterior glenohumeral instability. Which portion of the shoulder range of motion should the assistant expect the pain to be the **MOST** pronounced?

1. 70-80 degrees of lateral rotation
2. **80-90 degrees of lateral rotation**
3. 60-70 degrees of medial rotation
4. 70-80 degrees of medial rotation

Correct Answer: 2 (Dutton p. 607)

It is important for physical therapist assistants to collect as much information as possible about a patient's present pain. Many diagnoses have characteristic pain patterns.

1. 70-80 degrees of lateral rotation may have the potential to result in pain with active motion due to anterior glenohumeral instability, however, the portion of the range is not as provocative as 80-90 degrees of lateral rotation.

2. **80-90 degrees of lateral rotation places the greatest amount of pressure on the anterior structures, therefore, any level of inflammation, irritation or structural damage may be likely to produce pain with active motion.**

3. 60-70 degrees of medial rotation would be more likely to stress the posterior structures of the shoulder. Pain with medial rotation may be associated with posterior glenohumeral instability or suprahumeral impingement.

4. 70-80 degrees of medial rotation would be more likely to place additional stress on the posterior structures of the shoulder. Normal shoulder medial rotation is 0-70 degrees. This option would be more provocative to the posterior shoulder structures than option 3. Pain with medial rotation may be associated with posterior glenohumeral instability or suprahumeral impingement.

System: Musculoskeletal System
Content Outline: Diseases/Conditions that Impact Effective Treatment

➡ PTAEXAM THREE: QUESTION 122

A physical therapist assistant observes the gait of a child who has cerebral palsy. The assistant notes that the patient exhibits excessive lordosis during ambulation. Which of the following surgical procedures would **BEST** address this postural deformity?

1. Hamstring tendon lengthening
2. Adductor longus tendon lengthening
3. **Iliopsoas tendon lengthening**
4. Lumbar laminectomy

Correct Answer: 3 (Long p. 195)

Muscle tendon lengthening procedures are performed in children who have cerebral palsy to correct a deformity or muscle contracture. This procedure allows the muscle to return to its normal length and assists in correcting joint position. Children who have cerebral palsy can have prolonged or continuous spasticity which can lead to muscle shortening or contracture.

1. A hamstring tendon lengthening procedure will restore the length of the hamstring muscle. This procedure is used to reduce a knee flexion contracture and results in improved knee extension during gait. A hamstrings contracture is likely to result in a posterior pelvic tilt and reduced lumbar lordosis.

2. Lengthening of the adductor longus tendon is often performed with lengthening of the gracilis and iliopsoas in order to reduce hip subluxation in children with cerebral palsy. Lengthening of the adductor muscle group can result in reduction of a scissoring gait pattern.

3. **Contracture of the iliopsoas causes an excessive anterior pelvic tilt, which results in increased lordosis of the lumbar spine. Lengthening of the iliopsoas reduces the anterior pull on the pelvis and corrects the lordosis.**

4. A laminectomy is a surgical procedure that removes the lamina of a vertebra to relieve pressure on the spinal cord or nerves. The procedure is often performed in patients who have spinal stenosis. A laminectomy would not specifically address the muscular pull on the pelvis that is causing the excessive lordosis.

System: Musculoskeletal System
Content Outline: Diseases/Conditions that Impact Effective Treatment

 Level 2   p. 113

Level 2

PTAEXAM THREE: QUESTION 123

A physical therapist assistant completes a series of resisted movements on a patient who has a lower extremity injury. The patient denies pain initially, but reports increasing pain after performing a number of repetitions. This scenario is **MOST** consistent with which of the following conditions?

1. Complete rupture of a tendon
2. **Intermittent claudication**
3. Ligamentous laxity
4. Emotional hypersensitivity

Correct Answer: 2 (Roy p. 153)

Resistive movements attempt to identify the status of contractile tissue (i.e., muscles, tendons, associated attachments) and the nervous tissue supplying the contractile tissue.

1. A complete rupture of a tendon is characterized by significant muscle weakness. The onset of the weakness would be immediate.

2. **Intermittent claudication occurs as a result of insufficient blood supply and ischemia in active muscles. Symptoms most commonly include pain and cramping in muscles distal to the occluded vessel. Pain tends to progressively worsen with increasing activity.**

3. Ligamentous laxity would not significantly influence resistive movements. Ligamentous laxity is more commonly associated with excessive range of motion.

4. Emotional hypersensitivity may result in an exaggerated pain response with all forms of resistive movements. The exaggerated response would typically be evident immediately.

System: Musculoskeletal System
Content Outline: Diseases/Conditions that Impact Effective Treatment

PTAEXAM THREE: QUESTION 124

A physical therapist assistant reviews the findings of a research study in which a maximum oxygen consumption (VO_{2max}) assessment was completed on all subjects. Which of the following individuals should the assistant expect to have the largest maximum oxygen consumption?

1. **A 23-year-old male (weight: 240 pounds; height: 72 inches)**
2. A 25-year-old female (weight: 160 pounds; height: 66 inches)
3. A 53-year-old male (weight: 210 pounds; height: 69 inches)
4. A 47-year-old female (weight: 130 pounds; height: 62 inches)

Correct Answer: 1 (American College of Sports Medicine p. 58)

Maximum oxygen consumption (VO_{2max}) is generally considered the best indicator of cardiorespiratory endurance and aerobic fitness. Maximum oxygen consumption decreases with age at a rate of approximately 10% per decade after the age of 25.

1. **A 23-year-old male (weight: 240 pounds; height: 72 inches) would be expected to have the largest maximum oxygen consumption. Males have a higher maximum oxygen consumption than females and maximum oxygen consumption is directly proportional to height and weight.**

2. A 25-year-old female (weight: 160 pounds; height: 66 inches) would not be expected to have the largest maximum oxygen consumption of the presented options. This individual would, however, likely have a larger maximum oxygen consumption than the 47-year-old female since she is younger, heavier, and taller.

3. A 53-year-old male (weight: 210 pounds; height: 69 inches) would not be expected to have the largest maximum oxygen consumption of the presented options since the other male option is younger, heavier, and taller.

4. A 47-year-old female (weight: 130 pounds; height: 62 inches) would likely have the lowest maximum oxygen consumption of the presented options.

System: Cardiovascular and Pulmonary Systems
Content Outline: Physical Therapy Data Collection

Level 2

Level 2

➡ PTAEXAM THREE: QUESTION 125

A patient who has congestive heart failure starts to experience pain during an exercise session monitored by a physical therapist assistant. Which of the following actions is the **MOST** immediate for the assistant to take?

1. Notify the nursing staff to administer pain medication
2. Contact the referring physician
3. Discontinue the treatment session
4. **Ask the patient to describe the location and severity of the pain**

Correct Answer: 4 (Magee p. 8)

Congestive heart failure is characterized by the inability of the heart to maintain adequate cardiac output. Before the physical therapist assistant can adequately respond to the patient's report of pain, it is essential to gather additional information.

1. Administering pain medication is premature until more information is known about the pain. Once additional information is collected, the nursing staff will be able to make a more informed decision.

2. Contacting the physician is premature until more information is known about the location and severity of the pain. This type of detailed information is necessary to provide the physician with a better sense of what the patient is currently experiencing.

3. Discontinuing the treatment session based on a subjective report of pain is a viable option particularly given the patient's diagnosis, however, the physical therapist assistant would need to gather additional information about the pain prior to making a definitive decision.

4. **Having the patient describe the location and severity of the pain is the most immediate action the physical therapist assistant should take. The information can be collected in a timely manner and may be useful to determine the relative seriousness of the patient's subjective report of pain.**

System: Cardiovascular and Pulmonary Systems
Content Outline: Interventions

➡ PTAEXAM THREE: QUESTION 126

A physical therapist assistant reviews the medical record of a patient who has chronic obstructive pulmonary disease. The medical record indicates that the patient's current condition is consistent with chronic respiratory acidosis. Which of the following testing procedures was **MOST** likely used to identify this condition?

1. **Arterial blood gas analysis**
2. Pulmonary function testing
3. Graded exercise testing
4. Pulse oximetry

Correct Answer: 1 (Paz p. 64)

Arterial blood gas (ABG) analysis provides information on the functioning of the lungs (i.e., oxygenation and elimination of carbon dioxide). Respiratory acidosis is characterized by elevated $PaCO_2$ and below normal pH due to hypoventilation.

1. **Abnormal acid-base balance will result in respiratory alkalosis, respiratory acidosis, metabolic alkalosis or metabolic acidosis depending on the cause. These conditions can become life-threatening without intervention to normalize the pH within the body, which is typically 7.35-7.45. ABG analysis provides values for $PaCO_2$, PaO_2, O_2 saturation, and CO_2.**

2. Pulmonary function testing is a series of measurements that evaluates how well the lungs take in and release air and how well they move oxygen into and remove carbon dioxide from the blood. There are reference values based on height, weight, sex, and age and results are considered abnormal if they are not within 80% of these reference values for a given test.

3. Graded exercise testing is used to measure the response of the heart to a graded increase in oxygen demand. Exercise occurs using a systematic protocol that can assess other variables such as evaluation of arrhythmias, functional capacity, and significance of coronary artery disease.

4. An oximeter is a photoelectric device used to determine the oxygen saturation of blood. The device is most commonly applied to the finger or the ear. Oximetry is often used by physical therapist assistants to assess activity tolerance.

System: Cardiovascular and Pulmonary Systems
Content Outline: Diseases/Conditions that Impact Effective Treatment

⬤ Level 3

⬤ Level 2   p. 419

➡ PTAEXAM THREE: QUESTION 127

A physical therapist assistant observes a patient attempt to walk on their heels as part of a lower quarter screening. Which myotome would this activity **BEST** assess?

1. **L4**
2. L5
3. S1
4. S2

Correct Answer: 1 (Dutton p. 1461)

Involvement of a specific nerve root often results in predictable impairments including muscle weakness, diminished sensation, and impaired reflexes. Testing of the myotomes using functional activities such as walking on the heels allows the therapist to gain insight into the spinal level affected.

1. **The L4 myotome provides innervation for muscles such as the tibialis anterior. Heel walking relies to a large extent on the tibialis anterior being innervated and is therefore an effective test to assess the L4 myotome.**

2. The L5 myotome provides innervation for muscles such as the extensor hallucis and gluteus medius. The L5 myotome also provides innervation for muscles that promote heel walking, however, the L4 myotome would represent the primary innervation.

3. The S1 myotome provides innervation for muscles such as the hamstrings and plantar flexors. Toe walking would be a better functional test to assess the S1 and S2 myotomes.

4. The S2 myotome also provides innervation for muscles such as the hamstrings and plantar flexors.

System: Neuromuscular and Nervous Systems
Content Outline: Physical Therapy Data Collection

➡ PTAEXAM THREE: QUESTION 128

A physical therapist assistant treats a patient who has lower extremity weakness due to a laceration injury to the tibial nerve. Which movement would **LEAST** likely be affected by this nerve injury?

1. Plantar flexion of the ankle
2. **Extension of the great toe**
3. Flexion of the great toe
4. Flexion of toes 2-5

Correct Answer: 2 (Kendall p. 364)

The tibial nerve is a branch of the sciatic nerve that supplies innervation to the muscles of the posterior lower leg. In the foot, the tibial nerve branches into the medial and lateral plantar nerves.

1. Ankle plantar flexion is performed by several muscles that are innervated by the tibial nerve, including the gastrocnemius, soleus, plantaris, tibialis posterior, flexor hallucis longus, and flexor digitorum longus. A patient with a tibial nerve injury would have significant difficulty performing ankle plantar flexion.

2. **Extension of the great toe is performed by the extensor hallucis longus and extensor hallucis brevis. These muscles are innervated by the deep peroneal nerve, which is a branch of the common peroneal nerve. A patient with a tibial nerve injury would have no difficulty performing extension of the great toe.**

3. Flexion of the great toe is performed by the flexor hallucis longus and flexor hallucis brevis. These muscles are innervated by the tibial nerve. A patient with a tibial nerve injury would have significant difficulty performing flexion of the great toe.

4. Flexion of toes 2-5 is performed by the flexor digitorum longus and flexor digitorum brevis. These muscles are innervated by the tibial nerve. A patient with a tibial nerve injury would have significant difficulty performing flexion of toes 2-5.

System: Neuromuscular and Nervous Systems
Content Outline: Physical Therapy Data Collection

 Level 1   p. 71, 233

 Level 2   p. 228

➡ PTAEXAM THREE: QUESTION 129

A physical therapist assistant attempts to obtain the body temperature of a patient receiving oxygen by mask. Which method would be the **LEAST** appropriate to obtain the desired measurement?

1. Tympanic membrane temperature
2. Temporal artery temperature
3. **Oral temperature**
4. Axillary temperature

Correct Answer: 3 (Fairchild p. 51)

Body temperature represents a balance between the heat produced and the heat lost by the body. Body temperature is measured through a variety of methods including oral temperature, tympanic membrane temperature, temporal artery temperature, axillary temperature, and rectal temperature.

1. Tympanic membrane temperature reads the infrared heat waves released by the ear's tympanic membrane. An accurate measurement requires the examiner to pull the ear backward to straighten the ear canal.

2. Temporal artery temperature reads the infrared heat waves released by the temporal artery which runs across the forehead just below the skin. The temporal artery temperature is obtained by depressing a scan button while moving the thermometer across the forehead.

3. **Oral temperature is obtained by placing the tip of a thermometer under one side of the tongue towards the back of the oral cavity. The thermometer is held in place for three minutes with a glass thermometer and approximately 30 seconds with an electronic thermometer. Oral temperatures should not be assessed in patients receiving oxygen by mask because the time it takes to assess a temperature reading is likely to result in a significant drop in the patient's blood oxygen level.**

4. Axillary temperature is obtained by placing the tip of a thermometer in the armpit. The arm is then brought to the patient's side holding the elbow against the thorax for 4-5 minutes.

System: Non-Systems
Content Outline: Equipment, Devices, and Technologies; Therapeutic Modalities

➡ PTAEXAM THREE: QUESTION 130

A physical therapist assistant treats a patient who has a C6 spinal cord injury. Which of the following muscles would **NOT** be innervated based on the patient's level of injury?

1. Biceps
2. Deltoid
3. **Triceps**
4. Diaphragm

Correct Answer: 3 (Magee p. 25)

A patient with a C6 spinal cord injury would not possess motor, sensory or reflex function below the C6 level. As a result, any muscle or structure innervated below this level would not be active.

1. The biceps muscle is innervated by the musculocutaneous nerve (C5-C6).

2. The deltoid muscle is innervated by the axillary nerve (C5-C6).

3. **The triceps muscle is innervated by the radial nerve (C7-C8).**

4. The diaphragm is innervated by the phrenic nerve (C3, C4, C5).

System: Neuromuscular and Nervous Systems
Content Outline: Physical Therapy Data Collection

 Level 2   p. 608

Level 1   p. 267, 269-271

➡ PTAEXAM THREE: QUESTION 131

A physical therapist assistant assesses end-feel on a patient as part of a lower quarter screening. Assuming a normal end-feel, which of the following classifications should the assistant **MOST** expect with hip extension?

1. Soft
2. **Firm**
3. Hard
4. Empty

Correct Answer: 2 (Norkin p. 260)

End-feel is the type of resistance that is felt when passively moving a joint through the end range of motion.

1. A soft end-feel results in a yielding compression that halts further movement. An example of a soft end-feel would be associated with knee flexion secondary to compression of soft tissue.

2. **The end-feel most often associated with hip extension is firm due to tension in the anterior joint capsule and the iliofemoral ligament.**

3. A hard or bony end-feel results in an unyielding sensation most often caused by bone to bone contact. An example of a hard or bony end-feel would be elbow extension.

4. An empty end-feel results when pain prevents reaching the end of range of motion. Resistance is not felt, although protective muscle splinting or muscle spasm may be detected. An empty end-feel is always considered abnormal.

System: Musculoskeletal System
Content Outline: Physical Therapy Data Collection

➡ PTAEXAM THREE: QUESTION 132

A physical therapist assistant reviews the medical record of a patient who is in the intensive care unit and notices a physician order for arterial blood gas analysis six times daily. What type of indwelling line would be used to collect the necessary samples?

1. Intravenous
2. **Arterial**
3. Central venous
4. Pulmonary artery

Correct Answer: 2 (Fairchild p. 274)

Samples for blood gas analysis may be obtained from different regions of the vascular bed. Arterial samples are taken from either a needle puncture or indwelling catheter in a peripheral artery.

1. An intravenous line consists of a short catheter inserted through the skin into a peripheral vein. Intravenous lines are used as a route to administer medications or fluids.

2. **An arterial line consists of a catheter inserted through the skin into an artery connected to pressure tubing, a transducer, and a monitor. The device can be used for continuous direct blood pressure readings and to sample arterial blood for arterial blood gas analysis. The radial and brachial arteries are the most common sites for an arterial line.**

3. A central venous line consists of a catheter inserted through the skin into a large vein, usually the superior vena cava or inferior vena cava, or within the right atrium of the heart to measure right atrial pressure. The catheter also may be used as a route for medication or fluid administration, blood sampling, and emergency placement of a pacemaker.

4. A pulmonary artery line is a balloon-tipped catheter introduced via the internal jugular vein or subclavian vein passing through the right atrium, tricuspid valve, right ventricle, pulmonary valve, and into the pulmonary artery. It is used to monitor cardiovascular pressures and to sample mixed venous blood for gas analysis.

System: Cardiovascular and Pulmonary Systems
Content Outline: Diseases/Conditions that Impact Effective Treatment

 Level 2   p. 77

 Level 1   p. 608

➡ PTAEXAM THREE: QUESTION 133

A patient positioned in standing with the arm by the side and elbow flexed to 90 degrees completes shoulder medial and lateral rotation exercises using a piece of elastic tubing. What plane of the body is utilized with this activity?

1. Coronal
2. Frontal
3. Sagittal
4. **Transverse**

Correct Answer: 4 (Levangie p. 7)

Medial and lateral rotation with the arm positioned at the side with 90 degrees of elbow flexion occurs in a transverse plane.

1. The coronal plane divides the body into anterior and posterior sections. Motions in the coronal plane occur around an anterior-posterior axis.

2. The terms frontal and coronal are synonyms and describe the same plane of movement.

3. The sagittal plane divides the body into left and right halves. Motions in the sagittal plane occur around a medial-lateral axis.

4. **The transverse plane divides the body into upper and lower sections. Motions in the transverse plane occur around a vertical axis.**

System: Musculoskeletal System
Content Outline: Physical Therapy Data Collection

⊕ **Test Taking Tip:** A candidate should recognize that the frontal plane and the coronal plane are synonyms and as a result refer to the same plane of movement. Therefore, options 1 and 2 can be eliminated as potential answers to the question since they mutually exclude each other.

➡ PTAEXAM THREE: QUESTION 134

A physical therapist assistant works with a patient on therapeutic positioning. The patient has experienced a lengthy hospitalization, has significant weakness of the diaphragm, and is hypertensive. Which of the following positions should the assistant utilize to **INITIATE** treatment?

1. Prone
2. Supine
3. Trendelenburg
4. **Reverse Trendelenburg**

Correct Answer: 4 (Hillegass p. 537)

The reverse Trendelenburg position refers to a position in which the patient's head is elevated on an inclined plane in relation to the feet.

1. The prone position would be a difficult position in which to teach the patient diaphragmatic breathing since the weight of the abdominal contents on the diaphragm makes it more difficult for a weakened diaphragm to contract.

2. In supine, the weight of the abdominal contents on the diaphragm makes it more difficult for a weakened diaphragm to contract. The supine position can also reduce the functional residual capacity of the lungs by as much as fifty percent.

3. In the Trendelenburg position the patient's head is lower than their feet. The position is used to facilitate drainage from the lower lobes of the lungs and to increase blood pressure in hypotensive patients. The position would tend to increase the blood pressure of a patient that is already hypertensive.

4. **The reverse Trendelenburg position is recommended to reduce hypertension and facilitate movement of the diaphragm by using gravity to reduce the weight of the abdominal contents on the diaphragm.**

System: Other Systems
Content Outline: Interventions

 Level 1   p. 49-50

 Level 2   p. 394

▶ PTAEXAM THREE: QUESTION 135

A physical therapist assistant works with a patient who is HIV positive and has been admitted to the hospital for a course of intravenous antibiotics. The patient has been experiencing a persistent cough producing bloody sputum for four weeks and has been placed on airborne precautions. Which of the following rationales is the **MOST** likely reason for this level of precaution?

1. Decrease the risk of exposing the immunocompromised patient to pneumonia
2. Decrease the risk of exposing the immunocompromised patient to active tuberculosis
3. Decrease the risk of staff and visitor exposure to pneumonia
4. **Decrease the risk of staff and visitor exposure to active tuberculosis**

Correct Answer: 4 (Fairchild p. 34)

Standard precautions should be observed with all patients regardless of their reported medical history. Physical therapist assistants must also be aware of additional precautions which may be associated with more specific forms of infections. Airborne precautions typically include protection of respiratory pathways (e.g., wearing a mask or face shield) in order to prevent the risk of airborne transmission of infectious agents through evaporated droplets in air or dust particles.

1. Although it is important to protect a patient from exposure to potential sources of infection, airborne precautions are typically designated with the intent of preventing transmission of disease from the patient to others. Pneumonia is contracted via droplet transmission.

2. Neutropenic precautions may be instituted in addition to standard precautions for patients who are so immunocompromised that even a mild infection may be lethal. However, the patient's clinical presentation is consistent with active tuberculosis making it much more likely that the precautions have been instituted to protect others.

3. Pneumonia may produce symptoms similar to those described, however, the infection responsible is contracted via droplet transmission of an infectious virus, bacteria or fungi.

4. **Airborne precautions are typically instituted to protect staff and visitors from contracting an infection spread through airborne transmission. There is a significant prevalence of tuberculosis among patients who are HIV positive and the reported persistent cough and bloody sputum are consistent with the clinical presentation of the disease.**

System: Non-Systems
Content Outline: Safety and Protection; Professional
  Responsibilities; Research

▶ PTAEXAM THREE: QUESTION 136

A patient is examined by a physician after a recent onset of hand and finger weakness and muscular fasciculations. During the physician visit, the patient is informed that their medical condition is very serious and they have 2-5 years to live. Which of the following diseases is the **MOST** consistent with this scenario?

1. **Amyotrophic lateral sclerosis**
2. Multiple sclerosis
3. Parkinson's disease
4. Huntington's disease

Correct Answer: 1 (Goodman – Pathology p. 1455)

There are several degenerative diseases of the central nervous system, including amyotrophic lateral sclerosis, multiple sclerosis, Parkinson's disease, and Huntington's disease. These diseases are similar in that they affect the gray matter and/or white matter of the central nervous system. While there may be some overlap in symptoms between the varying diseases, they generally have their own unique clinical presentations.

1. **Amyotrophic lateral sclerosis (ALS) is a progressive motor neuron disease characterized by damage to both upper and lower motor neurons. Symptoms of ALS are wide-ranging and may include muscular atrophy and weakness, respiratory impairment, muscle fasciculations, cognitive impairments, and difficulty with speaking, chewing, and swallowing. Patients with ALS have a poor prognosis, with death usually occurring 2-5 years after diagnosis secondary to respiratory complications.**

2. Multiple sclerosis (MS) is a chronic disease caused by demyelination of the nerves within the brain and spinal cord. Symptoms of MS may include visual deficits, sensory changes, muscle weakness, fatigue, ataxia, and spasticity. Though patients with MS have a reduced life expectancy, they have a relatively normal life span.

3. Parkinson's disease (PD) is a chronic disease caused by degeneration of neurons within the basal ganglia. Symptoms of PD include tremors, rigidity, bradykinesia, akinesia, episodes of freezing, and balance impairments. A diagnosis of PD does not significantly affect a patient's life span.

4. Huntington's disease (HD) is a chronic hereditary disease that results in movement abnormalities. The primary symptom is chorea, a disorder characterized by abnormal, involuntary, jerky movements. A diagnosis of HD does not significantly affect a patient's life span.

System: Neuromuscular and Nervous Systems
Content Outline: Diseases/Conditions that Impact Effective
  Treatment

 Level 2   p. 674

 Level 1   p. 247, 292-293

➡ PTAEXAM THREE: QUESTION 137

A 12-month-old patient who has cerebral palsy demonstrates an abnormal persistence of the positive support reflex. During therapy this finding would **MOST** likely interfere with activities in which of the following positions?

1. Sitting
2. **Standing**
3. Prone on elbows
4. Supine

Correct Answer: 2 (Ratliffe p. 27)

The positive support reflex promotes extension of the lower extremities and trunk with weight bearing through the balls of the feet. If this reflex persists, it can interfere with standing, ambulation, balance reactions and weight shifting in standing, and can lead to plantar flexion contractures.

1. Sitting activities would not be influenced by the positive support reflex since there would not be stimulation to the ball of the foot. An infant is usually able to sit unsupported at six to seven months.

2. **The positive support reflex is elicited by contact of the ball of the foot with the floor surface when placed into a standing position. The reflex causes rigid extension of the lower extremities and trunk with weight bearing. This reflex is typically integrated at two to four months of age.**

3. Prone on elbows activities would not be influenced by the positive support reflex since there would not be stimulation to the ball of the foot. An infant is usually able to maintain the prone on elbows position at three to four months.

4. Supine activities would not be influenced by the positive support reflex since there would not be stimulation to the ball of the foot while in supine.

System: Neuromuscular and Nervous Systems
Content Outline: Interventions

➡ PTAEXAM THREE: QUESTION 138

A physical therapist assistant observes a patient running on a treadmill at an intensity of approximately 75 percent of their estimated maximum oxygen consumption. What is the **PRIMARY** source for the adenosine triphosphate (ATP) produced during this activity?

1. Amino acids
2. **Carbohydrates**
3. Fats
4. Proteins

Correct Answer: 2 (Nyland p. 36)

Assuming adequate availability of nutrients, carbohydrates and fats are the primary sources of energy production while proteins provide the raw materials for making hormones and muscle and facilitating numerous chemical processes. The percentage of carbohydrates and fats utilized are determined by a number of variables including intensity and duration of exercise.

1. Proteins consist of long chains of amino acids. The contribution of amino acids to the production of ATP is minimal during short-term exercise, but increases during prolonged activity.

2. **As exercise intensity increases (e.g., greater than 70% of maximum oxygen consumption), carbohydrates are responsible for the vast majority of ATP production. The transition from the use of fats to carbohydrates as the primary fuel source is referred to as the "crossover" concept. The rate of oxidation during exercise is a function of the rate of carbohydrate utilization and the availability of circulating fatty acids. If activity lasts for a long period of time (e.g., greater than one hour), fats play a greater role in energy metabolism.**

3. At lower levels of exercise intensity, the majority of ATP production comes from fats. As exercise intensity increases, the biochemical processes for fat metabolism are too slow to meet the needs for faster production of ATP, and carbohydrate utilization increases.

4. Proteins are used in ATP production as described in option 1. Protein can be metabolized in more significant amounts during long duration activity or long-term starvation.

System: Cardiovascular and Pulmonary Systems
Content Outline: Diseases/Conditions that Impact Effective Treatment

 Level 2   p. 277-278

 Level 2   p. 49

➡ PTAEXAM THREE: QUESTION 139

A patient treated in an acute care hospital one day ago is not able to attend a scheduled physical therapy session due to suspected critical limb ischemia. Which of the following symptoms is **MOST** commonly associated with this condition?

1. Severe pain in the legs and feet at rest
2. Increased temperature in the lower leg and foot
3. Bounding lower extremity peripheral pulses
4. Flaking skin on the legs with brownish discoloration

Correct Answer: 1 (Goodman – Pathology p. 641)

Critical limb ischemia refers to a severe obstruction of the arteries which markedly reduces blood flow to the extremities. The condition is considered the advanced stage of peripheral artery disease which results from a progressive buildup of plaque that narrows or blocks blood flow. Critical limb ischemia is a serious medical condition that potentially threatens the sustainability of the limb.

1. **Critical limb ischemia is characterized by severe pain in the legs and feet at rest. A patient often experiences the pain when in bed and may be able to diminish the intensity of pain by hanging the legs over the edge of the bed or getting up to walk around.**
2. Critical limb ischemia is characterized by a significant decrease in temperature of the lower legs and feet due to the significant decrease in blood flow.
3. A bounding pulse refers to a full and spring-like pulse on palpation as a result of cardiac contraction or excessive volume of circulating blood within the vascular system. Critical limb ischemia is characterized by absent or diminished peripheral pulses in the legs or feet.
4. Flaking skin on the legs with brownish discoloration is more characteristic of venous insufficiency. Critical limb ischemia is characterized by shiny, smooth, dry skin on the legs or feet.

System: Cardiovascular and Pulmonary Systems
Content Outline: Diseases/Conditions that Impact Effective
   Treatment

➡ PTAEXAM THREE: QUESTION 140

A patient who has muscle weakness and compromised balance uses a four-point gait pattern with two canes. The physical therapist assistant would like to instruct the patient to ascend and descend the stairs according to the normal flow of traffic. When ascending the stairs, which of the following methods is the **MOST** appropriate?

1. Use the handrail with the right hand and place the two canes in the left hand
2. Use the handrail with the left hand and place the two canes in the right hand
3. Place one cane in each hand and avoid using the handrail
4. Place the two canes in the left hand and avoid using the handrail

Correct Answer: 1 (Minor p. 428)

Since the normal flow of traffic assumes ascending on the right and descending on the left, the patient should grasp the railing with the right hand and use the two canes in the left hand when ascending and descending the stairs.

1. **Since the patient does not have unilateral weakness, it is most appropriate to ascend the stairs on the right in order to utilize the handrail and remain consistent with the normal flow of traffic.**
2. Since the normal flow of traffic assumes ascending on the right and descending on the left, the patient would be going against the normal flow of traffic by grasping the handrail with the left hand and using the two canes in the right hand.
3. The patient should use a handrail when available in order to improve stability and balance.
4. Failure to use the handrail would significantly increase the patient's relative risk of falling.

System: Non-Systems
Content Outline: Equipment, Devices, and Technologies;
   Therapeutic Modalities

 Level 2

 Level 2   p. 605-606

➡ PTAEXAM THREE: QUESTION 141

A physical therapist assistant treats a patient who has myasthenia gravis. Based on this diagnosis, which of the following clinical tests would **MOST** likely be abnormal?

1. Coordination testing

2. Sensory testing

3. Deep tendon reflex testing

4. **Endurance testing**

Correct Answer: 4 (Goodman – Pathology p. 1696)

Myasthenia gravis is an autoimmune disorder that disrupts neuromuscular transmission and results in muscle weakness and fatigability. The condition is characterized by weakness with repetitive activity that is restored quickly after a period of rest. Other neurologic findings typically are normal in patients with myasthenia gravis.

1. A patient with myasthenia gravis does not typically demonstrate coordination deficits and therefore would not exhibit abnormal findings with coordination testing. A patient with a cerebellar disorder would be more likely to exhibit abnormal findings with coordination testing.

2. A patient with myasthenia gravis does not typically demonstrate sensory deficits and therefore would not exhibit abnormal findings with sensory testing. A patient with a spinal cord injury would be more likely to exhibit abnormal findings with sensory testing.

3. A patient with myasthenia gravis does not typically demonstrate hyporeflexia or hyperreflexia and therefore would not exhibit abnormal findings with deep tendon reflex testing. A patient with a traumatic brain injury would be more likely to exhibit abnormal findings with deep tendon reflex testing.

4. **Myasthenia gravis is a condition that is characterized by muscle weakness and significant muscle fatigability. A patient with myasthenia gravis could demonstrate normal strength with manual muscle testing since it only requires a single muscle contraction. However, the patient would demonstrate significant weakness if required to perform repeated contractions. Endurance testing (e.g., treadmill testing, cycle ergometry) would likely be abnormal for this patient.**

System: Neuromuscular and Nervous Systems
Content Outline: Diseases/Conditions that Impact Effective
    Treatment

➡ PTAEXAM THREE: QUESTION 142

A physical therapist assistant treats a patient who has limited shoulder range of motion that the physical therapist determined is due to pain and not a specific tissue restriction. Which graded oscillation techniques would be the **MOST** appropriate to treat this patient?

1. **Grades I, II**

2. Grades II, III

3. Grades III, IV

4. Grades IV, V

Correct Answer: 1 (Kisner p. 135)

Graded oscillation techniques include grade I, II, III, IV, and V. The type of grade selected is dependent on the intended treatment objective.

1. **Grade I refers to small amplitude oscillations at the beginning of the range. Grade II refers to large amplitude oscillations performed within the range, but not reaching the limit of range. Grades I and II are primarily used to treat pain by stimulating mechanoreceptors.**

2. Grade II was previously defined. Grade III refers to large amplitude oscillations performed to the limit of available range and stressed into tissue resistance.

3. Grade III was previously defined. Grade IV refers to small amplitude oscillations performed at the limit of available range and stressed into the tissue resistance. Grades III and IV are primarily used as stretching maneuvers.

4. Grade IV was previously defined. Grade V refers to small amplitude, high velocity thrust techniques used to break up adhesions.

System: Musculoskeletal System
Content Outline: Interventions

 Level 2   p. 250, 328

Level 2   p. 104-105

➡ PTAEXAM THREE: QUESTION 143

A physical therapist assistant treats a patient who has lateral epicondylitis using iontophoresis. What type of current would the assistant use to administer this treatment?

1. Direct
2. Alternating
3. Pulsatile
4. Interferential

Correct Answer: 1 (Cameron p. 280)

Iontophoresis refers to the transcutaneous delivery of ions into the body for therapeutic purposes using an electrical current.

1. **Direct current is characterized by an uninterrupted flow of electrons toward the positive pole. This type of current is necessary to move the charged ions across the dermal barrier. Polarity remains constant and is determined based on treatment goals and the polarity of the chosen ion.**

2. Alternating current is characterized by the bidirectional (constantly changing) continuous flow of electrons. Electrons flowing in an alternating current move from the negative to positive pole, reversing direction when the polarity is reversed.

3. Pulsatile current is characterized by three or more pulses grouped together and may be unidirectional or bidirectional. A series of unidirectional pulses is known as monophasic pulsed current and a series of bidirectional pulses is known as biphasic pulsed current.

4. Interferential current combines two high frequency alternating waveforms that are biphasic. The two waveforms are delivered through two sets of electrodes through separate channels in the same stimulator.

System: Non-Systems
Content Outline: Equipment, Devices, and Technologies; Therapeutic Modalities

➡ PTAEXAM THREE: QUESTION 144

A physical therapist assistant treats a patient who has a cerebellar lesion. Which of the following clinical findings should the assistant **LEAST** expect to observe with this condition?

1. Athetosis
2. Dysmetria
3. Nystagmus
4. Dysdiadochokinesia

Correct Answer: 1 (O'Sullivan p. 211)

Athetosis is a term used to describe slow, writhing, and involuntary movements that may occur with damage to the basal ganglia.

1. **Athetosis is characterized by extraneous and involuntary movements, slowness of movement, and alterations in muscle tone. Athetoid movements may look "wormlike" with a rotatory component evident.**

2. Dysmetria occurs with cerebellar lesions and is defined as the inability to appropriately reach a target. The cerebellum is normally responsible for the timing, force, extent, and direction of the limb movement in order to correctly reach the target.

3. Nystagmus can occur with cerebellar lesions and is usually classified as gaze-evoked nystagmus. The patient will attempt to look toward an object in the periphery, but the eyes will drift involuntarily back to neutral. This may occur unilaterally or bilaterally depending on the cause of cerebellar dysfunction.

4. Dysdiadochokinesia occurs with cerebellar lesions and is defined as the inability to perform rapid alternating movements.

System: Neuromuscular and Nervous Systems
Content Outline: Diseases/Conditions that Impact Effective Treatment

 Level 1   p. 638-639, 644-646

 Level 2   p. 217, 238-239

SCOREBUILDERS

➡ PTAEXAM THREE: QUESTION 145

A physical therapist assistant administers strength testing after observing a patient exhibit a posterior trunk lean during gait. Which testing procedure would be **MOST** anticipated based on the observed finding?

1. Patient positioned in prone; downward pressure is applied to the posterior surface of the distal thigh

2. Patient positioned in sidelying; downward pressure is applied to the lateral ankle of the top leg

3. Patient positioned in prone; assistant passively brings the patient's heel towards their buttocks

4. Patient positioned in prone with knees flexed to 90 degrees; assistant medially rotates the hip

Correct Answer: 1 (Kendall p. 436)

Posterior trunk lean during gait is also known as gluteus maximus gait. This gait deviation is characterized by a posterior trunk lean between heel strike and foot flat and often occurs due to weakness of the gluteus maximus.

1. **The described scenario is consistent with muscle testing of the gluteus maximus. Weakness of the gluteus maximus can contribute to a posterior trunk lean between heel strike and foot flat, which is known as a gluteus maximus gait.**

2. The described scenario is consistent with muscle testing of the hip abductors. Weakness of the hip abductors is often associated with the presence of a Trendelenburg gait pattern. This type of gait pattern is not associated with a posterior trunk lean.

3. The described scenario is the testing procedure for Ely's test. A positive Ely's test may be indicative of a rectus femoris contracture and can contribute to an anterior pelvic tilt and increased lumbar lordosis with gait. A rectus femoris contracture is not associated with a posterior trunk lean.

4. The described scenario is the testing procedure for Craig's test which is used to assess the degree of femoral anteversion. Specifically, the assistant medially and laterally rotates the hip with the patient in prone with the knee flexed to 90 degrees. This test does not provide information about gluteus maximus strength.

System: Musculoskeletal System
Content Outline: Physical Therapy Data Collection

➡ PTAEXAM THREE: QUESTION 146

A physical therapist assistant measures 35 degrees of elbow flexion while a patient grasps the handgrip of a walker in standing. Which of the following statements **BEST** describes the height of the walker?

1. The walker height is too low for the patient

2. **The walker height is too high for the patient**

3. The walker height is appropriate for the patient

4. Not enough information is given to assess walker height

Correct Answer: 2 (Fairchild p. 221)

A patient using a properly fitting walker should exhibit 20–25 degrees of elbow flexion. This position of the elbow would allow the patient to most effectively use the upper extremities during ambulation. A walker can be used with all levels of weight bearing and offers a large base of support which promotes stability.

1. A walker height that is too low for the patient would result in elbow flexion less than the recommended 20-25 degrees. Any deviation from the recommended fit would decrease the efficiency of using the walker and increase the potential safety risk.

2. **A walker height that is too high for the patient would result in elbow flexion greater than the recommended 20-25 degrees.**

3. Elbow flexion of 35 degrees exceeds the upper limit of the acceptable range of elbow flexion (i.e., 20-25 degrees) when using a walker. As the height of the walker increases, the amount of elbow flexion will also increase.

4. The amount of elbow flexion is the primary indicator of the relative height of the walker. As a result, there is ample information provided to assess the height of the walker.

System: Non-Systems
Content Outline: Equipment, Devices, and Technologies; Therapeutic Modalities

---

 Level 3   p. 77-79

 Level 1   p. 602-603

SCOREBUILDERS

➡ PTAEXAM THREE: QUESTION 147

A physical therapist assistant attempts to assess the integrity of the L4 spinal level. Which deep tendon reflex would provide the assistant with the **MOST** useful information?

1. Lateral hamstrings
2. Medial hamstrings
3. **Patellar**
4. Achilles

Correct Answer: 3 (Magee p. 852)

Deep tendon reflexes are assessed to examine the integrity of the afferent and efferent peripheral nervous systems and the ability of the central nervous system to inhibit the reflex. The physical therapist assistant should attempt to assess the reflex by striking the tendon with the reflex hammer after placing the tendon on slight stretch.

1. The lateral hamstrings reflex is innervated at the S1-S2 spinal level.
2. The medial hamstrings reflex is innervated at the L5-S1 spinal level.
3. **The patellar reflex is innervated at the L3-L4 spinal level.**
4. The Achilles reflex is innervated at the S1-S2 spinal level.

System: Neuromuscular and Nervous Systems
Content Outline: Physical Therapy Data Collection

➡ PTAEXAM THREE: QUESTION 148

A physical therapist assistant completes a fitness screening on a 34-year-old patient prior to implementing an aerobic exercise program. What value **BEST** represents the patient's age-predicted maximal heart rate?

1. 168
2. 174
3. **186**
4. 196

Correct Answer: 3 (Minor p. 124)

Age-predicted maximal heart rate can be determined as follows: 220-age.

1. Based on the formula of 220-age, the rate of 168 is too low for this patient's age-predicted maximal heart rate.
2. Based on the formula of 220-age, the rate of 174 is too low for this patient's age-predicted maximal heart rate.
3. **Based on the formula of 220-age, the rate of 186 is equal to this patient's age-predicted maximal heart rate (220-34=186).**
4. Based on the formula of 220-age, the rate of 196 is too high for this patient's age-predicted maximal heart rate. This would be an unsafe rate for exercise.

System: Cardiovascular and Pulmonary Systems
Content Outline: Physical Therapy Data Collection

⇒ PTAEXAM THREE: QUESTION 149

During gait training of a patient, a physical therapist assistant observes that the patient's pelvis drops on the left during the left swing phase. The assistant should recognize that this gait deviation is **MOST** likely caused by weakness of which of the following muscles?

1. Left gluteus medius
2. **Right gluteus medius**
3. Left gluteus minimus
4. Right gluteus minimus

Correct Answer: 2 (Magee p. 1009)

A Trendelenburg gait pattern is characterized by excessive lateral trunk flexion and weight shifting over the stance leg. The gait pattern is often seen with lesions of the superior gluteal nerve, L5 radiculopathy, and poliomyelitis.

1. The gluteus medius acts to abduct the hip joint. The anterior fibers medially rotate and may assist in flexion of the hip joint. The posterior fibers laterally rotate and may assist in extension. Weakness of the left gluteus medius would be characterized by the pelvis dropping on the right during right swing phase.

2. **Weakness of the right gluteus medius would be characterized by the pelvis dropping on the left during left swing phase.**

3. The gluteus minimus acts to abduct and medially rotate the hip and may assist in hip flexion. Weakness of the left gluteus minimus would be identified by diminished strength in medial rotation and abduction of the left hip.

4. Weakness of the right gluteus minimus would be identified by diminished strength in medial rotation and abduction of the right hip.

System: Musculoskeletal System
Content Outline: Physical Therapy Data Collection

⇒ PTAEXAM THREE: QUESTION 150

A physical therapist assistant completes a sensory assessment on a patient who has multiple sclerosis. As part of the assessment, the assistant tests stereognosis, vibration, and two-point discrimination. What type of receptor is primarily responsible for generating the necessary information?

1. Deep sensory receptors
2. **Mechanoreceptors**
3. Nociceptors
4. Thermoreceptors

Correct Answer: 2 (O'Sullivan p. 97)

Mechanoreceptors generate information related to discriminative sensations. The information is then mediated through the dorsal column-medial lemniscal system. Examples of mechanoreceptors include free nerve endings, Merkel's disks, Ruffini endings, hair follicle endings, Meissner's corpuscles, and Pacinian corpuscles.

1. Deep sensory receptors are sensory receptors that are located in the muscles, tendons, and joints. Muscle and joint receptors are both classified as deep sensory receptors and include Golgi tendon organs, Pacinian corpuscles, muscle spindle, Ruffini endings, free nerve endings, and joint receptors. They evaluate position sense, proprioception, muscle tone, and movement.

2. **Mechanoreceptors are sensory receptors that respond to mechanical deformation of the area surrounding a receptor. They are cutaneous sensory receptors that are located at the terminal end of the afferent fibers. Certain areas of the body have a higher density of mechanoreceptors than others. Aggregately, they are responsible for sensations of touch, pressure, itch, tickle, vibration, and discriminative touch.**

3. Nociceptors are specialized peripheral free nerve endings that are found throughout different tissues within the body that respond to noxious stimuli and result in the perception of pain. A painful stimulus will ascend through the spinal cord via the lateral spinothalamic tract. Several areas of the brain provide specific responses to the painful stimulus.

4. Thermoreceptors are sensory receptors that respond to changes in temperature. Stimulation of the cold or warm receptors will ascend through the spinal cord via the lateral spinothalamic tract.

System: Neuromuscular and Nervous Systems
Content Outline: Physical Therapy Data Collection

 Level 2   p. 84, 101

 Level 2   p. 233

NOTES

Exam References,
Exam & Academic Review Indexes,
Motivational Moments and Resources

Insight PTAEXAM References

American College of Sports Medicine. *ACSM's Resource Manual for Guidelines for Exercise Testing and Prescription*. Seventh Edition. Lippincott Williams & Wilkins. 2014.

American Physical Therapy Association. *Code of Ethics*. HOD S06-09-07-12.

American Physical Therapy Association. *Criteria for Standards of Practice for Physical Therapy*. BOD S01-14-01-01. Updated: 04/15/14, web site 2017.

American Physical Therapy Association. *Defensible Documentation Elements*. Updated: 12/08/15, web site 2017.

American Physical Therapy Association. *Direction and Supervision of the Physical Therapist Assistant*. HOD P06-05-18-26. Updated: 08/07/12, web site 2017.

American Physical Therapy Association. *Guide for Conduct of the Physical Therapist Assistant*.

American Physical Therapy Association. *Guide to Physical Therapist Practice*. http://guidetoptpractice.apta.org/ APTA, 2014.

American Physical Therapy Association. *Guidelines: Physical Therapy Documentation of Patient/Client Management*. BOD G03-05-16-41. Updated: 05/19/2014, web site 2017.

American Physical Therapy Association. *Standards of Ethical Conduct for the Physical Therapist Assistant*.

Anemaet W, Moffa-Trotter M. *Home Rehabilitation: Guide to Clinical Practice*. Mosby. 2000.

Avers D, Brown M. Daniels and Worthingham's Muscle Testing: Techniques of Manual Examination and Performance Testing. Tenth Edition. Elsevier. 2019.

Bellew J, Michlovitz S, Nolan T. *Modalities for Therapeutic Intervention*. Sixth Edition. F.A. Davis Company. 2016.

Bickley L. *Bates' Guide to Physical Examination and History Taking*. Twelfth Edition. Wolters Kluwer. 2017.

Boissonnault W. *Primary Care for the Physical Therapist*. Second Edition. Elsevier. 2011.

Brannon F, Foley M, Starr J, Saul L. *Cardiopulmonary Rehabilitation: Basic Theory and Application*. Third Edition. F.A. Davis Company. 1998.

Brody L, Hall C. *Therapeutic Exercise: Moving Toward Function*. Fourth Edition. Lippincott Williams & Wilkins. 2018.

Brunnstrom S. *Movement Therapy in Hemiplegia*. Harper and Row Publishers Inc. 1992.

Cameron M. *Physical Agents in Rehabilitation: An Evidence-Based Approach to Practice*. Fifth Edition. Elsevier. 2018.

Cameron M, Monroe L. *Physical Rehabilitation: Evidence Based Examination, Evaluation, and Intervention*. W.B. Saunders Company. 2007.

Carr J, Shepherd R. *Neurologic Rehabilitation: Optimizing Motor Performance*. Churchill Livingstone. 2010.

Cech D, Martin S. *Functional Movement Development*. Third Edition. Elsevier. 2012.

Ciccone C. *Pharmacology for Rehabilitation*. Fifth Edition. F.A. Davis Company. 2016.

Coburn W, Malek K. *NSCA's Essentials of Personal Training*. Second Edition. Human Kinetics. 2012.

Cohen H. Neuroscience for Rehabilitation. J.B Lippincott Company. 1993.

Davenport T, Kulig K, Sebelski C, Gordon J, Watts H. Diagnosis for Physical Therapists: A Symptom-Based Approach. F.A. Davis Company. 2013.

DeMyer W. *Technique of the Neurologic Examination*. Fifth Edition. McGraw-Hill Company. 2004.

Dutton M. *Orthopaedic Examination, Evaluation, and Intervention*. Fourth Edition. McGraw-Hill Inc. 2017.

Dunleavy K, Slowik A. Therapeutic Exercise Prescription. Elsevier. 2019.

Edmond S. *Joint Mobilization/Manipulation*. Third Edition. Elsevier. 2016.

Ehrman J, Gordon P, Visich P, Keteyian S. *Clinical Exercise Physiology*. Second Edition. Human Kinetics. 2009.

Fairchild S, O'Shea R, Washington R. *Pierson and Fairchild's Principles and Techniques of Patient Care*. Sixth Edition. Elsevier. 2018.

Falvo D. *Effective Patient Education*. Fourth Edition. Jones and Bartlett Publishers. 2011.

Fell D, Lunnen K, Rauk R. Lifespan Neurorehabilitation: A Patient-Centered Approach from Examination to Interventions and Outcomes. F.A. Davis Company. 2018.

Frontera W, Silver J, Rizzor T. *Essentials of Physical Medicine and Rehabilitation: Musculoskeletal Disorders, Pain, and Rehabilitation*. Third Edition. Elsevier. 2015.

Frownfelter D, Dean E. *Cardiovascular and Pulmonary Physical Therapy: Evidence to Practice*. Fifth Edition. Mosby-Year Book. 2012.

Insight PTAEXAM References

Goodman C, Fuller K. *Pathology: Implications for the Physical Therapist*. Fourth Edition. Elsevier. 2015.

Goodman C, Heick J, Lazaro R. *Differential Diagnosis for Physical Therapists – Screening for Referral*. Sixth Edition. Elsevier. 2018.

Guccione A, Wong R, Avers D. *Geriatric Physical Therapy*. Third Edition. Mosby. 2011.

Gutman S. *Quick Reference Neuroscience for Rehabilitation Professionals*. Second Edition. Slack Inc. 2008.

Haines D. *Neuroanatomy in Clinical Context*. Ninth Edition. Wolters Kluwer. 2014.

Hertling D, Kessler R. *Management of Common Musculoskeletal Disorders*. Fourth Edition. Lippincott Williams & Wilkins. 2006.

Higgins, Michael. *Therapeutic Exercise: From Theory to Practice*. F.A. Davis Company. 2011.

Hillegass E, Sadowsky S. *Essentials of Cardiopulmonary Physical Therapy*. Fourth Edition. Elsevier. 2017.

Hoogenboom B, Voight M, Prentice W. *Musculoskeletal Interventions*: Techniques for Therapeutic Exercise. Third Edition. McGraw Hill Education. 2014.

Hoppenfeld S, Thomas H, Hutton R. *Physical Examination of the Spine and Extremities*. Prentice Hall. 1976.

Hurley W, Denegar C. *Research Methods: A Framework for Evidence-Based Practice*. Lippincott Williams & Wilkins. 2010.

Irwin S, Tecklin J. *Cardiopulmonary Physical Therapy: A Guide to Practice*. Fourth Edition. Mosby. 2004.

Johansson C, Chinworth S. Mobility in Context: Principles of Patient Care Skills. Second Edition. F.A. Davis Company. 2018.

Kauffman T, Scott R, Barr J, Moran M. *A Comprehensive Guide to Geriatric Rehabilitation*. Third Edition. Elsevier. 2014.

Kendall F, McCreary E. Provance P. *Muscles: Testing and Function with Posture and Pain*. Fifth Edition. Lippincott Williams & Wilkins. 2005.

Kisner C, Colby L, Borstad J. *Therapeutic Exercise Foundations and Techniques*. Seventh Edition. F.A. Davis Company. 2018.

La Baudour C, Bergeron J. *Emergency Medical Responder: First on Scene*. Ninth Edition. Pearson. 2012.

Levangie P, Norkin C. *Joint Structure and Function: A Comprehensive Analysis*. Fifth Edition. F.A. Davis Company. 2011.

Lewis C, Bottomley J: *Geriatric Rehabilitation: A Clinical Approach*. Third Edition. Prentice Hall. 2007.

Long T, Toscano K. *Handbook of Pediatric Physical Therapy*. Second Edition. Lippincott Williams & Wilkins. 2002.

Lundy-Ekman L. *Neuroscience: Fundamentals for Rehabilitation*. Fifth Edition. Elsevier. 2018.

Lusardi M, Milagros J, Nielsen C. *Orthotics and Prosthetics in Rehabilitation*. Third Edition. Elsevier. 2013.

Magee D. *Orthopedic Physical Assessment*. Sixth Edition. W.B. Saunders Company. 2014.

Martin S, Kessler M. *Neurologic Interventions for Physical Therapy*. Second Edition. 2007.

May B, Lockard M. *Prosthetics and Orthotics in Clinical Practice: A Case Study Approach*. F.A. Davis Company, 2011.

McKinnis L. *Fundamentals of Musculoskeletal Imaging*. Fourth Edition. F.A. Davis Company. 2014.

Means K, Kortebein P. *Geriatrics*. Demos Medical. 2013.

Minor M, Minor S. *Patient Care Skills*. Seventh Edition. Pearson Education, Inc. 2014.

Moore K. Dalley A. *Clinically Oriented Anatomy*. Seventh Edition. Lippincott Williams & Wilkins. 2013.

Myers D. *Psychology*. Ninth Edition. Worth Publishers. 2009.

Nichols-Larsen, Kegelmeyer D. *Neurologic Rehabilitation: Neuroscience and Neuroplasticity in Physical Therapy Practice*. McGraw Hill Education. 2016.

Norkin C, White D. *Measurement of Joint Motion: A Guide to Goniometry*. Fifth Edition. F.A. Davis Company. 2016.

Nosse L, Friberg D. *Managerial and Supervisory Principles for Physical Therapists*. Third Edition. Lippincott Williams & Wilkins. 2010.

Nyland J. *Clinical Decisions in Therapeutic Exercise: Planning and Implementation*. Pearson-Prentice Hall. 2006.

Osborne J. *Documentation for Physical Therapist Practice: A Clinical Decision-Making Approach*. Jones & Bartlett Learning. 2016.

O'Sullivan S, Schmitz T, Fulk G. *Physical Rehabilitation*. Sixth Edition. F.A. Davis Company. 2014.

Page C. *Management in Physical Therapy Practices*. Second Edition. F.A. Davis Company. 2015.

Palisano R, Orlin M, Shreiber J. *Campbell's Physical Therapy for Children*. Fifth Edition. Elsevier. 2017.

Insight PTAEXAM References

Paz J, West MP. *Acute Care Handbook for Physical Therapists*. Fourth Edition. W.B. Saunders Company. 2014.

Perry A, Potter P. *Clinical Nursing Skills and Techniques*. Eighth Edition. Mosby. 2013.

Plack M, Driscoll M. *Teaching and Learning in Physical Therapy: From Classroom to Clinic*. Slack Incorporated. 2011.

Porter R. *The Merck Manual*. Nineteenth Edition. Merck and Company, Inc. 2011.

Portney L, Watkins M. *Foundations of Clinical Research: Applications to Practice*. Third Edition. Prentice Hall. 2015.

Prentice W. *Therapeutic Modalities in Rehabilitation*. Fifth Edition. McGraw-Hill Inc. 2018.

Professional Guide to Diseases. Ninth Edition. Lippincott Williams & Wilkins. 2010.

Purtilo R, Haddad A. *Health Professional and Patient Interaction*. Eighth Edition. Elsevier. 2014.

Quinn L, Gordon J. *Functional Outcomes: Documentation for Rehabilitation*. Seventh Edition. W.B. Saunders Company. 2010.

Ratliffe KT. *Clinical Pediatric Physical Therapy: A Guide for the Physical Therapy Team*. Mosby. 1998.

Robnett R, Chop W. *Gerontology for the Healthcare Practitioner*. Third Edition. Jones & Bartlett Publishing. 2015.

Roy S, Wolf S, Scalzitti D. *The Rehabilitation Specialist's Handbook*. Fourth Edition. F.A. Davis Company. 2013.

Sadock B, Sadock V. *Kaplan & Sadock's Comprehensive Textbook of Psychiatry*. Ninth Edition. Lippincott Williams & Wilkins. 2009.

Sahrmann S. Diagnosis and Treatment of Movement Impairment Syndromes. Mosby. 2002

Sarwark J. *Essentials of Musculoskeletal Care*. American Academy of Orthopaedic Surgeons. Fourth Edition. 2010.

Scott R. *Promoting Legal and Ethical Awareness*. Mosby. 2009.

Seidel H, Ball J, Dains J, Benedict G. *Mosby's Guide to Physical Examination*. Fifth Edition. Mosby. 2003.

Seymour R. *Prosthetics and Orthotics: Lower Limb and Spinal*. Lippincott Williams & Wilkins. 2002.

Shamus E, Stern D. *Effective Documentation for the Physical Therapy Professional*. Second Edition. McGraw-Hill Inc. 2011.

Shamus E, Van Dujin A. *Manual Therapy of the Extremities*. Jones & Bartlett Learning. 2017.

Shumway-Cook A, Woollacott M. *Motor Control: Translating Research into Clinical Practice*. Fourth Edition. Lippincott Williams & Wilkins. 2011.

Smeltzer S, Bare B. Brunnert Suddarth's *Textbook of Medical-Surgical Nursing*. Wolters Kluwer Health. Twelfth Edition. 2010.

Smith D, Michael J, Bowker J. *Atlas of Amputations and Limb Deficiencies: Surgical, Prosthetic, and Rehabilitation Principles*. American Academy of Orthopaedic Surgeons. 2004.

Smolin L, Grosvenor M. *Nutrition: Science and Application*. Third Edition. 2013.

Straus S, Richardson W, Haynes R, Glasziou P. *Evidence-Based Medicine. How to Practice and Teach EBM*. Fourth Edition. Churchill Livingstone. 2011.

Sullivan P, Markos P. *Clinical Decision Making in Therapeutic Exercise*. Appleton & Lange. 1995.

Sussman C, Bates-Jensen B. *Wound Care: A Collaborative Practice Manual for Health Professionals*. Fourth Edition. Wolters Kluwer Health/Lippincott Williams & Wilkins. 2012.

Tan J. *Practical Manual of Physical Medicine and Rehabilitation*. Second Edition. Elsevier. 2006.

Tecklin J. *Pediatric Physical Therapy*. Fifth Edition. Lippincott Williams & Wilkins. 2015.

Thomas C. *Prevention Practice: A Physical Therapist's Guide to Health, Fitness, and Wellness*. Slack Inc. 2007.

Umphred D, Lazaro R, Roller M. *Neurological Rehabilitation*. Sixth Edition. Mosby. 2013.

Whalen K. *Pharmacology*. Sixth Edition. Lippincott Williams & Wilkins. 2014.

Wise C. *Orthopedic Manual Physical Therapy: From Art to Evidence*. F.A. Davis Company. 2015.

Insight Exam Index

Directions for Using the Insight Exams Index

The Insight Exam Index allows candidates to identify specific academic content in each of the three sample examinations. For example, consider the following entry: **Bronchial drainage 2:** 31; **3:** 97. The bold numbers represent the exam number and the non-bold numbers that follow represent the question number within the respective exam. Therefore, questions pertaining to bronchial drainage are located in Exam Two: Questions 31 and Exam Three: Question 97. The index provides candidates with an efficient and effective method to review selected academic content after completing each of the sample examinations.

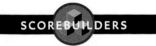

Insight Exam Index

Insight Exam Index

Insight Exam Index

Academic Review Index

Academic Review Index

Academic Review Index

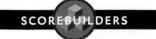

Academic Review Index

Academic Review Index

Academic Review Index

Academic Review Index

Academic Review Index

Academic Review Index

Academic Review Index

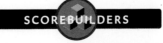

Academic Review Index

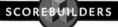

Academic Review Index

Academic Review Index

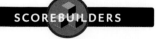

Academic Review Index

Academic Review Index

PTAEXAM: The Complete Study Guide

The new edition of **PTAEXAM: The Complete Study Guide** is the most comprehensive resource available for the NPTE-PTA. The resource is a virtual visual delight with full color and hundreds of images. The detailed academic review section includes chapter essentials and proficiency exercises to ensure student mastery of critical NPTE-PTA content.

Students are able to access our eLearning site called **Insight** using a unique registration code located on the inside front cover of the book. **Insight** contains 600 clinically-oriented questions with expansive explanations of the correct and incorrect answers. These questions are thought-provoking, challenging questions designed to be consistent with the specifications and rigor of the NPTE-PTA blueprint. A sophisticated performance analysis section allows students to identify their current strengths and weaknesses according to different system and content outline areas.

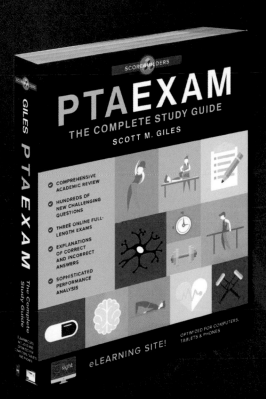

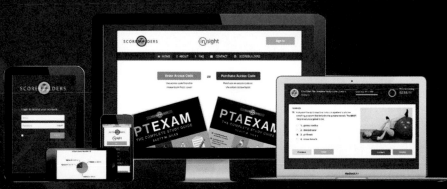

Author: Scott Giles PT, DPT, MBA
ISBN: 978-1-890989-41-5
Price: $85.00

Motivational Moment One

If it was easy, everyone would be a physical therapist assistant. Recognize that you still have some work left to do, but are incredibly close to achieving your goal!

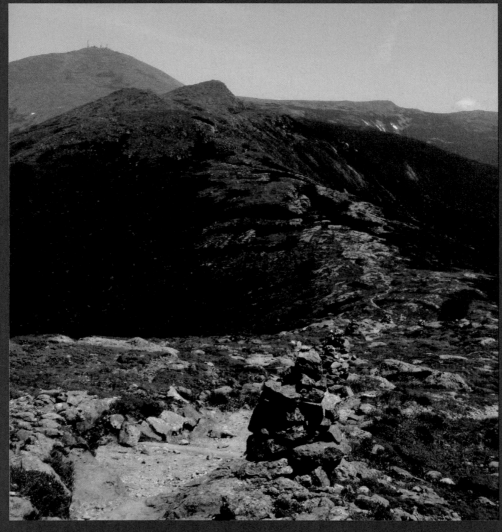

PHOTO BY BOB HOYT

Basecamp

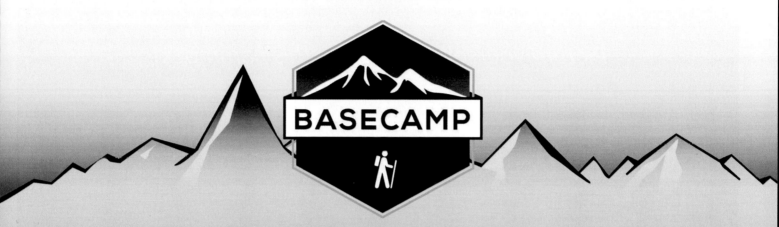

Basecamp takes students on a daily journey through five Mountains (Musculoskeletal, Neuromuscular, Cardiopulmonary, Other Systems, Non-Systems) and 120 Trails (e.g., Special Tests, Cardiac - Pathology, Motor Learning, Research Concepts). **Basecamp** collectively includes hundreds of academic assignments, 40 hours of videos, and 5,000 multiple-choice questions. Our new **Arena** app allows Basecamp users to access 5,000 content-based questions within our competitive games - **King of the Mountain** and **Climb**. Students purchase **Basecamp** for varying periods of time ranging from 30 days (Basecamp - Standard) to Forever (Basecamp - Lifetime).

Price:
Basecamp - Standard: $55.00
Basecamp - Annual: $85.00
Basecamp - Lifetime: $120.00

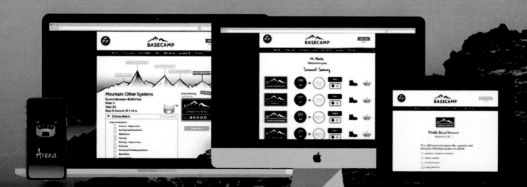

Better Products . . . Better Outcomes!

Motivational Moment Two

Picture yourself lounging in this hammock in a tropical oasis.
Make a list of other possible celebration activities after you pass the NPTE-PTA!

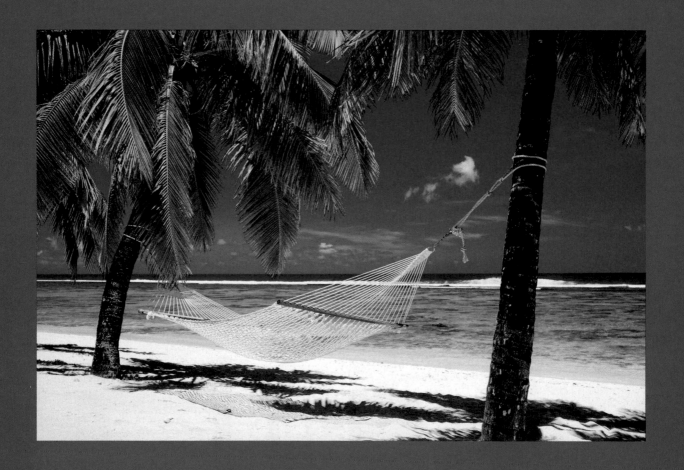

Online Advantage

Online Advantage offers students the opportunity to experience full-length web based exams weighted to the exact NPTE-PTA blueprint specifications. A sophisticated performance analysis offers Leaderboards, academic focus areas, and item analysis. See how your exam scores stack up to the competition!

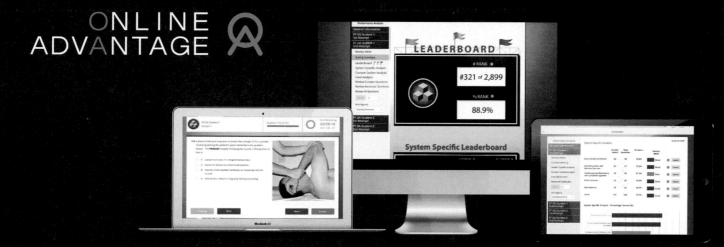

Online Advantage consists of two distinctly separate offerings:

Student version – The student version provides candidates with an ideal opportunity to assess their current examination performance relative to the performance of other licensing examination candidates. Comprehensive summary reports identify both areas of strength and weakness as well as offer specific suggestions for remedial activities.

Academic version – The academic version is designed to provide academic programs with the opportunity to administer a comprehensive examination to their graduating students. A detailed performance analysis section generates individual and group data and therefore is an ideal tool for individual and program assessment.

Price:
$35.00 for one examination
$50.00 for two examinations

* The questions utilized in **Online Advantage** are different than questions utilized in other Scorebuilders' products.

Better Products . . . Better Outcomes!

Motivational Moment Three

Studying for the NPTE-PTA is hard work, but you are only months away from experiencing something that you have not experienced in a very long time . . . Positive Cash Flow!

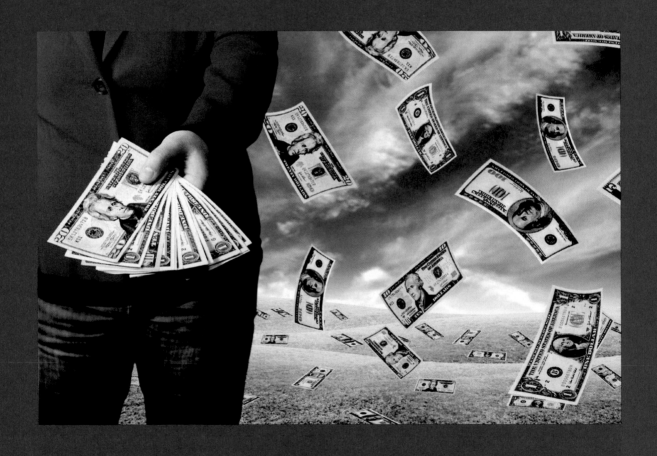

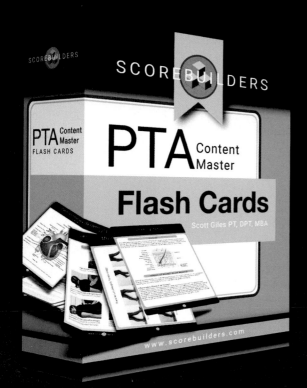
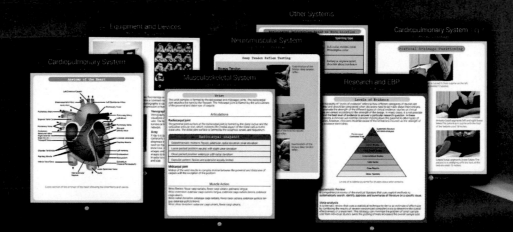

Motivational Moment Four

Imagine the impact you will make on the lives of your patients during a long and distinguished career as a physical therapist assistant!

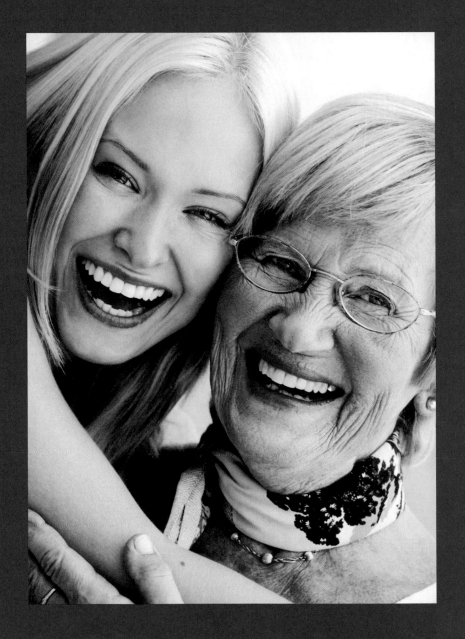

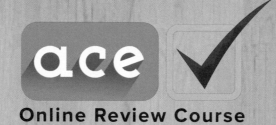
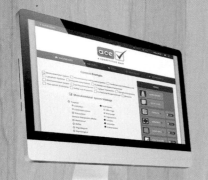
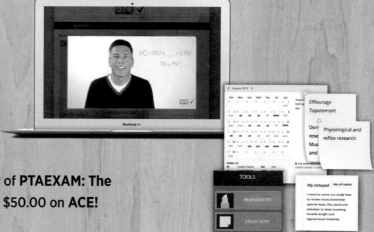
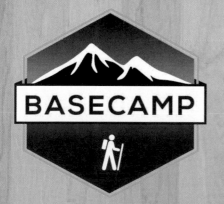
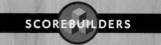

On-Campus Review Course

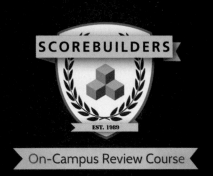

On-Campus Review Course

Our review course provides students with the most personal, effective, and efficient method to maximize performance on the NPTE-PTA. The course introduces students to challenging multiple-choice questions, recent examination trends, a myriad of study tools, and resources designed to increase mastery of essential exam content. Our goal is to maximize the efficiency of a student's study plan by focusing on critical exam content at an appropriate level of breadth and depth.

Scorebuilders offers over 260 review courses annually and is the largest provider of PT and PTA review courses in the United States. Our expert instructors are experienced educators who are superior teachers.

Participants attending our On-Campus Review Course will:

- Improve decision making skills when answering challenging multiple-choice questions.

- Develop a comprehensive study plan to maximize efficiency and performance.

- Identify indicators to determine readiness to take the examination.

All participants attending the course receive a 240 page detailed course manual that includes sample questions, assessment activities, study tools, and other valuable resources to improve performance on the NPTE-PTA.

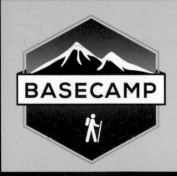

On-Campus Review Course participants receive free 30 Day **Basecamp - Standard** access ($55 value). **Basecamp** includes hundreds of academic assignments, 40 hours of videos, and 5,000 multiple-choice questions.

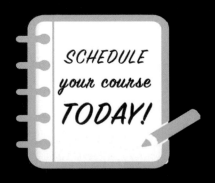

SCHEDULE your course TODAY!

Content Master

Content Master

Physical therapist assistants have the option of utilizing flash cards with an app. The app consists of a content review mode covering the same academic content as the traditional flash cards. Users rate their proficiency in selected content areas and create custom Study Stacks to improve academic mastery. This app also includes 600 multiple-choice questions designed to assess a candidate's knowledge of core academic content. Users take the multiple-choice questions in mini exams in unique systems and non-systems categories. A performance analysis section allows users to review questions and examine performance by category and over time. The questions are unique to the app and are not utilized in any other Scorebuilders' product.

Price: $29.99

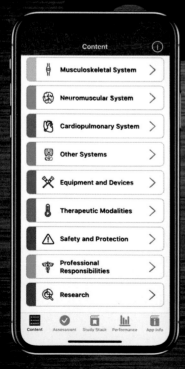
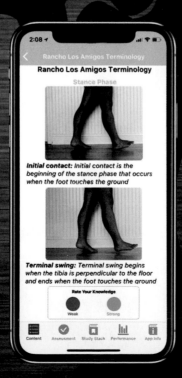
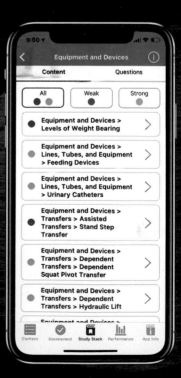

Available through the Apple App and Google Play Stores

PTA365

Seriously . . . this study app is FREE!

PTA365 provides users with a unique daily opportunity to assess their mastery of essential physical therapy content through multiple-choice questions. A complete explanation of both correct and incorrect options is offered for all questions. The app provides users with a method to track their individual performance over time and to compare their results to the relative performance of other physical therapist assistants.

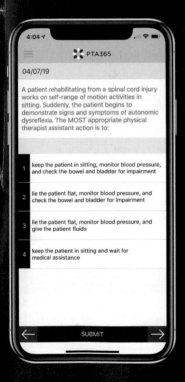
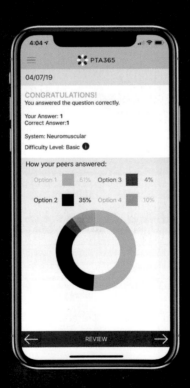
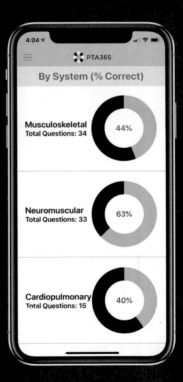

Available through the Apple App and Google Play Stores